Perioperative Medicine

Managing for Outcome

Perioperative Medicine
Managing for Outcome

Mark F. Newman, MD
Merel H. Harmel Professor and Chair
Department of Anesthesiology
Professor of Medicine
Duke University School of Medicine
Durham, North Carolina

Lee A. Fleisher, MD
Robert D. Dripps Professor and Chair
Department of Anesthesiology and Critical Care
Professor of Medicine
University of Pennsylvania School of Medicine
Philadelphia, Pennsylvania

Mitchell P. Fink, MD
Professor and Chairman
Department of Critical Care Medicine
Watson Professor of Surgery
University of Pittsburgh School of Medicine
Pittsburgh, Pennsylvania

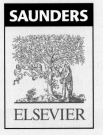

SAUNDERS

ELSEVIER

SAUNDERS
ELSEVIER

1600 John F. Kennedy Blvd.
Ste 1800
Philadelphia, PA 19103-2899

PERIOPERATIVE MEDICINE: MANAGING FOR OUTCOME   ISBN: 978-1-4160-2456-9

Notice

Knowledge and best practice in this field are constantly changing. As new research and experience broaden our knowledge, changes in practice, treatment, and drug therapy may become necessary or appropriate. Readers are advised to check the most current information provided (i) on procedures featured or (ii) by the manufacturer of each product to be administered, to verify the recommended dose or formula, the method and duration of administration, and contraindications. It is the responsibility of the practitioner, relying on his or her experience and knowledge of the patient, to make diagnoses, to determine dosages and the best treatment for each individual patient, and to take all appropriate safety precautions. To the fullest extent of the law, neither the Publisher nor the Editors assume any liability for any injury and/or damage to persons or property arising out of or related to any use of the material contained in this book.

The Publisher

Library of Congress Cataloging-in-Publication Data
Perioperative medicine : managing for outcome / [edited by] Mark F. Newman, Lee A. Fleisher, Mitchell P. Fink.—1st ed.
    p. ; cm.
  ISBN 978-1-4160-2456-9
  1. Therapeutics, Surgical.   2. Preoperative care.   3. Postoperative care.   4. Surgery—Complications—Prevention.   I. Newman, Mark F.   II. Fleisher, Lee A.   III. Fink, M. P. (Mitchell P.).
  [DNLM: 1. Perioperative Care—methods.   2. Intraoperative Complications—prevention & control.   3. Multiple Organ Failure—prevention & control.   4. Postoperative Complications—prevention & control.   5. Preoperative Care—methods. WO 178 P44512 2008]
  RD49.P463 2008
  617′.9192—dc22
                                                                        2006100962

Executive Publisher: Natasha Andjelkovic
Senior Developmental Editor: Ann Ruzycka Anderson
Publishing Services Manager: Tina K. Rebane
Senior Project Manager: Linda Lewis Grigg
Design Direction: Karen O'Keefe Owens

Printed in China

Last digit is the print number: 9   8   7   6   5   4   3   2   1

To our past, current, and future residents, fellows, and faculty, who, through their dedication, continue to advance the field of perioperative medicine and the care of our patients.

To our families, who have been so supportive:

To my wife, Susan, a partner, a friend, and, most important, a believer without whom I would be incomplete. To my mother and late father, who let me know that no matter what I accomplished it would be okay. And to my kids, Sarah, Jack, and Catherine, who remind me every day of the importance of what we do and what we learn.

Mark F. Newman

To my wife, Renee, who has been a partner and best friend for the past 16 years. To my children, Jessica and Matthew, for their unconditional love and support and constant reminder about the important things in life. Finally, to my parents and grandparents, who instilled in me the desire to always seek new knowledge.

Lee A. Fleisher

To my wife, Jan, who has been the love of my life for nearly 35 years. To my grown-up kids, Emily and Matt, who are both delightful, kind, and generous human beings. Finally, to my late parents, who both passed away during the past couple of years; they would have enjoyed leafing through this volume and reading this dedication.

Mitchell P. Fink

Contributors

Matthew Agnew, MD
Clinical Instructor
Department of Surgery
Division of Cardiothoracic Surgery
University of Washington School of Medicine
Seattle, Washington
Prevention of Ischemic Injury in Cardiac Surgery

Thomas Lloyd Archer, MD, MBA
Assistant Professor
Department of Anesthesiology
University of Texas School of Medicine at San Antonio
San Antonio, Texas
Economic Analysis of Perioperative Optimization

Lars M. Asmis, MD
Department of Anesthesiology
University Hospital of Zurich
Zurich, Switzerland
Hematologic Risk Assessment

Cecil O. Borel, MD
Associate Professor
Departments of Anesthesiology and Surgery
Duke University School of Medicine
Division Chief
Otolaryngology/Neuroanesthesia
Duke University Medical Center
Durham, North Carolina
Carotid and Intracranial Surgery; Neurosurgery

Martha Sue Carraway, MD
Associate Professor
Department of Medicine, Division of Pulmonary, Allergy, and Critical Care Medicine
Duke University School of Medicine
Durham, North Carolina
The Coagulation Cascade in Perioperative Organ Injury

Maurizio Cereda, MD
Clinical Assistant Professor
Department of Anesthesiology and Critical Care
University of Pennsylvania School of Medicine
Attending Physician
Department of Anesthesiology and Critical Care
Hospital of the University of Pennsylvania
Staff Anesthesiologist
Anesthesia Section
Philadelphia VA Medical Center
Philadelphia, Pennsylvania
Pulmonary Risk Assessment

Pierre-Guy Chassot, MD
Department of Anesthesiology
University Hospital of Lausanne
Lausanne, Switzerland
Hematologic Risk Assessment

Theodore G. Cheek, MD
Associate Professor of Anesthesia and Obstetrics and Gynecology
Department of Anesthesiology and Critical Care
University of Pennsylvania School of Medicine
Director
Obstetric Anesthesia
Hospital of the University of Pennsylvania
Philadelphia, Pennsylvania
Perioperative Protection of the Pregnant Woman

Albert T. Cheung, MD
Professor
Department of Anesthesiology and Critical Care
University of Pennsylvania School of Medicine
Staff Anesthesiologist
Department of Anesthesiology and Critical Care
University of Pennsylvania Health Systems
Hospital of the University of Pennsylvania and Presbyterian Medical Center
Philadelphia, Pennsylvania
Preservation of Spinal Cord Function

John L. Chow, MD, MS
Attending Anesthesiologist
Department of Anesthesia
St. Vincent Medical Center
Portland, Oregon
Risk Assessment and Perioperative Renal Dysfunction

Richard C. D'Alonzo, MD, PhD
Chief Resident
Department of Anesthesia
Duke University Medical Center
Durham, North Carolina
Perioperative Management of Bleeding and Transfusion

Clifford S. Deutschman, MS, MD, FCCM
Professor
Departments of Anesthesiology and Critical Care and Surgery
University of Pennsylvania School of Medicine
Philadelphia, Pennsylvania
The Inflammatory Response in Organ Injury

Christine A. Doyle, MD
Staff Physician
Department of Anesthesia
O'Connor Hospital
Partner Physician
Coast Anesthesia Medical Group
San Jose, California
Prevention and Treatment of Pulmonary Dysfunction

Kim A. Eagle, MD, FACC
Albion Walter Hewlett Professor of Internal Medicine
Clinical Director
Cardiovascular Center
University of Michigan Medical School
Ann Arbor, Michigan
Cardiac Risk Assessment in Noncardiac Surgery

Mitchell P. Fink, MD
Professor and Chairman
Department of Critical Care Medicine
Watson Professor of Surgery
Department of Surgery
University of Pittsburgh School of Medicine
Pittsburgh, Pennsylvania
Ischemia and Ischemia-Reperfusion–Induced Organ Injury

Lee A. Fleisher, MD
Robert D. Dripps Professor and Chairman
Department of Anesthesiology and Critical Care
Professor
Department of Internal Medicine
University of Pennsylvania School of Medicine
Chair of Anesthesiology and Critical Care
Hospital of the University of Pennsylvania
Philadelphia, Pennsylvania
Implications of Perioperative Morbidity on Long-Term Outcomes; Cardiac Risk Assessment in Noncardiac Surgery

Duane J. Funk, MD, FRCPC
Intensivist and Anesthesiologist
Department of Anesthesiology, Section of Critical Care Medicine
Duke University Medical Center
Durham, North Carolina
Prevention and Treatment of Gastrointestinal Morbidity; Endocrine and Electrolyte Disorders

Ronald A. Gabel, MD
Professor Emeritus
Department of Anesthesiology
University of Rochester School of Medicine and Dentistry
Rochester, New York
Pay for Performance: An Incentive for Better Outcomes

Robert R. Gaiser, MD
Professor
Department of Anesthesiology and Critical Care
University of Pennsylvania School of Medicine
Attending Anesthesiologist
Hospital of the University of Pennsylvania
Philadelphia, Pennsylvania
Preservation of Fetal Viability in Noncardiac Surgery

Tong J. Gan, MBBS, FRCA, FFARCS
Professor
Department of Anesthesiology
Duke University School of Medicine
Durham, North Carolina
Prevention and Treatment of Gastrointestinal Morbidity

Hilary P. Grocott, MD, FRCPC
Professor
Department of Anesthesiology
Duke University School of Medicine
Durham, North Carolina
Protecting the Central Nervous System during Cardiac Surgery

Jacob T. Gutsche, MD
Assistant Professor
Department of Anesthesiology and Critical Care
University of Pennsylvania School of Medicine
Philadelphia, Pennsylvania
Major Abdominal Surgery

Charles C. Hill, MD
Clinical Instructor in Cardiac Anesthesia
Department of Anesthesia
Stanford University School of Medicine
Stanford, California
Risk Assessment and Perioperative Renal Dysfunction

Steven E. Hill, MD
Associate Professor of Anesthesiology and Critical Care
Department of Anesthesiology
Duke University School of Medicine
Co-Medical Director
Acute Cardiothoracic Unit
Department of Anesthesiology
Co-Medical Director
Duke Center for Blood Conservation
Perioperative Services
Duke University Hospital
Durham, North Carolina
Perioperative Management of Bleeding and Transfusion

Katja Hindler, MD
Assistant Professor
Department of Anesthesiology and Intensive Care
University of Tübingen Medical School
Tübingen, Germany
Clinical Research Fellow
Department of Cardiovascular Anesthesia
Texas Heart Institute
St. Luke's Episcopal Hospital
Houston, Texas
Central Nervous System Risk Assessment

David T. Huang, MD, MPH
Visiting Assistant Professor
Department of Critical Care Medicine
University of Pittsburgh School of Medicine
Critical Care Physician
Abdominal Transplant ICU
Emergency Physician
Passavant Emergency Department
University of Pittsburgh Medical Center
Pittsburgh, Pennsylvania
Major Orthopaedic Surgery

Igor Izrailtyan, MD
Assistant Professor
Department of Anesthesiology
Stony Brook University School of Medicine
Attending Anesthesiologist
Stony Brook University Hospital
Stony Brook, New York
Perioperative Management of Valvular Heart Disease

Michael L. James, MD
Assistant Professor
Departments of Anesthesiology and Neurology
Duke University School of Medicine
Durham, North Carolina
Carotid and Intracranial Surgery; Neurosurgery

Per-Olof Jarnberg, MD, PhD
Professor of Anesthesiology
Vice Chairman of Clinical Affairs
Department of Anesthesiology and Peri-Operative Medicine
Oregon Health & Science University School of Medicine
Portland, Oregon
Perioperative Management of Renal Failure and Renal Transplant

Robert G. Johnson, MD, FACS, FCCP
C. Rollins Hanlon Professor and Chair
Department of Surgery
Saint Louis University School of Medicine
Chief
Department of Surgery
Saint Louis University Hospital
St. Louis, Missouri
Cardiovascular Risk Assessment in Cardiac Surgery

Carolyn E. Jones, MD
Assistant Professor of Surgery
University of Rochester School of Medicine and Dentistry
Staff Surgeon
Department of Surgery
University of Rochester Medical Center
Rochester, New York
Solid Organ Transplantation

Jagajan Karmacharya, MBBS, FRCS
Assistant Instructor in Surgery
University of Pennsylvania School of Medicine
Fellow in Vascular Surgery
Hospital of the University of Pennsylvania
Philadelphia, Pennsylvania
Prevention and Management of Deep Vein Thrombosis and Pulmonary Embolism

David C. Kaufman, MD, FCCM
Associate Professor of Surgery, Medicine, Anesthesia, and
  Medical Humanities
University of Rochester School of Medicine and Dentistry
Medical Director
Surgical Intensive Care Unit, Department of Surgery
University of Rochester Medical Center
Rochester, New York
Solid Organ Transplantation

John C. Keifer, MD
Associate Professor
Department of Anesthesiology
Duke University School of Medicine
Durham, North Carolina
Carotid and Intracranial Surgery

John A. Kellum, MD, FACP, FCCM, FCCP
Professor
Department of Critical Care Medicine
University of Pittsburgh School of Medicine
Critical Care Staff Intensivist
Liver Transplant ICU and Cardiothoracic ICU
Department of Critical Care Medicine
University of Pittsburgh Physicians/University of Pittsburgh
  Medical Center
Pittsburgh, Pennsylvania
Treatment of Acute Oliguria

Patrick K. Kim, MD, FACS
Assistant Professor of Surgery
Division of Traumatology and Surgical Critical Care
Department of Surgery
University of Pennsylvania School of Medicine
Attending Surgeon
Department of Surgery
Hospital of the University of Pennsylvania
Philadelphia, Pennsylvania
Multisystem Trauma

W. Andrew Kofke, MD, MBA, FCCM
Professor
Department of Anesthesiology and Critical Care
University of Pennsylvania School of Medicine
Staff Anesthesiologist
University of Pennsylvania Health System
Philadelphia, Pennsylvania
*Perioperative Management of Acute Central
Nervous System Injury*

Benjamin A. Kohl, MD
Assistant Professor
Department of Anesthesiology and Critical Care
University of Pennsylvania School of Medicine
Staff Physician
Department of Anesthesiology and Critical Care
Hospital of the University of Pennsylvania
Philadelphia, Pennsylvania
The Inflammatory Response in Organ Injury

Richard Kwon, MD
Clinical Lecturer
Department of Internal Medicine
University of Michigan Medical School
Ann Arbor, Michigan
Cardiac Risk Assessment in Noncardiac Surgery

Brain Lima, MD
Cardiothoracic Surgery Research Fellow
Department of Surgery
Duke University Medical Center
Durham, North Carolina
*Treatment of Perioperative Ischemia, Infarction, and
Ventricular Failure in Cardiac Surgery*

Alan Lisbon, MD, FCCM, FCCP
Associate Professor of Anaesthesia
Department of Anaesthesia
Harvard Medical School
Vice Chair for Critical Care
Department of Anesthesia, Critical Care and Pain Medicine
Beth Israel Deaconess Medical Center
Boston, Massachusetts
General Thoracic Surgery

Frederick W. Lombard, MBChB, FANZCA
Assistant Professor
Department of Anesthesiology
Duke University School of Medicine
Durham, North Carolina
Carotid and Intracranial Surgery

Alex Macario, MD, MBA
Professor of Anesthesia and Health Research and Policy
Department of Anesthesia
Stanford University School of Medicine
Stanford, California
Economic Analysis of Perioperative Optimization

G. Burkhard Mackensen, MD, PhD, FASE
Associate Professor
Department of Anesthesiology
Duke University School of Medicine
Durham, North Carolina
Cardiac Surgery

Michael D. Malinzak, BS, BA
MD/PhD Student
Department of Anesthesiology
Duke University School of Medicine
Durham, North Carolina
Sepsis and Septic Shock

Steve Mannis, MD, MBA
Assistant Clinical Professor
University of California, Davis, School of Medicine
Medical Director
Health South Surgery Centers
Sacramento, California
Economic Analysis of Perioperative Optimization

Carlo Enrique Marcucci, MD
Staff Member
Department of Anesthesiology
University Hospital Lausanne
Lausanne, Switzerland
Hematologic Risk Assessment

Joseph P. Mathew, MD
Associate Professor
Department of Anesthesiology
Duke University School of Medicine
Chief, Cardiothoracic Division
Department of Anesthesiology
Duke University Medical Center
Durham, North Carolina
Perioperative Management of Valvular Heart Disease

David L. McDonagh, MD
Assistant Professor, Departments of Anesthesiology and
  Neurology
Duke University School of Medicine
Program Training Director
Neurocritical Care
Duke University Medical Center
Durham, North Carolina
Carotid and Intracranial Surgery

Michael L. McGarvey, MD
Assistant Professor
Department of Neurology
University of Pennsylvania School of Medicine
Staff Neurologist
Hospital of the University of Pennsylvania
Philadelphia, Pennsylvania
Preservation of Spinal Cord Function

Mary K. McHugh, MD
Assistant Professor
Department of Anesthesiology and Critical Care
University of Pennsylvania School of Medicine
Attending Anesthesiologist
Hospital of the University of Pennsylvania
Philadelphia, Pennsylvania
Preservation of Fetal Viability in Noncardiac Surgery

Carmelo A. Milano, MD
Associate Professor
Department of Surgery
Duke University School of Medicine
Surgical Director for Cardiac Transplantation and
 Cardiothoracic Surgery
LVAD Programs
Duke University Medical Center
Durham, North Carolina
*Treatment of Perioperative Ischemia, Infarction, and
Ventricular Failure in Cardiac Surgery*

Christina T. Mora Mangano, MD, FAHA
Professor
Department of Anesthesia
Stanford University School of Medicine
Director
Division of Cardiovascular Anesthesiology
Stanford University Medical Center
Stanford, California
Risk Assessment and Perioperative Renal Dysfunction

Frederick A. Moore, MD, FACS
Head
Division of Surgical Critical Care and Acute Care Surgery
Department of Surgery
The Methodist Hospital
Houston, Texas
Acute Respiratory Failure

Eugene W. Moretti, MD, MHSc
Assistant Professor
Department of Anesthesiology
Duke University School of Medicine
Durham, North Carolina
Endocrine and Electrolyte Disorders

Carlene A. Muto, MD, MS
Assistant Professor
Department of Epidemiology and Medicine
Division of Infectious Diseases
University of Pittsburgh School of Medicine
Medical Director
Hospital Epidemiology and Infection Control
UPMC Presbyterian Hospital
System Medical Director
Infection Control
Center for Quality Improvement and Innovation
UPMC Hospital System
Pittsburgh, Pennsylvania
Prevention of Perioperative and Surgical Site Infection

**Patrick J. Neligan, MA, MB, BcH, FCARCSI,
DIBICM**
Assistant Professor
Department of Anesthesiology and Critical Care
University of Pennsylvania School of Medicine
Staff Physician
Hospital of the University of Pennsylvania
Philadelphia, Pennsylvania
Major Abdominal Surgery

Mark F. Newman, MD
Merel H. Harmel Professor and Chairman
Department of Anesthesiology
Professor of Medicine
Duke University School of Medicine
Durham, North Carolina
*Implications of Perioperative Morbidity on Long-Term
Outcomes*

Laura E. Niklason, MD
Assistant Professor
Departments of Anesthesiology and Biomedical Engineering
Yale University School of Medicine
New Haven, Connecticut
Sepsis and Septic Shock

Nancy A. Nussmeier, MD
Professor and Chair
Department of Anesthesiology
State University of New York Upstate Medical University
 College of Medicine
Chair
Department of Anesthesiology
University Hospital
Syracuse, New York
Central Nervous System Risk Assessment

Winston C. V. Parris, MD, FACPM
Professor
Department of Anesthesiology
Duke University School of Medicine
Medical Director and Chief
Pain and Palliative Clinic
Duke University Medical Center
Durham, North Carolina
Pain, Delirium, and Anxiety

Ronald G. Pearl, PhD, MD, FCCM
Professor and Chair
Department of Anesthesia
Stanford University School of Medicine
Chair of Anesthesia
Associate Director of Intensive Care
Department of Anesthesia
Stanford University Hospital and Clinics
Stanford, California
Prevention and Treatment of Pulmonary Dysfunction

Claude A. Piantadosi, MD
Professor of Medicine
Division of Pulmonary, Allergy, and Critical Care
Duke University School of Medicine
Durham, North Carolina
The Coagulation Cascade in Perioperative Organ Injury

Marian Pokrywka, MS, CIC
Infection Control Practitioner
Department of Infection Control and Hospital Epidemiology
University of Pittsburgh Medical Center
Pittsburgh, Pennsylvania
Prevention of Perioperative and Surgical Site Infection

Don Poldermans, MD, FESC
Professor of Anaesthesiology
Erasmus Medical College
Rotterdam, The Netherlands
Prevention of Ischemic Injury in Noncardiac Surgery

Patrick M. Reilly, MD, FACS
Associate Professor of Surgery
Department of Surgery
Division of Traumatology and Surgical Critical Care
University of Pennsylvania School of Medicine
Attending Surgeon
Hospital of the University of Pennsylvania
Philadelphia, Pennsylvania
Multisystem Trauma

Lesco L. Rogers, MD
Assistant Clinical Professor
Department of Anesthesiology
Division of Pain Management
Duke University School of Medicine
Durham, North Carolina
Pain, Delirium, and Anxiety

Stanley H. Rosenbaum, MD
Professor of Anesthesiology, Internal Medicine, and Surgery
Department of Anesthesiology
Yale University School of Medicine
Director of Perioperative and Adult Anesthesia
Department of Anesthesiology
Yale–New Haven Hospital
New Haven, Connecticut
The Value of Preoperative Assessment

Christopher T. Salerno, MD
Cardiovascular Surgeon
Corvasc MDs P.C.
Surgical Director
Heart Transplant Program
St. Vincent's Hospital
Indianapolis, Indiana
Prevention of Ischemic Injury in Cardiac Surgery

Babak Sarani, MD
Assistant Professor of Surgery
Department of Surgery
Division of Traumatology and Surgical Critical Care
University of Pennsylvania School of Medicine
Philadelphia, Pennsylvania
Major Orthopaedic Surgery

Todd W. Sarge, MD
Instructor in Anesthesia
Department of Anesthesia, Critical Care, and Pain Management
Harvard Medical School
Staff Anesthesiologist
Department of Anesthesia, Critical Care, and Pain Management
Beth Israel Deaconess Medical Center
Boston, Massachusetts
General Thoracic Surgery

David G. Silverman, MD
Professor and Director of Clinical Research
Department of Anesthesiology
Yale University School of Medicine
Attending Anesthesiologist
Medical Director of Pre-Admission Testing
Yale–New Haven Hospital
New Haven, Connecticut
The Value of Preoperative Assessment

Martin Slodzinski, MD, PhD
Assistant Professor
Department of Anesthesiology and Critical Care Medicine
Johns Hopkins University School of Medicine
Baltimore, Maryland
Prevention and Management of Perioperative Dysrhythmias

Donat R. Spahn, MD
Professor of Anesthesiology
University of Zurich School of Medicine
Chairman
Institute of Anesthesiology
University Hospital Zurich
Zurich, Switzerland
Hematologic Risk Assessment

Mark Stafford-Smith, MD, CM, FRCPC
Professor
Department of Anesthesiology
Duke University School of Medicine
Durham, North Carolina
Preservation of Renal Function

S. Rob Todd, MD, FACS
Medical Director
Surgical Intensive Care Unit
Associate Program Director
Surgical Critical Care and Acute Care Surgery
The Methodist Hospital
Houston, Texas
Acute Respiratory Failure

Ramesh Venkataraman, MD
Assistant Professor
Department of Critical Care Medicine
University of Pittsburgh School of Medicine
Pittsburgh, Pennsylvania
Treatment of Acute Oliguria

Gary A. Vercruysse, MD
Assistant Professor
Department of Surgery
Emory University School of Medicine
Co-Director
Burn Unit
Grady Memorial Hospital
Atlanta, Georgia
Acute Respiratory Failure

Edward D. Verrier, MD
William K. Edmark Professor of Cardiovascular
   Surgery
Department of Surgery
University of Washington School of Medicine
Chief, Cardiovascular Surgery
University of Washington Medical Center
Seattle, Washington
Prevention of Ischemic Injury in Cardiac Surgery

David S. Warner, MD
Professor of Anesthesiology, Surgery, and Neurobiology
Duke University School of Medicine
Vice Chairman
Department of Anesthesiology
Duke University Medical Center
Durham, North Carolina
Carotid and Intracranial Surgery

Robin V. West, MD
Assistant Professor
Department of Orthopaedics
University of Pittsburgh School of Medicine
Pittsburgh, Pennsylvania
Major Orthopaedic Surgery

Edward Y. Woo, MD
Assistant Professor
Department of Surgery
Division of Vascular Surgery
University of Pennsylvania School of Medicine
Attending Surgeon
Hospital of the University of Pennsylvania
Philadelphia, Pennsylvania
Prevention and Management of Deep Vein Thrombosis and Pulmonary Embolism

Foreword

Let us begin at the beginning. Patients who entrust their lives to us believe that we will provide care based on our years of investment in the development of education, knowledge, and skills. Our patients assume that we keep abreast of the information that exists through scientific study regarding the optimal approaches to patient care. They further expect us to apply this knowledge to them individually. In particular, patients and their families are aware of the amazing advancements in recent times in our understanding of the physiology of disease and its treatment.

Perioperative medicine, including anesthesiology, surgery, and critical care, has evolved rapidly, based on a broad range of information that has come from the combined knowledge from basic biology and the application of principles from the new science of clinical quality. The basis for clinical quality is the development of evidence about practice from pragmatic clinical trials, in which scientific principles are evaluated in the context of clinical practice to provide guidance on which practices improve patient outcomes and which practices are unnecessary or dangerous. Findings from this effort to define quality provide the basis for carefully written practice guidelines that consolidate the knowledge into translatable guidance in the form of clinical practice protocols.

Given this scientific progress, the editors of this text have been leaders in the increasing focus on evidence-based medicine. They have been prime movers in their field, stimulating efforts to improve our ability to apply our ever-increasing knowledge in the care of our patients, both globally and in the perioperative period. Indeed, we had the privilege of working with one of the grandfathers of rational perioperative care based on evidence, Dr. John Kirklin. We are sure that Dr. Kirklin would be honored to see the degree to which these concepts have been nurtured by Drs. Newman, Fleisher, and Fink as international leaders in the field of perioperative care.

Perioperative Medicine: Managing for Outcome is a sentinel step in attempting to collate the evidence as it relates to particular organ systems as well as different surgical interventions in the pre-, intra-, and post-operative periods. In contrast to much of the ongoing work focusing on process improvement to improve the efficiency of care associated with pay-for-performance, this text has attempted when possible to provide algorithms defining strategies to enhance the medical outcome of care from the perspective of the patient and health care providers.

The reason to call this text a sentinel step is obvious as you read and observe the many areas in which expert opinion alone drives our strategies. This first attempt toward focusing on managing for outcome in the perioperative period identifies not only opportunities for standardization of strategies, but also the need for further research to define strategies that are truly "best." This call for research focuses on improving the overall outcome for our patients, especially those who are at high risk for perioperative organ dysfunction. By organizing the knowledge base in this area with an emphasis on defining the level of evidence for improving outcomes, the editors and contributing authors have set the stage for an accelerated development of a knowledge system in perioperative care, and we will be watching with keen interest as it develops.

The recommended strategies will always be questioned, and it is clear that the editors have attracted authors who welcome these questions and welcome the investigation to enhance and improve strategies in the future as additional evidence becomes available. If the focus is on the outcomes for our patients, then the debate that begins here enhances the quantity and quality of life for the patients we care for every day. We congratulate the editors and authors on making this vital first step with the publication of a truly unique text that takes anesthesiology and perioperative medicine practitioners and investigators down the road to improved patient care.

J.G. Reves, MD
Vice-President of Medical Affairs and Dean
School of Medicine
Professor of Anesthesiology
Medical University of South Carolina

Robert Califf, MD
Vice-Chancellor for Health Affairs
Director, Duke Translational Research Institute
Professor of Medicine
Duke University Medical Center

Acknowledgment

We wish to express our gratitude to the numerous people who helped in the development and production of our book. First, the editorial assistants in our offices, Mark Colebrook, Donna Salvo, Kate Musselman, and Cheri Hepfl, were invaluable in multiple steps in the process. We are also indebted to our publisher, Natasha Andjelkovic, who believed in this book and helped develop the ideas and layout, as well as the Developmental Editor at Elsevier, Ann Ruzycka Anderson, and the Production Manager, Linda Lewis Grigg, who helped in the production of this book.

Contents

PART I

Introduction and Background

1 Implications of Perioperative Morbidity on Long-Term Outcomes

Lee A. Fleisher and Mark F. Newman

The practices of anesthesiology, surgery, and critical care have advanced greatly over the past 20 years. Through the efforts of experts in each field, an increasingly older population with progressive comorbidities now presents for surgery and anesthesia. This cohort of individuals grows as the population ages and the relative morbidity and mortality of surgery and anesthesia decline. Despite an enhanced ability to effectively care for this growing high-risk group, it remains at substantial risk for the development of perioperative organ dysfunction—myocardial, pulmonary, neurologic, and renal. The degree of dysfunction ranges from mild (sometimes silent) injury and enzyme leak to profound organ injury, coma, or death. The implications of the more immediate and severe injury occurring in the perioperative period have long been understood, but only recently has it been noted that injury thought to be transient may have long-term consequences. This realization is at the core of this book. In this chapter, we focus on reviewing perioperative management and guiding it on the basis of enhanced outcome. We describe studies that investigate perioperative organ injury and its implications for short- and long-term outcome, as well as current strategies that will be described further in later chapters.

■ PERIOPERATIVE MYOCARDIAL INJURY

The pioneering work of the Study of Perioperative Ischemia (SPI) group, and then the Multicenter SPI (McSPI) group, clearly shows that myocardial enzyme release occurs, at levels higher than previously understood, in cardiac and noncardiac major vascular surgery.[1-3] This finding indicates that greater levels of myocardial injury are associated with an increased probability of myocardial events including infarction and arrhythmia.[4,5] This work identified an important event rate, but substantial questions remain about the significance of these events relative to the patient, and whether they have a long-term impact on patient recovery.

Large prospective clinical trials investigating the ability of pharmaceutical interventions to reduce myocardial injury, morbidity, and mortality were some of the first trials with adequate power and long-term outcome assessment to lead to an understanding of the implications of perioperative injury. The GUARDIAN trial enrolled 5233 patients with an acute coronary syndrome at entry, 3439 patients scheduled for high-risk percutaneous coronary intervention (PCI), and 2918 clinically high-risk patients scheduled for coronary

artery bypass grafting (CABG) between May 1997 and November 1998.[6] The CABG cohort required urgent intervention (after a failed PCI) or a repeat CABG, or had a history of angina at rest or on minimal exercise within 4 weeks before randomization. In addition, these patients had two or more of the following risk factors: age greater than 65 years, female sex, diabetes mellitus, left ventricular ejection fraction of less than 35%, or left main or three-vessel coronary artery disease. Heart-muscle creatine kinase (CK-MB) levels were also collected at 8, 12, 16, and 24 hours after the procedure for CABG patients.[7] The peak CK-MB ratio was determined by dividing the peak CK-MB value by the upper limits of normal (ULN) for that laboratory, because the ULN for CK-MB and the type of assay used in different laboratories varied.

Findings for the CABG cohort indicate that patients without an increase in CK-MB (<1 ULN) had a significantly lower 6-month mortality than patients with a ULN of 10 or more (5.8 versus 12.0%, $P < .05$). The number of deaths occurring in the first 30 days after CABG was 64/119 (53.8%), and the number occurring between 30 days and 6 months was 55/119 (46.2%). Cumulative 6-month survival was inversely related to peak CK-MB ratio ($P < .0001$) (Fig. 1-1).

Like the GUARDIAN trial, the PRIMO-CABG trial was prospective, designed to test the value of C5 complement inhibition to reduce perioperative myocardial infarction and death.[8] A total of 3099 patients undergoing CABG surgery with or without valve surgery were enrolled between January 2002 and February 2003. Although the trial did not reach its primary efficacy endpoint, it did confirm the association between perioperative CK-MB release and mortality outlined in the GUARDIAN trial. The treatment-independent relationship between myocardial infarction (MI) through day 4 and mortality was determined (Fig. 1-2). The population of patients who did not have an MI through day 4 experienced mortality at 30, 90, and 180 days at 2.1%, 3.0%, and 4.0%, respectively. Among patients who had a clinically adjudicated MI through day 4, the mortalities at days 30, 90, and 180 were 10.9%, 14.6%, and 16.3%, respectively. Mortality incidences in the two populations were significantly different across the entire 6 months ($P < .001$, log-rank test).

The GUARDIAN and PRIMO-CABG I trials clearly defined the association between perioperative myocardial injury (enzyme leak) and the probability of mortality out to 6 months (see Figs. 1-1 and 1-2).[7,8] Although the Kaplan-Meier curves from the trials clearly show that mortality in the groups begins to differentiate early, indicating a higher incidence of acute morbidity and mortality, the curves continue to separate and remain different through 6 months, indicating that the degree of perioperative injury is associated with increased mortality in all time periods.[9] Clearly, the importance of the injury to further morbidity and mortality depends on the degree of the injury. Low levels of enzyme leak have little effect on long-term mortality, whereas greater levels produce an almost exponentially greater impact on mortality.

The final important factor in the association between perioperative myocardial injury and long-term morbidity and mortality comes from the results of the PRIMO-CABG trial and a smaller perioperative trial of beta-blocker therapy, which indicate that reducing perioperative injury could have positive long-term effects on outcome. In the PRIMO-CABG

I, pexelizumab reduced the incidence of severe CK-MB release, resulting in a strong trend toward improved survival in the treatment group (Figs. 1-3 and 1-4).[8] In a small-scale randomized trial in vascular surgery, Wallace and colleagues demonstrated that perioperative treatment with effective beta blockade reduced perioperative injury and, most importantly, that reduction in perioperative injury produced long-term benefit (Fig. 1-5).[10] Whether the benefit was produced by beta blockade in general or by the associated reduction in myocardial injury would require large-scale multicenter trials. Regardless of whether we can distinguish association from causality, we can, from a prediction standpoint, identify the individuals who are at greater risk and thus identify strategies to reduce the probability of later morbidity and mortality, and this would improve both quantity and quality of life for high-risk patients.

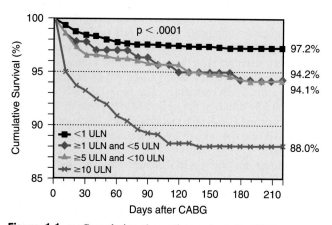

Figure 1-1 ■ Cumulative 6-month survival for 2332 coronary artery bypass grafting (CABG) patients by peak heart-muscle creatine kinase (CK-MB) enzyme ratio category (*P* < .0001). Pairwise comparisons between categories are significant for all groups except the <1 ULN group versus the ≥1 to <5 ULN group (*P* = .06) and the <1 ULN group versus the ≥5 to <10 ULN group (*P* = .98). ULN, upper limit of normal. *(From Gavard JA, Chaitman BR, Sakai S, et al: J Thorac Cardiovasc Surg 2003;126:807-813, with permission.)*

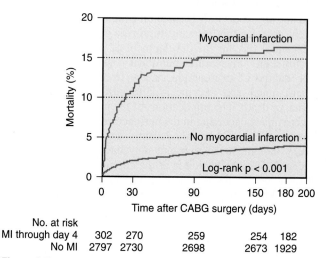

Figure 1-2 ■ Chart shows treatment-independent effect of adjudicated postoperative day 4 myocardial infarction on mortality after coronary artery bypass grafting (CABG). *(From Verrier ED, Shernan SK, Taylor KM, et al: JAMA 2004;291:2319-2327, with permission.)*

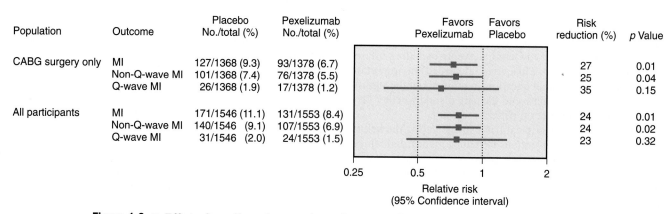

Figure 1-3 ■ Effect of pexelizumab on perioperative myocardial infarction (MI). CABG, coronary artery bypass grafting. *(From Verrier ED, Shernan SK, Taylor KM, et al: JAMA 2004;291:2319-2327, with permission.)*

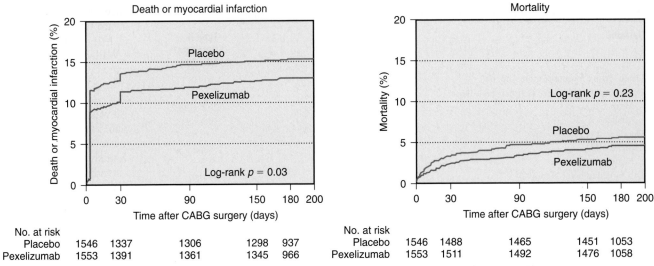

No. at risk
Placebo 1546 1337 1306 1298 937
Pexelizumab 1553 1391 1361 1345 966

No. at risk
Placebo 1546 1488 1465 1451 1053
Pexelizumab 1553 1511 1492 1476 1058

Figure 1-4 ■ Effect of pexelizumab on survival after coronary artery bypass grafting (CABG). Event-free *(left)* and 6-month survival *(right)*. *(From Verrier ED, Shernan SK, Taylor KM, et al: JAMA 2004;291:2319-2327, with permission.)*

Figure 1-5 ■ Overall mortality in atenolol trial as shown by Kaplan-Meier event curves for death. Patients were grouped according to the presence or absence of ischemia during the preoperative, intraoperative, and postoperative recording periods. The atenolol and placebo groups were combined. Only those patients with ischemia within the first 2 postoperative days were counted as ischemic. *(From Wallace A, Layug B, Tateo I, et al: Anesthesiology 1998;88:7-17, with permission.)*

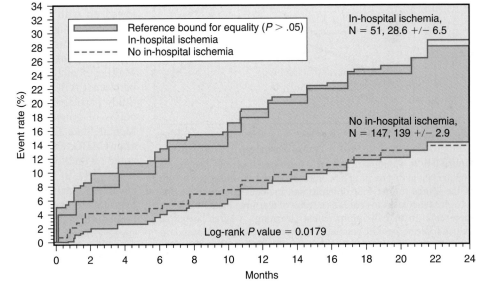

■ NEUROLOGIC INJURY

Perioperative neurologic injury ranges from frank stroke and coma to encephalopathy and neurocognitive dysfunction. The implications of perioperative injury to long-term morbidity and mortality are most clear with perioperative stroke. Stroke is the leading cause of severe disability today, and perioperative strokes (estimated to be 15% to 20% of all strokes) remain a significant contributor.[11,12] The estimated incidence of stroke is 500,000 per year, and another 200,000 recurrent strokes occur annually.[13] Among stroke survivors, 15% to 30% are permanently disabled.

Roach and colleagues defined the clinical and financial implications of perioperative stroke in their 1996 study, which demonstrated that patients who developed perioperative stroke not only had longer intensive care unit and hospital stays but also had a 10-fold increase of in-hospital mortality and approximately a fivefold increase in type II outcomes (encephalopathy) (Table 1-1).[14] These adverse consequences of perioperative neurologic injury did not end at the hospital door, however. Only 30% of the patients with perioperative stroke were discharged, compared with more than 90% of patients without a neurologic deficit. Even more surprising was the difference in discharge status of patients with encephalopathy: only 60% of these patients were discharged home, compared with more than 90% of those without adverse cerebral outcomes.[14]

Few would question the significance of perioperative stroke, but neurocognitive dysfunction has been thought of as a transient process without substantial long-term

| 1-1 | Mortality and Postoperative Resource Use According to Cerebral Outcome |

Variable	Type I Outcome (*N* = 66)	Type II Outcome (*N* = 63)	No Adverse Cerebral Event (*N* = 1979)
Death during hospitalization—no. (%)	14 (21)	6 (10)	38 (2)
Duration of postoperative hospital stay—days			
Mean ± SD	25.3 ± 22.2	20.5 ± 25.2	9.5 ± 12.4
Median	17.6	10.9	7.7
Duration of ICU stay—days			
Mean ± SD	11.1 ± 15.4	6.6 ± 7.9	2.6 ± 3.5
Median	5.8	3.2	1.9
Discharged to home—no. (%)*	21 (32)	38 (60)	1773 (90)

$P < .001$ for all comparisons among the groups.
*Patients not discharged to their homes either died or were discharged to intermediate- or long-term care facilities.
ICU, intensive care unit.
From Roach GW, Kanchuger M, Mangano CM, et al: N Engl J Med 1996;335:1857-1863, with permission.

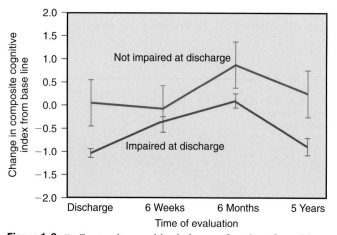

Figure 1-6 ■ Composite cognitive index as a function of cognitive impairment at discharge. The composite cognitive index is the sum of the scores for the four domains and includes cognitive decline as well as increases in scores as a result of learning. Positive change represents an overall improvement (learning), whereas negative values indicate overall decline. The *I* bars represent the standard error. *(From Newman MF, Kirchner JL, Phillips-Bute B, et al: N Engl J Med 2001;344:395-402, with permission.)*

implications. However, now several groups, including our own, have shown an association between the development of perioperative cognitive decline and long-term cognitive dysfunction.[15-17] This association indicates that those individuals exhibiting cognitive decline after surgery are more likely to go on to either continued or greater cognitive decline over time, even if they have improvement in the intervening period (Fig. 1-6).[15] There is substantial controversy as to whether this decline in function seen late—years after cardiac surgery—is associated with neurologic injury, thus mimicking a pattern of closed head injury with early improvement followed by late decline, or whether we have identified, through the use of more sophisticated testing, individuals who would have gone on to cognitive deterioration regardless of undergoing surgery and anesthesia.[18]

To understand the impact of CABG on long-term outcome, Lyketsos and colleagues performed a population-based cohort study involving participants in the Cache County Study of Memory Health and Aging.[19] At baseline, the study enrolled 5092 persons of age 65 and older and followed up with them 3 and 4 years later. Individuals who reported having undergone CABG surgery at study baseline or who had this surgery between follow-ups were compared with individuals who reported never having had the surgery. Multilevel models were used to examine the relationship between CABG surgery and cognitive decline over time. Study participants who had CABG surgery evidenced 0.95 points of greater decline relative to baseline on the Mini Mental State Examination at the first follow-up interview after CABG, and an average of 1.9 points of greater decline at the second follow-up interview, than those without CABG ($t^{1/4} = -2.51$, df = 2316, $P = .0121$), after adjusting for several covariates, including vascular conditions. This decline was restricted to individuals who were more than 5 years past the procedure, and it was not evident in the early years after the surgery. These results indicate that CABG surgery is associated with accelerated cognitive decline more than 5 years after the procedure in an older adult population.

Although cognitive decline after cardiac surgery has been investigated most, Monk and Phillips-Bute found that 2 years after major noncardiac surgery, 42% of older adult patients experienced a measurable cognitive decline.[20] Furthermore, they reported that 59% of patients experienced cognitive decline immediately after surgery. Their population included 354 patients scheduled to undergo major noncardiac surgery. The elective surgeries, requiring general anesthesia, were primarily orthopedic, including knee and joint replacements. The average age of patients was 69.5 years, 57% were women, and they had an average of 13.5 years of education. Each patient was given the same battery of tests at four different times: before surgery, at discharge, 3 months after surgery, and 2 years after surgery. The tests measured patients' abilities in four domains: psychomotor and mental speed, verbal learning, cognitive filtering, and attention/concentration. After determining the rates of cognitive decline, Monk and Phillips-Bute compared the outcomes of the 59% of patients who exhibited cognitive impairments at discharge with the outcomes of those who were not impaired. Although groups showed trends toward improvement at 3 months when compared with discharge, those who were impaired did not show as great an increase. After controlling for baseline cognitive scores, age, and years of education, it appeared that cognitive decline at discharge was the most significant predictor of decline at 2 years. The authors concluded that actions taken during surgery, including anesthetic management of the patients, could indeed have long-term implications for survival and quality of life.

Of particular interest is a recent report by Monk and colleagues that identifies an association between perioperative neurocognitive dysfunction and the mortality at 3 months and 1 year.[21] The investigative team completed a prospective assessment of 1200 patients undergoing elective noncardiac surgery, divided into groups of young (18 to 39 years old), middle-aged (40 to 59 years old), and older adults (60 years and older). A control group of primary family members was used to provide a change score similar to that used in the International Study for Postoperative Neurocognitive Dysfunction (ISPOCD). (Note that this produces a rate different from that quoted in the previous study.) Patients completed a neurocognitive battery at baseline (preoperatively), and at both 1 week and 3 months postoperatively. Patients were followed at 1 year to determine survival, but no additional neurocognitive assessments were undertaken at that time. A total of 61 (5.7%) patients died within 1 year of surgery, 16 within the first week, 20 in the 1-week to 3-month testing period, and 25 after the 3-month testing session. Patients who exhibited postoperative neurocognitive dysfunction at 1 week after surgery were more likely to die in the first year ($P = .01$). Likewise, there was increased incidence of death within the first year after surgery among those exhibiting postoperative neurocognitive dysfunction at 3 months postoperatively ($P = .01$).

The mechanism for the association between cognitive decline and 1-year mortality is not well defined. That the association between cognitive decline and mortality remains significant even when comorbidity is controlled (Charlson Comorbidity Score) may indicate that neurocognitive decline represents a sensitive marker for perioperative organ injury that results in long-term morbidity or specifically mortality.

Whether the defined association indicates that more severe perioperative injury causes greater long-term morbidity and mortality, or whether these individuals were at higher risk for going on to later decline or injury, it does show the significance of understanding risk and the potential to improve outcome. Strategies are needed to reduce long-term morbidity and mortality by reducing perioperative neurologic injury. Strategies to reduce overall organ injury would seem to have a strong probability of improving long-term outcome.

■ RENAL INJURY

Acute renal injury associated with high-risk cardiac and major vascular surgery increases the probability of morbidity and mortality, as well as the progression to frank renal failure requiring dialysis.[22,23] Although the incidence of renal failure requiring dialysis is small, acute renal injury, defined by increases in creatinine or reduced creatinine clearance, predicts marked increases in short-term morbidity and mortality.[23] The incidence of chronic renal insufficiency is low after routine cardiac surgery, but it is a major concern after heart transplant surgery. Since it was first reported, numerous studies have confirmed the presence of this complication in a high proportion of heart transplant recipients.[24-29] Greenberg and coworkers found that all patients had abnormal renal function 4 years after heart transplant surgery,[25] and 7% to 10% of these patients have been reported to progress to end-stage renal disease up to 8 years after heart transplant surgery.[27,29] A recent analysis of a national sample of heart transplant recipients found that the cumulative cost of treating end-stage renal disease after heart transplant surgery exceeds $13,000 over a 10-year period, representing an increase of over 9% in post-transplantation costs.[30] The cumulative 6-year risk for the development of end-stage renal disease after heart transplant surgery was estimated to be greater than 6%, with no evidence of a decreasing trend over the past 10 years despite the adoption of measures aimed at reducing risk.[30]

Progressive renal insufficiency after heart transplant surgery has been largely associated with the adverse side effects on the kidneys of the immunosuppressant drug cyclosporine.[25,26,31] Although acute nephrotoxicity attributable to cyclosporine has been well documented,[32,33] it is becoming clear that reducing the dose of cyclosporine or adopting a different immunosuppression strategy may not reduce the progression of chronic renal disease in these patients.[30,34,35] The association of postoperative acute renal insufficiency with greater risk of development of chronic renal disease independent of cyclosporine remains controversial.[25,36] The investigation of the possible impact of a perioperative event, such as acute renal injury, on long-term complications may lead to the development of interventional strategies to limit adverse outcomes.

Swaminathan and colleagues followed 298 consecutive primary heart transplant surgeries in adults, collecting serum creatinine values preoperatively, daily postoperatively, and at specified follow-up times for 3 years postoperatively.[37] Peak fractional change in postoperative serum creatinine (%ΔCr), defined as percent difference between preoperative serum creatinine (CrPre) and highest of the daily in-hospital postoperative values (Cr$_{max}$Post), was used to assess acute renal injury; this is a continuous variable that is generally unaffected by baseline renal function. The %ΔCr correlates with relative reductions in renal filtration, is independently associated with adverse outcomes after cardiac surgery including mortality, and has consistently been shown to be highly sensitive to perioperative renal insult. Using the Cockcroft-Gault equation, the preoperative creatinine clearance (CrClPre) was estimated from CrPre, and the lowest postoperative creatinine clearance (CrClPost) was estimated from Cr$_{max}$Post. The definitions of renal outcome were as follows:

- Acute renal failure (ARF), defined as a binary variable according to the Society of Thoracic Surgeons (STS)

National Database for postoperative ARF as the presence of one of the following[38]:

- $Cr_{max}Post$ of twice the CrPre value (i.e., $\%\Delta Cr >100$) and $Cr_{max}Post >2.0$ mg/dL
- New requirement for dialysis

- Acute renal injury (ARI), described as a continuous variable in terms of peak fractional change in postoperative serum creatinine ($\%\Delta Cr$), defined as stated in the preceding paragraph
- Chronic renal failure (CRF), the principal outcome for this study, was defined as a binary outcome using a modification of the National Kidney Foundation consensus guidelines (estimated CrCl <60 mL/min/1.73 m² for more than 3 months).[39] For purposes of this study, CRF was designated if any one of the following criteria was met:
  - CrCl <60 mL/min¹/1.73 m² at two consecutive follow-up times
  - Last recorded follow-up CrCl <60 mL/min¹/1.73 m²
  - Requirement for dialysis more than 3 months after surgery
- Chronic renal dysfunction (CRD), defined as a continuous outcome based on the percentage decrease in CrClPost more than 3 months after surgery relative to preoperative CrCl

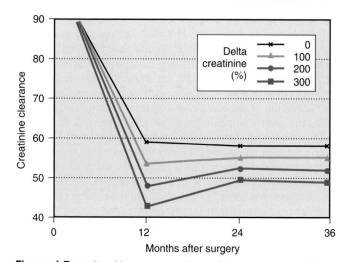

Figure 1-7 ■ Graphic representation of long-term creatinine clearance values in heart transplant recipients. *(From Swaminathan M, Roberts C, van Veeken K, et al: Ann Thorac Surg, 2007 [submitted].)*

In the study of Swaminathan and colleagues,[37] the $\%\Delta Cr$ was 57.7%. This value was observed to be higher than values reported in studies by our group looking at other forms of cardiac surgery. The primary multivariable logistic regression analysis revealed a significant independent association between ARF (STS definition) and CRF (defined as a binary outcome) ($P = .03$; odds ratio, 2.2). Advanced age, female sex, and weight were also independently associated with the development of CRF. The secondary repeated measures mixed-model analysis of variance revealed a significant independent association between increasing degrees of acute perioperative renal injury ($\%\Delta Cr$) and CRD ($\%\Delta CrCl$) ($P = .01$; F statistic, 6.2). Other independent factors were CrPre, follow-up time, age, female sex, and weight.

A graphic trend of long-term creatinine clearance values (Fig. 1-7)[37] over the 3-year follow-up period showed that patients with greater rises in $\%\Delta Cr$ after surgery have a sharper decline in creatinine clearance at 12 months after surgery than patients with smaller rises in $\%\Delta Cr$. The CrCl values tend to stabilize after the initial decline but do not reach baseline values again.

This study supports the hypothesis that acute perioperative renal injury is independently associated with chronic renal dysfunction after heart transplant surgery. In addition, it determined that increasing degrees of ARI are associated with worsening long-term renal function. This finding highlights the importance of an acute perioperative event and shows that it can produce an adverse long-term outcome. Preoperative risk profiling and prevention of acute perioperative renal injury may help reduce the incidence or progression of chronic renal disease in this vulnerable population.

■ ASSOCIATION VERSUS CAUSALITY

In each of the organ systems presented, perioperative organ injury is associated with a greater probability of long-term morbidity or mortality even if there is intervening recovery of function postoperatively. It would be simplest if we could identify that perioperative injury causes the morbidity and mortality that we see in our patients, but it would be difficult to justify this assertion from the statistical associations outlined. The difficulty that we face in recognizing individuals who have perioperative injury, many of whom recover acutely, is that this group very likely had significant pathology even before the procedure. As we look for an association, we need to identify what part of the increased morbidity and mortality after the operation is the result of the patient's own characteristics and other ongoing risk factors, and what part is related to further injury resulting from perioperative stress (e.g., inflammation, hemodilution, anesthesia).[18] Although this chapter highlights large-scale longitudinal trials assessing cognitive decline after surgery, other, smaller-scale trials with similarly diseased control groups have shown similar decline. Thus, severity of disease is the common thread, and the perioperative period is only a "stress test" predicting a higher probability of long-term morbidity and mortality if individuals fail. Large-scale longitudinal trials in high-risk patients are needed to illustrate how patient and procedure interact to define the probability of perioperative organ dysfunction and associated development of long-term organ-based morbidity and mortality. Despite the difficulty in defining the differences between association and causality for long-term decline, we must understand risk of injury if we hope to prevent it.

■ CONCLUSION

The association between perioperative injury and long-term outcome has important implications for the perioperative physician. First, if we identify the incidence and significance of this injury, we can focus on opportunities and strategies (as outlined in this book) to reduce that injury. Second, if we are able to identify the individuals with injuries who are at greater risk for postoperative morbidity and mortality, we may be able to intervene to reduce the probability that perioperative events will produce morbidity and mortality. Finally, and most importantly, as we recognize the associations, strategies can be developed that will reduce perioperative morbidity and mortality and improve the quantity and quality of life of our patients. Thus, we turn the focus of this book toward a strategy of perioperative medicine and managing for outcome.

■ REFERENCES

1. Smith RC, Leung JM, Mangano DT: Postoperative myocardial ischemia in patients undergoing coronary artery bypass graft surgery. S.P.I. Research Group. Anesthesiology 1991;74:464-473.
2. Hollenberg M, Mangano DT: Therapeutic approaches to postoperative ischemia. The Study of Perioperative Ischemia Research Group. Am J Cardiol 1994;73:30B-33.
3. Leung JM, Hollenberg M, O'Kelly BF, et al: Effects of steal-prone anatomy on intraoperative myocardial ischemia. The SPI Research Group. J Am Coll Cardiol 1992;20:1205-1212.
4. Mangano DT, Browner WS, Hollenberg M, et al: Long-term cardiac prognosis following noncardiac surgery. The Study of Perioperative Ischemia Research Group. JAMA 1992;268:233-239.
5. Leung JM, O'Kelly B, Browner WS, et al: Prognostic importance of postbypass regional wall-motion abnormalities in patients undergoing coronary artery bypass graft surgery. SPI Research Group. Anesthesiology 1989;71:16-25.
6. Theroux P, Chaitman BR, Danchin N, et al: Inhibition of the sodium-hydrogen exchanger with cariporide to prevent myocardial infarction in high-risk ischemic situations: Main results of the GUARDIAN trial. Guard during Ischemia Against Necrosis (GUARDIAN) Investigators. Circulation 2000;102:3032-3038.
7. Gavard JA, Chaitman BR, Sakai S, et al: Prognostic significance of elevated creatine kinase MB after coronary artery bypass surgery and after an acute coronary syndrome: Results from the GUARDIAN trial. J Thorac Cardiovasc Surg 2003;126:807-813.
8. Verrier ED, Shernan SK, Taylor KM, et al: Terminal complement blockade with pexelizumab during coronary artery bypass graft surgery requiring cardiopulmonary bypass: A randomized trial. JAMA 2004;291:2319-2327.
9. Goff DC Jr, Brass L, Braun LT, et al: Essential features of a surveillance system to support the prevention and management of heart disease and stroke: A scientific statement from the American Heart Association Councils on Epidemiology and Prevention, Stroke, and Cardiovascular Nursing and the Interdisciplinary Working Groups on Quality of Care and Outcomes Research and Atherosclerotic Peripheral Vascular Disease. Circulation 2007;115:127-155.
10. Wallace A, Layug B, Tateo I, et al: Prophylactic atenolol reduces postoperative myocardial ischemia. McSPI Research Group. Anesthesiology 1998;88:7-17.
11. Thom T, Haase N, Rosamond W, et al: Heart disease and stroke statistics—2006 update: A report from the American Heart Association Statistics Committee and Stroke Statistics Subcommittee. Circulation 2006;113:e85-151.
12. Morbidity and Mortality: 2004 Chart Book on Cardiovascular, Lung, and Blood Diseases. In Services UDoHaH (ed): Bethesda, National Institutes of Health; National Heart, Lung, and Blood Institute, 2004.
13. Rowe GG: Coronary vasodilator therapy for angina pectoris. Am Heart J 1964;68:691-696.
14. Roach GW, Kanchuger M, Mangano CM, et al: Adverse cerebral outcomes after coronary bypass surgery. Multicenter Study of Perioperative Ischemia Research Group and the Ischemia Research and Education Foundation Investigators. N Engl J Med 1996;335:1857-1863.
15. Newman MF, Kirchner JL, Phillips-Bute B, et al: Longitudinal assessment of neurocognitive function after coronary-artery bypass surgery. Neurological Outcome Research Group and CARE Investigators. N Engl J Med. 2001;344:395-402.
16. Stygall J, Newman SP, Fitzgerald G, et al: Cognitive change 5 years after coronary artery bypass surgery. Health Psychol 2003;22:579-586.
17. Newman MF, Grocott HP, Mathew JP, et al: Report of the substudy assessing the impact of neurocognitive function on quality of life five years after cardiac surgery. Neurologic Outcome Research Group and Cardiothoracic Anesthesia Research Endeavors (CARE) Investigators of the Duke Heart Center. Stroke 2001;32:2874-2881.
18. Mark DB, Newman MF: Protecting the brain in coronary artery bypass graft surgery. JAMA 2002;287:1448-1450.
19. Lyketsos CG, Toone L, Tschanz J, et al: A population-based study of the association between coronary artery bypass graft surgery (CABG) and cognitive decline: The Cache County study. Int J Geriatr Psychiatry 2006;21:509-518.
20. Monk TG, Phillips-Bute BG: Longitudinal assessment of neurocognitive function in elderly patients after major, noncardiac surgery. Anesthesiology 2004;101:A62.
21. Monk TG, Weldon BC, Garvan CW, et al: Predictors of cognitive dysfunction after major noncardiac surgery. Anesthesiology 2007 (in press).
22. Conlon PJ, Stafford-Smith M, White WD, et al: Acute renal failure following cardiac surgery. Nephrol Dial Transplant 1999;14:1158-1162.
23. Mangano CM, Diamondstone LS, Ramsay JG, et al: Renal dysfunction after myocardial revascularization: Risk factors, adverse out-comes, and hospital resource utilization. The Multicenter Study of Perioperative Ischemia Research Group. Ann Intern Med 1998;128:194-203.
24. Myers BD, Ross J, Newton L, et al: Cyclosporine-associated chronic nephropathy. N Engl J Med 1984;311:699-705.
25. Greenberg A, Egel JW, Thompson ME, et al: Early and late forms of cyclosporine nephrotoxicity: Studies in cardiac transplant recipients. Am J Kidney Dis 1987;9:12-22.
26. Greenberg A: Renal failure in cardiac transplantation. Cardiovasc Clin 1990;20:189-198.
27. Myers BD, Newton L, Oyer P: The case against the indefinite use of cyclosporine. Transplant Proc 1991;23(1 Pt 1):41-42.
28. Zietse R, Balk AH, vd Dorpel MA, et al: Time course of the decline in renal function in cyclosporine-treated heart transplant recipients. Am J Nephrol 1994;14:1-5.
29. Goldstein DJ, Zuech N, Sehgal V, et al: Cyclosporine-associated end-stage nephropathy after cardiac transplantation: Incidence and progression. Transplantation 1997;63:664-668.
30. Hornberger J, Best J, Geppert J, et al: Risks and costs of end-stage renal disease after heart transplantation. Transplantation 1998;66:1763-1770.
31. Greenberg A, Thompson ME, Griffith BJ, et al: Cyclosporine nephrotoxicity in cardiac allograft patients: A seven-year follow-up. Transplantation 1990;50:589-593.
32. Merli M, Milazzo F, Visigalli MM, et al: Renal function, early postoperatively, in patients undergoing heart transplantation: Experience with 61 patients. J Cardiothorac Anesth 1989;3(5 Suppl 1):62.
33. McGiffin DC, Kirklin JK, Naftel DC: Acute renal failure after heart transplantation and cyclosporine therapy. J Heart Transplant 1985;4:396-399.
34. Waser M, Maggiorini M, Binswanger U, et al: Irreversibility of cyclosporine-induced renal function impairment in heart transplant recipients. J Heart Lung Transplant 1993;12:846-850.
35. Sehgal V, Radhakrishnan J, Appel GB, et al: Progressive renal insufficiency following cardiac transplantation: Cyclosporine, lipids, and hypertension. Am J Kidney Dis 1995;26:193-201.

36. Miller LW, Pennington DG, McBride LR: Long-term effects of cyclosporine in cardiac transplantation. Transplant Proc 1990;22(3 Suppl 1):15-20.

37. Swaminathan M, Roberts C, van Veeken K, et al: Chronic renal failure after heart transplantation: Association with acute perioperative renal injury. Ann Thorac Surg 2007 (submitted).

38. Ferguson TB Jr, Dziuban SW Jr, Edwards FH, et al: The STS National Database: Current changes and challenges for the new millennium. Committee to Establish a National Database in Cardiothoracic Surgery, The Society of Thoracic Surgeons. Ann Thorac Surg 2000;69: 680-691.

39. Levey AS, Coresh J, Balk E, et al: National Kidney Foundation practice guidelines for chronic kidney disease: Evaluation, classification, and stratification. Ann Intern Med 2003;139:137-147.

Chapter

2 | Ischemia and Ischemia-Reperfusion–Induced Organ Injury

Mitchell P. Fink

■ A CELLULAR ENERGETICS PRIMER

The first law of thermodynamics states that the total amount of energy in a system remains constant before and after any sort of transforming event. The second law of thermodynamics states that even though the total amount of energy does not change after a transforming event, the total amount of usable energy—the Gibbs free energy (G)—always decreases. In accordance with the second law of thermodynamics, all reversible chemical reactions proceed in the direction that results in a net decrease in the Gibbs free energy for the system; in other words, the change in G (ΔG) is always less than zero. When cells in living systems need to carry out a reaction for which ΔG is positive, they couple the reaction to another reaction that is energetically favorable (i.e., characterized by a ΔG less than zero). If the algebraic sum of the ΔGs for the two coupled reactions is negative, then formation of the desired product can proceed. For example, the amidation of glutamate by ammonium ion to form glutamine is an *endergonic* reaction, meaning that ΔG is greater than zero. To drive this reaction toward the formation of glutamate, cells couple it to another reaction, the hydrolysis of adenosine triphosphate (ATP) to form adenosine diphosphate (ADP) and inorganic phosphate (Pi), which is *exergonic* (ΔG negative). The algebraic sum of the changes in Gibbs free energy for the two reactions is negative, and the coupled reactions proceed, yielding the products glutamine, ADP, Pi, and a hydrogen ion.

Within cells, hundreds of reactions would not proceed without this sort of coupling. And, in most cases, the exergonic reaction that drives formation of the desired product is hydrolysis of the terminal pyrophosphate ester linkage of ATP to yield ADP and Pi. The hydrolysis of ATP also drives other energy-requiring processes in cells, such as the active pumping of solutes against a concentration gradient across a membrane barrier. Thus, for proper functioning, all cells need a steady supply of ATP. Stated another way, ATP is the energy currency of the cell.

ATP can be generated in cells as a result of both aerobic and anaerobic processes. Anaerobic generation of ATP, or the energetically equivalent compound guanosine triphosphate (GTP), occurs in both the cytosol and the mitochondria as a result of the phosphorylation reactions that are catalyzed by the enzymes phosphoglycerate kinase, pyruvate kinase, and succinyl–coenzyme A (CoA) synthase. Aerobic generation of ATP occurs in the mitochondria as a result of a care-

fully orchestrated series of reactions that effectively couple the oxidation of substrates by molecular oxygen (O_2), on the one hand, to the phosphorylation of ADP to form ATP, on the other.

Good reducing agents are elements or compounds that have a strong propensity to donate electrons to another element or compound, whereas good oxidizing agents are elements or compounds that avidly accept electrons. O_2 is a very potent oxidizing agent. Two strong reducing agents—the reduced forms of nicotine adenine dinucleotide (NADH) and dihydroflavin adenine dinucleotide ($FADH_2$)—are produced in cells during glycolysis and the citric acid cycle. In mitochondria, these two reducing agents are oxidized by O_2, and the energy released during this process is used to drive the formation of ATP.

The reaction of a strong reducing agent, such as NADH, with a powerful oxidizing agent, such as O_2, releases a large amount of energy. To take optimal advantage of this highly exergonic redox reaction and capture as much of the energy released as possible in a usable form (i.e., as the high-energy terminal pyrophosphate bond in ATP), mitochondria "step down" the reducing potential of NADH (and $FADH_2$) in stages. Thus, the electrons are not transferred from NADH to O_2 all at once but rather are transferred through a series of intermediate compounds, called electron carriers, that have progressively lower reducing potentials. Several of the electron carriers involved in the mitochondrial respiratory chain are organized as complexes located within the inner mitochondrial membrane. These complexes use the energy released during electron transfer to actively pump protons from the mitochondrial matrix into the intermembrane space, thereby generating an electrochemical gradient across the inner mitochondrial membrane. The presence of this gradient drives hydrogen ions through a mitochondrial enzyme, the F_0F_1-ATPase, that catalyzes the formation of ATP from ADP and Pi.

For each mole of glucose metabolized to carbon dioxide and water, the net yield of ATP from substrate level (anaerobic) phosphorylation reactions is 4 moles of ATP, whereas the net yield of ATP from oxidative phosphorylation reactions is 32 moles of ATP. Thus, oxidative metabolism in normally functioning mitochondria is far more efficient at producing ATP than is anaerobic metabolism, and many cell types, such as hepatocytes, neurons, and cardiac myocytes, are dependent on a steady supply of O_2.

■ OXIDANT STRESS

Reactive Oxygen and Reactive Nitrogen Species

Reactive oxygen species (ROS) are reactive, partially reduced derivatives of O_2. Some important ROS in biological systems include superoxide radical anion ($O_2^-\cdot$), hydrogen peroxide (H_2O_2), and hydroxyl radical (OH·). Closely related are various so-called reactive nitrogen species (RNS), exemplified by the weak acid, peroxynitrous acid (ONOOH), and its anion, peroxynitrite (ONOO⁻). Free radicals are atoms or molecules that contain one or more unpaired electrons in outer (bonding) atomic or molecular orbitals. The presence of unpaired electron(s) usually renders these species extremely reactive. In biological systems, most free radicals are ROS; $O_2^-\cdot$ is a good example. By the same token, not all ROS or RNS are free radicals. For example, neither H_2O_2 nor ONOO⁻ is a free radical.

ROS are implicated as being important in the pathogenesis in a wide range of diseases or pathologic processes, including various forms of cancer, type 2 diabetes mellitus, atherosclerosis, chronic inflammatory conditions, ischemia-reperfusion injury, sepsis, and some neurodegenerative diseases.[1] Additionally, ROS are important under both physiologic and pathophysiologic conditions as key mediators in a number of different intracellular signaling cascades.[1]

Sources of ROS and RNS

Although many enzymatic processes can lead to the formation of ROS, the mitochondrial electron transport chain is thought to be the principal source of partially reduced forms of oxygen, at least in cell types such as neurons, cardiomyocytes, and hepatocytes, which are richly endowed with these organelles. Indeed, it is estimated that about 0.2% of the O_2 consumed by cells is converted into ROS, and 90% of the ROS generated are derived from mitochondria.[2]

In addition to intramitochondrial reactions, a variety of other enzymatic processes can generate ROS in mammalian cells. Principal among these are the reactions catalyzed by the enzymes nicotinamide adenine dinucleotide phosphate (NADPH) oxidase and xanthine oxidase (XO). NADPH oxidase catalyzes the one-electron reduction of O_2 to form $O_2^-\cdot$, using NADPH as the electron donor. NADPH oxidase is an enzyme complex that is assembled after the activation of phagocytes by microbes or microbial products (such as lipopolysaccharide [LPS]), various proinflammatory mediators (e.g., tumor necrosis factor), or exposure to ROS. In resting cells, the components of NADPH oxidase are present in the cytosol and the membranes of various intracellular organelles. When the cell is activated, the components are assembled on a membrane-bound vesicle, which then fuses with the plasma membrane, resulting in the release of $O_2^-\cdot$ outward into the extracellular milieu and inward into the phagocytic vesicle. The reaction catalyzed by NADPH oxidase is critical for the formation of ROS in macrophages and polymorphonuclear neutrophils (PMNs). NADPH oxidase, however, is also present in other cell types, including vascular smooth muscle cells, neurons, epithelial cells, and endothelial cells.[3-5]

XO catalyzes the oxidation of xanthine (or hypoxanthine) by O_2 to form uric acid and $O_2^-\cdot$. XO is a post-translationally modified form of another closely related enzyme, xanthine dehydrogenase (XD), which utilizes NAD^+ as a cofactor, and converts xanthine (or hypoxanthine) to uric acid without forming ROS. XD is rapidly converted to XO under a variety of physiologic and pathophysiologic conditions via (reversible) oxidation of critical cysteine residues or irreversible proteolytic cleavage of a segment of the protein. Conditions that are associated with XD-to-XO conversion include cellular hypoxia and exposure to various proinflammatory mediators.[6]

The enzyme nitric oxide synthase (NOS) is crucial for the formation of reactive nitrogen intermediates (RNI). NOS catalyzes the formation of a gaseous free radical, nitric oxide (NO·), and the amino acid L-citrulline, from the amino acid L-arginine, in a complex, five-electron redox reaction that requires O_2 and a number of other cofactors. If L-arginine availability is limiting, NOS can generate $O_2^-\cdot$.[7-9] At least three isoforms of NOS have been identified: NOS-1, or neuronal NOS (nNOS); NOS-3, or endothelial NOS (eNOS); and NOS-2, or inducible NOS (iNOS). Both nNOS and eNOS are constitutively expressed, and the production of NO· by these enzymes is tightly regulated by changes in intracellular Ca^{2+} concentration. In contrast, iNOS, which contains calmodulin as a tightly bound subunit even under nominally Ca^{2+}-free conditions, is expressed only after induction by various cytokines or LPS. A fourth form of NOS, mitochondrial NOS, has been postulated to exist, but the existence of this entity remains highly controversial.[10] Increased expression of iNOS is easily demonstrated when murine macrophages or PMNs are stimulated by LPS or various proinflammatory cytokines, such as interferon-γ (IFN-γ). It has been much harder to document iNOS induction in human phagocytic cells, but appropriately stimulated human macrophages are capable of producing NO· via an iNOS-dependent mechanism.[11] A variety of other human cell types, such as intestinal[12,13] and alveolar[14] epithelial cells, are also capable of producing large amounts of NO· via an iNOS-dependent mechanism.

The Central Role of Superoxide Radical Anion

Although intrinsically not exceptionally reactive, $O_2^-\cdot$ occupies a central place in the biochemistry of oxidant stress. The superoxide radical participates in the Haber-Weiss reaction ($O_2^-\cdot + H_2O_2 \rightarrow O_2 + OH\cdot + OH^-$), which combines a Fenton reaction ($Fe^{2+} + H_2O_2 \rightarrow Fe^{3+} + OH\cdot + OH^-$) and the reduction of Fe^{3+} by $O_2^-\cdot$, yielding Fe^{2+} and oxygen ($Fe^{3+} + O_2^-\cdot \rightarrow Fe^{2+} + O_2$).[15] The hydroxyl radical, OH·, is extremely reactive, combining within a very short period (~10^{-9} sec) with other molecules that are physically located close to its site of formation.[16] Under the conditions that are commonly associated with upregulated iNOS expression, cells are stimulated to produce not only NO· but also $O_2^-\cdot$. These two free radicals react with each other at diffusion-limited rates to produce the potent oxidizing and nitrosating agent, ONOO⁻.

The Molecular Targets for ROS and RNS

The general processes whereby ROS cause pathologic changes in cells and tissues are collectively referred to as oxidative (or oxidant) stress. Because ROS are continuously being produced in cells, oxidative stress occurs not as a result of the production of ROS per se but rather when the biosynthesis of ROS exceeds the capacity of various intrinsic antioxidant defense systems to detoxify these reactive species (see later).

At high concentrations, ROS can covalently modify most structures in the cell, including nucleic acids, lipids, and proteins.[17] The hydroxyl radical reacts with all components of the DNA molecule, damaging both the purine and pyrimidine bases and also the deoxyribose backbone.[17]

Single-strand breaks in nuclear DNA can activate an enzyme called poly(ADP-ribose)polymerase-1 (PARP-1). Activation of PARP-1 catalyzes the cleavage of NAD^+ into ADP-ribose and nicotinamide and the polymerization of the resultant ADP-ribose units into branching poly(ADP-ribose) homopolymers.[18,19] Simultaneously, poly-ADP ribose is degraded by various nuclear enzymes, especially poly(ADP-ribose) glycohydrolase.[19,20] The concurrent actions of PARP-1 and poly(ADP-ribose) glycohydrolase constitute the functional equivalent of an NADase. In states of acute inflammation or as a result of ischemia followed by reperfusion (see later), ROS and RNS, including H_2O_2 and $ONOO^-$ (and related oxidants), can induce single-strand breaks in nuclear DNA and thereby activate PARP-1. As a consequence, the $NAD^+/NADH$ content of cells can be depleted. Because NADH is the main reducing equivalent used to support oxidative phosphorylation, activation of PARP-1 can lead to a marked impairment in the ability of cells to utilize O_2 to support ATP synthesis.[21]

The notion that redox stress can lead to PARP-1 activation and metabolic inhibition on this basis was first articulated by Schraufstatter and colleagues.[22,23] Szabó and coworkers subsequently showed that exposure of cultured cells to physiologically relevant concentrations of $ONOO^-$ activated PARP-1 and, on this basis, resulted in impaired mitochondrial respiration.[24] Szabó and coworkers further showed that endogenously generated $ONOO^-$ was capable of activating PARP-1 and thereby inhibiting mitochondrial respiration in cultured immunostimulated macrophages[25] and vascular smooth muscle cells.[26]

ROS also attack carbon-carbon double bonds in the polyunsaturated fatty acid (PUFA) residues of phospholipids, leading to the formation of peroxyl radicals ($ROO\cdot$). The radicals that are thereby formed can attack other targets (e.g., another PUFA residue), leading to propagation of a chain reaction and widespread damage to cellular constituents. Additionally, ROS can oxidize the sulfhydryl (—SH) groups of cysteine residues in proteins, leading to the formation of intramolecular disulfides or mixed disulfides with other —SH-containing small molecules, notably the tripeptide glutathione (GSH). RNS, such as $ONOO^-$, can S-nitrosylate cysteine residues, leading to loss of function of key proteins.

Intrinsic Antioxidant Defense Mechanisms

In view of the myriad potential deleterious effects of ROS and RNS, it is not surprising that mammalian cells have evolved a number of different mechanisms for detoxifying these reactive species. A key compound in the cell's defenses against oxidant stress is GSH.[27] The oxidized form of glutathione is glutathione disulfide. GSH is highly abundant in the cytosol (1 to 11 mM), nuclei (3 to 15 mM), and mitochondria (5 to 11 mM) and is the major soluble antioxidant in these cellular compartments. GSH protects cells against redox stress in more than one way. First, GSH acts as a cofactor for several ROS detoxifying enzymes, such as glutathione peroxidase and glutathione transferase. Second, GSH directly scavenges certain highly reactive species (e.g., $OH\cdot$). And, third, GSH participates in the regeneration of other key endogenous antioxidants, such as ascorbate and vitamin E.

Another key group of endogenous ROS scavengers are isoforms of the enzyme superoxide dismutase (SOD). These enzymes react with $O_2^-\cdot$ and dismutate the radical to the nonradical products O_2 and H_2O_2, at rates that are faster than $O_2^-\cdot$ can react with other potential biological targets.[28] There are three known isoforms of SOD: the manganese-containing enzyme, SOD2, which is localized to mitochondria; the copper and zinc–containing enzyme, SOD1, which is localized to the cytosol; and SOD3, which is present in the extracellular milieu. Knocking out SOD2 is lethal in mice, emphasizing the critical importance of this SOD isoform.[28]

In addition to GSH-dependent and SOD-dependent mechanisms, other important cellular buffers against redox stress include various small molecules, such as ascorbate, vitamin E, carotenoids, and lipoic acid. Catalase, an enzyme that catalyzes the conversion of H_2O_2 to water and O_2, is also important.

■ ISCHEMIA

Tissues can be rendered ischemic as a result of a relatively localized derangement in perfusion, such as occurs during coronary thrombosis, or as a result of a more generalized derangement in cardiac output, such as occurs during hypovolemic shock. Both localized and generalized derangements in perfusion can be present simultaneously; an example might be hemorrhage, leading to a global embarrassment of cardiac output, in a patient with critical carotid stenosis caused by atherosclerotic vascular disease, precipitating a stroke. When tissues are ischemic, the supply of O_2 is inadequate to meet metabolic demand. Inevitably, during ischemia, there are a number of biochemical consequences, which vary somewhat, depending on the cell type that is affected. For example, some of the metabolic events in ischemic cardiomyocytes, which store energy not only as ATP but also as creatine phosphate, are different from those in ischemic hepatocytes, which lack the enzymatic machinery to make or store creatine phosphate. In cardiac and skeletal muscle cells, creatine phosphate serves as a temporary store of high-energy phosphate bonds.

Because O_2 is (totally or relatively) unavailable as a terminal electron acceptor, the flow of substrates through the mitochondrial tricarboxylic acid (TCA) cycle is inhibited, and little or no energy is available from oxidative phosphorylation. As a result, NADH accumulates in the cytosol and the $NADH/NAD^+$ ratio increases severalfold. In anoxia (with preserved blood flow), ATP levels can be partially defended by glycolysis, but during ischemia, glycolysis (of glucose derived from stored glycogen) is accompanied by accumulation of lactate and acidification of the cytoplasm. In this case, glycolysis is inhibited, further contributing to the cellular energy deficit.[29]

As the flow of electrons through the electron transport chain slows or ceases during ischemia, the inner mitochondrial membrane depolarizes, leading to accumulation of Pi, and to decreased synthesis of ATP. When the ATP level in the cell decreases, the phosphorylation potential (defined by the ratio of ATP concentration to ADP concentration) also decreases. As a consequence, cellular function is impaired. Furthermore, as intracellular pH (pH_i) decreases, mechanisms come into play that are designed to prevent excessive cellular acidification. Specifically, cells activate a cell membrane Na^+/H^+ antiporter, but this process leads to intracellular Na^+ accumulation, because the low phosphorylation potential (i.e., ATP deficit) limits functioning of the Na^+,K^+-ATPase that pumps Na^+ out of the cytosol. Consequently, the activity of the Na^+/Ca^{2+} antiporter, which usually pumps Ca^{2+} out of the cell, is reduced or reversed, and the cell becomes loaded with Na^+ and Ca^{2+}, leading to cellular swelling as well the toxic effects of an abnormally high intracellular ionized calcium concentration.

During prolonged cellular hypoxia, the decreased flow of electrons through the mitochondrial electron transport chain has another consequence in addition to those mentioned in the previous paragraph. Mitochondria generate relatively small quantities of ROS under normal conditions, but during episodes of cellular hypoxia, the production of ROS increases. Although this idea at first seems paradoxical, there are good data to suggest that mitochondrial $O_2^-\cdot$ production increases under hypoxic conditions.[30-32] On the basis of purely thermodynamic considerations, one would not predict that a decrease in substrate (O_2) concentration would cause an increase in the rate of a simple first-order reaction.

However, other factors are apparently involved. Guzy and Schumacker[33] have identified at least two potential mechanisms that can conceivably contribute to this paradoxical response. One hypothesis suggests that the interaction of O_2 with proteins or lipids at complex III modulates the lifetime of the free radical ubisemiquinone at this site. By prolonging the lifetime of the unstable ubisemiquinone molecule, the opportunity for $O_2^-\cdot$ production increases, despite the decreased availability of substrate (O_2). Another hypothesis suggests that hypoxia might increase the access of O_2 to ubisemiquinone at complex III. Thus, if the molecular structure of one or more of the proteins in complex III is affected by the O_2 concentration in the membrane such that the ability of O_2 to react with ubisemiquinone is improved under low-O_2 conditions, then this change would increase ROS production despite the decrease in the availability of O_2.

The Mitochondrial Permeability Transition Pore

Under normal physiologic conditions, the mitochondrial inner membrane is permeable to only a few selected metabolites and ions. However, under conditions of stress, a nonspecific pore known as the mitochondrial permeability transition pore (MPTP) opens in the mitochondrial inner membrane.

Opening of the MPTP allows free passage of any molecule smaller than about 1.5 kDa.[34] Two major consequences follow. First, although low-molecular-weight solutes move freely across the membrane, proteins do not. As a result, colloidal osmotic pressure causes mitochondria to swell. Although the unfolding of the cristae allows the matrix to expand without rupture of the inner membrane, the outer membrane breaks, permitting the release of proapoptotic proteins, such as cytochrome-*c,* from the intermembrane space into the cytosol. Second, the inner membrane becomes freely permeable to protons, leading to uncoupling of oxidative phosphorylation. Under these conditions, the F_0F_1-ATPase actually reverses direction and functions as an enzyme catalyzing the hydrolysis of ATP, rather than the synthesis of it. Accordingly, cellular ATP concentration decreases precipitously, leading to the disruption of ionic and metabolic homeostasis and the activation of degradative enzymes, such as phospholipases, nucleases, and proteases. Unless the MPTP closes, these changes lead to irreversible damage to the cell and necrotic death.

Opening of the MPTP is a complex process.[35] However, it is known that the key factor responsible for MPTP opening is mitochondrial calcium overload, especially when this is accompanied by oxidative stress, adenine nucleotide depletion, elevated Pi concentration, and mitochondrial depolarization. From the previous discussion, all the factors that promote opening of the MPTP are likely to occur during ischemia or, as will be discussed later, during the reperfusion that follows ischemia. In addition, ROS production can lead to irreversible damage to mitochondrial enzymes, including those in complexes I, II, and III and aconitase.

■ ISCHEMIA-REPERFUSION INJURY

Although essential to alleviate ischemic injury, reperfusion of ischemic tissues can paradoxically exacerbate damage, leading to cell death (via apoptosis or necrosis, or both) and dysregulated inflammation. Although extensively studied since ground-breaking work by Hearse and colleagues[36] and Granger and associates[37] several decades ago, the mechanisms whereby reperfusion exacerbates tissue injury remain incompletely understood.

The Role of Xanthine Oxidase

A considerable body of evidence suggests that XO-mediated formation of ROS is a critical early event in many forms of ischemia-reperfusion injury. During the period of ischemia, the breakdown of ATP results in the accumulation of hypoxanthine, a substrate for xanthine oxidase activity. Moreover, XD is irreversibly converted to XO during ischemia. XO-mediated ROS production, however, is delayed until reperfusion, because O_2 is an essential substrate for this reaction. Therefore, when blood flow is restored after a prolonged period of hypoperfusion, all the conditions are present to allow a burst of ROS production.

Although XO-mediated ROS formation is a critical early step in the pathogenesis of ischemia-reperfusion injury in some organs, such as the intestine,[37,38] the role of XO-dependent mechanisms in other organs, most notably the heart, is more controversial,[39,40] because human and rabbit cardiac tissue contain relatively small amounts of the XD gene product and yet are still susceptible to damage during the restoration of blood flow after a period of hypoperfusion. Current thinking generally supports the idea that human cardiac endothelial cells subjected to ischemia contain small but still biologically significant amounts of XO, and that XO-dependent ROS-mediated endothelial damage is an important early event in damage to the heart related to reperfusion.[41] In studies using human aortic or venous endothelial cells, XO-mediated ROS generation has been documented after postischemic reoxygenation.[42] Importantly, administration of allopurinol, a potent inhibitor of XO, has been shown to improve postoperative recovery and reduce lipid peroxidation in open-heart surgery patients.[43]

The Role of Neutrophils

The initial burst of oxidants during reperfusion (probably via an XO-dependent mechanism) can damage and/or activate capillary endothelial cells, leading to a multistep process that results in the accumulation of activated PMNs within the interstitium.[44,45] The first step is increased expression of a protein, P-selectin, on the surface of microvascular endothelial cells. When endothelial cells are activated by ROS (or various proinflammatory molecules that are released during reperfusion), P-selectin moves from an internal cell location to the cell surface. P-selectin interacts with a counter-receptor on PMNs called P-selectin glycoprotein 1 (PSGL-1). This initial low-affinity interaction results in intermittent leukocyte–endothelial binding, a phenomenon that induces a characteristic rolling of PMNs over the endothelium. This step is followed by firm adherence of PMNs to the endothelial surface as a result of the interaction of β_2-integrins (CD11a/CD18 and CD11b/CD18) on PMNs with endothelial intercellular adhesion molecule 1 (ICAM-1). Expression of ICAM-1 is upregulated on the surface of endothelial cells that have been activated by ROS or proinflammatory mediators. Leukocyte transmigration into the interstitial compartment is facilitated by platelet–endothelial cell adhesion molecule 1 (PECAM-1), which is constitutively expressed along endothelial cell–cell junctions. On reaching the extravascular compartment, activated PMNs release ROS as well as various proteases and elastases, resulting in increased microvascular permeability, edema, thrombosis, and parenchymal cell death. Accumulation of PMNs in the extravascular compartment is also facilitated by various chemotactic substances, including leukotriene B_4 and interleukin 8, which are released by activated cells.

The Role of Complement Activation

Oxidant stress results in complement activation and deposition of complement components on the vascular endothelium.[46] Furthermore, in experimental animals, both general depletion of complement and the pharmacologic blockade of specific complement components ameliorate tissue injury induced by ischemia and reperfusion.[46] Similarly beneficial effects are observed when complement activation is blocked in animals as a result of genetically induced deficiencies of key complement components. Blockade of complement after

oxidative stress decreases endothelial adhesion molecule expression, infiltration of PMNs, and the production of inflammatory mediators.

The Role of Mitochondrial Amplification of Oxidant Stress

Although normal mitochondrial respiration is associated with low-level ROS production, mitochondrial production of ROS is increased by exposure to oxidants. This phenomenon is termed ROS-induced ROS release (RIRR).[47] Two modes of RIRR have been described. The first mode is related to opening of the MPTP. Exposure of mitochondria to a level of oxidant stress that exceeds intrinsic detoxifying capacity leads to mitochondrial depolarization as a result of opening of the MPTP. In turn, mitochondrial depolarization promotes a burst of ROS production as a result of electron leakage from the electron transport chain.[47] The second mode of RIRR is MPTP independent, but it is related to opening of an inner mitochondrial membrane anion channel, resulting in a brief increase in ROS production from the electron transport chain.[48]

■ THERAPEUTIC CONSIDERATIONS

The best way to ameliorate tissue damage and organ dysfunction related to ischemia or ischemia-reperfusion is to prevent tissue hypoperfusion in the first place. In the context of perioperative medicine, this concept translates into the need to pay close attention to the adequacy of intravascular volume status and cardiac performance. However, in many circumstances, such as vascular reconstructive procedures, various cardiac operations, resuscitation from accidental trauma and hemorrhagic shock, and solid organ transplantation, episodes of tissue ischemia are unavoidable. Accordingly, there is enormous interest in developing improved pharmacologic strategies for ameliorating ischemia-induced and ischemia-reperfusion–induced tissue damage.

Although a wide variety of ROS scavengers have been evaluated in thousands of preclinical studies using experimental animals and in hundreds of clinical studies, this form of pharmacologic therapy remains largely experimental. One well-studied ROS scavenger, N-acetylcysteine (NAC), is widely used to ameliorate hepatic damage related to overdoses of acetaminophen,[49] a problem that is known to be caused by oxidant stress. Treatment with NAC has also been shown to prevent contrast-induced renal dysfunction, although the robustness of these data is very controversial.[50]

Various XO inhibitors, such as oxypurinol and allopurinol, have been studied for the treatment of a wide variety of acute and chronic conditions that are thought to be mediated, at least in part, by ROS-dependent mechanisms. Both positive[43,51,52] and negative[53,54] results have been reported.

Encouraging results were recently reported with nitrone-based free radical scavenger for the adjuvant treatment of acute stroke,[55] but these results will need to be validated in a larger, phase 3 clinical trial before the U.S. Food and Drug Administration (FDA) will approve this novel therapeutic agent for this indication. In contrast, discouraging results have been obtained in studies of pexelizumab, a monoclonal antibody against (complement component) C5.[56-58] Generally positive results, however, were obtained in studies of recombinant human C1-esterase inhibitor, which is a protein that blocks activation of the classical complement cascade.[59,60]

■ REFERENCES

1. Dröge W: Free radicals in the physiological control of cell function. Physiol Rev 2002;82:47-95.
2. Balaban RS, Nemoto S, Finkel T: Mitochondria, oxidants, and aging. Cell 2005;120:483-495.
3. Gill PS, Wilcox CS: NADPH oxidases in the kidney. Antioxid Redox Signal 2006;8:1597-1607.
4. Infanger DW, Sharma RV, Davisson RL: NADPH oxidases of the brain: Distribution, regulation, and function. Antioxid Redox Signal 2006;8:1583-1596.
5. Rokutan K, Kawahara T, Kuwano Y, et al: NADPH oxidases in the gastrointestinal tract: A potential role of Nox1 in innate immune response and carcinogenesis. Antioxid Redox Signal 2006;8:1573-1582.
6. Meneshian A, Bulkley GB: The physiology of endothelial xanthine oxidase: From urate catabolism to reperfusion injury to inflammatory signal transduction. Microcirculation 2002;9:161-175.
7. Fink MP: Role of reactive oxygen and nitrogen species in acute respiratory distress syndrome. Curr Opin Crit Care 2002;8:6-11.
8. Pou S, Pou WS, Bredt DS, et al: Generation of superoxide by purified brain nitric oxide synthase. J Biol Chem 1992;267:24173-24176.
9. Xia Y, Tsai AL, Berka V, et al: Superoxide generation from endothelial nitric-oxide synthase: A Ca^{2+}/calmodulin-dependent and tetrahydrobiopterin regulatory process. J Biol Chem 1998;273:25804-25808.
10. Jiang J, Kurnikov I, Belikova NA, et al: Structural requirements for optimized delivery, inhibition of oxidative stress and anti-apoptotic activity of targeted nitroxides. J Pharmacol Exp Ther 2007.
11. Nicholson SC, Bonecini-Almeida Mda G, Lapa e Silva JR, et al: Inducible nitric oxide synthase in pulmonary alveolar macrophages from patients with tuberculosis. J Exp Med 1996;183:2293-2302.
12. Perner A, Andresen L, Normark M, et al: Expression of inducible nitric oxide synthase and effects of L-arginine on colonic nitric oxide production and fluid transport in patients with "minimal colitis." Scand J Gastroenterol 2005;40:1042-1048.
13. Unno N, Hodin RA, Fink MP: Acidic conditions exacerbate interferon-gamma-induced intestinal epithelial hyperpermeability: Role of peroxynitrous acid. Crit Care Med 1999;27:1429-1436.
14. Okamoto T, Valacchi G, Gohil K, et al: S-nitrosothiols inhibit cytokine-mediated induction of matrix metalloproteinase-9 in airway epithelial cells. Am J Respir Cell Mol Biol 2002;27:463-473.
15. Liochev SI, Fridovich I: The Haber-Weiss cycle-70 years later: An alternative view. Redox Report 2002;7:55-57.
16. Pryor WA, Houk KN, Foote CS, et al: Free radical biology and medicine: It's a gas, man! Am J Physiol Regul Integr Comp Physiol 2006;291: R491-511.
17. Valko M, Leibritz D, Moncol J, et al: Free radicals and antioxidants in normal physiological functions and human disease. Int J Biochem Cell Biol 2007;39:44-84.
18. Lautier D, Lageux J, Thibodeau J, et al: Molecular and biochemical features of poly (ADP-ribose) metabolism. Mol Cell Biochem 1993;122: 171-193.
19. D'Amours D, Desnoyers S, D'Silva I, et al: Poly(ADP-ribosyl)ation reactions in the regulation of nuclear functions. Biochem J 1999;342: 249-268.
20. Ame JC, Jacobson EL, Jacobson MK: Molecular heterogeneity and regulation of poly(ADP-ribose) glycohydrolase. Mol Cell Biochem 1999;193:75-81.
21. Fink MP: Bench-to-bedside review: Cytopathic hypoxia. Crit Care 2002;6:491-499.
22. Schraufstatter IU, Hinshaw DB, Hyslop PA, et al: Oxidant injury of cells: DNA strand-breaks activate polyadenosine diphosphate-ribose polymerase and lead to depletion of nicotinamide adenine dinucleotide. J Clin Invest 1986;77:1312-1320.
23. Schraufstatter IU, Hyslop PA, Hinshaw DB, et al: Hydrogen peroxide-induced injury of cells and its prevention by inhibitors of poly(ADP-ribose) polymerase. Proc Natl Acad Sci U S A 1986;83:4908-4912.
24. Szabó C, Saunders C, O'Connor M, et al: Peroxynitrite causes energy depletion and increases permeability via activation of poly (ADP-ribose) synthetase in pulmonary epithelial cells. Am J Respir Cell Mol Biol 1997;16:105-109.
25. Zingarelli B, O'Connor M, Wong H, et al: Peroxynitrite-mediated DNA strand breakage activates poly-ADP ribosyl synthetase and causes cellular energy depletion in macrophages stimulated with bacterial lipopolysaccharide. J Immunol 1996;156:350-358.
26. Szabó C, Zingarelli B, O'Connor M, Salzman AL: DNA strand breakage, activation of poly-ADP ribosyl synthetase, and cellular energy depletion are involved in the cytotoxicity in macrophages and smooth muscle cells exposed to peroxynitrite. Proc Natl Acad Sci 1996;93: 1753-1758.
27. Masella R, Di Benedetto R, Vari R, et al: Novel mechanisms of natural antioxidant compounds in biological systems: Involvement of glutathione and glutathione-related enzymes. J Nutr Biochem 2005;16: 577-586.
28. Cuzzocrea S, Riley DP, Caputi AP, et al: Antioxidant therapy: A new pharmacological approach in shock, inflammation, and ischemia/reperfusion injury. Pharmacol Rev 2001;53:135-159.
29. Solaini G, Harris DA: Biochemical dysfunction in heart mitochondria exposed to ischaemia and reperfusion. Biochem J 2005;390:377-394.
30. Kulisz A, Chen N, Chandel NS, et al: Mitochondrial ROS initiate phosphorylation of p38 MAP kinase during hypoxia in cardiomyocytes. Am J Physiol Lung Cell Mol Physiol 2002;282:L1324-1329.
31. Guzy RD, Hoyos B, Robin E, et al: Mitochondrial complex III is required for hypoxia-induced ROS production and cellular oxygen sensing. Cell Metab 2005;1:401-408.
32. Park Y, Kehrer JP: Oxidative changes in hypoxic-reoxygenated rabbit heart: A consequence of hypoxia rather than reoxygenation. Free Radic Res Comm 1991;14:179-185.
33. Guzy RD, Schumacker PT: Oxygen sensing by mitochondria at complex III: The paradox of increased reactive oxygen species during hypoxia. Exp Physiol 2006;91:807-819.
34. Halestrap AP: The mitochondrial permeability transition: Its molecular mechanism and role in reperfusion injury. Biochem Soc Symp 1999;66:181-203.
35. Halestrap AP, Clarke SJ, Javadov SA: Mitochondrial permeability transition pore opening during myocardial reperfusion—a target for cardioprotection. Cardiovasc Res 2004;61:372-385.
36. Hearse DJ, Humphrey SM, Chain EB: Abrupt reoxygenation of the anoxic potassium-arrested perfused rat heart: A study of myocardial enzyme release. J Mol Cell Cardiol 1973;5:395-407.
37. Granger DN, Rutili G, McCord JM: Superoxide radicals in feline intestinal ischemia. Gastroenterology 1981;81:22-29.
38. Grisham MB, Hernandez LA, Granger DN: Xanthine oxidase and neutrophil infiltration in intestinal ischemia. Am J Physiol 1986;251: G567-574.
39. Terada LS, Rubinstein JD, Lesnefsky EJ, et al: Existence and participation of xanthine oxidase in reperfusion injury of ischemic rabbit myocardium. Am J Physiol 1991;260:H805-810.
40. Downey JM, Miura T, Eddy LJ, et al: Xanthine oxidase is not a source of free radicals in the ischemic rabbit heart. J Mol Cell Cardiol 1987;19:1053-1060.
41. Zweier JL, Talukder MA: The role of oxidants and free radicals in reperfusion injury. Cardiovasc Res 2006;70:181-190.
42. Zweier JL, Kuppusamy P, Lutty GA: Measurement of endothelial cell free radical generation: Evidence for a central mechanism of free radical injury in post-ischemic tissues. Proc Natl Acad Sci U S A 1988;85:4046-4050.
43. Coghlan JG, Flitter WD, Clutton SM, et al: Allopurinol pretreatment improves postoperative recovery and reduces lipid peroxidation in patients undergoing coronary artery bypass grafting. J Thorac Cardiovasc Surg 1994;107:248-256.
44. Vinten-Johansen J: Involvement of neutrophils in the pathogenesis of lethal myocardial reperfusion injury. Cardiovasc Res 2004;61: 481-497.
45. Eltzschig HK, Collard CD: Vascular ischaemia and reperfusion injury. Br Med Bull 2004;70:71-86.

46. Hart ME, Walsch MC, Stahl GL: Initiation of complement activation following oxidative stress: In vitro and in vivo observations. Mol Immunol 2004;41:165-171.

47. Zorov DB, Filburn CR, Klotz LO, et al: Reactive oxygen species (ROS)-induced ROS release: A new phenomenon accompanying induction of the mitochondrial permeability transition in cardiac myocytes. J Exp Med 2000;192:1001-1014.

48. Aon MA, Cortassa S, Marban E, et al: Synchronized whole cell oscillations in mitochondrial metabolism triggered by a local release of reactive oxygen species in cardiac myocytes. J Biol Chem 2003;278:44735-44744.

49. Kanter MZ: Comparison of oral and I.V. acetylcysteine in the treatment of acetaminophen poisoning. Am J Health Syst Pharm 2007;63:1821-1827.

50. Bagshaw SM, McAlister FA, Manns BJ, et al: Acetylcysteine in the prevention of contrast-induced nephropathy: A case study of the pitfalls in the evolution of evidence. Arch Intern Med 2006;166:161-166.

51. Guan W, Osanai T, Kamada T, et al: Effect of allopurinol pretreatment on free radical generation after primary coronary angioplasty for acute myocardial infarction. J Cardiovasc Pharmacol 2003;41:699-705.

52. Clancy RR, McGaurn SA, Goin JE, et al: Allopurinol neurocardiac protection trial in infants undergoing heart surgery using deep hypothermic circulatory arrest. Pediatrics 2001;108:61-70.

53. Gavin AD, Struthers AD: Allopurinol reduces B-type natriuretic peptide concentrations and haemoglobin but does not alter exercise capacity in chronic heart failure. Heart 2005;91:749-753.

54. Mosler P, Sherman S, Marks J, et al: Oral allopurinol does not prevent the frequency or the severity of post-ERCP pancreatitis. Gastrointest Endosc 2005;62:245-250.

55. Lees KR, Zivin JA, Ashwood T, et al: Stroke-Acute Ischemic NXY Treatment (SAINT I) Trial Investigators: NXY-059 for acute ischemic stroke. N Engl J Med 2006;354:588-600.

56. APEX AMI Investigators, Armstrong PW, Granger CB, et al: Pexelizumab for acute ST-elevation myocardial infarction in patients undergoing primary percutaneous coronary intervention: A randomized controlled trial. JAMA 2007;297:43-51.

57. Verrier ED, Shernan SK, Taylor KM, et al: Terminal complement blockade with pexelizumab during coronary artery bypass graft surgery requiring cardiopulmonary bypass: A randomized trial. JAMA 2004;291:2319-2327.

58. Mahaffey KW, Granger CB, Nicolau JC, et al: Effect of pexelizumab, an anti-C5 complement antibody, as adjunctive therapy to fibrinolysis in acute myocardial infarction: The COMPlement inhibition in myocardial infarction treated with thromboLYtics (COMPLY) trial. Circulation 2003;108:1176-1183.

59. Thielmann M, Marggraf G, Neuhauser M, et al: Administration of C1-esterase inhibitor during emergency coronary artery bypass surgery in acute ST-elevation myocardial infarction. Eur J Cardiothorac Surg 2006;30:285-293.

60. de Zwaan C, Kleine AH, Diris JH, et al: Continuous 48-h C1-inhibitor treatment, following reperfusion therapy, in patients with acute myocardial infarction. Eur Heart J 2002;23:1670-1677.

3 The Inflammatory Response in Organ Injury

Benjamin Kohl and Clifford S. Deutschman

The inflammatory response to anesthetized (e.g., from surgery) or unanesthetized (e.g., from trauma) injury is a predictable, well-orchestrated set of events that has evolved to maximize an organism's healing potential. It is not unique to humans but is found in all vertebrate animals. Although healthy patients with a normal, balanced, well-controlled inflammatory response usually recover uneventfully, there are two sets of conditions that may alter outcome. First, in patients with preexisting disease (e.g., chronic obstructive pulmonary disease, renal failure, congestive heart failure), recovery from surgery or trauma is influenced by the interaction of the inflammatory response and the preexisting condition. The reserve of a particular organ (i.e., its ability to respond normally in the face of injury) most likely dictates the contribution it can make to the inflammatory response. Organs with less reserve are less capable of producing the response necessary to ensure recovery. Second, outcome in patients with an unbalanced inflammatory response is determined by the type and extent of these abnormalities. For example, outcome after an exaggerated response (e.g., the systemic inflammatory response syndrome [SIRS] or sepsis) appears to be determined by the ability to support the cardiovascular and pulmonary systems through a period of hypermetabolism. Conversely, outcome after a suppressed response or after a prolonged illness that depletes the system reflects the ability to support the compromised organ systems through a period of impaired function.

This chapter will review the normal inflammatory response to injury, the nature and development of an unbalanced response, and the interaction of either with common disease states. Practitioners should not only understand the normal response but also be able to detect deviations and respond appropriately. The most common deviations seen in intensive care units (ICUs) result from sepsis. Thus, a discussion of SIRS and the septic syndrome is necessary. Finally, why do some patients spend weeks to months recovering from injury, whereas others improve in days? The answer to this question may lie in an impairment in the immune and endocrine systems that leads to a state of chronic critical illness. Thus, it is important to understand what happens when the inflammatory response triumphs over an organ's ability to recover. Specific disease states, such as the acute respiratory distress syndrome (ARDS) and renal failure, as well as immune and endocrine incompetence, will be discussed.

◼ THE STRESS RESPONSE

The normal inflammatory response, more commonly known as the stress response, was originally described by Sir David Cuthbertson and then detailed more elaborately by Francis Moore.[1-3] What both of these esteemed scientists observed was a biphasic immune, inflammatory, and metabolic response to injury (Fig. 3-1). The first phase (termed *ebb* by Cuthbertson) represents a coordinated response aimed at immediate survival. Most notably, there is profound peripheral vasoconstriction with concomitant hypothermia and shunting of blood and substrates to vital organs. This phase is more commonly termed *shock* and, while substrates are mobilized and delivered to vital organs, global resting energy expenditure (REE) decreases. From a teleologic standpoint, the mechanism of shock evolved to ensure survival immediately after injury. However, shock is a treatable disease and with appropriate management, this phase of the response can be limited to a short period. Once survival appears likely, a transition occurs into a second stage (termed *flow* by Cuthbertson). This hypermetabolic phase is driven by and is proportional to the degree of the initial injury. Despite variability in the intensity of the stress response, the timeline of events is usually predictable. Virtually all mediators of inflammation and metabolism peak at about post-injury day 2 and then return to baseline by post-injury day 6 to 7. Deviations from this time course represent the effects of preexisting medical illness, treatment, or postoperative/injury complications. A more detailed discussion of the stress response follows.

Hypermetabolic Phase of Acute Injury

The observed increase in REE after injury represents a small portion of the massive neurohormonal flux and organ hyperactivity that is occurring (Table 3-1). This response includes increases in heart rate, contractility, and cardiac output, and in minute ventilation, total body oxygen consumption, and carbon dioxide production.[4,5] The neuroendocrine system responds to injury by increasing the production and secretion of catecholamines, antidiuretic hormone (ADH), cortisol, insulin, glucagon, and growth hormone. The hemostatic system, including coagulation, fibrinolysis, and the complement cascade, becomes active. Cuthbertson postulated that all of these systems become hyperactive, peak, and then return to baseline, as illustrated in Figure 3-1. The peak of the catabolic, inflammatory phase is proportional to the

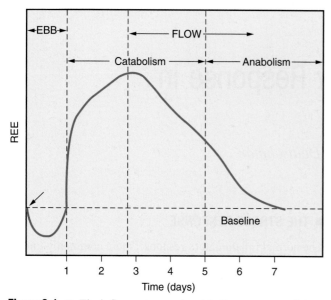

Figure 3-1 ■ The inflammatory and metabolic responses to injury are reflected in changes in resting energy expenditure (REE). Other indicators of stress (e.g., changes in cardiac output, heart rate, minute ventilation, plasma cytokine [interleukin] concentration, catecholamines) follow a similar time course. The *arrow* indicates the onset of injury (trauma or surgical incision).

3-1	Increases in Organ System Parameters after Major Surgery	

Organ System	Parameter
Cardiovascular	Cardiac output index
	Heart rate
	Systemic vascular resistance
Pulmonary	Minute ventilation (V_E)
	CO_2 production (V_{CO_2})
	Work of breathing
Nutritional/metabolic	Resting energy expenditure (REE)
	Inflammatory mediators
	Cytokines
	Interleukins
	Tumar necrosis factor (TNF)
	Oxygen consumption (V_{O_2})
	Lipolysis (respiratory quotient)
	Gluconeogenesis
	Glycogenolysis
Neuroendocrine	Catecholamines
	Corticosteroids
	Renin-angiotensin-aldosterone

The time course of these changes parallels that of the resting energy expenditure seen in Figure 3-1.

degree of injury. Key in this flow phase is the recruitment and migration of white blood cells (WBC). Macrophages migrate early in this response to afford the patient protection from microorganisms as well as to begin synthesis of collagen matrix as a barrier. At the same time, there is mobilization of hepatic glycogen stores (glycogenolysis), increased hepatic gluconeogenesis, lipolysis with mobilization of·free fatty acids, and skeletal and visceral muscle breakdown (providing substrates for gluconeogenesis). Recent studies have confirmed that body cell mass loss reflects a decrease in skeletal muscle mass and that total body water increases arise from resuscitation.[6] Thus, despite an often massive gain in weight, individuals lost an average of 16% of total body protein, 67% of which came from skeletal muscle. This hypermetabolic response ensures adequate quantities of substrates are supplied to key reparative cells—in particular, WBCs. Manifestations of this hypermetabolic phase can be seen clinically, metabolically, and physiologically (see Table 3-1).

The leukocytosis and hyperglycemia seen postoperatively are intimately related. White blood cells are obligate glutamine and glucose users and, thus, feed off the catabolism of skeletal and visceral muscles. Amino acids released into the circulation are taken up by the liver as substrates for gluconeogenesis and protein synthesis. The accumulation of substrates, however, is not sufficient for recovery. Nutrients must be delivered to the damaged tissue. This is no small feat given that most damaged tissue is relatively avascular (either iatrogenically by scalpel or via thrombosis of traumatized vessels). Although regional vasodilatation aids nutrient delivery, provision of substrates ultimately depends on development of a concentration gradient (i.e., mass action) and "vascular leak." Vascular leakage is seen clinically in every postoperative patient. The increased intravascular volume, along with greater arterial and venous capacitance, culminates in increased cardiac output. Patients are tachycardic, hyperthermic (representing hypermetabolism), hyperglycemic and leukocytotic (as a result of catabolism and repair), and edematous (from capillary leak).

In addition to the changes in hemodynamic parameters, indices of metabolism, such as REE, oxygen consumption, and carbon dioxide production, all increase in direct proportion to the magnitude of injury. This high rate of metabolism peaks between 48 and 72 hours and resolves by day 4 or 5. If allowed to go unchecked, this catabolic response would be disastrous. There must be some signal that indicates an end for the need of continued catabolism and high levels of substrate provision. For years, what initiated the transition from the peak of catabolism to a phase in which depleted endogenous stores were repleted (the "anabolic phase") remained a mystery. Although this question has not yet been definitively answered, research in wound healing may point in the right direction. Neovascularization (or angiogenesis) occurs between days 3 and 7 after an injury.[7,8] This time point coincides with a peak in vascular endothelial growth factor (VEGF) secretion.[9] Once angiogenesis has taken place and there is a mechanism to deliver substrates to damaged tissues, the need for high levels of catabolism abates. In particular, the body no longer needs to rely on a concentration gradient to deliver substrates to the site of injury. Future research into this area may have impact on development of novel therapeutics aimed at altering the stress response.

The changes in metabolism are paralleled and facilitated by alterations in physiologic responses. Thus, the cardiovascular system plays a critical role in the delivery of substrates (particularly amino acids and fatty acids) and oxygen to areas of damage. It also must ensure flow to areas where substrates are mobilized (e.g., skeletal muscle) and utilized (liver) and to "silent" regions during catabolism. Patients become tachycardic and hyperdynamic with an associated increase in myocardial oxygen consumption. Indeed, survival is associated with the ability to sustain this hypermetabolic state.[10-13] The capacity to maintain this hyperdynamic response depends on various intrinsic and extrinsic factors. The extrinsic factors include adequate volume resuscitation and maintenance of preload, afterload, and contractility. This concept of goal-directed therapy was first postulated by Shoemaker and Czer in 1979.[14] By maintaining a cardiac index of greater than 4.5 L/min/m^2, an oxygen delivery of greater than 600 mL/min/m^2, and an oxygen consumption of greater than 170 mL/min/m^2 (which were median values in a cohort of survivors of surgery), Shoemaker and colleagues demonstrated a reduction in mortality from 30% to 4%.[15] Details of more contemporary approaches to goal-directed therapy can be found elsewhere in this book.

In addition, pulmonary function must change to support inflammation. Increased excretion of carbon dioxide mandates an increase in minute ventilation. High levels of nitrogen mobilization, deamination, and excretion mandate an increase in renal blood flow and glomerular filtration rate. The liver must provide substrates through gluconeogenesis, detoxify nitrogenous waste via the synthesis of urea, and elaborate a series of acute-phase proteins that bind metabolic byproducts or contain proteolytic enzymes secreted by activated WBCs (α_1-antichymotrypsin or antitrypsin). Finally, the autonomic nervous system and the endocrine organs orchestrate the entire response.

■ INTERACTION OF INFLAMMATION AND COMMON DISEASES

Although the stress response as thus detailed is an expected and normal set of events following injury, the ability of patients to mount an appropriate reaction ultimately depends on organ reserve. Reserve is defined as the ability of a particular organ to respond normally in the face of injury. Thus, an organ with no reserve has no ability to adapt to, respond to, or recover from any physiologic perturbation. On the other hand, those organs (or cells) with high levels of reserve respond to injury in a manner that maintains physiologic homeostasis. Chronic and systemic diseases impact on a patient's ability to recover from surgery or injury by limiting overall reserve and negatively impacting on the capacity to mount a normal stress response. The following paragraphs will review three common disease states (coronary artery disease [CAD], chronic obstructive pulmonary disease [COPD], and diabetes mellitus) and the interaction they have with the inflammatory response.

Coronary Artery Disease

The ability of the physiologic system to support processes that contribute to hypermetabolism is exquisitely dependent on cardiac function. All indices of resting energy expenditure and basal metabolic rate rise postoperatively and usually peak between 48 and 72 hours (see Fig. 3-1). Therefore, CAD has a profound impact on the stress response to surgery or trauma. Myocardial ischemia or infarction in the postoperative period can be a result of coronary plaque disruption or myocardial oxygen demand/supply mismatch. Although usually thought of as mutually exclusive mechanisms, they are closely related, particularly during the stress response when inflammation is heightened. Patients can sustain myocardial infarctions (MIs) at different locations by different mechanisms. Most postoperative MIs occur in patients with significant coronary artery disease.[16] The peak incidence is on postoperative day 2, when cardiac output and thus myocardial oxygen demand are peaking. These MIs often present atypically. Chest pain may be absent or may be masked by postoperative pain or pain treatment. Most perioperative MIs are asymptomatic. The typical postoperative MI is characterized by the absence of Q waves. Perioperative MIs are frequently preceded by ST-segment depression rather than ST-segment elevation.[17-22] Whether a patient succumbs to the effects of CAD is highly dependent on coronary arterial anatomy, as well as on myocardial oxygen supply, delivery, and demand. Accordingly, there are a host of interventions that can limit the potential for an adverse myocardial event. These include maintenance of euvolemia, treatment of pain, prevention of anemia (although what level of hemoglobin is critical remains unclear), and prevention of tachycardia and hypotension. In patients with risk factors, perioperative beta-blockade has been shown to reduce cardiac morbidity and mortality.[23,24] Recent studies suggest a role for statin therapy and perhaps even angiotensin inhibition.[25-28]

Chronic Obstructive Pulmonary Disease

Patients with diagnosed COPD have a 2.7- to 4.7-fold increase in risk for postoperative pulmonary complications.[29-31] The ability to excrete CO_2 depends on sufficient pulmonary reserve. Postoperative pulmonary complications (PPCs) are common and have been documented to increase morbidity, mortality, and length of stay.[29,32] The anticipated surgical site is the most important risk factor for PPCs, and intrathoracic and abdominal surgeries carry the greatest risk for PPCs.[29,33,34] How intrinsic lung disease, such as COPD, impacts the postsurgical inflammatory response is not immediately apparent. However, because CO_2 production increases in the first 48 hours after surgery, impaired ventilation can be a problem for these patients. Increased CO_2 production (V_{CO_2}) is the main cause of increased minute ventilation (V_E) and thus respiratory demand in postoperative patients.[35] The primary pathophysiologic derangement in COPD is airflow obstruction, limiting expiratory flow. This flow limitation cannot be overcome by increased expiratory effort, which tends to collapse airways further. This effect is particularly exaggerated in patients with COPD. The only way to compensate for the increased demand in V_E is to increase inspiratory flow and lung volume. Thus, although the disease is primarily expiratory in origin, compensation occurs on the inspiratory limb. The increase in lung volume makes the diaphragm and chest wall muscles less efficient from a mechanical standpoint, placing these patients at very high risk for inspiratory fatigue.

Finally, CO_2 accumulation is sedating. This combination of increased VCO_2, decreased mechanical efficiency, and CO_2 narcosis dramatically increases the risk of primary respiratory failure. Data on appropriate treatment are lacking. However, it is reasonable to meticulously maintain pulmonary toilet and judiciously use bronchodilators.

Diabetes Mellitus

Hyperglycemia is common in the postoperative setting in both diabetics and nondiabetics.[36] The increase in blood sugar concentration is in part the result of catecholamine-, cortisol-, glucagon-, and cytokine-induced antagonism of peripheral insulin activity (particularly in the liver and skeletal muscles), as well as of a decrease in peripheral glucose uptake. Historically, stress-induced hyperglycemia was well regarded as a salutary response, and recommendations were to keep blood glucose between 160 and 200 mg/dL.[37] The untoward macrovascular and microvascular effects of chronic hyperglycemia in diabetic patients have long been appreciated. Diabetes is currently the sixth leading cause of death in the United States.[38] It is a disease associated with insulin dysregulation and excessive hepatic gluconeogenesis.[39-41] Patients with diabetes have more frequent admissions and greater lengths of stay, and they have increased morbidity and mortality compared with their nondiabetic counterparts. In addition to their inherent vascular disease, patients with diabetes are at particular risk for postoperative hyperglycemia. Recent investigations into outcome of hyperglycemic patients and the effect of maintaining euglycemia have had a profound impact on how we care for critically ill patients (particularly diabetics), patients with complications of CAD, and patients after cardiac surgery.[42-50] These data led the American Association of Clinical Endocrinologists to hold a consensus conference in 2003 specifically focusing on inpatient diabetes and metabolic control.[51] They concluded that blood sugar levels in diabetic patients should be maintained at less than 110 mg/dL in the ICU and that maximum levels should not exceed 180 mg/dL.

The effects of diabetes on the postoperative inflammatory response are not trivial. Patients are at high risk for hyperglycemia during this period, and studies have shown that maintenance of glucose levels below 150 mg/dL improves outcome in certain surgical populations.[48-50,52] However, important questions remain unanswered. Of key importance is the issue of timing. Hyperglycemia is essential for provision of glucose to relatively avascular tissues. Several days after injury, neovascularization should eliminate this requirement. In patients without diabetes, failure to normalize serum glucose levels may indicate a complication that results in prolonged hypermetabolism or endocrine dysfunction (see later). Efforts to normalize glucose, as well as to identify the cause of the abnormality, should be intensified. Diabetes, however, limits neovascularization and eliminates hyperglycemia as a marker of ongoing hypermetabolism. Thus, one is caught between the demands of white cells, which favor hyperglycemia, and the disease process, which demands tight control of serum glucose levels. The appropriate compromise has yet to be identified.

■ DEVIATIONS FROM THE NORMAL STRESS RESPONSE TO INJURY

Although the events just described represent a patient's normal response to injury in the presence of underlying pathology, some patients deviate. Some spend weeks, even months, recovering from their initial injury. The following discussion elaborates on those disease states that cause an abnormal response to tissue injury.

The Systemic Inflammatory Response Syndrome, Sepsis, and Hyperinflammation

The incidence of sepsis has increased dramatically over recent decades, primarily because of aging of the population, increases in the number of invasive procedures that are performed, and increases in the use of immunosuppressive agents.[53] Furthermore, of the approximately 750,000 annual cases of sepsis, at least one third are fatal.[54] Despite newer antimicrobial agents, a greater appreciation for sterility during invasive procedures, and newer technologies in advanced life support, the fatality rate for sepsis has remained unchanged.[54,55] Sepsis, however, comprises only a fraction of cases that, as a whole, are known as the systemic inflammatory response syndrome (SIRS). SIRS differs from the postoperative hypermetabolic response only in that it lasts longer. When caused by an infection, SIRS is called sepsis. In 1991, the American College of Chest Physicians (ACCP) and the Society for Critical Care Medicine (SCCM) established criteria for SIRS (Table 3-2).[56] Together, sepsis and SIRS are the most common reasons for admission into a surgical ICU.[56]

Persistent Hypermetabolism

As alluded to earlier, the first phase of the stress response (the ebb phase) ensures adequate blood flow to the brain and heart by peripheral vasoconstriction and deliberate shunting.[2] Once survival appears likely (i.e., in 12 to 24 hours, or after rapid resuscitation) a second, hypermetabolic (flow) phase begins. Differentiating this "normal" response from evolving SIRS/sepsis, however, requires an understanding and appreciation of the mechanism and time frame of both responses.

Multiple risk factors predispose patients to SIRS and increase the likelihood of the stress response becoming unabated and evolving into sepsis (Box 3-1). The combina-

3-2	**Criteria for Systemic Inflammatory Response Syndrome (SIRS)**
Fever or hypothermia	T > 38°C or T < 36°C
Tachycardia	HR > 90 bpm
Tachypnea or hyperventilation	RR > 20 breaths/min *or* $PaCO_2$ < 32 mm Hg
Leukocytosis or leukopenia	WBC > 12,000 or < 4000 cells/mm^3, *or* >10% immature bands

Patients with SIRS must meet at least two of the criteria. Patients with sepsis meet SIRS criteria in addition to having a documented infectious etiology.

bpm, beats per minute; HR, heart rate; RR, respiratory rate; T, temperature; WBC, white blood cells.

3-1	Risk Factors for Developing Systemic Inflammatory Response Syndrome

Inadequate or delayed resuscitation
Persistent inflammatory or infectious focus
Baseline organ dysfunction
Age >65 years
Immunosuppression
Steroids
Chemotherapy/cancer
Acquired immunodeficiency syndrome
Transplant patients
Asplenia
Alcohol abuse
Malnutrition
Invasive instrumentation

Adapted from Orbach S, Weiss YG, Deutschman CS: Care of the patient with sepsis or the systemic inflammatory response syndrome. In Murray MJ, Coursin DB, Pearl RG, Prough DS (eds): Critical Care Medicine: Perioperative Management. Philadelphia, Lippincott-Raven, 2002, pp 601-615.

tion of predisposing factors and severe injury may lead to a hormonal milieu that is favorable for continued inflammation and organ dysfunction. What differentiates sepsis from normal stress hypermetabolism is both the persistent time course and the evidence that dysfunction occurs at a cellular level.[57,58] This can be seen clinically, for example, as unresponsiveness to α_2-agonists (so-called vasoplegia), β-agonists, and peripheral insulin.[57,59,60]

Vasodilatory Shock

In most cases of shock (i.e., hemorrhagic, cardiogenic), the response to low-circulating volume or depressed cardiac function is peripheral vasoconstriction. In sepsis, however, vascular smooth muscle fails to constrict properly and frequently is resistant to vasopressors. Sepsis is the most common cause of vasodilatory shock. Other conditions, however, such as carbon monoxide poisoning may cause similar findings. Additionally, vasodilatory shock seems to be a final common pathway for other forms of shock.[61-64] Despite the profound vasodilation that is seen in vasodilatory shock, catecholamine concentrations remain increased and the renin-angiotensin system is activated.[65,66] Thus, at the tissue level (and particularly in vascular smooth muscle), there is resistance to endogenous vasoconstrictors. The likely reasons for this phenomenon are depletion of vasopressin stores and unregulated nitric oxide synthesis.[67-69] Furthermore, there is evidence that ionized calcium (which mediates the vasoconstrictor effects of norepinephrine and angiotensin II) is unable to enter the smooth muscle cell membranes as a result of nitric oxide–induced activation of potassium channels leading to hyperpolarization of the membrane.[70] Landry and coworkers showed that plasma vasopressin levels in septic shock were inappropriately low.[71] Furthermore, administration of vasopressin at 0.04 U/min in patients with septic shock increased arterial pressure from 92/52 mm Hg on average to 146/66 mm Hg on average, suggesting impaired baroreflex-mediated secretion.

Acute Lung Injury and Acute Respiratory Distress Syndrome

Both acute lung injury (ALI) and the acute respiratory distress syndrome (ARDS) represent the response of the lung to a local or remote injury. Initially, the inflammatory response leads to a diffuse capillary leakage in the lung, a phenomenon called noncardiogenic/nonhydrostatic pulmonary edema.[72] The result is ventilation–perfusion mismatching and hypoxemia. Patients become tachypneic in an effort to excrete the increased carbon dioxide produced by the hypermetabolic response to injury. In addition, the excess in lung water limits excursion with each tidal breath. The resulting decrease in the stimulation of stretch receptors in the lung parenchyma signals a need for increased minute ventilation.

The role of post-injury inflammation in the development of ALI and ARDS is poorly understood. Originally, atelectasis and pulmonary edema were the defining hallmarks of the syndrome.[73] Experiments with large-animal models of sepsis showed that lung vascular permeability increases, leading to protein-rich lung edema.[74-76] Fein and colleagues were the first to quantify this protein and show a consistently high ratio of protein in edema fluid to plasma protein concentration in patients with ARDS or ALI compared with the lower ratio in patients with heart failure.[77] Current hypotheses have incorporated these data and consider protein-rich edematous fluid within the alveoli as a hallmark of ALI and ARDS.[78] The cause of the increase in lung microvascular permeability is not clear. Early investigators knew that inflammation played a role, as they found leukocytes within the alveolar edema.[73] More recently, this has been confirmed by demonstration of increased numbers of polymorphonuclear cells (PMNs) and other leukocytes in bronchoalveolar lavage (BAL) samples from patients with ALI/ARDS. In addition, the injurious effects that PMN-derived oxidants and proteases have on the cells of the alveolar-capillary membrane[79-81] have been documented. Thus, inflammation mediated by PMNs is central to the development of ALI/ARDS.[72,82-85] In addition, it is apparent that PMNs do not act alone. In particular, lung macrophages, circulating monocytes, and other leukocytes have been implicated in the pathogenesis of ALI and ARDS. The role that platelets and other constituents of the coagulation system play in the development of ALI and ARDS is also being investigated.[86,87]

Despite all of our advances, an interdisciplinary group of investigators confirmed in 2002 that much is still unknown regarding the cause, consequence, and resolution of ALI and ARDS.[87] It has become evident that there are subgroups of individuals with ALI who progress to fibrosing alveolitis with alveolar and epithelial cell destruction and eventual multiple organ failure.[88,89]

Immunosuppression of Injury

The initial response to surgery or trauma, as well as the persistent state observed in SIRS, is characterized by a highly activated innate immune system that elaborates and secretes high levels of proinflammatory mediators. This rapidly gives way to a state of depressed immune function. As pointed out by Hotchkiss and Karl, patients with multiple organ dysfunction syndrome (MODS) may develop "a loss of delayed hypersensitivity, an inability to clear infection and a predisposition to nosocomial infection"[90] consistent with immunosuppression or anergy. Altered or impaired immune function has been demonstrated clearly by a number of investigators.[90-93] These studies reveal two possible patterns of response. In the first, a transition from hyperinflammation to immune depression in lymphocytes is paralleled by a change in the expression of surface antigens, cytokine elaboration patterns, and other aspects of cell function. This is consistent with a transition from a helper T cell 1 (Th1) to a Th2 phenotype, similar to but more pronounced than what occurs following a "normal" inflammatory response. Alternatively, lymphocyte dysfunction may present as a complete lack of response to external stimuli, that is, anergy. The net result is the development of sequential infections. As one is appropriately treated, another arises. The most common site for infection is the lung, where pneumonias with uncommon organisms become the rule. These infections prolong the hospital course. The pathophysiology may involve premature apoptosis of lymphocytes.[94]

■ ENDOCRINOPATHY OF SEPSIS AND "CHRONIC" CRITICAL ILLNESS

Somatotropic Axis

Enhanced proteolysis together with negative nitrogen balance are characteristic features of critical illness.[95] Indeed, continued proteolysis in critically ill patients can cause a loss of 10% of their muscle mass per week.[96] Both acute and chronic illness cause profound and distinct changes in the endocrine system.[97] These changes are both peripheral and central in origin. Normally, growth hormone (GH) is released from the anterior pituitary in a pulsatile fashion under the control of GH-releasing hormone (GHRH) and somatostatin. There is, however, a recently discovered third factor regulating GH secretion. This factor is an endogenous peptide, ghrelin, that is secreted by the stomach.[98] GH then has both direct and indirect effects. Directly, GH binds to peripheral receptors on target cells to maintain euglycemia and to stimulate protein anabolism and triglyceride metabolism. Indirectly, GH stimulates the liver and other tissues to secrete insulin-like growth factor-1 (IGF-1).

During the acute phase of critical illness or injury, circulating GH levels are elevated.[97,99] Growth hormone–binding protein (GHBP) levels decrease, reflecting reduced GH-receptor expression in peripheral tissues.[100] The combination of these changes leads to peripheral resistance to GH. Several investigators have hypothesized that these changes are a result of the release of cytokines, such as tumor necrosis factor-α (TNF-α), interleukin-1 (IL-1), and IL-6.[101,102]

As critical illness continues into the chronic phase, changes occur in the somatotropic axis again. First, there is a loss of periodicity to the pulsatile release of GH. Second, mean GH concentrations are substantially lower than in the acute phase of illness. Interestingly, this pattern appears to be independent of patient age, sex, or underlying disease.[97,103] Some have speculated that this relative GH deficiency con-

tributes to the wasting syndrome commonly seen in the chronic phase of critical illness.[104] Another hypothesis is that the pituitary, in general, is one of many organs involved in MODS. Regardless of the cause, GH deficiency and pituitary hypofunction are exquisitely responsive to GH-secretagogues such as GHRH and GH-releasing peptides (GHRPs). Indeed, GHRH and GHRP evoke a synergistic response suggesting that the blunted GH response in protracted critical illness is not due to decreased pituitary synthesis of GH or an irregularly high somatostatin-induced suppression of GH release.[105] As a result of these observations, a prospective, multicenter, double-blind, randomized, placebo-controlled study investigating high-dose GH in long-term (5 to 7 days) intensive care patients was initiated.[106] High doses of GH (mean daily dose, 0.10 ± 0.02 mg/kg) were associated with increased mortality (relative risk [RR], 2.4; confidence interval [CI], 1.6-3.5), increased length of hospital and ICU stay, and increased duration of mechanical ventilation. Although the authors did not have an explanation for the increase in morbidity and mortality, they postulated that GH-induced insulin resistance deprived cells of glucose. Furthermore, GH prevents the mobilization of glutamine from muscle and makes it less available for rapidly dividing cells such as leukocytes and enterocytes.[107]

Thyrotropic Axis

Soon after surgery or trauma, serum levels of triiodothyronine (T_3) drop precipitously and circulating concentrations of thyroxine, thyroid-stimulating hormone (TSH), and reverse T_3 increase. The decrease in T_3 most likely represents decreased peripheral conversion of thyroxine to T_4.[108] Although T_3 levels remain low throughout the acute phase of illness, levels of TSH inappropriately normalize, reflecting abnormal central feedback control.[109] The magnitude of the drop in T_3 within the first 24 hours of injury has been correlated with the severity of illness.[110] Many have advocated not treating the low T_3 levels, arguing that the change reflects an attempt to reduce energy expenditure.[111] Data to support this notion, however, are lacking. As the illness becomes chronic, changes in the thyrotropic axis tend to mimic those of the somatotropic axis. Mean TSH concentrations remain low and normal pulsatility is lost. Infusing thyroid-releasing hormone increases TSH (and peripheral thyroid hormone) consistent with a central origin of thyroid suppression.[97,112] The low T_3 syndrome, however, is not only central in origin, as peripheral metabolism changes also. Peeters and colleagues showed reduced type 1 deiodinase (the enzyme responsible for the peripheral conversion of thyroxine to T_3) activity in patients with prolonged critical illness.[113] The decrease in type 1 deiodinase activity may explain why administering thyroxine to critically ill patients fails to provide clinical change.[114] Thyroid hormone replacement during critical illness is beneficial in patients with a presumptive diagnosis of myxedema coma, although the optimal treatment regimen remains controversial.

Gonadal and Prolactin Axes

Prolonged critical illness is associated with hypogonadotropism and suppression of both the mean concentration and pulsatility of luteinizing hormone. As in other endocrine axes, hypoandrogenism and hypoprolactinemia result from combined central and peripheral defects.[115] A number of catabolic states are associated with low testosterone levels, including the postoperative phase, starvation, myocardial infarction, and chronic critical illness.[116-119] Suppression of prolactin secretion has been associated with altered immune function. Indeed, both T and B lymphocytes express receptors for prolactin. The fact that serum prolactin concentrations increase in acute illness has led many to hypothesize that this hormone serves as an initial activator of the immune cascade.[104] Similarly, blunted prolactin secretion in the chronic phase of illness may contribute to relative immune anergy and an increased susceptibility to infections.[120]

Pituitary-Adrenal Axis

Like other endocrine axes, the pituitary-adrenal axis reacts differently to acute and to chronic illness. The acute stress response is associated with high circulating levels of adrenocorticotropic hormone (ACTH) and cortisol, presumably driven by elevated hypothalamic cortisol-releasing hormone (CRH) levels. This hormonal milieu is associated with hyperinsulinemia, hyperglycemia, increased glycolytic rate, increased gluconeogenesis, lipolysis, and proteolysis. From a teleologic perspective, acute injury immediately prompts the body to search for repair and survival mechanisms. Modes of survival include diverting blood flow from the periphery to vital organs, limiting energy expenditure, slowing metabolism, and retaining fluid to maintain adequate intravascular volume. The glucose needed for these processes comes from hepatic gluconeogenesis, lipolysis to generate glycerol from triglycerides, and proteolysis to generate glucogenic amino acids from skeletal muscle. Normally, cortisol released from the adrenal cortex signals the pituitary and hypothalamus to attenuate secretion of ACTH and CRH, respectively. However, during acute injury, cytokines (e.g., IL-1, IL-6, TNF-α) inhibit this negative feedback. With prolonged critical illness, however, serum ACTH concentration decreases, whereas cortisol concentration remains elevated, suggesting that cortisol release is driven through an alternate, non-ACTH-mediated, pathway. Additionally, the pharmacokinetics of cortisol change during acute stress as the rate of hepatic cortisol extraction from the blood is decreased and the plasma half-life of cortisol is increased.[121] Additionally, cortisol-binding globulin (CBG) concentration and binding affinity for cortisol are decreased, increasing free and biologically active cortisol concentrations. Whether the hypercortisolism of critical illness is detrimental remains uncertain. Theoretically, hypercortisolism can contribute to impaired wound healing and myopathy. The chronic stage usually, however, leads to a recovery stage whereby pituitary hormone secretion normalizes as does peripheral feedback regulation, and anabolism ensues.[122]

Vasopressin

Vasopressin, commonly known as antidiuretic hormone (ADH), is necessary for vascular integrity and cardiovascular homeostasis. Historically, this hormone was used therapeutically for controlling bleeding resulting from gastrointestinal varices and reversing diabetes insipidus. Recently, however, vasopressin has been used to manage various forms of vasodilatory or redistributive shock. Studies by Landry and others have demonstrated that vasopressin deficiency develops early in critical illness (particularly septic shock) and is accompanied by an increase in receptor sensitivity.[71,123] Further investigations revealed that replacement with very low doses of vasopressin could reverse some of the vasoplegia noted in these patients.[124] These findings have been extended to other vasodilatory shock syndromes.[70,125] As a result, vasopressin in dosages ranging from 0.01 to 0.04 U/min is commonly used to increase blood pressure in septic or chronically critically ill patients.

■ SUMMARY/CONCLUSION

The nature and course of the inflammatory response determines outcome after surgical or traumatic injury. Otherwise healthy patients with a normal, balanced, well-controlled inflammatory response recover uneventfully from surgery or trauma. However, in patients with preexisting disease(s), recovery from surgery or trauma is determined by the interaction of normal inflammation and the preexisting condition. In those patients with an unbalanced inflammatory response from whatever cause, outcome is determined by the type and extent of the abnormal response. Thus, outcome after an exaggerated response (SIRS, sepsis, sepsis syndrome) is determined by the ability to support the cardiovascular and pulmonary systems throughout the period of hypermetabolism. Likewise, outcome after a suppressed response is determined by the ability to support the immune and endocrine systems through a period of hypoinflammation.

■ REFERENCES

1. Cuthbertson DP: Observations on the disturbances of metabolism produced by injury to the limbs. Q J Med 1932;1:233-244.
2. Cuthbertson D, Tilstone WT: Metabolism during the postinjury period. Adv Clin Chem 1969;12:1-55.
3. Moore FD, Olsen KH, McMurrey JD: The Body Cell Mass and Its Supporting Environment. Philadelphia, WB Saunders, 1978.
4. Cerra FB, Siegel JH, Border JR, et al: Correlations between metabolic and cardiopulmonary measurements in patients after trauma, general surgery and sepsis. J Trauma 1979;19:621-629.
5. Clowes GHA, O'Donnell TF, Blockburn GL, et al: Energy metabolism and proteolysis in traumatized and septic man. Surg Clin North Am 1976;56:1169-1184.
6. Monk DN, Plank LD, Franch-Arcas G, et al: Sequential changes in the metabolic response in critically injured patients during the first 25 days after blunt trauma. Ann Surg 1996;223:395-405.
7. Hunt TK, Knighton DR, Thakral KK, et al: Studies on inflammation and wound healing: Angiogenesis and collagen synthesis stimulated in vivo by resident and activated wound macrophages. Surgery 1984;96:48-54.
8. Knighton DR, Hunt TK, Scheuenstuhl H, et al: Oxygen tension regulates the expression of angiogenesis factor by macrophages. Science 1983;221:1283-1285.
9. Frank S, Hubner G, Breier G, et al: Regulation of vascular endothelial growth factor expression in cultured keratinocytes. J Biol Chem 1995;270:12607-12613.
10. Russell JA, Ronco JJ, Lockhat D, et al: Oxygen delivery and consumption and ventricular preload are greater in survivors than in non survivors of the adult respiratory distress syndrome. Am Rev Respir Dis 1990;141:659-665.

11. Shoemaker WC, Montgomery ES, Kaplan E, et al: Physiologic patterns in surviving and nonsurviving shock patients. Arch Surg 1973;106:630-636.

12. Hayes MA, Timmins AC, Yau EHS, et al: Oxygen transport patterns in patients with sepsis syndrome or septic shock: Influence of treatment and relationship to outcome. Crit Care Med 1997;25:926-936.

13. Hayes MA, Yau EHS, Timmins AC, et al: Response of critically ill patients to treatment aimed at achieving supranormal oxygen delivery and consumption: Relationship to outcome. Chest 1993;103:886-895.

14. Shoemaker WC, Czer LSC: Evaluation of the biologic importance of various haemodynamic and oxygen transport variables. Crit Care Med 1979;24:517-524.

15. Shoemaker WC, Appel PL, Kram HB, et al: Prospective trial of supranormal values of survivors as therapeutic goals in high risk surgical patients. Chest 1988;94:1176-1186.

16. Ellis SG, Hertzer NR, Young JR, et al: Angiographic correlates of cardiac death and myocardial infarction complicating major nonthoracic vascular surgery. Am J Cardiol 1996;77:1126-1128.

17. Badner NH, Knill RL, Brown JE, et al: Myocardial infarction after noncardiac surgery. Anesthesiology 1998;88:572-578.

18. Landesberg G, Luria MH, Cotev S, et al: Importance of long-duration postoperative ST-segment depression in cardiac morbidity after vascular surgery. Lancet 1993;341:715-719.

19. Landesberg G, Mosseri M, Wolf YG, et al: Perioperative myocardial ischemia and infarction: Identification by continuous 12-lead electrocardiogram with online ST-segment monitoring. Anesthesiology 2002;96:262-270.

20. McCann RL, Clements FM: Silent myocardial ischemia in patients undergoing peripheral vascular surgery: Incidence and association with perioperative cardiac morbidity and mortality. J Vasc Surg 1989;9:583-587.

21. Ouyang P, Gerstenblith G, Furman WR, et al: Frequency and significance of early postoperative silent myocardial ischemia in patients having peripheral vascular surgery. Am J Cardiol 1989;64:1113-1116.

22. Pasternak PF, Grossi EA, Baumann G, et al: The value of silent myocardial ischemia monitoring in the prediction of perioperative myocardial infarction in patients undergoing peripheral vascular surgery. J Vasc Surg 1989;10:617-625.

23. Mangano DT, Layug EL, Wallace A, et al: Effect of atenolol on mortality and cardiovascular morbidity after noncardiac surgery. Multicenter Study of Perioperative Ischemia Research Group. N Engl J Med 1996;335:1713-1720.

24. Poldermans D, Boersma E, Bax JJ, et al: The effect of bisoprolol on perioperative mortality and myocardial infarction in high-risk patients undergoing vascular surgery. N Engl J Med 1999;341:1789-1794.

25. O'Neil-Callahan K, Katsimaglis G, Tepper MR, et al: Statins decrease perioperative cardiac complications in patients undergoing noncardiac vascular surgery: The Statins for Risk Reduction in Surgery (StaRRS) study. J Am Coll Card 2005;45:336-342.

26. Lindenauer PK, Pekow P, Wang K, et al: Lipid-lowering therapy and in-hospital mortality following major noncardiac surgery. JAMA 2004;291:2092-2099.

27. Fox KM, EURopean trial On reduction of cardiac events with Perindopril in stable coronary Artery disease Investigators: Efficacy of perindopril in reduction of cardiovascular events among patients with stable coronary artery disease: Randomized, double-blind, placebo-controlled, multicentre trial (the EUROPA study). Lancet 2003;362:782-788.

28. Pepine CJ, Kowey PR, Kupfer S, et al: Predictors of adverse outcome among patients with hypertension and coronary artery disease. J Am Coll Card 2006;47:547-551.

29. Smetana GW: Preoperative pulmonary evaluation. N Engl J Med 1999;340:937-944.

30. Arozullah AM, Khuri SF, Henderson WG, Daley J: Development and validation of a multifactorial risk index for predicting postoperative pneumonia after major noncardiac surgery. Ann Intern Med 2001;135:847-857.

31. Trayner E Jr, Celli BR: Postoperative pulmonary complications. Med Clin North Am 2001;85:1129-1139.

32. Warner DO: Preventing postoperative pulmonary complications: The role of the anesthesiologist. Anesthesiology 2000;92:1467-1472.

33. Lawrence VA, Dhanda R, Hilsenbeck SG, et al: Risk of pulmonary complications after elective abdominal surgery. Chest 1996;110:744-750.

34. Brooks-Brunn JA: Predictors of postoperative pulmonary complications following abdominal surgery. Chest 1997;111:564-571.

35. Kiiski R, Takala J. Hypermetabolism and efficiency of CO_2 removal in acute respiratory failure. Chest 1995;108:290-292.

36. Mizock BA: Alterations in fuel metabolism in critical illness: Hyperglycaemia. Best Pract Res Clin Endocrinol Metab 2001;15:533-551.

37. Mizock BA: Alterations in carbohydrate metabolism during stress: A review of the literature. Am J Med 1995;98:75-84.

38. Center for Disease Control: National Vital Statistics Report. 2004;53: October. Available at www.cdc.gov/nchs/data/nvsr/nvsr53/nvsr53_05acc.pdf.

39. Weinstock RS: Treating type 2 diabetes mellitus: A growing epidemic. Mayo Clin Proc 2003;78:411-413.

40. Boord JB, Graber AL, Christman JW, et al: Practical management of diabetes in critically ill patients. Am J Respir Crit Care Med 2001;164:1763-1767.

41. Gerich JE: Contributions of insulin-resistance and insulin-secretory defects to the pathogenesis of type 2 diabetes mellitus. Mayo Clin Proc 2003;78:447-456.

42. Kagansky N, Levy S, Knobler H: The role of hyperglycemia in acute stroke. Arch Neurol 2001;58:1209-1212.

43. Capes SE, Hunt D, Malmberg K, et al: Stress hyperglycemia and increased risk of death after myocardial infarction in patients with and without diabetes: A systematic overview. Lancet 2000;355:773-778.

44. Capes SE, Hunt D, Malmberg K, et al: Stress hyperglycemia and prognosis of stroke in nondiabetic and diabetic patients: A systematic overview. Stroke 2001;32:2426-2432.

45. Malmberg K, Norhammer A, Wedel H, et al: Glycometabolic state at admission: Important risk marker of mortality in conventionally treated patients with diabetes mellitus and acute myocardial infarction: Long-term results from the Diabetes and Insulin-Glucose Infusion in Acute Myocardial Infarction (DIGAMI) study. Circulation 1999;99:2626-2632.

46. Gore DC, Chinkes D, Heggers J, et al: Association of hyperglycemia with increased mortality after severe burn injury. J Trauma 2001;51:540-544.

47. Norhammer AM, Ryden L, Malmberg K: Admission plasma glucose: Independent risk factor for long-term prognosis after myocardial infarction even in nondiabetic patients. Diabetes Care 1999;22:1827-1831.

48. Furnary AP, Gao G, Grunkmeier GL, et al: Continuous insulin infusion reduces mortality in patients with diabetes undergoing coronary artery bypass grafting. J Thorac Cardiovasc Surg 2003;125:1007-1021.

49. Van den Berghe G, Wouters P, Weekers F, et al: Intensive insulin therapy in critically ill patients. N Engl J Med 2001;345:1359-1367.

50. Van den Berghe G, Wilmer A, Hermans G, et al: Intensive insulin therapy in the medical ICU. N Engl J Med 2006;354:449-461.

51. Garbar AJ, Mohissi ES, Bransome ED, et al: American College of Endocrinology position statement on inpatient diabetes and metabolic control (presented at the National Press Club, Washington, DC, December 16, 2003). Endocr Pract 2004;10:77-82. Available at www.aace.com/pub/ICC/ACEPosiStat.pdf.

52. Finney SJ, Zekveld C, Elia A, Evans TW: Glucose control and mortality in critically ill patients. JAMA 2003;290:2041-2047.

53. Martin GS, Mannino DM, Eaton S, et al: The epidemiology of sepsis in the United States from 1979 through 2000. N Engl J Med 2003;348:1546-1554.

54. Angus DC, Linde-Zwirble WT, Lidicker J, et al: Epidemiology of severe sepsis in the United States: Analysis of incidence, outcome and associated costs of care. Crit Care Med 2001;29:1303-1310.

55. Friedman G, Silva E, Vincent JL: Has the mortality of septic shock changed with time? Crit Care Med 1998;26:2078-2086.

56. Bone RC, Balk RA, Cerra FB, et al: Definitions for sepsis and organ failure and guidelines for the use of innovative therapies in sepsis.

American College of Chest Physicians, Society of Critical Care Medicine Consensus Conference Committee. Chest 1992;101:1644-1655.

57. Clemens MG, Chaudry IH, Daineau N, Baue AE: Insulin resistance and depressed gluconeogenic capability during early hyperglycemic sepsis. J Trauma 1984;24:701-708.

58. Deutschman CS, De Maio A, Clemens MG: Sepsis-induced attenuation of glucagon and 8Br-cAMP modulation of phosphor enol pyruvate carboxykinase gene. Am J Physiol 1995;269:R584-591.

59. Breslow MJ, Miller CF, Parker SD, et al: Effect of vasopressors on organ blood flow during endotoxin shock in pigs. Am J Physiol 1987;252:H291-H300.

60. Ghosh S, Liu MS: Decrease in adenylate cyclase activity in dog livers during endotoxic shock. Am J Physiol 1983;245:R737-742.

61. Thiemermann C, Szabo C, Mitchell JA, et al: Vascular hyporeactivity to vasoconstrictor agents and hemodynamic decompensation in hemorrhagic shock is mediated by nitric oxide. Proc Natl Acad Sci U S A 1993;90:267-271.

62. Argenziano M, Choudhri AF, Oz MC, et al: A prospective randomized trial of arginine vasopressin in the treatment of vasodilatory shock after left ventricular assist device placement. Circulation 1997;96: II286-290.

63. Remington JW, Hamilton WF, Caddell HM, et al: Some circulatory responses to hemorrhage in the dog. Am J Physiol 1950;161:106-115.

64. Rutherford RB, Trow RS: The pathophysiology of irreversible hemorrhagic shock in monkeys. J Surg Res 1973;14:538-550.

65. Benedict CR, Rose JA: Arterial norepinephrine changes in patients with septic shock. Circ Shock 1992;38:165-172.

66. Cumming AD, Driedger A, McDonald JWD, et al: Vasoactive hormones in the renal response to systemic sepsis. Am J Kidney Dis 1988;11:23-32.

67. Tagawa T, Imaizumi T, Endo T, et al: Vasodilatory effect of arginine vasopressin is mediated by nitric oxide in human forearm vessels. J Clin Invest 1993;92:1483-1490.

68. Cines DB, Pollak ES, Buck CA, et al: Endothelial cells in physiology and in the pathophysiology of vascular disorders. Blood 1998;91: 3527-3561.

69. Holmes CL, Landry DW, Granton JT: Science review: Vasopressin and the cardiovascular system. Part 2—Clinical physiology. Crit Care 2004;8:15-23.

70. Landry DW, Oliver JA: The pathogenesis of vasodilatory shock. N Engl J Med 2001;345:588-595.

71. Landry DW, Levin HR, Gallant EM, et al: Vasopressin deficiency contributes to the vasodilation of septic shock. Circulation 1997;95:1122-1125.

72. Bernard G, Artigas A, Brigham K, et al: The American European Consensus Conference on ARDS. Am J Respir Crit Care Med 1994;149:818-824.

73. Ashbaugh DG, Bigelow DB, Petty TL, et al: Acute respiratory distress in adults. Lancet 1967;2:219-223.

74. Brigham KL, Woolverton WC, Blake LH, et al: Increased sheep lung vascular permeability caused by pseudomonas bacteremia. J Clin Invest 1974;54:792-804.

75. Ohkuda K, Nakahara K, Weidner WJ, et al: Lung fluid exchange after uneven pulmonary artery obstruction in sheep. Circ Res 1978;43: 152-161.

76. Brigham KL, Bowers R, Haynes J: Increased lung vascular permeability by *Escherichia coli* endotoxin. Circ Res 1979;45:292-297.

77. Fein A, Grossman RF, Jones JG, et al: The value of edema fluid protein measurement in patients with pulmonary edema. Am J Med 1979;67:32-38.

78. Ware LB, Matthay MA: The acute respiratory distress syndrome. N Engl J Med 2000;342:1334-1349.

79. Pittet JF, MacKersie RC, Martin TR, et al: Biological markers of acute lung injury: Prognostic and pathogenetic significance. Am J Respir Crit Care Med 1997;155:1187-1205.

80. Brigham KL: Mechanisms of lung injury. Clin Chest Med 1982;3: 9-24.

81. Cochrane CG, Spragg R, Revak SD: Pathogenesis of the adult respiratory distress syndrome: Evidence of oxidant activity in bronchoalveolar lavage fluid. J Clin Invest 1983;71:754-761.

82. Rinaldo JE, Rogers RM: Adult respiratory-distress syndrome: Changing concepts of lung injury and repair. N Engl J Med 1982;306: 900-909.

83. Kollef MH, Schuster DP: The acute respiratory distress syndrome. N Engl J Med 1995;332:27-37.

84. Matthay MA: Conference summary: Acute lung injury. Chest 1999;116:119S-126S.

85. Abraham E: Neutrophils and acute lung injury. Crit Care Med 2003;31: S195-199.

86. Zimmerman GA, Albertine KH, McIntyre TM: Pathogenesis of sepsis and septic-induced lung injury. In Lenfant C, Matthay MA (eds): Acute Respiratory Distress Syndrome. New York, Marcel Dekker, 2003, pp 245-287.

87. Matthay MA, Zimmerman GA, Esmon C, et al: Future research directions in acute lung injury: Summary of a National Heart, Lung, and Blood Institute working group. Am J Respir Crit Care Med 2003;167:1027-1035.

88. Albertine KH, Soulier MF, Wang Z, et al: Fas and fas ligand are up-regulated in pulmonary edema fluid and lung tissue of patients with acute lung injury and the acute respiratory distress syndrome. Am J Pathol 2002;161:1783-1796.

89. Tomashefski JF Jr: Pulmonary pathology of acute respiratory distress syndrome. Clin Chest Med 2003;21:435-466.

90. Hotchkiss RS, Karl IE: The pathophysiology and treatment of sepsis. N Engl J Med 2003;348:138-150.

91. Ayala A, O'Neill PJ, Uebele SA, et al: Mechanism of splenic immunosuppression during sepsis: Key role of Kupffer cell mediators. J Trauma 1997;42:882-888.

92. Oberholzer A, Oberholtzer C, Moldawer LL: Sepsis syndromes: Understanding the role of innate and acquired immunity. Shock 2001;16:83-96.

93. Shelley O, Murphy T, Paterson H, et al: Interaction between the innate and adaptive immune systems is required to survive sepsis and control inflammation after injury. Shock 2003;20:123-129.

94. Cobb JP, Hotchkiss RS, Karl IE, Buchman TG: Mechanisms of cell injury and death. Br J Anaesth 1996;77:3-10.

95. Rennie MJ: Muscle protein turnover and the wasting due to injury and disease. Br Med Bull 1985;41:257-264.

96. Gamrin L, Andersson K, Hultman E, et al: Longitudinal changes of biochemical parameters in muscle during critical illness. Metabolism 1997;46:756-762.

97. Van den Berghe G, de Zegher F, Bouillon R: Acute and prolonged critical illness as different neuroendocrine paradigms. J Clin Endocrinol Metab 1998;83:1827-1834.

98. Kojima M, Hosoda H, Date Y, et al: Ghrelin is a growth-hormone-releasing acylated peptide from stomach. Nature 1999;402: 656-660.

99. Ross R, Miell J, Freeman E, et al: Critically ill patients have high basal growth hormone levels with attenuated oscillatory activity associated with low levels of insulin-like growth factor-1. Clin Endocrinol 1991;35:47-54.

100. Hermansson M, Wickelgren RB, Hammerqvist F, et al: Measurement of human growth hormone receptor messenger ribonucleic acid by a quantitative polymerase chain reaction-based assay: Demonstration of reduced expression after elective surgery. J Clin Endocrinol Metab 1997;82:421-428.

101. Bentham J, Rodriguez-Arnao J, Ross RJ: Acquired growth hormone resistance in patients with hypercatabolism. Horm Res 1993;40: 87-91.

102. Timmins AC, Cotterill AM, Cwyfan Hughes SC, et al: Critical illness is associated with low circulating concentrations of insulin-like growth factors-I and -II, alterations in insulin-like growth factor binding proteins, and induction of an insulin-like growth factor binding protein-3 protease. Crit Care Med 1996;24:1460-1466.

103. Van den Berghe G, Baxter RC, Weekers F, et al: A paradoxical gender dissociation within the growth hormone, insulin-like growth factor I axis during protracted critical illness. J Clin Endocrinol Metab 2000;85:183-192.

104. Van den Berghe G: Endocrine evaluation of patients with critical illness. Endocrinol Metab Clin North Am 2003;32:385-410.

105. Van den Berghe G, de Zegher F, Bowers CY, et al: Pituitary responsiveness to growth hormone (GH) releasing hormone, GH-releasing

peptide-2, and thyrotropin releasing hormone in critical illness. Clin Endocrinol 1996;45:341-351.

106. Takala J, Ruokonen E, Webster NR, et al: Increased mortality associated with growth hormone treatment in critically ill adults. N Engl J Med 1999;341:785-792.

107. Biolo G, Iscra F, Toigo G, et al: Effects of growth hormone administration on skeletal muscle glutamine metabolism in severely traumatized patients: Preliminary report. Clin Nutr 1997;16:89-91.

108. Chopra IJ, Huang TS, Beredo A, et al: Evidence for an inhibitor of extrathyroidal conversion of thyroxine to 3,5,3'-triiodothyronine in sera of patients with non-thyroidal illness. J Clin Endocrinol Metab 1985;60:666-672.

109. Bacci V, Schussler GC, Kaplan TB: The relationship between serum triiodothyronine and thyrotropin during systemic illness. J Clin Endocrinol Metab 1982;54:1229-1235.

110. Rothwell PM, Lawler PG: Prediction of outcome in intensive care patients using endocrine parameters. Crit Care Med 1995;23:78-83.

111. Gardner DF, Kaplan MM, Stanley CA, et al: Effect of triiodothyronine replacement on the metabolic and pituitary responses to starvation. N Engl J Med 1979;300:579-584.

112. Fliers E, Wieringa WM, Swaab DF: Physiological and pathophysiological aspects of thyrotropin-releasing hormone gene expression in the human hypothalamus. Thyroid 1998;8:921-928.

113. Peeters RP, Wouters PJ, Kaptein E, et al: Reduced activation and increased inactivation of thyroid hormone in tissues of critically ill patients. J Clin Endocrinol Metab 2003;88:3202-3211.

114. Brent GA, Hershman JM: Thyroxine therapy in patients with severe non-thyroidal illnesses and low serum thyroxine concentrations. J Clin Endocrinol Metab 1986;63:1-7.

115. Van den Berghe G, Weekers F, Baxter RC, et al: Five-day pulsatile gonadotropin-releasing hormone administration unveils combined hypothalamic-pituitary-gonadal defects underlying profound hypoandrogenism in men with prolonged critical illness. J Clin Endocrinol Metab 2001;86:3217-3226.

116. Klibanski A, Beitens IZ, Badger TM, et al: Reproductive function during fasting in man. J Clin Endocrinol Metab 1981;53:258-266.

117. Wang C, Chan V, Yeung RTT: Effect of surgical stress on pituitary-testicular function. Clin Endocrinol 1978;9:255-266.

118. Wang C, Chan V, Tse TF, et al: Effect of acute myocardial infarction on pituitary testicular function. Clin Endocrinol 1978;9:249-253.

119. Van den Berghe G, de Zegher F, Lauwers P, et al: Luteinizing hormone secretion and hypoandrogenemia in critically ill men: Effect of dopamine. Clin Endocrinol 1994;41:563-569.

120. Devins SS, Miller A, Herndon BL, et al: Effects of dopamine on T-lymphocyte proliferative responses and serum prolactin concentrations in critically ill patients. Crit Care Med 1992;263:9682-9685.

121. Vermes I, Beishuizen A: The hypothalamic-pituitary-adrenal response to critical illness. Best Pract Res Clin Endocrinol Metab 2001;15:495-511.

122. Beishuizen A, Thijs LG, Haanen C, et al: Macrophage migration inhibitory factor and hypothalamo-pituitary-adrenal function during critical illness. J Clin Endocrinol Metab 2001;86:2811-2816.

123. Landry DW, Levin HR, Gallant EM, et al: Vasopressin pressor hypersensitivity in vasodilatory septic shock. Crit Care Med 1997;95:1122-1125.

124. Malay MB, Ashton RC Jr, Landry DW, Townsend RN: Low-dose vasopressin in the treatment of vasodilatory septic shock. J Trauma 1999;47:699-703.

125. Robin JK, Oliver JA, Landry DW: Vasopressin deficiency in the syndrome of irreversible shock. J Trauma 2003;54:S149-S154.

Chapter

4 The Coagulation Cascade in Perioperative Organ Injury

Martha Sue Carraway and Claude A. Piantadosi

Organ dysfunction is an important source of morbidity and mortality in the perioperative period.[1] Organ dysfunction may involve single or multiple organs, and the lungs, kidneys, and liver are commonly affected. The emergence of multiorgan dysfunction (MODS) after major surgery is uncommon and confounded by comorbid processes, but the syndrome has been increasingly recognized, and the mortality rate increases according to the number of organs involved. The pathogenesis of MODS in the perioperative period is not specifically known, but it appears to be linked to activation of the systemic inflammatory response syndrome. This may be related to variables in the operative procedure, including hypotension, hypovolemia, transient organ ischemia, multiple transfusions, use of extracorporeal membrane oxygenation, and sepsis, which is a major cause of perioperative morbidity and mortality.[2] The true incidence of perioperative organ dysfunction is uncertain, partly because of the lack of a uniform clinical definition.[3] Renal dysfunction and pulmonary complications (acute respiratory distress syndrome) are highly associated with certain operations such as coronary artery bypass grafting and abdominal vascular surgery, but they may occur after other types of surgery. Recent advances in our understanding of the pathogenesis of organ dysfunction in sepsis indicate that coagulation abnormalities contribute strongly to its evolution.[4,5] It is intriguing to postulate that similar coagulation abnormalities in the perioperative period play a role in the development of MODS in this setting.

The activities of the coagulation factors, and indeed the entire coagulation cascade, extend beyond the clotting function. Importantly, and relevant to perioperative stress, the coagulation proteins are linked to numerous proinflammatory signaling pathways.[6-8] The overall state of coagulation in the circulation depends on the balance between pro- and anticoagulant mechanisms.[4,5] When the balance is disrupted in favor of a procoagulant state, the proinflammatory signals of the coagulation proteins may be prevalent. Alternatively, disruption of coagulation leads to bleeding diatheses, which have major clinical importance in the operative setting. Impaired coagulation and the consequences of bleeding in the operative setting are well recognized[9]; this chapter is focused on procoagulant mechanisms that could impair organ function.

Activation of coagulation contributes to organ injury by several mechanisms, including small-vessel obstruction by thrombosis, extravascular fibrin deposition, and amplification of cellular inflammatory pathways.[4,5] The procoagulant state has been shown to be especially important in the pathogenesis of sepsis-associated MODS. Similar mechanisms are probably relevant to organ dysfunction in the perioperative period, where multiple proteins interact to alter the balance between procoagulant and anticoagulant.[10,11] Because the incidence of perioperative organ dysfunction is unknown and because it appears to vary between surgical sites and procedures, attributing organ dysfunction solely to a specific type of surgical procedure is problematic, especially in the presence of complications that may also affect organ function. Typically, these complications include postoperative sepsis and shock, which may produce abnormalities that are difficult to disassociate from the surgical event. The following paragraphs cover the basic coagulation and fibrinolytic functions, discuss alterations of these functions in the perioperative period, and review what is known about the role of coagulation abnormalities in organ dysfunction in other conditions and in relevant animal models.

■ OVERVIEW OF THE COAGULATION AND FIBRINOLYTIC CASCADES

Coagulation is initiated by the sequential activation of a group of serine proteases, leading ultimately to polymerization of the fibrin clot (Fig. 4-1). Extrinsic coagulation is initiated by cell surface expression of tissue factor (TF), which binds to activated factor VII (FVIIa) to form a complex. The TF-VIIa complex activates factor X to Xa, which cleaves prothrombin to thrombin (for review, see reference 9). Thrombin cleaves fibrinogen to fibrin, which becomes cross-linked to generate the fibrin clot. Natural anticoagulants balance the system—for example, to limit fibrin generation and deposition to specific sites of injury.[9] The natural anticoagulants include the tissue factor pathway inhibitor (TFPI), proteins C and S, and antithrombin III (ATIII).

Fibrinolytic proteins function to control fibrin accumulation. Tissue and urokinase plasminogen activators (TPA and UPA) activate plasminogen to plasmin, which directly degrades fibrin. The fibrinolytic system is regulated by plasminogen activator inhibitors (PAIs), which prevent the activity of TPA and UPA. Increased PAI expression occurs in several pathologic situations and results in impaired fibrinolysis. In general, in the normal host, the trauma of surgery favors the procoagulant state.

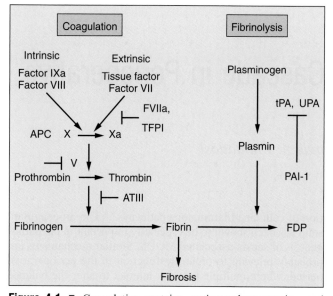

Figure 4-1 ■ Coagulation proteins, anticoagulant proteins, and fibrinolytic proteins. Coagulation proteases *(left)* are activated to lead to fibrin formation through a series of cleavage events. Naturally occurring anticoagulant systems balance procoagulant mechanisms. The role of fibrinolysis *(right)* is to resolve fibrin formation, and this is offset by plasminogen activator inhibitors (PAIs). APC, activated protein C; ATIII, antithrombin III; FDP, fibrin degradation products; TFPI, tissue factor pathway inhibitor; tPA, tissue plasminogen activator; UPA, urokinase plasminogen activator.

■ PERIOPERATIVE MONITORING OF COAGULATION

Coagulation can be monitored by measuring the levels of coagulation proteins and complexes, as well as by functional assays of clotting including the prothrombin time (PT) and the partial thromboplastin time (PTT).[12] Several other tests are not routinely available outside of research or academic settings. Caution should be used, however, in relating laboratory indices of hypercoagulability with thrombophilic events and organ injury, because most such associations have not been confirmed.

Routine coagulation parameters are insensitive to subtle alterations in thrombophilic tendency. PT and PTT assess the extrinsic and intrinsic coagulation cascades, respectively. D-dimer assays are widely available to detect fibrin degradation products, and their presence indicates activation of fibrinolysis, but the D-dimer is not necessarily a marker of increased fibrin formation. Levels of certain individual coagulation factors, such as factor VIII, can also be measured in the special hematology laboratory.

Other measurements are available to indicate activation of thrombin, which occurs beyond the convergence of the intrinsic and extrinsic pathways. Such tests, which are not rapidly or widely available, are used in research studies of hypercoagulability as outlined later. These include the thrombin–antithrombin complexes (TAT), and F1.2, a measurement of prothrombin fragments (indicating activated thrombin). Similarly, low levels of the anticoagulants ATIII

and protein C can reflect increases in coagulability, but these assays are often not available outside the research setting.

Functional measurements of clotting are more indicative of the integrated clotting response. The platelet function analyzer (PFA-100) measures platelet aggregation or plug time. The most widely used functional test for clotting is thromboelastography (TEG), which provides a comprehensive measurement of hemostatic function.[12] This test uses fresh blood to rapidly generate a thromboelastogram, which indicates time to initiation of clot formation (R), speed or rate of clot propagation (a), and clot strength (amplitude A, or shear elastic modulus G). The TEG takes into account both platelet function and fibrin–platelet interaction. Modifications of the method use inhibitors of platelet–fibrin interaction and inhibitors of platelet aggregation, and they can distinguish coagulation factor from platelet contributions to the clot formation.[13,14] Although the TEG does detect subtle changes in coagulation, studies that correlate changes in TEG with perioperative thrombosis or organ injury are lacking.

■ ALTERATION OF COAGULATION STATUS DURING THE PERIOPERATIVE PERIOD

The function of the coagulation system is altered during the perioperative period such that procoagulant mechanisms are activated, and anticoagulant and fibrinolytic mechanisms are depressed.[9] Multiple studies have demonstrated that these abnormalities occur in response to a variety of procedures. The primary outcomes and events measured for perioperative activation of coagulation are vascular thrombotic complications, including stroke, myocardial infarction, and venous thromboembolism. More subtle changes in regional organ function that result from clotting have only recently been suspected and have not yet been studied clinically in detail.

Specific pathways and mechanisms have been implicated in surgery-associated hypercoagulability. Extrinsic coagulation is activated by vascular injuries that expose or upregulate tissue factor on the endothelial surfaces, and by platelet thrombi at sites of injury that also generate fibrin clot formation.[9] Other surgical responses include increased levels of coagulation factors,[11] decreased levels and activity of endogenous anticoagulants such as activated protein C (APC) and ATIII,[15] and inhibition of fibrinolytic function.

Coagulation function is affected by several variables related to the immediate surgical procedure and concurrent interventions, as well as to postoperative complications. Several specific variables have been studied with respect to activation of procoagulant responses, but identifying the role of individual factors is difficult in the complex surgical setting. Variables that have been implicated include the pain or stress response, the mode of anesthesia, the type and quantity of intravenous fluid administration, body temperature, and the site of surgery.

Intraoperative Activation of Coagulation

Stress Response or Pain. Several studies have reported hypercoagulability as a part of a complex stress or pain response.[11,16] Enhanced coagulability developed over 15 minutes after insertion of a peripheral intravenous line in patients in the operative theatre before undergoing elective cesarean section.[16] This has been attributed to the stress response. This has also been inferred from other studies addressing effects of pain on coagulation parameters (see Pain Control, later).

Site of Surgery. Almost all surgical patients are at risk for thrombotic complications resulting from immobilization, although some procedures seem to have especially high rates of clot formation. Without prophylaxis, the incidence of deep vein thrombosis (DVT) is about 14% in gynecologic surgery, 22% in neurosurgery, 26% in abdominal surgery, and 45% to 60% in orthopedic surgery.[17] Although an increased likelihood of thrombotic complications is certainly influenced by the degree of immobilization required by the procedure, it may also reflect differential activation of coagulation related to operative location. Coagulation abnormalities have been demonstrated after a number of different types of surgical procedures.[17-20] After major abdominal surgery, such as Whipple's procedure, or pancreatic, gastric, or rectal resections, multiple signs of activation of both coagulation and fibrinolysis can be demonstrated by the end of the procedure, including decreased ATIII and fibrinogen and increased TAT and F1.2.[18] In addition, D-dimer and platelet aggregation are increased by 4 hours after surgery and remain elevated on the first postoperative day.

Although the available literature does not allow for comparison of coagulation parameters between different procedures, certain sites of surgery may be more apt to activate coagulation. For example, the brain is highly enriched in tissue factor (TF), and release of TF during parenchymal manipulation may explain an apparent increased susceptibility to thrombosis in neurosurgical patients undergoing craniotomy.[21-23] In the era before routine DVT prophylaxis, such patients had a 29% to 42% incidence of thrombotic complications. Vascular procedures are also likely to activate coagulation because of intravascular stimulation of tissue factor exposure.

Mode of Anesthesia. Several studies have shown that, compared with general anesthesia, epidural anesthesia reduces the incidence of thrombotic events[10,24] and is associated with beneficial effects on postoperative outcome.[25] Patients receiving epidural or spinal (neuraxial) anesthesia show diminished elaboration of procoagulants compared with those undergoing general anesthesia.[10] Other investigations have shown that after epidural anesthesia, patients appear to maintain adequate fibrinolysis, as evidenced by lower release of PAI-1[26] and enhanced release of plasminogen activators.[10,24] In addition, it is proposed that certain local anesthetic agents, such as lidocaine, may have anti-inflammatory actions,[27,28] which could potentially attenuate recruitment of procoagulant mechanisms. In a meta-analysis of studies of complications comparing general anesthesia alone with neuraxial anesthesia (epidural or spinal anesthesia), it was reported that in addition to having an overall mortality benefit, neuraxial blockade reduced the odds of thrombotic complications, including DVT and pulmonary embolism by 44% and 55%, respectively.[29] This meta-analysis is confounded by the inclusion of studies of multiple

surgical procedures and sites, which limits the conclusions. Moreover, in some of the studies reviewed, the use of general anesthesia was combined with neuraxial blockade for postoperative pain control. Thus, the effect of pain on coagulation was a confounding variable in the analysis. Subsequent randomized controlled trials have shown mixed results,[30,31] and it is not yet possible to recommend regional anesthesia specifically to prevent hypercoagulability.

Intravenous Fluid Administration. Fluid resuscitation with moderate to large volumes of fluid may be required during and after many surgical procedures because of vascular shifts, blood loss, and impaired autonomic tone. The resulting hemodilution appears to affect coagulation parameters, although this effect remains controversial. It has been predicted that extreme hemodilution results in a "dilutional coagulopathy," although recent studies in vitro and in vivo have indicated a procoagulant effect of hemodilution that is relevant to perioperative patients.[32,33] In vitro dilution of plasma results in altered TEG measurements that indicate hypercoagulability caused by disproportionate loss of ATIII activity, presumably due to a dilutional effect.[33] In surgical patients undergoing fluid resuscitation, decreased clot time and increased rate of clot formation were demonstrated after crystalloid fluid loading.[32] To directly study effects of fluid loading, a randomized controlled study was conducted to investigate the effect of acute crystalloid hemodilution on coagulation parameters in patients undergoing major hepatobiliary surgery.[34] In that study, the experimental group of patients had 30% of the blood volume withdrawn and replaced with saline over 30 minutes, and coagulation parameters in these patients were compared with the parameters in control surgical patients. Blood samples for TEG, complete blood count, coagulation profile, fibrinogen, antithrombin III, protein C, and thrombin–antithrombin complex concentrations demonstrated that the experimental group had increased coagulability by TEG, but the mechanism remained elusive, as the ATIII levels decreased in proportion to Hgb concentration. Although it is still controversial,[35] dilution has been postulated to play a role in perioperative thrombophilia.[32,33]

In addition to the considerations of hemodilution, the influence of specific fluid replacement therapies on coagulation parameters is also debatable. Intravenous fluid replacement is undertaken with crystalloid such as 0.9% sodium chloride or synthetic colloids such as dextran and hydroxyethyl starch (HES). Colloid plasma substitutes are thought to lead to hemostatic derangement independent of effects on hemodilution.[35] A meta-analysis of studies of colloids and hemostatic function concluded that these fluids are most likely to result in impaired coagulation when given in large volumes.[35] One study has shown that significant hemodilution with normal saline resulted in increases in procoagulant indices that were offset by use of HES at similar volume.[32] This finding also suggested a procoagulant effect of hemodilution and a possible anticoagulant effect of colloids.

Body Temperature. Hypothermia is encountered during surgical procedures, particularly following shock and massive resuscitation. Decreased body temperature may alter the coagulation and clotting function responses outlined earlier. Although long considered to have predominantly anticoagulant effects mediated through platelet dysfunction and impaired enzymatic activity of clotting factors, hypothermia is also postulated to lead to impaired fibrinolysis.[18] The overall balance of coagulation function relative to temperature remains undefined in the general surgical patient, although in trauma patients, hypothermic coagulopathy does occur at body temperatures below 34° C, with no effect on fibrinolytic activity.[36]

Postoperative Activation of Coagulation

Several important variables in the postoperative course have an impact on coagulation function and the possible risk of organ dysfunction. Increased coagulation parameters have been found to continue into the postoperative period.[18,25,37] Complications (such as sepsis and hypotension) and requirements for further fluid resuscitation appear to be major factors that perpetuate coagulation abnormalities during this time. Pain is one very important variable that is determined to contribute to coagulation abnormalities.

Pain Control. As mentioned previously (see Mode of Anesthesia), it has been suggested that local anesthetic agents may have biochemical effects that alter coagulation. It is also thought that improved pain control may have a beneficial effect on coagulation state, but available studies do not allow these effects to be delineated clearly.[10] One study compared postoperative pain control using epidural anesthesia with narcotic analgesia in patients undergoing major surgery for peripheral vascular disease under general anesthesia. Patients in the epidural analgesia group had lower activation of coagulation as evidenced by both thromboelastography and number of vascular events, including venous thromboembolism, myocardial infarction, and thrombosis of the vascular graft.[25] However, another group showed that in a large number of patients undergoing abdominal aortic surgery, there was no difference between the number of major organ failures in patients treated intensively with neuraxial pain control versus those treated with narcotic analgesia.[30]

▪ CONSEQUENCES OF DYSREGULATED COAGULATION

When coagulation balance is disrupted to favor procoagulant mechanisms, organ dysfunction is elicited by the deposition of fibrin in the vessel lumen and tissue parenchyma as well as by proinflammatory actions of coagulation proteins. The association between activation of coagulation and organ dysfunction is established in sepsis and other systemic inflammatory states. The following paragraphs briefly review these mechanisms and point out their potential relevance in perioperative organ dysfunction, which remains largely unexplored.

Proinflammatory Actions of Coagulation Proteases. Several key proteins in the extrinsic coagulation system are capable of generating intracellular signals. Tissue factor is an integral membrane glycoprotein with structural features of a class 2 cytokine receptor. TF is expressed on monocytes or macrophages and on endothelial cell surfaces, and after binding by circulating FVIIa, its interaction with other cell receptors or direct intracellular action leads to increased oxidant production, protein tyrosine phosphorylation, and calcium oscillations in human cells. Signal transduction pathways activated by the FVIIa/TF complex include p44/42 (ERK) and p38 mitogen-activated protein kinase (MAPK).[6-8] These signaling pathways activate inflammatory transcription factors and expression of proteins, such as interleukin (IL)-6 and vascular endothelial growth factor (VEGF), that further amplify inflammation and may promote capillary leak. These interactions are summarized in Figure 4-2.

Factor Xa and thrombin are serine protease components of extrinsic coagulation downstream from TF that have independent inflammatory signaling functions. FXa binds to a cell surface–based receptor, effector-cell protease receptor-1 (EPR-1), and thrombin binds to proteinase-activated receptor-1 (PAR-1).[6-8] As shown in Figure 4-2, multiple proinflammatory roles for EPR-1 and PAR-1 have been demonstrated, including nuclear factor (NF)-κB activation.

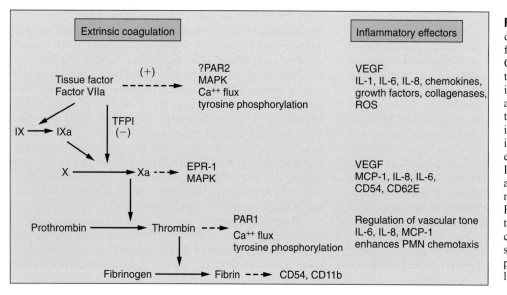

Figure 4-2 ▪ Interface between coagulation proteins and inflammatory signaling pathways. Coagulation proteins and receptors generate intracellular signals in inflammatory, parenchymal, and endothelial cells through the actions indicated. This results in elaboration of numerous inflammatory effectors. EPR-1, effector-cell protease receptor 1; IL, interleukin; MAPK, mitogen-activated protein kinase; MCP, monocyte chemotactic protein; PAR, protease-activated receptor; PMN, polymorphonuclear cells; ROS, reactive oxygen species; TFPI, tissue factor pathway inhibitor; VEGF, vascular endothelial growth factor.

Proliferative and proinflammatory responses to thrombin have been demonstrated in endothelial cells and macrophages, respectively. Finally, the terminal coagulation component, fibrin, promotes an acute cellular inflammatory response, contributes to surfactant inactivation in the lung, and provides a scaffold for collagen deposition in wounds and in the lung after acute lung injury.[4,38]

Relationship of Coagulation Abnormalities to Organ Dysfunction. Activation of coagulation is an important mechanism of injury to the lungs and other organs. In sepsis, the importance of coagulation to organ injury is well established in animal models. This also appears to be the case in human sepsis, where therapy with APC reduces mortality in severe sepsis.[39] Organ failure causality has also been suggested in human sepsis, where vascular and parenchymal fibrin deposition found in the lungs of septic patients is postulated to contribute to acute lung injury.[38] Fibrin deposition may also be a problem in acute renal failure in sepsis, where it is prominent in small arterioles.[40,41] Along with the endothelial damage that usually occurs during operative procedures, coagulation is activated by increased tissue factor expression on endothelial and inflammatory cells. This can lead to intravascular and extravascular fibrin deposition, leading to organ dysfunction by creating serious ischemic or distributive defects in microvascular blood flow.

Major organ dysfunction follows many types of surgery, as mentioned at the beginning of this chapter. Although a definitive role for relative hypercoagulability has not yet been demonstrated in perioperative organ dysfunction, further studies are warranted. Such an association is suggested by several studies. In one study, postoperative patients with disseminated intravascular coagulopathy had high rates of organ failure, and multiple microthrombi were found in tissues at autopsy.[42] In another study of patients undergoing major cardiac surgery, it was found that the odds ratio of developing renal failure was 2.5-fold higher in patients with substantial hemodilution.[43] Other groups have demonstrated similar findings (i.e., that changes in hematocrit alone do not explain the degree of renal dysfunction) and have postulated other mechanisms of hemodilution leading to renal failure.[44] Although coagulation parameters were not measured in these studies, it is intriguing to postulate a role for hypercoagulability induced by hemodilution.

■ SUMMARY AND RECOMMENDATIONS

The model of coagulation abnormalities leading to organ dysfunction in perioperative situations is a relatively new area of investigation. This idea has been well accepted in organ injury caused by sepsis, and it is quite likely relevant to perioperative conditions when coagulation abnormalities are present. In addition to the effects of operative trauma, many other variables are known to affect the evolution of coagulation abnormalities, including pain, fluid replacement, and anesthetic regimen. Of special interest as possible therapeutic targets are procoagulant aspects of hemodilution and anticoagulant effects of colloids, and anti-inflammatory and anticoagulant effects of local anesthetic agents. These factors correlate with changes in coagulation status, but much work

remains to be done to connect them causally to less obvious effects such as organ dysfunction. Furthermore, true incidences of organ dysfunction remain to be defined, as do special aspects related to the surgical procedure and perioperative care. Finally, much of the available data were obtained prior to or without regard to standard practices of postoperative thromboembolism prophylaxis. A modern approach to coagulation abnormalities in the postoperative setting needs to be developed to evaluate their effects on outcome, especially involving postoperative infection and organ failure. Recommendations for thromboembolism prophylaxis should be followed rigorously and organ function closely monitored in all postoperative patients at high risk for complications of hypercoagulability.

■ REFERENCES

1. Waydhas C, Nast-Kolb D, Trupka A, et al: Posttraumatic inflammatory response, secondary operations, and late multiple organ failure. J Trauma 1996;40:624-630.
2. Carmichael P, Carmichael AR: Acute renal failure in the surgical setting. Aust N Z J Surg 2003;73:144-153.
3. Novis BK, Roizen MF, Aronson S, Thisted RA: Association of preoperative risk factors with postoperative acute renal failure. Anesth Analg 1994;78:143-149.
4. Idell S, Koenig KB, Fair DS, et al: Serial abnormalities of fibrin turnover in evolving adult respiratory distress syndrome. Am J Physiol 1991;261:L240-L248.
5. Welty-Wolf KE, Carraway MS, Ortel TL, Piantadosi CA: Coagulation and inflammation in acute lung injury. Thromb Haemost 2002;88:17-25.
6. Cunningham MA, Romas P, Hutchinson P, et al: Tissue factor and factor VIIa receptor/ligand interactions induce proinflammatory effects in macrophages. Blood 1999;94:3413-3420.
7. Cirino G, Cicala C, Bucci M, et al: Factor Xa as an interface between coagulation and inflammation: Molecular mimicry of factor Xa association with effector cell protease receptor-1 induces acute inflammation in vivo. J Clin Invest 1997;99:2446-2451.
8. Johnson K, Choi Y, DeGroot E, et al: Potential mechanisms for a proinflammatory vascular cytokine response to coagulation activation. J Immunol 1998;160:5130-5135.
9. Roberts HR, Monroe DM, Escobar MA: Current concepts of hemostasis: Implications for therapy. Anesthesiology 2004;100:722-730.
10. Hahnenkamp K, Theilmeier G, Van Aken HK, Hoenemann CW: The effects of local anesthetics on perioperative coagulation, inflammation, and microcirculation. Anesth Analg 2002;94:1441-1447.
11. Collins GJ, Barber JA, Zajtchuk R, et al: The effects of operative stress on the coagulation profile. Am J Surg 1977;133:612-616.
12. Spiess BD: Coagulation monitoring in the perioperative period. Int Anesthesiol Clin 2004;42:55-71.
13. Tuman KJ, Spiess BD, McCarthy RJ, Ivankovich AD: Effects of progressive blood loss on coagulation as measured by thrombelastography. Anesth Analg 1987;66:856-863.
14. Gottumukkala VN, Sharma SK, Philip J: Assessing platelet and fibrinogen contribution to clot strength using modified thromboelastography in pregnant women. Anesth Analg 1999;89:1453-1455.
15. Andersson TR, Berner NS, Larsen ML, et al: Plasma heparin cofactor II and antithrombin in elective surgery. Acta Chir Scand 1987;153:291-296.
16. Gorton H, Lyons G, Manraj P: Preparation for regional anaesthesia induces changes in thrombelastography. Br J Anaesth 2000;84:403-404.
17. Bombeli T, Spahn DR: Updates in perioperative coagulation: Physiology and management of thromboembolism and haemorrhage. Br J Anaesth 2004;93:275-287.
18. Boldt J, Hüttner I, Suttner S, et al: Changes of haemostasis in patients undergoing major abdominal surgery: Is there a difference between elderly and younger patients? Br J Anaesth 2001;87:435-440.

19. Bradbury A, Adam D, Garrioch M, et al: Changes in platelet count, coagulation and fibrinogen associated with elective repair of asymptomatic abdominal aortic aneurysm and aortic reconstruction for occlusive disease. Eur J Vasc Endovasc Surg 1997;13:375-380.

20. Stern SH, Sharrock N, Kahn R, Insall JN: Hematologic and circulatory changes associated with total knee arthroplasty surgical instrumentation. Clin Orthop Rel Res 1994;299:179-189.

21. Heesen M, Kemkes-Matthes B, Deinsberger W, et al: Coagulation alterations in patients undergoing elective craniotomy. Surg Neurol 1997;47:35-38.

22. Powers SK, Edwards MSB: Prophylaxis of thromboembolism in neurosurgical patients: A review. Neurosurgery 1982;10:509-513.

23. Abrahams JM, Torchia MB, McGarvey M, et al: Perioperative assessment of coagulability in neurosurgical patients using thromboelastography. Surg Neurol 2002;58:5-11.

24. Modig J, Borg T, Bagge L, Saldeen T: Role of extradural and of general anaesthesia in fibrinolysis and coagulation after total hip replacement. Br J Anaesth 1983;55:625-629.

25. Tuman KJ, McCarthy RJ, March RJ, et al: Effects of epidural anesthesia and analgesia on coagulation and outcome after major vascular surgery. Anesth Analg 1991;73:696-704.

26. Rosenfeld BA, Beattie C, Christopherson R, et al: The effects of different anesthetic regimens on fibrinolysis and the development of postoperative arterial thrombosis. Perioperative Ischemia Randomized Anesthesia Trial Study Group. Anesthesiology 1993;79:435-443.

27. Beloeil H, Asehnoune K, Moine P, et al: Bupivacaine's action on the carrageenan-induced inflammatory response in mice: Cytokine production by leukocytes after ex-vivo stimulation. Anesth Analg 2005;100:1081-1086.

28. Honemann CW, Hahnenkamp K, Podranski T, et al: Local anesthetics inhibit thromboxane A2 signaling in *Xenopus* oocytes and human K562 cells. Anesth Analg 2004;99:930-937.

29. Rodgers A, Walker N, Schug S, et al: Reduction of postoperative mortality and morbidity with epidural or spinal anaesthesia: Results from overview of randomised trials. Br Med J 2000;321:1493.

30. Ganapathy S, McCartney JL, Beattie WS, Chan VWS: Best evidence in anesthetic practice: Prevention: Epidural anesthesia and analgesia does not reduce 30-day all-cause mortality and major morbidity after abdominal surgery. Can J Anesth 2003;50:143-146.

31. Fleron M-H, Weiskopf RB, Bertrand M, et al: A comparison of intrathecal opioid and intravenous analgesia for the incidence of cardiovascular, respiratory, and renal complications after abdominal aortic surgery. Anesth Analg 2003;97:2-12.

32. Ruttmann TG, James MFM, Aronson I: In vivo investigation into the effects of haemodilution with hydroxyethyl starch (200/0.5) and normal saline on coagulation. Br J Anaesth 1998;80:612-616.

33. Nielsen VG, Lyerly RT 3rd, Gurley WQ: The effect of dilution on plasma coagulation kinetics determined by thrombelastography is dependent on antithrombin activity and mode of activation. Anesth Analg 2004;99:1587-1592.

34. Ng KFJ, Lam CCK, Chan LC: In vivo effect of haemodilution with saline on coagulation: A randomized controlled trial. Br J Anaesth 2002;88:475-480.

35. de Jonge E, Levi M: Effects of different plasma substitutes on blood coagulation: A comparative review. Crit Care Med 2001;29:1261-1267.

36. Watts DD, Trask A, Soeken K, et al: Hypothermic coagulopathy in trauma: Effect of varying levels of hypothermia on enzyme speed, platelet function, and fibrinolytic activity. J Trauma 1998;44:846-854.

37. Ygge J: Changes in blood coagulation and fibrinolysis during the postoperative period. Am J Surg 1970;119:225-232.

38. Idell S: Anticoagulants for acute respiratory distress syndrome. Am J Respir Crit Care Med 2001;164:517-520.

39. Bernard GR, Vincent JL, Laterre PF, et al: Efficacy and safety of recombinant human activated protein C for severe sepsis. N Engl J Med 2001;344:699-709.

40. Welty-Wolf KE, Carraway MS, Miller DL, et al: Coagulation blockade prevents sepsis-induced respiratory and renal failure in baboons. Am J Respir Crit Care Med 2001;164:1988-1996.

41. Carraway MS, Welty-Wolf KE, Miller DL, et al: Tissue factor blockade: Treatment for organ injury in established sepsis. Am J Respir Crit Care Med 2003;167:1200-1209.

42. Ohsato K, Takaki A, Takeda S, et al: A clinical study on surgical patients with disseminated intravascular coagulation: With special reference to the occurrence of major organ failures. Nippon Geka Gakkai Zasshi 1983;84:860-864.

43. Karkouti K, Beattie WS, Wijeysundera DN, et al: Hemodilution during cardiopulmonary bypass is an independent risk factor for acute renal failure in adult cardiac surgery. J Thorac Cardiovasc Surg 2005;129:391-400.

44. Ranucci M, Menicanti L, Frigiola A: Acute renal injury and lowest hematocrit during cardiopulmonary bypass: Not only a matter of cellular hypoxemia. Ann Thorac Surg 2004;78:1880-1885.

PART II

Preoperative Assessment

Chapter

5 The Value of Preoperative Assessment

Stanley H. Rosenbaum and David G. Silverman

In most medical centers where major surgery is performed, patients are preoperatively assessed by a member of the department of anesthesiology. Although this preoperative assessment is modified for outpatient surgery and also before emergency surgery, when patients are not available before the surgery there is generally a presumption that the patient is optimally prepared for the planned surgery. Is preoperative assessment justified, or are the surgeon's preparations sufficient? Are the time, effort, and costs warranted?

Except for some special circumstances, there is a paucity of evidence (i.e., from controlled trials of comparable groups of patients, one group having undergone a preanesthetic evaluation and the other group not, when all other variables are held the same) of the efficacy of preoperative assessments.[1] However, such groups are unlikely to be analogous to a particular patient, which limits their value in addressing this question. There is always the occasional patient who has benefited from a preoperative evaluation, but do these occasional gains outweigh the costs, the annoyance, and the medical problems associated with delays or false-positive workups?

■ CASE DESCRIPTION

A 40-year-old woman arrives in the hospital for an elective hysterectomy for symptoms suggestive of uterine fibroids. Her general medical history, including several uncomplicated childbirths, is unremarkable; however, she has not had any medical care, except for her gynecologic visits, in several years. Because of scheduling problems, she was not seen for a preoperative evaluation. On arrival, her blood pressure is 150/115 mm Hg; laboratory tests and the electrocardiograph are all within normal limits. After discussion with her anesthesiologist and an internist, it is decided to reschedule the surgery until her blood pressure is under better control. The patient goes home and is followed in a medical clinic, where she has only borderline hypertension and her blood pressure is easily controlled on a low dose of a beta-adrenergic antagonist.

The patient is a single mother who requested that her sister take a vacation from her job and come in from another city to care for the patient's children during her hospitalization. With the cancellation of surgery, the sister's vacation is no longer suitably timed. The surgery is scheduled for 6 months later, when the sister can next take a vacation to care for the patient's family.

At surgery, the patient's blood pressure is ideal, but the surgeon finds a uterine malignancy with locally invasive

metastases. The patient's clinical prognosis was adversely affected by the surgical delay.

The case illustrates two issues that haunt perioperative medical care. (1) When should a medical concern (here, isolated hypertension) be regarded as sufficient to alter the surgery schedule? (2) Should more resources be devoted to ensure that patients undergo a preanesthetic evaluation, so that uncertainties can be addressed prior to the day of surgery? The day-of-surgery medical evaluation was unsatisfactory for this patient, and a preoperative evaluation might have prevented a potentially fatal delay. Perhaps preoperative evaluation can be justified by assuming that knowledge of the patient's medical issues is always valuable.

Four integrated processes occur prior to surgery. First, in the *diagnosis,* the clinical database for the patient is established. Judgments are made about further medical workup, factors that may directly affect the anesthesia or planned surgery, and, possibly, other medical issues that outweigh the importance of the planned procedure. When preparing a patient for surgery, the anesthesia and surgery teams must understand the patient's resilience to the stresses associated with anesthesia and surgery. Preoperative guidelines take these into account. The American College of Surgery and American Heart Association (ACC/AHA) guidelines[2] base recommendations for preoperative cardiology consultation on clinical risk factors and the anticipated cardiac risks of the particular surgery (Table 5-1). The American Society of Anesthesiologists (ASA) advisory for preanesthesia evaluation[1] recommends that patients be seen by a member of the anesthesia team prior to the day of surgery, not only if they have severe disease (as indicated by a high ASA physical status score[3,4]) but also if, despite a low severity of disease, they are undergoing a highly invasive procedure (as assessed by a classification system such as that proposed by Pasternak and colleagues[5] [Table 5-2]). More recently, Holt and Silverman recommended that a patient's medical history be described by system-specific scores for cardiac, respiratory, and endocrine conditions in accordance with the ASA 1-to-5 rankings of physical status (Table 5-3).[6] These system-specific scores can be added together, and they can also be integrated with the degree of surgical invasiveness, to generate assessments of resilience and risk.[6]

The second preoperative process is *optimization,* which involves efforts to ameliorate patient conditions that are less than optimal for surgery. For example, a patient with asthma might receive more aggressive bronchospasm prevention (e.g., with bronchodilators and steroids). Efforts might be made to control infection in the patient with bronchitis, to

| 5-1 | Summary of ACC/AHA Guidelines for Preoperative Cardiac Evaluation |

CARDIAC RISK FACTORS:	MAJOR*	INTERMEDIATE[†]		MINOR[‡]		NONE
Exercise Tolerance:	**Poor to Good**	**Poor[§]**	**Good[§]**	**Poor[§]**	**Good[§]**	**Poor to Good**
High-risk surgery: major or peripheral vascular; extensive intra-abdominal or intrathoracic with large fluid or blood loss; major emergency	Evaluate	Evaluate	Evaluate	Evaluate	—	—
Intermediate-risk surgery: carotid; uncomplicated head and neck, intra-abdominal or thoracic; hip and related orthopedic; prostate (lower end of this risk group)	Evaluate	Evaluate	—	—	—	—
Low-risk surgery: superficial, endoscopic	Evaluate	—	—	—	—	—

Exceptions: No interval change since cardiac evaluation within past 2 yr or revascularization within past 5 yr.

*Recent myocardial infarction, severe or unstable angina, uncontrolled congestive heart failure (CHF), significant arrhythmias (high-grade AV block, uncontrolled ventricular rate), critical valve disease.

[†]Stable "mild" angina, compensated or prior CHF, insulin-dependent diabetes mellitus with renal insufficiency (creatinine >2.0).

[‡]Advanced age, abnormal ECG (left ventricular hypertrophy, left bundle branch block, nonspecific ST, rhythm other than sinus [e.g., controlled atrial fibrillation]), low functional capacity, history of stroke, hypertension (if poorly controlled or with evidence of strain).

[§]According to the ACC/AHA guidelines, perioperative cardiac and long-term risk is increased in patients unable to meet a 4-MET (unit of metabolic activity) demand during most normal daily activities (e.g., walk around the house, light housework, walk one or two blocks on level ground at 2-3 mph). A reasonable cutoff may be the ability to climb two flights of stairs without significant shortness of breath or chest pain.

Based on ACC/AHA 2002 guideline update for perioperative cardiovascular evaluation for noncardiac surgery (see reference 2). Full text available on websites. http://www.americanheart.org/

| 5-2 | Classification of Surgical Severity |

Category	Description	Examples
1	Minimal risk to the patient independent of anesthesia; minimally invasive procedures with little or no blood loss	Breast biopsy; removal of minor skin or subcutaneous lesions; myringotomy tubes; hysteroscopy; cystoscopy; vasectomy; circumcision
2	Minimal to moderately invasive procedure; blood loss <500 mL; mild risk to patient independent of anesthesia	Diagnostic laparoscopy; laparoscopic cholecystectomy; laparoscopic lysis of adhesions; dilation & curettage; Fallopian tubal ligation; arthroscopy; inguinal hernia repair; tonsillectomy/adenoidectomy; umbilical hernia repair; septoplasty/rhinoplasty; percutaneous lung biopsy; extensive superficial procedures
3	Moderately to significantly invasive procedure; blood loss potential 500-1500 mL; moderate risk to patient independent of anesthesia	Thyroidectomy; hysterectomy; myomectomy; cystectomy; open cholecystectomy; laminectomy; hip/knee replacement; nephrectomy; major laparoscopic procedures; resection, reconstructive surgery of the digestive tract
4	Highly invasive procedure; blood loss >1500 mL; major risk to patient independent of anesthesia	Major orthopedic/spinal reconstruction; major reconstruction of the gastrointestinal tract; major genitourinary surgery (e.g., radical retropubic prostatectomy); major vascular repair without postoperative ICU stay
5	Highly invasive procedure; blood loss greater than 1500 mL; critical risk to patient independent of anesthesia; usual postoperative ICU stay with invasive monitoring	Cardiothoracic procedure; intracranial procedure

Based on descriptions in Pasternak LR: Preanesthesia evaluation of the surgical patient. Clin Anesth Updates 1995;6:1-12.[5]

protect the heart in the patient with coronary artery disease, to regulate glucose in the diabetic patient, and to control blood pressure in the patient with hypertension. Chronic conditions cannot be cured before surgery, so optimization is all that can be expected. The patient, anesthesiologist, and surgeon may have different views about what is optimal, and optimization may be limited by factors such as time constraints, resource availability, and financial issues. Nevertheless, care should be delivered in the best way possible.

The third preoperative process is *risk assessment*. When the surgeon first proposed surgery to the patient, the balance between risk and benefit was assessed. However, the risks are clearer after the processes of diagnosis and optimization are completed. Risk assessment integrates the status of the patient—at the current state of optimization—with the anticipated demands of surgery. Integration is an essential feature of the ACC/AHA guidelines for preoperative cardiac evaluation,[2] as well as for the ASA guidelines for preoperative

5-3 | **Comparison of Traditional Physical Status and Proposed System-Specific Status Classifications**

Score	Traditional ASA Physical Status	Proposed System-Specific* Status
1	Normal, healthy patient	Normal function, reserve, and resilience for the given system.
2	Mild systemic disease with no functional impairment	Early stage of dysfunction or compromise (of reserve or resilience) of the given system. Medically optimized disease, with limited impairment. Significant risk factors for dysfunction or compromise (e.g., smoking for pulmonary system).
3	Moderate systemic disease with functional limitations	Moderate disease of the given system, with measurable dysfunction or compromise. May benefit from optimization to minimize likelihood of perioperative morbidity.
4	Severe systemic disease that is a constant threat to life	Severe dysfunction or compromise of the given system that is a potential threat to life in the acute perioperative period.
5	Moribund; not expected to survive for 24 hr without surgical intervention	Acutely life-threatening dysfunction and/or compromise regardless of degree of upcoming surgical stress.

*For example, cardiac or respiratory.
ASA, American Society of Anesthesiologists.
From Holt N, Silverman DG: Modeling perioperative risk: Can numbers speak louder than words? Anesthesiol Clin North Am 2006;24:427-459.

evaluation.[1] When a scheduled surgical procedure is canceled or delayed for medical reasons, it has been determined that the risks are too high for the anticipated benefit, and further optimization or a reconsideration of the surgical plan may be needed.

Again, the patient, anesthesiologist, and surgeon may have different views of the risk. The patient must give consent for the procedure and thus can overrule the medical team, but it is the responsibility of the doctors to educate the patient. In some cases, the medical issues are conflicting. In the case history presented earlier, a minor cardiovascular issue disastrously interfered with an unappreciated life-threatening surgical problem. Established risk categorizations have statistical validity for groups of patients,[2,7-13] but for an individual patient they are helpful only as a crude assessment, because there are no evidence-based guidelines that are directly relevant to the particular setting.[14]

The fourth preoperative process is *perioperative planning,* which entails plans for perioperative care as well as medical and logistical instructions for the patient. Patients are educated about medications and diet, and about where, when, and with whom they must appear. There should be communication among perioperative care providers with respect to the anesthetic plan, special operating room requirements, special patient issues (e.g., latex allergies), and possible need for postoperative intensive care.

■ PATIENT SELECTION

It is not necessary for all patients scheduled for surgery to have a preoperative assessment by someone other than the primary surgeon. If, in the broad spectrum of surgical procedures, questions related to diagnosis, optimization, risk assessment, and planning are not relevant, preoperative assessment is not indicated. Similarly, if these issues are relatively minor and an up-to-date assessment (e.g., a recent medical workup by the patient's primary care provider) is available, the formal preoperative assessment is also not useful.[15,16] Because patient resilience is an essential aspect of the surgeon's decision to recommend surgery, the evidence may have already been gathered and the judgment made, making further consideration unnecessary. However, sometimes a careful medical review also provides preoperative preparation and teaching for the patient.

Each institution should have clear-cut criteria for the need for preoperative evaluation. These criteria are generally based on patient characteristics, on the nature of the proposed surgery, and on the anticipated anesthetic modality. A balance should be achieved between patient preference and availability, the stresses of the anesthesia and surgery, and the medical environment.[1] The *medical environment* includes local transportation, the likelihood that patients will have careful medical follow-up, and the availability of a suitable preoperative evaluation center.

Patient Characteristics

Most patient characteristics are valid considerations only when considered statistically. Nevertheless, in establishing policies, the age and weight of the patient, social factors (including tobacco or alcohol use), and readily ascertainable medical problems (e.g., diabetes or known heart disease) can be considered. As noted in Tables 5-1 and 5-3, these depend not only on the patient's medical condition but also on the surgical risk and complexity.[1,2] If it is the surgeon who decides to send the patient for a preoperative evaluation, subtle medical factors can be considered. If the decision is made by the automatic application of a policy, the factors must be simple enough to be entered clerically.

Surgical Factors

Although many aspects of a patient's physical condition are independent of the planned surgery, their impact on the patient's resilience depends on the nature and degree of perioperative stress. Thus the type of surgery guides the need for preoperative optimization, as well as intraoperative and postoperative planning. Therefore, many institutions base the policy regarding which patients receive preoperative evaluation on the nature of the surgery.

The surgeon often evaluates the patient's nonsurgical conditions. Some surgeons do such complete workups that referrals are needed only to subspecialists. Other surgeons refer all patients for a general medical assessment. Some bypass the formal preoperative evaluation system and obtain an assessment from a general internist, thereby obtaining a complete medical review but one that may fail to focus on specific anesthesia and perioperative issues. The relationship between the scale of the surgery and the patient's overall health often dictates the proper action.

Anesthesia Factors

The nature of the planned anesthetic also figures into the selection of patients for preoperative evaluation. Anesthetics range from local anesthesia for minor procedures, through various forms of intravenous sedation, to neuraxial regional anesthetics and general anesthetics. Even local anesthesia is not always a simple and safe technique, and it, too, depends on surgical and patient selection factors. However, there is some correlation between the extent of the anesthetic and the degree of surgical invasiveness, which may help guide policies for evaluation.

When policies based on patient selection, surgical procedure, or planned anesthetic do not encourage preoperative evaluation, it is the responsibility of the surgeon to focus on perioperative planning and patient education. The surgeon must also identify potential anesthesia problems (e.g., airway difficulty, aspiration risk, breastfeeding, and malignant hyperthermia) that may result in schedule delays or increased medical risk.

■ DIAGNOSIS

The preoperative evaluation is fundamentally a review of the patient's physical condition in preparation for surgery. It involves the establishment of a database cataloging factors that range from the simple demographics of age, height, and weight, to a full list of the patient's prior medical, surgical, and (when relevant) obstetric history, and relevant social factors. Social factors include alcohol and tobacco history, family history, family support, and relevant psychosocial, employment, and financial problems.

A key part of the evaluation is to recognize diagnoses that will need further treatment or optimization, special consultations that may be needed, and how these factors influence perioperative risk. The patient agrees to the surgery with the understanding that the care providers concur that the risks of the procedure are outweighed by the expected benefits. This calculation requires that the anesthesiologist and surgeon have sufficient knowledge about the patient to allow a reasonable estimation of the risks and benefits.

The preoperative database must include a complete list of the patient's medications, allergies, and relevant prior laboratory values. Despite the capacity of the medical system to provide innumerable laboratory and imaging studies, extensive routine testing is not medically or financially justifiable.[17-32] An aggressive search for preoperative diagnoses is not only time consuming and costly but also may produce false-positive results that lead to unwarranted additional assessments. If the probability of a diagnosis is greatly exceeded by the chance of a false-positive test, the test should be reconsidered.[33-35]

Most hospital, anesthesiology departments, and surgeons have guidelines to help them decide when further testing is appropriate. Relevant factors include patient age, the nature and complexity of the planned surgery, and the presence of comorbidities and their potential effect on perioperative resilience.

■ PREOPERATIVE CONSULTATION

Sometimes, a preoperative consultation with a medical subspecialist is indicated. A cardiologist might be asked for an assessment of potential cardiac ischemia and might recommend specialized diagnostic testing such as exercise stress testing or echocardiography. As noted by the ACC/AHA guidelines, the request to a consultant should be to make "recommendations concerning diagnosis and medical management" of the disorder in question and to "provide a clinical risk profile that can be used to make management decisions."[2] Similarly, pulmonary consultative help might be requested to clarify the diagnosis of chronic lung disease and to identify its fixed and reversible bronchospastic components. The goals of these consultations include guidance for medical optimization and insight into the surgical risks and potential postoperative problems.

Many patients do not have regular medical care. The specialty surgeon and the preoperative evaluation center necessarily focus on the immediate problem, but it may be an important part of patient care to consider matters related to the patient's overall health. Standard immunizations, tuberculin testing, routine gynecologic, breast, and prostate examinations, and dermatologic surveys for skin cancers are all medically important even though they are not part of the preoperative workup. A patient who receives a focused preoperative assessment might have the impression that all medical issues have been addressed and might therefore not seek evaluation for other conditions.

Anesthesiology issues may not be handled well by a general internist or even by an experienced surgeon. A potentially difficult airway can cause considerable risk if it is not diagnosed. An anesthesiologist can identify a patient who might not be readily ventilated by a bag-mask setup during the induction of anesthesia or who might have difficulty during endotracheal intubation. Patient preparation, operating room preparation, risk assessment, and the choice of anesthetic technique may all be affected if a difficult airway problem is foreseen. The anesthesiologist is also aware of subtle clues in the patient's history that might suggest a genetic defect that can lead to malignant hyperthermia. If the risk of this disorder is identified prior to surgery, a fatal outcome is generally avoidable.

Anesthetic drugs that can affect relatively obscure medical conditions might not be appreciated during an assessment performed by a subspecialist surgeon or a general internist. For example, barbiturates can cause neurologic problems in patients with inducible porphyrias (acute intermittent porphyria and variegate porphyria). Similarly, the propensity of the muscle relaxant succinylcholine to cause hyperkalemia can be a danger in some patients with upper motor neuron lesions, certain muscle disorders, or renal dysfunction.

■ OPTIMIZATION

The goal of preoperative care is to tilt the balance of surgical risk and benefit in the patient's favor. Although many medical conditions identified in a preoperative visit by a surgeon or a consultant cannot be cured or totally alleviated, there may be an opportunity to optimize them. Short-term therapeutic intervention is feasible for hypertension, heart rate control, diabetes mellitus, and some electrolyte imbalances. Of course, for many medical problems, intervention is not feasible. Tobacco and severe obesity lead to problems in the perioperative period, but elimination of their effects would require more time and interventional effort than is generally available preoperatively.

The initiation or adjustment of medications prior to surgery is one of the more important roles of the preoperative team. Medications can be started or stopped, either within a day of surgery or well in advance. Medications initiated to reduce perioperative morbidity include beta-adrenergic antagonists, statins, bowel preparations, antibiotics, and prophylactic medications to prevent aspiration and embolism. A decision to stop (for several days) or withhold (on the morning of surgery) must often find a balance between the medication's long-term benefit and its potential harm in the acute perioperative period. Medications stopped well in advance of surgery include antiplatelet agents such as clopidogrel, which, however, may be continued if there is pronounced concern about thrombosis. Medications stopped immediately prior to surgery include diuretics and oral hypoglycemics (Tables 5-4 and 5-5).

■ RISK ASSESSMENT

When the physicians and the patient have decided that the balance between risk and benefit is favorable, the patient must, except in the direst emergencies, sign an informed consent. However, an assessment of the degree of risk of the surgery and the anesthesia is very difficult to quantify precisely. For the patient, risk is a concept that is hard to imagine. Established risk scales provide guidelines that are useful for statistical cohorts but only roughly helpful for an individual patient.

Despite the theoretical difficulty, many attempts have been made to create numerically precise risk indexes. There are the relatively simple ASA physical status,[3] the rough classifications of the AHA,[2] and various quasi-numerical systems.[2,7,8,10-13] Although these latter systems (e.g., the Goldman, Eagle, and Detsky systems) do offer some help, precision is not possible. Strong and otherwise healthy patients have greater resilience in the face of surgical stress than the sick and frail. And the resilience of any patient may be sufficient for less stressful surgery but readily overcome by severe surgical insult.

As mentioned previously, our team at the Yale University School of Medicine has proposed a resilience score for organ systems jeopardized by an underlying condition (system-specific ASA physical status) and the severity of the upcoming surgery (rated 1 to 5).[6] An overall resilience score for a single organ system can be obtained by adding the standard ASA score and the surgical complexity score (to a maximum of 10). The higher the score, the more likely it is that the particular system will suffer injury or fail to meet the demands of the upcoming surgery. This system-specific score targets perioperative interventions and monitoring, and optimization can be directed to the system with the highest integrated score. Furthermore, the scores for each organ system assigned a score of 3 or more can then be added so as to more

5-4	**Medications Commonly Discontinued Several Days before Surgery**

Medication	Special Considerations and Comments
Tricyclic antidepressants	Continue for severe depression
Monoamine oxidase inhibitors (MAOIs)	Continue if severe condition (use MAOI-safe anesthetic that avoids meperidine)
Metformin	May stop 24-48 hr to ↓ risk of lactic acidosis
Birth control pills, estrogen replacement, tamoxifen	Prolonged risk of thromboembolism, especially after major oncologic and orthopedic surgery. Decision by surgeon or oncologist
Aspirin, clopidogrel (Plavix), cilostazol (Pletal), dipyridamole (Persantine)	May continue in patients with critical need for antithrombotic therapy and/or low risk of significant surgical bleeding. Duration of effect of cilostazol and dipyridamole < clopidogrel, aspirin, and ticlidopine. However, if major concern about intraoperative bleeding, stop for up to 10 days.
Warfarin (Coumadin)	Generally stop for 3-5 days. If high risk of thromboembolism, may replace with heparin or low-molecular-weight heparin
Nonsteroidal anti-inflammatory drugs	May continue for severe inflammatory disorder
Cyclooxygenase type 2 inhibitors	May continue to avoid flare-up (despite potential thrombosis or delayed healing).
Fish oil, vitamin E (>250 U/day), and many herbal medicinals	Potential multisystem (anticoagulant, cardiovascular) effects. Standard vitamins acceptable.

None of the recommendations is absolute; decisions are best made on an individual basis.

5-5 Medications Commonly Withheld on Morning of Surgery

Medication	Special Considerations and Comments
ACE inhibitors, angiotensin receptor blockers	Continue if refractory hypertension, fragile aneurysm, severe congestive heart failure (CHF), valvular insufficiency
Diuretics	May continue for CHF
Phosphodiesterase-5 inhibitors	May predispose to hypotension
Lithium	Interacts with anesthetic agents
Bupropion, trazodone	Predispose to exaggerated sympathetic response
Disulfiram (Antabuse)	Affects metabolism (e.g., phenytoin, warfarin)
Alendronate sodium (Fosamax)	Causes transient esophageal irritation
Particulate antacids	Cause pneumonitis if aspirated
Oral hypoglycemics	Risk of hypoglycemia in fasting patient
Long-acting insulin (no available IV access— e.g., day-of-surgery admission)	May also ↓ dose night before surgery if patient is prone to morning hypoglycemia. Initiate tighter control when IV access available
Rapidly acting insulin	Administer preoperatively only if hyperglycemia
Insulin pump	Withhold bolus; may continue basal rate
Pyridostigmine (for myasthenia gravis)	May complicate use of neuromuscular blocking drugs. Continue if risk of severe weakness or dysphagia
Low-molecular-weight heparin (enoxaparin)	Can replace warfarin; typically withhold for 12-24 hr

None of the recommendations is absolute; decisions are best made on an individual basis.

effectively reflect the impact of multisystem disease. For example, a patient who has level 4 respiratory disease and also has level 3 cardiac disease, renal disease, and diabetes would be assigned a cumulative resilience score of 13. This integrated resilience score helps overcome the limitation of two highly acclaimed means for preoperative assessment— the ASA physical status score[1,3,4] and the ACC/AHA classification of perioperative cardiac risk,[2] neither of which assigns a higher classification for multiple features within a given system or for comorbid diseases of multiple systems.

Sometimes a patient needs such extensive optimization for ideal surgical conditions that the surgery is delayed. Although the postponing of scheduled surgery might be viewed as inefficient, it is in fact a significant advantage of preoperative evaluation. Not only may it avert a bad outcome, but the cost savings resulting from rescheduling the surgery in advance of the planned date, as opposed to canceling it on the day of surgery, are considerable and may well justify the cost of the preoperative assessment.

■ PERIOPERATIVE PLANNING

Once a patient's diagnosis is known and surgery is agreed on, planning often adheres to standard practices for the specific institution. Practical considerations include, for example, arranging for presurgical bowel preparation, ensuring that appropriate antibiotics are given preoperatively, provision of aspiration prophylaxis and preoperative beta-blockade, and discontinuation of medications. Special instructions may be given to, for example, the nursing mother. Risk assessment may indicate variations in intraoperative and postoperative management, such as the combined administration of an epidural and general anesthetic and plans for postoperative intensive care.

Every plan requires communication between caregiver and patient and between caregivers. Because patients are

often overwhelmed in the days preceding surgery, they should be provided with printed instructions about eating and drinking; discontinuing, withholding, or initiating medications; jewelry, dentures, contact lenses, and continuous positive airway pressure masks; transportation on the day of surgery; and procedures to be followed after discharge.

■ REFERENCES

1. Practice Advisory for Preanesthesia Evaluation: A Report by the American Society of Anesthesiologists Task Force on Preanesthesia Evaluation. Anesthesiology 2000;96:485-496.
2. Eagle KA, Berger PB, Calkins H, et al: ACC/AHA guideline update for perioperative cardiovascular evaluation for noncardiac surgery-executive summary: A report of the American College of Cardiology/American Heart Association Task Force on Practice Guidelines (Committee to Update the 1996 Guidelines on Perioperative Cardiovascular Evaluation for Noncardiac Surgery). J Am Coll Cardiol 2002;39:542-553.
3. Keats AS: The ASA classification of physical status: A recapitulation. Anesthesiology 1978;49:233-236.
4. Saklad M: Grading patients for surgical procedures. Anesthesiology 1941;2:281-284.
5. Pasternak LR: Preanesthesia evaluation of the surgical patient. Clin Anesth Updates 1995;6:1-12.
6. Holt N, Silverman DG: Modeling perioperative risk: Can numbers speak louder than words? Anesthesiol Clin North Am 2006;24:427-459.
7. Detsky AS, Abrams HB, McLaughlin JR, et al: Predicting cardiac complications in patients undergoing non-cardiac surgery. J Gen Intern Med 1986;1:211-219.
8. Lee TH, Marcantonio ER, Mangione CM, et al: Derivation and prospective validation of a simple index for prediction of cardiac risk of major noncardiac surgery. Circulation 1999;100:1043-1049.
9. Auerbach AD, Goldman L: Beta-blockers and reduction of cardiac events in noncardiac surgery: Scientific review. JAMA 2002;287:1435-1444.
10. Goldman L, Caldera DL, Nussbaum SR, et al: Multifactorial index of cardiac risk in noncardiac surgical procedures. N Engl J Med 1977;297:845-850.

11. Eagle KA, Rihal CS, Mickel MC, et al: Cardiac risk of noncardiac surgery: Influence of coronary disease and type of surgery in 3368 operations. CASS Investigators and University of Michigan Heart Care Program. Coronary Artery Surgery Study. Circulation 1997;96:1882-1887.
12. Palda VA, Detsky AS: Perioperative assessment and management of risk from coronary artery disease. Ann Intern Med 1997;127:313-328.
13. Charlson ME, Pompei P, Ales KL, MacKenzie CR: A new method of classifying prognostic comorbidity in longitudinal studies: Development and validation. J Chron Dis 1987;40:373-383.
14. Tinetti ME, Bogardus ST Jr, Agostini JV: Potential pitfalls of disease-specific guidelines for patients with multiple conditions. N Engl J Med 2004;351:2870-2874.
15. Schein OD, Katz J, Bass EB, et al: The value of routine preoperative medical testing before cataract surgery. Study of Medical Testing for Cataract Surgery. N Engl J Med 2000;342:168-175.
16. Roizen MF: More preoperative assessment by physicians and less by laboratory tests. N Engl J Med 2000;342:204-205.
17. Fischer SP: Cost-effective preoperative evaluation and testing. Chest 1999;115(Suppl):96S-100S.
18. Golub R, Cantu R, Sorrento JJ, Stein HD: Efficacy of preadmission testing in ambulatory surgical patients. Am J Surg 1992;163:565-570.
19. Mancuso CA: Impact of new guidelines on physicians' ordering of preoperative tests. J Gen Intern Med 1999;14:166-172.
20. Smetana GW, Macpherson DS: The case against routine preoperative laboratory testing. Med Clin North Am 2003;87:7-40.
21. Marcello PW, Roberts PL: "Routine" preoperative studies: Which studies in which patients? Surg Clin North Am 1996;76:11-23.
22. Johnson H Jr, Knee-Ioli S, Butler TA, et al: Are routine preoperative laboratory screening tests necessary to evaluate ambulatory surgical patients? Surgery 1988;104:639-645.
23. Johnson RK, Mortimer AJ: Routine pre-operative blood testing: Is it necessary? Anaesthesia 2002;57:914-917.
24. Blery C, Charpak Y, Szatan M, et al: Evaluation of a protocol for selective ordering of preoperative tests. Lancet 1986;1:139-141.
25. Houry S, Georgeac C, Hay JM, et al: A prospective multicenter evaluation of preoperative hemostatic screening tests. The French Associations for Surgical Research. Am J Surg 1995;170:19-23.
26. Vogt AW, Henson LC: Unindicated preoperative testing: ASA physical status and financial implications. J Clin Anesth 1997;9:437-441.
27. Nardella A, Pechet L, Snyder LM: Continuous improvement, quality control, and cost containment in clinical laboratory testing: Effects of establishing and implementing guidelines for preoperative tests. Arch Pathol Lab Med 1995;119:518-522.
28. Larocque BJ, Maykut RJ: Implementation of guidelines for preoperative laboratory investigations in patients scheduled to undergo elective surgery. Can J Surg 1994;37:397-401.
29. Starsnic MA, Guarnieri DM, Norris MC: Efficacy and financial benefit of an anesthesiologist-directed university preadmission evaluation center. J Clin Anesth 1997;9:299-305.
30. Delahunt B, Turnbull PR: How cost effective are routine preoperative investigations? N Z Med J 1980;92:431-432.
31. Pasternak LR: Preoperative laboratory testing: General issues and considerations. Anesthesiol Clin North Am 2004;22:13-25.
32. Maurer WG, Borkowski RG, Parker BM: Quality and resource utilization in managing preoperative evaluation. Anesthes Clin North Am 2004;22:155-175.
33. Pauker SG, Kopelman RI: Interpreting hoofbeats: Can Bayes help clear the haze? N Engl J Med 1992;327:1009-1013.
34. Collen MF, Feldman R, Siegelaub AB, Crawford D: Dollar cost per positive test for automated multiphasic screening. N Engl J Med 1970;283:459-463.
35. Tape TG, Mushlin AI: How useful are routine chest x-rays of preoperative patients at risk for postoperative chest disease? J Gen Intern Med 1988;3:15-20.

6 Cardiac Risk Assessment in Noncardiac Surgery

Edward Kwon, Lee A. Fleisher, and Kim Eagle

The preoperative evaluation of a patient who is scheduled to undergo elective noncardiac surgery involves the study of multiple factors, including preexisting medical conditions, prior surgical history, and the risks associated with the surgery itself. Patients with risk factors or a known history of cardiovascular disease are shown to be at an increased risk of suffering significant cardiovascular morbidity and mortality during noncardiac surgery, not only during the immediate perioperative period but in the years following the procedure. Cardiac morbidity and mortality are among the most frequent adverse events occurring in noncardiac surgery, especially among high-risk groups undergoing major vascular surgery.[1] Underlying cardiac disease and perioperative adverse events have a variety of manifestations, including ischemic coronary disease, congestive heart failure, and valvular disease. Among the various categories of surgical procedures, three major groups are associated with a higher risk of adverse coronary events. The three include vascular, abdominal, and thoracic surgeries.[2] As the U.S. population continues to age, there is an increase in the rate of noncardiac surgery being performed, resulting in an increased rate of these adverse cardiac events. Also, relatively recent trends, including the expanding use of bariatric surgery, are expected to have a significant impact. The impact of cardiac events complicating these surgical procedures is significant, with up to 18% of patients having known coronary artery disease (CAD) or risk factors for CAD.[3]

In the clinical setting, patients too often receive a quick, cursory evaluation of their risk for perioperative cardiac events immediately before surgery, by a surgeon or an anesthesiologist. Many physicians consider this an insufficient approach to offer proper evaluation and maximal risk reduction for adverse events such as myocardial infarction (MI). They think that the purpose of a preoperative evaluation should not be simply to give medical clearance for surgery. A comprehensive algorithm should be developed that has multiple elements, including an evaluation of the patient's medical status. Based on this evaluation, it should be possible to make recommendations toward risk reduction and management of potential cardiac issues over the entire perioperative period. Furthermore, this system should provide a clinical risk profile that the patient, primary care physician, anesthesiologist, and surgeon can use in the generation of treatment decisions.

An increasing body of knowledge deals with the perioperative management of patients undergoing elective surgery, from the identification of those who may be at greatest risk for adverse cardiac events, to the formulation of strategies to help reduce that risk. Over the past few decades, numerous guidelines for cardiac evaluation prior to surgery have been developed. Most of the existing systems and guidelines have been derived from a body of evidence that is primarily nonsurgical in nature, based on selected populations of patients or expert consensus opinion. Many of the currently existing strategies of perioperative management include the same elements: history and physical examination, nonstress echocardiography, noninvasive cardiac stress testing, and invasive testing by either coronary angiography or electrophysiologic studies. The therapies aimed at reducing the incidence of perioperative cardiac complications fall into three general categories: preoperative coronary revascularization, perioperative medical therapy, and monitoring.[4] These guidelines are undergoing revision, but we continue to use the existing guidelines to aid in our clinical management and decision making, incorporating new knowledge when available.

■ PATIENTS WITH CARDIOVASCULAR DISEASE

Hypertension

Hypertension is a leading cause of death and disability in the majority of Western societies, and a common preoperative abnormality in surgical patients, with an overall prevalence of up to 20%. Chronic hypertension is associated with a greater incidence of CAD and MI in both the nonsurgical and surgical settings. The Study of Perioperative Ischemia Research Group trial demonstrated that a history of hypertension is one of five independent predictors of postoperative ischemia, and one of three independent predictors of increased postoperative mortality.[5]

Current practices based on nonsurgical literature dictate that elective surgery should not be postponed in patients with mild to moderate hypertension, and that any existing antihypertensive medications should be continued up to the day of surgery. A study of 989 chronically treated hypertensive patients without overt CAD who presented for noncardiac surgery with a diastolic blood pressure between 110 and 130 mm Hg were divided into two groups: those who had surgery postponed until receiving further treatment and those who proceeded with their surgery. No statistically significant differences in postoperative complications were found between these two arms of the study.[6] There is a recommendation that severe chronic or stage 3 hypertension, which is defined as a systolic blood pressure of greater than 180 mm Hg and/or a diastolic blood pressure of greater than 110 mm Hg, should always be controlled before any elective surgical procedure.[7] In this situation, if the patient is not on an existing antihypertensive regimen, one can be established with adequate blood pressure control in a matter of days to weeks. A hypertensive crisis is defined as a diastolic blood pressure of greater than 120 mm Hg, accompanied by evidence of end-organ damage and a high risk of MI or stroke. These episodes should be treated aggressively with the precipitants determined.

Coronary Ischemic Heart Disease

Myocardial ischemia is a pathologic state of the heart, often demonstrated in the setting of metabolic oxygen demand of myocardial tissues exceeding existing oxygen supply. This imbalance can be a result of a marked increase in metabolic demand, an abrupt reduction in the supply of oxygen, or a combination of the two, leading to infarction of myocardial tissue. MI is a common fatal complication of perioperative cardiovascular adverse events, accounting for up to 40% of postoperative deaths.[8] Although multiple causes can be attributed to this pathologic scenario, including severe hypertension, severe hypotension, tachycardia, coronary arterial vasospasm, hypovolemia, hypoxemia, anemia, and severe valvular disease, the most common cause of myocardial ischemia in Western societies is atherosclerotic disease of the coronary arteries. Current understanding of the pathophysiology of operative and nonoperative MI is based on the idea of coronary plaque rupture leading to vessel occlusion by the formation of a resulting thrombus.[9] Vessel occlusion is not only a result of thrombus formation but also of vessel spasm triggered by acute plaque rupture.[10,11] In the setting of perioperative MI, this abrupt loss of vital oxygen supply to a heart already enduring surgical stress leads to prolonged myocardial ischemia, resulting in tissue infarction, ventricular dysfunction, and, potentially, death. A study by Dawood, Eagle, and associates compared the pathophysiology of fatal postoperative MI to MI not related to surgery from both clinical and histopathologic standpoints.[12] Patients in this study were selected from a group of individuals who suffered a fatal myocardial infarction after elective or emergency noncardiac surgery between 1980 and 1990. Clinical criteria such as risk factors for infarction, associated medical problems, and diagnosis of MI based on laboratory parameters were used to select patients, as well as availability of complete histopathologic analysis of the coronary anatomy during the postmortem examination. Among the 41 patients who sustained a fatal perioperative MI in this study, 55% showed evidence of unstable plaques with disruption, and findings of plaque hemorrhage were discovered in 45% of the latter group. Severe and often multivessel disease, and coronary stenoses (left main, 20%; three vessel, more than 50%) were also prominent in this patient population.

The pathology of acute MI in the perioperative period appears to have the same elements seen in an acute MI that is unrelated to surgery: plaque hemorrhage, rupture, and occlusive thrombus formation leading to tissue ischemia.

Although some patients lack a history of known coronary disease, they may possess one of several clinical markers predictive of a future adverse cardiac event. Over the past several decades, various studies have related the presence of hypertension,[13] dyslipidemias,[14,15] smoking,[16,17] and diabetes mellitus[18,19] to an increased incidence of cardiovascular disease and adverse events such as MI. Tobacco use has been linked to heart disease since the first observational study in 1940.[20] Since then, multiple studies have confirmed the association between cigarette smoking and the increased incidence of MI.[16,17] Family history of cardiovascular disease has also been considered a strong risk factor for cardiac events, although the incidence of CAD or MI has been inconsistently associated with specific genetic groups.[21,22] Diabetes mellitus is a widespread disease affecting nearly 100 million people worldwide and has been found to increase the risk of CAD, stroke, peripheral vascular disease, and heart failure by two- to fourfold.[18] Not only has the presence of elevated low-density lipoprotein (LDL) levels been shown in epidemiologic studies to lead to increased rates of cardiovascular disease,[14,15] but clinical trials have shown beneficial effects of lipid-lowering therapy with 3-hydroxy-3-methylglutaryl-CoA (HMG-CoA) reductase inhibitor therapy in patients with a history of both MI and hyperlipidemia.[23,24] Recently, the INTER-HEART study looked at nine modifiable clinical risk factors, including apolipoprotein abnormalities, tobacco, hypertension, diabetes, abdominal obesity, psychosocial factors, fruit and vegetable consumption, alcohol use, and physical activity, relating them to the incidence of MI.[25] These various factors were collectively studied among patients from 52 different countries and found to have a strong relationship to the incidence of adverse coronary events, despite cultural and population differences. Smoking and lipid abnormalities accounted for nearly two thirds of the population-associated risk of an acute MI in this study.[25]

The presence of any number of these risks may prompt the need for further preoperative testing, although, except for diabetes mellitus, the presence of a solitary risk factor has not been associated with a marked increase in perioperative risk. Such testing, however, should not be performed unless the results are likely to impact a patient's perioperative management. If a history of known prior coronary disease exists, it must be investigated and evaluated to determine the severity and stability of disease and symptoms, the presence of a prior MI, and any prior workup and interventions performed. Patients with a history of mild stable angina, prior MI, and compensated congestive heart failure (CHF) are at an increased risk for perioperative events compared with patients with no existing cardiac disease. Patients with stable disease can present with a wide range of symptoms, from a complete lack of symptoms to significant dyspnea on exertion and angina after minimal physical activity. Those who demonstrate no symptoms or only minimal symptoms with regular activity generally do not require invasive procedures such as percutaneous intervention (PCI) and coronary artery bypass grafting (CABG), because the risks of the coronary procedure are higher than that of the noncardiac surgical procedure itself. However, additional cardiovascular testing, intervention, and monitoring should be considered for those who demonstrate symptoms indicative of extensive CAD. Patients who present at the extreme with unstable coronary syndrome or decompensated ischemic heart failure are in significant danger of suffering worsening disease in the perioperative period should surgery proceed. Unless the noncardiac surgery is truly emergent, postponing the procedure until cardiac issues can be stabilized is often warranted.[26]

Many changes have been made in the approach to patients with a history of known prior MI. In the past, a traditional waiting period of 6 months after an MI was observed before proceeding to an elective procedure, based on studies that demonstrated an increased incidence of recurrent MI if the surgery was performed within 6 months of the previous infarction.[27] This population of patients was further subdivided into high-risk patients who waited the full 6-month period, compared with lower-risk patients sustaining less complicated infarctions who waited only a 3-month interval before proceeding with surgery. Since that time, numerous clinical trials have suggested that separating patients into these 3- and 6-month intervals is unnecessary.[27,28] Despite the lack of clinical trials to support this, a waiting period of as short as 4 to 6 weeks after an MI has been deemed reasonable before proceeding with elective noncardiac surgery. From a pathophysiologic standpoint, the use of coronary reperfusion, widespread coronary revascularization, and multimedical coronary stabilization has changed the natural history of patients with a recent MI. At present, multiple systems of risk stratification exist for patients with known existing coronary disease, based on their clinical presentation and the presence of other comorbid factors. The purpose of all of these systems is to help guide treatment decisions that will minimize the risk of further ischemic events in the perioperative period.

Congestive Heart Failure

Another common condition is systolic or diastolic heart failure. Although most systolic heart failure has been linked with ischemic heart disease, the impairment of normal cardiac function is another strong contributor to perioperative cardiac mortality and to morbidity itself.[26] Systolic heart failure can be defined as the state in which the heart is unable to pump a sufficient amount of blood to meet the body's metabolic requirements. The left ventricle is most commonly involved, with secondary involvement of the right ventricle in many pathologic processes. Left ventricular dysfunction is often a result of ischemic coronary disease, but it can also be attributed to valvular abnormalities, arrhythmias, and pericardial disease. Diastolic dysfunction often displays symptoms of heart failure secondary to atrial hypertension, and although it can exist independently of systolic failure, it often exists concomitantly with systolic dysfunction. Like systolic failure, diastolic dysfunction can be brought about by systemic hypertension, ischemia, pericardial disease, and unique disease states like hypertrophic cardiomyopathy.

When a patient presents with symptoms related to heart failure, the underlying cause (or causes) of cardiac disease should be identified and treated prior to the start of any major noncardiac surgery. Goldman and coworkers demonstrated significant perioperative risk in the presence of a third heart sound or other signs of CHF during noncardiac surgery.[27] The presence of pulmonary edema is thought to be another indicator of increased cardiac morbidity and mortality.[29] Of the various causes of heart failure just listed, ischemic cardiomyopathy is usually of the greatest concern and places the patient at risk of developing further intraoperative ischemia. However, failure related to ischemia is managed in a very different fashion from other underlying causes of failure, such as dilated or hypertrophic cardiomyopathy.

Hypertrophic obstructive cardiomyopathy (HOCM) is a distinct entity that poses unique management issues in the perioperative setting. Reductions in venous return, lowered systemic vascular resistance (SVR), and increased venous capacitance can lead to a profound loss of left ventricular volume, resulting in an anatomic obstruction of left ventricular (LV) outflow with impairment of cardiac output delivery to the coronary and systemic circulation. The complexity of the underlying pathology has led to the belief that HOCM is a condition associated with a high risk of significant perioperative complications. Despite these existing beliefs, a small retrospective review of 35 patients by Cohn and Goldman suggested that the risk of general anesthesia, in combination with major noncardiac surgery, posed minimal additional cardiac risk to the patient, given careful intraoperative fluid and volume management. The study did suggest that the relative hypovolemia caused by a spinal anesthetic made this technique relatively contraindicated, although most clinicians do not adhere to this recommendation.[26] A retrospective study of 77 patients with asymmetrical septal hypertrophy undergoing major noncardiac procedures demonstrated a 40% incidence of adverse perioperative cardiac events, the majority of these events being episodes of CHF, suggesting that perioperative care of these patients can be performed safely.[30]

Valvular Disease

The presence of a cardiac murmur is common in patients who are scheduled to undergo elective noncardiac surgery. It should be determined whether this physical examination finding bears no clinical significance or indicates further evaluation. A consultant must distinguish between murmurs that are organic and those that are functional in nature, and must ascertain the clinical severity of any possible valvular dysfunction that may exist. Valvular pathology can range from innocent murmurs of no impact on perioperative management, to lesions requiring endocarditis prophylaxis, to the extreme scenario of critical aortic or mitral valve stenosis, which may lead to cancellation of the planned surgery until the lesion is repaired.

Aortic stenosis (AS) with a valve area of less than 0.7 cm^2 poses an extremely high cardiovascular risk to a patient facing noncardiac surgery. If the classic triad of symptoms (angina, syncope, heart failure) associated with AS is recognized during the preoperative evaluation, the procedure is usually postponed in lieu of further evaluation and interventions, including possible aortic valve replacement surgery. The biggest concern involving critical AS is the risk of severe acute cardiac decompensation under general or regional anesthesia, and this is followed by concern about the inability of the heart to compensate under the additional metabolic demands created by surgical stress. Case series do exist where patients with asymptomatic critical AS (valve areas <1 cm^2) have proceeded to necessary noncardiac surgery (usually because the patient refused cardiac surgery or had unacceptable comorbidities) with acceptable risk,[31] but these situations must be dealt with on an individual basis. If valve replacement surgery is not a reasonable option for patients because of time or necessity of the noncardiac procedure, percutaneous balloon valvuloplasty has been shown to be a helpful temporizing measure until they can receive a more definitive valve repair, albeit with a 10% risk of major periprocedural complications.[32]

Mitral stenosis (MS), although increasingly rare in Western societies, often warrants aggressive heart rate control to avoid tachycardia, which may lead to severe pulmonary congestion and inadequate filling of the left ventricle. Patients with severe MS benefit from balloon valvuloplasty or valve replacement surgery.[33] The presence of regurgitant valve disease for both the aortic and mitral valves is often better tolerated than their stenotic counterparts, and it can often be managed with similar strategies. This often includes aggressive medical therapy that involves careful volume control, afterload reduction with vasodilating drugs and diuretics, and the institution of bacterial endocarditis prophylaxis. In severe regurgitant diseases, measured LV ejection fraction (LVEF) may be a gross estimation of true EF. Patients who have mechanical prosthetic valves receive special consideration because of the issues of endocarditis prophylaxis and chronic anticoagulation.[34]

Arrhythmias and Conduction Disease

Cardiac arrhythmias and other conduction abnormalities are a common finding in the perioperative period and are particularly associated with advanced age and the presence of underlying cardiac disease.[35] To illustrate the potential danger of rhythm disturbances leading to perioperative cardiac complications, a prospective study of 4181 patients older than 50 years demonstrated a high rate of supraventricular arrhythmias during and after surgery. Such tachyarrhythmias place the patient at a significantly increased risk for ischemic events, from elevated metabolic demand to stroke, and particularly for atrial fibrillation with an uncontrolled rate.[36] Supraventricular tachyarrhythmias alone have been identified as an independent risk factor for perioperative coronary events.[7]

Traditionally, asymptomatic rhythm disturbances of a ventricular origin were viewed as a risk factor for adverse perioperative events. However, continued work in this area has not supported this notion, as studies have demonstrated that the presence of frequent premature ventricular contractions (PVC) and nonsustained ventricular tachycardia (VT) were not associated with any increased incidence of nonfatal MI or death in the perioperative period.[37] Although the presence of ventricular disturbances per se may not contribute to increased cardiac morbidity and mortality to a significant degree, these appearances during the preoperative evaluation period should spark a search for an underlying trigger, such as cardiopulmonary disease, infection, hypoxia, metabolic

derangements, and drug toxicities. Symptomatic ventricular arrhythmias should be controlled prior to elective noncardiac surgery.

Conduction abnormalities that involve the interruption of cardiac electrical impulses, especially second-degree Mobitz II atrioventricular blocks (AVB) and third-degree complete AV dissociation, require evaluation and some form of temporary or definitive treatment during the perioperative period. Unanticipated development of these conditions during surgery can lead to rapid hemodynamic deterioration unless intervention with a temporary pacemaker is implemented. Patients with existing implantable pacemakers and implantable cardioverter defibrillators (ICDs) should have their devices evaluated preoperatively by a specialist in arrhythmias, and they sometimes require magnet conversion to a default asynchronous mode during surgery and ICD deactivation or reactivation during the perioperative period to prevent any inappropriate discharges that can pose a danger to the patient or surgical team.

■ DEVELOPMENT OF A SYSTEM OF CARDIAC RISK INDEXING AND PREOPERATIVE TESTING

Over the past 25 years, many efforts have been made to develop systems of risk indexes, and algorithms have been developed on the basis of multivariate analyses, for the benefit of the physician involved in the perioperative care of a patient who is about to undergo noncardiac surgery. Many of these systems have been employed to assess the probability of cardiac complications, and the resulting data may be useful in determining the threshold for further evaluation or treatment. However, although cardiac risk can be measured, changes in management are often not performed in an appropriate manner. A preoperative evaluation should allow the physician responsible for the well-being of the patient scheduled for surgery to do the following: (1) clinically assess the patient's current medical status and provide a clinical risk profile, (2) decide whether further cardiac testing is indicated prior to surgery, and (3) make recommendations concerning the risk of perioperative cardiac complications and alter management with the purpose of lowering that risk.[26]

The Dripps–American Surgical Association (ASA) classification was initially developed and used through the late 1970s for the preoperative assessment of surgical risk.[38] The Dripps-ASA classification stratified patients into five classes based on general medical history and physical status, but it did not direct attention to elements of the patient history that were specific for different types of perioperative complications. The ASA classification gave clinicians a measure of predictive power for noncardiac perioperative complications, but it was found to be less reliable in helping anticipate the development of cardiac-specific adverse events. This weakness was attributed to its failure to incorporate clinical markers seen as risk factors unique to the prediction of cardiac-related complications. In 1977, Goldman and colleagues sought to address this issue with the development of a multifactorial index of cardiac risk specifically designed for patients scheduled to undergo noncardiac surgical procedures (Table 6-1).[27] This system looked at nine specific patient

6-1   Goldman Risk Index

Criteria*	Multivariate Discriminant-Function Coefficient	Points*
1. History		
a. Age > 70 yr	0.191	5
b. MI in previous 6 mo	0.384	10
2. Physical examination:		
a. S_2 gallop or JVD	0.451	11
b. Important VAS	0.119	3
3. Electrocardiogram:		
a. Rhythm other than sinus or PACs on last preoperative ECG	0.283	7
b. >5 PVCs/min documented at any time before surgery	0.278	7
4. General status:		
PO_2 <60 or PCO_2 >50 mm Hg; K <3.0 or HCO_3 <20 mEq/L; BUN >50 or Cr >3.0 mg/dL; abnormal SGOT; signs of chronic liver disease; or patient bedridden for noncardiac reasons	0.132	3
5. Procedure:		
a. Intraperitoneal, intrathoracic, or aortic procedure	0.123	3
b. Emergency procedure	0.167	4
Total possible	—	53

BUN, blood urea nitrogen; Cr, creatinine; ECG, electrocardiogram; HCO_3, bicarbonate; JVD, jugular-vein distention; K, potassium; MI, myocardial infarction; PACs, premature atrial contractions; PCO_2, partial pressure of CO_2; PO_2, partial pressure of O_2; PVCs, premature ventricular contractions; SGOT, serum glutamic oxaloacetic transaminase; VAS, valvular aortic stenosis.

characteristics, assigning a point value to each. On the basis of the cumulative score generated, a patient was assigned to one of four different classes. Through multivariate analyses, these classes were then correlated to a calculated range of risk for an adverse cardiac event occurring in the perioperative setting. The Goldman multivariate risk index was more objective in its cardiac assessment of a patient's risk level than the vague and poorly defined ASA classifications.

Although the Goldman risk index provided physicians a more powerful tool to help predict the occurrence of adverse cardiac events in noncardiac surgical patients, particularly those stratified into class III or IV, the study did not adequately assess the risk specific to the vascular surgery population.[39] The Goldman index also regarded CAD and MI in a very broad fashion, failing to look at other strong clinical markers associated with known or suspected coronary disease, such as severe angina. Modifications were performed on this risk index by other physicians, expanding the clinical factors to include symptoms of angina and CHF.[40] In 1999, Lee and associates reported a Revised Cardiac Risk Index (RCRI) consisting of six independent predictors of cardiac complications,[41] which included prior high-risk type of surgery, history of ischemic heart disease, history of CHF, history of cerebrovascular disease, preoperative treatment with insulin, and preoperative serum creatinine of greater than 2.0 mg/dL (Table 6-2). Patients who had two or more of these risk factors were felt to be at a higher risk of cardiac complications. Lee's risk index system was suggested as a simplified way for physicians to assess the risk of cardiac complications and help guide further decision making for testing and intervention, with a greater accuracy than previous risk indexes.[42] The RCRI is now commonly employed in many risk models. Although systems of risk prediction suggest that changes in patient management may be most appropriate in high-risk cohorts, the most effective means to lower risk have been less clearly defined.

The emphasis on risk assessment shifted from pure predictive risk indexes to comprehensive systems of patient evaluation, combined with appropriate management in the perioperative period. Studies by Eagle and colleagues[43] and

6-2   Rates of Major Cardiac Complications and Multivariate ORs* for Patients with Specified Risk Factors

Revised Cardiac Risk Index	Derivation Set (N = 2893)		Validation Set (N = 1422)	
	Crude Data	Adjusted OR (95% CI)	Crude Data	Adjusted OR (95% CI)
1. High-risk type of surgery	27/894 (3%)	2.8 (1.6, 4.9)	18/490 (4%)	2.6 (1.3, 5.3)
2. Ischemic heart disease	34/951 (4%)	2.4 (1.3, 4.2)	26/478 (5%)	3.8 (1.7, 8.2)
3. History of congestive heart failure	23/434 (5%)	1.9 (1.1, 3.5)	19/255 (7%)	4.3 (2.1, 8.8)
4. History of cerebrovascular disease	17/291 (6%)	3.2 (1.8, 6.0)	10/140 (7%)	3.0 (1.3, 6.8)
5. Insulin therapy for diabetes	7/112 (6%)	3.0 (1.3, 7.1)	3/59 (5%)	1.0 (0.3, 3.8)
6. Preoperative serum creatinine > 2.0 mg/dL	9/103 (9%)	3.0 (1.4, 6.8)	3/55 (5%)	0.9 (0.2, 3.3)

*Odds ratios based on logistic regression models including these six variables.
CI, confidence interval; OR, odds ratio.

Vanzetto and associates[44] helped determine that clinical variables could be used in guiding a clinician through the complex decision trees that lead to no testing, to noninvasive preoperative testing, or to invasive testing and intervention such as coronary revascularization. On the basis of these clinical variables, a physician could place a patient in a high-, intermediate-, or low-risk group for perioperative cardiac complications. Conventional practice prior to the release of national guidelines favored routine noninvasive cardiac testing in intermediate-risk patients while avoiding them in patients from the high-risk group.[43] This logic was based on the rationale that high-risk patients did not benefit from further noninvasive testing and would benefit only from intensive medical therapy or coronary angiography followed by possible coronary revascularization if interventions were contemplated. It was thought that noninvasive testing would help categorize intermediate-risk patients into high- and low-risk subcategories.[45] Patients in low-risk groups were thought to benefit little from noninvasive testing, as the likelihood of false-positive results would equal, if not exceed, that of true-positive test results.

A joint task force between the American College of Cardiology and the American Heart Association (ACC/AHA) led to the publication of practice guidelines for the perioperative cardiovascular evaluation of patients scheduled for noncardiac surgery.[7] The ACC/AHA guidelines were developed by a group of physicians from the specialties of cardiovascular medicine, anesthesia, and surgery, who examined evidence-based data on the most current medical literature of the time. These data were used to help formulate recommendations and strategies that would aid in all aspects of the perioperative management of the patient, including history taking, risk stratification, testing, intervention, and estimation of predicted health outcomes. The guidelines were developed to meet the needs of most patients in most clinical circumstances, but physicians were encouraged to make the final decisions concerning their individual patients. Two versions of the full-text guidelines are currently available on the websites of the American College of Cardiology (www.acc.org) and the American Heart Association (www.americanheart.org). A brief focused update on perioperative beta-blocker therapy has been released by the ACC, and the complete guidelines are currently being updated.

The ACC/AHA guidelines employ a classification scheme to help summarize the value of a particular diagnostic test or therapy:

Class I: Conditions for which there is evidence for and/or general agreement that a procedure be performed or a treatment is of benefit.

Class II: Conditions for which there is a divergence of evidence and/or opinion about the treatment.

Class III: Conditions for which there is evidence and/or general agreement that the procedure/treatment is not necessary.

The overriding theme of the 1996 guidelines, later affirmed in the 2002 update,[46] stressed that indications for further cardiac testing and treatment in high-risk patients about to undergo noncardiac surgery are identical to those for patients being treated in the nonsurgical setting. Performing coronary revascularization to help a patient simply "get through" noncardiac surgery is appropriate in only a small minority of high-risk patients. A conservative approach was recommended for the majority of patients facing surgery. This was confirmed by the recent Coronary Artery Revascularization Prophylaxis (CARP) study, in which prophylactic coronary revascularization beyond excellent medical therapy was not superior to medical outcomes at an average of 2.7 years after vascular surgery in nearly 500 patients with known stable coronary artery disease.[47]

A thorough preoperative clinical evaluation comprising a medical history, a physical examination, an electrocardiogram (ECG), and appropriate radiologic studies (chest radiograph) is paramount in any physician's decision-making algorithm. Such an evaluation should focus on the identification of existing or potentially existing cardiac disorders that would have a significant impact on the patient's perioperative course. Not only must the presence of cardiac disease be identified but also the severity and stability of disease and any known prior treatment must be assessed, in conjunction with other comorbid medical conditions and the type of surgery the patient is scheduled to receive.

Although there is a growing body of randomized controlled trials to identify which patients are most likely to benefit from preoperative coronary assessment and treatment, most clinicians still rely on the stepwise Bayesian strategy outlined in the ACC/AHA guidelines, which was developed through a combination of observational data and expert panel opinion (Fig. 6-1). This decision-making framework requires knowledge of clinical markers of cardiac risk, functional capacity of the patient, surgery-specific risks, and indications for coronary angiography. Proper use of this algorithm requires an appreciation of the different levels of risk attributable to these various clinical factors.

Clinical Markers

Clinical markers are divided into major, intermediate, and minor categories of predictors of cardiac risk (Box 6-1). Major clinical predictors of increased perioperative cardiovascular risk include unstable coronary syndromes, recent MI, unstable angina, decompensated CHF, significant arrhythmias (high-grade AV block, symptomatic arrhythmias in the presence of underlying heart disease, or supraventricular (SV) arrhythmias with uncontrolled ventricular rate), and severe valvular disease. The intermediate predictors of risk are mild angina pectoris, prior MI (>1 month before the planned surgery), compensated or prior CHF, and diabetes mellitus. The 2002 update included renal insufficiency (serum creatinine >2.0 mg/dL) as another intermediate risk factor based on the Revised Cardiac Risk Index. Advanced age, abnormal ECG, rhythm other than sinus, low functional capacity, poorly controlled systemic hypertension, and history of stroke are the minor predictors of risk. In contrast to the traditional 3- or 6-month interval between a prior MI and the surgery, these criteria list an MI that occurred less than 1 month before surgery as a major predictor of risk, and an MI that occurred more than a month prior as an intermediate predictor.

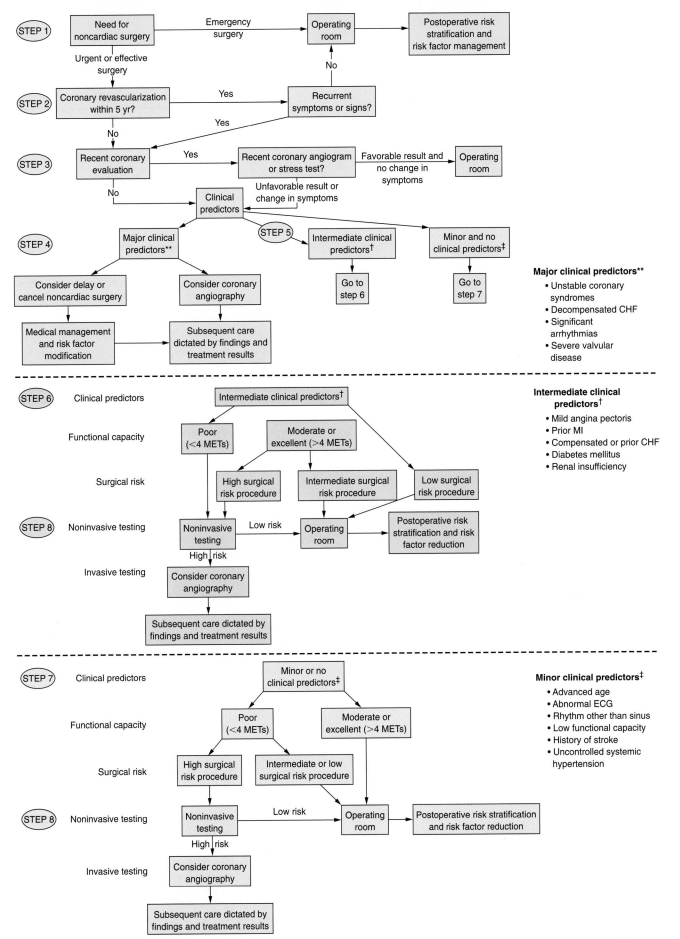

Figure 6-1 ■ Stepwise approach to preoperative cardiac assessment. METs, metabolic equivalents. (This article was published in *J Am Coll Cardiol*, 39, Eagle KA, Berger PB, Calkins H, Chaitman BR, Ewy GA, Fleischman KE, et al, ACC/AHA guideline update for perioperative cardiovascular evaluation for noncardiac surgery: a report of the American College of Cardiology/American Heart Association Task Force on Practice Guidelines (Committee to Update the 1996 Guidelines on Perioperative Cardiovascular Evaluation for Noncardiac Surgery), 542-553, Copyright Elsevier, 2002.)

6-1	**Clinical Predictors of Increased Perioperative Cardiovascular Risk***

Major

Unstable coronary syndromes
Recent myocardial infarction[†] (MI) with evidence of important ischemic risk by clinical symptoms or noninvasive study
Unstable or severe angina[‡] (Canadian class[§] III or IV)
Decompensated congestive heart failure
Significant arrhythmias
High-grade atrioventricular block
Symptomatic ventricular arrhythmias in the presence of underlying heart disease
Supraventricular arrhythmias with uncontrolled ventricular rate
Severe valvular disease

Intermediate

Mild angina pectoris (Canadian class[§] I or II)
Prior myocardial infarction by history or pathologic Q waves
Compensated or prior congestive heart failure
Diabetes mellitus

Minor

Advanced age
Abnormal ECG (left ventricular hypertrophy, left bundle branch block, ST-T abnormalities)
Rhythm other than sinus (e.g., atrial fibrillation)
Low functional capacity (e.g., inability to climb a flight of stairs with a bag of groceries)
History of stroke
Uncontrolled systemic hypertension

---

*Risk includes myocardial infarction, congestive heart failure, and death.
[†]The American College of Cardiology National Database Library defines recent MI as greater than 7 days but less than or equal to 1 month (30 days).
[‡]May include "stable" angina in patients who are unusually sedentary.
[§]See Campeau L: Grading of angina pectoris. Circulation 1976;54:522-523.
ECG, electrocardiogram.
Reprinted from Eagle KA, Brundage BH, Chaitman BR, et al: Guidelines for perioperative cardiovascular evaluation for noncardiac surgery. Report of the American College of Cardiology/American Heart Association Task Force on Practice Guidelines (Committee on Perioperative Cardiovascular Evaluation for Noncardiac Surgery). Circulation 1996; 93:1278-1317, with permission.

6-2	**Estimated Energy Requirements for Various Activities***

1 MET	Can you take care of yourself?
↓	Eat, dress, or use the toilet?
↓	Walk indoors around the house?
↓	Walk a block or two on level ground at 2 to 3 mph or 3.2 to 4.8 km/hr?
4 METs	Do light work around the house like dusting or washing dishes?
4 METs	Climb a flight of stairs or walk up a hill?
↓	Walk on level ground at 4 mph or 6.4 km/hr?
↓	Run a short distance?
↓	Do heavy work around the house like scrubbing floors or lifting or moving heavy furniture?
↓	Participate in moderate recreational activities like golf, bowling, dancing, doubles tennis, or throwing a baseball or football?
>10 METs	Participate in strenuous sports like swimming, singles tennis, football, basketball, or skiing?

MET, metabolic equivalent.
*Adapted from the Duke Activity Status Index and AHA Exercise Standards, and reprinted from Eagle KA, Brundage BH, Chaitman BR, et al: Guidelines for perioperative cardiovascular evaluation for noncardiac surgery. Report of the American College of Cardiology/American Heart Association Task Force on Practice Guidelines (Committee on Perioperative Cardiovascular Evaluation for Noncardiac Surgery). Circulation 1996;93:1278-1317, with permission,

Functional Capacity

A unit of metabolic equivalent, or MET, is defined as the number of calories consumed by a patient per minute in an activity, relative to the basal metabolic rate. Assuming 1 MET represents the metabolic demands of a human subject at rest, multiples of a patient's baseline MET value can be used to represent the aerobic demands for specific levels of activity, ranging from actions required to meet the basic needs of daily living to strenuous exercise and involvement in sports. The Duke Activity Status Index provides the clinician with a set of questions to determine a patient's functional status. As illustrated in Box 6-2, the basic activities of eating, dressing, using the toilet, walking indoors or one to two blocks outside on level ground, fall in the range of 1 to 4 METs. Climbing a flight of stairs, walking uphill, heavy housework involving lifting, and moderate recreational activities (golf, bowling, dancing) fall in the 4 to 10 MET range. Activities that require at least 10 METs include strenuous sports and exercise such as swimming, singles tennis, football, and running long distances. Patients who are unable to meet at least a 4-MET demand are known to be at increased risk of perioperative and long-term cardiac complications.[48,49]

Reilly and coworkers looked at the self-reported exercise tolerance of 600 outpatients scheduled for major noncardiac surgery, and those who were unable to walk four blocks or climb two flights of stairs were considered to have poor exercise tolerance.[48] This group of patients experienced a greater number of perioperative complications (20.4% versus 10.4%), including MI and neurologic events. Wiklund and colleagues examined the use of METs as a predictor of perioperative cardiac events after elective noncardiac surgical procedures.[50] METs for 5939 patients scheduled to undergo noncardiac surgery were calculated and compared with the incidence of cardiac events such as death, MI, acute CHF, severe hypertension, and other adverse endpoints. Age and physical status were significant predictors of adverse events ($P < .001$), but the use of METs ($P = .793$) as an index of cardiac risk was less reliable. Although estimated exercise capacity may be considered a vague estimate of perioperative risk, this quantification lends valuable information to the patient's overall health status, one that is often overlooked or downplayed in the preoperative evaluation.

Surgery-Specific Risks

Most of the focus of cardiovascular risk in surgery revolves around the patient's health, underlying cardiac disease, and other comorbid factors. Surgery-specific risk also plays a large role in overall risk assessment and is dependent on multiple factors, including the type of surgery, the degree of associated hemodynamic stress placed on the patient, and the degree of postoperative pain that the patient may experience. If two patients with a similar history of underlying cardiac disease were scheduled for two very different procedures, such as aortic aneurysm repair versus foot surgery, the wide disparity of stressors imposed on the patient can lead to very different outcomes and complications. Also, risk is associated not just with the specific procedure but also with the surgical volume at any given surgical center. Studies have demonstrated higher mortality rates of higher-risk procedures performed at medical centers with lower volumes, and with operators with lower volume. A survey of hospitals in Georgia examined the rate of stroke and death across various regional medical centers after carotid endarterectomy.[51] Hospitals that performed over 50 carotid procedures a year had less than a 3% rate of stroke or death, whereas hospitals that rarely performed the surgery saw postoperative stroke and death rates exceeding 5%. This institution-specific risk may be related to surgical, anesthesiologist, or perioperative nursing skill, and it could influence the caretaker's decision making for additional preoperative testing and intervention.

The ACC/AHA guidelines organize the wide array of surgical procedures into high-, intermediate-, and low-risk categories (with cardiac risks of >5%, 1% to 5%, and <1%, respectively) (Box 6-3). High-risk procedures include major emergency surgery, particularly in the elderly, aortic and other major vascular procedures, peripheral vascular surgery, and anticipated prolonged procedures associated with large fluid shifts or blood loss. Intermediate-risk procedures include intraperitoneal and intrathoracic surgery, carotid endarterectomy, head and neck surgery, orthopedic surgery, and prostate surgery. Bariatric surgery best fits in the intermediate-risk category along with other intra-abdominal operations.[52] Endoscopic, superficial procedures, cataract surgery, and breast surgery are found in the low-risk category. In defining the need for further evaluation at a given institution, local morbidity and mortality rates may have a greater impact than the general categories listed here.

Indications for Angiography

The ACC/AHA guidelines grouped indications for coronary angiography into class I, II, and III designations. Class I indications (meaning that angiography will be helpful) for patients with known or suspected CAD include high-risk results during noninvasive testing, angina pectoris unresponsive to medical therapy, unstable angina pectoris, and nondiagnostic or equivocal noninvasive test results in a high-risk patient scheduled for a high-risk surgery. Class II indications (angiography may be helpful) include intermediate-risk results during noninvasive testing, nondiagnostic or equivocal test results in a lower-risk patient undergoing a high-risk

6-3	Cardiac Risk* Stratification of Noncardiac Surgical Procedures

High (Reported Cardiac Risk Often >5%)

Emergent major procedures, particularly in older adults
Aortic and other major vascular procedures
Peripheral vascular procedures
Anticipated prolonged surgical procedures associated with large fluid shifts or blood loss

Intermediate (Reported Cardiac Risk Generally <5%)

Carotid endarterectomy
Head and neck procedures
Intraperitoneal and intrathoracic procedures
Orthopedic procedures
Prostate procedures

Low† (Reported Cardiac Risk Generally <1%)

Endoscopic procedures
Superficial procedure
Cataract procedure
Breast procedures

---

*Combined incidence of cardiac death and nonfatal myocardial infarction.
†Low-risk procedures do not generally require further preoperative cardiac testing.
Reprinted from Eagle KA, Brundage BH, Chaitman BR, et al: Guidelines for perioperative cardiovascular evaluation for noncardiac surgery. Report of the American College of Cardiology/American Heart Association Task Force on Practice Guidelines (Committee on Perioperative Cardiovascular Evaluation for Noncardiac Surgery). Circulation 1996; 93:1278-1317, with permission.

procedure, urgent noncardiac surgery in a patient recovering from a recent MI, and perioperative MI. Class III indications (angiography not necessary) include low-risk noncardiac surgery in patients with known CAD and low-risk results on noninvasive testing, screening for CAD without appropriate noninvasive testing, asymptomatic status after coronary revascularization with excellent exercise capacity, mild stable angina in patients with good LV function and low-risk noninvasive results, concomitant illness resulting in the patient's not being a candidate for revascularization, normal coronary angiogram within the last 5 years, and unwillingness of the patient to go through revascularization.

Figure 6-1 illustrates the stepwise process advocated by the ACC/AHA guidelines once the patient and surgical procedure have been stratified. An important distinction must be made as to whether the surgery is being performed on an urgent or an elective basis, as emergency surgery has been shown in various studies to carry a two- to fivefold increase in risk compared with an elective procedure.[7,53] Emergency procedures often do not allow the physician the opportunity to complete a more comprehensive evaluation prior to the procedure. If the noncardiac procedure is elective, then the next question to be asked is whether the patient had a coronary revascularization in the past 5 years or a coronary evaluation in the past 2 years. The presence of either in a clinically stable symptomatic or asymptomatic patient usually means that no further testing is needed at this point. If the patient does not meet these conditions, then further noninvasive testing and treatment should be considered prior to the elective surgery. The decision to proceed to noninvasive testing can be simplified if two of the three following factors are present: intermediate clinical predictors, poor functional capacity, or high-risk surgical procedure. Importantly, noninvasive testing should be performed only if the results will impact management. With the publication of the CARP trial (see later) the indications for invasive testing will most likely be further limited in the absence of overt symptoms. Rather, excellent medical therapy appears to be very protective in patients with stable CAD.

Since the publication of the original 1996 guidelines, several studies have been performed that support the notion that this stepwise approach to cardiovascular evaluation is both beneficial to the patient and cost effective.[54,55] An increased use of noninvasive stress testing followed by coronary revascularization was associated with a significant decrease in adverse perioperative cardiac events in a 4-year period after the publication of the guidelines, compared with a control period in the 4 years prior to the guidelines release.

When the ACC/AHA guidelines were updated in 2002, several additions were made to the 1996 recommendations. Perioperative beta-blocker therapy was recommended for patients in the following categories: (1) those who are currently on therapy to control angina, symptomatic arrhythmias, and hypertension, and (2) patients who are undergoing vascular surgery and are at high cardiac risk from ischemia on preoperative testing. Beta-blockers were suggested for patients with untreated hypertension (class IIa recommendations), known CAD, or those who have major risk factors for CAD. In 2006, a focused update on perioperative beta-blockade reinforced these recommendations (see www.acc.org). Although this has been adopted as standard practice, the evidence for the standardized use of perioperative beta-blockers for a more diverse group of patients undergoing noncardiac surgery has been less than compelling (see Chapter 10). With new evidence, the existing recommendations for coronary angiography were expanded, urging more judicious use of invasive testing.[56] An emphasis was put on the importance of maintaining normothermia during noncardiac surgery, and this was supported by studies that demonstrated a reduced incidence of perioperative cardiac events compared with routine care without temperature regulation.[57]

THE ROLE OF SEX IN THE ASSESSMENT OF PERIOPERATIVE CARDIAC RISK

In the assessment of a patient's perioperative cardiovascular risk status, the clinician must realize that the significance and relative weight of risk factors may be modified by sex. The data used in the publication of the 1996 ACC/AHA guidelines were derived from studies that grossly underrepresented female populations.[58] Lerner and associates performed a review of the Framingham Heart Study data that showed although men and women share many cardiovascular risk

factors, the relative significances of these factors were not necessarily identical.[59] CAD in women appeared to be more age dependent than in men, and for any given set of major, intermediate, or minor risk factors, women had a lower probability of having existing epicardial CAD. Women were found to be more prone to silent, uncomplicated, and unrecognized MI, making chest pain a less reliable indicator of CAD in this population. This alters the significance of unstable angina as a major clinical predictor, and of stable angina as an intermediate clinical predictor, as stated by the ACC/AHA guidelines.

Nonatherosclerotic causes of chest pain, including mitral valve prolapse and coronary artery spasm, were found to be more prevalent in women than in men. Large differences between the sexes were also seen in angiographic studies between men and women who were referred for chest pain. Women who presented with acute chest pain syndromes were more likely to have a negative angiogram than their male counterparts.[60] A retrospective study by Shackleford and associates[61] looked at perioperative cardiac morbidity in 206 patients receiving elective gynecologic surgery. The most useful predictors of cardiac adverse events in the postmenopausal subgroup were hypertension and a history of known CAD. This and other supporting studies may suggest that the presence of hypertensive disease plays a larger role in the development of perioperative cardiac events in women, as does "small-vessel" CAD, which is less readily apparent on coronary angiography.

NONINVASIVE TESTING FOR CARDIOVASCULAR DISEASE

Multiple modalities of noninvasive cardiac testing are available for the clinician performing a preoperative cardiovascular evaluation of a patient about to undergo noncardiac surgery. Tests can study cardiac function under resting conditions or settings of increased stress and oxygen demand. Various stress tests can be conducted with patient participation (exercise) or through passive pharmacologic-induced studies. As emphasized earlier, patients who report a high capacity for exercise tolerance in their daily activities usually gain little from additional testing. Some patients who would qualify for exercise testing lack the capacity to meet goal heart rates to produce valid test results and therefore may require further nonexercise stress imaging studies to help rule out MI.

Resting Echocardiography

Traditionally, measurements of the LVEF were thought to help identify patients at increased risk of postoperative cardiac complications. Multiple retrospective and prospective studies looked at the correlation between preoperative LV systolic function and the risk of postoperative cardiac morbidity and mortality.[62-65] The shared conclusion of these studies was that the greatest incidence of postoperative cardiac complications occurred in patients with an LVEF of less than 35%, linking poor ejection fraction to a higher incidence of postoperative ischemia, CHF, and death. Despite these data, a resting echocardiogram has never been unequivocally demonstrated to be a reliable predictor of perioperative ischemic events.[66,67]

Halm and associates released a study in 1996 that looked at 474 patients from the Veterans Affairs medical system with known high risk or presence of coronary disease who were scheduled to undergo elective noncardiac surgery.[66] Of the original 474 patients enrolled, 339 had transthoracic echocardiograms performed prior to surgery. Information about resting ejection fraction and wall motion did not identify those at high risk for adverse cardiac events such as sudden death, MI, or unstable angina. However, the study was underpowered to identify modest differences. Although the routine assessment of LV function as a part of preoperative screening is not advocated in all patients, an echocardiogram may provide useful information in patients with known or suspected LV dysfunction, as well as in those with existing comorbidities such as valvular disease and hypertrophic cardiomyopathy. Once the diagnosis and severity of these disorders is established by a resting echocardiographic study, the ACC/AHA guidelines recommend optimization by medical management of these various conditions prior to undertaking any elective noncardiac surgical procedure.[7]

Exercise Stress Testing

In ambulatory patients, treadmill or bicycle exercise stress testing is usually preferred over pharmacologic stress testing, as it gives the clinician an idea of myocardial capacity as well as a global picture of exercise tolerance. Many limitations may be encountered when attempting to administer exercise testing to patients at a high risk for perioperative events. Because of effort limitations or pharmacologic alterations from beta-blocker and calcium-channel blocker therapy, about half of the patients fail to achieve the age-predicted target heart rates necessary to rule out myocardial ischemia. Some patients are unable to exercise because of the primary disease that the noncardiac surgical procedure seeks to address, such as claudication in patients with vascular problems and severe degenerative joint disease in the orthopedic population. If an exercise stress test is performed, obtaining the details of the examination is critical. Peak heart rate, systolic blood pressure, number of METs achieved, predicted target heart rate, and presence of ECG changes or symptoms provide a better clinical picture to the caretaking physician than a simple "normal" or "abnormal." If ischemia is identified, noting the heart rate, blood pressure, and rate-pressure product at which it occurred may be useful for intraoperative and postoperative management.

Myocardial Perfusion Imaging

For patients who will gain more prognostic information from a nonexercise mode of testing, the choice between pharmacologic testing that can induce a hyperemic response (dipyridamole or adenosine) and testing that increases oxygen demand (dobutamine) should be based on factors specific to the patient as well as on the expertise in the clinician's institution.

Nuclear imaging tests using thallium or sestamibi look at changes in myocardial perfusion effected by pharmacologic vasodilatory agents such as dipyridamole or adenosine.

Coronary blood flow is increased in normal coronary circulation, but it is unchanged in occluded or severely stenotic vessels. Myocardial perfusion defects seen in the stress phase that subsequently improve on the resting/redistribution phase indicate stress-induced myocardial ischemia occurring in myocardial regions perfused by narrowed coronary arteries. Fixed defects that do not change after redistribution more likely represent myocardial scar from a prior infarction; they have less predictive value for a future perioperative ischemic event but indicate higher risk than do normal scan findings. The idea that cardiac risk increases with increasing size and number of reperfusion defects has been supported by multiple studies.[66,68] A system to quantify the degree of ischemic disease has been suggested to help improve the quality of risk assessment. Some groups of investigators have shown that scintigraphic results indicating low and high risk, particularly in the presence of increased lung uptake, may lead to an improved predictive value of perioperative events.[69,70]

Dobutamine Stress Echocardiography

The basis of stress echocardiography is a dynamic, real-time assessment of myocardial function in response to an exercise-induced or pharmacologically induced increase in inotropy and heart rate. The induction of wall motion defects under conditions of increased oxygen demand is believed to be an excellent predictor of increased short- and long-term cardiac risk.[71] Boersma and associates studied 1351 patients scheduled for major vascular surgery and found that those with a moderate number of defined cardiac risk markers benefited from the additional prognostic information provided by dobutamine stress echocardiography (DSE).[71] The presence of five or more segments (out of 16) denotes patients at greatest risk for perioperative cardiac complications. As a result of these data and other reports, the stress echocardiogram is a widely used preoperative test. It is generally contraindicated in patients with significant arrhythmias, marked hypertension or hypotension, and severe aortic stenotic disease. Beyond these cohorts, DSE provides an excellent alternative for patients who are unable to undergo exercise stress testing. Landesberg and colleagues followed the long-term survival rates of 502 patients undergoing 578 major vascular procedures retrospectively. Patients who demonstrated moderate to severe ischemia on preoperative thallium scanning had improved long-term survival after major vascular surgery if the surgery was preceded by coronary revascularization.[72] A meta-analysis conducted by Beattie and associates compared the abilities of stress echocardiography versus thallium imaging in predicting the risk of perioperative myocardial infarction in patients undergoing major noncardiac surgery and concluded that stress echocardiography had superior predictive capability for postoperative adverse cardiac events.[73]

■ PREOPERATIVE CORONARY REVASCULARIZATION

The need to further define cardiovascular risk through the use of noninvasive testing depends in part on the potential benefit of coronary revascularization as a means of reducing perioperative risk. Many clinicians agree, however, that coronary revascularization, whether it is coronary artery bypass grafting or percutaneous coronary intervention, should not be performed simply to help get a patient through the stress of a noncardiac surgical procedure.

Coronary Artery Bypass Grafting

Until recently, evidence-based decision making on this issue was hampered by the scarcity of randomized controlled trials studying the benefits of preoperative interventions in high-risk patients undergoing different types of noncardiac surgery. Retrospective data hinted at a possible benefit of revascularization in patients undergoing vascular surgery, including improvement in long-term outcomes.[74-76] One study showed some benefits in patients receiving preoperative CABG compared with those with equally severe, uncorrected disease (1.5% versus 3% to 14%); however, when coupled with the operative mortality from CABG alone, no short-term benefit was gained. The Coronary Artery Surgery Study (CASS) registry was a large database that enrolled patients from 1978 to 1981. It provided some of the strongest nonrandomized study evidence for the possible benefit of preoperative CABG in patients scheduled for elective vascular surgery. Initial studies of this patient database suggested a significant reduction of perioperative cardiac death, but there was no change in number of MIs between the patients who underwent preoperative CABG and those in the nonrevascularized group.[76] Another review of the CASS database revealed a lower rate of both death and perioperative MI in revascularized patients undergoing higher-risk noncardiac procedures, such as major vascular surgery.

Patients who received lower-risk noncardiac procedures (skin, breast, urologic, minor orthopedic procedures) did not appear to benefit from preoperative CABG, given the already low rates of perioperative cardiac adverse events. A protective benefit does exist for patients with a previous CABG who now are scheduled for noncardiac surgery. Assuming that the patient remains medically stable after revascularization, this protective effect is optimal over the first 4 to 6 years after CABG and then diminishes beyond this point.

Percutaneous Coronary Intervention

As is the case for preoperative CABG, there is not an abundance of randomized prospective data studying the benefit of PCI in high-risk patients prior to noncardiac surgery. Review of various studies with 50 patients or more undergoing noncardiac surgery after percutaneous transluminal coronary angioplasty (PTCA) demonstrated rates of perioperative mortality and MI that were not significantly better than rates in controls.[7] Another study showed a lower 30-day rate of cardiac complications in patients who received their PCI at least 90 days prior to noncardiac surgery, but this benefit was lost if the intervention was done within 90 days, suggesting that a prophylactic angioplasty does not necessarily improve postoperative outcome.[77] The ACC recommendation of a 1-week wait after balloon angioplasty to allow for healing of vessel injury illustrates that PCI is not a benign procedure and carries its own risks and morbidity.

The placement of coronary stents carries an even higher risk of postprocedure complications when combined with noncardiac surgery. One study observed that 40 patients who received PCI and stents placed less than 6 weeks before an elective noncardiac surgery had high rates of perioperative mortality, MI, and bleeding.[78] The majority of patients with catastrophic outcomes had had stents placed less than 14 days prior to surgery. Death was chiefly attributed to stent thrombosis in the first 2 weeks after placement. The authors recommended a minimum wait of 2 weeks, preferably 4 weeks, after stent placement before proceeding with a noncardiac procedure. A later study by Wilson and associates reexamined this question and suggested that surgery should be delayed at least 6 weeks after stent placement, providing optimal time for coronary endothelial healing and the discontinuation of required antiplatelet agents.[79] Vincenzi and colleagues studied 103 patients from three institutions who had coronary stent placement within 1 year of noncardiac surgery.[80] Given the high risk of death associated with surgery performed within 6 weeks of coronary stenting, the safety of balloon angioplasty alone was revisited in a study by Brilakis and associates, who collected data on the adverse events of 350 patients who underwent noncardiac surgery within 2 months of angioplasty without stenting.[81] Once again, balloon angioplasty was shown to be a relatively safe form of intervention in patients who required surgery in as little as 2 weeks after PCI. A new innovation in PCI and stenting involved the introduction of drug-eluting coronary stents designed to further minimize the rate of in-stent restenosis after intervention. Costa and coworkers conducted a study of 42 patients with known coronary lesions, comparing the efficacy of everolimus-eluting stents versus non–drug-impregnated stents in the prevention of restenosis at 1 and 6 months after PCI.[82] Although the sample size was small, the drug-eluting stents were found to be safe and effective in the treatment of coronary lesions and in reducing intimal proliferation, compared with plain metal stents.

Coronary Artery Bypass Grafting versus Percutaneous Coronary Intervention

Conventional practice guidelines use the number of coronary occlusions or the anatomic location of the lesions to determine which type of revascularization is needed. CABG has been traditionally indicated when there are three or more correctable occlusions and/or left main coronary artery disease. If these criteria are not met, then PCI intervention is often the method of choice, if it is technically feasible. Sometimes, a patient with known uncorrected multivessel coronary disease is scheduled for surgery. For such a case, the relative benefits of PCI and CABG were not studied until 2001, when the Bypass Angioplasty Revascularization Investigation (BARI) was conducted.[83] Patients had previously received either PCI or CABG and the two groups had similar rates of perioperative MI and cardiac death (1.6%), with maximal benefit gained if revascularization was done within 4 years of noncardiac surgery.

Coronary Artery Revascularization Prophylaxis Trial

In late 2004, the results of the Coronary Artery Revascularization Prophylaxis (CARP) trial were released.[47] The CARP trial is currently the only randomized study of the benefit of coronary revascularization before elective major vascular surgery. This population of patients was chosen for the study on the basis of prior literature illustrating rates of CAD as high as 50%,[74] and on the basis of the high incidence of perioperative cardiac events.[29] Of the 5859 patients scheduled for vascular surgery across 18 different Veterans Affairs medical centers, 510 were enrolled in this study and randomly assigned to either medical therapy and coronary revascularization before surgery or medical therapy and no revascularization. The indications for vascular surgery in this group of 500 patients included peripheral vascular disease (67%) and abdominal aortic aneurysm (33%). Not only were patients required to be scheduled for these specific procedures to be eligible for the study, but they also needed the results of a coronary angiogram showing one or more major coronary arteries with a 70% or greater stenosis amenable to revascularization. Clinical exclusion criteria for these patients included a need for urgent or emergency surgery, severe coexisting illness, and prior known revascularization without evidence of recurrent ischemia. Anatomic exclusion criteria

from the study included the presence of left main coronary stenosis greater than 50%, an LV ejection fraction of less than 20%, and severe aortic stenosis. About 80% of the enrolled patients were initially excluded from this study on the basis of these criteria.

Results at 30 days after vascular surgery showed no significant difference in occurrence of postoperative MI (12% in the intervention group versus 14% in the nonintervention group), and mortality rates were nearly identical 2.7 years out from the initial randomization (Table 6-3). The authors concluded that a strategy of coronary artery revascularization before major cardiac surgery in stable cardiac patients being treated medically is not recommended. This conclusion was based on the lack of improvement in short- or long-term postoperative outcomes such as MI, death, or length of hospital stay. Perioperative medical therapy was maximized in these patients, leading to a conclusion that careful assessment of the patient's health status and appropriate treatment with beta-blockers and statins must be addressed

6-3 Outcomes of Elective Major Vascular Surgeries with and without Revascularization Pretreatment

Characteristic	Revascularization (N = 225)	No Revascularization (N = 237)	P Value
Surgical Management			
Abdominal surgery [no. (%)]*	89 (39.9)	99 (42.1)	.89
Urgent or emergency status [no. (%)]	13 (5.8)	14 (5.9)	.90
General anesthesia [no. (%)]	180 (80.0)	199 (84.0)	.50
Altered surgical procedure [no. (%)]	33 (14.7)	27 (11.4)	.30
Days after randomization	—	—	<.001
Median	54	18	—
Interquartile range	28-80	7-42	—
Perioperative Medications [no. (%)]			
Beta-adrenergic blockers	188 (83.6)	204 (86.1)	.45
Aspirin[†]	168 (76.7)	165 (70.2)	.12
Statin[‡]	121 (53.8)	122 (54.0)	.93
Heparin[§]	209 (93.7)	219 (93.2)	.82
Intravenous nitroglycerin	63 (28.0)	87 (36.7)	.05
Postoperative Events (within 30 days)			
Death [no. (%)]	7 (3.1)	8 (3.4)	.87
Myocardial infarction[¶]			
Enzymes [no. (%)]	26 (11.6)	34 (14.3)	.37
Enzymes and ECG [no. (%)]	19 (8.4)	20 (8.4)	.99
Stroke [no. (%)]	1 (0.4)	2 (0.8)	.59
Loss of leg [no. (%)]	1 (0.4)	5 (2.1)	.11
Renal dialysis [no. (%)]	1 (0.4)	1 (0.4)	.97
Reoperation [no. (%)]	17 (7.6)	18 (7.6)	.99
Total days in the intensive care unit	—	—	.25
Median	2.0	2.0	—
Interquartile range	1-3	1-4	—
Total days in the hospital	—	—	.29
Median	6.5	7.0	—
Interquartile range	4-10	5-12	—

*No information was available for two patients in each group.
†An altered surgical procedure is a surgical procedure (abdominal or infrainguinal) that differed from the procedure that was planned before randomization.
‡No information was available for six patients in the revascularization group and two in the no-revascularization group.
§No information was available for 11 patients in the no-revascularization group.
¶Myocardial infarction was defined by any elevation in cardiac enzymes after surgery, as well as by any elevation in cardiac enzymes with ischemic changes on the electrocardiogram (ECG).

Reprinted from McFalls EO, Ward HB, Moritz TE, et al: Coronary-artery revascularization before elective major vascular surgery. N Engl J M 2004;351:2795-2804.

before proceeding with a high-risk vascular procedure. Landesberg and colleagues pointed out that the criteria for selection of CARP study patients did not match those of the ACC/AHA guidelines concerning selection of patients for revascularization after demonstration of moderate-to-severe inducible ischemia by noninvasive stress testing.[84] Only 44.3% of the 510 patients studied had moderate to large defects on myocardial perfusion studies, and only 33.3% of patients had triple-vessel disease. With a significant portion of the study group demonstrating only low to moderate risk for adverse coronary events, the question of the benefit of preoperative coronary revascularization in the moderate- to high-risk groups still remains in question. Importantly, patients with left main coronary artery stenosis, severe aortic stenosis, and severe left ventricular function were excluded. Thus, the CARP trial was not a study of a screening strategy but rather of treatment in a very well-defined cohort. Nevertheless, the results of this study help illustrate the consensus opinion that preoperative revascularization should be reserved for those patients who demonstrate unstable cardiac symptoms, or for stable coronary patients when a known survival benefit from such interventions has been demonstrated.

■ SUMMARY

Successful preoperative evaluation of high-risk cardiac patients who are about to undergo noncardiac surgery requires an organized and logical approach. This requires careful attention and clear communication between the physicians involved in the patient's perioperative care, including the primary care physician, anesthesiologist, consultants, and surgeon. A focused algorithm should be based on the growing body of evidence that better defines the indications and benefits of specific modes of perioperative testing and treatment on specific subsets of patients. A single style of preoperative cardiovascular testing and risk assessment can no longer be applied to all patients scheduled for major surgery. It is increasingly evident that the potential benefits of cardiac ischemic stress testing and revascularization are applicable to a shrinking subset of symptomatic patients; this knowledge helps eliminate an unnecessary workup while generating an accurate and useful cardiac risk profile for any individual who may undergo noncardiac surgery. Combined with selective testing, intervention with optimal medical therapy may provide an ideal model of evaluation for the reduction not only of cardiac risk but also of other forms of perioperative morbidity and mortality.

■ REFERENCES

1. Kertai MD, Boersma E, Klein J, et al: Optimizing the prediction of perioperative mortality in vascular surgery by using a customized probability model. Arch Intern Med 2005;165:898-904.
2. Eagle KA, Rihal CS, Mickel MC, et al: Cardiac risk of noncardiac surgery: Influence of coronary disease and type of surgery in 3368 operations. CASS Investigators and University of Michigan Heart Care Program. Coronary Artery Surgery Study. Circulation 1996; 96:1882-1887.
3. Mangano DT, Layug EL, Wallace A, et al: Effect of atenolol on mortality and cardiovascular morbidity after noncardiac surgery: Multicenter Study of Perioperative Ischemia Research Group. N Engl J Med 1996;335:1713-1720.
4. Fleisher LA, Eagle KA: Clinical practice. Lowering cardiac risk in noncardiac surgery. N Engl J Med 2001;345:1677-1682.
5. Hollenberg M, Mangano DT, Browner WS, et al: Predictors of postoperative myocardial ischemia in patients undergoing noncardiac surgery. The Study of Perioperative Ischemia Research Group. JAMA 1992;268:205-209.
6. Weksler M, Klein M, Szendro G, et al: The dilemma of immediate preoperative hypertension: To treat and operate, or to postpone surgery? J Clin Anesth 2003;15:179-183.
7. Eagle KA, Brundage BH, Chaitman BR, et al: Guidelines for perioperative cardiovascular evaluation for noncardiac surgery. Report of the American College of Cardiology/American Heart Association Task Force on Practice Guidelines (Committee on Perioperative Cardiovascular Evaluation for Noncardiac Surgery). Circulation 1996;93: 1278-1317.
8. Mangano DT: Perioperative cardiac morbidity. Anesthesiology 1990; 72:153-184.
9. Poldermans D, Boersma E, Bax JJ, et al: Correlation of location of acute myocardial infarct after noncardiac vascular surgery with preoperative dobutamine echocardiographic findings. Am J Cardiol 2001;88: 1413-1414.
10. Hellstrom HR: Evidence in favor of the vasospastic cause of coronary artery thrombosis. Am Heart J 1979;97:449-452.
11. Kalsner S, Richards R: Coronary arteries of cardiac patients are hyperactive and contain stores of amines: A mechanism for coronary spasm. Science 1984;223:1435-1437.
12. Dawood MM, Gutpa DK, Southern J, et al: Pathology of fatal perioperative myocardial infarction: Implications regarding pathophysiology and prevention. Int J Cardiol 1996;57:37-44.
13. The fifth report of the Joint National Committee on Detection, Evaluation, and Treatment of High Blood Pressure (JNC V). Arch Intern Med 1993;153:154-183.
14. Castelli WP, Anderson K, Wilson PW, et al: Lipids and risk of coronary heart disease. Framingham Study. Ann Epidemiol 1992;2:23-28.
15. Assmann G, Schulte H, von Eckardstein A: Hypertriglyceridemia and elevated lipoprotein(a) are risk factors for major coronary events in meddle-aged men. Am J Cardiol 1996;77:1179-1184.
16. Centers for Disease Control: Reducing the Health Consequences of Smoking: 25 Years of Progress: A Report of the Surgeon General. Rockville, Md, US Dept Health and Human Services, Public Health Service. CDC publication 89-8411, 1989.
17. Willett WC, Green A, Stampfer MJ, et al: Relative and absolute excess risks of coronary heart disease among women who smoke cigarettes. N Engl J Med 1987;317:1303-1309.
18. Kannel WB, McGee DL: Diabetes and cardiovascular disease. The Framingham Study. JAMA 1979;241:2035-2038.
19. Haffner SM, Lehto S, Ronnemaa T, et al: Mortality from coronary heart disease in subjects with type 2 diabetes and in nondiabetic subjects with and without prior myocardial infarction. N Engl J Med 1998;339: 229-234.
20. English JP, Willius FA, Berkson J: Tobacco and coronary disease. JAMA 1940;115:1327-1329.
21. Marenberg ME, Risch N, Berkman LF, et al: Genetic susceptibility to death from coronary heart disease in a study of twins. N Engl J Med 1994;330:1041-1046.
22. Lloyd-Jones DM, Nam BH, D'Agostino RB, et al: Parental cardiovascular disease as a risk factor for cardiovascular disease in middle-aged adults: A prospective study of parents and offspring. JAMA 2004;291: 2204-2211.
23. Prevention of cardiovascular events and death with pravastatin in patients with coronary heart disease and a broad range of initial cholesterol levels. The Long-term Intervention with Pravastatin in Ischaemic Disease (LIPID) Study Group. N Engl J Med 1998;339: 1349-1357.
24. EUROASPIRE. A European Society of Cardiology survey of secondary prevention of coronary heart disease: Principal results. EUROASPIRE Study Group. European Action of Secondary Prevention through Intervention to Reduce Events. Eur Heart J 1997;18:1569-1582.
25. Yusuf S, Hawken S, Ounpuu S, et al: Effect of potentially modifiable risk factors associated with myocardial infarction in 52 countries

(the INTERHEART study): Case controlled study. Lancet 2004;364: 937-952.

26. Cohn SL, Goldman L: Preoperative risk evaluation and perioperative management of patients with coronary artery disease. Med Clin North Am 2003;87:111-136.

27. Goldman L, Caldera DL, Nussbaum SR, et al: Multifactorial index of cardiac risk in noncardiac surgical procedures. N Engl J Med 1977;297:845-850.

28. Tarhan S, Moffitt EA, Taylor WF, et al: Myocardial infarction after general anesthesia. JAMA 1972;220:1451-1454.

29. Detsky AS, Abrams HB, McLaughlin JR, et al: Predicting cardiac complications in patients undergoing non-cardiac surgery. Ann Intern Med 1989;110:859-866.

30. Haering JM, Comunale ME, Parker RA, et al: Cardiac risk of noncardiac surgery in patients with asymmetric septal hypertrophy. Anesthesiology 1996;85:254-259.

31. Torsher LC, Shub C, Rettke SR, et al: Risk of patients with severe aortic stenosis undergoing noncardiac surgery. Am J Cardiol 1998;81: 448-452.

32. Otto C, Mickel M, Kennedy J, et al: Three-year outcome after balloon aortic valvuloplasty: Insights into prognosis of valvular aortic stenosis. Circulation 1994;89:642-650.

33. Reyes VP, Raju BS, Wynne J, et al: Percutaneous balloon valvuloplasty compared with open surgical commissurotomy for mitral stenosis. N Engl J Med 1994;331:961-967.

34. Dajani AS, Bisno AL, Chung KJ, et al: Prevention of bacterial endocarditis: Recommendations by the American Heart Association. JAMA 1990;264:2919-2922.

35. Goldman L, Caldera DL, Southwick FS, et al: Cardiac risk factors and complications in non-cardiac surgery. Medicine 1978;57:357-370.

36. Amar D: Perioperative atrial tachyarrhythmias. Anesthesiology 2002;97:1618-1623.

37. O'Kelly B, Browner WS, Massie B, et al: Ventricular arrhythmias in patients undergoing noncardiac surgery. The Study of Perioperative Ischemia Research Group. JAMA 1992;268:217-221.

38. Dripps RD, Lamont A, Eckenhoff JE: The role of anesthesia in surgical mortality. JAMA 1961;178:261-266.

39. Jeffrey CC, Kunsman J, Cullen DJ, et al: A prospective evaluation of cardiac risk index. Anesthesiology 1983;58:462-464.

40. Detsky AS, Abrams HB, McLaughlin JR, et al: Predicting cardiac complications in patients undergoing non-cardiac surgery. J Gen Intern Med 1986;1:211-219.

41. Lee TH, Marcantonio ER, Mangione CM, et al: Derivation and prospective validation of a simple index for prediction of cardiac risk of major noncardiac surgery. Circulation 1999;100:1043-1049.

42. Kumar R, McKinney WP, Raj G, et al: Adverse cardiac events after surgery: Assessing risk in a veteran population. J Gen Intern Med 2001;16:507-518.

43. Eagle KA, Coley CM, Newell JB, et al: Combining clinical and thallium data optimizes preoperative assessment of cardiac risk before major vascular surgery. Ann Intern Med 1989;110:859-866.

44. Vanzetto G, Machecourt J, Blendea D, et al: Additive value of thallium single-photon emission computed tomography myocardial imaging for prediction of perioperative events in clinically selected high cardiac risk patients having abdominal aortic surgery. Ann Intern Med 1989;110:859-866.

45. L'Italien GJ, Paul SD, Hendel RC, et al: Development and validation of a Bayesian model for perioperative cardiac risk assessment in a cohort of 1,081 vascular surgical candidates. J Am Coll Cardiol 1996;27: 779-786.

46. Eagle KA, Berger PB, Calkins H, et al: ACC/AHA guideline update for perioperative cardiovascular evaluation for noncardiac surgery: Executive summary. J Am Coll Cardiol 2002;39:542-553.

47. McFalls EO, Ward HB, Moritz TE, et al: Coronary-artery revascularization before elective major vascular surgery. N Engl J Med 2004;351:2795-2804.

48. Reilly DF, McNeely MJ, Doerner D, et al: Self-reported exercise tolerance and the risk of serious perioperative complications. Arch Intern Med 1999;159:2185-2192.

49. Older P, Hall A, Hader R: Cardiopulmonary exercise testing as a screening test for perioperative management of major surgery in the elderly. Chest 1999;116:355-362.

50. Wiklund RA, Stein HD, Rosenbaum SH: Activities of daily living and cardiovascular complications following elective, noncardiac surgery. Yale J Biol Med 2001;74:75-87.

51. Karp HR, Flanders WD, Shipp CC, et al: Carotid endarterectomy among Medicare beneficiaries: A statewide evaluation of appropriateness and outcome. Stroke 1998;29:46-52.

52. Buchwald H, Avidor Y, Braunwald E, et al: Bariatric surgery: A systematic review and meta-analysis. JAMA 2004;292:1724-1737.

53. Mangano DT, Goldman L: Preoperative assessment of patients with known or suspected coronary disease. N Engl J Med 1995;333: 1750-1756.

54. Bartels C, Bechtel J, Hossmann V, et al: Cardiac risk stratification for high-risk vascular surgery. Circulation 1997;95:2473-2475.

55. Froehlich JB, Karavite D, Russman PL, et al: American College of Cardiology/American Heart Association preoperative assessment guidelines reduce resource utilization before aortic surgery. J Vasc Surg 2002;36:758-763.

56. Kaluza GL, Joseph J, Lee JR, et al: Catastrophic outcomes of noncardiac surgery soon after coronary stenting. J Am College Cardiol 2000;35:1288-1294.

57. Frank SM, Fleisher LA, Breslow MJ, et al: Perioperative maintenance of normothermia reduces the incidence of morbid cardiac events: A randomized clinical trial. JAMA 1997;227:1127-1134.

58. Liu LL, Wiener-Kronish JP: Preoperative cardiac evaluation of women for noncardiac surgery. Cardiol Clin 1998;16:59-66.

59. Lerner DJ, Kannel WB: Patterns of coronary heart disease morbidity and mortality in the sexes: A 26-year follow-up of the Framingham population. Am Heart J 1986;111:383-390.

60. Welch CC, Proudfit WL, Sheldon WC: Coronary arteriographic findings in 1,000 women under age 50. Am J Cardiol 1975;35:211-215.

61. Shackleford DP, Hoffman MK, Kramer PR Jr, et al: Evaluation of preoperative cardiac risk index values in patients undergoing vaginal surgery. Am J Obstet Gynecol 1995;173:80-84.

62. Pasternack PF, Imparato AM, Riles TS, et al: The value of the radionuclide angiogram in the prediction of perioperative myocardial infarction in patients undergoing lower extremity revascularization procedures. Circulation 1985;72:3-7.

63. Fletcher JP, Antico VF, Gruenewald S, et al: Risk of aortic aneurysm surgery as assessed by preoperative gated heart pool scan. Br J Surg 1989;76:26-28.

64. Pedersen T, Kelbaek H, Munck O: Cardiopulmonary complications in high-risk surgical patients: The value of preoperative radionuclide cardiography. Acta Anaesthesiol Scand 1990;34:183-189.

65. Lazor L, Russell JC, DaSilva J, et al: Use of the multiple uptake gated acquisition scan for the preoperative assessment of cardiac risk. Surg Gynecol Obstet 1988;167:234-238.

66. Halm EA, Browner WS, Tubau JF, et al: Echocardiography for assessing cardiac risk in patients having noncardiac surgery. Study of Perioperative Ischemia Research Group. Ann Intern Med 1996;125: 433-441.

67. Brown KA, Rowen M: Extent of jeopardized viable myocardium determined by myocardial perfusion imaging best predicts perioperative cardiac events in patients undergoing noncardiac surgery. J Am Coll Cardiol 1993;21:325-330.

68. Hendel RC, Whitfield SS, Villegas BJ, et al: Prediction of late cardiac events by dipyridamole thallium imaging in patients undergoing elective vascular surgery. Am J Cardiol 1992;70:1243-1249.

69. Fleisher LA, Rosenbaum SH, Nelson AH, et al: Preoperative dipyridamole thallium imaging and Holter monitoring as a predictor of perioperative cardiac events and long term outcome. Anesthesiology 1995;83:906-917.

70. Poldermans D, Arnese M, Fioretti PM, et al: Improved cardiac risk stratification in major vascular surgery with dobutamine-atropine stress echocardiography. J Am Coll Cardiol 1995;26:648-653.

71. Boersma E, Poldermans D, Bax JJ, et al: Predictors of cardiac events after major vascular surgery: Role of clinical characteristics, dobutamine echocardiography, and beta-blocker therapy. JAMA 2001;285: 1865-1873.

72. Landesberg G, Mosseri M, Wolf YG, et al: Preoperative thallium scanning, selective coronary revascularization, and long-term survival after major vascular surgery. Circulation 2003;108:177-183.

73. Beattie WS, Abdelnaem E, Wijeysundera DN, et al: A meta-analytic comparison of preoperative stress echocardiography and nuclear scintigraphy imaging. Anesth Analg 2006;102:8-16.

74. Hertzer NR, Beven EG, Young EG, et al: Coronary artery disease in peripheral vascular patients: A classification of 1000 coronary angiograms and results of surgical management. Ann Surg 1984;199: 223-233.

75. Hertzer NR, Young JR, Beven EG, et al: Late results of coronary bypass in patients with peripheral vascular disease: II. Five year survival according to sex, hypertension and diabetes. Cleve Clin J Med 1987;54:15-23.

76. Foster ED, Davis KB, Carpenter JA, et al: Risk of noncardiac operation in patients with defined coronary disease: The Coronary Artery Surgery Study (CASS) registry experience. Ann Thorac Surg 1986;41:42-50.

77. Posner KL, Van Norman GA, Chan V: Adverse cardiac outcomes after noncardiac surgery in patients with prior percutaneous transluminal coronary angioplasty. Anesth Analg 1999;89:553-560.

78. Kaluza GL, Joseph J, Lee JR, et al: Catastrophic outcomes of noncardiac surgery soon after coronary stenting. J Am College Cardiol 2000;35:1288-1294.

79. Wilson SH, Fasseas P, Orford JL, et al: Clinical outcome of patients undergoing noncardiac surgery after coronary stenting. J Am Coll Cardiol 2003;42:234-240.

80. Vincenzi MN, Meislitzer T, Heitzinger B, et al: Coronary artery stenting and non-cardiac surgery: A prospective outcome study. Br J Anaesth 2006;96:686-693.

81. Brilakis ES, Orford JL, Fasseas P, et al: Outcome of patients undergoing balloon angioplasty in the two months prior to noncardiac surgery. Am J Cardiol 2005;96:512-514.

82. Costa RA, Lansky AJ, Mintz GS, et al: Angiographic results of the first human experience with everolimus-eluting stents for the treatment of coronary lesion (the FUTURE I trial). Am J Cardiol 2005; 95:113-116.

83. Hassan SA, Hlatky MA, Boothroyd DB, et al: Outcomes of noncardiac surgery after coronary bypass surgery or coronary angioplasty in the Bypass Angioplasty Revascularization Investigation (BARI). Am J Med 2001;110:260-266.

84. Landesberg G, Mosseri M, Fleisher L: Coronary revascularization before vascular surgery. N Engl J Med 2005;352:1492-1493.

Chapter

7 | Cardiovascular Risk Assessment in Cardiac Surgery

Robert G. Johnson

Chapter 6 examined cardiac risk assessment in patients undergoing noncardiac surgery. The assessment of cardiovascular risk in patients considered for cardiac operations differs, however, because cardiac disease has already been demonstrated in this population. Indeed, some of these patients are evaluated for cardiac surgery because their risk assessment prior to noncardiac surgery showed that they have potentially treatable cardiac disease.

■ THE VALUE OF RISK ASSESSMENT BEFORE CARDIAC SURGERY

Preoperative risk assessment has four overlapping uses: (1) it provides an estimate of an individual patient's risk-to-benefit ratio; (2) it suggests the potential for modifying an individual's operative risk by altering the timing of the surgery or by using some other intervention before an index surgery; (3) it has been used increasingly in the past decade to assess the quality of individual providers and of care systems, by accounting for patient-specific factors and random variations that contribute to postoperative outcome[1,2]; and (4) its techniques provide a foundation for research and lead to improved care delivery and treatment options. Simply sharing risk-adjusted data with providers is associated with improvement in patient outcome, mortality, and morbidity, within a care system.[3-5] Optimal use of risk-assessment techniques and data prior to cardiac surgery requires an understanding of their inherent strengths and weaknesses.

Much of the information about preoperative assessment of independent organ systems that is presented in later chapters pertains to patient assessment prior to cardiac surgery as well. Risk assessment in patients prior to cardiac surgery differs from that in patients having noncardiac surgery for two major reasons: (1) patients in the former group have extant cardiac disease, and (2) many, if not most, of them will require cardiopulmonary bypass during their surgery. Risks of morbidity for cardiac surgical patients include central nervous system,[6] pulmonary,[7,8] renal,[9,10] and hematologic[11] complications. Although this chapter focuses primarily on the overall mortality risk assessment of patients prior to cardiac surgery, postoperative cardiac-related deaths account for most of the mortality after cardiac surgery.[12]

■ COLLECTION OF PATIENT DATA IN CARDIAC SURGERY

The widespread adoption of coronary artery bypass grafting (CABG) in the 1970s laid the foundation for collecting outcomes data on a large number of patients having cardiac surgery. These patients were undergoing a narrow variety of procedures (solitary CABG, CABG plus one or more valves, and isolated valve surgeries) usually with extracorporeal circulation in a relatively few centers. Because mortality is a clear outcome that occurs with some regularity after cardiac surgery, and because that morbidity is reasonably definable, the acquisition of data in large institutional, regional, and national databases was promoted. These accumulated data permitted outcome analyses that generated multiple risk-assessment tools and models. Some of these outcomes analyses have been mandated publicly but most have been voluntary and scholarly.

The data and analyses from these models display a number of characteristics. Although administrative data are still occasionally the foundation of analyses by government or third-party payers, their use for risk assessment was discredited 2 decades ago. These data are collected by nonclinician coders whose focus is hospital reimbursement and who often use nonclinical terminology. Furthermore, it is usually not possible to differentiate a condition that existed prior to surgery from one that developed afterward.[13] The collection flaws of administrative data combined with the lack of reliable risk-adjustment render any comparative use of the data largely meaningless.[2]

The ideal database collection is the automated entry of real-time clinical data. Electronic medical record and laboratory reporting increasingly make that ideal possible. However, until real-time data collection can include postoperative outcomes, some form of patient record abstraction is necessary. Such data should be collected as concurrently as possible, by dedicated, objective clinicians (usually research nurses) not directly responsible for the care delivered. When the individuals collecting data are distracted by a bias stemming from their primary responsibility, inconsistencies can corrupt the data within an institution or practice. Databases must have clear, concisely written definitions that are reviewed regularly by the data collectors for their consistent applicability. Fewer data fields with mostly menu-driven options increase the reliability of collection, but the statistical analysis of these more parsimonious models is controversial.[2,14,15] For example, a number of well-recognized national databases have no mechanism for decreasing interobserver variation. Regular national phone conferences among collectors, or, better yet, site visits with data-collection review, minimize the data flaws associated with multiple sites and multiple collectors. Reliable data collection, absent electronic direct real-time population of data fields, is resource intensive, but most major institutions with cardiac surgical programs have come to recognize that participation in a major regional or national database is essential.

CREATING RISK-ASSESSMENT MODELS FOR CARDIAC SURGERY

Although consistent and objective data collection is the foundation of an outcomes/risk-assessment model, the statistical analysis that allows risk adjustment is critical. Factors to be considered in risk model development depend on the population selected and include the following: (1) the type of surgery (e.g., all cardiac surgery, CABG only, valve only, valve and CABG, off-pump CABG), (2) geography (single institution, multi-institution, state, regional, or national), (3) the outcomes to be predicted (short-term mortality, long-term mortality, specific morbidities such as stroke or renal failure), and (4) the statistical methods to be employed (with or without univariate selection of factors and the choice of multivariate analytical techniques: logistic regression, stepwise logistic regression, or Bayesian analysis).

Unlike in data collection, parsimony of well-collected data fields may be a disadvantage in model development.[14] If more risk factors are inserted into a model, especially if they are inconsistently defined or subjectively determined, then the model's validity can be jeopardized as a result of inclusion of covariates and collinear factors.[2,16] Evaluation of multiple models suggests that relatively few, discrete factors account for most of the variation in outcome prediction.[17] Indeed, the design of a risk assessment model has many pitfalls, but they can be avoided if the intent of the risk model is determined a priori. For example, a model might be used for individual patient predictions, provider comparisons, or system improvement. The population of patients from which a model is derived requires a sufficient number of patients with and without the given outcomes to be risk-adjusted. Finally, appropriate statistical methods are required not only to select the variables to be thrust into a model, but also to ascertain that the model meets the initially established intent.[2,18]

Because a majority of the variation in outcomes can be predicted on the basis of a few preoperative factors, independent risk factors can be identified by multivariable analysis that accounts for most of the variability in the outcome under evaluation.[2,17] This does not diminish, however, a clinician's need to know the predictive value of a specific preoperative factor in an individual patient (univariate analysis). The specific preoperative factor might actually contribute very little

to a comprehensive model (accounting for little of the overall variability in an outcome by multivariable analysis), but that relates to the infrequency of a given preoperative risk factor in the cardiac surgical population.

Risk factors not represented explicitly in a model may be represented implicitly through other variables. For example, in one Bayesian model (Merged Cardiac Registry–HDR), female sex is associated with poorer outcomes after CABG, but if body surface area is included, then female sex no longer significantly contributes to the predictive model. On the other hand, a clinically relevant preoperative factor may not be reflected in the prediction model at all; this problem often occurs because of the difficulty in consistent data collection. For example, few models include more than the most obvious data on cardiac/coronary anatomy (left main coronary artery stenosis is most commonly included), and where included, these data seem to minimally impact on the predictive model. Nevertheless, surgeons may subjectively predict increased risk for an individual patient with diffuse coronary disease poorly amenable to bypass, or for a patient with extensive perivalvular calcification prior to aortic or mitral surgery. Neither diffuse disease nor extensive calcification is a factor in well-established predictive models. Although a provider or care system can derive significant benefit from data collection, analysis, and risk assessment, it is important to understand the limitations and the value of a particular risk assessment model as it relates to individual patients and their preoperative condition.

ESTABLISHED RISK-ASSESSMENT MODELS IN CARDIAC SURGERY

The dynamic nature of cardiac surgery risk assessment and the need for some accepted risk-assessment standard and the benefit of simplicity are illustrated by the Parsonnet scoring system first described in 1989[19] from a relatively narrow experience. This linear, additive risk score was simple to use and became widely adopted as an objective, independent method to quantify a published cohort's operative risk. Twice revised to improve its accuracy, a logistic risk-assessment model was published[16] in 2000, along with a simple additive model employing risk score-categories. This model was derived from 10,703 CABG, valve, and combination surgeries performed at 10 contributing New Jersey centers over a 2-year period (1994-1995). Forty-seven risk factors were forced into this logistic regression analysis (not stepwise regression or the result of univariate selection), and Table 7-1 shows the 10 highest-ranked factors for this all-cardiac surgery population (CABG, valve, and combined procedures). The receiver operating characteristic (ROC), or c-statistic, reflects the model's ability to discriminate for the outcome (death); 1.0 is perfect. For this model, the c-statistic is reported as 0.811 for the training set and 0.785 for the test set.[16]

Models also have been developed from large voluntary, multisite databases in the United States. These include the databases of the Society of Thoracic Surgeons (STS),[10,20] the Veterans Affairs (VA),[21] the Merged Cardiac Registry,[22] and

7-1   Parsonnet and Bernstein's Logistic Model

Top 10 Factors (from among 47*)	Coefficient Rank	Percent of Test Population
Second or subsequent cardiac reoperation	1.9914	0.41
Dialysis dependency	1.3662	0.93
Cirrhosis	1.2679	0.27
Age 79 yr	1.1052	7.88
Pulmonary hypertension	1.0831	10.72
First cardiac reoperation	1.0216	7.06
Ejection fraction <30%	0.7802	8.40
Age 75-79 yr	0.6861	13.76
Ejection fraction 30% to 49%	0.6687	38.62
Female sex	0.6180	31.34

*Excluding high-coefficient factors present in <0.5% of the test population, including refusal of blood products, idiopathic thrombogenic purpura, acquired immunodeficiency syndrome (not merely positive for human immunodeficiency virus), and active untreated endocarditis.

the Northern New England Cardiovascular Disease Study Group (NNE).[23,24] State-mandated outcomes databases include the New York State registry.[25] From the data of each of these, a model of mortality prediction has been developed. In each case, a training cohort was separated out (e.g., every other patient or every third patient) to derive risk factors from which a model was developed, and then this model was tested on another population (the remaining patients, those not selected for the training set, are the test cohort). Nearly all predictive models were initially based on patients having solitary coronary artery bypass surgery, but most of the various databases have derived models for different valve surgeries as well.

Table 7-2 contrasts solitary CABG mortality prediction models and their odds ratios (ORs) for several voluntary databases. Each of these models reports c-statistics (ROC curves) demonstrating acceptable discrimination for the outcome, ranging from 0.73 to 0.81. The ORs express the increased likelihood of an outcome in individuals in a population with a particular risk factor, compared with those without. For example, an OR of less than 1.0 for being male would mean an OR of greater than unity for being female. An OR of 1.2 for females would mean that females (not any given female) are 20% more likely than males to experience a given outcome. Confidence intervals (CIs) define the increased likelihood within some range, usually 90% or 95%. For a given characteristic to be statistically significant, its CI must not cross unity, as that would mean that there is an equal chance the factor would decrease or increase the chance of the event.

Given the relatively similar discrimination (c-statistic) between these models, it is interesting to note the many differences and some similarities among the factors determined to be important to the respective models. Contrast, for example, the parsimonious VA dataset with the inclusive STS set. Interestingly, the VA dataset performs well on the STS population.[5] In each model, much depends on how certain factors were defined, and more importantly on which factors were considered for the given model. Age, female sex, some

measure of left ventricle (LV) function, recent myocardial infarction (MI), renal dysfunction, and reoperation are consistent predictors of mortality after CABG across the different models and, among these, reoperation has the greatest weight in these predictors of mortality after CABG.

Models for prediction of postoperative mortality after valve surgery have been developed from these databases as well. The STS model[26] included two multivariate analyses, one for isolated aortic valve repair (AVR) or mitral valve repair (MVR) (49,073 patients), and one for CABG combined with either of these (43,463 patients), entered from 1994 to 1997. The c-statistics for these two models were 0.77 and 0.74, respectively. The NNE[27] logistic model for aortic valve mortality found independent predictors of in-hospital mortality to include older age, smaller body surface area, prior cardiac surgery, increased creatinine level, New York Heart Association (NYHA) class IV, congestive heart failure (CHF) and atrial fibrillation, urgent or emergent priority, concomitant CABG, and earlier year of surgery (ROC = 0.75). Independent predictors for in-hospital mortality after mitral surgery included female sex, older age, diabetes, coronary artery disease, prior stroke, increased creatinine level, NYHA class IV, CHF, urgent or emergent priority, and replacement rather than repair of the mitral valve (ROC = 0.79). A report from the VA database showed that the predictors for acute mortality after CABG were very similar to the predictors of acute mortality after valve replacement, with the exception of compromised preoperative functional (completely or partially dependent) status as an additional predictor for valve mortality (OR 1.64 for AVR patients, 95% CI = 1.29-2.09, and 2.21 OR for MVR patients, 95% CI 1.48-3.30). Previous cardiac surgery and NYHA functional status were more predictive for CABG alone than they were for the valve surgery.[28] The similarities in the derived models for valve and CABG are consistent with the fact that combined models such as EuroSCORE[29] and Parsonnet use a single model that predicts well for all cardiac surgery. The similarities of different models for the different surgeries (same outcome: mortality) does not diminish the fact that development of, or search for, different prediction models may aid in an understanding of the differing risks for the patient populations undergoing different surgeries, even if the ultimate predictive discrimination is equivalent.

The EuroSCORE model depicted in Table 7-3 shows the factors determined to be important in predicting mortality after cardiac surgery in eight European states. This well-studied model includes a quick additive method for individual prediction of risk. That these two methods do not predict risk equally across risk groups is an example of poorer calibration in the additive model.[30] The EuroSCORE model has discrimination characteristics on the training and test sets equivalent to those of the U.S. models, and its application to patients from the STS database reveals it to function satisfactorily for patients in the United States as well.[31]

■ LIMITATIONS OF RISK-ASSESSMENT MODELS

Even with appropriate data collection and statistical analysis techniques, risk-assessment models have genuine limitations.

7-2   **Solitary CABG Mortality Prediction Models: Inputs and Their Odds Ratios**

Inputs/Predictors	Odds Ratios (95% Confidence Interval)	Inputs/Predictors	Odds Ratios (95% Confidence Interval)
Northern New England Cardiovascular Disease Study Group[23,24] (NNE)*		Left main coronary artery disease ≥50%	1.18
		Male sex	0.84
Age: < 55; 55-59; 60-64; 65-69; 70-74; >75	1; 1.5; 2; 2.6; 3.4; 4.7	Mitral insufficiency (MI)	1.22
Female sex	1.2	Multiple reoperations	4.19
BSA: >2; 1.8-1.99; 1.6-1.79; <1.6	1; 1.3; 1.8; 2.4	NYHA functional class IV	1.15
Charlson comorbidity score 0; 1; ≥2	1; 1.5; 2.3	Race: other	1.12
Prior CABG	3.6	Prior MI	1.18
Ejection fraction: ≤ 60; 50-59; 40-49; <40	1; 1.4; 1.6; 1.9	Percutaneous transluminal coronary angioplasty <6 hr	1.32
LVEDP (mm Hg): ≥14; 15-18; 19-22; >22	1; 1.3; 1.6; 2.1	Peripheral or central vascular disease	1.29
Priority of surgery: elective; urgent; emergent	1; 2.1; 4.4	Renal failure/dialysis	1.88
Left main stenosis: <50%; 50%-89%; ≥90%	1; 1; 1	Shock	2.04
Diseased coronary arteries (no.): 1; 2; 3	1; 1.3; 1.6	Emergency status	1.96
		Triple-vessel disease	1.21
Veteran's Affairs[21] (VA)†			
Serum creatinine >3 mg/dL	4.7	**Health Data Research[22] (HDR)§**	
Previous cardiac operation	2.7	Age: 18-55; 56-64; 65-74; 75-80; 81-100	0.37; 0.72; 0.97; 1.6; 2.56
Preoperative intra-aortic balloon pump	2.6		
Age (decade increments)	1.6	BSA: BMI from 7-20	12.6
Peripheral vascular disease	1.6	BSA: 0.5-1.5; 1.5-1.7; 1.7-1.9; 1.9-2.1; 2.1-4	2.15; 1.38; 1.17; 0.83; 0.64
Chronic obstructive pulmonary disease	1.3		
Canadian Heart Association class III or IV	1.3	BSA: male; female	0.83; 1.47
Priority of operation elective	0.8	History of cancer	1.04
		CNS: prior stroke; carotid disease; other CNS history; no CNS	1.71; 1.39; 1.25; 0.93
Society of Thoracic Surgery[10,20] (STS)‡		Chronic obstructive pulmonary disease	1.61
Age (per year)	1.05	DM/HTN: both; DM only; HTN only; neither	1.25; 0.9; 1.0; 0.78
Aortic stenosis	1.40	LVEF: >49; 40-49; 30-39; 20-29; <20	0.67; 0.99; 1.54; 2.5; 6.63
Race: black	1.34		
BSA (per 0.1 unit change)	0.91	Left ventricular hypertrophy	1.16
Chronic lung disease	1.41	MI: 0-6 hr; >6 hr; never	4.58; 1.32; 0.69
Cerebrovascular accident	1.10	Surgical status: elective/urgent; emergency; desperate	0.8; 3.18; 20.43
Diabetes; oral treatment	1.15		
Ejection fraction >50%	0.98	Race: white; black; other	0.92; 1.41; 1.12
First reoperation	2.76	Peripheral vascular disease	1.89
Race: Hispanic	1.04	Reoperation: 1; 2; 3; no reoperation	1.69; 2.71; 2.06; 0.92
Hypercholesterolemia	0.82	Renal failure: dialysis; Cr >1.5%; renal failure; none	3.94; 2.5; 2.19; 0.82
Hypertension	1.12		
Intra-aortic balloon pump	1.46		
Immunosuppressive therapy	1.75		
Insulin	1.50		

Each of the following models can be updated from more recent test and training cohorts; for this table, the most recent published or commercially available prediction model was used for each database.

*The NNE, a regional database coordinated by a Dartmouth outcomes research group, includes all cardiac surgery centers in northern New England. Their data and analytical teams have fostered group-driven investigations producing many excellent subpopulation analyses[23] of preoperative factors and prediction models for a variety of morbidities.

†The national database of VA cardiac centers was the genesis of the VA's more comprehensive National Surgical Quality Improvement Project. It has been compared favorably with the larger, private, and less male STS database.

‡The STS is the national database with the largest number of contributors and the source of multiple other predictive models based on operation type (valves) and outcome (morbidities such as renal failure requiring dialysis; stroke).

§HDR's Merged Cardiac Registry includes member centers from across the United States and a few international contributors. Their Bayesian model is updated annually and available in palm or laptop versions as Cardiac Risk Predictor software.

BMI, body mass index; BSA, body surface area; CABG, coronary artery bypass grafting; CNS, central nervous system; Cr, creatinine; DM/HTN, diabetes mellitus/hypertension; LVEDP, left ventricular end-diastolic pressure; MI, myocardial infarction.

For all the benefit they provide, they can still account for only a portion of the variability in actual outcomes. The discrimination of a model is its ability to separate, to discriminate, any pair into two distinct outcomes (mortality, for example, discriminates between the living and the dead). This model characteristic is described by the c-statistic (originally from the world of early radar evaluation—discriminating a plane from a cloud, for example). As noted, the established models described have ROC values in the 0.73 to 0.81 range (1.0 is perfect, and >0.70 to 0.80 is useful). The discrimination of most models is far from perfect in associating preoperative characteristics with a postoperative outcome in a given patient. Calibration is another property of a prediction model. This characteristic is often described by the Hosmer-

7-3	EuroScore: Factors Important for Predicting Mortality after Cardiac Surgery

All-Cardiac-Surgery Mortality Model Inputs/Predictors	Odds Ratios (95% Confidence Interval)
Age (continuous)	1.1
Female sex	1.4
Serum creatinine	1.9
Extracardiac arteriopathy	1.9
Pulmonary disease	1.6
Neurologic dysfunction	2.3
Previous cardiac surgery	2.6
Recent myocardial infarction	1.6
Left ventricular ejection fraction: 40%-50%; <30%	1.5; 2.5
Chronic congestive heart failure	1.5
Systolic pulmonary hypertension	2
Active endocarditis	2.5
Unstable angina	1.5
Surgery timing: urgent; emergency	1.6; 2.8
Critical preoperative state	2.2
Ventricular septal rupture	3.8
Noncoronary surgery	1.6
Thoracic aortic surgery	3.2

EuroSCORE[29]: 128 European centers contributed 19,030 patients having cardiac surgery dataset during 1995. The association of preoperative ($n = 68$) and operative ($n = 29$) factors with mortality was assessed by univariate selection into a logistic model with a c-statistic of 0.79. A simple additive model has also been developed and widely used,[30] and its variation from the logistic model is well detailed.

Lemeshow goodness-of-fit statistic. This property is the one that allows a model to appropriately predict the percentage of patients with a given outcome. Patients are segregated into categories of risk. The ability of the model to predict the actual percentage of those in each category with an outcome should not be different (P value should be nonsignificant) across the risk categories, if the model is well calibrated.[32] Calibration can usually be adjusted or accounted for in a model, but discrimination cannot. These are just two of many important statistical considerations in the assessment and use of these various models. Perhaps most important is their applicability to a given test population. A model's reported c-statistic or Hosmer-Lemeshow goodness-of-fit statistic describes its ability to discriminate and calibrate risk for the population from which it was derived[18] (given the segregation of a test and training set as described previously). Increasingly, as these models are applied to populations[29,33] that are different from those from which they were derived, we are able to increase, or decrease, confidence in their risk-assessment utility.

The outcome to be predicted by a model may be a limitation in itself. Although mortality seems binary, its definition has been the subject of some debate. The general contemporary notion is that mortality means "in-hospital death" or death within 30 days out of the hospital. However, the use of extended care may cloud this endpoint. Increasingly, death in the first year[34] after a procedure is considered to be a more important endpoint. In this regard, a researcher might have to choose between a more identifiable (and thus collectable) endpoint (i.e., short-term mortality) and a clearly valuable and socially desirable, but less definable, endpoint (i.e., longer-term mortality). Furthermore, if mortality as an endpoint is problematic, morbidity is even more so. The collection of data and the definition of morbidity are critical to the validity of any model, as are sample size and incidence of the morbidity outcome. A limitation of the models is illustrated by the variety of predictive factors shown in Tables 7-1 through 7-3; no model can base an outcome prediction on a factor that was not given a chance to be included in the model itself.[2]

Importantly, all the models are derived from experiences that are at least a couple of years old at the time of analysis. By the time a model is published or employed, it may be less valid in predicting outcomes for a contemporary population of patients having treatments that evolved since the data were collected. As new procedures are developed and adopted, such as off-pump CABG, risk models are necessarily tested on these new populations[35] and newer specific models will be developed. Thus evolution of patient selection and treatment are a limitation of prediction models. Improvements in technique are anticipated to positively exaggerate the difference between observed performance and the outcome estimated by a model based on a system prior to improvements. Still, despite these limitations, prediction models have been enormously useful. As an understanding of the pitfalls of risk assessment increases, and real-time data acquisition becomes more common, these prediction models and the risk adjustment they provide will continue to improve.

■ CARDIAC-SPECIFIC RISK FACTORS

When assessing cardiovascular risk in the cardiac surgical patient, the cardiac-specific factors identified in the models discussed here should be considered, along with a factor that is less well represented—that is, cardiac, and particularly coronary, anatomy. Left main coronary artery disease and sometimes the observation of one-, two-, or three-vessel involvement are included, but none of these factors is a strong predictor of overall mortality in any model or across the models. For example, the NNE model shows no increased OR for increasing left main stenosis, and there is no coronary anatomy factor in the VA and EuroSCORE models at all. The role of coronary anatomy may be limited partly because this parameter is hard to quantify. Also, surgeons are adept at overcoming any discernible negative prognostic factors, at least in the short term. In a study separate from their CABG mortality model, the NNE[36] identified coronary diameter as a negative prognostic sign among patients undergoing CABG. Even controlling for body size and age, women had smaller arteries (mid left anterior descending) than men, which at least partially explained a female mortality disadvantage that extends beyond body surface area. More sophisticated quantification of coronary anatomy has yet to find its way into mortality prediction models. Specific valve mortality models include valve location (mitral or aortic) but not anatomic factors (e.g., calcification), but such determinations are neither well quantified nor common.

Most important in the objective assessment of cardiac-specific risk in cardiac surgery is the anticipation of postoperative cardiac failure. O'Connor and colleagues of the Northern New England Cardiovascular Disease Study Group showed[12] that unanticipated heart failure accounts for the greatest proportion of variability in the mortality rates of different individual surgeons. In 1996, David and colleagues identified the following predictors of low cardiac output after cardiac surgery: low left ventricular ejection fraction (EF) (<20%), prior surgery, emergency timing, female sex, diabetes, age (>70), left main coronary artery disease, recent MI, and triple-vessel coronary involvement.[37] Five years later, the NNE followed their 1998 modes-of-death[12] study with a multivariate analysis that identified female sex, prior CABG surgery, EF less than 40%, urgent or emergency surgery, advanced age (70 to 79 years, and older than 80 years), peripheral vascular disease, diabetes, dialysis-dependent renal failure, and three-vessel coronary disease[38] as significant predictors of cardiac failure after cardiac surgery. The similarity between the two sets of factors is logical and striking. The ability to modify such factors is restricted to patient preparation and selection of operative timing. Surgery in an emergency setting is universally identified as carrying a significantly increased risk of mortality.[10,21,22,24,29] However, this acute operative risk must be balanced with the risk of preoperative death without the emergency surgery.[39]

The NNE postoperative heart failure risk-assessment model has been transduced into a simple scoring tool for predicting heart failure after cardiac surgery.[35] This paper-and-pencil tool allows stratification of patients according to their risk of heart failure after cardiac surgery and thereby permits different monitoring and treatment for those at low risk as opposed to those at high risk for heart failure after cardiac surgery. Monitoring differences might include the use of pulmonary artery catheters and transesophageal echocardiography only in high-risk patients. Treatment differences could include more aggressive use of intra-aortic balloon pumps, inotropes, and myocardial protection alterations in the higher risk patients. At present, the evidence to support such selective monitoring and treatment is not substantial.

Timing of a CABG after infarction remains controversial. The evidence is consistent that stabilization of patients prior to cardiac surgery and an increasing time interval between an acute infarction and surgery are associated with lower mortality than is seen in unstable patients or those receiving surgery soon (e.g., 6 days) after infarction. Prospective studies of postinfarction patients comparing a planned delay versus no delay are lacking, and a humane study design is difficult to envision, so the literature is retrospective with respect to timing. Consistent with prior data, Lee and coworkers observed a continuum of decreased CABG mortality from 1 hour to 14 days after infarction, with a distinct drop after 3 days.[40]

■ EVIDENCE FOR CLINICAL APPLICATION OF RISK-ASSESSMENT TOOLS

Risk models can be used clinically in individual patients, heeding the caveats cited earlier, to prospectively provide guidance as to operative timing and preparation. A prediction derived from such a model may inform the patient's informed consent, and it is commonly used to do so, but it is not well evaluated in terms of contributing to an improved outcome. Prediction models are not able to predict with a high degree of certainty the outcome in a given patient. Patients and referring physicians have long expected surgeons and anesthesiologists to provide some semiquantitative estimate of morbidity and mortality risk. Subjective estimates by experienced surgeons in an established system are about as accurate as any available model.[41] Surgeons' subjective estimates, although not well studied, probably vary widely across practitioners and may offer less information to a patient than data from an objective model. The value of risk-assessment models in educating patients is real, but the benefit is poorly defined (Table 7-4).

The use of cardiac risk assessment for modification of risk is also more attractive than it is demonstrably beneficial. Although it is appealing to consider that identification of risk factors could lead to adjustments that would prevent a predicted negative outcome, there is little evidence that outcomes have been improved by altering specific risk factors. Of course, many of these factors, such as age and sex, cannot be modified, but others, such as interval to surgery after an MI, can be.[38,39] Chapter 6 on cardiac risk assessment in the noncardiac patient illustrates this in the discussion of coronary revascularization before major vascular surgery.[42,43] Specific morbidity prediction models[10,38,44] clearly offer the opportunity for potential clinical benefit and investigation of the impact of intervention. Risk-assessment outcome predictions may be the foundation of interventional trials (without concomitant controls) that seek a significant, positive variance in actual, observed outcomes compared with expected, predicted outcomes. This rapid-cycle improvement technique is promoted by such organizations as the Institute for Healthcare Improvement. Such efforts (essentially using statistical historical controls) do not provide highly regarded evidence, nor are they favorably reviewed by peer-reviewed journals, despite the fact that they may provide the opportunity for rapid clinical change.

Currently, the highest level of evidence for individual preoperative and operative risk modification comes from appropriately designed prospective trials. An excellent guideline for patients having CABG has been published and was updated in 2004 by a joint group of the American Heart Association and the American College of Cardiology. These authors summarized and graded a very large number of relevant clinical trials.[40] Familiarity with this guideline is fundamental for practitioners of surgical revascularization. A similar guideline exists for valve disease.[45] Although its focus is broader than surgery, it is still highly relevant to preoperative assessment of the patient with valve disease.

The value of risk assessment for a care system is far better supported by evidence than its value for the individual patient. Although the political and external use of risk adjustment is beyond the scope of this chapter, this is a potential benefit as risk assessment is transformed into risk adjustment.[46,47] Individual providers and care systems are more fairly evaluated by external nonclinicians using outcomes

| 7-4 | Key Points and Their Graded Risk: Benefit and Evidence Support | | | |

Key Points and Their Graded Risk: Benefit and Evidence Support	Benefit Is Significantly Greater than Risk: Procedure/Treatment SHOULD Be Performed/Administered	Benefit Is Greater than Risk: Procedure/Treatment IS REASONABLE	Benefit Is Greater than or Equal to Risk: Procedure/Treatment MAY BE CONSIDERED	Risk Is Greater than or Equal to Benefit: Procedure/Treatment IS NOT HELPFUL AND MAY BE HARMFUL
Level of Evidence: Low	Preoperative stabilization of patients requiring emergency operation whenever possible [39, 40]	Use of risk-assessment models in informing patients [52] Use of risk assessment in modifying operative risks	Use of risk assessment in interventional trials for risk modification. Public and payer use of risk-adjusted outcomes data [49, 51]	
Level of Evidence: Medium	Use of risk-assessment models for provider and system improvement [3, 21, 5, 53, 54, 55]			Use of risk-assessment models that are derived from administrative data [13, 48]
Level of Evidence: High	Use of AHA/ACC guidelines in coronary and valve patients [39, 45]			

databases and risk-adjustment methods that do not rely on administrative data and analysis.[13,48] Nevertheless, the evidence that thoughtful use of risk-adjusted data or "report cards" is used by insurers and patients is lacking.[49-51]

However, appropriate risk-assessment models have improved care when they have been employed in an informative, collaborative manner.[3,20,52] This has been true in the Northern New England experience, in the VA system, and in the Society of Thoracic Surgeons as a whole. This has also been cited by mandated reporting systems with administrative risk-adjustment[53] in New York State. Importantly, these outcomes improvements may be further extended by low-cost, highly informational interventions. A nationwide STS initiative showed improvement from baseline after mammary artery graft use and beta-blocker use after encouraging providers to contrast their use with nationwide benchmarks.[54] A statewide effort to improve cardiac surgery processes and outcomes involved mostly education and collaboration of best practices to achieve improvements in mammary artery graft use (similar to the national trend but better than another state control), aspirin use, and incidence of intubation of less than 6 hours.[55] Cardiovascular risk assessment prior to cardiac surgery has many applications, but the most evident one is improvement in the quality of patient care.

■ REFERENCES

1. Iezzoni LI: Using risk-adjusted outcomes to assess clinical practice: An overview of issues pertaining to risk adjustment. Ann Thorac Surg 1994;58:1822-1826.
2. Shahian DM, Blackstone EH, Edwards FH, et al: Report from the STS Workforce on Evidence Based Surgery. Cardiac surgery risk models: A position article. Ann Thorac Surg 2002;74:1749.
3. O'Connor GT, Plume SK, Olmstead EM, et al: A regional intervention to improve the hospital mortality associated with coronary artery bypass graft surgery. The Northern New England Cardiovascular Disease Study Group. JAMA 1996;275:841-846.
4. Khuri SF, Daley J, Henderson WG: The comparative assessment and improvement of quality of surgical care in the Department of Veterans Affairs. Arch Surg 2002;137:20-27.
5. Grover FL, Shroyer AL, Hammermeister K, et al: A decade's experience with quality improvement in cardiac surgery using the Veterans Affairs and Society of Thoracic Surgeons national databases. Ann Surg 2001;234:464-472.
6. Charlesworth DC, Likosky DS, Marrin CA, et al: Development and validation of a prediction model for strokes after coronary artery bypass grafting. Ann Thorac Surg 2003;76:436-443.
7. Milot J, Perron J, Lacasse Y, et al: Incidence and predictors of ARDS after cardiac surgery. Chest 2001;119:884-888.
8. Canver CC, Chanda J: Intraoperative and postoperative risk factors for respiratory failure after coronary bypass. Ann Thorac Surg 2003;75:853-857.
9. Wang F, Dupuis JY, Nathan H, Williams K: An analysis of the association between preoperative renal dysfunction and outcome in cardiac surgery: Estimated creatinine clearance or plasma creatinine level as measures of renal function. Chest 2003;124:1852-1862.
10. Shroyer ALW, Coombs LP, Peterson ED, et al: The Society of Thoracic Surgeons: 30-day operative mortality and morbidity risk models. Ann Thorac Surg 2003;75:1856-1865.
11. Despotis GJ, Filos KS, Zoys TN, et al: Factors associated with excessive postoperative blood loss and hemostatic transfusion requirements: A multivariate analysis in cardiac surgical patients. Anesth Analg 1996;82:13-21.
12. O'Connor GT, Birkmeyer JD, Dacey LJ, et al: Results of a regional study of modes of death associated with coronary artery bypass grafting. Northern New England Cardiovascular Disease Study Group. Ann Thorac Surg 1998;66:1323-1328.
13. Mack MJ, Herbert M, Prince S, et al: Does reporting of coronary artery bypass grafting from administrative databases accurately reflect actual clinical outcomes? J Thorac Cardiovasc Surg 2005;129:1309-1317.
14. Nowicki ER: What is the future of mortality prediction models in heart valve surgery? Ann Thorac Surg 2005;80:396-398.
15. Tu JV, Sykora K, Naylor CD: Assessing the outcomes of coronary artery bypass graft surgery: How many risk factors are enough? Steering Committee of the Cardiac Care Network of Ontario. J Am Coll Cardiol 1997;30:1317-1323.

16. Bernstein AD, Parsonnet V: Bedside estimation of risk as an aid for decision-making in cardiac surgery. Ann Thorac Surg 2000;69:823-828.
17. Jones RH, Hannan EL, Hammermeister KE, et al: Identification of preoperative variables needed for risk adjustment of short-term mortality after coronary artery bypass graft surgery. The Working Group Panel on the Cooperative CABG Database Project. J Am Coll Cardiol 1996;28:1478-1487.
18. Omar RZ, Ambler G, Royston P, et al: Cardiac surgery risk modeling for mortality: A review of current practice and suggestions for improvement. Ann Thorac Surg 2004;77:2232-2237.
19. Parsonnet V, Dean D, Bernstein AD: A method of uniform stratification of risk for evaluating the results of surgery in acquired heart disease. Circulation 1989;79(Suppl 1):3-12.
20. The Society of Thoracic Surgeons: Available at www.sts.org/sections/stsnationaldatabase.
21. Grover FL, Shroyer AL, Hammermeister K, et al: A decade's experience with quality improvement in cardiac surgery using the Veterans Affairs and Society of Thoracic Surgeons national databases. Ann Surg 2001;234:464-472.
22. Health Data Research: Available at www.healthdataresearch.com/mcr_file.htm.
23. O'Connor GT, Plume SK, Olmstead EM, et al: Multivariate prediction of in-hospital mortality associated with coronary artery bypass graft surgery. Northern New England Cardiovascular Disease Study. Circulation 1992;85:2110-2118.
24. The Northern New England Cardiovascular Disease Study Group: Available at www.nnecdsg.org/pub_lit_2.htm.
25. Hannan EL, Kumar D, Racz M, et al: New York State's Cardiac Surgery Reporting System: Four years later. Ann Thorac Surg 1994;58:1852-1857.
26. Edwards FH, Peterson ED, Coombs LP, et al: Prediction of operative mortality after valve replacement surgery. J Am Coll Cardiol 2001;37:885-892.
27. Nowicki ER, Birkmeyer NJ, Weintraub RW, et al: Multivariable prediction of in-hospital mortality associated with aortic and mitral valve surgery in northern New England. Ann Thorac Surg 2004;77:1966-1977.
28. Gardner SC, Grunwald GK, Rumsfeld JS, et al: Comparison of short-term mortality risk factors for valve replacement versus coronary artery bypass graft surgery. Ann Thorac Surg 2004;77:549-556.
29. Roques F, Nashef SAM, Michel P, et al: Risk factors and outcome in European cardiac surgery: Analysis of the EuroSCORE multinational database of 19030 patients. Eur J Cardiothorac Surg 1999;15:816-823.
30. Zingone B, Pappalardo A, Dreas L: Logistic versus additive EuroSCORE: A comparative assessment of the two models in an independent population sample. Eur J Cardiothorac Surg 2004;26:1134-1140.
31. Nashef SA, Roques F, Hammill BG, et al: EuroSCORE Project Group. Validation of European System for Cardiac Operative Risk Evaluation (EuroSCORE) in North American cardiac surgery. Eur J Cardiothorac Surg 2003;24:336-337.
32. Grunkemeier GL, Jin R: Receiver operating characteristic curve analysis of clinical risk models. Ann Thorac Surg 2001;72:323-326.
33. Jin R, Grunkemeier GL, Starr A: Validation and refinement of mortality risk models for heart valve surgery. Ann Thorac Surg 2005;80:471-479.
34. Edwards MB, Taylor KM: Is 30-day mortality an adequate outcome statistic for patients considering heart valve replacement? Ann Thorac Surg 2003;76:482-485.
35. Wu Y, Grunkemeier GL, Handy JR: Coronary artery bypass grafting: Are risk models developed from on-pump surgery valid for off-pump surgery? J Thorac Cardiovasc Surg 2004;127:174-178.
36. O'Connor NJ, Morton JR, Birkmeyer JD, et al: Effect of coronary artery diameter in patients undergoing coronary bypass surgery. Northern New England Cardiovascular Disease Study Group. Circulation 1996;93:652-655.
37. Rao V, Ivanov J, Weisel RD, et al: Predictors of low cardiac output syndrome after coronary artery bypass. J Thorac Cardiovasc Surg 1996;112:38-51.
38. Surgenor SD, O'Connor GT, Lahey SJ, et al: Northern New England Cardiovascular Disease Study Group. Predicting the risk of death from heart failure after coronary artery bypass graft surgery. Anesth Analg 2001;92:596-601.
39. Eagle KA, Guyton RA, and the ACC/AHA Task Force on Practice Guidelines: ACC/AHA 2004 Guideline Update for Coronary Artery Bypass Graft Surgery—Summary Article: A Report of the American College of Cardiology/American Heart Association Task Force on Practice Guidelines. Circulation 2004;110:1168-1176.
40. Lee DC, Oz MC, Weinberg AD, Ting W: Appropriate timing of surgical intervention after transmural acute myocardial infarction. J Thorac Cardiovasc Surg 2003;125:115-120.
41. Johnson RG, Thurer R, Sellke FW, et al: A comparison of objective versus subjective post-CABG mortality predictions. Chest 2000;118(Suppl 4):86S.
42. Landesberg G, Mosseri M, Fleisher LA, et al: Coronary revascularization before vascular surgery. N Engl J Med 2005;352:1492-1495.
43. McFalls EO, Ward HB, Moritz TE, et al: Coronary-artery revascularization before elective major vascular surgery. N Engl J Med 2004;351:2795-2804.
44. Charlesworth DC, Likosky DS, Marrin CA, et al: Development and validation of a prediction model for strokes following coronary artery bypass grafting. Ann Thorac Surg 2003;76:436-443.
45. Bonow RO, Carabello B, de Leon AC Jr, et al: Guidelines for the management of patients with valvular heart disease: Executive summary. A report of the American College of Cardiology/American Heart Association Task Force on Practice Guidelines (Committee on Management of Patients with Valvular Heart Disease). Circulation 1998;98:1949-1984.
46. Shahian DM, Normand SL, Torchiana DF, et al: Cardiac surgery report cards: Comprehensive review and statistical critique. Ann Thorac Surg 2001;72:2155-2168.
47. Bridgewater B, Grayson AD, Jackson M, et al: North West Quality Improvement Programme in Cardiac Interventions. Surgeon specific mortality in adult cardiac surgery: Comparison between crude and risk stratified data. BMJ 2003;327:13-17.
48. Geraci JM, Johnson ML, Gordon HS, et al: Mortality after cardiac bypass surgery: Prediction from administrative versus clinical data. Med Care 2005;43:149-158.
49. Erikson LC, Torchiana DF, Schneider EC, et al: The relationship between managed care insurance and use of lower-mortality hospitals for CABG surgery. JAMA 2000;283:1976-1982.
50. Ireson CL, Ford MA, Hower JM, Schwartz RW: Outcome report cards: Necessity in the health care market. Arch Surg 2002;137:46-51.
51. Shahian DM, Yip W, Westcott G, Jacobson J: Selection of a cardiac surgery provider in the managed care era. J Thorac Cardiovasc Surg 2000;120:978-989.
52. Nugent W: Collaborative practice: A personal journey. Ann Thorac Surg 2001;71:765.
53. Hannan EL, Kilburn H, Racz M, et al: Improving the outcomes of coronary artery bypass surgery in New York State. JAMA 1994;271:761-766.
54. Ferguson TB Jr, Society of Thoracic Surgeons: Continuous quality improvement in medicine: Validation of a potential role for medical specialty societies. Am Heart Hosp J 2003;1:264-272.
55. Holman WL, Allman RM, Sanso M, et al, for the Alabama CABG Study Group: Alabama Coronary Artery Bypass Grafting Project: Results of a statewide quality improvement initiative. JAMA 2001;285:3003-3010.

8 Central Nervous System Risk Assessment

Katja Hindler and Nancy A. Nussmeier

Stroke is the third leading cause of death in the United States, and it will continue to be a major health problem as the population ages.[1] Perioperative stroke is a particularly debilitating and tragic complication of otherwise successful surgery. Although this chapter will focus primarily on stroke in patients who undergo cardiac surgery, where the incidence is fairly high (1% to 8%),[2-4] the patient risk factors for central nervous system (CNS) complications are relevant to all types of surgery. These factors include advanced age, genetic predisposition, female gender,[5] hypertension, diabetes, cerebrovascular disease, and aortic atherosclerosis.

■ CARDIAC SURGERY

Certain perioperative risk factors are unique to cardiac surgery, including cardiopulmonary bypass (CPB) itself. Debate about the potential deleterious effects of CPB revolves around temperature management, the inflammatory response to CPB, optimal mean arterial pressure, hemodilution, nonpulsatile CPB, acid–base management, and microembolic phenomena. However, the alternative—off-pump cardiac surgery—is not risk free either, and it cannot be used with patients undergoing cardiac surgical procedures that combine coronary artery bypass grafting (CABG) and intracardiac surgery (e.g., valve repair or replacement). Other operations, including CABG combined with carotid endarterectomy, carry unique neurologic risks related to inherent patient factors, complications of the surgical procedures, or both.

In cardiac and other surgical settings, identification of patients at highest risk for cerebral injury is a necessary first step in investigating new methods of mitigating such injury. Strategies may focus on prevention or on acute post-injury intervention with pharmacologic agents or other treatments.

Patient Risk Factors

Advanced Patient Age

Advanced patient age, particularly an age of 70 years or more, is a significant risk factor for postoperative cognitive dysfunction. Improvements in anesthetic and surgical techniques, as well as in postoperative monitoring and management, have made it possible to perform cardiac operations on a greater proportion of older adult patients, with a reasonable assurance of good outcome. Currently, approximately 35% of patients undergoing cardiac surgery are older than 70 years (W. K. Vaughn, unpublished data, September 2005). Yet, the risk for neurologic complications in this population increases with age (Fig. 8-1), rising at a higher rate than the risk for cardiac complications. Historically, the frequency of stroke

in patients undergoing CABG surgery has been 0.4% or lower in patients less than 50 years of age, almost 5% in patients more than 70 years of age, and nearly 9% in patients older than 75 years.[6] A recent multicenter follow-up study of CABG patients revealed a stroke rate of 4.7% in octogenarians, but only 1.6% in patients less than 80 years old.[7] Furthermore, octogenarians who have a stroke after CABG surgery have mortality rates as high as 38%—5 to 10 times higher than the mortality of patients who did not have postoperative strokes.[8]

The incidence of cognitive or neuropsychological decline is also much higher in patients aged 70 years or more than in younger patients, and the recovery rate from cognitive decline is lower in the older patients. For example, one study found that patients in their 50s who develop neuropsychological deficits after cardiac surgery have a 67% chance of recovering after 1 month, whereas this chance is less than 60% in patients over 70.[9]

The association between advanced age and a higher risk for overt stroke and neuropsychological decline after cardiac surgery may be due to several mechanisms. First, advanced age is a marker for morbidities such as hypertension, unstable angina, heart failure, and history of pulmonary disease. Second, older adult patients with coronary disease are usually referred for surgical intervention later in the course of their disease and have less functional reserve than younger patients. Third, aging is associated with atherosclerosis and an increased risk for various types of embolism, as well as with changes in the cerebral vasculature and in the autoregulation of blood flow. Fourth, when acute cerebral injury occurs in older adult patients, it is superimposed on a decreased functional baseline. Fifth, the possible consequences of being in a hospital environment, such as sleep deprivation, immobility, dehydration, and sensory overload, as well as being out of the home environment, are implicated in the genesis of older adult patients' neuropsychological deficits.

Genetic Predisposition

Neuropsychological testing has shown that some patients have a genetic predisposition toward cognitive decline after cardiac surgery. In particular, the Typ4 allele of the apolipoprotein E (APOE) gene is associated with postoperative cognitive decline in older adults and in patients with lower educational levels.[10] For example, Tardiff and colleagues[11] found a significant association between the APOE Typ4 allele and low scores on tests of short-term memory conducted 6 weeks after surgery. Alzheimer's patients, who are predisposed to develop cognitive decline, also show mutations of the APOE allele.[10,12] Although studies comparing

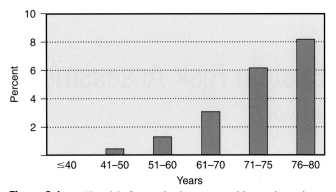

Figure 8-1 ■ The risk for stroke increases with age in patients undergoing coronary artery bypass grafting. *(Data from Gardener et al, 1985. Redrawn from Nussmeier NA: J Cardiothorac Vasc Anesth 1994;8(1 Suppl 1):13-18, with permission.)*

cognitive dysfunction in vascular dementia and Alzheimer's disease are controversial, changes in semantic, verbal, and nonverbal memory described after cardiac operations seem similar to those seen in the early stages of chronic dementias. However, episodic memory is more likely to be impaired in Alzheimer's patients, whereas executive processing is impaired in patients with vascular dementia.[10] Because the APOE Typ4 protein is involved in the repair of neuronal injuries, variations in the APOE gene may contribute to a lack of CNS reserve or homeostatic reparative mechanisms, making Typ4 carriers more prone to cognitive dysfunction after CPB. The complex relationship between genetic variation and the effects of cardiac surgery on cerebral function has not yet been investigated in detail. In the future, genetic screening of patients before cardiac surgery may improve assessments of patients' risk for adverse neurologic outcomes.

Female Sex

Women are more likely than men to suffer cerebral injury during CABG surgery (3.8% versus 2.4%).[3] This higher risk for neurologic events in women may partially explain the higher operative mortality of female CABG patients. In fact, in a study by Hogue and colleagues,[13] a postoperative neurologic event increased the risk for death to a greater degree in women than in men (33% versus 28%). A subsequent study by this group showed that a history of stroke was the strongest predictor of new stroke for both men and women.[14]

Women have several risk factors that may contribute to their higher post-CABG neurologic morbidity and mortality. First, women are more likely than men to present urgently or emergently for CABG surgery.[15-17] This may be because physicians are less likely to suspect coronary artery disease (CAD) in women than in men, so that physicians often fail to identify significant CAD in women and refer them for proper treatment. Second, women who undergo CABG tend to be older and to have more comorbidities than do male CABG patients. For example, female CABG patients are more likely to have hypertension, diabetes, peripheral vascular disease, and prior strokes than are male CABG patients.[18-20] Female CABG patients are also more likely to

have a history of severe or unstable angina or congestive heart failure.[21] Third, women are significantly smaller than men in height, weight, body surface area, and body mass index.[22,23] Smaller body size is positively associated with adverse outcomes because smaller people generally have narrower arteries than do larger people, presenting a greater technical challenge for surgeons performing CABG or carotid surgery.

However, female CABG patients' increased susceptibility to neurologic events cannot be fully explained by these risk factors. Other factors, including hormonal ones, may be involved. One somewhat enigmatic piece of evidence for hormonal involvement is the apparently higher postoperative mortality of premenopausal women who undergo CABG as compared with men of similar age.[24,25] This finding raises the question of whether premenopausal women who develop atherosclerosis have inadequate estrogen or abnormalities of the estrogen receptor, compared with other premenopausal women.

Estrogen is known to modify the inflammatory response to the reperfusion of ischemic tissues[26,27] and to inhibit neointimal formation and subsequent thrombosis in animal models of vascular injury.[26-30] However, a large prospective study of participants in the Women's Health Initiative, who were not undergoing a surgical procedure, noted an excess risk for stroke in women taking estrogen plus progestin for more than 1 year (hazard ratio, 1.41 [1.07-1.85]).[31] Furthermore, in a retrospective study of women undergoing carotid endarterectomy, the perioperative stroke rate was numerically, but not significantly, higher in women receiving hormone replacement therapy.[32] Further study is needed to determine whether perioperative hormone replacement therapy has a positive or negative effect on the incidence of perioperative stroke.

Hypertension

Frye and coworkers[33] found that in primary CABG patients, history of hypertension was a powerful predictor of stroke within 1 year after hospital discharge. Several studies in patients undergoing cardiac surgery have noted that patients who took antihypertensive medication preoperatively were at greater risk for postoperative stroke than those who did not.[8,34,35] Patients with a history of hypertension may be at greater risk if they have high systolic blood pressure (>145 mm Hg) at hospital admission.[4] Additionally, Reich and colleagues[36] found that diastolic arterial hypertension during CPB independently predicted stroke in patients undergoing cardiac surgery (odds ratio, 5.4). Preoperative hypertension has also been identified as a significant risk factor for mortality after stroke in patients who have undergone CABG.[37]

Hypertension is associated with an increased incidence of hemorrhagic, ischemic, and lacunar stroke because it causes marked adaptive changes in the cerebral circulation. Antihypertensive treatment reduces the risk for all of these types of strokes and for transient ischemic attacks (TIAs), possibly because antihypertensive medications are neuroprotective themselves.[38,39] Lowering blood pressure reduces stroke risk by up to 40% in all hypertensive populations.[40] However, overzealous antihypertensive treatment may cause cerebral ischemia, especially in the initial treatment of severe hypertension.

Intraoperative blood pressure deviations may add risk beyond that of the underlying condition of essential hypertension. Multiple studies have shown that patients with chronic hypertension have an elevated cerebral autoregulatory pressure threshold.[41-43] This heightened limit is probably largely a result of thickening of the walls (i.e., hyaline arteriosclerosis) of the resistance vessels.

In summary, hypertension contributes to patients' risk for adverse neurologic outcomes in cardiac surgery patients. Careful perioperative blood pressure management may reduce the effect of hypertension in such patients, particularly those with a previous history of severe hypertension.

Diabetes

Approximately 20% of CABG patients have diabetes mellitus, which makes them an important subgroup of the CABG population. These patients are unusually vulnerable to a variety of morbid events, including neurologic complications, and numerous studies show that diabetes is an independent risk factor for cerebral injury after CABG. Indeed, the incidence of perioperative and postoperative neurologic complications is significantly higher in diabetic than in nondiabetic CABG patients. One study found that the rate of post-CABG strokes was 6.3% in diabetic patients and 2.5% in nondiabetic patients.[43a] Another trial showed that diabetic patients had a 3.5-fold higher risk for neurologic dysfunction after cardiac surgery with CPB.[43b]

In general, diabetic patients tend to be older and have a higher incidence of comorbidities, such as hypertension, class II to IV angina, and low ejection fraction. Diabetic patients also have an increased risk for accelerated arteriosclerotic disease.[44] Endothelial hyperplasia and thickening basement membranes affect both the microvasculature and the macrovasculature. Additionally, considerable evidence suggests that the endothelial cells of diabetic patients generate more oxygen free radicals than do the endothelial cells of nondiabetic patients. These oxygen free radicals not only destroy nitric oxide, a vasodilator, but also are potent vasoconstrictors themselves. Other mechanisms that may contribute to endothelial dysfunction in diabetic patients include the release of potent vasoconstrictors, such as prostanoids and endothelin-1, and increased activation of protein kinase C, which causes abnormalities in cell signal transduction. These functional and morphologic changes in the cerebral vasculature make vascular disease more severe, diffuse, and accelerated in diabetic patients than in nondiabetic patients.

In addition, diabetic patients appear to lose the ability to regulate cerebral blood flow (CBF) adequately during CPB.[45] An intact CBF autoregulation system is essential to match CBF with metabolism, because CPB involves rapid changes in temperature, systemic perfusion rates, and systemic blood pressure. Unlike nondiabetic patients, diabetic patients do not show increased CBF in response to rising CO_2 levels. Also, there is a roughly linear relationship between CBF and mean arterial blood pressure in diabetic patients. Thus, CBF during CPB may be more pressure-dependent in this patient population than it is in nondiabetic patients. Furthermore, in diabetic patients, CBF does not increase with the temperature-associated increase in the cerebral metabolic rate for oxygen ($CMRO_2$) during post-CPB rewarming. Diabetic patients compensate for these imbalances in oxygen delivery by increasing the amount of oxygen extracted from cerebral blood.

Conflicting clinical data exist regarding the association between hyperglycemia (blood glucose greater than 200 mg/dL) during CPB and neurologic outcome after cardiac surgery. Several factors, such as hormone-induced alterations in glucose homeostasis, as well as reduced peripheral glucose utilization, contribute to perioperative hyperglycemia. Additionally, the inflammatory "stress response" to extracorporeal circulation, glucose-pump prime solutions, and administration of glucocorticosteroids aggravate an intraoperative hyperglycemic state.

Generally, hyperglycemia may worsen the neurologic outcome of global or focal ischemia during CPB by increasing lactate production. The resulting lactic acidosis aggravates ischemic damage. In addition, hyperglycemia prevents the increase in brain adenosine that is normally triggered by ischemia and that promotes vasodilatation. However, two studies noted no neurologic injury in patients managed with glucose levels as high as 700 mg/dL during bypass, and showed that the majority of post-CPB cognitive changes are not associated with blood glucose levels.[46,47] This may be because the potential negative impact of hyperglycemia during cerebral ischemia is attenuated by hypothermia during CPB, thereby mitigating any correlation between blood glucose levels during CPB and adverse neurologic outcomes. Furthermore, there is now growing evidence that the use of glucose-containing crystalloid priming (GCP) solutions during intracardiac or extracardiac surgery is not a risk factor per se for cerebral injury in diabetic or nondiabetic patients. Metz and Keats[46] showed that glucose-treated patients required significantly less fluid and weighed 3 kg less on the fifth postoperative day than patients not receiving glucose.

On the other hand, perioperative hypoglycemia (blood glucose levels below 40 mg/dL) may worsen neurologic function after CPB. "Tight control" of intraoperative blood glucose in nondiabetic patients undergoing cardiac surgery may initiate postoperative hypoglycemia.[48] Unfortunately, signs and symptoms of hypoglycemia are difficult to detect during general anesthesia. Therefore, it is mandatory to determine serial blood glucose levels perioperatively in patients at high risk for hypoglycemia (e.g., insulin-dependent diabetic patients, including children, and patients who are taking medications or have diseases associated with hypoglycemia).

In summary, discoveries about the adverse impact of hypoglycemia on the brain have tempered aggressive approaches to the control of hyperglycemia in patients at risk for cerebral ischemia. Should blood glucose control be implemented, it is essential to monitor blood glucose levels frequently and to adjust insulin dosages immediately to prevent hypoglycemia. If frequent glucose level monitoring is not feasible, then aggressive control of hyperglycemia is not recommended.

Cerebrovascular Disease

Patients' risk for carotid artery disease is positively correlated with their risk for CAD. Carotid artery stenosis (assessed by extracranial duplex ultrasound) is found in 5% to 15% of adult cardiac surgery patients. Its frequency increases with the number of coronary vessels involved. The likelihood of carotid stenosis also increases with age: carotid stenosis of 50% or greater is detected in 4% of CABG patients who are 60 years old or younger, in 11% of CABG patients more than 60 years old, and in 15% of CABG patients more than 70 years old.[49-51]

Cardiac surgery patients with significant carotid disease are at substantial risk of developing neurologic deficits during or after surgery.[51] Naylor and coworkers[52] reported that CABG patients with carotid bruit were almost four times more likely to have a perioperative stroke than CABG patients with no bruit. Similarly, in a study of CABG patients older than 60 years, the risk for postoperative stroke was 15% in patients with carotid stenosis of 75% or more, whereas this risk was only 0.6% in patients with no carotid stenosis.[53]

Previously, it was assumed that most strokes and TIAs associated with CABG surgery resulted from cerebral hypoperfusion caused by cerebrovascular disease or hypotension during CPB. Therefore, it was thought that maintaining a higher arterial pressure (> 90 mm Hg) during CPB in patients with known cerebral artery occlusion of less than 75% could improve regional CBF and oxygenation, resulting in smaller cerebral infarcts.[54] Additionally, patients with known carotid bruit were scheduled for carotid endarterectomy (CEA) before cardiac surgery to prevent hypoperfusion related to carotid stenosis.[55]

There is growing evidence that the presence of a carotid bruit is an important marker of advanced vascular disease in general, and aortic arch disease in particular, and that embolic phenomena cause most strokes. Carotid bruit seems to be the only significant preoperative predictor of severe aortic arch atheroma, a major risk factor for stroke in CABG patients.[56] Carotid disease or aortic disease, or both, may therefore cause neurologic deficits. Thus, it is now suggested that cardiac surgery patients benefit from CEA only if they have neurologic symptoms resulting from carotid stenosis.

In general, a history of neurologic symptoms such as TIA or stroke indicates an increased risk for acute perioperative stroke during or after CABG surgery.[57] Approximately 7% of CABG patients have a history of stroke or TIA.[58,59] The risk for perioperative stroke is significantly higher in patients with prior cerebral events than in neurologically asymptomatic patients.[14,34,60] For example, Hogue and colleagues[14] found that among cardiac surgery patients, the rate of perioperative stroke was much higher in those with a history of stroke (50% in women and 83.3% in men) than in patients with no history of stroke (6.5% in women and 5.6% in men). Clearly, factors predictive of an increased risk for post-CABG stroke include both the presence of carotid artery disease and preexisting neurologic symptoms.

Asymptomatic Carotid Stenosis

About 95% of patients with carotid bruit are asymptomatic.[52] The incidence of perioperative stroke is relatively low in these patients: about 3% in those with unilateral stenosis and 7% in those with bilateral disease.[52] This may be because asymptomatic carotid stenosis does not limit CBF during CPB. In patients with asymptomatic carotid stenosis, stroke during cardiac surgery is more likely to result from cerebral emboli secondary to an atherosclerotic aorta than from hemispheric hypoperfusion.[61] Because it is probably atheroemboli from the aorta, not the carotids, that is responsible for acute neurologic injury in these patients, prophylactic CEA may have little value for them.[61,62] A clinical trial conducted by Terramani and coworkers[63] showed no significant decrease in the risk for perioperative stroke in patients with asymptomatic carotid stenosis when CEA was performed concomitantly with cardiac surgery.

It may be that patients with cerebrovascular disease are at an increased risk of developing long-term neurologic deficits after cardiac surgery. Two studies have found that cardiac surgery patients with carotid stenosis greater than 70% (even those without preoperative neurologic symptoms) have a markedly greater risk of developing postoperative cerebral deficits than patients with less carotid stenosis.[64,65] Nevertheless, prophylactic CEA for cardiac surgery patients with asymptomatic carotid stenosis has not been shown to reduce long-term stroke risk.

Symptomatic Carotid Stenosis

Neurologically symptomatic CABG patients with severe carotid stenosis (>80%) have a high risk of developing new perioperative neurologic deficits.[52,66-68] Naylor and colleagues[52] noted that the risk for perioperative stroke is about 18% in symptomatic patients with severe unilateral stenosis and 26% in those with bilateral stenoses. Furthermore, 38% of such patients have mobile aortic atheroma in addition to their severe cerebrovascular disease.[56] Together, severe cerebrovascular disease and mobile aortic atheroma result in an extraordinarily high risk for neurologic injury from cerebral hypoperfusion or atherosclerotic emboli, or both, in the carotids or the aorta during cardiac surgery.

Patients with previous neurologic symptoms have less functional reserve, because they usually have some degree of permanent deficit even if their symptoms appear to have resolved.[69] Thus, previously neurologically symptomatic patients are more likely to be affected by a new neurologic insult. Symptomatic carotid artery stenosis at the time of cardiac surgery is an accepted indication for CEA before or during CABG, because this practice has been shown to improve neurologic outcome in neurologically symptomatic patients with carotid stenosis greater than 70%.[70] Therefore, every neurologically symptomatic patient scheduled for cardiac surgery should undergo preoperative carotid examination and, if necessary, CEA.

Clinical Management of Carotid Stenosis

The degree of carotid stenosis can be assessed easily with duplex ultrasound scanning. With color imaging that shows the flow pattern of blood in the obstructed vessel, duplex ultrasound has become a very accurate means of evaluating carotid disease. In fact, duplex ultrasound is 90% more sensitive than angiography for detecting carotid stenosis.[71]

The severity of both carotid and cardiac disease in a given patient should determine whether CABG and CEA should be simultaneous or staged. Patients with less severe cardiac disease (i.e., stable coronary disease and a good ejection fraction) and symptomatic carotid disease seem to benefit from CEA before CABG is performed.[72,73] However, the risk for perioperative myocardial infarction (MI) posed by preexisting coronary artery disease in this population should not be disregarded. In high-risk patients, simultaneous CEA and CABG surgery does not significantly increase the risk for perioperative stroke.[62] Furthermore, whether CEA is performed before or after the start of CPB does not appear to affect outcome. A systematic review of 94 series (describing 7863 procedures) of simultaneous CEA and CABG concluded that the best results were obtained when CEA was performed first, followed by off-pump CABG without aortic cross-clamping.[74] In summary, combined CEA and CABG is certainly an option for symptomatic patients.

Aortic Atherosclerosis

Prevalence and Clinical Importance

Moderate or severe atherosclerosis of the ascending aorta is among the most powerful predictors of stroke in cardiac surgery patients, and adverse cerebral outcome is closely associated with the presence of aortic atheroma.[75] Wolman and coworkers[4] reported a 15.7% incidence of overt neurologic injury in cardiac surgery patients with documented aortic atherosclerosis.

The prevalence of proximal aortic atherosclerosis increases with age. It is approximately 20% in CABG patients aged 50 to 59, 60% in those aged 60 to 69, and almost 80% in those aged 75 or older.[76] As the mean age of coronary revascularization patients increases, the clinical importance of thoracic aortic burden also increases.

Many authors cite the form, size, location, and other characteristics of aortic atheromas as important predictors of embolic events.[77,78] Greater plaque thickness (>4 mm), surface irregularity, and mobility of superimposed or noncalcified thrombi are associated with a high risk for embolism during surgery.[77] Cerebral emboli are more often associated with atheroma in the transverse aortic arch (31%) than with atheroma in the ascending (3%) or descending (17%) thoracic aorta.[78] Furthermore, the higher incidence of stroke in the left hemisphere than in the right suggests that emboli frequently originate in the aortic arch and move in the direction of blood flow to the downstream carotid vessel.[79]

Detecting Aortic Atherosclerosis

If moderate or severe aortic atherosclerosis is present, it is essential to detect it before or during surgery. Surgical palpation is the traditional intraoperative technique for assessing the ascending aorta. However, in a group of 50 cardiac surgery patients, visual inspection and palpation detected atherosclerotic aortic disease in only 12 patients, whereas ultrasonic imaging detected it in 29 patients.[80] Visual inspection and palpation, therefore, underestimate the prevalence and severity of aortic atherosclerosis. Still, this method of assessment is valuable, because the risk for perioperative stroke is four times higher in patients with palpable atheroma than in patients without palpable disease.[2]

Newer assessment techniques, such as transesophageal echocardiography (TEE), allow high-resolution imaging of the aortic wall, more accurate grading of atheromatous disease, and calculation of the atheroma burden as the percentage of the viewed aortic lumen area that is occupied by the plaques (Fig. 8-2). Additionally, TEE can detect far more emboli than is possible with transcranial Doppler ultrasonography (TCD), which used to be a standard technique for monitoring cerebral emboli in the middle cerebral arteries during CABG surgery.[81] (The lower number of emboli detected by TCD might be explained by the fact that only a fraction of the aortic emboli enter the cerebral circulation.) Nonetheless, the scope of TEE is limited by the interposition of the trachea and the left mainstem bronchus, which makes it impossible to completely visualize the area where the ascending aorta meets the arch—the most common site of atheroma and the usual site for aortic cannulation and cross-clamping. In general, TEE can be used to image the ascending aorta to a mean distance of 7.4 cm from the aortic annulus.

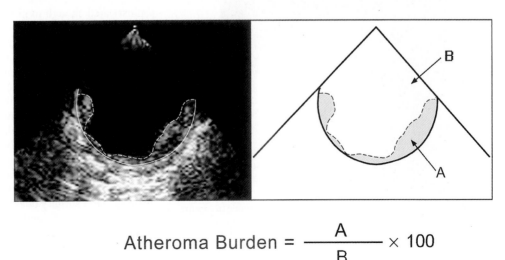

Figure 8-2 ■ The aortic atheroma burden is calculated from the transesophageal echocardiographic cross-section of the aorta. A, atherosclerotic plaques; B, aortic lumen area. (Reprinted from *Bar-Yosef S, Anders M, Mackensen GB, et al: Ann Thorac Surg 2004;78:1556-1563.* Copyright 2004, with permission from *Society of Thoracic Surgeons.*)

$$\text{Atheroma Burden} = \frac{A}{B} \times 100$$

In a retrospective analysis conducted by Fanshawe and coworkers,[82] up to 42% of the length of the ascending aorta could not be visualized with multiplane TEE, even though multiplane TEE produced more detailed views of the aorta than biplane TEE.

These limitations inspired the development of a new imaging modality: linear and phased-array direct epiaortic ultrasound (EAU). A high-frequency (5- or 7-MHz) transducer placed directly on the aorta provides multiple views of the distal ascending aorta (from the aortic annulus to the innominate artery) with far better resolution than that of TEE. This technique is even more sensitive than preoperative computed tomography and is, at present, the method of choice for gauging the severity of aortic arch atherosclerosis.[83] In clinical situations, a combination of TEE and EAU may be the most accurate means of assessing aortic atherosclerosis.[84] If TEE does not detect significant lesions in the descending aorta, there is a low likelihood of significant ascending aortic disease. However, a finding of atheroma in the descending aorta with TEE warrants further examination of the ascending aorta with EAU.

Preventing Embolization Related to Aortic Atherosclerosis

Most emboli detected by TCD occur near the start or end of CPB (i.e., during aortic cannulation, clamping, and declamping).[81,85-89] Various devices have been developed to catch or divert different types of potentially embolic aortic debris. For example, intra-aortic filters capture and extract fibrous atheromas and other particulate debris from the circulation before they can travel distally and occlude important cerebral blood vessels (Fig. 8-3). The filter is deployed into the aorta immediately before cross-clamp release and remains in place until the patient is weaned from bypass. Multiple trials have shown that intra-aortic filtration reduces the rate of cerebral events (e.g., stroke, TIA, and memory deficit) by 50% to 70% in CABG patients, especially those at high risk.[4,90,91] Additionally, Schmitz and colleagues[92] showed that an 80-year-old

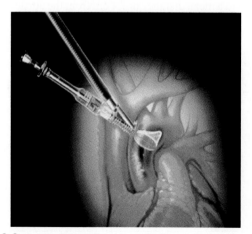

Figure 8-3 ■ The Embol-X intra-aortic filter is designed to capture emboli released during cardiac surgery. (Reprinted from *Banbury MK, Kouchoukos NT, Allen KB, et al: Ann Thorac Surg 2003;76:508-515.* Copyright 2003, with permission from *Society of Thoracic Surgeons.*)

patient with the filter has the same risk of developing an adverse neurologic event as a 55-year-old patient without the filter. Therefore, intra-aortic filtration may be especially beneficial for older adult patients.

Another device, the Cobra, is a dual-lumen aortic catheter that, when placed in the ascending aorta, profoundly reduces brain and ocular embolism while allowing independent temperature control in the aortic arch and descending aorta.[93,94] An inflatable wing shunts the emboli down the descending aorta by blocking the vessels that the emboli would normally enter. A study of the Cobra catheter in a porcine model of CABG showed a 90% reduction in cerebral embolism.[95]

Aortic manipulation, such as cross-clamping, side-clamping for proximal graft anastomosis, clamp removal, and aortic and cardioplegia cannula insertion, is integral to on-pump CABG. All of these actions can dislodge an atherosclerotic plaque or thrombus, causing embolism and ischemic damage to the brain.[96] Figure 8-4 shows the percentage of the total number of emboli detected in patients during each phase of CABG.[97] More than 50% of the signals produced by emboli could be attributed to a corresponding surgical manipulation. The remaining miscellaneous signals were often spontaneous and were of a lower magnitude. The majority of procedure-related emboli were detected during the clamping periods: 18.7% during cross-clamping and 22.4% during side-clamping. Therefore, cannulation options for CPB other than aortic cannulation should be considered. By using femoral or axillary cannulation, it is possible to avoid manipulating the atherosclerotic aorta, which is the main source of cerebral emboli.

Additionally, studies have shown that removing the "partial occluding" or "side-biting" clamp, in particular, is one of the three surgical maneuvers (along with cannulation and cardiac manipulation) that generate the most microemboli.[88,98] Therefore, using a single aortic cross-clamp, rather than both an aortic cross-clamp and a side-biting clamp, to avoid manipulating and clamping suspected emboligenic areas may reduce the risk for stroke.[98,99] Although single-clamp techniques require longer cross-clamp and bypass times, current techniques of myocardial preservation are sophisticated enough to minimize the additional risk.

Furthermore, placing proximal anastomoses on the subclavian vein or using internal mammary artery grafts and free conduits as sequential or Y-grafts may allow surgeons to perform complete revascularization without touching the ascending aorta or the aortic arch.[100] Another solution is off-pump coronary revascularization, which does not require cannulation and cross-clamping.[101] This procedure completely avoids aortic manipulation and, consequently, reduces the rate of cerebral emboli originating from aortic atheroma plaques. Thus, high-risk patients with proven aortic atheroma burden may especially benefit from off-pump CABG.

In contrast, prophylactic aortic arch endarterectomy during CABG surgery does not reduce the incidence of intraoperative stroke. Indeed, a clinical study has associated aortic arch endarterectomy with a 3.6-fold increase in the incidence of neurologic events in patients undergoing cardiac surgery.[102]

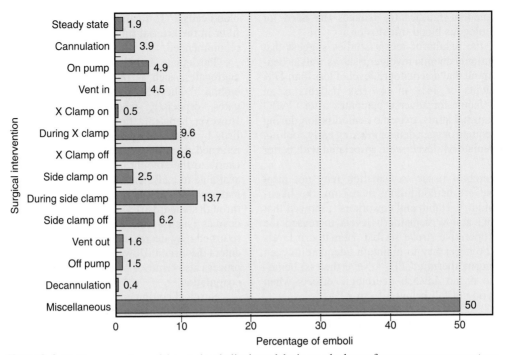

Figure 8-4 ■ The percentage of detected emboli released during each phase of on-pump coronary artery bypass surgery. *(Redrawn from Stump DA, Jones TJ, Rorie KD: J Cardiothorac Vasc Anesth 1999;13:600-613, with permission.)*

Perioperative Risk Factors

Cardiopulmonary Bypass

Cerebral Blood Flow

Despite significant technical and technological improvements, CPB itself remains a nonphysiologic procedure that causes significant pathologic changes. All circulating blood components are vulnerable to trauma associated with extracorporeal circulation, especially when artificial blood pumps are operated at high flow rates. The currently accepted CPB flow rate is 2.0 to 2.4 L/m^2/min, which is lower than the normal awake physiologic blood flow rate of about 3.2 L/m^2/min.

Several factors enable the brain to tolerate these lower flow rates. First, hypothermia during CPB reduces oxygen requirements; at 20°C, body oxygen consumption is reduced from its normothermic (37°C) rate of about 120 mL/m^2/min to about 33 mL/m^2/min. Second, reducing the blood flow rate does not have much effect on CBF, which is approximately 40 to 60 mL/100 g/min under normal conditions and about 20 to 60 mL/100 g/min during CPB. Third, the brain itself is relatively tolerant of reductions in CBF. Under normothermic conditions, ischemic brain-cell death occurs only when CBF is less than 10 mL/100 g/min; during hypothermia, the threshold is even lower.[103] Because conventional CPB does not produce such low levels of CBF, it is difficult to argue that a global reduction in cerebral perfusion is the cause of brain injury during extracorporeal circulation.

Pulsatile versus Nonpulsatile Perfusion

Currently, CPB is most often performed with nonpulsatile perfusion provided by either a roller pump or a centrifugal pump. Nonpulsatile perfusion causes an increase in vascular resistance that is presumably mediated by chemical vasoconstrictors. Nonetheless, whether nonpulsatile CPB compromises cerebral circulation and contributes to neurologic injury is unclear.

What is somewhat clear is that pulsatile perfusion improves CBF during CPB. A study of CBF in dogs on CPB showed that CBF was 19% higher in nonischemic brains and 55% higher in ischemic brains when pulsatile perfusion was used instead of nonpulsatile perfusion.[104] In humans, pulsatile perfusion during hypothermic bypass increases CBF by about 15%.[105,106] However, there are no data showing that the use of pulsatile CPB improves neurologic outcome. This may be because the relatively small aortic cannulas used in human CPB markedly dampen pulsatile waveforms.

Furthermore, pulsatile pumping systems require greater technological sophistication and thus are more expensive than common nonpulsatile pumping systems. Therefore, unless more data are produced to support it, expanded use of pulsatile flow is not likely.

Hemodilution

Inducing hemodilutional anemia (i.e., lowering hematocrit levels to approximately 20%) is a common practice in hypothermic CPB. The resulting reduction in blood viscosity is believed to reduce the risk for adverse outcomes caused by arterial hypertension (e.g., aortic dissection). Additionally, low hematocrit levels (<20%) have been assumed to minimize microcirculatory disturbances during CPB and, thereby, to improve cerebral perfusion and oxygen delivery.[107] Also, when combined with crystalloid priming techniques, induced hemodilutional anemia significantly reduces the need for intraoperative autologous blood transfusion.[108]

Nonetheless, the results of recent studies suggest that induced hemodilutional anemia involves risks as well as benefits. One study found that a hematocrit level of less than 17% in high-risk patients or 14% in low-risk patients is an independent risk factor for adverse outcomes after CABG surgery.[109] In an animal study, extreme hemodilution during CPB caused inadequate oxygen delivery during early cooling, whereas higher hematocrit levels were associated with better cerebral recovery.[110]

Generally, cerebral tissue oxygenation may not meet demand during severe hemodilution, increasing the likelihood of cerebral injury. Habib and coworkers[111] showed that performing CABG at low hematocrit levels increased the incidence of postoperative stroke sixfold. Hematocrit levels above 18% may be necessary to maintain adequate oxygen delivery during normothermic CPB.[112] Nevertheless, hemodilution has little or no adverse neurologic effects when hematocrit levels do not fall below 21% to 22%.[111]

Embolization during Cardiopulmonary Bypass

Embolic cerebral injury during CPB is caused by either macroembolism or microembolism. These two categories refer to the size of the occluded vessels: a macroembolism occludes a vessel greater than 200 μm in diameter, whereas a microembolism occludes a vessel less than 200 μm in diameter. These two types of embolism have different clinical manifestations: a single macroembolus can cause hemiplegia, whereas a solitary microembolus usually has no noticeable effect on neurologic outcome (except when it occludes a vessel in a very susceptible area, such as the retina). On the other hand, large numbers of microemboli can produce diffuse cerebral injury.

The size of an embolus is unrelated to its composition, which can be of several types. Gaseous emboli consist of air or anesthetic gas, particularly nitrous oxide. A large amount of air is introduced into the surgical field when a cardiac chamber is opened—for example, during valve repair or replacement. One possible way to reduce the number of emboli from this source is to flood the surgical field with CO_2 during cardiac procedures. The CO_2 is used to replace air in the operative field because the more soluble carbon dioxide may reduce the number and sequelae of gaseous emboli.

Air introduced through the arterial line can cause either microembolism or macroembolism. Changes in the partial pressure of blood gases (which is temperature dependent) can cause bubbles to form, especially during the rewarming phase of CPB. Historically, gaseous microemboli produced by bubble oxygenators were an important source of diffuse cerebral injury.[113] These microemboli formed because of the turbulence created by the bubbling of gas in blood. The use of in-line arterial filtration with bubble oxygenators reduces the number of these emboli, thereby reducing postoperative neurologic impairment. Nonetheless, membrane oxygenators are used more commonly today. They are thought to produce better neurologic outcomes than bubble oxygenators, because the oxygen diffuses passively through a semipermeable membrane, which prevents turbulence and the disruption of

blood cells.[113] To further reduce embolus formation, use of a filter in the arterial tubing of membrane oxygenators is also recommended.[114]

Particulate emboli most commonly consist of biologic aggregates, such as thrombi, platelet aggregates, and lipid emboli.[115] The CPB circuit generates platelet–fibrin aggregates, especially when heparinization is inadequate.[115] However, heparinization itself may contribute to lipid embolism by stimulating endothelial lipoprotein lipase. Blood returned from the surgical field can also contribute significantly to the amount of particulate or lipid-loaded material available to cause embolization. It is likely that most of this material is small enough or deformable enough to pass through standard arterial line filters. The use of blood salvage devices (such as cell-savers) to process blood before it is returned may decrease the amount of particulate matter that enters the circuit. However, the cell-saver's intrinsic washing process also removes platelets and clotting factors, impairing coagulation.

Surgical equipment may also be a source of emboli. For example, embolization by polyvinyl chloride or silicone tube fragments generated by the pump has been described.[116] Fortunately, several technical improvements made in recent years have reduced these hazards. Use of improved hemocompatible extracorporal circuits and membrane oxygenators with in-line arterial filtration has minimized the microembolic risk during CPB. Therefore, it is doubtful whether extracorporeal circulation per se still contributes importantly to cerebral injury after cardiac surgery.[117] Currently, most clinically overt cerebral emboli are related to atheroembolism rather than to CPB, as previously noted.

Mean Arterial Pressure during Cardiopulmonary Bypass

Autoregulation keeps CBF relatively constant over a wide range of arterial blood pressures. CBF is approximately 50 mL/100 g/min and depends mainly on the cerebral perfusion pressure (CPP), which is calculated as the mean arterial pressure (MAP) minus the intracranial pressure (ICP). Although the ICP is not commonly measured during cardiac surgery, CBF can be estimated indirectly by measuring the central venous pressure. In general, CPP and CBF remain relatively constant over a wide range of MAP levels because of autoregulation. In patients not undergoing CPB, perfusion-pressure autoregulation is less certain when MAP is less than 50 mm Hg or greater than 150 mm Hg, when CBF becomes pressure dependent. In patients with chronic hypertension and increased sympathetic tone, autoregulation may actually shift the pressure–flow relationship to the right (i.e., to higher pressures).

However, during CPB with moderate hypothermia and hemodilution, perfusion pressure seems not to be an important predictor of clinically apparent cerebral dysfunction. Of the many published studies of the influence of MAP or hypoperfusion during CPB on neurologic outcome, the majority show little or no relationship.[118,119] Additionally, one study found an association between lower arterial pressure during CPB (MAP <50 mm Hg) and lower risk for neurologic injury.[47] In summary, the preponderance of data suggests that during cardiac surgery, mechanisms other than hypoperfusion during CPB—primarily embolic phenomena—are responsible for most overt postoperative neurologic injury. Therefore, it is probably unnecessary to maintain a specific "high" arterial pressure during nonpulsatile, hypothermic, hemodiluted CPB.

In contrast, results of a study by Gold and coauthors[120] suggest that the MAP may influence neurologic outcome in some CABG patients. Notably, the authors pooled the mortality and the neurologic and cardiac outcome data to show that the combined morbidity and mortality was significantly lower in the high-pressure group than in the low-pressure one. An analysis by Hartman and colleagues[85] of data from a subset of Gold and colleagues' patient population revealed a trend indicating that patients with documented high-grade atherosclerosis had fewer strokes when relatively high mean arterial pressures (80 to 100 mm Hg) were maintained during CPB.

In cardiac surgery and other settings, it is possible that hypoperfusion and cerebral embolism often coexist and that their pathophysiology may be interactive.[121] Cerebral emboli may impair CBF autoregulation, making CBF more dependent on the MAP.[122] Also, reduced perfusion limits the ability of the bloodstream to "wash out" emboli and reduces the available blood flow to regions rendered ischemic by emboli that block nutrient arteries.[121] The brain border zones (i.e., the watershed areas) are a frequent destination for microemboli that are not cleared by the bloodstream.[89] Therefore, impaired washout may be an important but neglected phenomenon that is intertwined with hypoperfusion, embolization, and brain infarction. In conclusion, although embolization (from the atherosclerotic aorta or the carotids, or both) is probably the cause of most overt cerebral injury during cardiac surgery, maintaining collateral perfusion during CPB, after CPB, and throughout the postoperative period may be an effective way of reducing the severity of cerebral infarction.

Acid–Base Management

In general, hypercapnia causes cerebral vasodilation, whereas hypocapnia causes cerebral vasoconstriction. However, the solubility of carbon dioxide is dependent on temperature during hypothermic CPB. Decreasing body core temperature increases carbon dioxide solubility and, accordingly, reduces blood $PaCO_2$ levels, although the total amount of carbon dioxide remains constant.

General acid–base balance is defined as a pH of 7.4 and an arterial $PaCO_2$ of 40 mm Hg at normothermia (37°C). The two most commonly used methods of maintaining this balance during CPB are pH-stat management and α-stat management. In pH-stat management, blood gases are temperature corrected, and the arterial pH is maintained at 7.4 during CPB regardless of the core temperature. As blood pH rises during induced hypothermia, pH stability is maintained by reducing the total gas inflow rate to the oxygenator (i.e., the sweep speed) using two ventilating gases, O_2 and air. In contrast, in α-stat management, blood gases are not temperature corrected, the ratio (α) of dissociated to nondissociated imidazole groups of the histidine buffer system is kept constant, and no adjustment of CO_2 is required during hypothermic CPB.

Proponents of pH-stat management argue that it is more physiologic because it is similar to the way some animals adapt to temperature changes, as seen in poikilothermic animals and hibernating mammals.[123] Hypothermia shifts the oxyhemoglobin dissociation curve to the left; this shift may be aggravated by the alkalosis induced by α-stat management, so that oxygen delivery at the tissue level is impaired severely enough to cause tissue hypoxia and N-methyl-D-aspartate (NMDA) receptor activation.[124]

Maintaining normal or increased cerebral blood flow with the pH-stat strategy results in more homogeneous brain cooling and consequent greater reduction of oxygen consumption, better cerebral tissue oxygenation, less significant derangements in cerebral metabolism, and better behavioral recovery and survival in animal models than α-stat management.[107,125,126] A study of adult patients on CPB found that, compared with α-stat, the pH-stat strategy promoted an increase in the saturation of jugular venous oxygen ($SjVO_2$) and a decrease in arteriovenous oxygen and glucose differences.[127] Furthermore, evidence that infants undergoing deep hypothermic CPB have better postoperative overt neurologic outcomes and less morbidity with pH-stat management has led to the adoption of this strategy by most pediatric cardiac centers.[128]

However, although greater CBF indicates better cerebral perfusion, it may also cause more emboli. Proponents of α-stat management have asserted that reduced CBF during hypothermia with α-stat management reduces the delivery of emboli to the brain and may improve neuropsychological outcomes.[129] However, although animal studies have showed a decreased embolic load with α-stat management,[130] this finding has not been duplicated in prospective human studies.[131] Proponents of α-stat management also argue that it preserves cerebral flow–metabolism coupling and autoregulation of cerebral vasculature better than pH-stat management (although autoregulation is not eliminated with the pH-stat strategy).[132-134] At this time, no studies in the adult patient population have shown a clear advantage in morbidity or mortality outcomes for one blood gas management strategy over the other, although the majority of cardiac centers use α-stat management in adults undergoing CPB.

Inflammatory Response

Cardiopulmonary bypass is a form of extracorporeal circulation that uses circuits made from synthetic materials. Contact between the patient's circulating blood and the foreign surfaces of the CPB circuit causes a systemic inflammatory response that includes a coagulation cascade and the activation of fibrinolytic and complement pathways.[135] Inflammatory activity is also part of the body's normal response to the ischemia caused by embolization and hypoperfusion during cardiac surgery. The activation of the inflammatory cascade involves platelets, neutrophils, coagulation factors, kinins, and other vasoactive and inflammatory mediators and can result in either cellular repair or neuronal destruction.

It has been shown that this systemic inflammatory response is closely linked to the use of CPB in cardiac operations. Furthermore, cerebral magnetic resonance imaging of patients after cardiac surgical procedures has shown substantial diffuse brain swelling resulting in the loss of the normal appearance of the sulci and gyri.[136] This cerebral edema is presumably caused by an increase in capillary permeability, which is a feature of the systemic inflammatory response.

In contrast, none of this inflammatory activity appears to have detectable effects on postoperative neurologic function. Recent trials have not revealed any overall relationship between inflammatory mediators and postoperative neuropsychological changes in CABG patients. Additionally, there is no indication that inflammatory response contributes directly to cognitive decline after CPB. A prospective study of neurologic outcomes in CABG patients by Westaby and coworkers[137] found no association between elevated inflammatory markers and cerebral dysfunction. Studies comparing on-pump and off-pump cardiac surgery show that they are associated with similar incidences of postoperative neuropsychological dysfunction despite the significantly smaller inflammatory responses of the off-pump patients.[5,138-140] These findings suggest that it is unlikely that the inflammatory response to CPB is itself the cause of postoperative cognitive decline.

Temperature Control

Deliberate hypothermia is known to be a reliable method of neuroprotection during CABG, reducing the effects of cerebral ischemic injury from any cause. As shown in animal models, even mild hypothermia (as little as $1^\circ C$ to $2^\circ C$) minimizes the severity of cerebral ischemia. Additionally, inducing delayed mild hypothermia as late as 1 hour after the ischemic event is effective in postponing neuronal injury.

Various mechanisms, mostly studied in animal models, underlie the protective effects of hypothermia (Table 8-1). First, hypothermia may attenuate the effects of cerebral ischemia by creating a favorable balance between oxygen supply and demand, thereby decreasing $CMRO_2$. The relationship between temperature and metabolic activity can be expressed as Q10, which represents the amount by which global brain metabolism decreases for each $10^\circ C$ reduction in temperature.[141,142] The median value of Q10 has been reported as 2.8, but the relationship between temperature and metabolic rate really depends on the particular range of temperatures within which temperature change takes place.[143] Between $27^\circ C$ and $37^\circ C$, the mean Q10 value is 2.23. This value doubles to 4.53

at temperatures below $27^\circ C$. Therefore, the relationship between temperature and $CMRO_2$ is neither linear nor exponential. Furthermore, the reduction in metabolic rate does not correlate with the degree of cerebral protection provided by hypothermia.[143]

Other evidence suggests that hypothermia reduces not only the metabolic rate but also the delayed release of excitatory amino acids, neurotransmitters that play an important role in the process of neuronal death.[144] Additionally, lowering brain temperature is crucial to preventing blood–brain barrier dysfunction. Hypothermia reduces the permeability of brain arterioles and thus stabilizes these blood vessels' barrier function.[145] Furthermore, hypothermia may also interfere with the inflammatory response by suppressing polymorphonuclear leukocyte cell adhesion in the damaged region.[146,147]

In contrast, both intra-ischemic and delayed postischemic hyperthermia exacerbates the severity of neurologic injury. Even elevation of body temperature by as little as $2^\circ C$ has deleterious effects on cerebral protection and decreases cerebral tolerance to ischemia. As shown in several studies, hyperthermia delays neuronal metabolic recovery and increases excitotoxic neurotransmitter release, oxygen free radical production, intracellular acidosis, and blood–brain barrier permeability, causing multifocal breakdown at sites in the thalamus, hippocampus, and striatum (see Table 8-1).[148,149] Hyperthermia also affects protein kinase activity and destabilizes the cytoskeleton. Additionally, in hospitalized stroke patients, body temperature is associated with infarct size and mortality. Fever and hyperthermia worsen the prognosis; fever has been shown to independently predict poor outcome in stroke patients.[150]

In patients undergoing CPB, hypothermia is always initiated after aortic cannulation and the onset of bypass, but macroembolization of the brain is unlikely during this period because the heart is excluded from the circulation by the aortic cross-clamp. Thus, temperature management during this period minimally affects neurologic outcome. Rather, the two periods of highest risk for micro- and macroembolization occur near the start and the end of the CPB period. Near the start of CPB, aortic cannulation and cross-clamping are performed even though the brain is not yet cold. Near the end of CPB, the aortic cross-clamp is removed, usually after the patient has been rewarmed. Unfortunately, as many as half of all overt strokes associated with cardiac surgery may occur at the time of cross-clamp removal.[151]

During the rewarming period, cerebral hyperthermia aggravates any cerebral injury that has occurred.[152] Aggressive rewarming is commonly practiced to avoid the afterdrop in temperature that usually occurs after CPB is discontinued, but excessive rewarming during this period can cause cerebral hyperthermia at the exact moment when cerebral embolization is most likely. Therefore, rewarming should be started early enough to achieve stability of the desired temperature before CPB is terminated.

Awareness of the limitations of any temperature monitoring site is also crucial to successful temperature management. Brain parenchymal temperature cannot be directly measured during cardiac surgery; rather, it must be estimated

8-1	**Protective Effects of Hypothermia and Deleterious Effects of Hyperthermia on Cerebral Ischemia**

Hypothermia	Hyperthermia
Favorable balance between O_2 supply and demand	Imbalance between O_2 supply and demand
↓ Excitotoxic neurotransmitter release	↑ Excitotoxic neurotransmitter release
↓ Blood–brain barrier permeability	↑ Blood–brain barrier permeability
↓ Inflammatory response	↑ Inflammatory response
	↑ Free radical production
	↑ Intracellular acidosis
	Destabilizes cytoskeleton

from tympanic, nasopharyngeal, esophageal, rectal, bladder, or jugular venous bulb temperature. However, there is poor concordance between cerebral temperature and temperatures measured at most of these sites. The jugular bulb temperature should be considered the gold standard—the proximity of the jugular bulb to the carotid origins and the aortic cannula makes jugular bulb temperature the most similar to brain temperature.[153,154] For example, nasopharyngeal and esophageal temperatures are consistently lower (by as much as 2°C) than jugular venous bulb temperature during rewarming.[155] Bladder and rectal temperatures exhibit even larger differences from jugular bulb temperature throughout rewarming: more than 4°C for bladder (making bladder temperature virtually useless) and nearly 3°C for rectal temperature.[156] In summary, temperatures measured at the nasopharyngeal, esophageal, bladder, or rectal sites underestimate jugular bulb temperature during rewarming (Fig. 8-5), and bladder and rectal temperatures should never be used to guide rewarming.[153] Because monitoring jugular bulb temperature is not usually feasible, however, the temperature of the blood in the arterial line that exits the oxygenator provides a better indication of CBF during rewarming and a reasonable approximation of global brain temperature.[157]

When nasopharyngeal temperature is monitored, it should not be allowed to exceed 36.5°C to 37.0°C. (Both jugular bulb temperature and brain temperature are higher than nasopharyngeal temperature.) This practice prevents cerebral overheating and, consequently, avoids the exacerbation of recent brain injury. Some clinicians advocate weaning high-risk patients from CPB at a temperature that is slightly lower than normal (approximately 35°C to 36°C).[158] In a randomized controlled study, Nathan and colleagues[159] showed that patients rewarmed to a lower-than-normal temperature (34°C) were significantly less likely to have postoperative cognitive deficits than patients rewarmed to 37°C.[159]

Although this approach has advantages, the potential risks posed by postoperative hypothermia should not be disregarded. These include coagulopathy, hemodynamic instability, bleeding, and shivering, which increases myocardial oxygen consumption.[160,161] All of these factors must be considered in selecting the best rewarming technique for an individual patient.

Hyperthermia that develops after surgery may be just as hazardous as intraoperative hyperthermia. Temperatures exceeding 38.5°C are common during the first 48 hours after cardiac surgery, occurring in nearly 40% of patients.[162] This postoperative hyperthermia is known to be correlated with increased cognitive dysfunction 6 weeks after cardiac surgery.[163] Therefore, hyperthermia in the postoperative period should be treated with antipyretics and, if necessary, active body surface cooling.

In summary, patients on CPB should be rewarmed early and slowly. In patients at high risk for adverse neurologic outcomes, limited rewarming (up to 36°C) followed by gradual (i.e., 4-hour) surface warming to 37.0°C can prevent cerebral hyperthermia while minimizing the risk for postoperative hypothermia.[164]

Off-Pump Surgery

The possibility that CPB causes neurologic damage (through the mechanisms of nonpulsatile perfusion, increased inflammatory activity, platelet and complement activation, or embolus release as described earlier) helped to spur the development of off-pump coronary artery bypass grafting (OPCAB). OPCAB may have a significant impact on some of these risk factors. For example, OPCAB avoids the whole issue of appropriate temperature management during and after CPB. Additionally, OPCAB avoids the need for cannulation and cross-clamping, and, when internal mammary artery grafts are performed, there is no need to use a partially

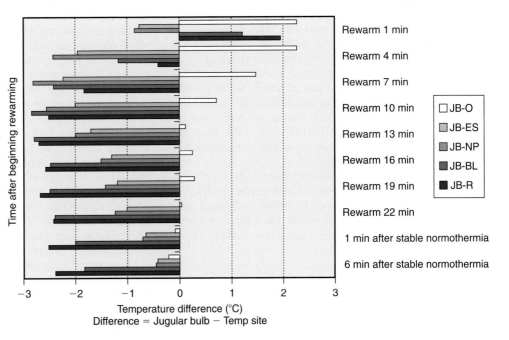

Figure 8-5 ■ Temperature differences between the jugular bulb (JB) and other sites during the rewarming phase of cardiopulmonary bypass. The number of subjects in the study was 28. BL, bladder; ES, esophagus; NP, nasopharynx; O, arterial outlet of the membrane oxygenator; R, rectum. *(Redrawn from Nussmeier NA, Li S, Strickler AG, et al: Temperature measurement during cardiopulmonary bypass. Anesth Analg 2002;94:35, with permission.)*

occluding or side-biting clamp while the proximal anastomoses are being made.[101] Thus, it is possible to avoid releasing aortic atherosclerotic debris that can cause embolism. In a prospective cohort study conducted by Watters and colleagues,[165] transcranial Doppler imaging detected more cerebral emboli in patients undergoing revascularization with CPB (median, 79; range, 38-876) than in patients having OPCAB (median, 3; range, 0-18). However, no postoperative neurologic deficits were seen in either of the study groups.

OPCAB has a few important disadvantages with regard to neuropsychological outcome. First, OPCAB depends on the use of internal mammary artery grafts, which makes it difficult to achieve complete revascularization in certain patients. This may be why Khan and coworkers[166] found poorer graft patency in OPCAB patients than in on-pump CABG patients 3 months after surgery. Second, OPCAB may itself pose unique risks to the brain because it often involves a relatively low MAP, use of the Trendelenburg position, and some degree of venous occlusion, all of which contribute to a relatively low cerebral perfusion pressure. Third, like on-pump CABG, OPCAB requires the use of sternotomy and heparin, so the inflammatory response is not completely avoided.

In some studies, when compared with conventional CABG with CPB, OPCAB improved in-hospital and 30-day mortality and reduced postoperative cognitive decline.[167,168] Murkin and colleagues[129] reported that OPCAB surgery resulted in a lower incidence of cognitive dysfunction at both short-term and mid-term postoperative follow-up than did conventional CABG. Additionally, Bucerius and coworkers[34] found that the use of OPCAB instead of conventional CABG might protect against postoperative delirium.

Other studies, however, show no particular advantage of OPCAB over CABG with CPB. A prospective study conducted by Taggart and colleagues[138] showed similar patterns of early decline and late recovery of cognitive function in patients undergoing CABG with and without CPB, suggesting that CPB is not an important cause of postoperative cognitive impairment. Another prospective study also detected no significant influence of CPB on the incidence of postoperative neuropsychological decline in bypass surgery patients.[5] Furthermore, a randomized, prospective study by Lloyd and coworkers[169] found that although S-100 protein concentrations were briefly elevated after CPB—indicating that the brain or the blood–brain barrier, or both, may be more adversely affected by CABG with CPB than by OPCAB—this elevation was not associated with detectable neuropsychological deterioration.

Unfortunately, no large, prospective trials have yet been conducted to investigate the potential benefits of OPCAB surgery for neurologic outcome. Therefore, individual surgeons must decide whether or not to use CPB in a given patient, taking all potential risk factors and adequacy of revascularization into account.

Intracardiac Surgery

Historically, intracardiac operations, such as valve replacements, carried a higher risk (4.2% to 13%) of overt cerebral injury than CABG procedures (0.6% to 5.2%).[170] However,

at least one study has reported that the incidence of CNS complications is higher in CABG surgery patients (11%) than in patients who undergo surgical valve repair or replacement (7%).[171] Apparently, the incidence of overt stroke during valve surgery has decreased during the past 2 decades, from approximately 4% in the 1980s to 2.6% in the late 1990s, whereas risk in CABG patients has increased because of older age and more severe atherosclerotic disease.[4,171,172]

Macroembolization by air or particulate matter from the surgical field is believed to be the main cause of CNS complications in intracardiac surgery patients.[170] Air embolism is more likely after open-chamber procedures, because large bubbles can remain trapped in the heart long after it is closed. In addition, patients who undergo open-chamber procedures usually have some valve calcification, valve vegetation, or intracardiac thrombus, all of which increase the risk for severe particulate embolization. As a result, the number of emboli detected by TCD during surgery is significantly higher in valve surgery patients than in CABG surgery patients.[171] However, one study found that valve repair surgery patients did not differ significantly from multiple-graft CABG patients in their incidences of neuropsychological deficit in the immediate postoperative period, although 6 months after surgery, the degree of improvement in neuropsychological status was greater in the CABG surgery patients.[5]

Combined Intracardiac Surgery and CABG

More than 100,000 combined cardiac procedures, such as CABG plus intracardiac surgery, are performed annually throughout the world. The incidence of concurrent CABG and mitral valve replacement has increased significantly in the past decade.[173]

There is considerable evidence that patients who undergo combined intracardiac procedures and CABG are at a particularly high risk for adverse neurologic outcomes. The incidence of overt stroke in patients who undergo concomitant CABG and intracardiac surgery is more than double that observed in patients who have isolated CABG surgery.[4] Additionally, patients who undergo combined elective mitral valve replacement and CABG have a significantly higher incidence of postoperative stroke (8.4%) than patients who undergo isolated mitral valve repair (3.4%).[174] In one study, 16% of patients who underwent combined cardiac procedures suffered an overt postoperative neurologic injury—fatal stroke, nonfatal stroke, or detectable deterioration in intellectual function.[4] Patients with postoperative stroke had a fourfold higher risk for hospital mortality than patients without neurologic deficit, and two thirds of these patients had to be discharged to rehabilitation facilities.

Several factors may contribute to the elevated risk for CNS complications seen in patients who have undergone combined procedures. For example, compared with patients who undergo isolated cardiac surgery, patients who undergo concomitant procedures tend to be older and are more likely to have cardiac valve calcification, moderate or severe aortic atherosclerosis, and other serious comorbidities. Combined procedures also require longer CPB and aortic cross-clamp durations than isolated procedures. In other words, patients undergoing combined procedures have all the cerebral risks inherent to each separate procedure, making their risk extraordinary.

In contrast, a study of CAD patients with mild-to-moderate aortic stenosis or regurgitation found that 14.5% of those who underwent CABG alone required reoperation, whereas only 6.5% of those who underwent combined CABG and valve replacement needed reoperation during a follow-up period of 3 years.[175] Although the patients in that study were not randomly assigned, the results show that a combined procedure might have advantages for patients with mild or moderate aortic stenosis. The decision to perform combined or separate procedures on a given patient should take into account all factors that may increase the patient's overall risk, such as left ventricular dysfunction, New York Heart Association class IV, history of congestive heart failure or myocardial infarction, and urgent surgery.[176]

Atrial Fibrillation

A number of cardiac surgery patients experience delayed strokes late in the postoperative period after an initial, neurologically uneventful recovery from anesthesia. In a retrospective study by Hogue and colleagues,[3] the overall stroke rate of patients undergoing cardiac surgery was 1.8%, and 65% of these were delayed strokes. The mechanisms responsible for these postoperative strokes are not well delineated. However, the occurrence of atrial fibrillation (AF) after cardiac surgery is increasingly recognized as a cause of delayed stroke. Cerebral embolism is a known complication of sustained AF in the nonsurgical setting, and even brief periods of AF can lead to left atrial thrombus formation.[177] A study of patients who had postoperative AF that lasted less than 48 hours found a 14% incidence of left atrial thrombus on transesophageal echocardiograms.[178]

In cardiac surgery patients, AF is a frequent complication in the postoperative period and is strongly linked with an increased risk for congestive heart failure, renal insufficiency, stroke, and prolonged hospitalization.[179,180] The incidence of AF is about 32% after CABG surgery, 42% after mitral valve replacement, 49% after aortic valve replacement, and 62% after combined CABG and valve procedures.[181] Additionally, as the mean age of cardiac surgical patients increases, so does the frequency of AF. Because cardiac surgical patients are in a hypercoagulable state during and after surgery, AF could easily predispose them to atrial thrombogenesis and subsequent embolization. Thus, AF probably plays a role in strokes that follow cardiac surgery and may cause as many as one third of postoperative strokes in CABG patients. A mean of 2.5 episodes of AF precedes the occurrence of stroke in these patients.[182] Another study found that AF was associated with a sixfold increase in the risk for postoperative stroke, and that AF preceded more than 50% of all postoperative strokes.[183] The majority of cardiac surgery patients who experienced a stroke had had a previous AF arrhythmic period (continuous or intermittent) of more than 48 hours.[183]

Even when it is hemodynamically tolerated, postoperative AF is associated with an increased stroke risk, especially when associated with low cardiac output syndrome.[3] Prior history of AF and low postoperative cardiac output are

independent risk factors for postoperative AF.[3,184] Other risk factors for AF include age-related structural changes in the atrium, such as dilation, muscle atrophy, decreased conduction tissue, and fibrosis. Additionally, inadequate cooling of the atria during hypothermic CPB and an early return of atrial electrical activity during aortic cross-clamping are associated with atrial conduction abnormalities and subsequent AF.[185] The electrophysiologic mechanism of postoperative AF is believed to derive from dissimilar atrial refractoriness after CPB. Alterations of atrial refractoriness by the autonomic nervous system that result in tachycardia or brief episodes of AF promote the maintenance of AF.[186]

The primary goals of AF treatment are ventricular rate control, anticoagulation, and conversion to sinus rhythm. β-Adrenergic receptor or calcium channel blockers can restore heart rate control in AF patients. In situations where these drugs are contraindicated, digoxin may be useful for slowing heart rate. The use of anticoagulation therapy must be balanced against the individual patient's risk for pericardial hemorrhage; anticoagulation is recommended for cardiac surgery patients with postoperative AF only when the arrhythmia is persistent or is associated with impaired left ventricular function. Early electrical cardioversion is indicated whenever AF is linked with hemodynamic deterioration. Antiarrhythmic drugs, such as amiodarone, procainamide, and propafenone, may convert post-CABG AF to sinus rhythm. β-Blockers are effective as prophylaxis for postoperative AF, reducing the incidence by 50% or more, whereas calcium channel blockers or procainamide do not appear to prevent postoperative AF.[187] Amiodarone, which has predominantly class III antiarrhythmic effects, has also been tested as a means of AF prophylaxis.[179]

■ NONCARDIAC SURGERY

Intraoperative and postoperative neurologic complications are most common in the cardiac surgical population, with a reported incidence of approximately 1% to 8%.[2-4] Most patients who undergo cardiac surgery have multiple preoperative risk factors, and the use of CPB may contribute additional risk (see Cardiac Surgery, earlier). Nonetheless, these patients are not the only population at risk for CNS complications. For example, patients undergoing carotid endarterectomy have a similar (i.e., 2% to 6%) reported risk for perioperative stroke.[188,189] Additionally, patients undergoing neurosurgery, including surgery for cerebral aneurysm or arteriovenous malformation, are at risk for cerebral ischemia.[190] As with cardiac surgical patients, identification of perioperative risk factors (as well as intraoperative management of arterial pressure, blood glucose, $PaCO_2$, and body temperature) is important in patients undergoing other types of surgical intervention.

Advanced Age

In older adult patients, prolonged postoperative cognitive dysfunction is relatively common, regardless of the type of surgery.[191,192] One study found that 5% of total knee replacement patients who were older than 70 years still had cognitive dysfunction 6 months after surgery.[193] Another prospective study of patients undergoing major noncardiac surgery noted persistent cognitive deficit 3 months postoperatively in 14% of patients who were older than 70.[192]

Age-related morphologic and biochemical changes may account for these findings. Neuronal size and number, as well as the number of synapses, decline with age, and this decline accelerates after the age of 60.[194,195] Hippocampal cholinergic neurons and Purkinje cells are reduced, and neurotransmitter systems (such as the central cholinergic system) are also altered during aging.[196] These age-related changes in the brain make older adult patients more susceptible to cognitive dysfunction after surgeries involving certain anesthetic agents, including meperidine (odds ratio, 2.7) and benzodiazepine (odds ratio, 3.0).[197] Additionally, anticholinergic agents such as atropine and scopolamine, which are commonly used during anesthesia, may aggravate a preexisting cholinergic deficit and cause postoperative cognitive dysfunction.[198]

Interestingly, the type of anesthesia administered (i.e., general or spinal/epidural) does not influence the risk for postoperative cognitive dysfunction. A randomized prospective trial investigated the effect of epidural versus general anesthesia on postoperative cognitive function in older patients undergoing orthopedic surgery.[193] Assessment of memory, psychomotor, and language skills 1 week and 6 months after surgery revealed no significant differences between the two groups. Moreover, the findings of a systematic review of 19 randomized and four nonrandomized trials support the hypothesis that spinal/epidural anesthetic techniques are not associated with better postoperative cognitive function than general anesthetic techniques. This lack of difference is due in part to the concomitant use of intravenous sedation during regional anesthesia.[199]

Mean Arterial Pressure

Cerebral blood flow is autoregulated by cerebral perfusion pressure, which ranges from 60 to 150 mm Hg, as described under Cardiac Surgery, earlier. A minimal CPP of 60 mm Hg can usually ensure maintenance of adequate CBF during surgery. However, during cerebral ischemia, autoregulation is attenuated or abolished in the ischemic region. Under these circumstances, a CPP of 60 mm Hg may or may not be sufficient for adequate cerebral perfusion. In one study of patients with severe head injury, increasing CPP from 60 to 70 mm Hg improved cerebral oxygen delivery (indicated by a significant rise in jugular bulb venous oxygen saturation and a reduction in the cerebral arteriovenous oxygen difference).[200] However, further augmentation of CPP beyond 70 mm Hg produced no additional improvement in cerebral oxygen delivery, suggesting that autoregulation became the main determinant of adequate cerebral perfusion above this threshold. Another prospective trial measured the effects of induced hypertension on cerebral perfusion in patients with ischemic stroke.[201] An increase in MAP from approximately 80 to 110 mm Hg was associated with an increase in CPP from approximately 70 to 100 mm Hg, without a clinically significant rise in intracranial pressure.[201] Moreover, in other studies, inducing arterial hypertension (i.e., increasing

arterial systolic pressure by 20%, without exceeding 200 mm Hg) in patients suffering from acute stroke apparently improved neurologic outcome without significantly increasing the risk for cardiac arrhythmia or cerebral hemorrhage.[202,203] Nonetheless, the increased risk for cerebral bleeding associated with elevated blood pressure should not be underestimated. Therefore, blood pressure should be increased gradually in patients with acute stroke.

Certainly, hypotension can increase cerebral infarct volume and, thus, increase the risk for adverse outcome in patients with stroke or head injury.[204] Firm guidelines, including a target threshold for CPP, have yet to be established. Therefore, appropriate blood pressure management must be individually determined for each patient.

Blood Glucose Management

Intraoperative hyperglycemia increases the supply of glucose to the brain, which can cause significant lactic acid production and metabolic acidosis when cerebral hypoperfusion is present. Several studies suggest a close relationship between decreased blood pH (caused by metabolic acidosis) and the degree of subsequent neuronal damage.[205-207] In a rat model, preexisting hyperglycemia aggravated neuronal brain damage caused by an ischemic event.[205] In contrast, pre-ischemic normoglycemia was associated with less hippocampal damage. In humans, differences have been noted between diabetic and nondiabetic patients who were hospitalized for ischemic stroke.[208] Diabetic patients with stroke had a significantly worse neurologic outcome, including a greater number of stroke-related deaths ($P < .05$).[208] Furthermore, although randomized prospective trials are pending, the results of a retrospective study indicate that hyperglycemia (plasma glucose concentration >140 mg/dL) may independently predict poor prognosis after stroke.[209]

Intraoperative hypoglycemia is also associated with neuronal brain damage. Blood glucose levels below 40 mg/dL cause electroencephalographic suppression and aggravate seizure activity. Furthermore, severe hypoglycemia (blood glucose level <20 mg/dL) causes neuronal necrosis by damaging the neuronal cell membrane, particularly in the superficial layers of the cortex and in the hippocampal region.[210] Hence, target blood glucose levels between 100 and 140 mg/dL are recommended for patients at risk for cerebral ischemia.[211] Maintaining this level necessitates frequent intraoperative monitoring of blood glucose levels.

Acid–Base Management

As described earlier under Cardiac Surgery, arterial carbon dioxide concentration and CBF are closely linked. Hyperventilation-induced hypocapnia reduces CBF and thereby minimizes intracranial volume and pressure. Thus, patients with elevated intracranial pressures (e.g., patients with expanding cerebral masses) might benefit from short-term intraoperative hyperventilation. However, a prospective randomized trial found that, in patients with severe head injury, intraoperative hyperventilation was associated with poorer neurologic outcome 3 and 6 months after trauma.[212] Based on these findings, guidelines prepared by the Brain Trauma

Foundation suggest that hyperventilation should be avoided during the first 5 days after traumatic head injury.[213]

Furthermore, intraoperative hypocapnia in patients with ischemic cerebral lesions can enhance neuronal damage.[214-216] In one study, hyperventilation in patients with cerebral infarction reduced regional CBF, but primarily in brain regions not affected by ischemic injury.[217] These findings suggest that there is abnormal arterial vasoconstriction at baseline in ischemia-injured brain regions, which may result from decreased metabolic function and reduced ability of the arterial endothelium to extract CO_2. As a result, arterial vessels cannot further constrict in response to hypocapnia. However, CBF reactivity to hypercapnia increases markedly in ischemic areas of the brain.[217] In summary, clinicians should be aware that the application of prophylactic intraoperative hyperventilation may aggravate cerebral injury in patients with ischemic or traumatic brain lesions.

Temperature Control

There is an inverse relationship between the brain's tolerance to ischemia and brain temperature. Neuronal damage occurs after 5 minutes of cerebral ischemia during normothermia, whereas hypothermia with a temperature of $16°C$ enables the brain to tolerate ischemia for up to 30 minutes.[218] For this reason, moderate or deep hypothermia is sometimes used during cardiopulmonary bypass, as described earlier under Cardiac Surgery. However, there is growing evidence that even a small reduction in body temperature (i.e., to $33°C$ to $34°C$) markedly improves the brain's tolerance to intraoperative ischemia.[219-221] For example, in a study in which the middle cerebral arteries of rats were temporarily occluded, measured ischemic infarct volume was 48% less in rats maintained at $33°C$ than in rats maintained at $37°C$.[221] However, hypothermia did not reduce infarct volume when the cerebral vessel was permanently occluded.

The efficacy of intraoperative mild hypothermia in humans remains controversial.[222] A recent randomized study found that, in patients undergoing cerebral aneurysm clipping after acute subarachnoid aneurysmal hemorrhage, neurologic outcome was no better with intraoperative hypothermia (in which surface cooling techniques were used to lower esophageal temperature to a target temperature of $33.5°C$) than with normothermia (target temperature of $36.5°C$).[223] On the other hand, intraoperatively induced mild hypothermia during neurosurgery does not appear to increase morbidity or mortality.[224] Hence, the therapeutic use of mild intraoperative hypothermia may be considered when prolonged temporary cerebral occlusion is required (e.g., in patients with high-grade cerebral aneurysms). Certainly, any increase in brain temperature during or after cerebral ischemia may aggravate neuronal damage and should be avoided.[225]

■ CONCLUSION

Great strides have been made in recent decades toward the prevention of perioperative strokes, particularly in cardiac surgery patients. Nonetheless, although many strokes may be preventable, they are not entirely predictable or readily diagnosed in the anesthetized patient. Furthermore, no magic bullet for amelioration has been developed. Finally, the etiologies, neuropathologic evidence, and long-term importance of the more subtle neuropsychological deficits that are present in many patients after cardiac surgery are uncertain. Clearly, protection of the central nervous system remains a fertile field for further research.

■ ACKNOWLEDGMENT

We thank Stephen N. Palmer, PhD, ELS, for providing editorial support.

■ REFERENCES

1. American Heart Association: Heart Disease and Stroke Statistics—2005 update. Dallas, American Heart Association, 2004.
2. Roach GW, Kanchuger M, Mangano CM, et al: Adverse cerebral outcomes after coronary bypass surgery. Multicenter Study of Perioperative Ischemia Research Group and the Ischemia Research and Education Foundation Investigators. N Engl J Med 1996;335:1857-1863.
3. Hogue CW Jr, Murphy SF, Schechtman KB, Davila-Roman VG: Risk factors for early or delayed stroke after cardiac surgery. Circulation 1999;100:642-647.
4. Wolman RL, Nussmeier NA, Aggarwal A, et al: Cerebral injury after cardiac surgery: Identification of a group at extraordinary risk. Multicenter Study of Perioperative Ischemia Research Group (McSPI) and the Ischemia Research Education Foundation (IREF) Investigators. Stroke 1999;30:514-522.
5. Andrew MJ, Baker RA, Bennetts J, et al: A comparison of neuropsychologic deficits after extracardiac and intracardiac surgery. J Cardiothorac Vasc Anesth 2001;15:9-14.
6. Nussmeier NA: Neuropsychiatric complications of cardiac surgery. J Cardiothorac Vasc Anesth 1994;8(Suppl 1):13-18.
7. Baskett R, Buth K, Ghali W, et al: Outcomes in octogenarians undergoing coronary artery bypass grafting. Can Med Assoc J 2005;172:1183-1186.
8. McKhann GM, Goldsborough MA, Borowicz LM Jr, et al: Predictors of stroke risk in coronary artery bypass patients. Ann Thorac Surg 1997;63:516-521.
9. Hammon JW Jr, Stump DA, Kon ND, et al: Risk factors and solutions for the development of neurobehavioral changes after coronary artery bypass grafting. Ann Thorac Surg 1997;63:1613-1618.
10. Graham NL, Emery T, Hodges JR: Distinctive cognitive profiles in Alzheimer's disease and subcortical vascular dementia. J Neurol Neurosurg Psychiatry 2004;75:61-71.
11. Tardiff BE, Newman MF, Saunders AM, et al: Preliminary report of a genetic basis for cognitive decline after cardiac operations. The Neurologic Outcome Research Group of the Duke Heart Center. Ann Thorac Surg 1997;64:715-720.
12. Traykov L, Baudic S, Thibaudet MC, et al: Neuropsychological deficit in early subcortical vascular dementia: Comparison to Alzheimer's disease. Dement Geriatr Cogn Disord 2002;14:26-32.
13. Hogue CW Jr, Barzilai B, Pieper KS, et al: Sex differences in neurological outcomes and mortality after cardiac surgery: A Society of Thoracic Surgery national database report. Circulation 2001;103:2133-2137.
14. Hogue CW Jr, De Wet CJ, Schechtman KB, Davila-Roman VG: The importance of prior stroke for the adjusted risk of neurologic injury after cardiac surgery for women and men. Anesthesiology 2003;98:823-829.
15. Edwards FH, Carey JS, Grover FL, et al: Impact of gender on coronary bypass operative mortality. Ann Thorac Surg 1998;66:125-131.
16. Herlitz J, Brandrup-Wognsen G, Karlson BW, et al: Mortality, risk indicators of death, mode of death and symptoms of angina pectoris during 5 years after coronary artery bypass grafting in men and women. J Intern Med 2000;247:500-506.

17. Abramov D, Tamariz MG, Sever JY, et al: The influence of gender on the outcome of coronary artery bypass surgery. Ann Thorac Surg 2000;70:800-805.

18. Aldea GS, Gaudiani JM, Shapira OM, et al: Effect of gender on postoperative outcomes and hospital stays after coronary artery bypass grafting. Ann Thorac Surg 1999;67:1097-1103.

19. Williams MR, Choudhri AF, Morales DL, et al: Gender differences in patients undergoing coronary artery bypass surgery, from a mandatory statewide database. J Gend Specif Med 2000;3:41-48.

20. Woods SE, Noble G, Smith JM, Hasselfeld K: The influence of gender in patients undergoing coronary artery bypass graft surgery: An eight-year prospective hospitalized cohort study. J Am Coll Surg 2003;196:428-434.

21. Mendes LA, Jacobs AK, Davidoff R, Ryan TJ: The gender paradox. Rev Port Cardiol 1999;18(Suppl 3):III21-24.

22. Fisher LD, Kennedy JW, Davis KB, et al: Association of sex, physical size, and operative mortality after coronary artery bypass in the Coronary Artery Surgery Study (CASS). J Thorac Cardiovasc Surg 1982;84:334-341.

23. Habib RH, Zacharias A, Schwann TA, et al: Worse early outcomes in women after coronary artery bypass grafting: Is it simply a matter of size? J Thorac Cardiovasc Surg 2004;128:487-488.

24. Vaccarino V, Lin ZQ, Kasl SV, et al: Sex differences in health status after coronary artery bypass surgery. Circulation 2003;108:2642-2647.

25. Vaccarino V, Lin ZQ, Kasl SV, et al: Gender differences in recovery after coronary artery bypass surgery. J Am Coll Cardiol 2003;41:307-314.

26. Bakir S, Mori T, Durand J, et al: Estrogen-induced vasoprotection is estrogen receptor dependent: Evidence from the balloon-injured rat carotid artery model. Circulation 2000;101:2342-2344.

27. Mori T, Durand J, Chen Y, et al: Effects of short-term estrogen treatment on the neointimal response to balloon injury of rat carotid artery. Am J Cardiol 2000;85:1276-1279.

28. Li G, Chen YF, Kelpke SS, et al: Estrogen attenuates integrin-beta-dependent adventitial fibroblast migration after inhibition of osteopontin production in vascular smooth muscle cells. Circulation 2000;101:2949-2955.

29. Oparil S, Chen SJ, Chen YF, et al: Estrogen attenuates the adventitial contribution to neointima formation in injured rat carotid arteries. Cardiovasc Res 1999;44:608-614.

30. White CR, Shelton J, Chen SJ, et al: Estrogen restores endothelial cell function in an experimental model of vascular injury. Circulation 1997;96:1624-1630.

31. Rossouw JE, Anderson GL, Prentice RL, et al: Risks and benefits of estrogen plus progestin in healthy postmenopausal women: Principal results from the Women's Health Initiative randomized controlled trial. JAMA 2002;288:321-333.

32. Lane JS, Shekherdimian S, Moore WS: Does female gender or hormone replacement therapy affect early or late outcome after carotid endarterectomy? J Vasc Surg 2003;37:568-574.

33. Frye RL, Kronmal R, Schaff HV, et al: Stroke in coronary artery bypass graft surgery: An analysis of the CASS experience. The participants in the Coronary Artery Surgery Study. Int J Cardiol 1992;36:213-221.

34. Bucerius J, Gummert JF, Borger MA, et al: Stroke after cardiac surgery: A risk factor analysis of 16,184 consecutive adult patients. Ann Thorac Surg 2003;75:472-478.

35. Engelman DT, Cohn LH, Rizzo RJ: Incidence and predictors of TIAs and strokes following coronary artery bypass grafting: Report and collective review. Heart Surg Forum 1999;2:242-245.

36. Reich DL, Bodian CA, Krol M, et al: Intraoperative hemodynamic predictors of mortality, stroke, and myocardial infarction after coronary artery bypass surgery. Anesth Analg 1999;89:814-822.

37. Ali Ozatik M, Kamil Gol M, Fansa I, et al: Risk factors for stroke following coronary artery bypass operations. J Card Surg 2005;20:52-57.

38. Amory DW, Grigore A, Amory JK, et al: Neuroprotection is associated with beta-adrenergic receptor antagonists during cardiac surgery: Evidence from 2,575 patients. J Cardiothorac Vasc Anesth 2002;16:270-277.

39. Savitz SI, Erhardt JA, Anthony JV, et al: The novel beta-blocker, carvedilol, provides neuroprotection in transient focal stroke. J Cereb Blood Flow Metab 2000;20:1197-1204.

40. Amenta F, Mignini F, Rabbia F, et al: Protective effect of antihypertensive treatment on cognitive function in essential hypertension: Analysis of published clinical data. J Neurol Sci 2002;203-204:147-151.

41. Ogunniyi A, Talabi O: Cerebrovascular complications of hypertension. Niger J Med 2001;10:158-161.

42. Toyoda K, Fujii K, Ibayashi S, et al: Attenuation and recovery of brain stem autoregulation in spontaneously hypertensive rats. J Cereb Blood Flow Metab 1998;18:305-310.

43. Strandgaard S, Paulson OB: Cerebral blood flow in untreated and treated hypertension. Neth J Med 1995;47:180-184.

43a. Herlitz J, Wognsen GB, Emanuelsson H, et al: Mortality and morbidity in diabetic and nondiabetic patients during a 2-year period after coronary artery bypass grafting. Diabetes Care 1996;19:698-703.

43b. Morricone L, Ranucci M, Denti S, et al: Diabetes and complications after cardiac surgery: Comparison with a non-diabetic population. Acta Diabetol 1999;36:77-80.

44. Pallas F, Larson DF: Cerebral blood flow in the diabetic patient. Perfusion 1996;11:363-370.

45. Croughwell N, Lyth M, Quill TJ, et al: Diabetic patients have abnormal cerebral autoregulation during cardiopulmonary bypass. Circulation 1990;82(5 Suppl):IV407-412.

46. Metz S, Keats AS: Benefits of a glucose-containing priming solution for cardiopulmonary bypass. Anesth Analg 1991;72:428-434.

47. van Wermeskerken GK, Lardenoye JW, Hill SE, et al: Intraoperative physiologic variables and outcome in cardiac surgery: Part II. Neurologic outcome. Ann Thorac Surg 2000;69:1077-1083.

48. Chaney MA, Nikolov MP, Blakeman BP, Bakhos M: Attempting to maintain normoglycemia during cardiopulmonary bypass with insulin may initiate postoperative hypoglycemia. Anesth Analg 1999;89:1091-1095.

49. Hirotani T, Kameda T, Kumamoto T, et al: Stroke after coronary artery bypass grafting in patients with cerebrovascular disease. Ann Thorac Surg 2000;70:1571-1576.

50. D'Agostino RS, Svensson LG, Neumann DJ, et al: Screening carotid ultrasonography and risk factors for stroke in coronary artery surgery patients. Ann Thorac Surg 1996;62:1714-1723.

51. Rath PC, Agarwala MK, Dhar PK, et al: Carotid artery involvement in patients of atherosclerotic coronary artery disease undergoing coronary artery bypass grafting. Indian Heart J 2001;53:761-765.

52. Naylor AR, Mehta Z, Rothwell PM, Bell PR: Carotid artery disease and stroke during coronary artery bypass: A critical review of the literature. Eur J Vasc Endovasc Surg 2002;23:283-294.

53. Faggioli GL, Curl GR, Ricotta JJ: The role of carotid screening before coronary artery bypass. J Vasc Surg 1990;12:724-729.

54. Chi OZ, Wei HM, Tse J, et al: Cerebral microregional oxygen balance during chronic versus acute hypertension in middle cerebral artery occluded rats. Anesth Analg 1996;82:587-592.

55. Hertzer NR, Ouriel K: Results of carotid endarterectomy: The gold standard for carotid repair. Semin Vasc Surg 2000;13:95-102.

56. Demopoulos LA, Tunick PA, Bernstein NE, et al: Protruding atheromas of the aortic arch in symptomatic patients with carotid artery disease. Am Heart J 1995;129:40-44.

57. Rorick MB, Furlan AJ: Risk of cardiac surgery in patients with prior stroke. Neurology 1990;40:835-837.

58. Almassi GH, Sommers T, Moritz TE, et al: Stroke in cardiac surgical patients: Determinants and outcome. Ann Thorac Surg 1999;68:391-397.

59. Rao V, Christakis GT, Weisel RD, et al: Risk factors for stroke following coronary bypass surgery. J Card Surg 1995;10(4 Suppl):468-474.

60. Ghosh J, Murray D, Khwaja N, et al: The influence of asymptomatic significant carotid disease on mortality and morbidity in patients undergoing coronary artery bypass surgery. Eur J Vasc Endovasc Surg 2005;29:88-90.

61. Hines GL, Scott WC, Schubach SL, et al: Prophylactic carotid endarterectomy in patients with high-grade carotid stenosis undergoing coronary bypass: Does it decrease the incidence of perioperative stroke? Ann Vasc Surg 1998;12:23-27.

62. Ricotta JJ, Char DJ, Cuadra SA, et al: Modeling stroke risk after coronary artery bypass and combined coronary artery bypass and carotid endarterectomy. Stroke 2003;34:1212-1217.

63. Terramani TT, Rowe VL, Hood DB, et al: Combined carotid endarterectomy and coronary artery bypass grafting in asymptomatic carotid artery stenosis. Am Surg 1998;64:993-997.

64. Rockman CB, Su W, Lamparello PJ, et al: A reassessment of carotid endarterectomy in the face of contralateral carotid occlusion: Surgical results in symptomatic and asymptomatic patients. J Vasc Surg 2002;36:668-673.

65. Rockman CB, Riles TS, Lamparello PJ, et al: Natural history and management of the asymptomatic, moderately stenotic internal carotid artery. J Vasc Surg 1997;25:423-431.

66. Suematsu Y, Nakano K, Sasako Y, et al: Strategies for CABG patients with carotid artery disease and perioperative neurological complications. Heart Vessels 2000;15:129-134.

67. Blaser T, Hofmann K, Buerger T, et al: Risk of stroke, transient ischemic attack, and vessel occlusion before endarterectomy in patients with symptomatic severe carotid stenosis. Stroke 2002;33:1057-1062.

68. Yoon BW, Bae HJ, Kang DW, et al: Intracranial cerebral artery disease as a risk factor for central nervous system complications of coronary artery bypass graft surgery. Stroke 2001;32:94-99.

69. Cramer SC: Functional imaging in stroke recovery. Stroke 2004;35(11 Suppl 1):2695-2698.

70. Rothwell PM, Eliasziw M, Gutnikov SA, et al: Endarterectomy for symptomatic carotid stenosis in relation to clinical subgroups and timing of surgery. Lancet 2004;363:915-924.

71. Belsky M, Gaitini D, Goldsher D, et al: Color-coded duplex ultrasound compared to CT angiography for detection and quantification of carotid artery stenosis. Eur J Ultrasound 2000;12:49-60.

72. Stoneburner JM, Nishanian GP, Cukingnan RA, Carey JS: Carotid endarterectomy using regional anesthesia: A benchmark for stenting. Am Surg 2002;68:1120-1123.

73. Brown KR: Treatment of concomitant carotid and coronary artery disease: Decision-making regarding surgical options. J Cardiovasc Surg (Torino) 2003;44:395-399.

74. Naylor R, Cuffe RL, Rothwell PM, et al: A systematic review of outcome following synchronous carotid endarterectomy and coronary artery bypass: Influence of surgical and patient variables. Eur J Vasc Endovasc Surg 2003;26:230-241.

75. Djaiani G, Fedorko L, Borger M, et al: Mild to moderate atheromatous disease of the thoracic aorta and new ischemic brain lesions after conventional coronary artery bypass graft surgery. Stroke 2004;35: e356-358.

76. Wareing TH, Davila-Roman VG, Barzilai B, et al: Management of the severely atherosclerotic ascending aorta during cardiac operations: A strategy for detection and treatment. J Thorac Cardiovasc Surg 1992;103:453-462.

77. Sheikhzadeh A, Ehlermann P: Atheromatous disease of the thoracic aorta and systemic embolism: Clinical picture and therapeutic challenge. Z Kardiol 2004;93:10-17.

78. Trehan N, Mishra M, Kasliwal RR, Mishra A: Reduced neurological injury during CABG in patients with mobile aortic atheromas: A five-year follow-up study. Ann Thorac Surg 2000;70:1558-1564.

79. Mackensen GB, Ti LK, Phillips-Bute BG, et al: Cerebral embolization during cardiac surgery: Impact of aortic atheroma burden. Br J Anaesth 2003;91:656-661.

80. Marshall WG Jr, Barzilai B, Kouchoukos NT, Saffitz J: Intraoperative ultrasonic imaging of the ascending aorta. Ann Thorac Surg 1989; 48:339-344.

81. Barbut D, Yao FS, Hager DN, et al: Comparison of transcranial Doppler ultrasonography and transesophageal echocardiography to monitor emboli during coronary artery bypass surgery. Stroke 1996;27:87-90.

82. Fanshawe M, Ellis C, Habib S, et al: A retrospective analysis of the costs and benefits related to alterations in cardiac surgery from routine intraoperative transesophageal echocardiography. Anesth Analg 2002;95:824-827.

83. Sylivris S, Calafiore P, Matalanis G, et al: The intraoperative assessment of ascending aortic atheroma: Epiaortic imaging is superior to both transesophageal echocardiography and direct palpation. J Cardiothorac Vasc Anesth 1997;11:704-707.

84. Wilson MJ, Boyd SY, Lisagor PG, et al: Ascending aortic atheroma assessed intraoperatively by epiaortic and transesophageal echocardiography. Ann Thorac Surg 2000;70:25-30.

85. Hartman GS, Yao FS, Bruefach M III, et al: Severity of aortic atheromatous disease diagnosed by transesophageal echocardiography predicts stroke and other outcomes associated with coronary artery surgery: A prospective study. Anesth Analg 1996;83:701-708.

86. van der Linden J, Casimir-Ahn H: When do cerebral emboli appear during open heart operations? A transcranial Doppler study. Ann Thorac Surg 1991;51:237-241.

87. Barbut D, Hinton RB, Szatrowski TP, et al: Cerebral emboli detected during bypass surgery are associated with clamp removal. Stroke 1994;25:2398-2402.

88. Clark RE, Brillman J, Davis DA, et al: Microemboli during coronary artery bypass grafting: Genesis and effect on outcome. J Thorac Cardiovasc Surg 1995;109:249-257.

89. Barbut D, Grassineau D, Lis E, et al: Posterior distribution of infarcts in strokes related to cardiac operations. Ann Thorac Surg 1998;65: 1656-1659.

90. Wimmer-Greinecker G: Reduction of neurologic complications by intra-aortic filtration in patients undergoing combined intracardiac and CABG procedures. Eur J Cardiothorac Surg 2003;23:159-164.

91. Schmitz C, Blackstone EH: International Council of Emboli Management (ICEM) Study Group results: Risk adjusted outcomes in intraaortic filtration. Eur J Cardiothorac Surg 2001;20:986-991.

92. Schmitz C, Weinreich S, White J, et al: Can particulate extraction from the ascending aorta reduce neurologic injury in cardiac surgery? J Thorac Cardiovasc Surg 2003;126:1829-1838.

93. Cook DJ, Orszulak TA, Zehr KJ, et al: Effectiveness of the Cobra aortic catheter for dual-temperature management during adult cardiac surgery. J Thorac Cardiovasc Surg 2003;125:378-384.

94. Slater JM, Orszulak TA, Zehr KJ, Cook DJ: Use of the Cobra catheter for targeted temperature management during cardiopulmonary bypass in swine. J Thorac Cardiovasc Surg 2002;123:936-942.

95. Cook DJ, Zehr KJ, Orszulak TA, Slater JM: Profound reduction in brain embolization using an endoaortic baffle during bypass in swine. Ann Thorac Surg 2002;73:198-202.

96. Kapetanakis EI, Stamou SC, Dullum MK, et al: The impact of aortic manipulation on neurologic outcomes after coronary artery bypass surgery: A risk-adjusted study. Ann Thorac Surg 2004;78:1564-1571.

97. Stump DA, Jones TJ, Rorie KD: Neurophysiologic monitoring and outcomes in cardiovascular surgery. J Cardiothorac Vasc Anesth 1999;13:600-613.

98. Tsang JC, Morin JF, Tchervenkov CI, et al: Single aortic clamp versus partial occluding clamp technique for cerebral protection during coronary artery bypass: A randomized prospective trial. J Card Surg 2003;18:158-163.

99. Grega MA, Borowicz LM, Baumgartner WA: Impact of single clamp versus double clamp technique on neurologic outcome. Ann Thorac Surg 2003;75:1387-1391.

100. Menkis AH: Management of the ascending aorta in routine cardiac surgery. Semin Cardiothorac Vasc Anesth 2004;8:19-24.

101. Gaudino M, Glieca F, Alessandrini F, et al: The unclampable ascending aorta in coronary artery bypass patients: A surgical challenge of increasing frequency. Circulation 2000;102:1497-1502.

102. Stern A, Tunick PA, Culliford AT, et al: Protruding aortic arch atheromas: Risk of stroke during heart surgery with and without aortic arch endarterectomy. Am Heart J 1999;138(4 Pt 1):746-752.

103. Hossmann KA: Viability thresholds and the penumbra of focal ischemia. Ann Neurol 1994;36:557-565.

104. Tranmer BI, Gross CE, Kindt GW, Adey GR: Pulsatile versus nonpulsatile blood flow in the treatment of acute cerebral ischemia. Neurosurgery 1986;19:724-731.

105. Murkin JM, Martzke JS, Buchan AM, et al: A randomized study of the influence of perfusion technique and pH management strategy in 316 patients undergoing coronary artery bypass surgery: I. Mortality and cardiovascular morbidity. J Thorac Cardiovasc Surg 1995;110: 340-348.

106. Murkin JM: The role of CPB management in neurobehavioral outcomes after cardiac surgery. Ann Thorac Surg 1995;59:1308-1311.

107. Duebener LF, Sakamoto T, Hatsuoka S, et al: Effects of hematocrit on cerebral microcirculation and tissue oxygenation during deep hypothermic bypass. Circulation 2001;104(12 Suppl 1):I260-I264.

108. Habib RH, Zacharias A, Schwann TA, et al: Role of hemodilutional anemia and transfusion during cardiopulmonary bypass in renal injury after coronary revascularization: Implications on operative outcome. Crit Care Med 2005;33:1749-1756.

109. DeFoe GR, Ross CS, Olmstead EM, et al: Lowest hematocrit on bypass and adverse outcomes associated with coronary artery bypass grafting. Northern New England Cardiovascular Disease Study Group. Ann Thorac Surg 2001;71:769-776.

110. Shin'oka T, Shum-Tim D, Jonas RA, et al: Higher hematocrit improves cerebral outcome after deep hypothermic circulatory arrest. J Thorac Cardiovasc Surg 1996;112:1610-1620.

111. Habib RH, Zacharias A, Schwann TA, et al: Adverse effects of low hematocrit during cardiopulmonary bypass in the adult: Should current practice be changed? J Thorac Cardiovasc Surg 2003;125: 1438-1450.

112. Liam BL, Plochl W, Cook DJ, et al: Hemodilution and whole body oxygen balance during normothermic cardiopulmonary bypass in dogs. J Thorac Cardiovasc Surg 1998;115:1203-1208.

113. Turri F, Della Volpe A, Leirner AA: Clinical comparison of blood oxygenators: A retrospective study. Artif Organs 1995;19:263-266.

114. Whitaker DC, Newman SP, Stygall J, et al: The effect of leucocyte-depleting arterial line filters on cerebral microemboli and neuropsychological outcome following coronary artery bypass surgery. Eur J Cardiothorac Surg 2004;25:267-274.

115. Blauth CI: Macroemboli and microemboli during cardiopulmonary bypass. Ann Thorac Surg 1995;59:1300-1303.

116. Gourlay T: Biomaterial development for cardiopulmonary bypass. Perfusion 2001;16:381-390.

117. Nollert G, Reichart B: Cardiopulmonary bypass and cerebral injury in adults. Shock 2001;16(Suppl 1):16-19.

118. Newman MF, Kramer D, Croughwell ND, et al: Differential age effects of mean arterial pressure and rewarming on cognitive dysfunction after cardiac surgery. Anesth Analg 1995;81:236-242.

119. Slogoff S, Reul GJ, Keats AS, et al: Role of perfusion pressure and flow in major organ dysfunction after cardiopulmonary bypass. Ann Thorac Surg 1990;50:911-918.

120. Gold JP, Charlson ME, Williams-Russo P, et al: Improvement of outcomes after coronary artery bypass: A randomized trial comparing intraoperative high versus low mean arterial pressure. J Thorac Cardiovasc Surg 1995;110:1302-1311.

121. Caplan LR, Hennerici M: Impaired clearance of emboli (washout) is an important link between hypoperfusion, embolism, and ischemic stroke. Arch Neurol 1998;55:1475-1482.

122. Sungurtekin H, Boston US, Orszulak TA, Cook DJ: Effect of cerebral embolization on regional autoregulation during cardiopulmonary bypass in dogs. Ann Thorac Surg 2000;69:1130-1134.

123. Lutz PL, Nilsson GE: Mechanisms of brain anoxia tolerance. In Lutz PL, Nilsson GE (eds): The brain without oxygen: Causes of failure and mechanisms for survival, ed 2. Austin, Tex, RG Landes, 1997, pp 103-164.

124. Giffard RG, Monyer H, Christine CW, Choi DW: Acidosis reduces NMDA receptor activation, glutamate neurotoxicity, and oxygen-glucose deprivation neuronal injury in cortical cultures. Brain Res 1990;506:339-342.

125. Kurth CD, O'Rourke MM, O'Hara IB: Comparison of pH-stat and alpha-stat cardiopulmonary bypass on cerebral oxygenation and blood flow in relation to hypothermic circulatory arrest in piglets. Anesthesiology 1998;89:110-118.

126. Pokela M, Dahlbacka S, Biancari F, et al: pH-stat versus alpha-stat perfusion strategy during experimental hypothermic circulatory arrest: A microdialysis study. Ann Thorac Surg 2003;76:1215-1226.

127. Kiziltan HT, Baltali M, Bilen A, et al: Comparison of alpha-stat and pH-stat cardiopulmonary bypass in relation to jugular venous oxygen saturation and cerebral glucose-oxygen utilization. Anesth Analg 2003;96:644-650.

128. du Plessis AJ, Jonas RA, Wypij D, et al: Perioperative effects of alpha-stat versus pH-stat strategies for deep hypothermic cardiopulmonary bypass in infants. J Thorac Cardiovasc Surg 1997;114:991-1000.

129. Murkin JM, Martzke JS, Buchan AM, et al: A randomized study of the influence of perfusion technique and pH management strategy in 316 patients undergoing coronary artery bypass surgery: II. Neurologic and cognitive outcomes. J Thorac Cardiovasc Surg 1995;110: 349-362.

130. Plochl W, Cook DJ: Quantification and distribution of cerebral emboli during cardiopulmonary bypass in the swine: The impact of $PaCO_2$. Anesthesiology 1999;90:183-190.

131. Plochl W, Krenn CG, Cook DJ, et al: Can hypocapnia reduce cerebral embolization during cardiopulmonary bypass? Ann Thorac Surg 2001;72:845-849.

132. Murkin JM, Farrar JK, Tweed WA, et al: Cerebral autoregulation and flow/metabolism coupling during cardiopulmonary bypass: The influence of $PaCO_2$. Anesth Analg 1987;66:825-832.

133. Patel RL, Turtle MR, Chambers DJ, et al: Alpha-stat acid-base regulation during cardiopulmonary bypass improves neuropsychologic outcome in patients undergoing coronary artery bypass grafting. J Thorac Cardiovasc Surg 1996;111:1267-1279.

134. Stephan H, Weyland A, Kazmaier S, et al: Acid-base management during hypothermic cardiopulmonary bypass does not affect cerebral metabolism but does affect blood flow and neurological outcome. Br J Anaesth 1992;69:51-57.

135. Holmes JH, Connolly NC, Paull DL, et al: Magnitude of the inflammatory response to cardiopulmonary bypass and its relation to adverse clinical outcomes. Inflamm Res 2002;51:579-586.

136. Restrepo L, Wityk RJ, Grega MA, et al: Diffusion- and perfusion-weighted magnetic resonance imaging of the brain before and after coronary artery bypass grafting surgery. Stroke 2002;33:2909-2915.

137. Westaby S, Saatvedt K, White S, et al: Is there a relationship between cognitive dysfunction and systemic inflammatory response after cardiopulmonary bypass? Ann Thorac Surg 2001;71:667-672.

138. Taggart DP, Browne SM, Halligan PW: Neurocognitive function after coronary-artery bypass surgery. N Engl J Med 2001;345:544-545.

139. Gu YJ, Mariani MA, Boonstra PW, et al: Complement activation in coronary artery bypass grafting patients without cardiopulmonary bypass: The role of tissue injury by surgical incision. Chest 1999;116:892-898.

140. Ascione R, Lloyd CT, Underwood MJ, et al: Inflammatory response after coronary revascularization with or without cardiopulmonary bypass. Ann Thorac Surg 2000;69:1198-1204.

141. Michenfelder JD, Milde JH: The relationship among canine brain temperature, metabolism, and function during hypothermia. Anesthesiology 1991;75:130-136.

142. Skaryak LA, Chai PJ, Kern FH, et al: Blood gas management and degree of cooling: Effects on cerebral metabolism before and after circulatory arrest. J Thorac Cardiovasc Surg 1995;110:1649-1657.

143. Steen PA, Newberg L, Milde JH, Michenfelder JD: Hypothermia and barbiturates: Individual and combined effects on canine cerebral oxygen consumption. Anesthesiology 1983;58:527-532.

144. Fujisawa H, Koizumi H, Ito H, et al: Effects of mild hypothermia on the cortical release of excitatory amino acids and nitric oxide synthesis following hypoxia. J Neurotrauma 1999;16:1083-1093.

145. Dietrich WD, Busto R, Halley M, Valdes I: The importance of brain temperature in alterations of the blood-brain barrier following cerebral ischemia. J Neuropathol Exp Neurol 1990;49:486-497.

146. Chen H, Chopp M, Welch KM: Effect of mild hyperthermia on the ischemic infarct volume after middle cerebral artery occlusion in the rat. Neurology 1991;41:1133-1135.

147. Chen Z, Chen H, Rhee P, et al: Induction of profound hypothermia modulates the immune/inflammatory response in a swine model of lethal hemorrhage. Resuscitation 2005;66:209-216.

148. Castillo J, Davalos A, Noya M: Aggravation of acute ischemic stroke by hyperthermia is related to an excitotoxic mechanism. Cerebrovasc Dis 1999;9:22-27.

149. Madl JE, Allen DL: Hyperthermia depletes adenosine triphosphate and decreases glutamate uptake in rat hippocampal slices. Neuroscience 1995;69:395-405.

150. Azzimondi G, Bassein L, Nonino F, et al: Fever in acute stroke worsens prognosis: A prospective study. Stroke 1995;26:2040-2043.

151. Osguthorpe SG: Hypothermia and rewarming after cardiac surgery. AACN Clin Issues Crit Care Nurs 1993;4:276-292.

152. Ginsberg MD, Busto R: Combating hyperthermia in acute stroke: A significant clinical concern. Stroke 1998;29:529-534.

153. Johnson RI, Fox MA, Grayson A, et al: Should we rely on nasopharyngeal temperature during cardiopulmonary bypass? Perfusion 2002;17:145-151.

154. Ohsumi H, Kitaguchi K, Nakajima T, et al: Internal jugular bulb blood velocity as a continuous indicator of cerebral blood flow during open heart surgery. Anesthesiology 1994;81:325-332.

155. Grocott HP, Newman MF, Croughwell ND, et al: Continuous jugular venous versus nasopharyngeal temperature monitoring during hypothermic cardiopulmonary bypass for cardiac surgery. J Clin Anesth 1997;9:312-316.

156. Grocott HP, Nussmeier NA: Neuroprotection in cardiac surgery. Anesthesiol Clin North Am 2003;21:487-509.

157. Nussmeier NA, Li S, Strickler AG, et al: Temperature measurement during cardiopulmonary bypass. Anesth Analg 2002;94:35.

158. Nathan HJ, Parlea L, Dupuis JY, et al: Safety of deliberate intraoperative and postoperative hypothermia for patients undergoing coronary artery surgery: A randomized trial. J Thorac Cardiovasc Surg 2004;127:1270-1275.

159. Nathan HJ, Wells GA, Munson JL, Wozny D: Neuroprotective effect of mild hypothermia in patients undergoing coronary artery surgery with cardiopulmonary bypass: A randomized trial. Circulation 2001;104(12 Suppl 1):I85-91.

160. Insler SR, O'Connor MS, Leventhal MJ, et al: Association between postoperative hypothermia and adverse outcome after coronary artery bypass surgery. Ann Thorac Surg 2000;70:175-181.

161. Frank SM, Fleisher LA, Breslow MJ, et al: Perioperative maintenance of normothermia reduces the incidence of morbid cardiac events: A randomized clinical trial. JAMA 1997;277:1127-1134.

162. Thong WY, Strickler AG, Li S, et al: Hyperthermia in the forty-eight hours after cardiopulmonary bypass. Anesth Analg 2002;95:1489-1495.

163. Grocott HP, Mackensen GB, Grigore AM, et al: Postoperative hyperthermia is associated with cognitive dysfunction after coronary artery bypass graft surgery. Stroke 2002;33:537-541.

164. Bar-Yosef S, Mathew JP, Newman MF, et al: Prevention of cerebral hyperthermia during cardiac surgery by limiting on-bypass rewarming in combination with post-bypass body surface warming: A feasibility study. Anesth Analg 2004;99:641-646.

165. Watters MP, Cohen AM, Monk CR, et al: Reduced cerebral embolic signals in beating heart coronary surgery detected by transcranial Doppler ultrasound. Br J Anaesth 2000;84:629-631.

166. Khan NE, De Souza A, Mister R, et al: A randomized comparison of off-pump and on-pump multivessel coronary-artery bypass surgery. N Engl J Med 2004;350:21-28.

167. Puskas JD, Winston AD, Wright CE, et al: Stroke after coronary artery operation: Incidence, correlates, outcome, and cost. Ann Thorac Surg 2000;69:1053-1056.

168. Sharony R, Bizekis CS, Kanchuger M, et al: Off-pump coronary artery bypass grafting reduces mortality and stroke in patients with atheromatous aortas: A case control study. Circulation 2003;108(Suppl 1):II15-20.

169. Lloyd CT, Ascione R, Underwood MJ, et al: Serum S-100 protein release and neuropsychologic outcome during coronary revascularization on the beating heart: A prospective randomized study. J Thorac Cardiovasc Surg 2000;119:148-154.

170. Nussmeier NA: Adverse neurologic events: Risks of intracardiac versus extracardiac surgery. J Cardiothorac Vasc Anesth 1996;10:31-37.

171. Kuroda Y, Uchimoto R, Kaieda R, et al: Central nervous system complications after cardiac surgery: A comparison between coronary artery bypass grafting and valve surgery. Anesth Analg 1993;76:222-227.

172. Borger MA, Ivanov J, Weisel RD, et al: Decreasing incidence of stroke during valvular surgery. Circulation 1998;98(19 Suppl):II137-143.

173. Karp RB, Mills N, Edmunds LH Jr: Coronary artery bypass grafting in the presence of valvular disease. Circulation 1989;79(6 Pt 2):I182-184.

174. Thourani VH, Weintraub WS, Craver JM, et al: Influence of concomitant CABG and urgent/emergent status on mitral valve replacement surgery. Ann Thorac Surg 2000;70:778-783.

175. Hochrein J, Lucke JC, Harrison JK, et al: Mortality and need for reoperation in patients with mild-to-moderate asymptomatic aortic valve disease undergoing coronary artery bypass graft alone. Am Heart J 1999;138(4 Pt 1):791-797.

176. Brunvand H, Offstad J, Nitter-Hauge S, Svennevig JL: Coronary artery bypass grafting combined with aortic valve replacement in healthy octogenarians does not increase postoperative risk. Scand Cardiovasc J 2002;36:297-301.

177. Wolf PA, Abbott RD, Kannel WB: Atrial fibrillation as an independent risk factor for stroke: The Framingham Study. Stroke 1991;22:983-988.

178. Stoddard MF, Dawkins PR, Prince CR, Ammash NM: Left atrial appendage thrombus is not uncommon in patients with acute atrial fibrillation and a recent embolic event: A transesophageal echocardiographic study. J Am Coll Cardiol 1995;25:452-459.

179. Hill LL, De Wet C, Hogue CW Jr: Management of atrial fibrillation after cardiac surgery—part II: Prevention and treatment. J Cardiothorac Vasc Anesth 2002;16:626-637.

180. Mathew JP, Fontes ML, Tudor IC, et al: A multicenter risk index for atrial fibrillation after cardiac surgery. JAMA 2004;291:1720-1729.

181. Creswell LL, Schuessler RB, Rosenbloom M, Cox JL: Hazards of postoperative atrial arrhythmias. Ann Thorac Surg 1993;56:539-549.

182. Lahtinen J, Biancari F, Salmela E, et al: Postoperative atrial fibrillation is a major cause of stroke after on-pump coronary artery bypass surgery. Ann Thorac Surg 2004;77:1241-1244.

183. Murdock DK, Rengel LR, Schlund A, et al: Stroke and atrial fibrillation following cardiac surgery. WMJ 2003;102:26-30.

184. Amar D, Shi W, Hogue CW Jr, et al: Clinical prediction rule for atrial fibrillation after coronary artery bypass grafting. J Am Coll Cardiol 2004;44:1248-1253.

185. Mullen JC, Khan N, Weisel RD, et al: Atrial activity during cardioplegia and postoperative arrhythmias. J Thorac Cardiovasc Surg 1987;94:558-565.

186. Hogue CW Jr, Filos KS, Schuessler RB, Sundt TM III: Sinus nodal function and risk for atrial fibrillation after coronary artery bypass graft surgery. Anesthesiology 2000;92:1286-1292.

187. Bert AA, Reinert SE, Singh AK: A beta-blocker, not magnesium, is effective prophylaxis for atrial tachyarrhythmias after coronary artery bypass graft surgery. J Cardiothorac Vasc Anesth 2001;15:204-209.

188. Sullivan TM: Current indications, results, and technique of carotid angioplasty/stenting. Semin Vasc Surg 2005;18:87-94.

189. Barnett HJ, Meldrum HE, Eliasziw M: The appropriate use of carotid endarterectomy. Can Med Assoc J 2002;166:1169-1179.

190. Ross IB, Dhillon GS: Complications of endovascular treatment of cerebral aneurysms. Surg Neurol 2005;64:12-18.

191. Merchant RA, Lui KL, Ismail NH, et al: The relationship between postoperative complications and outcomes after hip fracture surgery. Ann Acad Med Singapore 2005;34:163-168.

192. Moller JT, Cluitmans P, Rasmussen LS, et al: Long-term postoperative cognitive dysfunction in the elderly ISPOCD1 study. ISPOCD investigators. International Study of Post-Operative Cognitive Dysfunction. Lancet 1998;351:857-861.

193. Williams-Russo P, Sharrock NE, Mattis S, et al: Cognitive effects after epidural vs general anesthesia in older adults: A randomized trial. JAMA 1995;274:44-50.

194. Brody H: The aging brain. Acta Neurol Scand Suppl 1992;137:40-44.

195. Selkoe DJ: Aging brain, aging mind. Sci Am 1992;267:134-142.

196. Mrak RE, Griffin ST, Graham DI: Aging-associated changes in human brain. J Neuropathol Exp Neurol 1997;56:1269-1275.

197. Marcantonio ER, Juarez G, Goldman L, et al: The relationship of postoperative delirium with psychoactive medications. JAMA 1994;272:1518-1522.

198. Parikh SS, Chung F: Postoperative delirium in the elderly. Anesth Analg 1995;80:1223-1232.

199. Wu CL, Hsu W, Richman JM, Raja SN: Postoperative cognitive function as an outcome of regional anesthesia and analgesia. Reg Anesth Pain Med 2004;29:257-268.

200. Chan KH, Dearden NM, Miller JD, et al: Multimodality monitoring as a guide to treatment of intracranial hypertension after severe brain injury. Neurosurgery 1993;32:547-552.

201. Schwarz S, Georgiadis D, Aschoff A, Schwab S: Effects of induced hypertension on intracranial pressure and flow velocities of the middle cerebral arteries in patients with large hemispheric stroke. Stroke 2002;33:998-1004.

202. Rordorf G, Koroshetz WJ, Ezzeddine MA, et al: A pilot study of drug-induced hypertension for treatment of acute stroke. Neurology 2001; 56:1210-1213.

203. Marzan AS, Hungerbuhler HJ, Studer A, et al: Feasibility and safety of norepinephrine-induced arterial hypertension in acute ischemic stroke. Neurology 2004;62:1193-1195.

204. Chambers IR, Kirkham FJ: What is the optimal cerebral perfusion pressure in children suffering from traumatic coma? Neurosurg Focus 2003;15:E3.

205. Warner DS, Gionet TX, Todd MM, McAllister AM: Insulin-induced normoglycemia improves ischemic outcome in hyperglycemic rats. Stroke 1992;23:1775-1780.

206. Ekholm A, Katsura K, Siesjo BK: Coupling of energy failure and dissipative K^+ flux during ischemia: Role of preischemic plasma glucose concentration. J Cereb Blood Flow Metab 1993;13:193-200.

207. Siesjo BK, Katsura K, Mellergard P, et al: Acidosis-related brain damage. Prog Brain Res 1993;96:23-48.

208. Pulsinelli WA, Levy DE, Sigsbee B, et al: Increased damage after ischemic stroke in patients with hyperglycemia with or without established diabetes mellitus. Am J Med 1983;74:540-544.

209. Weir CJ, Murray GD, Dyker AG, Lees KR: Is hyperglycaemia an independent predictor of poor outcome after acute stroke? Results of a long-term follow up study. BMJ 1997;314:1303-1306.

210. Auer RN: Hypoglycemic brain damage. Metab Brain Dis 2004;19:169-175.

211. Wass CT, Lanier WL: Glucose modulation of ischemic brain injury: Review and clinical recommendations. Mayo Clin Proc 1996;71: 801-812.

212. Muizelaar JP, Marmarou A, Ward JD, et al: Adverse effects of prolonged hyperventilation in patients with severe head injury: A randomized clinical trial. J Neurosurg 1991;75:731-739.

213. The Brain Trauma Foundation, the American Association of Neurological Surgeons, the Joint Section on Neurotrauma and Critical Care: Hyperventilation. J Neurotrauma 2000;17:513-520.

214. Miyamoto E, Tomimoto H, Nakao Si S, et al: Caudoputamen is damaged by hypocapnia during mechanical ventilation in a rat model of chronic cerebral hypoperfusion. Stroke 2001;32:2920-2925.

215. Ohyu J, Endo A, Itoh M, Takashima S: Hypocapnia under hypotension induces apoptotic neuronal cell death in the hippocampus of newborn rabbits. Pediatr Res 2000;48:24-29.

216. Ravussin P, Moeschler O, Graftieaux JP, De Tribolet N: [Relaxation and protection of the brain on the operating table]. Neurochirurgie 1994;40:359-362.

217. Takano T, Nagatsuka K, Ohnishi Y, et al: Vascular response to carbon dioxide in areas with and without diaschisis in patients with small, deep hemispheric infarction. Stroke 1988;19:840-845.

218. Kurihara E, Ishikawa A, Tamaki N, Okada Y: The protective effect of hypothermia on the recovery of neural activity after deprivation of oxygen and glucose: Study of slices from the hippocampus and superior colliculus. Neurosci Lett 1996;204:197-200.

219. Busto R, Dietrich WD, Globus MY, et al: Small differences in intraischemic brain temperature critically determine the extent of ischemic neuronal injury. J Cereb Blood Flow Metab 1987;7: 729-738.

220. Minamisawa H, Smith ML, Siesjo BK: The effect of mild hyperthermia and hypothermia on brain damage following 5, 10, and 15 minutes of forebrain ischemia. Ann Neurol 1990;28:26-33.

221. Ridenour TR, Warner DS, Todd MM, McAllister AC: Mild hypothermia reduces infarct size resulting from temporary but not permanent focal ischemia in rats. Stroke 1992;23:733-738.

222. Olsen TS, Weber UJ, Kammersgaard LP: Therapeutic hypothermia for acute stroke. Lancet Neurol 2003;2:410-416.

223. Todd MM, Hindman BJ, Clarke WR, Torner JC: Mild intraoperative hypothermia during surgery for intracranial aneurysm. N Engl J Med 2005;352:135-145.

224. Hindman BJ, Todd MM, Gelb AW, et al: Mild hypothermia as a protective therapy during intracranial aneurysm surgery: A randomized prospective pilot trial. Neurosurgery 1999;44:23-32.

225. Wass CT, Lanier WL, Hofer RE, et al: Temperature changes of ≥1° C alter functional neurologic outcome and histopathology in a canine model of complete cerebral ischemia. Anesthesiology 1995;83: 325-335.

9 Risk Assessment and Perioperative Renal Dysfunction

Christina T. Mora Mangano, Charles C. Hill, and John L. Chow

All patients undergoing surgery—from simple surgery to an extremely complex operative procedure—suffer some perturbation in oxygen delivery to the kidneys. Postoperative renal dysfunction (of new onset or exacerbated from the preoperative state) portends an increase in overall morbidity, mortality, and hospital resource utilization. Thus, the identification of patients with an increased risk for postoperative renal dysfunction is critical. The prognosis of renal dysfunction for a particular patient scheduled for a specific operative intervention will (1) assist the patient and the family in the decision to undergo a particular operation, and (2) permit optimization of preoperative, intraoperative, and postoperative renal homeostasis. Several investigations suggest that the anticipation of renal dysfunction and the early diagnosis of acute renal insufficiency are critical to the effective treatment of renal compromise and the avoidance of temporary or chronic renal replacement therapies. Patient characteristics (e.g., young versus advanced age), the type of operative procedure (e.g., endoscopic cholecystectomy versus aortic arch replacement) and its specific characteristics (e.g., the duration of hypotension or suprarenal cross-clamp placement, circulatory arrest), and concomitant renal insults (aminoglycoside or radiocontrast dye) all affect the risk of developing postoperative renal dysfunction (Box 9-1).

Several chapters in this book address the subject of the kidney and surgery; the specific goal of this chapter is to provide clinicians with methods to identify patients at an increased risk for postoperative renal dysfunction or failure. First, an outline of the intrinsic effects of surgery and anesthesia on renal physiology illustrates why *all* patients suffer renal compromise in the perioperative setting. Second, we discuss patient characteristics that are associated with an increase in postoperative renal dysfunction. Third, we detail three types of surgical interventions—extracorporeal circulation, profound hypothermic circulatory arrest (HCA), and suprarenal aortic occlusion—that mechanically and profoundly reduce normal renal perfusion during an operative procedure. (Although this is not an exhaustive list of the mechanical perturbations that can affect renal blood flow during an operative procedure, these interventions are chosen because they are used in a number of common procedures.) Fourth, because preexisting renal impairment is associated with an increased risk for postoperative dysfunction, we present strategies to identify occult dysfunction or quantify

the magnitude of renal compromise. We conclude the chapter with a review of existing renal risk scoring systems and their respective utilities.

EFFECTS OF SURGERY AND ANESTHESIA ON RENAL PERFUSION

The kidney is an elegant system of integrated processes that maintain fluid homeostasis. Although the kidney requires only 10% of the total corporeal oxygen consumption, the renal cortex receives 90% of the total renal blood flow (RBF) and extracts only 18% of the oxygen delivered. In contrast, the renal medulla receives only 10% of the RBF to the kidney, and it is the site of the costly energy- and oxygen-consuming processes that are responsible for reabsorbing tubular sodium and water. In the medulla, 79% of the oxygen delivered is extracted, resulting in a high arteriovenous oxygen gradient in this region of the kidney. Thus, the medulla is exquisitely sensitive to reductions in RBF. A 40% reduction in RBF may lead to acute tubular necrosis, especially in the presence of other renal insults. Interventions that improve RBF (increased cardiac output, fluid replacement) or reduce medullary oxygen consumption also improve the tolerance to intermittent ischemia.[1] Other phenomena, including exposure to radiocontrast dyes and an increased bilirubin or myoglobinuria, exacerbate the adverse response to renal hypoxia by increasing the osmotic load to the nephron and further increasing oxygen requirements.

Several types of drugs can cause nephrotoxicity through a variety of mechanisms. The perioperative use of aminoglycosides or nonsteroidal anti-inflammatory drugs (NSAIDs) may precipitate renal dysfunction in the hypoxic kidney. The chronic use of angiotensin-converting enzyme (ACE) inhibitors may lead to an attenuation of the normal compensatory response to a decrease in renal perfusion. Aprotinin is an anti-inflammatory serine protease inhibitor that is used intraoperatively to reduce blood loss, especially in cardiac and orthopedic surgery patients. Aprotinin is concentrated in the kidney, and data suggest that its use is associated with postoperative renal dysfunction and failure.[2-4] One group of investigators reported that ACE inhibitors and aprotinin have a synergistic adverse effect on postoperative renal function in patients undergoing cardiac surgery with cardiopulmonary bypass (CPB).[5]

9-1	Factors Associated with an Increased Risk of Postoperative Renal Dysfunction

Patient Characteristics

- Advanced age
- Diabetes
- Compromised ventricular function
- Peripheral vascular disease
- Renovascular disease
- Sepsis
- Hepatic failure

Operative Procedure

- Aortic surgery
- Cardiopulmonary bypass
- Trauma surgery
- Liver transplant
- Renal transplant

Perioperative Renal Insults

- Prolonged dehydration
- Prolonged bladder obstruction
- Hypoxia
- Hypotension
- Aminoglycoside exposure
- Myoglobin or hemoglobin in the urine
- Radiology study dyes

Anesthesia (both general and regional) and surgery, independently and synergistically, impair renal homeostasis during operative procedures. Both types of anesthesia cause some magnitude of peripheral vasodilation and perhaps third-spacing, thus reducing circulating blood volume and renal perfusion. Vasodilation and the resultant reduction in RBF is particularly a problem in the patient who has abstained from food or fluids for 8 or more hours, was prescribed chronic diuretics or ACE inhibitors, has suffered recent vomiting or gastric emptying, has undergone a recent bowel preparation, or is actively bleeding. No studies have demonstrated that general anesthetic technique is better than regional in limiting the likelihood of postoperative renal dysfunction. Neither anesthetic approach impairs the normal compensatory responses to hypovolemia and decreases in RBF.[6]

Much research has focused on the potential adverse renal effects of fluoride ions on the metabolism of potent volatile anesthetic drugs. Of the clinically used inhalational agents, sevoflurane and enflurane release the greatest number of fluoride moieties. However, the pharmacokinetics of these drugs greatly limits the likelihood of renal dysfunction secondary to fluoride exposure. Sevoflurane interacts with soda lime or barium hydroxyl carbon dioxide absorbers to produce a potentially nephrotoxic haloalkene known as compound A. However, the human metabolic pathways for this compound limit the likelihood of compound A–induced nephrotoxicity. Indeed, there are no published reports of renal dysfunction associated with exposure to sevoflurane in surgical patients.

■ PATIENT CHARACTERISTICS AND THE RISK OF POSTOPERATIVE RENAL DYSFUNCTION

Patient-specific factors (identifiable in the preoperative period) that are associated with postoperative renal disease (RD) or failure and dialysis fall generally into one of three categories: (1) patient characteristics suggesting impaired renal functional reserve, (2) physiologic findings associated with impaired renal perfusion, or (3) pathophysiologic processes that cause renal toxicity. Potential risk factors include advanced age, abnormal serum creatinine values, diabetes mellitus, and any sign, symptom, or factor indicative of a reduced cardiac output (CO) and thus compromised renal perfusion. However, the low incidence of postoperative RD necessitating renal replacement intervention (<2.0% even in high-risk populations) and the lack of sensitive, routine laboratory studies that reveal RD even when it does not result in an increase in creatinine or blood urea nitrogen (BUN), have challenged investigators to identify factors that are associated with postoperative renal disease or failure.

Patient Characteristics Associated with Reduced Renal Reserve

With advancing age, renal mass and overall function deteriorate. By age 70, the number of functioning nephrons is reduced by half. Novis and colleagues[7] reviewed 28 studies assessing risk factors for RD after surgery. Four of the five largest studies identified increasing age as a risk for postoperative RD. In a study of 2400 patients undergoing elective coronary revascularization, Mangano and associates[8] found that patients between 70 and 80 years old and those over 80 years old suffered a twofold or fourfold increase in the risk for postoperative RD, respectively. Similarly, Chertow and colleagues, in their study of 42,723 U.S. Department of Veterans Affairs (VA) cardiac surgery patients found that 1.5% and 1.8% of CABG patients between 70 and 80 years old, and older than 80 years, respectively, required postoperative dialysis. In comparison, only 0.5% and 0.9% of patients 50 to 59 and 60 to 69 years of age, respectively, required renal replacement therapy. However, in the multivariate model, after adjusting for peripheral vascular disease, prior cardiac surgery, and other related variables, advanced age did not remain a significant variable. This outcome highlights the difficulty of separating the many related phenomena associated with reduced renal reserve.

Patients with diabetes mellitus (DM), especially those suffering longstanding disease managed with insulin, have reduced renal reserve. Type I DM and preoperative glucose values greater than 300 mg% were significantly and independently associated with postoperative RD in the multicenter study by Mangano and coworkers.[8] Those patients with type I DM and those with hyperglycemia suffered a relative risk of 1.8 and 3.7, respectively, for developing postoperative RD. Although some investigators have failed to demonstrate an independent association between DM and RD, many others have developed risk score indices that include DM as a variable.

Reduced renal functional reserve is best identified by measures of glomerular filtration. However, most studies rely on serum creatinine values as a measure of renal reserve. Because creatinine values are substantially affected by non-renal factors, they are inadequate measures of glomerular filtration. Some studies have used the Cockcroft-Gault equation to estimate glomerular filtration rate (GFR).[9] Studies using serum creatinine values, derived values for GFR, or true creatinine clearance assessments have, almost uniformly, identified reduced preoperative renal reserve, manifested as an increase in creatinine or as a reduction in GFR, as the most common and one of the most important patient characteristics associated with postoperative renal dysfunction (Table 9-1).

Several studies have emphasized the importance of even mild preoperative renal dysfunction on postoperative RD. Weerasinghe and colleagues studied 1427 patients with no known renal disease who were scheduled for elective primary coronary artery bypass graft (CABG) surgery.[10] They reported that patients with a minimal elevation in creatinine values (Cr >130 μmol/L) had a substantial increase in the need for postoperative mechanical renal support (relative risk, 24.3).

Patient Characteristics Suggesting Reduced Renal Blood Flow

Many patients presenting for surgery—particularly cardiac or major vascular surgery—have signs and symptoms that suggest a reduced CO and thus reduced RBF. Such signs and symptoms include rales, rhonchi, edema, jugular venous distention, abnormal heart sounds, a need for pharmacologic or mechanical myocardial support, and laboratory evidence of a reduced ejection fraction (<35%). Even in the absence of apparent renal dysfunction (i.e., with normal creatinine values), these patients may have a greatly reduced ability to maintain normal GFR and fluid homeostasis, especially with the additional insults of surgery and other interventions.

The study by Chertow and colleagues[11] of more than 42,000 cardiac surgery patients and the report by Thakar and associates[12] of more than 33,000 cardiac surgery patients both emphasize the prognostic value of signs, symptoms, interventions, and laboratory assessments indicating compromised myocardial performance and thus compromised renal perfusion. The preoperative presence of any of these factors may be considered a potential risk factor for postoperative RD.

Several studies assessed the association of postoperative RD with factors that might be expected to be associated with reduced renal blood flow, such as renal artery stenosis.[13,14] In one of the studies, Conlon and colleagues assessed the association of preexisting renal artery stenosis (>50% stenosis) with postoperative RD, but found no correlation between the two variables.[13] In a prospective study of 564 cardiac surgery patients, Chew and colleagues found that patients with apolipoprotein (APL) E4 alleles, compared with those with APL E2 or E3 alleles, were less likely to suffer an increase in postoperative serum creatinine.[15] This report was the first study that permits preoperative risk stratification for renal dysfunction based on genetic characteristics.

Other Preoperative Patient Variables Associated with Renal Toxicity

A patient may suffer various pathophysiologic processes in the preoperative period that expose the kidney to toxic insults, thus stressing renal reserve. These phenomena cause an increase in renal oxygen demand. For example, hepatic failure or obstruction leads to an increase in bilirubin and other incompletely metabolized moieties. As these metabolites accumulate, the renal parenchyma compensates for hepatic insufficiency and must detoxify, excrete, concentrate, or secrete these toxic substances. This increase in oxygen demand may limit the kidney's ability to withstand the further renal insults inflicted during the perioperative period. Similarly, patients suffering massive trauma, hemorrhage, or extensive burn injuries have increased renal oxygen requirements, as the kidneys must filter increased plasma levels of myoglobin and hemoglobin. Both sepsis and gut ischemia are associated with endotoxin release and may lead to a reduction in renal perfusion and perhaps, more importantly, an accelerating inflammatory response. In an inflammatory response, the kidney is recruited to help manage many of the inflammatory kinins, and it is exposed to activated leukocytes. Filtered inflammatory mediators may be tubulotoxic. Hypotension reduces GFR, and efferent arterioles constrict to compensate. Ultimately, the hypotension, the medullary ischemia, and the sludging of activated neutrophils lead to an increased neutrophil adhesion potential. Adherent neutrophils release vasoconstrictive and tubulotoxic mediators,

9-1	Risk of Renal Dysfunction According to Renal Reserve				
Renal Reserve	Remaining Nephrons (%)	Glomerular Filtration Rate (mL/min)	Signs/Symptoms	Laboratory Abnormalities	Risk of Dysfunction or Failure
Normal	>50	125	None	None	Minimal
Decreased renal reserve	40	50-80	None	None	Mild
Renal insufficiency	20-40	20-50	Nocturia	Moderate increase in BUN/creatinine, unless stressed	Moderate
Uremia	5-10	<20	Uremic syndrome	Multiple	Severe

BUN, blood urea nitrogen.
From Prough DS, Foreman AS: Anesthesia and the renal system. In Barash PG, Stoelting R, Cullen G (eds): Clinical Anesthesia, ed 2. Philadelphia, Lippincott Williams & Wilkins, 1992, pp 1125-1156, with permission.

further increasing renal oxygen demand and reducing oxygen delivery.

Other Preoperative Patient Factors Associated with Postoperative Renal Dysfunction

Other patient factors including previous cardiac surgery, peripheral vascular disease, hypertension, and chronic obstructive pulmonary disease have been identified by some investigators as prognostic for postoperative RD. These factors, which have not been uniformly accepted as risk factors, are discussed in the following paragraphs.

■ SURGICAL INTERVENTIONS ASSOCIATED WITH SUBSTANTIAL INTRAOPERATIVE RENAL ISCHEMIA

Cardiopulmonary Bypass

Renal dysfunction after CPB is a well-recognized phenomenon. There is, however, a lack of consensus on the definition of renal dysfunction (Table 9-2).[7,8,11,16-28] In most studies, it is defined on the basis of the elevation of serum creatinine level from its baseline value (i.e., an increase of 0.5 mg/dL, or

>50%) and the need for postoperative renal replacement therapy.[29] The Society of Thoracic Surgeons Database defines renal dysfunction as a postoperative serum creatinine level of greater than 2.0 mg/dL associated with a doubling of the preoperative creatinine level. However, the use of serum creatinine values is increasingly discredited as an appropriate measure of renal dysfunction (see later).

The incidence of renal dysfunction after cardiac surgery ranges from 2% to 28.1%, with approximately 0.4% to 4.7% patients who developed acute renal failure (ARF) requiring dialysis (see Table 9-3). In a landmark study of 42,773 patients by Chertow and coworkers, dialysis-dependent ARF occurred in 1.1% of patients with a 63.7% associated mortality—alarming when compared with the 4.3% mortality for those who did not require dialysis after cardiac surgery.[11] Postoperative ARF heralds a poor prognosis with increasing complications and mortality, especially for patients with postoperative respiratory failure, hypotensive episodes, bleeding, atrial fibrillation, or other end-organ dysfunction.[8,11,30-32]

These patients remain in the intensive care unit and hospital for greater durations and are more likely to require specialized long-term care.[8,10,11,22] The overall mortality for

9-2	**Studies of Renal Dysfunction after Cardiopulmonary Bypass Surgery**							
Author (ref. no.)	**Number of Patients**	**Study Design**	**Definition of Renal Dysfunction**	NONDIALYSIS OUTCOME		DIALYSIS OUTCOME	
				Incidence (%)	**Mortality (%)**	**Incidence (%)**	**Mortality (%)**
Yeboah et al. (16)	428	—	—	26	38	4.7	70
Abel et al. (17)	500	Prospective	Cr >1.5 mmol/L	21.6	13.8	3	100
Bhat et al. (18)	490	Retrospective	Cr ≥1.6 mmol/L*	28.1	10.9	2.2	45
McLeish et al. (19)	1542	Retrospective	—	Not reported	Not reported	1.3	35
Hilberman et al. (20)	204	Case control	BUN ≥30 mmol/L†	2.5	60	2.5	60‡
Gailunas et al. (21)	752	Retrospective	Cr >1.5 mmol/L	17	Not reported	1.5	27
Lange et al. (22)	2959	—	—	Not reported	Not reported	1.2	53
Corwin et al. (23)	572	Case control	$Cr_{postop} \geq 1.5 \, Cr_{preop}$	6.3	Not reported	1	33
Slogoff et al. (24)	504	—	Cr ≥1.5 mmol/L§	2.4	0.2	0.4	0
Zanardo et al. (25)	775	Prospective	Cr ≥1.5 mmol/L	15.1	9.5	0.5	44
Mangano/McSPI (8)	2417	Prospective	Cr ≥2.0 mmol/L	7.7	19	1.4	40
Abrahamov et al. (26)	2214	Retrospective	CrCl <40 mL/min/ 1.73 m²¶	2.1	Not reported	1%	30
Grayson et al. (27)	5132	Retrospective	Cr >2.0 mmol/L	2	Not reported	0.9	32.9 or 46.2¶
Antunes et al. (28)	2455	Prospective	Cr ≥2.1 mmol/L**	5.6	5.8	0.6	33.3

*Also, $Cr_{postop} - Cr_{preop} \geq 0.4$ mmol/L (mg/dL).
†Or inulin or creatinine clearance ≤50 mL/min/1.73 m².
‡Mortality is combined for dialysis and nondialysis patients.
§And fractional excretion of sodium >1% or total urinary sodium >20 μg/L or urine with casts, epithelial cells, or cellular debris.
¶Creatinine clearance at least a 15-mL/min decline from preoperative level.
¶Depending on the type of surgery (32.9% after coronary artery bypass graft (CABG); 46.2% after valve operation with or without CABG)).
**Plus an increased creatinine level of ≥0.9 mmol/L from preoperative to maximum postoperative values.
BUN, blood urea nitrogen; Cr, creatinine; CrCl, creatinine clearance; Cr_{postop}, postoperative creatinine; Cr_{preop}, preoperative creatinine; V, valve.

patients who developed ARF requiring renal replacement therapy ranges from 27% to 100%. The economic impact of renal complication in cardiac surgery patients is considerable. In fact, it is estimated that nationally, the direct hospital cost of caring for patients with post-CPB renal failure is approaching $645 million.[33]

Renal functional impairment after CPB is generally characterized as acute tubular necrosis (ATN) and acute or chronic renal dysfunction.[20] The latter is usually the result of acute renal ischemia superimposed on older adult patients with limited renal reserve.[8,34] Factors suggestive of compromised renal perfusion are associated with an increased risk for renal dysfunction and failure. Predictive risk factors for ARF include advanced age (>70 years old), preoperative left ventricular dysfunction, atherosclerotic vascular disease, decreased renal reserve, diabetes, prior myocardial revascularization, intraoperative bypass time (>3 hours), complexity of the operation (e.g., valvular surgery), perioperative use of nephrotoxic agents (e.g., radiocontrast dyes), and postoperative low CO.[8,16,24,26,27,29,35-39]

Historically, extracorporeal circulation was thought to be associated with multiple perturbations in renal physiology and function. During CPB, there are substantive decreases (25% to 75%) in RBF and GFR and increases in renal vascular resistance. These physiological perturbations are likely sequelae of the loss of pulsatile blood flow,[40] increases in circulating catecholamines and inflammatory mediators,[41] macroembolic and microembolic insults to the kidney (organic and inorganic debris),[42] release of free hemoglobin from traumatized red blood cells,[43] decrease in flow rates and mean arterial pressure during CPB.[1,16,17,44] In addition, extreme hemodilution and deep hypothermic circulatory arrest have been associated with a significantly greater likelihood of postoperative renal dysfunction.[45] However, several studies have found no effects of noncirculatory arrest hypothermia,[46-48] pulsatile perfusion,[49,50] pH management,[50] or membrane oxygenators[51] on renal function after CPB. Lema and colleagues studied the GFR and effective renal plasma flow of patients with a creatinine level of less than 1.5 mg/dL undergoing hypothermic CPB and found that renal function was not adversely affected by CPB.[36]

The widely used off-pump coronary artery bypass (OPCAB) approach to coronary revascularization was expected to substantially reduce the incidence of end-organ dysfunction (e.g., renal, cerebral) observed in patients undergoing coronary surgery with CPB. However, over the past decade, a substantial number of retrospective and prospective studies comparing the adverse outcome rates associated with off- and on-pump strategies have failed to show a superiority of an off-pump technique. Although studies of patients undergoing OPCAB revealed significantly fewer changes in microalbuminuria, fractional extraction of sodium, free water clearance, free hemoglobin, and N-acetyl-beta-D-glucosaminidase,[52] OPCAB is not associated with a reduction in postoperative renal impairment.[53-55] In patients with preoperative nondialysis-dependent renal insufficiency, however, the OPCAB surgery appears to lower the incidence of postoperative renal failure, need for renal replacement therapy,

and mortality.[56-58] McCreath and associates suggested that a port access minithoracotomy approach to mitral valve surgery may confer a reduction in the incidence of ARF when compared with a median sternotomy approach.[59]

Pharmacologic approaches to reduce post-CPB renal dysfunction have been studied extensively in recent years. Although most of these pharmacologic agents appeared to promote urine output in the perioperative period, intraoperative urine output had no correlation with postoperative renal function, especially when diuretics were used intraoperatively.[60] Dopamine (DA) at low doses activates the DA-1 receptor and has the theoretical benefits of renal artery dilation, natriuresis, and diuresis. Although DA was once shown to increase renal plasma flow, GFR, and urinary sodium excretion,[61] these dopaminergic effects were not observed in patients with impaired renal function (GFR < 50 mL/min/1.73 m^2), probably because of a lack of renal reserve capacity in response to the effects of dopamine.[62] Randomized controlled trials with cardiac surgery patients have not demonstrated that prophylactic low-dose dopamine can preserve renal function, reduce the development of ARF,[63-66] and decrease mortality. In addition, the positive inotropic and chronotropic effects of dopamine could lead to the development of perioperative arrhythmias and an increase in myocardial oxygen consumption that are potentially deleterious to cardiac surgery patients.[67] Furthermore, the use of dopamine to promote diuresis in patients who are hypovolemic is likely to exacerbate renal failure.[68] In view of the lack of proven benefits and the potential harm, routine use of dopamine to promote diuresis in the perioperative setting is not recommended.

Mannitol is a hyperosmotic agent that increases GFR during periods of renal hypoperfusion, augments renal cortical and medullary blood flow, and promotes scavenging of reactive hydroxyl free radicals. It reduces renal oxygen consumption during periods of ischemia and enhances diuresis of intraluminal debris. However, the prophylactic use of mannitol in patients undergoing CPB has not produced convincing improvement in renal function and mortality outcome.[69,70]

Loop diuretics such as furosemide offer benefits similar to those of mannitol in reducing oxygen consumption and improving diuresis by preventing the accumulation of obstructive casts. In two separate prospective randomized studies, the use of furosemide during and after CPB was found to have no clinical benefits and to be potentially detrimental to renal function.[71,72] Although dopamine, mannitol, and furosemide can convert oliguric to nonoliguric renal failure and facilitate management of fluids and electrolytes, in the absence of evidence that forced diuresis translates to mortality benefit, the routine use of these medications is not encouraged.

A selective DA-1 receptor agonist, fenoldopam, has the theoretical advantages of decreasing renal vascular resistance and increasing RBF and GFR.[73] Caimmi and coworkers studied patients with a preoperative creatinine level of greater than 1.5 mg/dL and found that infusion of fenoldopam (0.1 to 0.3 µg/kg/min) during CPB and the early postoperative period is associated with an improvement in postoperative creatinine level and creatinine clearance.[74] In a prospective, multicenter, cohort study of high-risk patients with renal failure, prophylactic infusion of fenoldopam was associated with a 50% reduction of ARF and a decrease in mortality from 15.7% to 6.5%.[75] These clinical benefits are based on a preliminary experience with fenoldopam and should be confirmed by larger-scale prospective randomized trials before using it routinely.

Vasodilators such as calcium channel blockers (e.g., nifedipine, diltiazem) have been shown to improve GFR in patients undergoing CPB.[76-79] However, clinically significant improvement in morbidity and mortality endpoints are lacking to advocate its routine practice.

Clonidine is a nonselective alpha-adrenergic agonist that may prevent renal hypoperfusion by inhibiting stress-induced catecholamine–mediated vasoconstriction. Kulka and associates found that in patients with normal risk for postoperative renal dysfunction, clonidine at 4 μg/kg prevented the deterioration of creatinine clearance after cardiac surgery better than placebo.[80] However, the long-term benefit and mortality outcome in high-risk patients have not been fully evaluated.

Atrial natriuretic peptide (ANP) is important in intravascular fluid and circulatory regulation. It promotes diuresis and natriuresis, increases GFR, reverses afferent renal vasoconstriction and efferent renal dilation, and inhibits sodium reabsorption.[81,82] Intraoperative volume loading has been shown to regulate ANP release, and its concentrations may predict long-term outcome after CABG.[83,84] In recent studies, intraoperative infusion of ANP has been shown to decrease central venous pressure, pulmonary capillary wedge pressure, pulmonary vascular resistance, peripheral vascular resistance, and the renin-angiotensin-aldosterone system, as well as increasing RBF, GFR, and diuresis.[85-87] The precise effects of these natriuretic peptides on post-CPB renal function and their potential role in curtailing renal failure and its associated mortality have not yet been determined.

Urodilatin is a natriuretic peptide that exerts its effects by promoting RBF and by its action on the distal collecting tubules. In a small-sample-size ($N = 7$) study of patients who developed oliguria or anuria refractory to conventional nondialysis-dependent treatment after cardiac surgery, Wiebe and colleagues showed that infusion of urodilatin at 2 ng/kg/min was effective in reversing oliguric ARF and preventing the need for renal replacement therapy.[88] Further studies are needed to elucidate the clinical efficacy in a larger patient population.

Two studies that examined the institution of early renal replacement therapy in the form of continuous venovenous hemodiafiltration in patients with established postoperative ARF found a statistically significant reduction in overall mortality outcome.[89,90]

In summary, the effects of CPB on the renal system have significant health and economic impacts. However, despite intensive investigation into the pathogenesis and prevention of renal failure, there has been only limited progress in the development of effective protective strategies. As intravascular volume depletion and hypoperfusion can lead to exacerbation of renal ischemia and accentuate the risk for postoperative ARF, avoidance of nephrotoxic agents and close attention to maintenance of intravascular volume, blood pressure, and CO are central in the effort to reduce the occurrence of ARF after cardiac surgery.[91] Genetic screening for specific inflammatory markers (interleukin-6 gene promoter polymorphism, apolipoprotein E) to determine predisposition may be an additional means of identifying patients at risk for renal dysfunction.[92,93] In recent years, kidney-specific proteins measured perioperatively have been correlated with prolonged CPB time and may help predict renal injury after CPB.[94]

Major Aortic Surgery

Patients undergoing major aortic surgery with or without hypothermic circulatory arrest are particularly vulnerable to perioperative renal injury and dysfunction. These patients are typically of advanced age and have atherosclerosis of the central circulation and end-organ (heart, brain, kidney) vasculature beds. Thus, vasculature surgery patients have many of the characteristics that are prognostic for postoperative renal dysfunction in cardiac surgery patients. Review of the literature suggests that the presence of preoperative RD is the most consistent predictor for postoperative RD following major vascular surgery.[95-104] However, because each type of major vascular surgery is associated with a significant mechanical perturbation that interferes with RBF—cross-clamping of the aorta, left-heart bypass, renal artery reimplantation or surgery, or CPB with or without hypothermic circulatory arrest—the type and duration of the particular mechanical intervention render other potential variables less important predictors of postoperative RD.

The reported incidences of RD and dialysis after major aortic surgery vary substantially (Table 9-3).[100-116] The reported incidences of postoperative renal dysfunction and renal failure range between 5% and 29% and 1.6% and 22.2%, respectively. This reflects the nonuniform definitions of preoperative and postoperative renal dysfunction but also, and perhaps more importantly, the underlying potential for significant, potentially life-threatening differences in patient characteristics and management strategies in this eclectic group of patients.

Most clinicians caring for patients with an abdominal aortic aneurysm (AAA) recognize the critical nature of the decisions regarding the intraoperative position of the aortic cross-clamp. Cardiovascular anesthesiologists encourage their surgical colleagues to consider infrarenal cross-clamp placement (if at all possible) in patients undergoing AAA surgery. Studies by Breckwoldt and coworkers[105] and Johnston[106] emphasize the importance of infrarenal versus suprarenal cross-clamp placement on the development of postoperative RD (see Table 9-4). In a study of 205 patients with AAA, Breckwoldt and colleagues found that the patients managed with an infrarenal clamp ($n = 39$) were much less likely to develop postoperative dysfunction than patients requiring suprarenal occlusion of the aorta ($n = 166$). The multicenter study by Johnston[106] included 666 patients managed with an infrarenal or suprarenal aortic cross-clamp and confirmed the findings of Breckwoldt's group (see Fig. 9-1).

| 9-3 | Studies of Renal Dysfunction after Vascular Surgery |

Surgery	Study Author (ref. no.)	Postoperative Renal Dysfunction (%)	Postoperative Dialysis Required (%)	Risk Factors for Renal Failure
Infrarenal	Powell (116a)	–	8-9*	Preoperative RD
Infrarenal vs. suprarenal	Breckwoldt et al. (105)	Infrarenal 13.9	1.80	No single factor
		Suprarenal 38.5	2.60	
AAA infrarenal + suprarenal	Johnston (106)	5.0-33.0	0.4-6.0	Preoperative RD, AX site, RV ligation, RA bypass
	Shepard (116b)	14	1.18	
Renal involvement	Hallett (116c)	22	9.0-35.0	—
	Chaikof et al. (107)	4.0	18.3	Preoperative RD
	Nypaver et al. (99)	16.98	5.66	RA bypass/endarterectomy, any postoperative complication
	Allen et al. (108)	12.3	3.08	Preoperative RD
	Cambria et al. (109)	9.0	15.0	Preoperative RD
	Acher et al. (110)	19.0*	2.0-71.0	Preoperative RD
Aortic rupture	Panneton et al. (111)	27.7	6.3	Preoperative RD
	Bauer et al. (112)	29.0	—	AX time/site, preoperative RD, age, hypotension
	Hajarizaden et al. (113)	11.43	18.1	–
	Berisa et al. (114)	16.0	84.0	Preoperative RD
Thoracoabdominal	Crawford et al. (100)	–	5.0-17.0	Preoperative renal dysfunction
	Schepens et al. (101)	–	11.9-14.1	Age, preoperative creatinine, CAD, DM
	Svensson et al. (102)	15.87	13	Repair of visceral artery, preoperative RD, and postoperative complication
	Godet (116d)	17.26	8	Age > 50 yr, preoperative RD, LRA, ischemic time, transfusion
	Safi et al. (103)	2.5	15	LRA reattachment, preoperative RD, visceral perfusion, simple cross-clamp technique
Endovascular	White et al. (115)	14.29	21.43	—
	Sharma et al. (116)	3.7*	11.1*	Aortoiliac source of embolus

AAA, abdominal aortic aneurysm; AX, aortic cross-clamp; CAD, coronary artery disease; DM, diabetes mellitus; LRA, left renal artery; RA, renal artery; RD, non–dialysis-dependent renal failure; RV, renal vein.
*If preoperative CR > 1.5 mg%.

Surgical patients with thoracoabdominal aneurysmal disease may suffer the greatest perturbations to perioperative renal homeostasis. A variety of approaches are used to limit the ischemic time and overall insult to the kidneys; hypothermic circulatory arrest, left heart bypass, and renal "plegia" are measures to reduce renal metabolism or limit actual interruption of RBF.[100-105] However, most patients continue to be at risk for profound kidney damage, because several common intraoperative events further perturb renal metabolism. Substantial blood loss, visceral ischemia and endotoxemia, requirements for massive blood product transfusions, and renal ischemia all portend postoperative renal dysfunction.

There is debate in the surgical community about the optimal set of approaches for operative management of extensive aortic disease. Some clinicians claim that hypothermic circulatory arrest is superior to left-heart bypass in preserving renal function. Soukiasian and colleagues reviewed all of their cases of thoracoabdominal aneurysms between 1989 and 2001.[117] In 1994, they changed their practice paradigm to include circulatory arrest for this type of patient rather than left-heart bypass. In the first group of 20 patients, the rate of renal failure was 15%, and it was 0% in the 39 patients managed with HCA. Comments published with the article essentially dismissed these findings and quoted work from Crawford, Cosseli, and others that counter these findings.[100] Importantly, this high-risk group of patients is managed differently by different surgeons and in different institutions. It represents an extremely confounded environment. It is difficult to distill the true driving factors for postoperative renal dysfunction, and prospective, randomized studies to define the risk factors associated with renal dysfunction are lacking. However, most studies suggest that preexisting renal dysfunction, aortic rupture, and the requirement for renal reconstruction are associated with an increase in renal morbidity.

One of the most promising developments in the management of aortic disease is the introduction of stent grafts,[118-122] and the techniques are rapidly evolving. Several types of grafts are approved for use in the descending thoracic and abdominal aorta. Some centers use multiple stent grafts to reconstruct the thoracoabdominal aorta. The Stanford group

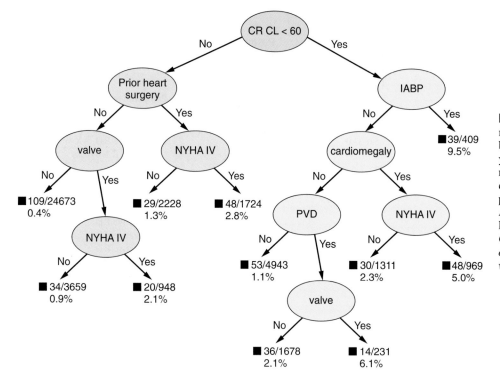

Figure 9-1 ■ Preoperative renal risk algorithm. Classification tree based on recursive partitioning analysis. Next to the *solid boxes* are the risk categories. CR CL, creatinine clearance; IABP, intra-aortic balloon pump; NYHA, New York Heart Association; PVD, peripheral vascular disease. *(Adapted from Chertow GM, Lazarus JM, Christiansen CL, et al: Circulation 1997;95:878-884, with permission.)*

may use a combined "open-and-closed" approach: open access is achieved (limiting the source of one of the most common adverse events associated with stent grafts), and a stent is used where adequate "landing zones" can be identified.

Black and colleagues reported on 29 consecutive patients treated with endovascular occlusion and open visceral revascularization for management of thoracoabdominal aneurysms.[122] Five of the patients had known renal insufficiency. Postoperatively, four patients suffered renal dysfunction, with two requiring temporary dialysis. The group concluded that they would manage all Crawford types I, II, and III thoracoabdominal aneurysms with this approach. As in other work in the surgical management of thoracoabdominal aortic disease, no prospective randomized studies have defined the difference in risk between open and stent graft repairs in regard to a number of adverse outcomes, including renal dysfunction.

In summary, vascular surgery patients represent an eclectic group with multiple intrinsic and extrinsic potential risk factors for renal dysfunction. However, the magnitude of the morbid intraoperative events (cross-clamp placement, HCA, left-heart bypass) associated with these vascular procedures is likely to be the greatest determinant of perioperative risk for renal adverse events.

■ PERIOPERATIVE TESTING OF RENAL FUNCTION

Although there is improvement in the ability to identify patients at risk for perioperative acute renal dysfunction or failure, the methods to detect and quantify both

9-2	**Renal Function Tests Available for Clinical Use**

- Urine volume
- Urine specific gravity
- Urine osmolality
- Serum creatinine and blood urea nitrogen
- Urine to plasma creatinine ratio
- Urine to plasma urea ratio
- Urinary sodium excretion
- Fractional excretion of sodium
- Free water clearance
- Creatinine clearance
- Renal blood flow

From Sear JW: Br J Anaesth 2005;95:20-32, with permission.

deteriorations and subsequent improvement in renal function require further refinement.

Although many renal function tests are available and each examines a different aspect of the kidney's physiologic function (Box 9-2),[6] GFR remains the most important indicator of renal function. GFR is most frequently estimated by creatinine clearance, a value obtained from a 24-hour urine collection (Table 9-4).[123] Although some authors have investigated a creatinine clearance estimate based on a 2-hour standard, a 24-hour creatinine clearance estimate of GFR is, at present, the best predictive marker of changes in renal function and the potential development of perioperative dysfunction.

9-4	Comparison* of Methods for Determination of Glomerular Filtration Rate		
Clearance Method	**Testing Complexity**	**Accuracy**	**Clinical Usefulness**
Classic insulin clearance	++++	++++	+
Radioisotope clearance	+++	+++½	++
Radioisotope plasma disappearance	+++	+++	++
Creatinine clearance	++	++	+++
Nomogram creatinine clearance	+½	+½	+++
Serum creatinine	+	+	++++

*Rated from high (++++) to low (+).
From Mehta RL, Chertow GM: J Am Soc Nephrol 2003;14:2178-2187, with permission.

Historically, serum creatinine (sCr) and urine output (UO) have been the most clinically accessible means to assess and follow renal function. In spite of their practicality, they are highly dependent values. Normal sCr values vary as a function of age, sex, race, body habitus, and diet.[124] Changes in sCr are not specific and do not reveal the etiology, site, and extent of injury. Also, sCr changes are insensitive to changes in GFR and may be delayed for several days. UO and sCr may be altered by diuretics and dialysis and other preventative and treatment modalities. Furthermore, many studies have shown a variable correlation between sCr and UO and the risk of developing perioperative ARF. There is also no clear association between changes in sCr and morbidity or the prognosis for long-term recovery. Additionally, definitions of ARF based on initial and subsequent changes in sCr have varied widely.[123]

Much of the recent literature has focused on the application of the modified Cockcroft-Gault equation to estimate creatinine clearance (CrCl), which is an alternative measure of renal function with improved accuracy and estimation of renal reserve.[9] The equations in men and women are as follows:

$$CrCl \text{ (in men)} = ([140 - age] \times weight \times 1.2) \div sCr$$

$$CrCl \text{ (in women)} = ([140 - age] \times weight) \div sCr$$

A recent study by Wijeysundera and colleagues found that a combination of sCr and CrCl allowed identification of patients they designated as having occult renal insufficiency, defined as a normal sCr with a CrCl of 60 mL/min or less.[125] They found that approximately 13% of patients with a normal sCr had occult renal insufficiency, which was independently associated with the need for postoperative renal replacement therapy in cardiac surgery patients.

A more recent method of estimating GFR involves measurement of serum cystatin C, an alkaline nonglycosylated protein.[125,126] Cystatin C is produced by virtually all nucleated cells and is freely filtered through the glomerular membrane and nearly completely reabsorbed and degraded by the proximal tubular cells. The reference-range values for cystatin C

are the same for men, women, and children, and they are not dependent on muscle mass or diet. A recent meta-analysis by Dharnidharka and coworkers, which compared serum cystatin C levels with CrCl values, suggested that cystatin C is a better surrogate of GFR and one that reflects changes in GFR more rapidly.[127]

Recent elucidations of the pathophysiology of ARF have revealed the need for earlier detection of both deterioration and improvement in renal function. Newer techniques are now being investigated that could provide more detailed assessment of both the nature and timing of injury. These could allow for earlier diagnosis, identification of specific time points for intervention, and quantifiable measurements for therapeutic effectiveness.

One emerging field is urinary proteomics. Clinical proteomics, or urinary protein profiling, has brought about the discovery of novel protein biomarkers for renal diseases.[128] One application of urinary proteomics involves the use of surface-enhanced laser desorption/ionization time-of-flight mass spectrometry (SELDI-TOF-MS), which has emerged as one of the preferred methods of urinary protein profiling. SELDI-TOF-MS allows rapid profiling of multiple urine samples and detects low-molecular-weight biomarkers that are often missed by other methods.

Nguyen and colleagues recently used SELDI-TOF-MS technology.[128] They prospectively enrolled all patients undergoing CPB who had congenital heart disease between January and November of 2004 in their institution. Fifteen patients (25%) developed ARF in the immediate postoperative period. Using 2- and 6-hour post-CPB urine samples, the investigators found three urinary biomarkers that were both 100% sensitive and 100% specific for predicting the development of ARF. The use of SELDI-TOF-MS and urinary proteomics is an emerging field with the potential to greatly enhance our current ability to diagnose and treat perioperative ARF.[128]

Several other new techniques are also being investigated and are ready to be adapted for human studies. KIM-1 may be an early marker for renal tubule injury, and a cysteine-rich protein (CYP 61) has been found in the urine after ischemia-reperfusion injury. Newer contrast agents used with magnetic resonance imaging are being tested in experimental ARF models and may provide insight into intrarenal hemodynamics, the level and extent of proximal tubule injury, and the presence of inflammation.[123]

■ PERIOPERATIVE RENAL RISK SCORING ALGORITHMS

The development of numerous scoring systems based on well-defined risk factors has provided greater insight into which patients are at greatest risk for perioperative renal dysfunction. Most of the indices include many of the risk factors discussed in this chapter.

Chertow's proposed algorithm to predict postoperative renal failure and dialysis after cardiac surgery was developed on a robust database of over 42,000 VA patients.[11] He identified 10 clinical variables related to baseline cardiovascular disease and renal function (Box 9-3). On the basis of these variables, he divided renal risk into three categories—low risk (<0.4%), medium risk (0.9% to 2.8%), and high risk (>5.0%). His group used recursive partitioning to identify 11 separate groups based on interactions among key discriminating variables. For example, primary CABG surgery patients with essentially normal preoperative renal function have a less than 0.4% risk of requiring postoperative dialysis. In contrast, valvular heart surgery patients with preoperative renal dysfunction, class IV heart failure, and intra-aortic balloon pump (IABP) counter-pulsation support have a greater than 5.0% risk for postoperative renal failure and dialysis (Fig. 9-1).

Thakar and coworkers created an ARF score for postoperative dialysis based on over 33,000 cardiac surgery patients at the Cleveland Clinic Foundation (Table 9-5).[12] This score included 13 preoperative variables assigned point values of 1 or 2. Patients could have a score of zero to a maximum of 17. The four risk categories were assigned point values of 0 to 2, 3 to 5, 6 to 8, and 9 to 13 (Fig. 9-2). The frequency of dialysis ranged between 0.5% and 21.1%. The model was consistent for both the test and validation data sets, with an area under the curve of 0.82 in both cases.

Mangano and the McSPI research group[8] reported probabilities for developing postoperative renal dysfunction based on their multivariate logistic model of preoperative risk factors (Table 9-6). For example, patients 70 to 79 years of age who had preoperative heart failure, renal dysfunction, and a previous CABG had a 33.3% chance of developing postoperative renal dysfunction. Their data set was not sufficiently robust to develop a risk score for the 1.7% of the patients in their study who required postoperative renal replacement therapy. Interestingly, the risks for dialysis after heart surgery in the Chertow,[11] Thakar,[12] Mangano,[8] and Aronson[129] studies were equal (approximately 1.7%).

A scoring system cannot answer whether a particular patient should undergo a cardiac procedure. However, it provides an objective assessment of the risk of developing a morbid event that will be associated with a protracted hospital stay and that will place the patient at an increased risk for

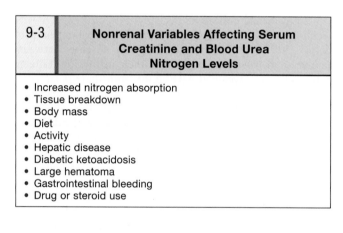

9-3	**Nonrenal Variables Affecting Serum Creatinine and Blood Urea Nitrogen Levels**

- Increased nitrogen absorption
- Tissue breakdown
- Body mass
- Diet
- Activity
- Hepatic disease
- Diabetic ketoacidosis
- Large hematoma
- Gastrointestinal bleeding
- Drug or steroid use

9-5	**Acute Renal Failure Score***

Risk Factor	Points
Female sex	1
Congestive heart failure	1
Left ventricular ejection fraction <35%	1
Preoperative use of IABP	2
COPD	1
Insulin-dependent diabetes	1
Previous cardiac surgery	1
Emergency surgery	2
Valve surgery only (compared with CABG)	1
CABG + valve surgery (compared with CABG)	2
Other cardiac surgeries	2
Preoperative creatinine 1.2 to <2.1 mg/dL (compared with 1.2)	2
Preoperative creatinine ≥2.1 mg/dL (compared with 1.2)	5

*Minimum total score, 0; maximum total score, 17.
From Thakar CV, Arrigain S, Worley S, et al: J Am Soc Nephrol 2005;16:162-168, with permission.

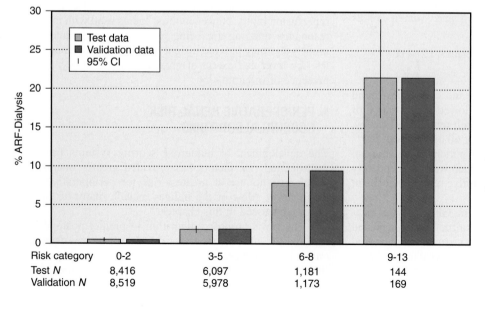

Figure 9-2 ■ The acute renal failure (ARF) risk categories. CI, confidence interval. *(Adapted from Thakar CV, Arrigain S, Worley S, et al: J Am Soc Nephrol 2005;16:162-168, with permission.)*

9-6 Preoperative Risk Factors and Predicted Probabilities of Renal Dysfunction

Number of Risk Factors	Risk Factor				Age <70 Years		Age 70-79 Years		Age 80-95 Years	
	Congestive Heart Failure	Redo CABG	Type 1 Diabetes	Preoperative Creatinine Level >124 μmol/L	Observed	Predicted (95% CI)	Observed	Predicted (95% CI)	Observed	Predicted (95% CI)
					n (%)	%	n (%)	%	n (%)	%
0	No	No	No	No	909 (1.9)	3.0 (2.3-4.0)	330 (7.0)	5.3 (3.9-7.2)	68 (11.8)	9.9 (6.1-15.6)
1	No	No	No	Yes	80 (5.0)	6.7 (4.5-9.8)	76 (18.4)	11.5 (8.0-16.3)	16 (12.5)	20.3 (12.6-31.1)
	No	No	Yes	No	68 (5.9)	6.0 (3.8-9.5)	21 (4.8)	10.5 (6.4-16.8)	1 (0.0)	18.6 (10.1-31.8)
	No	Yes	No	No	130 (6.2)	7.8 (5.4-11.1)	56 (14.3)	13.3 (9.2-18.9)	4 (25.0)	23.1 (13.9-36.0)
	Yes	No	No	No	144 (7.6)	7.3 (5.1-10.2)	73 (12.3)	12.5 (8.8-17.4)	17 (29.4)	21.8 (13.7-32.8)
2	No	No	Yes	Yes	9 (22.2)	13.0 (7.9-20.7)	7 (0.0)	21.4 (13.3-32.6)	0	—
	No	Yes	No	Yes	25 (20.0)	16.4 (10.8-24.1)	13 (30.8)	26.3 (18.3-36.4)	0	—
	No	Yes	Yes	No	8 (37.5)	15.0 (9.0-24.0)	3 (33.3)	24.3 (14.7-37.5)	1 (0.0)	38.6 (21.9-58.4)
	Yes	No	No	Yes	19 (47.4)	15.4 (10.3-22.4)	26 (7.7)	24.9 (17.8-33.7)	9 (44.4)	39.3 (26.5-53.8)
	Yes	No	Yes	No	27 (25.9)	14.1 (9.0-21.3)	11 (18.2)	23.0 (14.7-33.9)	0	—
	Yes	Yes	No	No	19 (31.6)	17.7 (11.9-25.6)	14 (7.1)	28.1 (19.5-38.7)	1 (100.0)	43.3 (28.3-59.7)
3	No	Yes	Yes	Yes	1 (100.0)	29.1 (17.9-43.6)	1 (100.0)	42.8 (28.1-58.8)	0	—
	Yes	No	Yes	Yes	12 (8.3)	27.6 (18.0-39.8)	4 (25.0)	40.9 (28.4-54.8)	1 (0.0)	57.5 (39.9-73.5)
	Yes	Yes	No	Yes	2 (0.0)	33.3 (22.8-45.9)	9 (33.3)	47.6 (35.5-60.1)	2 (0.0)	64.0 (47.4-77.8)
	Yes	Yes	Yes	No	3 (33.3)	31.0 (19.8-45.0)	0	—	0	—
4	Yes	Yes	Yes	Yes	2 (50.0)	51.1 (35.7-66.3)	0	—	0	—

For "Observed" columns, n = observed number of patients with risk factor combinations and % = observed proportion of patients with renal dysfunction among those with the specified risk factor combination. For the "Predicted" columns, % = predicted probability of renal dysfunction derived from the multivariate logistic regression model of preoperative factors. CABG, coronary artery bypass graft.

From Mangano CM, Diamondstone LS, Ramsay JG, et al: Ann Intern Med 1998;128:194-203, with permission.

perioperative death. Although some preoperative risk factors (e.g., advanced age, previous cardiac surgery) cannot be altered, others might be controlled or ameliorated. Cardiac function should be optimized and renal perfusion enhanced. Hyperglycemia should be treated aggressively. Therapy with nephrotoxic medications should be avoided or minimized. Identification of a high-risk group of patients allows individuals and their families a more comprehensive informed consent about their decision to pursue health-care alternatives.

■ CONCLUSION

The problem of renal dysfunction occurring after major cardiac and vascular surgery is likely to increase in the next decade. Patients presenting for surgery are increasingly older and more likely to have a decrement in renal function, increasing their vulnerability to serious adverse renal events after an operative procedure. Hypertension and diabetes also are more prevalent in our culture, increasing renal risk in operative patients. Finally, physicians are more aggressive in treating life-threatening illness (major aortic pathology, poor myocardial performance), and patients expect advanced therapies. Unfortunately, few approaches can obviate the problem of renal dysfunction in at-risk patients. Indeed, the prevalence of renal dysfunction and failure after AAA has not changed in 3 decades. Because we have a more complete understanding of the pathophysiology of perioperative renal dysfunction and can identify at-risk patients, we have the opportunity to identify new interventions to decrease the prevalence of postoperative renal dysfunction.

■ REFERENCES

1. Ramsay JG: The respiratory, renal, and hepatic systems: Effects of cardiac surgery and cardiopulmonary bypass. In Mora C (ed): Cardiopulmonary Bypass. New York, Springer Verlag, 1995, p 147.
2. Mangano DT, Tudor IC, Dietzel C, for the Multicenter Study of Perioperative Ischemia (McSPI) Research Group and the Ischemia Research and Education Foundation: The risk associated with aprotinin in cardiac surgery. N Engl J Med 2006;354:353-365.
3. Kramer HJ, Moch T, von Sicherer L, Dusing R: Effects of aprotinin on renal function and urinary prostaglandin excretion in conscious rats after acute salt loading. Clin Sci (Lond) 1979;56:547-553.
4. Rustom R, Grime JS, Maltby P, et al: Observations on the early renal uptake and later tubular metabolism of radiolabeled aprotinin (Trasylol) in man: Theoretical and practical considerations. Clin Sci (Lond) 1993;84:231-241.
5. Kincaid EH, Ashburn DA, Hoyle JR, et al: Does the combination of aprotinin and angiotensin-converting enzyme inhibitor cause renal failure after cardiac surgery? Ann Thorac Surg 2005;80:1388-1393.
6. Sear JW: Kidney dysfunction in the postoperative period. Br J Anaesth 2005;95:20-32.
7. Novis BK, Roizen MF, Aronson S, Thisted RA: Association of preoperative risk factors with postoperative acute renal failure. Anesth Analg 1994;78:143-149.
8. Mangano CM, Diamondstone LS, Ramsay JG, et al: Renal dysfunction after myocardial revascularization: Risk factors, adverse outcomes, and hospital resource utilization. The Multicenter Study of Perioperative Ischemia Research Group. Ann Intern Med 1998;128:194-203.
9. Cockcroft DW, Gault MH: Prediction of creatinine clearance from serum creatinine. Nephron 1976;16:31-41.
10. Weerasinghe A, Hornick P, Smith P, et al: Coronary artery bypass grafting in non-dialysis-dependent mild-to-moderate renal dysfunction. J Thorac Cardiovasc Surg 2001;121:1083-1089.
11. Chertow GM, Lazarus JM, Christiansen CL, et al: Preoperative renal risk stratification. Circulation 1998;95:878-884.
12. Thakar CV, Arrigain S, Worley S, et al: A clinical score to predict acute renal failure after cardiac surgery. J Am Soc Nephrol 2005;16:162-168.
13. Conlon PJ, Crowley J, Stack R, et al: Renal artery stenosis is not associated with the development of acute renal failure following coronary artery bypass grafting. Ren Fail 2005;27:81-86.
14. Erentug V, Bozbuga N, Polat A, et al: Coronary bypass procedures in patients with renal artery stenosis. J Card Surg 2005;20:345-349.
15. Chew ST, Newman MF, White WD, et al: Preliminary report on the association of apolipoprotein E polymorphisms with postoperative peak serum creatinine concentrations in cardiac surgical patients. Anesthesiology 2000;93:325-331.
16. Yeboah ED, Petrie A, Pead JL: Acute renal failure and open heart surgery. Br Med J 1972;1:415-418.
17. Abel RM, Buckley MJ, Austen WG, et al: Etiology, incidence, and prognosis of renal failure following cardiac operations: Results of a prospective analysis of 500 consecutive patients. J Thorac Cardiovasc Surg 1976;71:323-333.
18. Bhat JG, Gluck MC, Lowenstein J, Baldwin DS: Renal failure after open heart surgery. Ann Intern Med 1976;84:677-682.
19. McLeish KR, Luft FC, Kleit SA: Factors affecting prognosis in acute renal failure following cardiac operations. Surg Gynecol Obstet 1977;145:28-32.
20. Hilberman M, Myers BD, Carrie BJ, et al: Acute renal failure following cardiac surgery. J Thorac Cardiovasc Surg 1979;77:880-888.
21. Gailiunas P Jr, Chawla R, Lazarus JM, et al: Acute renal failure following cardiac operations. J Thorac Cardiovasc Surg 1980;79:241-243.
22. Lange HW, Aeppli DM, Brown DC: Survival of patients with acute renal failure requiring dialysis after open heart surgery: Early prognostic indicators. Am Heart J 1987;113:1138-1143.
23. Corwin HL, Sprague SM, DeLaria GA, Norusis MJ: Acute renal failure associated with cardiac operations: A case-control study. J Thorac Cardiovasc Surg 1989;98:1107-1112.
24. Slogoff S, Reul GJ, Keats AS, et al: Role of perfusion pressure and flow in major organ dysfunction after cardiopulmonary bypass. Ann Thorac Surg 1990;50:911-918.
25. Zanardo G, Michielon P, Paccagnella A, et al: Acute renal failure in the patient undergoing cardiac operation: Prevalence, mortality rate, and main risk factors. J Thorac Cardiovasc Surg 1994;107:1489-1495.
26. Abrahamov D, Tamariz M, Fremes S, et al: Renal dysfunction after cardiac surgery. Can J Cardiol 2001;17:565-570.
27. Grayson AD, Khater M, Jackson M, et al: Valvular heart operation is an independent risk factor for acute renal failure. Ann Thorac Surg 2003;75:1829-1835.
28. Antunes PE, Prieto D, Ferrao de Oliveira J, et al: Renal dysfunction after myocardial revascularization. Eur J Cardiothorac Surg 2004;25:597-604.
29. Swaminathan M, Phillips-Bute BG, Conlon PJ, et al: The association of lowest hematocrit during cardiopulmonary bypass with acute renal injury after coronary artery bypass surgery. Ann Thorac Surg 2003;76:784-791.
30. Anderson RJ, O'Brien M, MaWhinney S, et al: Renal failure predisposes patients to adverse outcome after coronary artery bypass surgery. VA Cooperative Study #5. Kidney Int 1999;55:1057-1062.
31. Anderson RJ, O'Brien M, MaWhinney S, et al: Mild renal failure is associated with adverse outcome after cardiac valve surgery. Am J Kidney Dis 2000;35:1127-1134.
32. Albahrani MJ, Swaminathan M, Phillips-Bute B, et al: Postcardiac surgery complications: Association of acute renal dysfunction and atrial fibrillation. Anesth Analg 2003;96:637-643.
33. Callahan M, Battleman DS, Christos P, et al: Economic consequences of renal dysfunction among cardiopulmonary bypass surgery patients: A hospital-based perspective. Value Health 2003;6:137-143.

34. Koning HM, Koning AJ, Defauw JJ: Optimal perfusion during extra-corporeal circulation. Scand J Thorac Cardiovasc Surg 1987;21:207-213.
35. Brosius FC III, Hostetter TH, Kelepouris E, et al: Detection of chronic kidney disease in patients with or at increased risk of cardiovascular disease: A science advisory from the AHA Kidney and Cardiovascular Disease Council; the Councils on High Blood Pressure Research, Cardiovascular Disease in the Young, and Epidemiology and Prevention; and the Quality of Care and Outcomes Research Interdisciplinary Working Group: Developed in collaboration with the National Kidney Foundation. Circulation 2006;114:1083-1087.
36. Lema G, Meneses G, Urzua J, et al: Effects of extracorporeal circulation on renal function in coronary surgical patients. Anesth Analg 1995;81:446-451.
37. Davila-Roman VG, Kouchoukos NT, Schechtman KB, et al: Atherosclerosis of the ascending aorta is a predictor of renal dysfunction after cardiac operations. J Thorac Cardiovasc Surg 1999;117:111-116.
38. Provenchere S, Plantefeve G, Hufnagel G, et al: Renal dysfunction after cardiac surgery with normothermic cardiopulmonary bypass: incidence, risk factors, and effect on clinical outcome. Anesth Analg 2003;96:1258-1264.
39. Swaminathan M, Phillips-Bute BG, et al: The association of lowest hematocrit during cardiopulmonary bypass with acute renal injury after coronary artery bypass surgery. Ann Thorac Surg 2003;76:784-791.
40. Mori A, Watanabe K, Onoe M, et al: Regional blood flow in the liver, pancreas and kidney during pulsatile and nonpulsatile perfusion under profound hypothermia. Jpn Circ J 1988;52:219-227.
41. Reves JG, Karp RB, Buttner EE, et al: Neuronal and adrenomedullary catecholamine release in response to cardiopulmonary bypass in man. Circulation 1982;66:49-55.
42. Blauth CI: Macroemboli and microemboli during cardiopulmonary bypass. Ann Thorac Surg 1995;59:1300-1303.
43. Donohoe JF, Ventatachalam MA, Bernard DB, Levinsky NG: Tubular leakage and obstruction after renal ischemia: Structural functional correlations. Kidney Int 1978;13:208-222.
44. Yeh TJ, Brackney EL, Hall DP, et al: Renal complications of open-heart surgery: Predisposing factors, prevention, and management. J Thorac Cardiovasc Surg 1964;47:79-97.
45. Mora Mangano CT, Neville MJ, Hsu PH, et al: Aprotinin, blood loss, and renal dysfunction in deep hypothermic circulatory arrest. Circulation 2001;104:I276-I281.
46. Regragui IA, Izzat MB, Birdi I, et al: Cardiopulmonary bypass perfusion temperature does not influence perioperative renal function. Ann Thorac Surg 1995;60:160-164.
47. Swaminathan M, East C, Phillips-Bute B, et al: Report of a substudy on warm versus cold cardiopulmonary bypass: Changes in creatinine clearance. Ann Thorac Surg 2001;72:1603-1609.
48. Harrington DK, Lilley JP, Rooney SJ, et al: Nonneurologic morbidity and profound hypothermia in aortic surgery. Ann Thorac Surg 2004;78:596-601.
49. Hickey PR, Buckley MJ, Philbin DM: Pulsatile and nonpulsatile cardiopulmonary bypass: Review of a counterproductive controversy. Ann Thorac Surg 1983;36:720-737.
50. Badner NH, Murkin JM, Lok P: Differences in pH management and pulsatile/nonpulsatile perfusion during cardiopulmonary bypass do not influence renal function. Anesth Analg 1992;75:696-701.
51. Hessel EA II, Johnson DD, Ivey TD, et al: Membrane versus bubble oxygenator for cardiac operations. A prospective randomized study. J Thorac Cardiovac Surg 1980;80:111-122.
52. Loef BG, Epema AH, Navis G, et al: Off-pump coronary revascularization attenuates transient renal damage compared with on-pump coronary revascularization. Chest 2002;121:1190-1194.
53. Jarvinen O, Laurikka J, Tarkka MR: Off-pump versus on-pump coronary bypass. Comparison of patient characteristics and early outcomes. J Cardiovasc Surg 2003;44:167-172.
54. Schwann NM, Horrow JC, Strong MD 3rd, et al: Does off-pump coronary artery bypass reduce the incidence of clinically evident renal dysfunction after multivessel myocardial revascularization? Anesth Analg 2004;99:959-964.
55. Berson AJ, Smith JM, Woods SE, et al: Off-pump versus on-pump coronary artery bypass surgery: Does the pump influence outcome? J Am Coll Surg 2004;199:102-108.
56. Ascione R, Nason G, Al-Ruzzeh S, et al: Coronary revascularization with or without cardiopulmonary bypass in patients with preoperative nondialysis-dependent renal insufficiency. Ann Thorac Surg 2001;72:2020-2025.
57. Beauford RB, Saunders CR, Niemeier LA, et al: Is off-pump revascularization better for patients with non-dialysis-dependent renal insufficiency? Heart Surg Forum 2004;7:E141-E146.
58. Bucerius J, Gummert JF, Walther T, et al: On-pump versus off-pump coronary artery bypass grafting: Impact on postoperative renal failure requiring renal replacement therapy. Ann Thorac Surg 2004;77:1250-1256.
59. McCreath BJ, Swaminathan M, Booth JV, et al: Mitral valve surgery and acute renal injury: Port access versus median sternotomy. Ann Thorac Surg 2003;75:812-819.
60. Hilberman M, Derby GC, Spencer RJ: Sequential pathophysiological changes characterizing the progression from renal dysfunction to acute failure following cardiac operations. J Thorac Cardiovacu Surg 1980;79:838-844.
61. Horwitz D, Fox SM D, Goldberg LI: Effects of dopamine in man. Circ Res 1962;10:237-243.
62. ter Wee PM, Smit AJ, Rosman JBZ, et al: Effect of intravenous infusion of low-dose dopamine on renal function in normal individuals and in patients with renal disease. Am J Nephrol 1986;6:42-46.
63. Myles PS, Buckland MR, Schenk NJ, et al: Effect of "renal-dose" dopamine on renal function following cardiac surgery. Anaesth Intensive Care 1993;21:56-61.
64. Lassnigg A, Donner E, Grubhofer G, et al: Lack of renoprotective effects of dopamine and furosemide during cardiac surgery. J Am Soc Nephrol 2000;11:97-104.
65. Woo EB, Tang AT, el-Gamel A, et al: Dopamine therapy for patients at risk of renal dysfunction following cardiac surgery: Science or fiction? Eur J Cardiothorac Surg 2002;22:106-111.
66. Carcoana OV, Mathew JP, Davis E, et al: Mannitol and dopamine in patients undergoing cardiopulmonary bypass: A randomized clinical trial. Anesth Analg 2003;97:1222-1229.
67. Chiolero R, Borgeat A, Fisher A: Postoperative arrhythmias and risk factors after open heart surgery. Thorac Cardiovasc Surg 1991;39:81-84.
68. Tang AT, el-Gamel A, Keevil B, et al: The effect of "renal-dose" dopamine on renal tubular function following cardiac surgery: Assessed by measuring retinal binding protein (RBP). Eur J Cardiothorac Surg 1999;15:717-721.
69. Better OS, Rubinstein I, Winaver JM, et al: Mannitol therapy revisited (1940-1997). Kidney Int 1997;52:886-894.
70. Ip-Yam PC, Murphy S, Baines M, et al: Renal function and proteinuria after cardiopulmonary bypass: The effects of temperature and mannitol. Anesth Analg 1994;78:842-847.
71. Lassnigg A, Donner E, Grubhofer G, et al: Lack of renoprotective effects of dopamine and furosemide during cardiac surgery. J Am Soc Nephrol 2002;11:97-104.
72. Lim E, Ali ZA, Attaran R, et al: Evaluating routine diuretics after coronary surgery: A prospective randomized controlled trial. Ann Thorac Surg 2002;73:153-155.
73. Singer I, Epstein M: Potential of dopamine A-1 agonists in the management of acute renal failure. Am J Kidney Dis 1998;31:743-755.
74. Caimmi PP, Pagani L, Micalizzi E, et al: Fenoldopam for renal protection in patients undergoing cardiopulmonary bypass. J Cardiothorac Vasc Anesth 2003;17:491-494.
75. Ranucci M, Soro G, Barzaghi N, et al: Fenoldopam prophylaxis of postoperative acute renal failure in high-risk cardiac surgery patients. Ann Thorac Surg 2004;78:1332-1337.
76. Bertolissi M, Antonucci F, De Monte A, et al: Effects on renal function of a continuous infusion of nifedipine during cardiopulmonary bypass. J Cardiothorac Vasc Anesth 1996;10:238-242.
77. Zanardo G, Michielon P, Rosi P, et al: Effects of a continuous diltiazem infusion on renal function during cardiac surgery. J Cardiothorac Vasc Anesth 1993;7:711-716.

78. Amano J, Suzuki A, Sunamori M, et al: Effect of calcium antagonist diltiazem on renal function in open heart surgery. Chest 1995;107:1260-1266.

79. Bergman AS, Odar-Cederlof I, Westman L, et al: Diltiazem infusion for renal protection in cardiac surgical patients with preexisting renal dysfunction. J Cardiothorac Vasc Anesth 2002;16:294-299.

80. Kulka PJ, Tryba M, Zenz M: Preoperative alpha2-adrenergic receptor agonists prevent the deterioration of renal function after cardiac surgery: Results of a randomized, controlled trial. Crit Care Med 1996;24:947-952.

81. McIntyre RW, Schwinn DA: Atrial natriuretic peptide. J Cardiothorac Anesth 1989;3:91-98.

82. Espiner EA, Richards AM: Effects of atrial natriuretic peptide in normal and hypertensive humans. In Samson WK, Quirion R (eds): Atrial Natriuretic Peptides. Boca Raton, Fla, CRC Press, 1990, pp 243-260.

83. Hynynen M, Tikkanen I, Salmenpera M, et al: Plasma atrial natriuretic peptide concentrations during induction of anesthesia and acute volume loading in patients undergoing cardiac surgery. J Cardiothorac Anesth 1987;1:401-407.

84. Berendes E, Schmidt C, Van Aken H, et al: A-type and B-type natriuretic peptides in cardiac surgical procedures. Anesth Analg 2004;98:11-19.

85. Ohki S, Ishikawa S, Ohtaki A, et al: Hemodynamic effects of alpha-human atrial natriuretic polypeptide on patients undergoing open-heart surgery. J Cardiovasc Surg (Torino) 1999;40:781-785.

86. Sezai A, Shiono M, Orime Y, et al: Low-dose continuous infusion of human atrial natriuretic peptide during and after cardiac surgery. Ann Thorac Surg 2000;69:732-738.

87. Sward K, Valson F, Ricksten SE: Long-term infusion of atrial natriuretic peptide (ANP) improves renal blood flow and glomerular filtration rate in clinical acute renal failure. Acta Anaesthesiol Scand 2001;45:536-542.

88. Wiebe K, Meyer M, Wahlers T, et al: Acute renal failure following cardiac surgery is reverted by administration of urodilatin (INN: Ularitide). Eur J Med Res 1996;1:259-265.

89. Demirkilic U, Kuralay E, Yenicesu M, et al: Timing of replacement therapy for acute renal failure after cardiac surgery. J Card Surg 2004;19:17-20.

90. Stevens LM, El-Hamamsy I, Leblanc M, et al: Continuous renal replacement therapy after heart transplantation. Can J Cardiol 2004;20:619-623.

91. Ronco C, Bellomo R: Prevention of acute renal failure in the critically ill. Nephron Clin Pract 2003;93:C13-20.

92. Gaudino M, Di Castelnuovo A, Zamparelli R, et al: Genetic control of postoperative systemic inflammatory reaction and pulmonary and renal complications after coronary artery surgery. J Thorac Cardiovasc Surg 2003;126:1107-1112.

93. MacKensen GB, Swaminathan M, Ti LK, et al: Preliminary report on the interaction of apolipoprotein E polymorhism with aortic atherosclerosis and acute nephropathy after CABG. Ann Thorac Surg 2004;78:520-526.

94. Boldt J, Brenner T, Lehmann A, et al: Is kidney function altered by the duration of cardiopulmonary bypass? Ann Thorac Surg 2003;75:906-912.

95. Ellenberger C, Schweizer A, Diaper J, et al: Incidence, risk factors and prognosis of changes in serum creatinine early after aortic abdominal surgery. Intensive Care Med 2006;32:1808-1816.

96. Kertai MD, Boersma E, Bax JJ, et al: Comparison between serum creatinine and creatinine clearance for the prediction of postoperative mortality in patients undergoing major vascular surgery. Clin Nephrol 2003;59:17-23.

97. Wahlberg E, DiMuzio PJ, Stoney RJ: Aortic clamping during elective operations for infrarenal disease: The influence of clamping time on renal function. J Vasc Surg 2002;36:13-18.

98. Kudo FA, Nishibe T, Miyazaki K, et al: Postoperative renal function after elective abdominal aortic aneurysm repair requiring suprarenal aortic cross-clamping. Surg Today 2004;34:1010-1013.

99. Nypaver TJ, Shepard AD, Reddy DJ, et al: Repair of pararenal abdominal aortic aneurysms: An analysis of operative management. Arch Surg 1993;128:803-811; discussion 811-813.

100. Crawford ES, Crawford JL, Safi HJ, et al: Thoracoabdominal aortic aneurysms: Preoperative and intraoperative factors determining immediate and long-term results of operations in 605 patients. J Vasc Surg 1986;3:389-404.

101. Schepens MA, DeFauw JJ, Hamerlijnck RP, Vermeulen FE: Risk assessment of acute renal failure after thoracoabdominal aortic aneurysm surgery. Ann Surg 1994;219:400-407.

102. Svensson LG, Crawford ES, Hess KR, et al: Thoracoabdominal aortic aneurysms associated with celiac, superior mesenteric, and renal artery occlusive disease: Methods and analysis of results in 271 patients. J Vasc Surg 1992;16:378-338; discussion 89-90.

103. Safi HJ, Harlin SA, Miller CC, et al: Predictive factors for acute renal failure in thoracic and thoracoabdominal aortic aneurysm surgery. J Vasc Surg 1996;24:338-344; discussion 344-345.

104. Carrel TP, Berdat PA, Robe J, et al: Outcome of thoracoabdominal aortic operations using deep hypothermia and distal exsanguination. Ann Thorac Surg 2000;69:692-695.

105. Breckwoldt WL, Mackey WC, Belkin M, O'Donnell TF Jr: The effect of suprarenal cross-clamping on abdominal aortic aneurysm repair. Arch Surg 1992;127:520-524.

106. Johnston KW: Multicenter prospective study of nonruptured abdominal aortic aneurysm: Part II. Variables predicting morbidity and mortality. J Vasc Surg 1989;9:437-447.

107. Chaikof EL, Smith RB 3rd, Salam AA, et al: Ischemic nephropathy and concomitant aortic disease: A ten-year experience. J Vasc Surg 1994;19:135-146; discussion 146-148.

108. Allen BT, Anderson CB, Rubin BG, et al: Preservation of renal function in juxtarenal and suprarenal abdominal aortic aneurysm repair. J Vasc Surg 1993;17:948-958; discussion 958-959.

109. Cambria RP, Brewster DC, L'Italien GJ, et al: Renal artery reconstruction for the preservation of renal function. J Vasc Surg 1996;24:371-380; discussion 380-382.

110. Acher CW, Belzer FO, Grist TM, et al: Late renal function in patients undergoing renal revascularization for control of hypertension and/or renal preservation. Cardiovasc Surg 1996;4:602-606.

111. Panneton JM, Lassonde J, Laurendeau F: Ruptured abdominal aortic aneurysm: Impact of comorbidity and postoperative complications on outcome. Ann Vasc Surg 1995;9:535-541.

112. Bauer EP, Redaelli C, von Segesser LK, Turina MI, Heartcenter Bodensee Kreuzlingen, Switzerland: Ruptured abdominal aortic aneurysms: Predictors for early complications and death. Surgery 1993;114:31-35.

113. Hajarizadeh H, Rohrer MJ, Herrmann JB, Cutler BS: Acute peritoneal dialysis following ruptured abdominal aortic aneurysms. Am J Surg 1995;170:223-226.

114. Berisa F, Beaman M, Adu D, et al: Prognostic factors in acute renal failure following aortic aneurysm surgery. Q J Med 1990;76:689-698.

115. White RA, Donayre CE, Walot I, et al: Preliminary clinical outcome and imaging criterion for endovascular prosthesis development in high-risk patients who have aortoiliac and traumatic arterial lesions. J Vasc Surg 1996;24:556-569; discussion 569-571.

116. Sharma PV, Babu SC, Shah PM, Nassoura ZE: Changing patterns of atheroembolism. Cardiovasc Surg 1996;4:573-579.

116a. Powell RJ, Roddy SP, Meier GH, et al: Effects of renal insufficiency on outcome following infrarenal surgery. Am J Surg 1997;174:126-130.

116b. Shepard AD, Tollefson DFJ, Reddy DJ, et al: Left flank retroperitoneal exposure: A technical aid to complex aortic reconstruction. J Vasc Surg 1991;14:238-291.

116c. Hallett JW Jr, Textor SC, Kos PB, et al: Advanced renovascular hypertension and renal insufficiency: Trends in medical comorbidity and surgical approach from 1970 to 1993. J Vasc Surg 1995;21:750-760.

116d. Godet G, Fleron M-H, Vicaut E, et al: Risk factors for acute postoperative renal failure in thoracic or thoracoabdominal aortic surgery: A prospective study. Anesth Analg 1997;85:1227-1232.

117. Soukiasian HJ, Raissi SS, Kleisli T, et al: Total circulatory arrest for the replacement of the descending and thoracoabdominal aorta. Arch Surg 2005;140:394-398.

118. Leurs LJ, Bell R, Degrieck Y, et al: Endovascular treatment of thoracic aortic diseases: Combined experience from the EUROSTAR and United Kingdom Thoracic Endograft registries. J Vasc Surg 2004;40:670-679; discussion 679-680.

119. Makaroun MS, Dillavou ED, Kee ST, et al: Endovascular treatment of thoracic aortic aneurysms: Results of the phase II multicenter trial of the GORE TAG thoracic endoprosthesis. J Vasc Surg 2005;41:1-9.

120. Ranucci M, Romitti F, Isgro G, et al: Oxygen delivery during cardio-pulmonary bypass and acute renal failure after coronary operations. Ann Thorac Surg 2005;80:2213-2220.

121. Resch TA, Greenberg RK, Lyden SP, et al: Combined staged procedures for the treatment of thoracoabdominal aneurysms. J Endovasc Ther 2006;13:481-489.

122. Black SAB, Wolfe JHN, Clark M, et al: Complex thoracoabdominal aortic aneurysms: Endovascular exclusion with visceral revascularization. J Vasc Surg 2006;43:1081-1089.

123. Mehta RL, Chertow GM: Acute renal failure definitions and classification: Time for change? J Am Soc Nephrol 2003;14:2178-2187.

124. Levey AS, Bosch JP, Lewis JB, et al: A more accurate method to estimate glomerular filtration rate from serum creatinine: A new prediction equation—Modification of Diet in Renal Disease study group. Ann Intern Med 1999;130:461-470.

125. Wijeysundera DN, Karkouti K, Beattie WS, et al: Improving the identification of patients at risk of postoperative renal failure after cardiac surgery. Anesthesiology 2006;104:65-72.

126. Finney H, Newman DJ, Gruber W, et al: Initial evaluation of cystatin C measurement by particle-enhanced immunonephelometry on the Behring nephelometer systems (BNA, BN II). Clin Chem 1997;43:1016-1022.

127. Dharnidharka VR, Kwon C, Stevens G: Serum cystatin C is superior to serum creatinine as a marker of kidney function: A meta-analysis. Am J Kidney Dis 2002;40:221-226.

128. Nguyen MT, Ross GF, Dent CL, Devarajan P: Early prediction of acute renal injury using urinary proteomics. Am J Nephrol 2005;25:318-326.

129. Aronson S, Fontes ML, Miao Y, Mangano DT: Risk index for perioperative renal dysfunction/failure: Critical dependence on pulse pressure hypertension. Circulation 2007;115:733-742.

130. Prough DS, Foreman AS: Anesthesia and the renal system. In Barash PG, Stoelting R, Cullen G (eds): Clinical Anesthesia, ed 2. Philadelphia, Lippincott Williams & Wilkins, 1992, pp 1125-1156.

Chapter

10 Pulmonary Risk Assessment

Maurizio Cereda

The pulmonary risk assessment of the operative candidate is guided by relatively weak evidence, particularly compared with the large volume of literature generated by the interest in the preoperative cardiac evaluation.[1,2] However, postoperative pulmonary complications (PPCs) have an undeniable clinical relevance, as they are frequent and they impose a significant financial burden.[3] PPCs appear to have a higher incidence than cardiac complications[4] and, based on known rates, it has been estimated that more than 1 million surgical patients have a PPC each year in the United States.[5] The effect of these complications on relevant outcomes has been reported by more than one study, and their onset is associated with an increased duration of hospital stay.[6] A prospective cohort study on patients undergoing nonthoracic surgery showed that patients who developed a PPC had a mean hospital stay of 27.9 days, as opposed to a mean stay of 4.5 days in patients who did not have a PPC.[5] Mortality rates are also higher in patients who have a PPC[7] or postoperative pneumonia.[8]

Pulmonary risk assessment should follow the general principles that guide the preoperative evaluation of the surgical patient. Data should be obtained in a timely and cost-efficient manner and should help estimate the probability of a pulmonary complication in the individual patient. Modifiable and unmodifiable risk factors should be identified and used to help determine the patient's eligibility for a specific procedure and to guide the choice of risk-reduction strategies. The main difficulty in pulmonary risk assessment is that it is not entirely clear how well the information obtained can be used. To date, there are no definite cutoff variables that indicate a prohibitive risk for PPCs requiring denial of a procedure. Although the risk for PPCs can be high in certain populations and for certain procedures, this risk can still be considered acceptable by the patient and by the physicians involved. Additionally, continuing evolution of surgical and perioperative care invalidates cutoffs suggested by past studies. Finally, the evidence supporting most of the available risk-reduction interventions is still relatively weak.

An additional difficulty in performing pulmonary risk assessment is that there has been conflicting evidence on which variables are predictors of complications. In fact, several possible risk factors have been identified, but only a few of them have been found to be independent predictors of PPCs in more than one study. The reason for these discrepancies is probably that only a minority of the available studies fulfilled the standards for high-quality prognostic studies,[9] such as a prospective design, the use of a blinded evaluator of the postoperative outcomes, the use of strict outcome definitions, and the adoption of multivariate analysis to account for coexisting factors. Additionally, most of the studies available evaluated small patient populations, and they differed considerably in the definitions chosen for variables and complications.[10] Only more recently have higher-quality studies been conducted, and, based on their results, it is now possible to make a few suggestions on pulmonary risk assessment.[4,5,11-15] The available data suggest that the risk for PPCs can be determined in a relatively simple and inexpensive manner. For a long time, laboratory and instrumental data, specifically pulmonary function tests (PFTs), have been considered to be very important in the preoperative pulmonary evaluation. However, the role of testing in nonthoracic surgery has been reduced because there is adequate evidence that pulmonary risk can be estimated through patient history and physical examination.[1] Thoracic surgery, and particularly lung resection, constitutes a particular case in which instrumental testing is used to determine how much lung tissue can be removed without causing intolerable functional impairment.

■ EPIDEMIOLOGY

The reported incidence of PPCs varies considerably among studies. The most likely reason for this discrepancy is a lack of agreement on what defines a pulmonary complication. As a consequence, past reports have not distinguished between clinical events with questionable effects on outcome, such as intraoperative bronchospasm or low-grade fever, and significant events such as pneumonia and respiratory failure.[1] A more systematic approach should evaluate only those complications that are likely to affect mortality, prolong hospital stay, or require specific treatment (Table 10-1). These clinical entities should be defined by criteria as stringent and unequivocal as possible, such as the criteria for nosocomial pneumonia.[16] This approach to the study of PPCs has been adopted by investigators only in relatively recent times, and it has resulted in an improved understanding of the risk factors associated with these complications.[10] However, the reported rate of pulmonary complications is variable even when stricter criteria for the diagnosis of PPCs are used, probably because of the heterogeneity of the populations studied and the surgical procedures performed (Table 10-2).

Pneumonia, respiratory failure, and atelectasis are the most frequent PPCs.[4,14] In particular, pneumonia is probably the single most important pulmonary complication, because it has a definite impact on outcomes. Postoperative pneumonia has been detected in 18.6% of 140 patients undergoing major surgery[8] and is associated with mortality rates as high as 21%.[11] Perioperative bronchospasm seems to occur in a surprisingly small portion of the population even when patients with asthma are considered.[17] However, broncho-spasm was the most frequent complication in smokers with evidence of airway obstruction by spirometry.[18]

■ ETIOLOGY AND PATHOPHYSIOLOGY

The mechanisms that lead to PPCs are complex and only partially understood. Clearly, factors related to preexisting diseases, surgical trauma, and anesthesia interact in pre-disposing a patient to the development of PPCs (Fig. 10-1). Perioperative loss of lung volumes with consequent forma-tion of atelectasis is widely accepted as one of the most important mechanisms that create PPCs. Atelectasis is initiated by general anesthesia itself, and may deteriorate gas exchange intraoperatively and in the early postoperative period.[19] Using computerized tomography (CT) scans of the chest, Hedenstierna and associates observed small areas of alveolar collapse shortly after the induction of general anes-thesia in healthy subjects,[20] but they could not demonstrate the same phenomenon in patients receiving epidural anesthesia.[21]

The causes of the formation of atelectasis during general anesthesia are multiple. Lung tissue has a natural tendency toward gravity-dependent alveolar collapse during mechani-cal ventilation, as suggested by the fact that atelectasis is located in the recumbent parts of the lungs[22] (Fig. 10-2). Mechanical ventilation and muscle relaxation cause cephalad

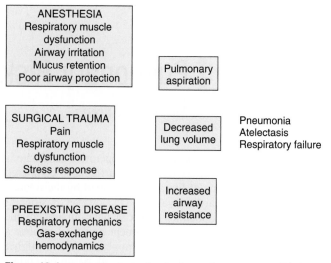

Figure 10-1 ■ Mechanisms that lead to pulmonary complications in the surgical patient.

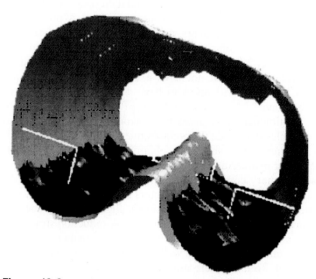

Figure 10-2 ■ Three-dimensional reconstruction of computed tomography chest scans performed on an anesthetized and para-lyzed patient. *(Reprinted with permission from Hedenstierna G: Clin Physiol Funct Imaging 2003;23:123-129.)*

10-1	Criteria That Define Relevant Postoperative Pulmonary Complications
Complication	**Criteria**
Pneumonia	Clinical diagnostic criteria for nosocomial pneumonia*
Respiratory failure	Requires invasive or noninvasive mechanical ventilation
Atelectasis	Requires intervention (bronchoscopy, postural therapy)
Pleural effusion	Requires drainage
Pneumothorax	Requires drainage
Bronchospasm	Requires bronchodilator therapy

*Diagnostic criteria for nosocomial pneumonia from Garner JS, Jarvis WR, Emori TG, et al: Am J Infect Control 1988;16:128-140.

10-2	Reported Rates of Postoperative Pulmonary Complications (PPC)		
Author, Year (Ref.)	**PPC Rate (%)**	**Patients (N)**	**Type of Surgery**
Hall et al., 1991 (7)	23	1000	Abdominal
Lawrence et al., 1995 (4)	9.6	2291	Abdominal
Wong et al., 1995 (49)	37	105	Nonthoracic (in patients with COPD)
Hall et al., 1996 (45)	12	456	Abdominal
Brooks-Brunn, 1997 (48)	22.5	400	Abdominal
McAlister et al., 2003 (13)	8	272	Nonthoracic
Warner et al., 1996 (17)	1.7	706	General (asthma)
Williams-Russo et al., 1992 (55)	6	278	General
McAlister et al., 2005 (5)	2.7	1005	Nonthoracic
Mitchell et al., 1998 (15)	11	148	General

COPD, chronic obstructive pulmonary disease.

displacement and decreased respiratory excursion of the posterior part of the diaphragm, a finding that explains the mainly caudal distribution of the areas of atelectasis (Fig. 10-3).[23,24] Even when spontaneous breathing is allowed, general anesthetic agents may cause lung volume loss, because they induce impaired coordination between respiratory muscle groups, causing inspiratory activation of expiratory muscles and an inward motion of the ribcage during inspiration.[25]

Reabsorption of intra-alveolar gas is another mechanism of atelectasis formation during anesthesia, when the inspired fraction of oxygen (FIO_2) is close to 1.0.[26] However, this mechanism is probably not important when a lower FIO_2 is used, as suggested by a study in which two groups of patients randomized to receive either 0.8 or 0.3 FIO_2 during anesthesia and surgery had comparable postoperative atelectasis and gas exchange.[27] Intraoperative atelectasis also very likely has a role in the genesis of hypoxemia in the later postoperative period. This is suggested by a study where patients who were hypoxemic during anesthesia had an increased rate of hypoxemia in the first 4 postoperative days, compared with patients who were intraoperatively normoxemic.[28]

Other factors besides anesthesia cause lung volume loss in the postoperative period. Functional residual capacity (FRC) declines after surgery, and the observed changes are bigger when the site of surgical incision is closer to the diaphragm.[29] Consequently, the incidence of postoperative hypoxemia is increased after surgery to the chest and the upper abdomen compared with peripheral surgeries.[30] Pain and surgical trauma lead to limitation of inspiratory excursion and are important contributors to postoperative lung volume loss. There is also evidence that surgical manipulation of upper abdominal viscera results in a reflex dysfunction of the diaphragm muscle that is not related to pain, as shown in patients after laparoscopic cholecystectomy.[31] However, the existence of postoperative diaphragm dysfunction has been questioned, because the studies that detected it may have misinterpreted findings caused by inspiratory activation of the abdominal muscles rather than by diaphragm dysfunction.[32]

Atelectasis is considered a relevant complication in itself, because it can cause hypoxemia and respiratory failure, and also because it is thought to predispose to pneumonia. However, a causative link between atelectasis and pneumonia

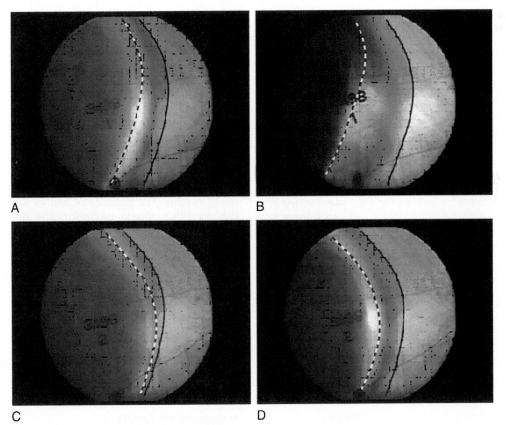

Figure 10-3 ■ Lateral views of the diaphragm at end inspiration *(stippled line)* and at end expiration *(thick line)* in a healthy subject during spontaneous breathing (**A** and **B**) and during mechanical ventilation (**C** and **D**). The area between the two lines represents diaphragm excursion. Inspirations with baseline tidal volumes (**A** and **C**) and with large tidal volumes (**B** and **D**) are shown. Overall diaphragm excursion was reduced during mechanical ventilation at both tidal volumes. The posterior *(inferior parts of the pictures)* portion of the diaphragm had the greatest reduction in tidal excursion. *(Reprinted with permission from Kleinman BS, Frey K, VanDrunen M, et al: Anesthesiology 2002;97:298-305.)*

has not been convincingly demonstrated. Only recently, experimental data demonstrated that eliminating atelectasis limited bacterial growth in an animal model of pneumonia, suggesting that collapsed alveoli provide a favorable environment for infection.[33]

In addition to volume loss, other factors play a role in the genesis of PPCs and of postoperative pneumonia. An important factor is probably mucus retention caused by decreased coughing from pain and medications, and by dysfunction of mucociliary transport in the airway mucosa. Mucociliary transport is an important mechanism of pulmonary defense, and its velocity is decreased by anesthesia and endotracheal intubation with a cuffed tube (Fig. 10-4).[34,35] Smokers have a decreased mucociliary transport velocity during anesthesia compared with nonsmokers,[36] a finding that may help to explain the high rate of PPCs in these patients. It is not clear how long this functional impairment of mucus transport lasts after the end of anesthesia and extubation. However, prolonged endotracheal intubation with cuffed endotracheal tubes also causes significant structural damage to the tracheal mucosa, with loss of cilia and epithelial cells,[37] which could have longer-lasting effects on mucus excretion.

Aspiration of contaminated oropharyngeal secretions is thought to be a prominent mechanism leading to nosocomial and postoperative pneumonia.[8] Aspiration may occur during the intubation maneuver and anesthesia, but undetected aspiration is probably frequent after surgery. Prolonged endotracheal intubation predisposes to aspiration of oropharyngeal material and puts the patient at risk for ventilator-associated pneumonia, a complication that doubles the risk for mortality.[38] Oropharyngeal and laryngeal protective mechanisms can be transiently decreased after surgery and may also predispose the nonintubated patient to pneumonia. Nasogastric intubation is likely to decrease airway protective mechanisms and predispose to occult aspiration. Residual subclinical muscle relaxation has been detected in patients who received long-acting muscle relaxants, and it was associated with an increased rate of pulmonary complications.[39] Poor airway protection and aspiration of secretions is probably even more common after certain procedures, such as transhiatal esophagectomy,[40] explaining the 28.5% rate of postoperative pulmonary complications observed after this surgery.[41]

Airway manipulation during intubation triggers reflex bronchospasm that can complicate intraoperative management and potentially prolong intubation and mechanical ventilation. Smokers have an increased sensitivity to airway irritants,[42] which may explain why these patients are more prone than nonsmokers to events such as laryngospasm and bronchospasm.[43]

Finally, chronic pulmonary disease causes gas exchange and respiratory mechanics abnormalities that reduce the patients' ability to tolerate superimposed acute lung disease, and render them prone to respiratory failure. Additionally, patients with chronic obstructive pulmonary disease (COPD) have dysfunction of the respiratory muscles because of chest wall deformation and myopathy.[44] These patients may be unable to withstand the increased ventilatory demand and the higher work of breathing required in the postoperative period, and they may require ventilatory support earlier than patients with normal muscle function.

■ PREOPERATIVE EVALUATION

The preoperative pulmonary evaluation is an integral part of the general preoperative risk assessment. The evaluator should start by collecting information on the patient's general history and overall health status, and then focus on the respiratory system. The presence of factors known to affect the risk for PPCs should be specifically investigated during history taking and the physical examination. Particular attention should be paid to the type of procedure that will be performed and its expected duration.

Most patients undergoing nonthoracic procedures, regardless of the type, are not likely to benefit from instrumental testing and may proceed to have surgery without further pulmonary evaluation. For patients undergoing thoracic surgery, the preoperative evaluation assesses the patient's eligibility for the procedure. The evaluation of the patient who is a candidate for pulmonary resection is discussed later.

Medical History

Extrapulmonary Factors

A review of the patient's general history increases the accuracy of the preoperative pulmonary evaluation, because several extrapulmonary factors have been found to correlate with the probability of PPCs (Box 10-1). Although advanced age is probably an important risk factor for PPCs, its significance has been questioned because earlier studies reporting

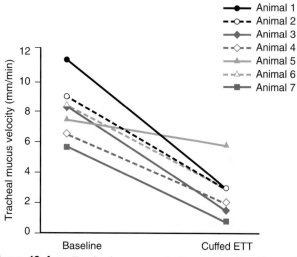

Figure 10-4 ■ Tracheal mucus velocity measured radiographically from displacement of metal disks insufflated in the distal trachea of anesthetized sheep. Mucus velocity decreased dramatically after insertion of a cuffed endotracheal tube in the proximal trachea. *Point A,* before insertion; *point B,* after insertion. (*Redrawn from Trawoger R, Kolobow T, Cereda M, Sparacino ME: Anesthesiology 1997;86:1140-1144.*)

10-1	Historical Factors Likely to Be Independent Predictors of Pulmonary Complications

- Advanced age (refs. 5, 13, 7, 45-48)
- Smoking history (refs. 13, 48, 11, 12)
- History of lung disease (refs. 11, 12, 45)
- High body weight (refs. 7, 48)
- Increased sputum production (ref. 15)
- Neurologic impairment (refs. 11, 12, 48)
- Exercise intolerance or dyspnea (refs. 11, 12, 55)
- ASA status (refs. 7, 45, 49)
- Functionally dependent status (refs. 11, 12)
- Malnutrition (refs. 11, 12)
- History of cancer (ref. 48)
- Preoperative hospital stay (ref. 7)
- Obstructive sleep apnea (ref. 64)

an increased rate of PPCs in older patients did not account for the presence of coexisting diseases by multivariate analysis and were thus flawed.[1] Later studies that did account for the effects of other conditions confirmed that an association between age and PPCs exists.[7,45-47] McAlister and colleagues found that age greater than 65 years was an independent predictor of PPCs in two studies where patients undergoing nonthoracic surgery were evaluated with a blinded prospective design.[5,13] These studies used multivariate analysis and fulfilled the criteria of a high-quality design for the evaluation of prognostic variables. Arozullah and coworkers detected an independent association of advanced age with both postoperative ventilatory failure and postoperative pneumonia, using prospectively collected data from the Department of Veteran Affairs National Surgical Quality Improvement Program (NSQIP).[11,12]

Other nonpulmonary factors have been found to be associated with the risk for PPCs. In the NSQIP population, Arozullah and colleagues reported that indexes of a poor nutritional status, such as a low serum albumin concentration and a history of weight loss, and indexes of an altered blood volume status, such as abnormal blood urea nitrogen (BUN) concentration, were all associated with postoperative respiratory failure and with pneumonia.[11,12] In these same studies, an increased probability of PPCs was also observed in patients who had a history of dependent functional status, recent alcohol use, diabetes, congestive heart failure, and renal failure. Preoperative neurologic impairment and history of stroke have also been reported to be independent predictors of PPCs in more than one study,[11,12,48] probably because of an increased occurrence of aspiration of gastric or pharyngeal secretions.

The American Society of Anesthesiologists (ASA) classification is a good instrument to evaluate the patient's overall physical condition, and its score is related to the overall incidence of postoperative complications. Multiple studies have detected a correlation between the ASA score and PPCs. An ASA score of higher than 2 has been found to be predictive of pulmonary complications after abdominal surgery,[7,45] and an ASA score of ≥4 was an independent predictor of PPCs in patients with severe COPD.[49] In a prospective longitudinal

study by Hall and coworkers,[7] the coexistence of advanced age and an ASA score of greater than 1 identified the majority (88%) of the patients who developed any PPC. Other health classification systems that are not specifically focused on the respiratory system may be useful in the pulmonary evaluation. Both the Goldman cardiac risk index and the Charlson comorbidity index have been reported to be associated with the incidence of PPCs.[14]

It is common to assume that patients who are obese are at high risk of having pulmonary complications, but this belief has been questioned since some studies failed to detect a correlation between obesity and PPCs. For example, a study on patients undergoing thoracotomy[50] and a study on patients receiving laparoscopic cholecystectomy[51] did not find a higher risk for PPCs in obese patients. However, factors related to the type of surgery and to patient selection in these studies might explain these results, because other studies did detect a correlation between obesity and PPCs. In fact, an elevated body mass index (BMI) was an independent predictor of PPCs by multivariate analysis in at least two studies.[7,48] In the prospective blinded study by McAlister and colleagues, a BMI of greater than 30 was associated with an increased risk for PPCs by univariate analysis,[5] although the correlation was not significant by multivariate analysis.

Pulmonary Factors

After an evaluation of the overall health status, history taking should elicit specific pulmonary risk factors (see Box 10-1), such as a history of chronic or acute pulmonary diseases, a smoking history, or sleep-related breathing disorders.

The presence of COPD was associated with an increased risk for PPCs in many studies.[5,7,13,45,46,52] In the NSQIP population, a previous diagnosis of COPD was an independent risk factor for both postoperative pneumonia (odds ratio [OR], 1.72) and for respiratory failure (OR, 1.81).[11,12] Even when a history of COPD is not documented, its presence can be suspected on the basis of elements of history, such as elevated sputum production. In a prospective study of 148 veterans undergoing nonthoracic surgery, the presence of high preoperative sputum production was an independent predictor of PPCs by multivariate analysis.[15] Similar results were reported by Barisione and colleagues.[53]

It is unclear whether a history of asthma is associated with increased rates of clinically significant pulmonary complications. In a review of the records of 706 patients with asthma undergoing surgery, Warner and coworkers reported a small incidence (1.7%) of bronchospasm during or after surgery. The rate of this event was higher in patients who had a recent asthma exacerbation.[17] However, the incidence of more severe complications and of postoperative respiratory failure was negligible in this study. In both prospective studies by McAlister and colleagues, a history of asthma was not associated with a higher risk for pulmonary complications.[5,13]

The onset of an acute pulmonary process or a recent exacerbation of preexisting lung disease are considered important risk factors for developing PPCs, and their presence is thought to be an adequate reason to postpone surgery, if possible. In the NSQIP study, the presence of preexisting pneumonia had an OR of 1.7 for developing postoperative respiratory failure.[12] For patients who have a recent or ongoing upper respiratory infection, postponing the operation is probably appropriate in the setting of elective surgery, but the evidence supporting this decision is relatively weak. For example, a recent upper respiratory infection significantly complicates the postoperative course in children and after cardiac surgery,[54] but there is little evidence that this problem also occurs in adults. In the study by Warner and coworkers, asthmatic patients with recent upper respiratory infections were not at increased risk for PPCs compared with the rest of the population.[17] In a prospective study, a history of upper or lower respiratory infection was not associated with a higher risk for PPCs.[48] Similarly, recent upper respiratory infections were not associated with PPCs in both studies by McAlister and colleagues.[5,13] The presence of dyspnea and exercise intolerance should be investigated during the preoperative evaluation, because these symptoms have been related to the risk for PPCs.[12,52,55] However, the association between dyspnea and PPCs was not confirmed in all studies.[5]

Having a history of tobacco use is probably the most solid risk factor for PPCs, because smoking has been established to be an independent predictor of PPCs by several studies.[5,11-23,48,56] In patients who are not current smokers, the risk of contracting a PPC decreases with time from smoking cessation, but it is unclear how much time is required for this risk to decrease optimally. Warner and coworkers reported that patients who quit smoking less than 8 weeks before surgery had a higher rate of PPCs than patients who quit earlier.[57] However, a longer smoke-free period seems to be needed to reduce the risk for PPCs to the level of the nonsmoking population, as suggested by the study by Arozullah and colleagues, which showed that having smoked within a year before surgery increased the risk for pneumonia[12] compared with the remaining patients. Based on study results, it has been suggested that smokers who do not quit entirely,[56] or who quit less than 8 weeks before surgery,[57] may have an increased risk for PPCs, not only compared with the nonsmoking population but also compared with patients who did continue to smoke. However, these results may have been affected by methodological flaws, because they have not been confirmed by more recent studies. A prospective observational study on thoracotomy patients did not detect an increase in the rate of PPCs in patients who quit smoking only within 8 weeks before the surgery, compared with patients who did not quit at all.[58] The results of the studies by McAlister and coworkers suggested that the extent of previous tobacco consumption may be a more important risk factor for PPCs than the timing of smoking cessation. In fact, these authors observed that the probability of PPCs was related to the number of pack-years smoked[5] and that having smoked more than 40 pack-years (the lifetime equivalent of a pack a day for at least 40 years) was an independent predictor of PPCs,[13] but they did not detect an independent association between recent smoking (within 2 weeks) and the incidence of PPCs.

Obstructive sleep apnea (OSA) is a sleep-related breathing disorder with a relatively high prevalence in the population and with a significant impact on health. The prevalence of symptomatic OSA has been estimated to be around 5%, whereas the prevalence of asymptomatic OSA is likely to be near 20%.[59] Sleep-related breathing disorders are diagnosed and graded by measuring the apnea-hypopnea index (AHI) by polysomnography. However, only a minority of patients with OSA present with a previous instrumental diagnosis. In the remaining patients, OSA can be suspected on the basis of key history elements such as snoring, witnessed apneas, restlessness during sleep, and daytime somnolence.[60] Unfortunately, the sensitivity and specificity of these variables in the diagnosis of OSA are probably low.

The presence of sleep apnea may be associated with an increased rate of perioperative complications. In fact, OSA is accompanied by a cluster of comorbidities that can affect surgical outcomes. These include systemic and pulmonary hypertension, right heart failure, diabetes, obesity, and stroke.[61] However, it is also a common perception that OSA per se may independently increase the risk for complications of surgery and anesthesia. Patients with sleep-related breathing disorders have decreased control of airway muscle tone and ventilation during sleep, which is exacerbated by long-acting narcotics and residual anesthetic effects in the postoperative period.[62] Thus, airway problems, postoperative hypoxemia, and ventilatory failure are possible and have been documented in patients with OSA who undergo upper airway surgery. In this setting, the frequency of adverse respiratory events is related to the severity of OSA.[63] There is still little evidence showing an independent association between sleep apnea and perioperative morbidity outside of upper airway surgery. In a retrospective case-control study on patients who underwent joint replacement, a diagnosis of OSA was associated with a significantly higher combined rate of complications and with prolonged hospital stay compared with controls.[64] However, the rate of pulmonary complications did not differ between the two groups.

Physical Examination

Physical examination is another important tool in the preoperative evaluation of the patient's pulmonary status, because it may allow the detection of unrecognized preexisting pulmonary disease. Although the diagnosis of chronic lung disease is often made by instrumental testing, a combination of data from patient history and physical examination has reasonable accuracy in predicting the presence of COPD.[65] Lawrence and colleagues documented that having an abnormal thoracic physical examination was an independent predictor of PPCs; however, they did not specify the types of abnormalities detected, thus decreasing the practical usefulness of their results.[14] The studies by McAlister and associates[5,13] are more informative, as they rigorously evaluated specific physical findings and detected significant correlations between these and the risk for PPCs (Table 10-3). In these studies, multiple physical findings correlated with the incidence of PPCs, and two of them were independent predictors of complications: decreased laryngeal height[13] and positive cough test.[5] The presence of wheezing on standard auscultation is usually considered an important physical sign, but it was not significantly associated with a higher risk for PPCs in these studies. This result is in agreement with a

10-3	**Physical Findings Associated with Increased Risk of Postoperative Pulmonary Complications**		
Finding	**Technique**	**Odds Ratio (95% CI)**	**P Value**
Positive cough test	Coughing once after deep inspiration triggers recurrent coughing.	4.3 (1.5-12.3)*	.01
		3.84 (1.51-9.80)†	.01
Positive wheeze test	Wheezing after five deep inspirations/expirations	3.4 (1.2-9.4)*	.04
		0.94 (0.12-7.08)†	1.00
Forced expiratory time ≥9 sec	Duration of forced exhalation after one deep inspiration	5.7 (2.3-14.2)*	.0002
		4.28 (1.22-15.02)†	.04
Maximum laryngeal height ≤4 cm	Distance between the sternal notch and the top of the thyroid cartilage at end expiration	6.9 (2.7-17.4)*	<.0001
		1.17 (0.44-3.12)†	.79
Wheezing on standard auscultation	Presence or absence of wheezing on standard thoracic exam	3.1 (0.9-10.0)*	.13
		2.39 (0.54-10.51)†	.23

*Data from McAlister FA, Khan NA, Straus SE, et al: Am J Respir Crit Care Med 2003;167:741-744.
†Data from McAlister FA, Bertsch K, Man J, et al: Am J Respir Crit Care Med 2005;171:514-517.

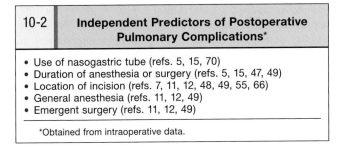

10-2	**Independent Predictors of Postoperative Pulmonary Complications***

- Use of nasogastric tube (refs. 5, 15, 70)
- Duration of anesthesia or surgery (refs. 5, 15, 47, 49)
- Location of incision (refs. 7, 11, 12, 48, 49, 55, 66)
- General anesthesia (refs. 11, 12, 49)
- Emergent surgery (refs. 11, 12, 49)

*Obtained from intraoperative data.

previous study in which decreased laryngeal height was an independent predictor of the presence of COPD as diagnosed by spirometry, whereas wheezing was not.[65] These results combined suggest that simple findings obtained through a methodic physical examination may help in the prediction of the probability of PPCs.

Operative Factors

Evaluation of operative data should be part of the pulmonary risk assessment, because multiple studies have reported correlations between these factors and the incidence of PPCs (Box 10-2). The type of the surgery and the location of the incision are probably important contributors to the pulmonary risk. In the studies by Arozullah and coworkers, abdominal aortic, thoracic, and upper abdominal surgery were the strongest of all independent predictors of PPCs, because they had the highest odds ratios for respiratory failure and pneumonia.[11,12] Other studies have reported an increased risk for PPCs during abdominal surgery,[49] and particularly after upper abdominal incisions. In fact, the risk for PPCs is higher when the incision is closer to the diaphragm.[7,48,66] McAlister and colleagues also detected a correlation between the rate of PPCs and abdominal surgery.[5] However, having abdominal surgery was not confirmed to be an independent risk factor for PPCs by univariate analysis. This discrepancy with previous studies may be explained by the fact that only a minority of the study patients underwent upper abdominal surgery in McAlister's study. Performance of surgery under emergent conditions has been reported to be associated with a higher risk for PPCs.[11,12,49] In the NSQIP studies, both neurologic and neck surgery were associated with increased risk

for respiratory failure and pneumonia, suggesting a role of poor airway protection in the genesis of PPCs, although the odds ratios were not as high as for thoracoabdominal surgery.[11,12]

The planned choice of surgical approach may significantly affect the risk for PPCs. There is some evidence that performing laparoscopic surgery is associated with decreased pulmonary complications, as shown by Hall and coworkers.[67] In a randomized study, patients undergoing laparoscopic fundoplication had better respiratory function and a shorter hospital stay than patients who had an open procedure.[68] The advent of endovascular aneurysm repair is probably going to have an effect on pulmonary complications. In fact, a randomized trial comparing open with endovascular abdominal aortic aneurysm repair detected a significantly smaller risk for severe pulmonary complications in the patients who received the endovascular repair (2.9% versus 10.9%, with a risk ratio of 3.7).[69]

Among the intraoperative factors, the duration of anesthesia and of surgery is probably one of the strongest predictors of PPCs. This association has been detected by more than one study.[47-49,66] McAlister and associates reported that a duration of anesthesia longer than 2.5 hours was an independent predictor of PPCs, with an OR of 3.3.[5] Duration of anesthesia was also an independent risk factor for PPCs in a prospective study by Mitchell and colleagues.[15] It is not clear, however, whether the duration of the procedure has an effect on PPCs independent of the complexity and type of the procedure itself. Concerning the anesthetic technique, there is conflicting evidence on the importance of the type of anesthesia as a risk factor for PPCs. In the NSQIP studies, general anesthesia was associated with higher risk for ventilatory failure and pneumonia, with ORs of 1.91 and 1.56, respectively.[11,12] However, in both studies by McAlister and coworkers, general anesthesia had no correlation at all with the risk for PPCs.[5,13] The evaluation of the type of anesthesia as a risk factor for PPCs through observational studies is complicated by the fact that the effect of anesthesia is not easily distinguishable from the effect of the site of surgery. In fact, general anesthesia is more frequent in surgeries at high risk for PPCs, such as thoracoabdominal surgery, and relatively less frequently selected for peripheral surgeries.

The use of a perioperative gastric tube is another important risk factor for the development of PPCs. At least two prospective studies[5,15] and one retrospective study[70] have reported that the perioperative use of nasogastric tubes was an independent predictor of pulmonary complications. This correlation was confirmed by multivariate analysis, which suggests that gastric suctioning per se, and not its use in high-risk procedures, causes pulmonary complications. The mechanism of causation of PPCs by nasogastric tube is likely to be decreased airway protection and aspiration of pharyngeal secretions.

Preoperative Testing

Preoperative testing is valuable only if it provides data that cannot be obtained from the history and physical examination, and if it helps determine the probability of a complication in patients who are known to have risk factors. Preoperative tests that are typically ordered as part of a pulmonary risk assessment include pulmonary function tests, arterial blood gases, chest radiographs, and, less commonly, exercise testing. However, it is unclear which, if any, of these tests adds useful information to the preoperative evaluation.

PFTs have been used to screen for unknown pulmonary disease and to risk-stratify patients, assuming a relationship between the severity of PFT abnormalities and the probability of PPCs. On the basis of currently available evidence, PFTs are unlikely to fulfill either of these purposes. They are probably not indispensable for the identification of patients with pulmonary disease, as suggested by recent studies in which history taking and physical examination had a reasonable accuracy in the diagnosis of COPD.[65,71] When present together, a history of smoking, advanced age, and laryngeal height shorter than 4 cm greatly increased the probability of detecting obstructive airway disease.[71]

The performance of PFTs as a risk-stratification tool is also very questionable.[72] They have been used for this purpose for many years, because past studies showed that patients who had abnormal PFT results had a higher risk for PPCs.[72] However, the validity of the evidence supporting this practice has been revisited and found to be methodologically flawed.[1,73] Studies that showed a correlation between PFT abnormalities and PPCs probably did so because they relied only on univariate analysis and did not account for concomitant risk factors. More recent and rigorous studies either failed to demonstrate a correlation between PFTs and the incidence of PPCs or could not confirm by multivariate analysis that PFT data are independent predictors of PPCs. In a case-control study by Lawrence and colleagues, comorbidity indexes and abnormal chest examination were independently associated with PPCs, whereas PFT results were not.[14] Mitchell and coworkers showed that, in patients undergoing general elective surgery, PFT results had no significant correlation with PPCs, unlike preoperative sputum production, duration of the procedure, and use of nasogastric tubes.[15] A possible explanation of these results is that other factors, such as the overall physical status and nonpulmonary comorbidities, may be more important than the degree of airway obstruction in predisposing to PPCs. Other studies also suggest that

pulmonary and nonpulmonary data collected through clinical evaluation contain most of the information necessary to make a risk prediction, rendering the information obtained from PFTs superfluous. In the studies by McAlister and colleagues, PFT data were significantly associated with the incidence of PPCs. However, none of the PFT variables were found to be independent predictors of PPCs by multivariate analysis, whereas variables such as smoking history, duration of anesthesia, and selected physical examination findings were independently related to PPCs.

The implication of these results is that no information is added by routinely performing PFTs as part of the clinical evaluation of patients undergoing nonthoracic surgery. Therefore, PFTs should be used only within the context of a diagnostic workup to confirm a diagnosis of pulmonary disease in patients who have findings suggesting its presence, or in patients with known chronic pulmonary disease whose symptoms suggest a superimposed exacerbation. The 1990 consensus statement of the American College of Physicians (ACP) limited the use of PFTs in nonthoracic surgery to patients undergoing upper abdominal surgery who had a history of smoking or dyspnea, and to patients undergoing more peripheral surgeries who had unexplained pulmonary symptoms[74.] (Box 10-3). In 1995, it was estimated that 39% of preoperative PFTs performed did not fulfill the ACP recommendations.[75] Based on this estimate, a cost analysis performed in 1997 described an annual excess expenditure of several million dollars resulting from unneeded PFTs.[76] It is possible that compliance with ACP guidelines has improved in the past few years, with substantial financial savings. However, it may be argued that the use of PFTs should be even more restricted than suggested by the ACP. No strong evidence supports the routine use of preoperative PFTs for high-risk nonthoracic surgeries and in high-risk patients. In a study by Warner and coworkers, 135 patients with moderate to severe flow limitation according to PFTs were compared with a group of patients with similar characteristics but without obstructive disease.[18] The group with obstructive disease had increased frequency of bronchospasm, but the rates of more significant complications were similar in the two groups. In particular, there was no difference in the incidence of prolonged intubation. In a study by Wong and colleagues, patients with severe COPD had a high (37%) risk of developing any PPCs.[49] By multivariate analysis, it was

---

10-3	**Guidelines for Preoperative Use of Pulmonary Function Tests**

- Patients undergoing cardiac or upper abdominal surgery with a history of smoking or dyspnea
- Patients undergoing lower abdominal surgery if dyspnea or history of smoking indicates prolonged surgery
- Patients undergoing orthopedic surgery with uncharacterized lung disease
- All patients undergoing lung resection

From American College of Physicians: Ann Intern Med 1990;112: 793-794.

possible to determine that, although a lower forced expiratory volume in 1 second (FEV_1) was associated with PPCs, nonpulmonary factors such as anesthesia duration and scoring systems such as the ASA's were better predictors of PPCs.

Arterial blood gas analyses, like PFTs, have been used in the past for the preoperative evaluation of nonthoracic surgery patients despite the lack of strong evidence suggesting their value. Hypercapnia with $PaCO_2$ higher than 45 mm Hg has been considered an important risk factor for PPCs and mortality.[77] Similarly, arterial hypoxemia has been considered an important risk factor for PPCs and a contraindication for surgery. These blood gas alterations may help in the risk–benefit assessment of a certain procedure, because their presence is associated with significantly shortened life expectancy in patients with COPD.[78] However, neither hypercapnia nor hypoxemia has been shown to be an independent predictor of the risk for PPCs.[5,13]

Chest radiographs are still routinely performed preoperatively in older patients, in patients with known pulmonary disease, and in patients who smoke. Although this practice is deeply rooted, there is little or no evidence that routine chest radiographs affect the perioperative management or outcomes in any way.[79] In patients who are asymptomatic or have no risk factors for pulmonary disease, chest radiographs are unlikely to reveal new information,[80] and they are likely to lead to unnecessary further testing in case of false-positive results. Patients who have risk factors for pulmonary disease are more likely to have abnormal findings. However, it is not clear whether chest radiographs add any information to the pulmonary risk stratification in patients who have stable symptoms or no symptoms at all.[79] The only reasonable use of chest radiology may be for patients with new or unexplained pulmonary symptoms, where radiography may uncover unknown pulmonary disease requiring further workup, or for those with an acute process, such as a pneumonia, in which case it may be prudent to postpone elective surgery.

Two studies support exercise testing as a useful tool to identify patients at risk for PPCs in nonthoracic surgery. Gerson and coworkers reported that a decreased exercise tolerance, evaluated by bicycle ergometry, was an independent predictor of cardiac, pulmonary, and combined cardiopulmonary complications in a group of patients undergoing both thoracic and nonthoracic surgeries.[81] The test had a negative predictive value of 0.91, but a low positive predictive value of 0.42. Girish and colleagues performed exercise testing prior to high-risk surgeries, including thoracotomy, by simply measuring the number of flights of stairs that the patients were capable of climbing.[82] A poor performance on this simple test was an independent risk factor for combined cardiopulmonary complications, whereas PFT results, age, weight, and preexisting pulmonary disease were not. The inability to climb more than two flights of stairs had a positive predictive value of 0.8 and a negative predictive value of 0.82 for postoperative cardiopulmonary complications. This study suggests that this simple test of exercise tolerance may be adopted in the clinical evaluation of patients scheduled to undergo high-risk surgeries.[82] However, there is still inadequate evidence to recommend routine exercise testing for the preoperative assessment of nonthoracic surgery patients.

Pulmonary hypertension is relatively common in patients with COPD or other types of chronic pulmonary diseases. The prevalence of pulmonary hypertension in patients with severe COPD ranges between 5% and 10%.[83] The detection of pulmonary hypertension has important prognostic value and may help in patient selection, because the presence of this condition is associated with significant life-span shortening in patients with COPD.[84] In thoracic surgery, pulmonary hypertension is used as a criterion to deny certain procedures, such as lung reduction surgery.[85] Pulmonary hypertension and right ventricular failure can significantly complicate intraoperative and postoperative management of patients undergoing high-risk surgeries, and it can be hypothesized that patients who tolerate moderate hypertension at rest may become acutely decompensated in the perioperative period. There should be awareness of the possible presence of these conditions when evaluating patients who have chronic pulmonary diseases and who need to undergo major surgery. Their existence can be suspected from clinical evaluation, but the accuracy of history and physical examination in the diagnosis of pulmonary hypertension is probably low.

Echocardiography is commonly used in the evaluation of patients with suspected right ventricular compromise or pulmonary hypertension. Pulmonary artery pressure is quantified by evaluation of tricuspid regurgitation, whrease right ventricular size and contractility are qualitatively assessed.[86] However, the quality of echocardiography studies is often poor, and their diagnostic accuracy is inferior to pulmonary artery catheterization in patients with COPD who have hyperinflated lungs.[87] To date, there is no evidence supporting the routine use of echocardiography to detect pulmonary hypertension in the preoperative evaluation for nonthoracic surgery, even of patients with advanced pulmonary disease. Although recommendations cannot be made, it may be reasonable to obtain echocardiography studies in those patients with severe lung disease who have signs compatible with right heart dysfunction, or who have significant exercise intolerance.

■ RISK SCORES

Risk scores can be useful clinical tools if they provide a reasonably accurate estimate of the probability of complications, and if the information can be used to guide therapeutic choices. Additionally, risk scores can provide some insight into the most important factors contributing to the genesis of a certain outcome. Although cardiac risk scores such as the Goldman index[88] have been in use for several years, pulmonary evaluation has lacked a valid risk index until very recently.

In two companion cohort studies, Arozullah and coworkers built and validated multifactorial risk score systems to predict postoperative pneumonia[11] and respiratory failure.[12] The studies were conducted at separate times and both used patient data from the department of Veterans Affairs NSQIP. The intent of the NSQIP was to provide tools to assess the quality of surgical care while adjusting for the patient's baseline risk for mortality and morbidity. Study patients underwent a variety of noncardiac procedures, including lung resections. Only transplants and surgeries with negligible mortality rates were excluded. Outcomes were tightly defined: pneumonia was diagnosed according to the Centers for Disease Control (CDC) criteria,[16] and respiratory failure was defined as a need for mechanical ventilation for more than 48 hours after surgery, or as a need for reintubation and ventilation after postoperative extubation. Data were analyzed by logistic regression, and variables that were independently related to the outcomes were used to develop the two scoring systems. In the scores, each variable was assigned a value depending on the regression coefficients: variables with higher values had more significant weights in the determination of the outcomes (Tables 10-4 and 10-5). The type of surgery was the strongest predictor of both pneumonia and respiratory failure. Interestingly, most factors identified as predictors of pneumonia were also predictors of respiratory failure, suggesting that the risk for these two complications can probably be assessed in a unified manner. Finally, based on the final risk scores, patients were assigned to five risk classes and, for each of these, the accuracy of risk prediction was validated in independent cohorts of patients, confirming that the models had adequate performance (Table 10-6).

The strengths of these two studies were the size of the populations investigated (a total of 500,000 patients) and the prospective cohort design, although data were collected through review of medical records and in an unblinded manner. Other weaknesses of these studies are related to the particular population investigated, which was mainly composed of male subjects with significant comorbidities, limiting somewhat the ability to extrapolate the results to the general population. Neither blood gases nor PFTs were included in the models, because of difficulties in obtaining these data, and this may be considered another weakness of the study. However, given what is currently known about the poor predictive power of PFTs and blood gas analysis, it is unlikely that their presence would have substantially changed

---

10-4   Respiratory Failure Risk Index

Preoperative Predictor	Point Value
Type of surgery	
Abdominal	27
Thoracic	21
Neurosurgery, upper abdominal, peripheral vascular	14
Neck	11
Emergency surgery	11
Albumin <3 g/dL	9
Blood urea nitrogen >30 mg/dL	8
Partially or fully dependent functional status	7
History of chronic obstructive pulmonary disease	6
Age (years)	
>70	6
60-69	4

Adapted with permission from Arozullah AM, Daley J, Henderson WG, Khuri SF: Ann Surg 2000;232:242-253.

10-5   Risk Index for Postoperative Pneumonia

Preoperative Risk Factor	Point Value
Type of surgery	
Abdominal aortic	15
Thoracic	14
Upper abdominal	10
Neck	8
Neurosurgery	8
Vascular	3
Age	
>80	17
70-79	13
60-69	9
50-59	4
Functional status	
Totally dependent	10
Partially dependent	6
Weight loss >10% in past 6 months	7
History of chronic obstructive pulmonary disease	5
General anesthesia	4
Impaired sensorium	4
History of cerebrovascular accident	4
Blood urea nitrogen level	
<8 mg/dL	4
22-30 mg/dL	2
>30 mg/dL	3
Transfusion >4 units	3
Emergency surgery	3
Steroid use for chronic condition	3
Current smoker within 1 year	3
Alcohol intake > two drinks/day in past 2 weeks	2

Adapted from Arozullah AM, Khuri SF, Henderson WG, Daley J: Ann Intern Med 2001;135:847-857.

10-6   Risk Categories for Respiratory Failure and Pneumonia

Class	Postoperative Respiratory Failure Risk Index (Point Total)	Probability of Respiratory Failure (%)	Postoperative Pneumonia Risk Index (Point Total)	Probability of Pneumonia (%)
1	0-10	0.5	0-15	0.2
2	11-19	2.2	16-25	1.2
3	20-27	5.0	26-40	4.0
4	28-40	11.6	41-55	9.4
5	>40	30.5	>55	15.3

Adapted from Arozullah AM, Khuri SF, Henderson WG, Daley J: Ann Intern Med 2001;135:847-857, and Arozullah AM, Daley J, Henderson WG, Khuri SF: Ann Surg 2000;232:242-253.

the performance of these models. Additionally, most of the information needed to formulate a risk prediction with the two models by Arozullah and colleagues can be relatively easily obtained, and this adds appeal to these risk-prediction indexes. A recent review by Smetana and coworkers auspicated that these indexes will be incorporated in the clinical practice.[89]

An evaluation algorithm for nonthoracic surgery is given in Figure 10-5. A thorough history and physical examination should be obtained, with particular attention to pulmonary and nonpulmonary factors that have been shown to be independent predictors of PPCs. In patients who have recent or ongoing respiratory infections, delay of surgery for 2 to 3 weeks should be considered, if acceptable from the surgical point of view. Patients with known chronic lung disease and with worse symptoms, or patients who have no known respiratory disease but who have a new onset of symptoms, should receive further evaluation, and involvement of a pulmonary specialist may be considered. Chest radiography and PFTs may be considered as well. In patients who have stable pulmonary symptoms but who are undergoing a high-risk procedure (upper abdominal surgery, major vascular surgery, surgery of probable duration longer than 2.5 hours, likely use of gastric suctioning), a further attempt at risk stratification using the postoperative pneumonia and respiratory failure risk indexes (see Tables 10-4 and 10-5) can be performed. In patients with a high score and a high probability of PPCs (see Table 10-6), risk-reduction strategies, alternative surgical approaches, or nonsurgical management may be considered.

■ EVALUATION OF THE LUNG RESECTION CANDIDATE

The preoperative evaluation of the candidate for lung resection surgery is particularly important. In fact, pulmonary complications are relatively common after lung resection, with rates reported to be 25% overall[90] and 49% after pneumonectomy.[91] This is probably because thoracic surgery patients have a unique cluster of comorbidities and risk factors predisposing them to PPCs, including cardiovascular diseases, smoking history, COPD, and advanced age. Additionally, lung resection decreases postoperative lung function, putting patients with poor functional reserve at risk for complications and disability. Therefore, the aim of the preoperative evaluation is not only to assess the risk for PPCs but also to determine whether a patient is a candidate for surgery and to establish the amount of pulmonary tissue that can be resected without causing intolerable functional impairment.

The risk assessment of these patients is complicated by the fact that evolution in perioperative care has improved short-term mortality and morbidity. Thus, selection criteria that were considered valid in the past are now questioned.[92] For example, advanced age used to be considered a major contraindication to extensive lung resection. However, recent guidelines indicate that patients younger than 80 years should receive lung resections, if indicated.[93] Age should be factored into the decision to operate only in those patients who are older than 80, or who need pneumonectomy, because patients in these groups seem to have an increased incidence of complications compared with younger populations.

The preoperative evaluation for lung resection should start with the identification of pulmonary and nonpulmonary risk factors for PPCs, by physical examination and by history taking, as discussed for nonthoracic surgery. Factors shown to be related to PPCs in thoracic surgery patients include cardiovascular disease, smoking history, and ASA status.[90] Intraoperative factors that have been shown to affect the rate of PPCs in patients undergoing lung resection are duration of procedure,[90] blood loss, and the amount of intravenous fluids administered.[91]

The preoperative assessment of lung resection candidates, unlike assessment of those undergoing nonthoracic surgery, relies heavily on instrumental testing. The evaluation algorithm for thoracic surgery has recently been re-evaluated by the British Thoracic Society (BTS).[93] The BTS guidelines recommend only tests that are supported by adequate clinical evidence and, based on favorable study results, those that place particular emphasis on the prediction of postoperative pulmonary function and the use of exercise testing. According to the BTS guidelines, all lung resection candidates should receive spirometry in their initial evaluation. Surgery can be performed with no further evaluation in pneumonectomy patients who have an FEV_1 of greater than 2 L, or greater than 80% of predicted, and in lobectomy patients who have an FEV_1 of greater than 1.5 L.

The BTS guidelines suggest that the diffusing capacity of the lung for carbon monoxide (DLCO) can be used in a complementary manner with spirometry, particularly for those patients who have symptoms not entirely explained by spirometry results. According to a prospective study, patients in whom both FEV_1 and DLCO are higher than 80% of predicted can undergo pneumonectomy with an acceptable risk for complications.[94] All patients whose spirometry and DLCO do not meet these initial evaluation criteria should undergo further tests to predict postoperative pulmonary reserve. The goal of this approach is to identify patients who are likely to have excessive respiratory dysfunction after the surgery. Predicted postoperative FEV_1 (ppoFEV_1) and predicted postoperative DLCO (ppoDLCO) can be estimated if the preoperative values and the planned extent of the lung resection are known. The latter can be estimated using radionuclide lung perfusion scans, or simply by counting and adding the segments that will be removed. Good correlations have been shown between actual values of postoperative pulmonary function and the predicted ones. The use of perfusion scans to predict postoperative lung function is recommended for pneumonectomies, whereas for lobectomies, using the segment count method is probably sufficiently accurate.[95] Patients who have ppoFEV_1 and ppoDLCO higher than 40% of predicted have an acceptable risk for postoperative complications, whereas all other patients should be considered at higher risk. A ppoFEV_1 lower than 30% seems to indicate a very high postoperative risk and, in these cases, nonoperative management should at least be considered.[92] However, acceptable mortality and morbidity rates have been reported even in patients who had low predicted postoperative pulmonary function.[96]

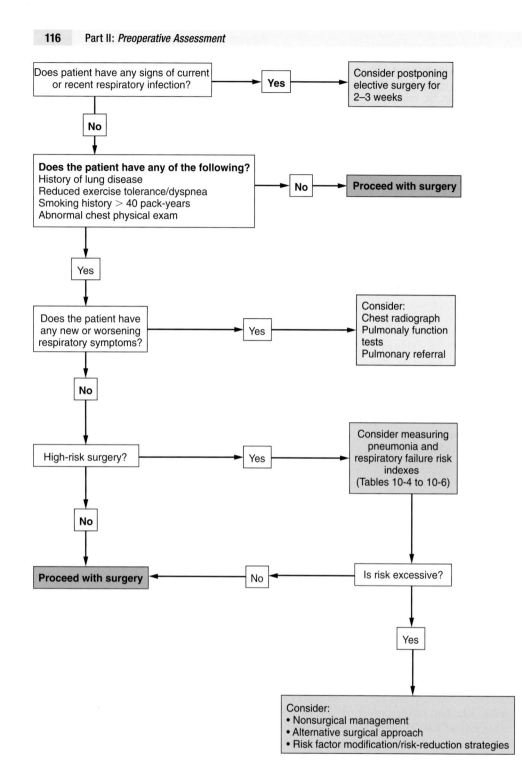

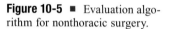

Figure 10-5 ■ Evaluation algorithm for nonthoracic surgery.

Additionally, it has been suggested that preoperative PFTs overestimate postoperative loss in exercise ability, particularly after lobectomy.[97] Therefore, the BTS guidelines recommend further evaluation through exercise testing in patients with poor predicted postoperative lung function.

Exercise testing is valuable for this purpose, as it provides a reasonably accurate assessment of a patient's cardiopulmonary functional status and ability to tolerate perioperative stress. Exercise ability can be evaluated by

formal cardiopulmonary exercise testing, where the maximal oxygen consumption (VO_{2max}) is calculated. Patients with a VO_{2max} greater than 15 mL/kg/min do not have a high risk for morbidity and mortality, whereas patients with a VO_{2max} less than 10 mL/kg/min have a high risk and should be considered for nonsurgical treatment.[98] Exercise testing can be combined with radionuclide lung scanning to obtain predicted postoperative VO_{2max} ($ppoVO_{2max}$). In a small prospective study by Bolliger and colleagues,[97] all patients with a $ppoVO_{2max}$ lower than 10 mL/kg/min died. When formal exercise testing is not available, exercise ability can be evaluated with alternative tests, such as stair climbing and shuttle walking. Although stair climbing is not well standardized, patients who can climb more than five flights of stairs can be assumed to have a VO_{2max} of greater than 20 mL/kg/min, whereas patients who cannot climb one flight of stairs probably have a VO_{2max} of less than 10 mL/kg/min.[99]

Although exercise testing for the evaluation of lung resection patients has been recommended by the BTS guidelines and by other authors,[92] other studies suggested that exercise testing results may not be independent predictors of PPCs. In a study by Epstein and coworkers, VO_{2max} was not independently related to the frequency of postoperative complications, whereas a combined cardiopulmonary risk score obtained from clinical data was.[100] In 137 patients undergoing lung resections from segmentectomy to pneumonectomy, Wyser and colleagues prospectively tested an algorithm incorporating exercise testing and estimated postoperative pulmonary function. The use of this algorithm identified a population with low morbidity and mortality rates. However, these rates were low only as compared with a series of historic controls from the same institutions prior to algorithm implementation, and a prospective comparison of a pathway including these tests is still missing.[94]

■ REFERENCES

1. Smetana GW: Preoperative pulmonary evaluation. N Engl J Med 1999;340:937-944.
2. Arozullah AM, Conde MV, Lawrence VA: Preoperative evaluation for postoperative pulmonary complications. Med Clin North Am 2003;87:153-173.
3. Warner DO: Preventing postoperative pulmonary complications: The role of the anesthesiologist. Anesthesiology 2000;92:1467-1472.
4. Lawrence VA, Hilsenbeck SG, Mulrow CD, et al: Incidence and hospital stay for cardiac and pulmonary complications after abdominal surgery. J Gen Intern Med 1995;10:671-678.
5. McAlister FA, Bertsch K, Man J, et al: Incidence of and risk factors for pulmonary complications after nonthoracic surgery. Am J Respir Crit Care Med 2005;171:514-517.
6. Kozlow JH, Berenholtz SM, Garrett E, et al: Epidemiology and impact of aspiration pneumonia in patients undergoing surgery in Maryland, 1999-2000. Crit Care Med 2003;31:1930-1937.
7. Hall JC, Tarala RA, Hall JL, Mander J: A multivariate analysis of the risk of pulmonary complications after laparotomy. Chest 1991;99:923-927.
8. Ephgrave KS, Kleiman-Wexler R, Pfaller M, et al: Postoperative pneumonia: A prospective study of risk factors and morbidity. Surgery 1993;114:815-819; discussion 819-821.
9. Lijmer JG, Mol BW, Heisterkamp S, et al: Empirical evidence of design-related bias in studies of diagnostic tests. JAMA 1999;282:1061-1066.
10. Fisher BW, Majumdar SR, McAlister FA: Predicting pulmonary complications after nonthoracic surgery: A systematic review of blinded studies. Am J Med 2002;112:219-225.
11. Arozullah AM, Khuri SF, Henderson WG, Daley J: Development and validation of a multifactorial risk index for predicting postoperative pneumonia after major noncardiac surgery. Ann Intern Med 2001;135:847-857.
12. Arozullah AM, Daley J, Henderson WG, Khuri SF: Multifactorial risk index for predicting postoperative respiratory failure in men after major noncardiac surgery. The National Veterans Administration Surgical Quality Improvement Program. Ann Surg 2000;232:242-253.
13. McAlister FA, Khan NA, Straus SE, et al: Accuracy of the preoperative assessment in predicting pulmonary risk after nonthoracic surgery. Am J Respir Crit Care Med 2003;167:741-744.
14. Lawrence VA, Dhanda R, Hilsenbeck SG, Page CP: Risk of pulmonary complications after elective abdominal surgery. Chest 1996;110:744-750.
15. Mitchell CK, Smoger SH, Pfeifer MP, et al: Multivariate analysis of factors associated with postoperative pulmonary complications following general elective surgery. Arch Surg 1998;133:194-198.
16. Garner JS, Jarvis WR, Emori TG, et al: CDC definitions for nosocomial infections, 1988. Am J Infect Control 1988;16:128-140.
17. Warner DO, Warner MA, Barnes RD, et al: Perioperative respiratory complications in patients with asthma. Anesthesiology 1996;85:460-467.
18. Warner DO, Warner MA, Offord KP, et al: Airway obstruction and perioperative complications in smokers undergoing abdominal surgery. Anesthesiology 1999;90:372-379.
19. Strandberg A, Tokics L, Brismar B, et al: Atelectasis during anaesthesia and in the postoperative period. Acta Anaesthesiol Scand 1986;30:154-158.
20. Hedenstierna G, Tokics L, Strandberg A, et al: Correlation of gas exchange impairment to development of atelectasis during anaesthesia and muscle paralysis. Acta Anaesthesiol Scand 1986;30:183-191.
21. Reber A, Bein T, Högman M, et al: Lung aeration and pulmonary gas exchange during lumbar epidural anaesthesia and in the lithotomy position in elderly patients. Anaesthesia 1998;53:854-861.
22. Hedenstierna G: Alveolar collapse and closure of airways: Regular effects of anaesthesia. Clin Physiol Funct Imaging 2003;23:123-129.
23. Kleinman BS, Frey K, VanDrunen M, et al: Motion of the diaphragm in patients with chronic obstructive pulmonary disease while spontaneously breathing versus during positive pressure breathing after anesthesia and neuromuscular blockade. Anesthesiology 2002;97:298-305.
24. Reber A, Nylund U, Hedenstierna G: Position and shape of the diaphragm: Implications for atelectasis formation. Anaesthesia 1998;53:1054-1061.
25. Warner DO, Warner MA, Ritman EL: Human chest wall function while awake and during halothane anesthesia: I. Quiet breathing. Anesthesiology 1995;82:6-19.
26. Joyce CJ, Williams AB: Kinetics of absorption atelectasis during anesthesia: A mathematical model. J Appl Physiol 1999;86:1116-1125.
27. Akca O, Podolsky A, Eisenhuber E, et al: Comparable postoperative pulmonary atelectasis in patients given 30% or 80% oxygen during and 2 hours after colon resection. Anesthesiology 1999;91:991-998.
28. Wetterslev J, Hansen EG, Kamp-Jensen M, et al: PaO_2 during anaesthesia and years of smoking predict late postoperative hypoxaemia and complications after upper abdominal surgery in patients without preoperative cardiopulmonary dysfunction. Acta Anaesthesiol Scand 2000;44:9-16.
29. Latimer RG, Dickman M, Day WC, et al: Ventilatory patterns and pulmonary complications after upper abdominal surgery determined by preoperative and postoperative computerized spirometry and blood gas analysis. Am J Surg 1971;122:622-632.
30. Xue FS, Li BW, Zhang GS, et al: The influence of surgical sites on early postoperative hypoxemia in adults undergoing elective surgery. Anesth Analg 1999;88:213-219.
31. Sharma RR, Axelsson H, Oberg A, et al: Diaphragmatic activity after laparoscopic cholecystectomy. Anesthesiology 1999;91:406-413.
32. Drummond GB: Diaphragmatic dysfunction: An outmoded concept. Br J Anaesth 1998;80:277-280.
33. van Kaam AH, Lachmann RA, Herting E, et al: Reducing atelectasis attenuates bacterial growth and translocation in experimental pneumonia. Am J Respir Crit Care Med 2004;169:1046-1053.
34. Trawoger R, Kolobow T, Cereda M, Sparacino ME: Tracheal mucus velocity remains normal in healthy sheep intubated with a new endotracheal tube with a novel laryngeal seal. Anesthesiology 1997;86:1140-1144.
35. Sackner MA, Hirsch J, Epstein S: Effect of cuffed endotracheal tubes on tracheal mucous velocity. Chest 1975;68:774-777.

36. Konrad FX, Schreiber T, Brecht-Kraus D, Georgieff M: Bronchial mucus transport in chronic smokers and nonsmokers during general anesthesia. J Clin Anesth 1993;5:375-380.

37. Reali-Forster C, Kolobow T, Giacomini M, et al: New ultrathin-walled endotracheal tube with a novel laryngeal seal design. Anesthesiology 1996;84:162-172.

38. Safdar N, Dezfulian C, Collard HR, Saint S: Clinical and economic consequences of ventilator-associated pneumonia: A systematic review. Crit Care Med 2005;33:2184-2193.

39. Berg H, Roed J, Viby-Mogensen J, et al: Residual neuromuscular block is a risk factor for postoperative pulmonary complications: A prospective, randomised, and blinded study of postoperative pulmonary complications after atracurium, vecuronium and pancuronium. Acta Anaesthesiol Scand 1997;41:1095-1103.

40. Heitmiller RF, Jones B: Transient diminished airway protection after transhiatal esophagectomy. Am J Surg 1991;162:442-446.

41. Atkins BZ, Shah AS, Hutcheson KA, et al: Reducing hospital morbidity and mortality following esophagectomy. Ann Thorac Surg 2004; 78:1170-1176; discussion 1170-1176.

42. Erskine RJ, Murphy PJ, Langton JA: Sensitivity of upper airway reflexes in cigarette smokers: Effect of abstinence. Br J Anaesth 1994;73:298-302.

43. Schwilk B, Bothner U, Schraag S, Georgieff M: Perioperative respiratory events in smokers and nonsmokers undergoing general anaesthesia. Acta Anaesthesiol Scand 1997;41:348-355.

44. Skeletal muscle dysfunction in chronic obstructive pulmonary disease: A statement of the American Thoracic Society and European Respiratory Society. Am J Respir Crit Care Med 1999;159(4 Pt 2): S1-40.

45. Hall JC, Tarala RA, Hall JL: Respiratory insufficiency after abdominal surgery. Respirology 1996;1:133-138.

46. Pedersen T, Eliasen K, Henriksen E: A prospective study of risk factors and cardiopulmonary complications associated with anaesthesia and surgery: Risk indicators of cardiopulmonary morbidity. Acta Anaesthesiol Scand 1990;34:144-155.

47. Pereira ED, Fernandes AL, da Silva Ancao M, et al: Prospective assessment of the risk of postoperative pulmonary complications in patients submitted to upper abdominal surgery. Sao Paulo Med J 1999;117:151-160.

48. Brooks-Brunn JA: Predictors of postoperative pulmonary complications following abdominal surgery. Chest 1997;111:564-571.

49. Wong DH, Weber EC, Schell MJ, et al: Factors associated with postoperative pulmonary complications in patients with severe chronic obstructive pulmonary disease. Anesth Analg 1995;80:276-284.

50. Dales RE, Dionne G, Leech JA, et al: Preoperative prediction of pulmonary complications following thoracic surgery. Chest 1993; 104:155-159.

51. Phillips EH, Carroll BJ, Fallas MJ, Pearlstein AR: Comparison of laparoscopic cholecystectomy in obese and non-obese patients. Am Surg 1994;60:316-321.

52. Kroenke K, Lawrence VA, Theroux JF, et al: Postoperative complications after thoracic and major abdominal surgery in patients with and without obstructive lung disease. Chest 1993;104:1445-1451.

53. Barisione G, Rovida S, Gazzaniga GM, Fontana L: Upper abdominal surgery: Does a lung function test exist to predict early severe postoperative respiratory complications? Eur Respir J 1997;10:1301-1308.

54. Khongphatthanayothin A, Wong PC, Samara Y, et al: Impact of respiratory syncytial virus infection on surgery for congenital heart disease: Postoperative course and outcome. Crit Care Med 1999; 27:1974-1981.

55. Williams-Russo P, Charlson ME, MacKenzie CR, et al: Predicting postoperative pulmonary complications: Is it a real problem? Arch Intern Med 1992;152:1209-1213.

56. Bluman LG, Mosca L, Newman N, Simon DG: Preoperative smoking habits and postoperative pulmonary complications. Chest 1998;113: 883-889.

57. Warner MA, Offord KP, Warner ME, et al: Role of preoperative cessation of smoking and other factors in postoperative pulmonary complications: A blinded prospective study of coronary artery bypass patients. Mayo Clin Proc 1989;64:609-616.

58. Barrera R, Shi W, Amar D, et al: Smoking and timing of cessation: Impact on pulmonary complications after thoracotomy. Chest 2005; 127:1977-1983.

59. Young T, Peppard PE, Gottlieb DJ: Epidemiology of obstructive sleep apnea: A population health perspective. Am J Respir Crit Care Med 2002;165:1217-1239.

60. den Herder C, Schmeck J, Appelboom DJ, de Vries N: Risks of general anaesthesia in people with obstructive sleep apnoea. BMJ 2004; 329:955-959.

61. Yaggi HK, Concato J, Kernan WN, et al: Obstructive sleep apnea as a risk factor for stroke and death. N Engl J Med 2005;353:2034-2041.

62. Loadsman JA, Hillman DR: Anaesthesia and sleep apnoea. Br J Anaesth 2001;86:254-266.

63. Kim JA, Lee JJ, Jung HH: Predictive factors of immediate postoperative complications after uvulopalatopharyngoplasty. Laryngoscope 2005;115:1837-1840.

64. Gupta RM, Parvizi J, Hanssen AD, Gay PC: Postoperative complications in patients with obstructive sleep apnea syndrome undergoing hip or knee replacement: A case-control study. Mayo Clin Proc. 2001;76:897-905.

65. Straus SE, McAlister FA, Sackett DL, Deeks JJ: The accuracy of patient history, wheezing, and laryngeal measurements in diagnosing obstructive airway disease. CARE-COAD1 Group: Clinical Assessment of the Reliability of the Examination-Chronic Obstructive Airways Disease. JAMA 2000;283:1853-1857.

66. Kroenke K, Lawrence VA, Theroux JF, Tuley MR: Operative risk in patients with severe obstructive pulmonary disease. Arch Intern Med 1992;152:967-971.

67. Hall JC, Tarala RA, Hall JL: A case-control study of postoperative pulmonary complications after laparoscopic and open cholecystectomy. J Laparoendosc Surg 1996;6:87-92.

68. Nilsson G, Larsson S, Johnsson F: Randomized clinical trial of laparoscopic versus open fundoplication: Blind evaluation of recovery and discharge period. Br J Surg 2000;87:873-878.

69. Prinssen M, Verhoeven EL, Buth J, et al: A randomized trial comparing conventional and endovascular repair of abdominal aortic aneurysms. N Engl J Med 2004;351:1607-1618.

70. Bullock TK, Waltrip TJ, Price SA, Galandiuk S: A retrospective study of nosocomial pneumonia in postoperative patients shows a higher mortality rate in patients receiving nasogastric tube feeding. Am Surg 2004;70:822-826.

71. Straus SE, McAlister FA, Sackett DL, Deeks JJ: Accuracy of history, wheezing, and forced expiratory time in the diagnosis of chronic obstructive pulmonary disease. J Gen Intern Med 2002;17:684-688.

72. Stein M, Cassara EL: Preoperative pulmonary evaluation and therapy for surgery patients. JAMA 1970;211:787-790.

73. Lawrence VA, Page CP, Harris GD: Preoperative spirometry before abdominal operations: A critical appraisal of its predictive value. Arch Intern Med 1989;149:280-285.

74. American College of Physicians: Preoperative pulmonary function testing. Ann Intern Med 1990;112:793-794.

75. Hnatiuk OW, Dillard TA, Torrington KG: Adherence to established guidelines for preoperative pulmonary function testing. Chest 1995; 107:1294-1297.

76. De Nino LA, Lawrence VA, Averyt EC, et al: Preoperative spirometry and laparotomy: Blowing away dollars. Chest 1997;111:1536-1541.

77. Tisi GM: Preoperative evaluation of pulmonary function: Validity, indications, and benefits. Am Rev Respir Dis 1979;119:293-310.

78. Hodgkin JE: Prognosis in chronic obstructive pulmonary disease. Clin Chest Med 1990;1:555-569.

79. Joo HS, Wong J, Naik VN, Savoldelli GL: The value of screening preoperative chest x-rays: A systematic review. Can J Anaesth 2005;52:568-574.

80. Rucker L, Frye EB, Staten MA: Usefulness of screening chest roentgenograms in preoperative patients. JAMA 1983;250:3209-3211.

81. Gerson MC, Hurst JM, Hertzberg VS, et al: Prediction of cardiac and pulmonary complications related to elective abdominal and noncardiac thoracic surgery in geriatric patients. Am J Med 1990;88: 101-107.

82. Girish M, Trayner E Jr, Dammann O, et al: Symptom-limited stair climbing as a predictor of postoperative cardiopulmonary complications after high-risk surgery. Chest 2001;120:1147-1151.

83. Naeije R: Pulmonary hypertension and right heart failure in chronic obstructive pulmonary disease. Proc Am Thorac Soc 2005;2:20-22.

84. Weitzenblum E, Hirth C, Ducolone A, et al: Prognostic value of pulmonary artery pressure in chronic obstructive pulmonary disease. Thorax 1981;36:752-758.

85. The National Emphysema Treatment Trial Research Group: Rationale and Design of the National Emphysema Treatment Trial: A prospective randomized trial of lung volume reduction surgery. Chest 1999;116:1750-1761.

86. Higham MA, Dawson D, Joshi J, et al: Utility of echocardiography in assessment of pulmonary hypertension secondary to COPD. Eur Respir J 2001;17:350-355.

87. Arcasoy SM, Christie JD, Ferrari VA, et al: Echocardiographic assessment of pulmonary hypertension in patients with advanced lung disease. Am J Respir Crit Care Med 2003;167:735-740.

88. Goldman L, Caldera DL, Nussbaum SR, et al: Multifactorial index of cardiac risk in noncardiac surgical procedures. N Engl J Med 1977;297:845-850.

89. Smetana GW, Cohn SL, Lawrence VA: Update in perioperative medicine. Ann Intern Med 2004;140:452-461.

90. Stephan F, Boucheseiche S, Hollande J, et al: Pulmonary complications following lung resection: A comprehensive analysis of incidence and possible risk factors. Chest 2000;118:1263-1270.

91. Patel RL, Townsend ER, Fountain SW: Elective pneumonectomy: Factors associated with morbidity and operative mortality. Ann Thorac Surg 1992;54:84-88.

92. Beckles MA, Spiro SG, Colice GL, Rudd RM: The physiologic evaluation of patients with lung cancer being considered for resectional surgery. Chest 2003;123:105S-114S.

93. British Thoracic Society, Society of Cardiothoracic Surgeons of Great Britain and Ireland Working Party: BTS guidelines: Guidelines on the selection of patients with lung cancer for surgery. Thorax 2001;56:89-108.

94. Wyser C, Stulz P, Soler M, et al: Prospective evaluation of an algorithm for the functional assessment of lung resection candidates. Am J Respir Crit Care Med 1999;159:1450-1456.

95. Bolliger CT, Guckel C, Engel H, et al: Prediction of functional reserves after lung resection: Comparison between quantitative computer tomography, scintigraphy, and anatomy. Respiration 2002;69:482-489.

96. Ribas J, Diaz O, Barbera JA, et al: Invasive exercise testing in the evaluation of patients at high risk for lung resection. Eur Respir J 1998;12:1429-1435.

97. Bolliger CT, Jordan P, Soler M, et al: Pulmonary function and exercise capacity after lung resection. Eur Respir J 1996;9:415-421.

98. Bolliger CT, Jordan P, Soler M, et al: Exercise capacity as a predictor of postoperative complications in lung resection candidates. Am J Respir Crit Care Med 1995;151:1472-1480.

99. Pollock M, Roa J, Benditt J, et al: Estimation of ventilatory reserve by stair climbing. Chest 1993;104:1378-1383.

100. Epstein SK, Faling LJ, Daly BD, Celli BR: Predicting complications after pulmonary resection: Preoperative exercise testing vs a multifactorial cardiopulmonary risk index. Chest 1993;104:694-700.

11 Hematologic Risk Assessment

Carlos Marcucci, Pierre-Guy Chassot, Lars M. Asmis, and Donat R. Spahn

Hematologic risk assessment (HRA) is essential for patients refusing the transfusion of blood and blood products for religious beliefs (e.g., Jehovah's Witnesses), in patients for whom no or an insufficient number of red blood cell (RBC) units are available, in patients with a history of a bleeding disorder or preoperative laboratory evidence of compromised blood coagulation, and, last but not least, in patients on antiplatelet drugs (Box 11-1). The goal of HRA is to minimize transfusion needs and preventable complications such as hemorrhage and thrombosis, and the ability to do this depends on the clinical setting. Efficient collaboration and communication among surgeons, anesthesiologists, and at times, other specialists are prerequisites to successful perioperative patient management, which includes HRA.

■ RED BLOOD CELL TRANSFUSION

Jehovah's Witnesses claim a strict obedience to the precepts of the Bible, where it is said that the soul abides in the blood. Therefore, they refuse the transfusion of whole blood, blood cells, and plasma.[1] The refusal or acceptance of what they call the "minor" components of the blood (e.g., albumin, coagulation factors) is left up to the individual patient. Substances produced by genetic engineering are accepted. Moreover, the integrity of the vascular tree must be safeguarded, because the blood—that is, the soul—cannot remain outside the body: Jehovah's Witnesses reject autologous blood donation, but they accept cardiopulmonary bypass or normovolemic hemodilution as long as the continuity of the blood circulation is preserved. In Western countries, the respect of individual thought is at the core of the Charter of Human Rights. The principle of patient autonomy, which prevails in this situation, requires that the beliefs of the patient be respected, provided the patient clearly understands the risks.[2] Therefore, the refusal of blood must be respected in adults with proper judgment. Nevertheless, a refusal of one therapeutic option does not release the physician from exploring all other possibilities of care.[3,4]

Patients who have received multiple transfusions in the past or reacted to unusual antigens with elaboration of antibodies may develop antibodies directed against relevant red cell surface antigens, leading to multiple incompatibilities. Some patients raise a high level of a clinically important alloantibody that is directed against a very common antigen (e.g., present in more than 90% of individuals). It might then become almost impossible to find blood units to which they do not react, or not enough for a proposed surgery.

If a patient refuses RBC transfusion, or if an insufficient number of RBC units is available, the maximum allowable blood loss (mABL) must be estimated (Fig. 11-1). This can be done by the following formula, assuming that normovolemia is maintained[5]:

$$\text{mABL} = \text{BV} \cdot \ln(\text{Hb}_0/\text{Hb}_{\text{MIN}}),$$

where BV is blood volume, Hb_0 is preoperative hemoglobin concentration (Hb), and Hb_{MIN} is the lowest tolerable Hb. Blood volume is 70 to 75 mL/kg in male and 60 to 65 /kg in female non-obese patients. A 70-kg male patient with an initial hemoglobin concentration of 14 /dL and a Hb_{MIN} of 6 g/dL thus can tolerate a blood loss of 4.4 L. However, with a borderline anemia of 12 g/dL and a (cardiac) comorbidity requiring a Hb_{MIN} of 8 g/dL,[6] the mABL is only 2.1 L. In a 70-kg female patient with a borderline anemia of 11 g/dL and a Hb_{MIN} of 8 g/dL, the mABL is even smaller, only 1.3 L.

The next step is to compare the mABL with the historical perioperative blood loss for the planned operation performed by the local surgical team. This comparison should be with the historical perioperative blood loss rather than the intraoperative blood loss, because for many operations the postoperative blood loss is significant.[7] If the mABL is considerably greater than the historical perioperative blood loss, no further measures are necessary and the surgery can be performed safely, even in the absence of RBCs. However, if the mABL is similar to or smaller than the expected perioperative blood loss, additional measures are required.

First, the endogenous RBC mass should be increased by preoperative erythropoietin and/or iron therapy if time allows (Box 11-2). The goal of the erythropoietin and iron therapy is to increase the Hb level by 1 g/dL each week. In anemic patients (hematocrit <39%), this therapy increases hematocrit (Ht) up to 45% and clearly reduces the need for allogeneic blood transfusions (average reduction is 30%).[8] In addition, it allows preoperative autologous blood donation (PABD) despite anemia,[9] and it increases the amount of blood collected by intraoperative isovolemic hemodilution.[10] Erythropoietin and iron therapy have been used successfully in individual cases where blood transfusion was refused or impossible.

In the early 1990s, PABD of 1 to 2 units of blood 2 to 4 weeks before surgery represented 8.5% of all transfused units, but this has declined to 4.7% in recent years.[11] However, in many cases, PABD is no more than simple hemodilution, because only a fraction of the donated erythrocytes are regenerated preoperatively[12]; moreover, approximately half of all PABD units are never transfused. PABD should therefore be considered only if large blood losses are expected (>2000 mL) and if the likelihood of transfusion exceeds 50%.[13] To maximize the advantages of PABD, a longer

11-1	Situations Requiring Hematologic Risk Assessment

Patients refusing red blood cell (RBC) transfusions
No or insufficient number of RBCs available
Patients with a history of a bleeding disorder
Patients with a prolonged prothrombin time (PT)
Patients with a prolonged activated partial thromboplastin time (aPTT)
Patients with a low platelet count
Patient with a platelet function defect
Patient on antiplatelet drugs

11-2	Blood-Sparing Strategies

Preoperative Pharmacologic Preparation

- Erythropoietin (EPO), 150-300 IU kg^{-1}, six doses in 3 weeks (Alternative: 600 IU kg^{-1}, three doses in 7-10 days)
- Iron, 100-300 mg/day, IV or PO
- Folic acid, 5 mg/day
- Vitamin B$_{12}$, 15-30 µg/day

Preoperative Autologous Blood Donation (PABD)

Intraoperative Alternatives to Blood Transfusions

- Acute normovolemic hemodilution
- Cell salvage and retransfusion techniques (Cell-Saver)

Anesthesia Technique

- Intraoperative normothermia
- Maintained normovolemia with crystalloids ± colloids
- Hyperoxic ventilation (FiO$_2$ 1.0)
- Deep anesthesia with muscle relaxation

Pharmacologic Treatment

- Antifibrinolytic substances (aprotinin, ε-aminocaproic acid, tranexamic acid)
- Desmopressin (Minirin)
- Coagulation factors (fresh-frozen plasma, fibrinogen, factors II, VII, IX, X)
- Factor VIIa (NovoSeven)

Artificial O$_2$ Carriers (Not Yet in Clinical Use)

- (Fluorocarbon, hemoglobin solution)

Acceptance of Minimal Hb Values

- 6 /dL in healthy individuals
- 8 g/dL in aged or compromised patients

Adaptation of Surgical Procedure

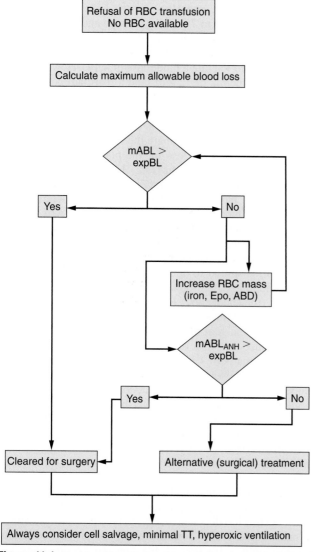

Figure 11-1 ■ Algorithm for perioperative management of red blood cell (RBC) transfusion and cell salvage in patients for whom homologous blood transfusion is contraindicated. ABD, autologous blood donation; Epo, erythropoietin; mABL, maximal allowable blood loss; mABL$_{ANH}$, mABL after acute normovolemic hemodilution; expBL, expected blood loss; TT, therapy.

interval before surgery or the use of erythropoietin and iron is required to allow regenerative erythropoiesis.

If PABD is not an option, or if the patient does not respond to combined erythropoietin and iron therapy, preoperative acute normovolemic hemodilution (ANH) and cell saving should be considered (see Fig. 11-1).[14,15] ANH can be performed until the Hb$_{MIN}$ is reached; most often, however, it is performed only to Hb levels of 8 to 9 g/dL.[16] The Hb that is mass harvested during ANH (HbM$_{ANH}$) can be calculated as follows:

$$HbM_{ANH} = (BV/100) \cdot (Hb_{pre-ANH}/Hb_{post-ANH}),$$

where Hb$_{pre-ANH}$ is the Hb concentration prior to ANH, and Hb$_{post-ANH}$ is the Hb concentration after ANH. After ANH, the patient is thus bleeding with a Hb between Hb$_{post-ANH}$ and Hb$_{MIN}$. Accordingly, the maximum allowable blood loss after ANH (mABL$_{ANH}$) is calculated as follows:

$$mABL_{ANH} = (HbM_{ANH} \cdot 100)/Hb_{post-ANH}.$$

mABL$_{ANH}$ is larger than mABL, and the difference, which depends on the initial RBC mass,[5,17] is in the order of magnitude of 250 to 1000 mL.

Another option, in selected cases, is lowering Hb$_{MIN}$, particularly in conjunction with pure oxygen ventilation; this technique has been shown to reverse ANH-induced myocardial ischemia[18] and cognitive dysfunction[19] and allows hemodilution of animals beyond the critical Hb found at room air ventilation.[20] This simple option is useful when the actual blood loss is significantly greater than the expected blood loss. Also, it allows for a longer waiting period before the retransfusion of autologous RBCs, including ANH blood, ideally until the surgical blood loss has stopped.

The lower the Hb, the more important it is to maintain normovolemia (see Box 11-2). Only at normovolemia are the compensatory mechanisms maximally efficacious.[21] Therefore, large amounts of crystalloids and colloids should be infused during surgeries with a large blood loss. The mixture of crystalloids and colloids selected should produce the smallest possible effect on blood coagulation, so highly substituted, high-molecular-weight hydroxyethyl starch solutions should be avoided.[22] The alternatives are gelatin, albumin, and fresh-frozen plasma.[23] In addition, maintaining normothermia and avoiding hypothermia is of great importance.[24]

If the preoperative treatment cannot augment the RBC mass sufficiently, and the mABL becomes greater than the expected blood loss, and if the combined use of ANH and cell saving cannot cover the difference, alternative treatment strategies, including less invasive and nonsurgical treatment modalities, must be considered (see Box 11-2).

■ HEMOSTASIS

Hemostasis is a complex mechanism involving the vessel wall, circulating cellular elements (particularly platelets), and circulating soluble factors such as coagulation factors. The characteristics of blood flow (laminar versus turbulent, flow velocity, pressure gradients, wall tension, and elasticity) define vascular bed specificity, which describes how different aspects of hemostasis can be relevant in different vascular beds. Hemostasis in general can be described by four phases:

1. *Vasoconstriction.* When the vessel wall is damaged, the vessel diameter reduces, thereby diminishing the size of the breach and bringing the circulating elements of coagulation into proximity to the endothelium.
2. *Primary hemostasis.* Circulating platelets adhere to the subendothelial structures, secrete mediators of platelet activation, aggregate, and fuse to form a primary hemostatic plug that can subsequently be consolidated by secondary hemostasis.
3. *Secondary hemostasis.* The various coagulation factors and cofactors interact on the platelets' surfaces to form insoluble fibrin strands that will mediate clot retraction and result in formation of a stable thrombus.
4. *Recanalization.* After the endothelial continuity has been reestablished, the blood clot is broken down by the fibrinolytic system, and blood flow is restored through the vessel.

Primary Hemostasis

Immobilized von Willebrand factor (VWF) that adheres to exposed subendothelial collagen mediates the adhesion of circulating platelets through the interaction with the platelets' glycoprotein receptor (GP) Ib and VWF. In the subsequent process of platelet activation, thrombocytes change from discoid to spherical, form pseudopods, and secrete multiple factors that enhance further platelet activation and coagulation. In the next step of activation, GPIIb/IIIa-receptors and negatively charged phospholipids are expressed on the platelets' surface. The GPIIb/IIIa receptors are the anchors by which platelets adhere to one another; and phospholipids provide the negatively charged surface necessary for the assembly and interaction of coagulation factors of secondary hemostasis.

Secondary Hemostasis

On the surface of activated platelets, circulating coagulation factors now start a chain reaction, resulting in the formation of fibrin strands (Fig. 11-2). The traditional division of this reaction into an extrinsic, an intrinsic, and a common pathway is a simplification of a complex series of interactions. The simplification is useful to illustrate the underlying mechanisms of common coagulation tests (e.g., prothrombin time [PT] and activated partial thromboplastin time [aPTT]), but it is not a valid model of coagulation in vivo. A more recent view, the cellular model of hemostasis, attributes to tissue factor (TF) the role of initiating coagulation in vivo, and it subdivides secondary hemostasis into four sequences: initiation, propagation, termination, and elimination.

Initiation

Circulating factor VII (FVII) forms a complex with TF, a membrane protein expressed by fibroblasts in the subendothelium and possibly in the endothelium. The formation of the TF-FVII complex leads to structural alterations that lead to activation of FVII. Alternatively, freely circulating FVIIa binds to TF, as it is not rapidly inactivated in circulation. However, without the cofactor TF, FVII is not capable of initiating the procoagulant chain reactions. The association of the FVIIa-TF complex with the platelet phospholipid membrane constitutes the procoagulant complex known as extrinsic tenase. It is called *extrinsic* because it contains TF, a protein that is normally not found in blood, and *tenase* because the complex transforms factor X into its active form Xa. The latter will form the second procoagulant complex, prothrombinase, which requires activated FVa and phospholipids as cofactors. Prothrombinase catalyses the transformation of prothrombin (factor II) to thrombin (FIIa), the key enzyme of the coagulation cascade. At this stage, the amount of FIIa produced depends on the amount of TF available. Extrinsic tenase, however, is also capable of activating factor IX to factor IXa, which will form the third procoagulant complex, intrinsic tenase, which requires FVIIIa and phospholipid as cofactors. All the constituents of intrinsic tenase, as its name implies, are normally present in blood. It catalyses the conversion of factor X to factor Xa and thus amplifies the production of thrombin. Factor IX can also be activated by another pathway, known as the intrinsic pathway, which involves circulating elements such as kallikrein, high-molecular-weight kininogen, and factor XII, which activates factor XI to FXIa, which in turn activates factor IX to form

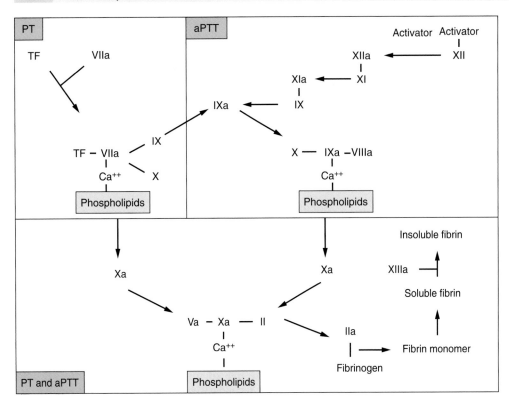

Figure   11-2 ■ Coagulation pathways and specificity of different coagulation assays. aPTT, activated partial thromboplastin time; PT, prothrombin time; TF, tissue factor.

the intrinsic tenase. The role of this pathway in vivo is unclear, but its integrity can be tested in vitro by adding an activator of factor XII (e.g., kaolin or celite) to plasma.

Propagation

The rapidly increasing amount of thrombin on the platelets' surface further enhances its own production by several feedback loops, activates factor XIII, and transforms fibrinogen into fibrin monomers. These assemble to form soluble fibrin polymers, which are rendered insoluble by factor XIIIa, a transglutaminase that cross-links the fibrin molecules, thus stabilizing the platelet clot.

Termination

Several enzymatic processes inhibit the coagulation reactions to prevent unimpeded progression of intravascular coagulation. One of these processes, the activation of protein C, is initiated by the coagulation cascade itself, and the two others depend on circulating inhibitors known as tissue factor pathway inhibitor and antithrombin.

Elimination

The fibrinolytic process that degrades the thrombus and restores blood flow in the vessel is catalyzed by plasmin. Plasminogen, the precursor of plasmin, circulates freely in plasma. It is incorporated in the thrombus as the latter starts to form. Tissue plasminogen activator (tPA) and urokinase-type plasminogen activator (uPA), known activators of plasminogen, are secreted by vascular cells.

■ PREOPERATIVE RISK ASSESSMENT

Two strategies are applied to preoperatively identify patients at risk for bleeding complications. The first is to screen all patients preoperatively. Tests include assessments for primary hemostasis (primarily platelet count [PC]), and for secondary hemostasis, PT, and aPTT, in various combinations. However, none of these purely laboratory-based strategies has been shown prospectively to be efficient or cost effective in identifying patients at risk.

The second, more recent, strategy involves identifying patients at risk by their medical history and a physical examination, and then performing laboratory tests in that subpopulation (Fig. 11-3). The risk-assessment strategy proposed by Koscielny and colleagues[25] involves an extensive bleeding history utilizing a standardized questionnaire (Box 11-3). The patients identified as being at risk by this test are then submitted to further laboratory testing that includes PT, aPTT, PC, platelet function testing utilizing the Platelet Function Analyzer (PFA-100), and a functional von Willebrand factor assay. This strategy was shown to be capable of identifying patients at risk and to reduce transfusional needs when applied in combination with a standardized therapeutic regimen.

Medical History and Physical Examination

Clinical examination is one of the best tools to identify patients at risk for bleeding.[26] The patient's personal and family history can provide important clues to the presence

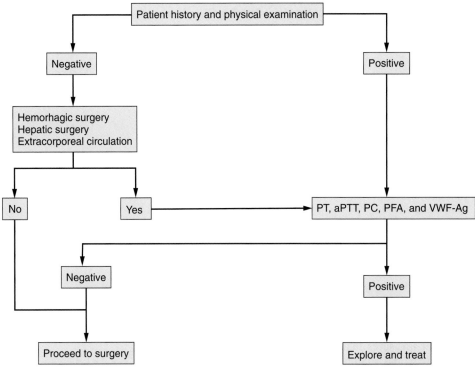

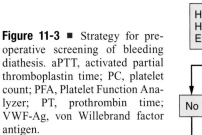

Figure 11-3 ■ Strategy for preoperative screening of bleeding diathesis. aPTT, activated partial thromboplastin time; PC, platelet count; PFA, Platelet Function Analyzer; PT, prothrombin time; VWF-Ag, von Willebrand factor antigen.

11-3	Questionnaire for Detecting an Increased Bleeding Risk

1. Have you ever experienced strong nose bleeding without prior reason?
2. Did you ever have—without trauma—"blue spots" (hematoma) or "small bleedings" (at the torso or other unusual regions of the body)?
3. Did you ever have bleeding of the gums without apparent reason?
4. How often do you have bleedings or "blue spots" (hematoma): more than 1 or 2 times a week or 1 to 2 times a week?
5. Do you have the impression that you have prolonged bleedings after minor wounds (e.g., razor cuts)?
6. Did you have prolonged or grave bleedings during or after operations (e.g., tonsillectomy, appendectomy, or during labor)?
7. Did you ever have prolonged or grave bleedings after a tooth extraction?
8. Did you ever receive blood packs or blood products during an operation? If so, please define the operation(s).
9. Is there a history of bleeding disorders in your family?
10. Do you take analgesic drugs or drugs against rheumatic disease? If so, please specify.
11. Do you take other drugs? If so, please specify.
12. Do you have the impression that you have prolonged menstruation (>7 days) or a high frequency of tampon change? (to be answered only by women)

From Koscielny J, Ziemer S, Radtke H, et al: Clin Appl Thromb Hemost 2004;10:195-204, with permission.

11-1	Characteristics of Acquired and Hereditary Bleeding Disorders

Acquired Bleeding Disorders	Hereditary Bleeding Disorders
Negative family history	More than one patient in family is affected
Presence of associated diseases	
Variable in time	Hereditary pattern
Variable in aspect and type	Rather fixed pattern of bleeding
Onset usually in middle age or later	History of blood transfusion
	Onset at early age

From Girolami A, Luzzatto G, Varvarikis C, et al: Haemophilia 2005;11:193-202, with permission.

and type of bleeding disorder. Several questionnaires have been published. The Koscielny questionnaire (see Box 11-3) was established retrospectively and later validated in a prospective study, each study including more than 5000 patients.[25,27] Using this questionnaire, 5021 out of 5649 patients (88.8%) were identified as having a negative bleeding history. Subsequent laboratory tests showed a prolonged aPTT in only nine of these patients, all of which were caused by a lupus anticoagulant. No other test found any bleeding disorder in any of these patients. The most reliable questions in the list were related to bleeding of minor wounds (sensitivity, 85%), frequent bruising (sensitivity, 73%), and use of nonsteroidal anti-inflammatory drugs (NSAIDs) (sensitivity, 67.2%). The positive predictive value was greater than 99% if these four questions were answered in the affirmative.

Elements that can help discriminate between hereditary and acquired bleeding disorders are listed in Table 11-1. If a

11-2 **Clinical Presentation of the Major Bleeding Disorders**

Disorder	GI	Joints	Cerebral	Muscular	Skin and Mucosae	Urinary Tract
Congenital						
Fibrinogen	+	+	++	+	+	++
Factors II, VII, X	+	+	++++	++	+	++
Hemophilia A and B	+	++++	++	++	+	++
Von Willebrand's disease	+++	+	±	+	+++	+
Acquired						
Coumarin	+	±	++	++	++	++
Heparin	++	±	++	+++	+++	++
Liver failure	++++	±	±	++	+++	+
Thrombocytopenia	++	±	+	++	++++	+
Hyperfibrinolysis	++	−	++++	++	++	++

±, possible; +, rare; ++, frequent; +++, usual; ++++, always present.
From Girolami A, Luzzatto G, Varvarikis C, et al: Haemophilia 2005;11:193-202, with permission.

positive family history is present, the patient is asked about the intensity and type of bleeding and the hereditary pattern. If a bleeding tendency is present, recent medication that might interfere with normal coagulation (e.g., NSAIDs, aspirin) or measures that may have been taken to stop the bleeding (e.g., nasal tamponade, vitamin K), recent illnesses, and recent transfusion should all be asked about. All patients with liver disease, renal failure, hypersplenism, or hematologic disease must be questioned, and their files must be examined. Physical signs that can indicate pathologic states associated with increased bleeding include purpura, hematomas, jaundice, hepatomegaly, splenomegaly, and adenopathy.

The clinical presentation of bleeding diatheses varies, and different signs can be related to different disorders. The most frequent manifestations are cutaneous and mucosal bleeding. Oozing, hemarthrosis, and muscular hematomas are other types of bleeding that can be found in several bleeding disorders. The clinical presentations of the major bleeding disorders are listed in Tables 11-2 and 11-3.

Cutaneous bleeding, or purpura, can be subdivided into petechiae, purpuric lesions, and ecchymosis. Petechiae are small lesions, less than 2 mm in diameter, and are mainly caused by thrombocytopenia. Purpuric spots are 3 to 6 mm in diameter and are most frequently caused by Henoch-Schönlein purpura and cryoglobulinemia. Ecchymoses are large dermal extravasations of blood with a diameter exceeding 6 to 7 mm. They appear most often on exposed body parts and are caused by thrombocytopenia, cortisone therapy, or erythrocyte autosensitization. *Easy bruising* defines the tendency of a patient to have variable skin lesions such as ecchymoses and hematomas after minor trauma. Often, the patient cannot recall the trauma that caused the bruising. Usually there is an underlying thrombocytopenia or coagulation disorder. Senile vessel fragility and Cushing's syndrome can also cause easy bruising of the skin. Oozing is a special feature of cutaneous bleeding. It can be defined by the continuing loss of blood at puncture sites or wounds. The underlying disorder can be hypofibrinogenemia, hyperfibrinolysis, thrombocytopenia, or factor XIII deficiency. Newborns with

11-3 **Clinical Presentation of Major Bleeding Disorders**

Disorder	Findings
Conjunctival ecchymosis	Hypertension
	Thrombocytopenia
	Circulating anticoagulants
Petechiae	Thrombocytopenia
Mucosal	Rendu-Osler-Weber syndrome
	Von Willebrand's disease
	Platelet disorders
Hematomas	Single-factor congential deficiency
	Circulating anticoagulants
	Traumas
Hemarthrosis	Hemophilia A and B
	FII, FVII, FX deficiency
Easy bruising	Thrombocytopenia
	Cushing's disease

From Girolami A, Luzzatto G, Varvarikis C, et al: Haemophilia 2005;11:193-202, with permission.

factor XIII deficiency or afibrinogenemia often present with oozing at the umbilical stump.

Mucosal bleeding can occur at any organ covered with mucosa: the gastrointestinal, respiratory, urinary, and uterovaginal tracts, and the eyes. It is frequently seen in cases of thrombocytopenia and von Willebrand's disease (VWD). It also can be caused by a variety of non–coagulation-related disorders such as Rendu-Osler-Weber syndrome, gastrointestinal ulcers, malignancies, infections, and varicose veins. Menorrhagia and metrorrhagia are frequent in thrombocytopenia and VWD. Minor uterovaginal bleeding ("breakthrough bleeding") is often the result of hormonal imbalance, but it may be caused by congenital factor deficiencies (factors II, V, and X). Conjunctival ecchymosis can be found in hypertension, thrombocytopenia, and anticoagulant use. Hematuria is most often caused by non–coagulation-related disorders.

Intramuscular and intra-articular bleeding occur frequently in patients with hemophilia. Hemarthrosis has also been described in factor II, VII, and X deficiencies.

These patients are particularly prone to intracerebral hemorrhages.

Tests of Primary Hemostasis

Absolute preoperative platelet count is a highly reliable and reproducible test, but it gives information only about the number of platelets circulating, not about their function. Alone, it is not an efficient predictor of perioperative bleeding, but in conjunction with other tests, it is included by many authors in a preoperative screening regimen.[25,28] A patient presenting with a PC of less than 100 g/L should be investigated. The main causes for low platelet count are listed in Box 11-4. Thrombocytopenia can be congenital or it can be caused by low platelet production, peripheral platelet destruction, or dilution. The perioperative management for different types of thrombocytopenia is depicted in Figure 11-4. The use of antiplatelet drugs is the most frequent cause of platelet dysfunction. Recent developments and insights into cardiovascular treatments make the perioperative use of antiplatelet drugs a very important issue (see Management of Patients under Antiplatelet Therapy, later).

11-4	**Causes of Low Platelet Count**

Pseudothrombocytopenia

Impaired Production

- Congenital thrombocytopenia
- Acute leukemia
- Myelodysplasia
- Osteopetrosis
- Toxins (e.g., chemotherapy, alcohol)
- Infection (e.g., human immunodeficiency virus)

Peripheral Consumption

- Autoimmune
  - Primary (e.g., idiopathic thrombocytopenic purpura)
  - Secondary
- Disseminated intravascular coagulation
- Thrombotic thrombocytopenic purpura
- Hemolytic-uremic syndrome

Redistribution and Dilution

- Massive transfusion
- Splenomegaly

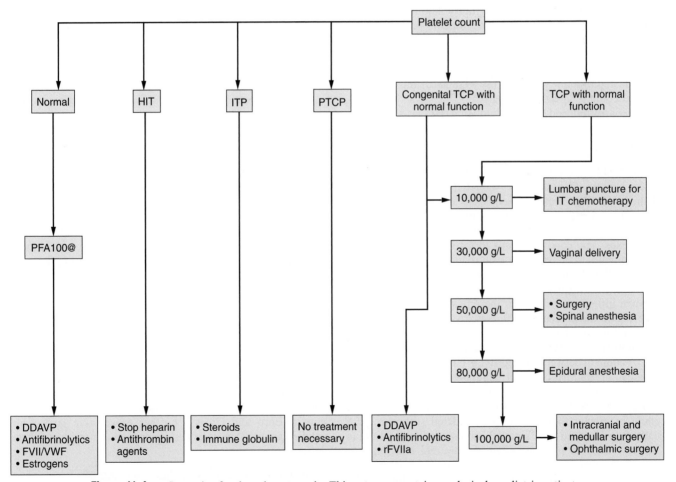

Figure 11-4 ■ Strategies for thrombocytopenia. This category contains exclusively pediatric patients undergoing lumbar puncture for intrathecal (IT) chemotherapy. Lumbar puncture for other reasons or spinal anesthesia requires 50,000 μg/L. DDAVP, desmopressin; HIT, heparin-induced thrombocytopenia; ITP, idiopathic thrombocytopenic purpura; PTCP, pseudothrombocytopenia; rFVIIa, recombinant activated factor VII; TCP, thrombocytopenia; VWF, von Willebrand factor.

Pseudothrombocytopenia is the result of suppress by the agglutination of thrombocytes in vitro, causing a falsely low PC without the clinical bleeding tendency. It occurs in 0.2% of the general population and in 1.9% of hospitalized patients,[29-31] and it accounts for up to 15% of low PCs in hospital laboratories. It is caused by an antibody with affinity for antigens expressed by the thrombocytes in vitro. The use of ethylenediamine tetra-acetic acid (EDTA) as an anticoagulant in test tubes strongly enhances pseudothrombocytopenia. The GP IIb/IIIa inhibitor abciximab can induce an antibody-mediated, clinically important thrombocytopenia and has been shown to induce a pseudothrombocytopenia in 2% of patients undergoing coronary interventions through a related mechanism.

Congenital thrombocytopenia (CTP) accounts for a very small number of the low PCs encountered. CTP is a heterogeneous group of disorders with variable bleeding tendencies. The management of patients with CTP who are bleeding or scheduled for surgery is not well defined. The available options include desmopressin (DDAVP), antifibrinolytics, platelet transfusion, and recombinant factor VIIa (rFVIIa).[33]

Immune thrombocytopenia is caused by antibodies to circulating platelets. It can be a primary autoimmune disorder, known as idiopathic thrombocytopenic purpura (ITP), or secondary to infections (e.g., human immunodeficiency virus infection), systemic lupus erythematosus, antiphospholipid syndrome, and B-cell malignancies. ITP is treated with steroids and immune globulins (IVIG, anti-D, anti-CD 20) if platelet count is lower than 20 g/L.[34]

Heparin-induced thrombocytopenia (HIT) is a particular form of immune thrombocytopenia related to prolonged (minimum, 5 days) heparin infusion.[35] Its pathogenesis is based on the binding of the heparin molecule with circulating factor 4 (PF4), a protein stored in platelet alpha-granules. These heparin–PF4 complexes induce the production of antibodies that form immune complexes and activate platelets with their Fc fragment. The activated platelets release additional PF4, enhancing the formation of the immune complexes. The condition leads to thrombocytopenia and a prothrombotic state. HIT is a serious and unpredictable complication that should be suspected in every patient who shows a drop in PC of greater than 50% of baseline after 5 days of heparin infusion, or sooner if there has been heparin exposure within the preceding 100 days.[36] HIT can be treated by interrupting the heparin infusion and administering antithrombin agents such as argatroban and lepirudin.

A count of between 20 and 100 g/L may lead to increased surgical or traumatic hemorrhage but normally does not result in spontaneous bleeding, which can occur if the count drops to less than 20 g/L.[37] If platelet function is normal, a count of greater than 50 g/L is considered sufficient for a patient to undergo any kind of surgery, including cardiac surgery. Only in procedures where minimal bleeding can have deleterious consequences (e.g., neurosurgery and ophthalmic surgery) should the lower limit of 100 g/L be respected.[38] Platelet transfusion can be indicated if a PC is less than 100 g/L and intraoperative or postoperative microvascular bleeding is present.[14] In obstetrics, gestational thrombocytopenia is a benign condition that does not require

platelet transfusion.[39] Thrombocytopenia associated with preeclampsia and hemolysis, elevated liver enzymes and low platelets (HELLP), however, requires close follow-up and transfusion of platelets if the count drops to less than 30 g/L for a vaginal delivery, and to less than 50 g/L in the case of a cesarean section.[38] After central venous catheter placement, oozing at the puncture site is reported if the platelet count is less than 50 g/L.[40] On the other hand, based on an evaluation of 5000 procedures involving 958 consecutive children, Howard and colleagues decided that lumbar puncture for intrathecal chemotherapy in pediatric patients can safely be performed if the platelet count is 10 g/L or greater.[41,42] For spinal anesthesia, a lower limit of 50 g/L is advocated, whereas for epidural anesthesia a PC of 80 g/L has been recommended because of the higher risk for spinal hematoma.[38]

In vivo testing of platelet function can be performed with the bleeding time, but this test is influenced by so many variables that it cannot be reliably reproduced. It has poor discriminating power in predicting operative blood loss,[43,44] and it is poorly related to platelet count.[45] In 1998, the American Society of Pathologists stated that bleeding time cannot be used as a predictor for surgical hemorrhage, that a normal bleeding time does not exclude excessive hemorrhage, and that bleeding time cannot reliably distinguish between patients who have recently ingested aspirin and those who have not.[46] Bleeding time is thus abandoned as a preoperative test to evaluate bleeding tendency or to predict surgical blood loss.

More recent preoperative screening strategies include platelet function testing and a test for von Willebrand factor antigen. The PFA-100 is sensitive for platelet function and von Willebrand factor activity.[47] In this test, whole blood is aspirated through a collagen-coated membrane in a 150-μm aperture. Platelet activation is stimulated by adding either epinephrine or adenosine diphosphate. The time for the aperture to close as a result of platelet aggregation is measured and compared with control values. Use of the PFA-100 appears justified, as of the 5649 patients tested in the Koscielny study, 628 had a positive bleeding history, and of these 628 patients, 256 (40.8%) had abnormal screening tests. Of those patients with abnormal bleeding tests, 250 (98%) had impaired platelet function, as measured with PFA-100, and 39 (15%) had reduced VWF antigen levels. The majority of thrombocytopathies were drug-induced platelet dysfunction that responded well to perioperative DDAVP treatment. In contrast, only 9% and 4% had altered aPTT and PT, respectively. Other methods available to assess platelet function include thromboelastography with platelet mapping, the Plateletworks analyzer, the Multiplate analyzer, the cone and plate analyzer system, and traditional aggregometry according to Born and Cross.[48] Further prospective large-scale studies are still necessary to determine the utility of these latter assays.

Tests of Secondary Hemostasis: PT and aPTT

Many tests of secondary hemostasis have been evaluated for their capacity to predict bleeding. Preoperative PT or aPTT, for example, have been shown not to predict hemorrhagic complications in gynecologic oncology surgery,[49] abdominal and thyroid surgery,[50] dental surgery,[51] liver biopsy,[52] thoracocentesis and paracentesis,[53,54] transbronchial lung biopsy,[55] renal biopsy,[56] angiographic procedures,[57] and central venous catheter insertion.[56,58] However, in a population at risk as identified by the Koscielny algorithm, such tests may prove useful in identifying patients with underlying bleeding disorders.

The fibrin monomer test is an interesting candidate test, as it did show a correlation with bleeding complications in a relatively small prospective study.[59] Further studies are necessary to define the optimal spectrum of tests for preoperative screening.

The PT and aPTT are in vitro coagulation tests designed to detect deficiencies of coagulation factors. In the PT, tissue factor and calcium are added to citrated plasma and the time

needed for a clot to form is measured and compared with control values. In the aPTT, an activator of factor XII is added to plasma, and time to clot formation is expressed in seconds. Thus, PT specifically tests the integrity of the extrinsic pathway, and aPTT tests the intrinsic pathway. Both tests are abnormal if the coagulopathy impairs the common pathway (see Fig. 11-2). Clotting times are prolonged in the presence of disseminated intravascular coagulation (DIC), liver disease, coumarin therapy, heparin therapy, vitamin K deficiency, congenital factor deficiencies, dysfibrinogenemia, factor VIII deficiency secondary to VWD, specific coagulation factor inhibitors, or lupus anticoagulant or anticardiolipins. These different states and their influence on clotting tests are discussed later. Strategies for perioperative care in these patients are depicted in Figure 11-5.

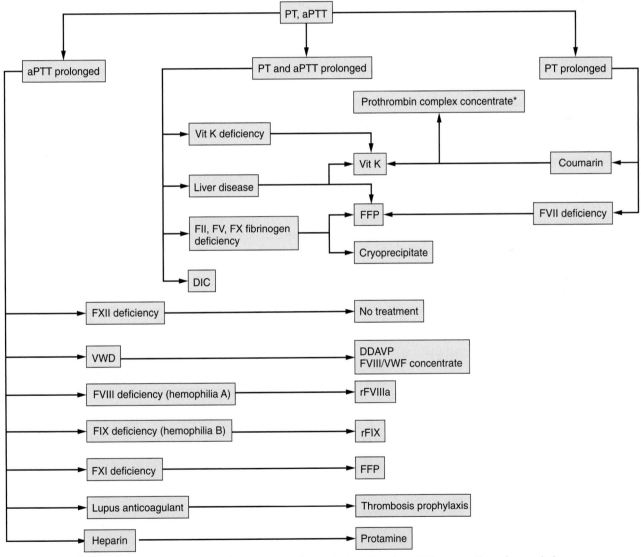

Figure 11-5 ■ Strategies for the treatment of coagulation disorders. *The correction of coagulation disorders by the administration of vitamin K takes 2 to 3 days. If urgent correction is necessary, Prothromplex or fresh-frozen plasma (FFP) is necessary. aPTT, activated partial thromboplastin time; DDAVP, desmopressin; DIC, disseminated intravascular coagulation; F, factor; PT, prothrombin time; rF, recombinant factor; Vit K, vitamin K; VWD, vow Willebrand's disease; VWF, von Willebrand factor.

DIC is a severe coagulopathy associated with advanced disease states such as sepsis, burns, massive transfusion, and shock. It is unlikely that prolonged PT or aPTT will uncover an otherwise unsuspected DIC.

Liver disease has to be in an advanced and clinically apparent state before the reduced hepatic production of coagulation factors leads to coagulopathies. Factors V, VII, and X have to fall below 50% of normal values and prothrombin levels have to be less than 30% before the PT prolongs. The aPTT stays within normal limits until the activity of the factors of the intrinsic pathway is less than 30%.[37]

Vitamin K deficiency can be suspected in cases of malnutrition or malabsorption, but it may be uncovered by a pathologic PT or, if very severe, a prolonged aPTT.

Congenital factor VII deficiency leads to a prolongation of PT without affecting aPTT; it is a very rare condition that leads to variable bleeding tendency, from mild to life-threatening. Deficiencies in the factors II, V, and X lead to abnormal PT and aPTT, but these are very rare,[37,60] and the cost to detect this condition by routine testing of the surgical population is unjustifiable.

Dysfibrinogenemia is caused by a variety of structural abnormalities in the fibrinogen molecule.[61] It can be inherited or acquired. The prevalence of the inherited forms is unknown; its hereditary pattern is usually autosomal dominant, and the clinical presentation can be either a bleeding or a thrombosis tendency. Both features can be present in the same patient, and most patients are asymptomatic. The disease is suspected on the basis of a bleeding or thrombosis tendency, which is not explained by other more common entities, and by a pathologic PT that may be prolonged or shortened. Other tests, such as reptilase time and fibrinogen analysis, are needed for confirmation. Acquired dysfibrinogenemia is caused by diseases of the liver or biliary tract (cirrhosis, liver failure, acetaminophen overdose, obstructive jaundice). It can also be a paraneoplastic phenomenon in the case of hepatoma or renal malignancies. It is unknown if acquired dysfibrinogenemia is an independent risk factor for bleeding or thrombosis.

The aPTT is prolonged by deficiencies of factors XII, XI, IX, and VIII, by lupus anticoagulant, and by VWD. Congenital factor XII deficiency is relatively frequent in Asians, but it does not lead to increased bleeding, even in the total absence of the factor. Factor XI deficiency is generally a rare disorder (1 in 1 million) except in the population of Ashkenazic Jews, where the prevalence is 12%.[62] It is an autosomal recessive bleeding disorder detectable by a prolongation of aPTT characterized by injury-related hemorrhage.[63] It is one of the very few conditions that may go unnoticed until excessive bleeding during surgery occurs. Preoperative transfusion of fresh-frozen plasma can prevent hemorrhage. Deficiencies of factors VIII and IX are known as hemophilia A and B, respectively. These patients have a longstanding history of bleeding complications and are extremely unlikely to be first diagnosed by a routine preoperative screening. VWD leads to factor VIII deficiency, because VWF serves as a carrier protein for this factor and prevents it from destruction by circulating inhibitors. VWD results in a prolonged aPTT, with variable bleeding tendency, depending on the amount and function of circulating VWF.[64] It is the most frequent inherited bleeding disorder, with a prevalence as high as 2% in the general population according to some studies.[65] Based on patients referred for bleeding, on the other hand, the prevalence has been estimated to be 30 to 100 cases per million.[64] In types 1 and 2, the bleeding tendency varies strongly and may even go unnoticed; in type 3 (complete or near-complete absence of the factor), bleeding is severe and present in the very early stages of life. Lupus anticoagulant can cause a prolongation of the aPTT but normally does not affect PT.[37] Paradoxically, these patients have an increased risk for thrombotic complication and do not show increased bleeding risk unless thrombocytopenia or decreased thrombin levels are present. In this case, the PT is also prolonged.

In summary, if both medical history and physical examination are negative, it is very unlikely that further laboratory testing will uncover unsuspected factor deficiencies or bleeding tendencies. Moreover, because of their design, PT and aPTT are poor predictors of surgical blood loss, even if their values are abnormal. Thus, the routine screening of a surgical population with PT and aPTT tests is not justified. At best, routine use of these tests leads to confusing results, repetition of tests, and unjustified cancellation or postponing of surgery. However, when coagulation abnormalities are expected as a result of the surgical procedure itself (major hepatic surgery, extracorporeal circulation, massive blood loss and transfusion), preoperative baseline PT and aPTT values must be obtained to be able to interpret intraoperative and postoperative values.

In patients with a positive bleeding history, laboratory tests can differentiate disorders of primary and secondary coagulation. Platelet function analysis by means of PFA-100 and VWF antigen tests are much more likely to detect an underlying coagulopathy than PT, aPTT, and PC. Most of the underlying pathologies are acquired platelet dysfunction.

Whether drug-induced coagulopathies should be corrected preoperatively depends on several factors, such as the patient's cardiovascular risk profile and the severity of expected surgical bleeding complications.

■ MANAGEMENT OF PATIENTS UNDER ANTIPLATELET THERAPY

Antiplatelet drugs offer a high degree of protection against myocardial infarction, stroke, and peripheral vascular occlusion. Three classes of antiplatelet agents are currently used: acetylsalicylic acid (ASA), adenosine-5′-diphospate (ADP) receptor antagonists (thienopyridines), and glycoprotein (GP) IIb/IIIa receptor antagonists.[66]

- ASA irreversibly acetylates platelet cyclooxygenase-1 (COX-1), inhibiting the synthesis of the potent platelet aggregator and vasoconstrictor thromboxane A_2. Restoration of platelet COX-1 activity depends on the generation of fresh platelets, because the inhibition of COX-1 is irreversible. There is no antidote to ASA except platelet transfusion. However, platelet replacement is rarely indicated because ASA induces only a weak inhibition of platelet function. ASA does not usually prolong the bleeding time.

- The only thienopyridine currently in use is clopidogrel, which irreversibly inhibits platelet aggregation. It prolongs bleeding time 1.5- to 3-fold of baseline after 3 to 7 days of treatment. After clopidogrel cessation, platelet function recovers gradually and reaches normal values 7 days after the last dose.
- The GPIIb/IIIa receptor antagonists are potent antiplatelet agents that are usually administered intravenously after percutaneous coronary interventions (PCI) to block platelet aggregation and prevent early acute stent thrombosis. Three substances are in clinical use: abciximab, eptifibatide, and tirofiban. Abciximab has a half-life of 23 hours; its molecules are redistributed among circulating, newly formed, and probably transfused platelets. Eptifibatide and tirofiban have considerably lower affinity for the GPIIb/IIIa receptor. Their action is characterized by rapid plasma clearance; platelet aggregation recovers 50% of its activity after 6 and 4 hours, respectively. To prevent massive blood losses, platelet transfusions are necessary in case of surgery within 24 hours of abciximab administration.[67] In contrast, 6 hours after administration of tirofiban or eptifibatide, the hemorrhagic risk is no longer increased.[68,69]

Lifelong ASA therapy is a grade 1A recommendation for chronic coronary artery disease (CAD) and acute coronary syndromes (ACS), for cerebrovascular disease, and for peripheral arterial disease.[70] In primary and secondary prevention, ASA reduces myocardial ischemic events by 34%

to 50%.[71,72] In the secondary prevention of stroke, the risk for subsequent stroke is decreased by 25% and the risk for vascular death by 15%.[71] According to a decision analysis model, continued aspirin use decreases perioperative mortality by 27% in vascular surgery.[73] The optimal dosage range for ASA is 75 to 150 mg/day. Higher dosages do not increase protection but may increase the risk for major extracranial hemorrhage.[74] The combination of ASA and clopidogrel is a grade 1A recommendation in patients after PCI, with unstable CAD, or with chronic stable CAD and a high risk for developing acute myocardial infarction (MI).[70] Clopidogrel (75 mg/day) is more efficacious in the prevention of ischemic stroke (30% reduction), MI, and vascular death (55% to 70% reduction) than ASA alone (Table 11-4).[75-77] However, dual antiplatelet therapy results in a higher incidence of spontaneous major hemorrhage compared with ASA (3.7% versus 2.7%) or clopidogrel (8% versus 3%) monotherapy.[77,78]

Clopidogrel, in addition to ASA, is mandatory in patients with unstable coronary disease and after PCI, because of the highly thrombogenic lesion created by the interruption of endothelial continuity. After PCI, the duration of dual treatment depends on the procedure performed (see Table 11-4), as follows:

- In simple dilatation without placement of an intracoronary stent, 2 weeks is considered sufficient.
- When a bare metal stent is deployed, the process of reendothelialization takes 6 to 8 weeks[79,80]; dual antiplatelet therapy is recommended for at least 4 to 6 weeks.

11-4 | **Indications for Use of Antiplatelet Agents, and Treatment Information**

Situation	Aspirin (ASA)	Clopidogrel	ASA + Clopidogrel
Chronic coronary artery disease	Lifelong 75-150 mg/day RRR MI: 50% (1°), 33% (2°) LR: 1A	Throughout surgery 75 mg/day RRR MI: 19% (2°) LR: 2B	Throughout surgery — RRR MI: 50% (2°) LR: 2B
Acute coronary syndromes	LD: 250 mg IV 75-150 mg/day RRR MI: 46% (2°) LR: 1A	LD: 300 mg 75 mg/day — LR: 1A (if ASA not possible)	— — — LR: 1A
Percutaneous coronary intervention (PCI), no stent	Lifelong 75-150 mg/day RRR MI: 60% LR: 1A	2 wk 75 mg/day RRR MI + death: 31% LR: 1A	2 wk — — LR: 1A
PCI, bare-metal stent	Lifelong RRR MI: 60% LR: 1A	4-8 wk RRR MI + death: 31% LR: 1A	4-8 wk — LR: 1A
PCI, drug-eluting stent	Lifelong —	12 mo LR: 1A (LE: 1B)	3-6 mo (12 mo) RRR MI + death: 27%
Coronary artery bypass graft	Lifelong RRR MI + stroke: 48%	Lifelong RRR MI + stroke: 29%	— —
Stroke	Lifelong RRR: 25% (2°)	Throughout surgery RRR: 25%-30% (2°)	Throughout surgery RRR: 25%-30% (2°)
Peripheral arterial disease	Lifelong RRR: MI, stroke + death: 23%	Throughout surgery RRR: MI, stroke + death: 24%	— —

1°, primary prevention; 2°, secondary prevention; LD, loading dose; LR, level of recommendation (class 1, clearly indicated; A, indication based on large trials with clear-cut results; B, indication based on smaller trials or with less clear results; class 2, good supportive evidence); MI, myocardial infarction; RRR, relative risk reduction; LE, level of evidence.
From references 70-72, 75-77, 81, 107-110.

- Drug-eluting stents, which slowly release antimitogen drugs and inhibit cell proliferation in the adjacent coronary artery wall, delay the process of reendothelialization, thus prolonging the period during which the patients is at high risk for in-stent thrombosis. Dual antiplatelet therapy is recommended for up to 12 months after stenting with drug-eluting stents.

Because the long-term incidence of cardiovascular death, stroke, MI, or urgent revascularization after PCI is significantly reduced in ASA-clopidogrel patients compared with patients under ASA alone,[76] a consensus conference has recommended a 12-month therapy of clopidogrel in addition to the lifelong treatment with ASA.[81]

Interruption of antiplatelet agents used for prevention of cardiovascular and cerebrovascular diseases places patients at high risk for arterial thrombosis, with possible dramatic outcomes. Withdrawal of aspirin in patients with stable CAD has been shown to be associated with a fourfold increase in the rate of death compared with patients appropriately treated.[82] ASA withdrawal precedes 10% of all acute cardiovascular syndromes.[83] The outcomes of patients who stopped ASA within 2 weeks before an ACS, compared with those who did not interrupt antiplatelet therapy, reveals a twofold increase in mortality (19.2% versus 9.9%) and myocardial infarction rate (21.9% versus 12.4%) in the withdrawer group, even if a replacement with low-molecular-weight heparin was initiated.[84] Cessation of antiplatelet therapy is the major independent predictor of stent occlusion. It is associated with a twofold to fivefold increase in mortality and infarction rate, a 20% incidence of thrombosis in uncoated stents, and 20% to 45% mortality in drug-eluting stents.[85-87] Thrombotic stent occlusion resulting in myocardial infarction after aspirin cessation has been reported as late as 15 months after PCI with drug-eluting stents.[88]

Combined with the increased platelet adhesiveness and decreased fibrinolysis characteristic of the intraoperative and postoperative situations, these data plead in favor of continuing the antiplatelet treatment through the perioperative period. Unfortunately, because this treatment is known to increase the risk for bleeding and proscribes neuraxial blockade, it has been standard practice to interrupt it 7 to 10 days before the intervention, the aim being to minimize perioperative blood loss and/or to perform regional anesthesia. But how real is this hemorrhagic risk?

Few randomized controlled studies have addressed this topic in noncardiac surgery. With ASA alone, they have shown no increase of operative blood loss, or an increase with little clinical relevance because it ranges from 2.5% to 10%,[73,89-91] and meanwhile, a significant reduction in myocardial infarctions and cerebrovascular accidents was noted.[90,91] The bleeding rate is variable according to the type of surgery. There is no significant increase in surgical hemorrhage during breast biopsies, ophthalmologic procedures, airway and gastrointestinal endoscopies, or different types of digestive and vascular surgery, but the rate of transfusions or reoperation for hemostasis is increased after tonsillectomy and transurethral prostatectomy.[83,92] In orthopedic surgery, the results are controversial; for example, one large trial[93] has

shown an increase in bleeding and transfusion in patients with hip fractures under ASA therapy (odds ratio, 1.5), but two other studies failed to identify aspirin as a risk factor in spine surgery and femoral neck fractures.[94,95] Bleeding-related fatalities after aspirin ingestion have been reported only in intracranial neurosurgery and transurethral prostatectomy.[96,97]

With dual antiplatelet therapy (ASA plus clopidogrel), the average increase in surgical bleeding is 25%,[77] and the rate of major bleedings rises from 0.7% in controls to 1.13% in treated patients.[71] However, recent studies have ruled out any significant increase in bleeding after hemorrhagic procedures such as colonoscopic polypectomy, transbronchial lung biopsy, or different types of major surgery.[92,98,99] In cardiac surgery with cardiopulmonary bypass (CPB) and full heparinization, on the other hand, the surgical bleeding, chest tube drainage, transfusion rate, and length of hospital stay are increased by about 50% under dual antiplatelet therapy.[100] The effect of clopidogrel cannot easily be interrupted or antagonized if a hemorrhagic operation requires reversing its action. Therefore, some surgeons prefer to operate on patients treated by heparin instead of antiplatelet agents. Unfortunately, heparin is a poor choice as a monotherapy because of its unpredictability in the individual patient. Heparin alone is not recommended by the American College of Chest Physicians guidelines as a therapy for ACS.[81] Only a combination of heparin and aspirin adjusted to an aPTT between 1.5 and 2 times the control value (50 to 70 seconds) has given results similar to dual antiplatelet therapy.[76,101]

For each 1000 patients treated with dual antiplatelet therapy, there is an increase of 13 patients with significant bleeding.[78] But among 1000 patients with MI who were given aspirin for 2 years, 40 could be expected to avoid a serious cardiovascular event during the first month and another 40 could be expected to avoid a cardiovascular event in the next 2 years.[71] With an incidence of approximately 20% of mortality and 40% of permanent disability, the consequences of arterial thromboembolism are dismal compared with a fatality rate of less than 3% for major operative bleeding.[102] Therefore, the cessation of antiplatelet agents to minimize bleeding is unjustified for almost all surgical procedures in patients with severe or unstable CAD, high-risk vascular situations, or threatening stroke. Maintenance of clopidogrel is acceptable for abdominal, thoracic, or orthopedic surgery, but it might be excessive for some endoscopic resections with high bleeding risks and poorly controllable hemostasis, and for intracranial surgery, where even minor hemorrhagic complications can lead to dramatic outcomes. For these groups of patients, interruption of clopidogrel is indicated, but aspirin alone can probably be safely continued, although no studies are available to prove this choice (Fig. 11-6). In cardiac surgery with CPB, clopidogrel should also be interrupted because there is a major increase in bleeding. The anesthesiologist and the surgeon should decide what is best for the patient in each situation, by pondering the risk for bleeding versus the risk for coronary or cerebral thrombosis. The evidence collected in the recent literature supports the continuation of antiplatelet drugs even at the cost of a slightly elevated

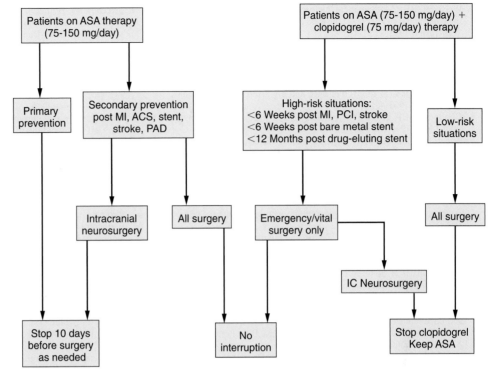

Figure 11-6 ■ Decisional algorithm for patients receiving antiplatelet therapy. ACS, acute coronary syndrome; ASA, acetylsalicylic acid; IC, intracranial; MI, myocardial infarction; PAD, peripheral arterial disease; PCI, percutaneous coronary intervention.

risk for bleeding and transfusion. One or 2 units of transfused blood may be less deleterious than acute MI or stroke.

A second important aspect of antiplatelet therapy is its impact on neuraxial blockade, because keeping the protecting effect of clopidogrel precludes the benefit of the sympatholytic and analgesic effects of epidural or combined anesthesia. However, the neuraxial sympatholysis is beneficial to the ischemic myocardium as long as the cardiac nerves are blocked; therefore, the reduction in the incidence of intraoperative ischemia and postoperative MI is significant only with high thoracic epidural anesthesia, where it has been recorded to be as high as 40%.[103,104] It does not reach significance with low thoracic or lumbar epidural anesthesia, nor with an intrathecal technique.[103,105,106] Epidural anesthesia, alone or in combination with general anesthesia, does not modify mortality or infarction rate in a meta-analysis of 11 randomized trials, despite its slight antithrombotic effect (total 1173 patients).[103] Unfortunately, the outstanding analgesia of epidural anesthesia is possible only at the cost of withdrawing the antiplatelet agents 7 to 10 days before the surgery. In ACS and during the reendothelialization phase of coronary stents, this withdrawal is associated with a twofold to fivefold increase in mortality and infarction rate.[84-87] This is much higher than the 40% decrease in MI observed with high thoracic, and only high thoracic, epidurals. It has not been proven yet that the antithrombotic effect of epidural anesthesia might be superior to the effect of clopidogrel and aspirin. Therefore, it seems safer to continue aspirin and clopidogrel throughout the operative period and to forgo using neuraxial blockade. An equipotent intraoperative sympatholysis can be realized as well with intravenous substances such as beta-blockers, alpha-2 agonists, and higher dosages

of opioids. The only real disadvantage is a lack of equivalence in the quality of postoperative analgesia.

In conclusion, present data show that the cardiovascular and neurologic risks of withdrawing low-dose aspirin before an operation are greater than the risks of hemorrhage and transfusion caused by the increase in blood loss. Aspirin withdrawal is dangerous mainly in secondary prevention, and it can be stopped in the case of primary prevention if surgically indicated. If clopidogrel is indicated to prevent coronary thrombosis after an acute coronary syndrome or after coronary stenting, it should not be interrupted in the perioperative period of noncardiac surgery, except in the case of intracranial neurosurgery. Because clopidogrel is of the utmost importance during the first 6 to 12 weeks after PCI, only emergency operations can be carried out during this period. Clopidogrel significantly increases the surgical blood loss and the transfusion rate in cardiac surgery on CPB and full heparinization; in this case, it is better to stop it before the surgery, as long as the coronary circulation is not compromised.

■ **REFERENCES**

1. Singelenberg R: The blood transfusion taboo of Jehovah's Witnesses: Origin, development and function of a controversial doctrine. Soc Sci Med 1990;31:515-523.
2. Beauchamp T, Childress J: Principles of Biomedical Ethics. New York, Oxford University Press, 1994.
3. Finfer S, Howell S, Miller J, et al: Managing patients who refuse blood transfusions: An ethical dilemma. BMJ 1994;308:1423-1426.
4. Ward M: Management of Anaesthesia for Jehovah's Witnesses. London, Association of Anaesthetists of Great Britain and Ireland, 1999.

5. Weiskopf RB: Mathematical analysis of isovolemic hemodilution indicates that it can decrease the need for allogeneic blood transfusion. Transfusion 1995;35:37-41.

6. Spahn DR, Dettori N, Kocian R, Chassot PG: Transfusion in the cardiac patient. Crit Care Clin 2004;20:269-279.

7. Rosencher N, Kerkkamp HE, Macheras G, et al: Orthopedic Surgery Transfusion Hemoglobin European Overview (OSTHEO) study: Blood management in elective knee and hip arthroplasty in Europe. Transfusion 2003;43:459-469.

8. Goodnough LT, Monk TG, Andriole GL: Erythropoietin therapy. N Engl J Med 1997;336:933-938.

9. Price TH, Goodnough LT, Vogler WR, et al: The effect of recombinant human erythropoietin on the efficacy of autologous blood donation in patients with low hematocrits: A multicenter, randomized, double-blind, controlled trial. Transfusion 1996;36:29-36.

10. Sowade O, Warnke H, Scigalla P, et al: Avoidance of allogeneic blood transfusions by treatment with epoetin beta (recombinant human erythropoietin) in patients undergoing open-heart surgery. Blood 1997;89:411-418.

11. Brecher ME, Goodnough LT: The rise and fall of preoperative autologous blood donation. Transfusion 2001;41:1459-1462.

12. Monk TG, Goodnough LT, Brecher ME, et al: A prospective randomized comparison of three blood conservation strategies for radical prostatectomy. Anesthesiology 1999;91:24-33.

13. Birkmeyer JD, Goodnough LT, AuBuchon JP, et al: The cost-effectiveness of preoperative autologous blood donation for total hip and knee replacement. Transfusion 1993;33:544-551.

14. Spahn DR: Strategies for transfusion therapy. Best Pract Res Clin Anaesthesiol 2004;18:661-673.

15. Waters JH, Lee JS, Karafa MT: A mathematical model of cell salvage compared and combined with normovolemic hemodilution. Transfusion 2004;44:1412-1416.

16. Matot I, Scheinin O, Jurim O, Eid A: Effectiveness of acute normovolemic hemodilution to minimize allogeneic blood transfusion in major liver resections. Anesthesiology 2002;97:794-800.

17. Weiskopf RB: Efficacy of acute normovolemic hemodilution assessed as a function of fraction of blood volume lost. Anesthesiology 2001;94:439-446.

18. Meier J, Kemming GI, Kisch-Wedel H, et al: Hyperoxic ventilation reduces 6-hour mortality at the critical hemoglobin concentration. Anesthesiology 2004;100:70-76.

19. Weiskopf RB, Feiner J, Hopf HW, et al: Oxygen reverses deficits of cognitive function and memory and increased heart rate induced by acute severe isovolemic anemia. Anesthesiology 2002;96:871-877.

20. Meier J, Kemming G, Meisner F, et al: Hyperoxic ventilation enables hemodilution beyond the critical myocardial hemoglobin concentration. Eur J Med Res 2005;10:462-468.

21. Jamnicki M, Kocian R, van der Linden P, et al: Acute normovolemic hemodilution: Physiology, limitations, and clinical use. J Cardiothorac Vasc Anesth 2003;17:747-754.

22. Strauss RG, Pennell BJ, Stump DC: A randomized, blinded trial comparing the hemostatic effects of pentastarch versus hetastarch. Transfusion 2002;42:27-36.

23. Egli GA, Zollinger A, Seifert B, et al: Effect of progressive haemodilution with hydroxyethyl starch, gelatin and albumin on blood coagulation. Br J Anaesth 1997;78:684-689.

24. Spahn DR, Casutt M: Eliminating blood transfusions: New aspects and perspectives. Anesthesiology 2000;93:242-255.

25. Koscielny J, Ziemer S, Radtke H, et al: A practical concept for preoperative identification of patients with impaired primary hemostasis. Clin Appl Thromb Hemost 2004;10:195-204.

26. Girolami A, Luzzatto G, Varvarikis C, et al: Main clinical manifestations of a bleeding diathesis: An often disregarded aspect of medical and surgical history taking. Haemophilia 2005;11:193-202.

27. Koscielny J, von Tempelhoff GF, Ziemer S, et al: A practical concept for preoperative management of patients with impaired primary hemostasis. Clin Appl Thromb Hemost 2004;10:155-166.

28. Robinson KL, Marasco SF, Street AM: Practical management of anticoagulation, bleeding and blood product support for cardiac surgery. Part 1. Bleeding and anticoagulation issues. Heart Lung Circ 2001;10:142-153.

29. Sweeney JD, Holme S, Heaton WA, et al: Pseudothrombocytopenia in plateletpheresis donors. Transfusion 1995;35:46-49.

30. Vicari A, Banfi G, Bonini PA: EDTA-dependent pseudothrombocytopaenia: A 12-month epidemiological study. Scand J Clin Lab Invest 1988;48:537-542.

31. Payne BA, Pierre RV: Pseudothrombocytopenia: A laboratory artifact with potentially serious consequences. Mayo Clin Proc 1984;59:123-125.

32. Sane DC, Damaraju LV, Topol EJ, et al: Occurrence and clinical significance of pseudothrombocytopenia during abciximab therapy. J Am Coll Cardiol 2000;36:75-83.

33. Cines DB, Bussel JB, McMillan RB, Zehnder JL: Congenital and acquired thrombocytopenia. Hematology Am Soc Hematol Educ Program 2004:390-406.

34. Cines DB, Bussel JB: How I treat idiopathic thrombocytopenic purpura (ITP). Blood 2005;106:2244-2251.

35. Davoren A, Aster RH: Heparin-induced thrombocytopenia and thrombosis. Am J Hematol 2006;81:36-44.

36. Warkentin TE: Heparin-induced thrombocytopenia: Pathogenesis and management. Br J Haematol 2003;121:535-555.

37. Cobas M: Preoperative assessment of coagulation disorders. Int Anesthesiol Clin 2001;39:1-15.

38. Samama CM, Djoudi R, Lecompte T, et al: Perioperative platelet transfusion: Recommendations of the Agence Francaise de Securite Sanitaire des Produits de Sante (AFSSaPS) 2003. Can J Anaesth 2005;52:30-37.

39. Anteby E, Shalev O: Clinical relevance of gestational thrombocytopenia of <100,000/microliters. Am J Hematol 1994;47:118-122.

40. Fisher NC, Mutimer DJ: Central venous cannulation in patients with liver disease and coagulopathy: A prospective audit. Intensive Care Med 1999;25:481-485.

41. Howard S, Gajjar A, Cheng C, et al: Risk factors for traumatic and bloody lumbar puncture in children with acute lymphoblastic leukemia. JAMA 2002;288:2001-2007.

42. Howard S, Gajjar A, Ribeiro RC, et al: Safety of lumbar puncture for children with acute lymphoblastic leukemia and thrombocytopenia. JAMA 2000;284:2222-2224.

43. Barber A, Green D, Galluzzo T, Ts'ao CH: The bleeding time as a preoperative screening test. Am J Med 1985;78:761-764.

44. Simon TL, Akl BF, Murphy W: Controlled trial of routine administration of platelet concentrates in cardiopulmonary bypass surgery. Ann Thorac Surg 1984;37:359-364.

45. Rodgers RP, Levin J: A critical reappraisal of the bleeding time. Semin Thromb Hemost 1990;16:1-20.

46. Peterson P, Hayes TE, Arkin CF, et al: The preoperative bleeding time test lacks clinical benefit: College of American Pathologists' and American Society of Clinical Pathologists' position article. Arch Surg 1998;133:134-139.

47. Harrison P: The role of PFA-100 testing in the investigation and management of haemostatic defects in children and adults. Br J Haematol 2005;130:3-10.

48. Born GV, Cross MJ: The aggregation of blood platelets. J Physiol 1963;168:22-42.

49. Myers ER, Clarke-Pearson DL, Olt GJ, et al: Preoperative coagulation testing on a gynecologic oncology service. Obstet Gynecol 1994;83:438-444.

50. Eika C, Havig O, Godal HC: The value of preoperative haemostatic screening. Scand J Haematol 1978;21:349-354.

51. Redding SW, Olive JA: Relative value of screening tests of hemostasis prior to dental treatment. Oral Surg Oral Med Oral Pathol 1985;59:34-36.

52. Ewe K: Bleeding after liver biopsy does not correlate with indices of peripheral coagulation. Dig Dis Sci 1981;26:388-393.

53. McVay PA, Toy PT: Lack of increased bleeding after paracentesis and thoracentesis in patients with mild coagulation abnormalities. Transfusion 1991;31:164-171.

54. Webster ST, Brown KL, Lucey MR, Nostrant TT: Hemorrhagic complications of large volume abdominal paracentesis. Am J Gastroenterol 1996;91:366-368.

55. Kozak EA, Brath LK: Do "screening" coagulation tests predict bleeding in patients undergoing fiberoptic bronchoscopy with biopsy? Chest 1994;106:703-705.

56. Jouet P, Meyrier A, Mal F, et al: Transjugular renal biopsy in the treatment of patients with cirrhosis and renal abnormalities. Hepatology 1996;24:1143-1147.

57. Darcy MD, Kanterman RY, Kleinhoffer MA, et al: Evaluation of coagulation tests as predictors of angiographic bleeding complications. Radiology 1996;198:741-744.

58. Mumtaz H, Williams V, Hauer-Jensen M, et al: Central venous catheter placement in patients with disorders of hemostasis. Am J Surg 2000;180:503-505; discussion 506.

59. Korte W, Gabi K, Rohner M, et al: Preoperative fibrin monomer measurement allows risk stratification for high intraoperative blood loss in elective surgery. Thromb Haemost 2005;94:211-215.

60. Acharya SS, Coughlin A, Dimichele DM: Rare Bleeding Disorder Registry: Deficiencies of factors II, V, VII, X, XIII, fibrinogen and dysfibrinogenemias. J Thromb Haemost 2004;2:248-256.

61. Cunningham MT, Brandt JT, Laposata M, Olson JD: Laboratory diagnosis of dysfibrinogenemia. Arch Pathol Lab Med 2002;126:499-505.

62. Fujikawa K: Historical perspective of factor XI. Thromb Res 2005;115:441-450.

63. Seligsohn U: Factor XI deficiency. Thromb Haemost 1993;70:68-71.

64. Mannucci PM: Treatment of von Willebrand's disease. N Engl J Med 2004;351:683-694.

65. Werner EJ, Broxson EH, Tucker EL, et al: Prevalence of von Willebrand disease in children: A multiethnic study. J Pediatr 1993;123:893-898.

66. Harder S, Klinkhardt U, Alvarez JM: Avoidance of bleeding during surgery in patients receiving anticoagulant and/or antiplatelet therapy: Pharmacokinetic and pharmacodynamic considerations. Clin Pharmacokinet 2004;43:963-981.

67. Juergens CP, Yeung AC, Oesterle SN: Routine platelet transfusion in patients undergoing emergency coronary bypass surgery after receiving abciximab. Am J Cardiol 1997;80:74-75.

68. Dyke CM, Bhatia D, Lorenz TJ, et al: Immediate coronary artery bypass surgery after platelet inhibition with eptifibatide: Results from PURSUIT. Platelet Glycoprotein IIb/IIIa in Unstable Angina: Receptor Suppression Using Integrelin Therapy. Ann Thorac Surg 2000;70:866-871; discussion 871-872.

69. Genoni M, Zeller D, Bertel O, et al: Tirofiban therapy does not increase the risk of hemorrhage after emergency coronary surgery. J Thorac Cardiovasc Surg 2001;122:630-632.

70. Harrington RA, Becker RC, Ezekowitz M, et al: Antithrombotic therapy for coronary artery disease: The Seventh ACCP Conference on Antithrombotic and Thrombolytic Therapy. Chest 2004;126(3 Suppl):513S-548S.

71. Antithrombotic Trialists' Collaboration: Collaborative meta-analysis of randomised trials of antiplatelet therapy for prevention of death, myocardial infarction, and stroke in high risk patients. BMJ 2002;324:71-86.

72. Pearson TA, Blair SN, Daniels SR, et al: AHA Guidelines for Primary Prevention of Cardiovascular Disease and Stroke: 2002 Update: Consensus Panel Guide to Comprehensive Risk Reduction for Adult Patients without Coronary or Other Atherosclerotic Vascular Diseases. American Heart Association Science Advisory and Coordinating Committee. Circulation 2002;106:388-391.

73. Neilipovitz DT, Bryson GL, Nichol G: The effect of perioperative aspirin therapy in peripheral vascular surgery: A decision analysis. Anesth Analg 2001;93:573-580.

74. Peters RJ, Mehta SR, Fox KA, et al: Effects of aspirin dose when used alone or in combination with clopidogrel in patients with acute coronary syndromes: Observations from the Clopidogrel in Unstable Angina to Prevent Recurrent Events (CURE) study. Circulation 2003;108:1682-1687.

75. CAPRIE: A randomised, blinded, trial of clopidogrel versus aspirin in patients at risk of ischaemic events (CAPRIE). CAPRIE Steering Committee. Lancet 1996;348:1329-1339.

76. Mehta SR, Yusuf S, Peters RJ, et al: Effects of pretreatment with clopidogrel and aspirin followed by long-term therapy in patients undergoing percutaneous coronary intervention: The PCI-CURE study. Lancet 2001;358:527-533.

77. Yusuf S, Zhao F, Mehta SR, et al: Effects of clopidogrel in addition to aspirin in patients with acute coronary syndromes without ST-segment elevation. N Engl J Med 2001;345:494-502.

78. Bezerra DC, Bogousslavsky J: Antiplatelets in stroke prevention: The MATCH trial. Some answers, many questions and countless perspectives. Cerebrovasc Dis 2005;20(Suppl 2):109-118.

79. Eagle KA, Berger PB, Calkins H, et al: ACC/AHA guideline update for perioperative cardiovascular evaluation for noncardiac surgery: Executive summary a report of the American College of Cardiology/American Heart Association Task Force on Practice Guidelines (Committee to Update the 1996 Guidelines on Perioperative Cardiovascular Evaluation for Noncardiac Surgery). Circulation 2002;105:1257-1267.

80. Ueda Y, Nanto S, Komamura K, Kodama K: Neointimal coverage of stents in human coronary arteries observed by angioscopy. J Am Coll Cardiol 1994;23:341-346.

81. Popma JJ, Berger P, Ohman EM, et al: Antithrombotic therapy during percutaneous coronary intervention: The Seventh ACCP Conference on Antithrombotic and Thrombolytic Therapy. Chest 2004;126(3 Suppl):576S-599S.

82. Allen LaPointe NM, Kramer JM, DeLong ER, et al: Patient-reported frequency of taking aspirin in a population with coronary artery disease. Am J Cardiol 2002;89:1042-1046.

83. Burger W, Chemnitius JM, Kneissl GD, Rucker G: Low-dose aspirin for secondary cardiovascular prevention: Cardiovascular risks after its perioperative withdrawal versus bleeding risks with its continuation—Review and meta-analysis. J Intern Med 2005;257:399-414.

84. Collet JP, Montalescot G, Blanchet B, et al: Impact of prior use or recent withdrawal of oral antiplatelet agents on acute coronary syndromes. Circulation 2004;110:2361-2367.

85. Ferrari E, Benhamou M, Cerboni P, Marcel B: Coronary syndromes following aspirin withdrawal: A special risk for late stent thrombosis. J Am Coll Cardiol 2005;45:456-459.

86. Iakovou I, Schmidt T, Bonizzoni E, et al: Incidence, predictors, and outcome of thrombosis after successful implantation of drug-eluting stents. JAMA 2005;293:2126-2130.

87. Sharma AK, Ajani AE, Hamwi SM, et al: Major noncardiac surgery following coronary stenting: When is it safe to operate? Catheter Cardiovasc Interv 2004;63:141-145.

88. McFadden EP, Stabile E, Regar E, et al: Late thrombosis in drug-eluting coronary stents after discontinuation of antiplatelet therapy. Lancet 2004;364:1519-1521.

89. Horlocker TT, Wedel DJ, Schroeder DR, et al: Preoperative antiplatelet therapy does not increase the risk of spinal hematoma associated with regional anesthesia. Anesth Analg 1995;80:303-309.

90. Lindblad B, Persson NH, Takolander R, Bergqvist D: Does low-dose acetylsalicylic acid prevent stroke after carotid surgery? A double-blind, placebo-controlled randomized trial. Stroke 1993;24:1125-1128.

91. McCollum C, Alexander C, Kenchington G, et al: Antiplatelet drugs in femoropopliteal vein bypasses: A multicenter trial. J Vasc Surg 1991;13:150-161; discussion 161-162.

92. Wilson SH, Fasseas P, Orford JL, et al: Clinical outcome of patients undergoing non-cardiac surgery in the two months following coronary stenting. J Am Coll Cardiol 2003;42:234-240.

93. PEP: Prevention of pulmonary embolism and deep vein thrombosis with low dose aspirin: Pulmonary Embolism Prevention (PEP) trial. Lancet 2000;355:1295-1302.

94. Nuttall GA, Horlocker TT, Santrach PJ, et al: Predictors of blood transfusions in spinal instrumentation and fusion surgery. Spine 2000;25:596-601.

95. Manning BJ, O'Brien N, Aravindan S, et al: The effect of aspirin on blood loss and transfusion requirements in patients with femoral neck fractures. Injury 2004;35:121-124.

96. Thurston AV, Briant SL: Aspirin and post-prostatectomy haemorrhage. Br J Urol 1993;71:574-576.

97. Palmer JD, Sparrow OC, Iannotti F: Postoperative hematoma: A 5-year survey and identification of avoidable risk factors. Neurosurgery 1994;35:1061-1064; discussion 1064-1065.

98. Hui AJ, Wong RM, Ching JY, et al: Risk of colonoscopic polypectomy bleeding with anticoagulants and antiplatelet agents: Analysis of 1657 cases. Gastrointest Endosc 2004;59:44-48.

99. Wahidi MM, Garland R, Feller-Kopman D, et al: Effect of clopidogrel with and without aspirin on bleeding following transbronchial lung biopsy. Chest 2005;127:961-964.

100. Chu MW, Wilson SR, Novick RJ, et al: Does clopidogrel increase blood loss following coronary artery bypass surgery? Ann Thorac Surg 2004;78:1536-1541.

101. Oler A, Whooley MA, Oler J, Grady D: Adding heparin to aspirin reduces the incidence of myocardial infarction and death in patients with unstable angina: A meta-analysis. JAMA 1996;276:811-815.

102. Kearon C, Hirsh J: Management of anticoagulation before and after elective surgery. N Engl J Med 1997;336:1506-1511.

103. Beattie WS, Badner NH, Choi P: Epidural analgesia reduces postoperative myocardial infarction: A meta-analysis. Anesth Analg 2001;93:853-858.

104. Park WY, Thompson JS, Lee KK: Effect of epidural anesthesia and analgesia on perioperative outcome: A randomized, controlled Veterans Affairs cooperative study. Ann Surg 2001;234:560-569; discussion 569-571.

105. Norris EJ, Beattie C, Perler BA, et al: Double-masked randomized trial comparing alternate combinations of intraoperative anesthesia and postoperative analgesia in abdominal aortic surgery. Anesthesiology 2001;95:1054-1067.

106. O'Hara DA, Duff A, Berlin JA, et al: The effect of anesthetic technique on postoperative outcomes in hip fracture repair. Anesthesiology 2000;92:947-957.

107. Diener HC, Bogousslavsky J, Brass LM, et al: Aspirin and clopidogrel compared with clopidogrel alone after recent ischaemic stroke or transient ischaemic attack in high-risk patients (MATCH): Randomised, double-blind, placebo-controlled trial. Lancet 2004;364:331-337.

108. Lee T: Guidelines for unstable angina. In Zipes DP, Libby P, Bonow RO, Braunwald E (eds): Braunwald's Heart Disease, ed 7. Philadelphia, Elsevier Saunders, 2005, p 1276.

109. Lee T: Guidelines for chronic stable angina. In Zipes DP, Libby P, Bonow RO, Braunwald E (eds): Braunwald's Heart Disease, ed 7. Philadelphia, Elsevier Saunders, 2005, p 1351.

110. Mangano D: Multicenter Study of Perioperative Ischemia Research Group. Aspirin and mortality from coronary artery bypass. N Engl J Med 2002;347:1309-1317.

PART III

Preservation of Organ Function and Prevention and Management of Perioperative Organ Dysfunction

Cardiovascular System

Chapter

12 Prevention of Ischemic Injury in Cardiac Surgery

Matthew Agnew, Christopher Salerno, and Edward Verrier

The development by John and Mary Gibbon of the heart-lung machine a half century ago ushered in the modern era of cardiac surgery. Prior to 1953, the emerging field of heart surgery was limited primarily to brief operations conducted on the aorta, great vessels, pericardium, and cardiac surface, all of which were performed without interrupting cardiac function; valvular repairs were often performed with a blind sweep of the surgeon's finger. The introduction of the Gibbon oxygenator made possible the bloodless, motionless field necessary to perform anything beyond the simplest of cardiac repairs.[1-3] In the previous decades, advances in the commercial production of the natural anticoagulant heparin had made that drug safe, inexpensive, and readily available. Together, these two developments provided the foundation for the modern surgical treatment of cardiovascular disease.[4]

Interestingly, despite his initial success with extracorporeal oxygenation (repair of an atrial septal defect in an 18-year-old woman),[1] Gibbon's next three patients all died, and he never again used the machine. Clearly, oxygenating the blood was only a fraction of the battle, and strategies needed to be developed to keep the patient safe while on the heart-lung machine. This chapter is an attempt to summarize the major developments in myocardial protection. Some, such as hypothermia, trace their history back to the early days of the field. Others, such as preconditioning, remain to be translated from the experimental stage to the clinical realm. Taken together, these strategies have led to tremendous decreases in the morbidity and mortality associated with heart surgery, and they have enabled cardiac surgery, particularly coronary artery bypass grafting (CABG), to become one of the most widely and successfully performed procedures in the world.

Despite the myriad advancements in the prevention of ischemia during cardiac surgery, no universally applicable myocardial protection technique has been identified,[5] and the ideal method for myocardial protection still remains to be established.[6] In part, this may be due to the overall success of four generations of cardiac surgeons in reducing the morbidity and mortality associated with cardiac surgery to very low levels, which makes demonstrating a significant difference between one technique and another more challenging. A greater part of the explanation stems from our relatively recent acknowledgment of the fact that each cardiac surgery patient is unique, and thus a given patient's response to cardiac surgery, including, in particular, cardiopulmonary bypass (CPB), reflects individual biological variability. Thus, no single intervention or strategy or protocol in isolation can be expected to succeed for every patient.[7]

A third reason for the many ongoing controversies in myocardial protection is the uniqueness of each operating surgeon. In the past 2 decades, medical societies and institutions the world over have attempted a paradigm shift in which practice patterns are grounded in evidence-based medicine. This model deemphasizes intuition and unsystematic clinical experience as sufficient grounds for clinical decision making and stresses the examination of evidence from rational, hypothesis-driven clinical and experimental research.[8] However, recent surveys of practice patterns in the United States[9] and Great Britain[10] belie the fact that, to a great degree, cardiac surgery is still as much an art as it is a science. Indeed, a cursory review of the Cochrane Library, an internationally recognized evidence-based health-care database, reveals minimal information on CABG. Similarly, Claus Bartels and colleagues recently conducted a study of the scientific evidence supporting 48 major principles that are currently applied for CABG performance, and their evaluation found that the data concerning the effectiveness and safety of every one of these key principles was insufficient in both amount and quality to serve as a basis for practical, evidence-based guidelines.[11]

Nevertheless, despite the significant variation that exists between different countries, between different institutions, and even between individuals within institutions, some universally accepted tenets can be identified. Recognizing that an efficiently executed and technically superior operation performed on an appropriate patient under the right circumstances is perhaps the greatest form of myocardial protection, in this chapter we shall attempt to highlight these protective strategies, and the data (or lack thereof) supporting them, in an effort to develop an evidence-based approach to prevention of ischemic injury during cardiac surgery.

■ PERIOPERATIVE ISCHEMIA PREVENTION STRATEGIES

The success of any operation requires a coordinated plan of care that begins prior to the patient entering the operating room and continues throughout the postoperative period. As with surgical intervention, the ideal medical management of stable and unstable coronary artery disease, heart failure, and acute myocardial infarction continues to evolve and improve, as does the care of the postoperative cardiac patient. The appropriate use of medicines such as beta-blockers, afterload-reducing agents, statins, and antiplatelet agents is essential, but pharmacotherapy is just one facet of cardiac care. Inadequate attention to patient-controlled factors such as dietary modification, smoking cessation, glucose control, and exercise may doom a technically perfect operation, hastening the onset of graft failure and the recurrence of ischemia, and thus these lifestyle issues are of equal importance in determining the success or failure of any procedure. A vast literature and numerous large, well-conducted clinical trials are available to guide the internist, cardiologist, or intensive care specialist who may be primarily responsible for directing care of the cardiac patient outside of the operating room, and a detailed discussion of the perioperative management of ischemic heart disease is beyond the scope of this chapter. However, there are strategies in which the surgical team plays a central role, and which therefore merit brief discussion here.

Optimal Timing of Cardiac Surgery after Acute Myocardial Infarction

The appropriate timing of revascularization surgery in the setting of acute myocardial infarction (MI) has been the subject of uncertainty since the earliest days of CABG. In contrast to the patient with stable coronary artery disease or unstable angina, to whom the general rule of "sooner is better" applies, the conventional wisdom for patients who have experienced MI is to delay surgical intervention if possible. For patients with evidence of valvular or papillary muscle dysfunction, ongoing ischemia despite maximal medical therapy, or cardiogenic shock, high mortality in the absence of surgery warrants the risk of immediate surgical intervention, either CABG or implantation of a ventricular assist device (see Chapter 14). Less clear is the best course of action to take with the relatively stable patient who has just experienced acute MI.

Over the past 30 years, numerous attempts have been made to identify the appropriate timing of operative intervention after MI. As long ago as 1974, Cooley and colleagues noted a striking difference in in-hospital mortality of CABG patients after MI. When CABG was performed within 7 days of MI, mortality was 38%; when performed 31 to 60 days after MI, mortality fell to 6%.[12] This study and others performed in the early 1970s[13,14] led to a generation of cardiac surgeons' delaying operative management of the acute MI patient. As the management of acute MI evolved in the 1980s and 1990s, particularly with the advent of new thrombolytic therapy, platelet inhibitors, percutaneous transluminal coronary angioplasty, coronary stenting, and intra-aortic balloon pumps (IABPs), a number of investigators attempted again to identify the optimal timing of surgery after MI. Although new data suggest that perhaps such a long delay between MI and CABG is not necessary, few of these studies were randomized, and results have been disparate.[15-20] Several large retrospective data analyses have been used to create risk models that suggest that, when possible, waiting 7 days after MI may lead to improved outcomes.[21-23] Other investigators have argued that in the setting of a nontransmural (non–Q-wave) MI, patients may undergo CABG relatively safely at any time; and that even in the case of a transmural (Q-wave) infarct, a delay of 48 to 72 hours may be sufficient.[24-26] At present, therefore, although no firm conclusion can be made regarding the optimal timing of CABG in the setting of acute MI, the available evidence suggests that a delay of 3 to 7 days is appropriate. As mechanical assist devices increase physicians' abilities to manage the sequelae of MI, particularly cardiogenic shock, new questions have arisen as to whether the initial surgical intervention should be definitive revascularization or insertion of an assist device to lengthen the window of time between MI and surgery.

■ INTRAOPERATIVE ISCHEMIA-PREVENTION STRATEGIES

Nonoperative Strategies

Anesthesia Considerations

The concept of cardiac anesthesia has been in development since the introduction of the cardiopulmonary bypass machine in the 1950s, and the modern cardiac anesthesiologist is an indispensable member of the cardiac surgery team. Because the focus of the cardiac surgeon while in the operating room must be devoted to the performance of a technically superior operation, the cardiac anesthesiologist, whose tasks include surveying numerous monitors and ongoing laboratory results, is in perhaps the best position to identify the subtle changes in a patient's status that may signify ischemia or other impending pathophysiology. We shall now review a number of the specific tools that may be used to identify ischemia, as well as some of the nonoperative remedies employed to prevent or treat ischemia in the setting of cardiac surgery.

Monitoring for Ischemia

Routine intraoperative monitoring during CABG includes temperature monitoring, pulse oximetry, capnography, surface electrocardiography (ECG), and noninvasive blood pressure monitoring. More invasive monitoring typically employed during cardiac surgery includes an arterial line for continuous blood pressure monitoring and repeated blood sampling, a central venous catheter to measure central venous pressure, and use of a pulmonary artery catheter (PAC). Although ECG changes are the classic mode of monitoring for ischemia, newer technologies such as the PAC and transesophageal echocardiography may provide superior ischemia detection.

The PAC provides potentially valuable information regarding pulmonary arterial pressure, "wedge pressure" (as a surrogate of left-sided filling pressure), cardiac output, mixed venous saturation, and both systemic and vascular resistance, all of which can be used to guide management directed at improving perfusion.[27] Nevertheless, use of the PAC has been a topic of great debate ever since its introduction into clinical practice, and the controversy continues to rage today.[28] Almost 20 years ago, several published studies failed to detect a benefit from the use of PACs in the setting of acute myocardial ischemia/infarction.[29,30] Similarly, in 1989, Tuman and colleagues published their study showing no differences in outcome when PACs were used during CABG.[31,32] In 1996, the SUPPORT trial reported that PAC use was associated with longer hospital and intensive care unit (ICU) stays, significantly increased costs, and increased mortality, including a 1.5-fold increase in the relative risk of death in postoperative patients.[33] In the ensuing discussions, some called for a moratorium on continued use of the PAC.[34] However, attachment to the device by most practitioners proved strong, and, with evidence that the PAC was a useful tool for identifying perioperative ischemia,[35,36] a more measured approach was adopted. Nevertheless, even the staunchest of PAC supporters recognized that nonselective, routine use of the PAC was not justified.[27]

Throughout the 1990s, use of the PAC in the setting of CABG became more selective, and today its use varies widely by institution. Still, at the year 2000, 1 to 2 million PACs were being placed annually in the United States, at an estimated cost of $2 billion.[37] A retrospective study published in 2000 that surveyed facilities from around the country where CABG is routinely performed found that approximately 60% of patients undergoing CABG also receive a PAC, and 40% of institutions recorded greater than 85% of patients receiving PACs.[38] This same study reported that in the setting of nonemergent CABG surgery, PAC was associated with an increased risk of in-hospital mortality, greater length of stay, and higher total costs. In 2002, Schwann and colleagues published their experience with 2684 consecutive patients using a highly selective approach to the use of the PAC.[39] Their combined (both planned and unplanned) use of the PAC was only 9%; nevertheless, they found that this highly selective use did not increase operative risk or adversely affect outcomes. They further suggested that consideration of ejection fraction, Society of Thoracic Surgeons risk level, use of an IABP, presence of congestive heart failure, reoperation, or New York Heart Association class IV allows a prediction with high sensitivity of those patients who may require PAC insertion.[39]

One alternative to the PAC is transesophageal echocardiography (TEE). Advocates of TEE point to the fact that it is safer and that it can provide nearly all the same data as the PAC, plus additional information on wall motion, ejection fraction, stroke volume, overall volume status, and valvular function not ascertainable by any other method.[40] Small, nonrandomized studies of TEE in the setting of CABG have shown that TEE may be more important than PAC in guiding interventions involving fluid administration, vasoactive medications, and other anti-ischemia therapies,[41] and that among high-risk patients undergoing CABG, data provided by TEE affected anesthetic or surgical management of 50%.[42]

The reported safety and benefits of TEE notwithstanding, debate similar to that surrounding the PAC has emerged. Critics of TEE point to studies suggesting that unsuspected TEE findings of major significance occur in less than 2% of cases,[43] that intraoperative interpretation by cardiac anesthesiologists is widely variable and often does not concur with later interpretation by cardiologists,[41,44] and that, like PAC, TEE has not been shown to improve outcomes.[45] Critics also point to the fact that performing TEE may divert the anesthesiologist from performing other critical tasks; in one study, anesthesiologists' response time to an alarm light was 10 times slower when performing TEE than during monitor observation.[46]

In sum, a range of modalities to detect ischemia are available to the modern cardiac anesthesiologist, and the wealth of information provided by them is undisputed. In valvular cardiac surgery, the importance of TEE is well established. However, in the setting of myocardial revascularization, serious questions remain unanswered as to whether the information these devices provide, and the way that clinical care is guided by that information, is helpful as determined by measuring important outcome variables such as morbidity, mortality, and cost. Thus, judicious rather than routine use is warranted.

Anesthetic Agents

The goals of cardiac anesthesia are to maintain hemodynamic stability and myocardial oxygen balance, minimize the incidence and severity of ischemic episodes, and facilitate prompt and uncomplicated separation from cardiopulmonary bypass and assisted ventilation.[47] Throughout the relatively short history of cardiac surgery, numerous anesthetic regimens have been developed, each with its own proponents and each with purported advantages and shortcomings. To date, however, no evidence exists that any one technique can be claimed to be superior for patients with cardiovascular disease.[48]

Anesthesia during the early years of cardiac surgery consisted primarily of high-dose opioids, first morphine, and later, synthetic opioids. In the 1970s, fentanyl gained widespread acceptance for both induction and maintenance of anesthesia because of its improved hemodynamic stability. Because opiate-alone anesthesia was associated with an unacceptably high risk of patient awareness (which can lead to hypertension, tachycardia, and an attendant increase in myocardial oxygen consumption), benzodiazepines were added. More recently, propofol and volatile anesthetics have become a mainstay in both the induction and maintenance of cardiac anesthesia. Although some centers have gone to an all-intravenous anesthetic technique, the reported preconditioning protection provided by inhaled anesthetics[49,50] has led some to advocate their continued and routine use. In practice, the importance of anesthesia in minimizing ischemic risk is perhaps most evident during induction, when the potentially wide variation in blood pressure may put overwhelming strain on an already stressed heart. Standard therapy in the modern era, therefore, may include preinduction use of beta-blockade in addition to anxiolytics. Typical induction agents include a combination of paralytic, analgesic, and anesthetic agents. Anesthesia is maintained with a combination of analgesics and anesthetic agents.

Thoracic Epidural Anesthesia
In addition to the ongoing development of new anesthetic agents, changes in the method of delivery are occurring. Thoracic epidural analgesia has been investigated in relation to its potential role in preventing ischemic injury. Unfortunately, studies examining the issue have produced conflicting results[51-53]; thus, it remains to be determined whether this mode of anesthetic delivery may provide a greater degree of protection than the traditional inhalation or intravenous routes.

Metabolic Considerations

Systemic Temperature
With the passing of Wilfred Gordon Bigelow in 2005, cardiac surgery lost the man referred to as "the father of heart surgery in Canada."[54] After training at Johns Hopkins, Bigelow returned to the University of Toronto and the Banting Research Institute in 1947, where over the next 2 decades, he and his colleagues performed much of the initial research that identified hypothermia as a practical means by which the body could be protected during the brief periods of circulatory arrest required for relatively simple cardiac repairs. Prior to his investigations, heart surgery was performed in an environment approaching normothermia. The early cardiopulmonary bypass circuits did not include a heat exchanger, and most of the temperature change that did occur was passive. Indeed, if any attempt was made to regulate the patient's body temperature, it was to maintain normothermia. Hypothermia was seen as the enemy to sick and wounded patients because of its detrimental effects on coagulation and because metabolic rates were actually known to increase as patients got colder, largely caused by shivering. Bigelow's systematic studies of surface-induced hypothermia, primarily using a canine model, were the first to show that with shivering controlled by adequate anesthesia, metabolism actually decreased in a linear relationship to core body temperature, with each $10°C$ temperature drop corresponding to a roughly 50% reduction in oxygen consumption.[55-57]

Although metabolism could be essentially halted at low enough temperatures, providing excellent protection for the brain, temperatures below $28°C$ to $32°C$ led to cardiac and pulmonary failure, limiting the early use of hypothermic protection alone to cases requiring only very brief periods of

cardiac arrest. With the advent of cardiopulmonary bypass, however, temperatures could be reduced to $10°C$, thereby lengthening the window of protection. Following these early observations on systemic hypothermia, numerous others expanded on the use of hypothermia and its application in cardiac surgery. Shumway and colleagues soon demonstrated the additional benefit gained by topical cooling of the heart using ice cold saline.[58,59] Other advances, including introduction of the heat exchanger in the cardiopulmonary bypass circuit, made hypothermia a mainstay of myocardial protection in the early years of cardiac surgery.

Despite significant advances in our understanding of the molecular processes involved in tissue metabolism, hypothermia continues to be a central component of myocardial protection strategies, particularly in the transplant realm.[60,61] The use of hypothermia, however, remains very individual to the surgeon or institution. Some centers actively cool the body systemically; others simply let the patient's temperature drift downward. Almost all centers cool the heart, although since the early 1990s some investigators have advocated "warm heart surgery."[62-64]

Although significant debate persists, consensus is building that rather than the creation of severe hypothermia or active maintenance of normothermia, the appropriate temperature both for the systemic circulation and for cardioplegia infusion may be mild to moderate hypothermia (approximately $20°C$ to $32°C$). A number of studies suggest that such a tepid strategy provides the best level of myocardial protection without the consequences of hypothermia.[65-75]

Myocardial Acid–Base Management
The influence of intraoperative systemic pH status on CABG outcomes has been studied primarily in relation to its influence on neuroprotection. Most cardiac surgeons, and certainly cardiac anesthesiologists, are familiar with the concept of α-stat versus pH-stat management strategies, a detailed discussion of which is beyond the scope of this chapter. Less well understood is the relationship between ischemia, myocardial acid–base management, and non-neurologic outcomes.

Normal myocardial pH (7.2) is lower than systemic,[76] and various studies have demonstrated that mild acidosis (6.8 to 7.0) may actually protect the myocardium during ischemia by decreasing cardiomyocyte energy demands.[77,78] However, myocardial pH during CABG may be much more severe, with typical measurements of pH 6.5 or lower, and may trigger cell death via apoptosis.[79,80] Decreased myocardial pH is a consequence of inadequate coronary blood flow—low flow leads to decreased oxygen delivery, decreased washout of hydrogen ions, and an attendant rise in myocardial tissue P_{CO_2}—and as such may be used as a surrogate marker for myocardial ischemia. During cardiac surgery, low coronary flow may occur as a result of preexisting severe coronary artery stenosis, ineffective cardioplegia during cardiopulmonary bypass, or inadequate revascularization.[81] Myocardial acidosis may be the sentinel event in a potentially devastating cycle in which inadequate oxygen delivery leads to depressed myocardial function, which in turn necessitates the use of inotropes, which in turn leads to increased myocardial oxygen consumption.[82]

As an indicator of underlying ischemia, measurement of myocardial acidosis—like the ECG, pulmonary artery catheter, and transesophageal echocardiography—represents a potentially valuable monitoring tool for guiding the care of the cardiac surgery patient. Regular, repeated arterial blood gas measurements are standard practice in cardiac surgery, but they represent only static images of a constantly changing landscape and may not accurately reflect the condition of the myocardium. Current myocardial protection strategies based on these intermittent measurements may be insufficient.[83] Many attempts have therefore been made to develop real-time, continuous myocardial pH measuring devices.[84] Continuous blood gas monitors, for example, have been credited with decreasing the need for intraoperative pacing and cardioversion, decreasing the length of postoperative mechanical ventilation, and decreasing the length of ICU stay.[85]

In a series of studies over the past 30 years, Khuri and colleagues have perhaps done more than any other to increase our understanding of the potential importance of myocardial pH management. These investigators have developed a system using electrodes implanted in the ventricular wall that allow continuous pH measurements to monitor for regional myocardial ischemia and decreased coronary perfusion. Their retrospective analyses conclude that low myocardial pH can predict clinically relevant outcomes ranging from an increased need for inotropic support[82] to an increased risk of 30-day adverse events[86] to decreased long-term survival.[81] On the basis of their findings, they have developed a series of recommendations aimed at keeping myocardial pH in a safe range throughout all aspects of any cardiac surgery procedure.[76] Though compelling, these data and recommendations require prospective, randomized examination and external validation before they can be widely recommended.

Blood Glucose

Diabetes mellitus has long been considered an established risk factor both for the development of cardiovascular disease[87] and for significant perioperative morbidity and mortality associated with cardiac surgery.[88-92] Even after adjusting for other confounding risk factors such as age, hypertension, hypercholesterolemia, and smoking, diabetes has been shown in numerous studies to be a significant independent predictor of both short- and long-term survival after coronary artery bypass grafting.[93-96] The data are not all consistent, as some studies have not identified diabetes as an independent predictor of mortality.[97] Nevertheless, because diabetes now affects almost one third of patients undergoing bypass surgery, optimal perioperative glucose management must be a goal of all cardiac surgeons.

Although the mechanism of diabetes-related cardiac pathophysiology is multifactorial, patients with more severe forms of the disease (i.e., those who require preoperative insulin therapy), and by extension those with higher blood glucose levels, have a poorer prognosis.[94] Both acute and chronic hyperglycemia increase the risk of ischemic myocardial injury through a number of mechanisms, all of which

may come into play during cardiac surgery. These include a decrease in coronary collateral blood flow, endothelial dysfunction, and attenuation of the protective effects of inhaled anesthetics and other pharmacologic preconditioning agents.[98,99] The association of higher blood glucose and increased morbidity and mortality has shifted the focus of research in this area away from characterizing the risk from diabetes per se, to the role of elevated blood glucose in cardiac pathophysiology. In the absence of intervention, serum glucose concentrations in the intraoperative and perioperative periods often become elevated far above the normal range, even in nondiabetic patients. The cause of this elevation, which is similar to that which occurs in other forms of surgery and is in response to stress such as trauma or infection, reflects a combination of acute glucose intolerance in the form of insulin suppression, stress-hormone–induced gluconeogenesis, and impaired glucose excretion as a consequence of enhanced renal tubular resorption.[100] The metabolic effects of diabetes and elevated blood glucose have been shown to be similarly wide ranging and include a higher incidence of left ventricular dysfunction, more diffuse coronary artery disease, altered endothelial function, and abnormal fibrinolytic and platelet function.[101]

Maintenance of normal glucose levels during the intraoperative and perioperative periods is difficult, even in nondiabetic patients, and carries with it the risk for potentially life-threatening iatrogenic hypoglycemia.[102] Nevertheless, Furnary and colleagues have performed a series of studies investigating the feasibility of tight perioperative glycemic control and its effects on the important outcomes of sternal wound infection and death.[103] An initial study of 1585 diabetic patients undergoing cardiac surgery demonstrated that elevated blood glucose levels (>200 mg/dL) on the first and second postoperative days were associated with a higher incidence of deep sternal wound infection, and that in fact the average blood glucose level over those 2 days was the strongest predictor of deep sternal wound infection in a diabetic patient.[103] On the basis of these findings, these investigators hypothesized that tight glycemic control would decrease the incidence pf postoperative sternal wound infections. A prospective study of 2467 diabetic patients undergoing cardiac surgery was performed, in which maintaining serum glucose at a level of less than 200 mg/dL was the goal. The control group (968 patients) was treated with intermittent doses of subcutaneous insulin, with administration based on a sliding scale; the study group (1499 patients) was treated with a continuous intravenous insulin infusion in an attempt to maintain a blood glucose level of less than 200 mg/dL. Continuous intravenous insulin infusion resulted in better glycemic control and a significant reduction in the incidence of deep sternal wound infection (0.8%) compared with the intermittent subcutaneous insulin injection group (2.0%, $P = .01$).[104] A subsequent retrospective review of 3554 diabetic patients undergoing isolated CABG demonstrated once again that continuous insulin infusion resulted in better glycemic control. Furthermore, improved glycemic control led to a 57% reduction in mortality, with this reduction being accounted for by cardiac-related deaths.[105] Based on these results, the authors concluded that diabetes mellitus per se is not a true risk factor for death after CABG, and that continuous insulin infusion should become the standard of care for glucose control in diabetic patients undergoing CABG. On reviewing the available data, other investigators have also reached the conclusion that hyperglycemia, not the diagnosis of diabetes, significantly increases the risk of adverse clinical outcomes, longer hospitalizations, and increased health care costs for cardiac surgery patients.[106] Additional compelling evidence comes from a prospective study involving 1548 critically ill patients in the surgical intensive care unit, in which even tighter control (a serum glucose level goal of between 80 and 110 /dL, versus 180 to 200 mg/dL) was associated with significantly improved mortality (4.6% versus 8.0%, $P < .04$).[107] From these data, it seems reasonable to conclude that tight glycemic control may be beneficial to all patients undergoing cardiac surgery.

Transfusion Strategy

Despite the development of national consensus guidelines for blood transfusion in the 1980s,[108-110] as recently as 2002 it was estimated that some 20% of all allogeneic blood transfusions in the United States were associated with cardiac surgery.[111] National guidelines notwithstanding, a number of studies have demonstrated that transfusion practices vary dramatically across institutions, with some centers transfusing less than 5% of patients and others transfusing nearly all patients.[112-115] Different transfusion practices even within the same institution[116] highlight the lack of agreed-on transfusion thresholds.

The myocardium relies on either increased blood flow or increased oxygen content to satisfy increased oxygen demand.[117] One of the primary rationales for blood transfusions in the setting of cardiac ischemia, therefore, is to increase oxygen-carrying content to the stressed myocardium. Unfortunately, very little evidence exists to support this rationale. On the contrary, some degree of anemia is required during hypothermic cardiopulmonary bypass to reduce blood viscosity and allow adequate flow without excessive arterial blood pressure. Furthermore, a number of large studies have concluded that blood transfusion is associated with increased short- and long-term mortality,[118,119] including transfusions in the setting of CABG.[120]

Decreased hematocrit is one of the prime drivers of the decision to transfuse, but management of hematocrit during cardiopulmonary bypass is controversial. Multiple studies have demonstrated that normovolemic anemia is well tolerated in cardiac patients, even at levels as low as 14%.[121] Spiess and colleagues analyzed more than 2200 bypass patients and found that high hematocrit (34% or greater) on entry to the ICU was associated with a significantly higher rate of myocardial infarction than was low hematocrit (less than 24%), leading them to conclude that low hematocrit might be protective against perioperative MI.[122] In contrast, Klass and colleagues performed their own study of 500 CABG patients and found no association between perioperative MI rate and hematocrit value on entry into the ICU.[123] Habib and colleagues examined 5000 operations using cardiopulmonary bypass and found that a number of clinically significant outcomes, including stroke, MI, cardiac failure, renal failure,

pulmonary failure, and mortality, were all increased if the lowest intraoperative hematocrit value was less than 22%.[124] Similarly, DeFoe and colleagues have demonstrated that low hematocrit during CABG is associated with perioperative cardiac failure and increased in-hospital mortality.[125] Each of these studies suffers from being retrospective in design, and significant differences in patient populations and other key factors make direct comparisons difficult. Until a well-designed prospective study is performed, the optimal hematocrit value on cardiopulmonary bypass will remain undetermined, leaving the evaluation of this key indicator of the need to transfuse to the discretion of the physician.

Although the optimal hematocrit during CABG surgery is the subject of continued debate, accumulating data are providing an increasingly clear picture of the deleterious effects of blood transfusion. Numerous studies have demonstrated the proinflammatory properties of transfused blood.[126,127] In addition, the immunomodulatory effects of transfusion have been known for more than 2 decades,[128] and blood transfusion has been associated with increased risk of bacterial as well as viral infection.[129-132] A number of blood conservation strategies have been designed with the specific intent of decreasing the need for transfusion, including technical modifications to the bypass circuit and the use of various drugs, including aprotinin. For those patients in whom transfusion cannot be avoided, the use of leuko-reduced blood is gaining favor as a method of minimizing the detrimental effects of transfused blood. A national universal leuko-reduction program in Canada has been credited with decreasing mortality and antibiotic use in high-risk patients.[133] In the setting of CABG, the role of transfusing leuko-reduced blood is unsettled. At least two studies have shown that leuko-reduction is not associated with a decrease in postoperative infections, as one might expect.[134,135] However, in a well-conducted, prospective trial, Furnary and colleagues have shown that transfusing leuko-reduced blood confers a survival advantage that is present at 1 month and persists up to a year.[135]

In sum, despite the regular occurrence of blood transfusion in cardiac surgery patients, the indications, goals, effectiveness, and safety of this common clinical practice remain uncertain. Clinician preference and habit therefore continue to be the prime determinants of many blood transfusion strategies.[136] Results of numerous studies are mixed but, as one prominent expert in the field has concluded, the predominance of data regarding red blood cell transfusion does not support the premise that it improves outcome.[137] Thus, until the appropriate patients and circumstances of transfusion are better defined, it is a practice to be avoided.

Operative Strategies to Prevent Ischemia and Ischemia-Reperfusion Injury

For an operation that is performed safely more than a million times annually worldwide, CABG is an incredibly complex procedure. The use of a cardiopulmonary bypass machine to pump artificially oxygenated blood to the rest of the body means that essentially every organ and every physiologic system in the body is affected. Accordingly, strategies aimed at minimizing the morbidity and mortality associated with heart surgery are equally broad in scope. Although overlap exists, conceptually one may divide these efforts into two broad categories, strategies to protect the myocardium itself and strategies to protect against the effects of CPB. In addition, a third category is emerging that includes newer techniques that are a combination of the two and thus do not fall easily into either of the first two categories.

Myocardial Protection Strategies

Cardioplegia

Generally agreed-on characteristics of the ideal cardioplegia solution are that it will (1) arrest the heart rapidly, (2) minimize energy requirements while the heart is arrested, (3) prevent damage caused by the absence of coronary blood flow, and (4) prevent ischemia-reperfusion (I/R) injury when blood flow is restored.[138] The earliest cardioplegia solutions contained a high (2.5%) concentration of potassium citrate.[139,140] Although this solution was effective in achieving chemical cardiac arrest, it was abandoned after only several years when the high potassium concentration was shown to induce myocardial necrosis.[141] In the mid 1960s, several new cardioplegia solutions were introduced, and they were the forerunners of solutions still in use today. The most popular of these were Bretschneider's intracellular crystalloid solution,[142-144] St. Thomas' Hospital extracellular crystalloid solution,[145] and several solutions developed by American researchers.[146-149] These new solutions continued to rely on hyperkalemia to induce cardiac arrest, although at much lower levels than the previous solutions. By the late 1970s, use of potassium-based cold crystalloid cardioplegia had become common practice in the United States. Since that time, efforts to improve on cardioplegia have focused on composition of the solution, temperature, the route of delivery, and the use of special additives.

Cardioplegia Composition: Blood versus Crystalloid. Asanguineous crystalloid solutions have been shown to provide good protection against ischemia, even in cases with prolonged bypass times[150]; however, their poor oxygen-carrying capacity may give rise to oxygen debt. This problem may be overcome, in part, by reducing myocardial metabolism via hypothermia, by oxygenating the crystalloid solution,[151] or by using blood as the cardioplegia vehicle.

Potassium-based blood cardioplegia, introduced in the late 1970s, was shown experimentally to provide better protection than either blood alone or crystalloid cardioplegia.[152] Work by Buckberg and colleagues demonstrated that blood cardioplegia could be performed safely in humans and with good results.[153,154] Laks and associates provided similar positive results in 1979.[155] Since that time, a number of studies have shown that blood cardioplegia may lead to decreased creatine kinase-MB enzyme release and improved postoperative ventricular function,[156,157] and that it may be of particular benefit to patients with unstable angina[158] or reduced left ventricular function.[159,160]

The preponderance of evidence suggests that use of blood cardioplegia is superior to use of crystalloid; however, no large-scale, randomized trial has ever been undertaken to provide a more definitive answer. Despite these limitations, over the past 20 years blood cardioplegia has become the preferred means of myocardial protection for most cardiac surgeons,[161] an adaptation that seems justified by the available evidence.

Cardioplegia Temperature: Warm versus Cold. For 4 decades, hypothermia was considered a fundamental need in cardiac surgery. However, in the early 1990s, Lichtenstein and colleagues published the earliest reports describing the use of retrograde continuous normothermic cardioplegia.[62,63] This study compared 121 consecutive patients undergoing CABG with normothermic cardioplegia to 133 historical controls, and it showed significant improvement in perioperative myocardial infarction rate (1.7% versus 6.8%, $P < .05$), decreased use of IABP (0.9% versus 9.0%, $P < .005$), and decreased prevalence of low output syndrome (13.5% versus 3.3%, $P < .005$).[62] In 1994, the Warm Heart Investigators Trial reported the initial results of a study involving more than 1700 patients randomized either to continuous warm-blood cardioplegia (systemic temperature 33°C to 37°C) or cold-blood cardioplegia (systemic temperature 25°C to 30°C). This study again demonstrated decreased evidence of enzymatic myocardial infarction using normothermia (warm 12.3% versus cold 17.3%, $P < .001$) and decreased incidence of postoperative low output syndrome in warm patients (6.1% versus 9.3%, $P < .01$).[64] A subsequent prospectively designed subanalysis of this study demonstrated that warm cardioplegia significantly reduced the overall prevalence of morbidity and mortality (warm 15.9% versus cold 25.2%, $P < .01$); this protection was seen across all risk groups.[162]

Cardioplegia Route of Delivery: Antegrade versus Retrograde. Retrograde delivery of cardioplegia offers a number of potential advantages over antegrade perfusion, including the ability to perfuse regions of the myocardium that would not be reached via antegrade infusion because of occlusion of coronary arteries,[163-165] and the ability to maintain continuous cardioplegia. Disadvantages include the fact that it is technically more difficult than cannulation of the aorta, that retrograde flow provides less homogeneous distribution of cardioplegic solution,[166] and that the right ventricle and posterior ventricular septum are less well protected.[167-169] Despite these limitations, a number of investigators have demonstrated good outcomes using retrograde cardioplegia.[170-172] Numerous attempts have been made to determine whether antegrade or retrograde cardioplegia provides superior protection. No definitive conclusion has been reached, but many investigators have determined that a combined approach is likely to yield the greatest success, and that high-risk patients with severe coronary artery occlusion and/or left ventricular dysfunction, or patients undergoing repeat coronary revascularization, stand to benefit the most from retrograde delivery of cardioplegia.[160,173-175]

Cardioplegia Metabolic Enhancements. The combination of glucose-insulin-potassium (GIK) has been studied in the setting of myocardial ischemia for 4 decades.[176] In animal models, GIK administration has been shown to decrease infarct size, improve ventricular function, and decrease ventricular arrhythmias.[177,178] Early studies in humans were equally promising.[179-182] Unfortunately, two large clinical trials failed to show any significant benefit of GIK administration in cardiac surgery patients.[183,184]

The addition of beta-blockade to cardioplegia solutions is a relatively new protective strategy. First reported by Sweeney and Frazier in 1992,[185] the strategy relies on continuous infusion of beta-blockade to slow, rather than arrest, the heart. Creation of such a hypocontractile state decreases myocardial work and oxygen demand while at the same time avoiding ischemia and allowing continuous infusion of substrate-enhanced cardioplegia.[185] Small randomized studies in humans have shown that beta-blockade cardioplegia decreases biochemical indices of myocardial injury when compared to cold crystalloid cardioplegia[186] or cold blood cardioplegia,[187] but clinical outcomes were unaffected. In emergent CABG patients, beta-blockade resulted in improved outcomes when compared with cold crystalloid cardioplegia, including a reduction in the incidence of perioperative MI, decreased need for inotropic support, and decreased length of stay.[188] These results, although intriguing, await validation in the form of a large, well-designed clinical trial prior to widespread implementation.

Noncardioplegia Myocardial Protection Strategies

Hypothermia. Of all the noncardioplegia-based myocardial protection strategies, hypothermia has been used most widely and with the most consistent benefit. As we have learned more about the potential negative consequences of lowered body temperature, and as other protection strategies have been developed, the role of hypothermia has become less central in myocardial protection. Nevertheless, its importance in the history of cardiac surgery cannot be overemphasized, and even today deep systemic hypothermia may be the strategy of choice in special situations.[189]

Arrest Variations. Cardiac arrest serves the dual purpose of greatly reducing the metabolic demand of the myocardium while providing the motionless field necessary to complete many surgical maneuvers. As discussed earlier, potassium-based depolarizing chemical cardioplegia has been the mainstay of cardiac arrest mechanisms since the late 1960s. However, a number of alternative techniques have been employed, many of which may be used in conjunction with chemical cardioplegia. These include hypothermia[55,58] and intermittent aortic cross-clamping with electrically induced ventricular fibrillation.[190] Newer strategies such as polarized arrest[191] and "electroplegia"[192] have yet to be tested in large clinical studies. Of the accepted arrest techniques, cold crystalloid cardioplegia and intermittent aortic cross-clamping are used most widely. Proponents of intermittent cross-clamping cite its simplicity and the reduced cumulative ischemia in comparison with cardioplegia, but head-to-head comparative studies have failed to demonstrate the superiority of either strategy.[193-195]

Cannulation Techniques. The modern technique of placing a patient on cardiopulmonary bypass is remarkably similar to the technique employed by pioneers in the field 50 years ago.[196] Both the venous and arterial systems are cannulated as they enter and exit the heart, respectively. When the venae cavae and aorta are then clamped, blood flow is diverted to the bypass machine, effectively excluding the heart and lungs. Cardiac venting is typically required to remove blood that enters the heart from noncoronary collateral flow such as the bronchial arteries and thebesian veins. In addition to improving operative visibility, effective drainage prevents distention of the ventricles. Alternatives to the most common forms of venous drainage (cavoatrial and bicaval cannulation) and arterial perfusion (ascending aortic cannulation) exist and may be particularly useful in certain circumstances, but no technique has been demonstrated to have a significant impact on prevention of ischemic or inflammatory injury.

One cannulation technique that has been shown to decrease the inflammatory response to cardiac surgery is biventricular bypass, in which the patient's own lungs are used for gas exchange instead of the traditional oxygenator in the cardiopulmonary bypass circuit.[197] This method, also referred to as the Drew-Anderson technique, was originally described in the 1950s[198,199] but has been the focus of renewed interest in recent years.[200] The technique, which requires double arterial cannulation (in the aorta and in the pulmonary artery) and double atrial cannulation (in the left and right atria), has two theoretical advantages over standard CPB. First, keeping the lungs constantly perfused may minimize pulmonary I/R injury. Second, by reducing contact of blood with the foreign surface of the oxygenator, the inflammatory response is greatly diminished. As one contemporary of Drew observed, "Certainly the organism's own lung is an ideal oxygenator."[201]

In a canine experimental model comparing biventricular bypass to standard cardiopulmonary bypass, biventricular bypass resulted in improved pulmonary performance and preservation of leukocytes and platelets.[202] Several small randomized controlled human trials have shown that the biventricular bypass technique leads to decreased pulmonary leukocyte sequestration,[203] reduced levels of proinflammatory cytokines such as interleukin (IL)-6 and IL-8,[204,205] and reduced platelet and leukocyte activation.[205] Of greater clinical import is that time to extubation, postoperative blood loss, and transfusion requirements were all reduced in biventricular bypass patients.[204] In sum, this resurrected technique shows promise in ameliorating the ischemic and inflammatory consequences of CPB, but additional prospective, large-scale studies are needed to validate these preliminary findings and to identify the appropriate clinical circumstances in which biventricular bypass should be used.

Strategies to Prevent CPB-Associated Inflammation and I/R Injury

As noted, the potential negative consequences of heart surgery with cardiopulmonary bypass have been apparent since its introduction. The well-recognized inflammatory response associated with extracorporeal circulation has been the subject of extensive investigation,[197,206-210] and a detailed discussion is outside the scope of this review. Although once thought to be almost exclusively the result of blood coming into contact with the foreign (i.e., nonphysiologic) surface of the bypass circuit, it is now known that many circuit-independent factors also contribute to CPB-associated inflammation, including the surgical trauma itself, aortic cross-clamping, variations in body temperature, alteration of blood flow, metabolic perturbations, endotoxemia, and a cascade of endogenously mediated events initiated at reperfusion (e.g., production of reactive oxygen intermediates and upregulation of proinflammatory cytokines). Nevertheless, passage of blood through the bypass circuit represents a profound deviation from normal and is in all likelihood the greatest contributor to CPB-associated inflammation—it is certainly the most studied of all these factors. Numerous cell types, including neutrophils, monocytes, platelets, endothelial cells, and cardiomyocytes are involved, and together with activation of the contact and complement systems, they affect nearly every organ in the body and contribute to alterations in the regulation of such key processes as vasomotor tone, membrane permeability, and coagulation.

In addition to the inflammatory cascades set in motion by CPB, heart surgery with the use of bypass necessarily creates a period of global myocardial hypoxia/ischemia followed, on recirculation, by reperfusion. Although it is the most effective method to prevent ischemic injury, reperfusion may paradoxically lead to an exacerbation of, rather than an improvement in, hypoxic injury. In the setting of CPB, this clinical phenomenon has been variously described as sick heart syndrome, postcardiotomy shock, no-reflow phenomenon, postpump syndrome, low output syndrome, myocardial stunning, systemic inflammatory response syndrome, or simply ischemia-reperfusion injury. Extensive investigations into the cellular and molecular mechanisms of I/R injury undertaken over the past 3 decades reveal a complex process involving multiple cell types and numerous mediators. We now understand that CPB, hypoxia, and I/R all trigger endothelial cell activation, which in turn initiates a host of pathophysiologic responses, including altered vasomotor control, hypercoagulability, fibrinolysis, increased expression of cell surface molecules, and upregulation of numerous inflammatory cytokines and chemokines.[208,211-224] These changes lead to an influx of effector cells such as neutrophils and macrophages, as well as to a further increase the inflammatory cytokine production. At the organ level, I/R injury may manifest in a reversible form (e.g., hibernating or stunned myocardium) or the damage may be more permanent (i.e., infarction).[219,225-229] Although hypoxia alone leads to myocardial cell death, reperfusion has been shown to extend this region of infarction. The relative importance of necrosis versus apoptosis remains undetermined,[230-234] but these two very different mechanisms of cellular death—the former generally associated with unregulated cellular damage and extension of the infarct zone, and the latter thought to be a controlled, adaptive response—highlight the importance of altered gene expression caused by I/R.

Strategies to ameliorate the pathophysiologic responses to CPB fall under two main categories, those that involve technical alterations in the bypass circuit itself and those that are aimed at reducing inflammation, the latter being primarily in the form of pharmacotherapy.

Cardiopulmonary Bypass Circuit Modifications

Since its introduction, the cardiopulmonary bypass circuit has undergone numerous advances, each of which has contributed to declining morbidity and mortality associated with cardiac surgery. The many and varied challenges posed by use of CPB has made it one of the most researched areas of cardiovascular medicine.[235]

Heparin-Bonded Circuits. To minimize the systemic inflammatory response to the CPB circuit, a number of strategies have been implemented in an attempt to make the circuit more biocompatible. By far the best studied molecule used in these modified circuits is heparin. In theory, a layer of heparin molecules lining the CPB circuitry may mimic the heparan sulfate that coats endothelial cells in vivo, thereby reducing the pathophysiologic response that occurs when blood cells come into contact with the foreign surface.[236] Gott and colleagues first reported the binding of heparin to artificial surfaces in 1963.[237] Since that time, heparin-bonded circuits have been tested extensively, and abundant experimental and clinical evidence suggests that heparin-bonded circuits do in fact attenuate the activation of leukocytes,[238,239] platelets,[240] and complement[241-243]; decrease release of inflammatory cytokines[244]; and diminish the formation of thromboembolic debris[245] during CPB. Although evidence exists that heparin-bonded circuits may not actually decrease thrombogenesis,[246] several controlled studies suggest that the level of anticoagulation can be safely decreased when heparin-bonded circuits are used.[247-249] Work from our institution has demonstrated that a strategy that combines heparin-bonded circuits and low-dose heparinization as part of a comprehensive blood conservation strategy decreases the inflammatory response and need for transfusion more than any single measure in isolation.[250]

Cardiotomy Suctioning. The possible negative consequences of infusion of cardiotomy suction blood have been recognized for decades. As early as 1963, it was demonstrated that neurologic complications associated with CPB could be ameliorated by discarding shed blood rather than returning it to the patient,[251] and diffuse cerebral intravascular fat emboli have been observed in patients who die of neurologic complications in the perioperative period.[252] To minimize this potentially disastrous complication, a defoaming chamber is incorporated into the cardiotomy reservoir, and various filtration systems have been implemented. Recent evidence suggests that use of a cell saver may be an even more effective method of recycling shed mediastinal blood. Cell savers have been shown to reduce the lipid burden from shed blood before it is returned to the patient and to reduce the number of lipid microemboli.[253,254] An additional advantage of a cell saver is that it removes leukocytes from the shed blood, which may help to minimize the inflammatory reaction.

Less readily apparent than the threat of embolism but perhaps equally detrimental are the significant metabolic and proinflammatory effects that are associated with reinfusion of cardiotomy suction blood. Paradoxically, attempts to minimize transfusion requirements by salvaging shed mediastinal blood may be offset by heightened inflammation, vasomotor dysfunction, and altered coagulation. In an observational study involving 12 academic medical centers and more than 600 patients, Body and colleagues concluded that autotransfusion of shed mediastinal blood was ineffective as a blood conservation strategy, and that it may be associated with an increased risk of wound infection.[255]

Open versus Closed Circuit. Contact with air and filters is known to contribute to blood activation. The conventional CPB circuit includes an *open* venous reservoir, which collects both venous return and cardiotomy blood; blood in this open reservoir is exposed to the air and must pass through an integrated filter. A *closed* reservoir is independent from the cardiotomy reservoir, is never exposed to the air, and does not require a filter. Use of closed reservoirs has been shown to decrease fibrin deposition[256] and decrease the expression of a number of inflammatory mediators, including complement levels, the proinflammatory cytokine IL-8, thromboxane, elastase, and tissue plasminogen activator antigen.[257,258] More important, closed reservoirs have been shown to decrease blood loss, decrease the need for blood transfusion, and decrease the length of stay.[257,259] Although limited to only a few studies, these data are promising, and use of closed reservoirs should be expected to increase in the coming years, as a result of solid evidence of their efficacy.

Pump Type. Currently, two types of pump, roller and centrifugal, are used in the vast majority of cardiac surgery cases with CPB. For many years, CPB was performed with the only type of pump readily available, the continuous roller pump. Hemolysis, the risk of pumping large volumes of air, and spallation (the release of particles from the tubing surface) are known consequences of the roller pump[196]; however, its simplicity of design and implementation, as well as relatively low cost, are used to justify its continued use. Reported advantages of a centrifugal pump are improved blood handling, elimination of the risk of overpressurization, and decreased spallation.[260,261] In vitro analysis has demonstrated reduced hemolysis using centrifugal pumps[262]; however, two small studies have shown that terminal complement levels, the proinflammatory cytokines IL-6 and IL-8, neutrophil count, and elastase levels are all higher when using centrifugal pumps.[263,264] Clinical outcomes, including chest tube drainage, transfusion requirements, and length of hospital stay may be improved through the use of centrifugal pumps,[265] although clinical benefit has not been shown in all studies.[266,267]

Both roller and centrifugal pumps generate continuous, nonpulsatile blood circulation. In the 1950s, Wesolowski and Welch published a series of reports based on more than 20 years spent developing an artificial pump.[201,268] Their studies, using a canine model, indicated that a short term (up to 6 hours) of nonpulsatile flow had no apparent effect on pulmonary, cardiac, renal, or central nervous system physiology. Limited evidence accumulated since that time suggests that the flow characteristics do have physiologic consequences,[269] and small studies have demonstrated that pulsatile CPB may reduce endothelial damage, suppress cytokine activation, and prevent increases in endogenous endotoxin levels.[270,271] Taylor and coworkers have suggested that pulsatile flow may provide significant clinical benefit, including improved postoperative ventricular function and reduced mortality.[272] However, these positive findings have not been universal.[273] The effects of pulsatility have been the subject of several recent reviews.[274-276] In short, the impact of nonpulsatile flow

is not fully known. In the absence of more convincing data, no definitive recommendation can be made regarding the preferred pump type.

Blood Filtration: Leukocyte Depletion. The central role of leukocytes, particularly neutrophils, in the inflammatory response to CPB and I/R injury is well established. Like many other strategies, leukocyte depletion seems to be fairly effective in reducing inflammatory cells and mediators involved in the response to CPB,[277-283] but clinically relevant data have been inconsistent.[284-291] A number of investigators have noted that leukocyte depletion may be beneficial only in certain populations, such as children,[292,293] patients with impaired cardiac function,[279,282,294-296] and patients undergoing emergent CABG.[297]

Pharmacologic Protection Strategies

Just as numerous modifications to the CPB circuit have been devised to combat the complexity of the endogenous response to cardiac surgery, numerous pharmacologic interventions have been studied as well. Taking a broad view of the data regarding pharmacologic anti-inflammatory strategies, two conclusions emerge. First, a common feature of many of these drugs is that although experimentally each may significantly reduce the biochemical markers of infection, their clinical import has been questionable. With notable exceptions (e.g., aprotinin, pexelizumab), most have not undergone the sort of large, prospective, double-blinded, randomized trial that would enable some measure of certainty on their efficacy. Second, as more is learned about the inflammatory mechanisms initiated by cardiac surgery and the unique response of each cardiac surgery patient to those mechanisms, it is becoming clear that no single therapy, in isolation, is effective or appropriate for all situations in all patients. Thus, future investigations must be designed to determine the most beneficial combination of anti-inflammatory strategies, so that treatment can be tailored accordingly.

Corticosteroids. Experimentally, corticosteroids have been shown to decrease the levels of numerous proinflammatory cytokines and chemokines, to reduce complement levels, to prevent the production of thromboxane and prostaglandins, and to inhibit the activation of inflammatory cells, including macrophages and neutrophils.[298,299] The effectiveness of corticosteroids in the setting of CPB has been studied by a number of investigators. General agreement exists that at the molecular level, corticosteroids are effective in minimizing the inflammatory response to CPB. Various studies have demonstrated reductions in the release of proinflammatory cytokines IL-6 and IL-8,[300-302] complement levels,[303,304] tumor necrosis factor α (TNFα),[302,305-307] cellular adhesion molecules,[307,308] and neutrophil activation and sequestration.[309,310] At the same time, the anti-inflammatory cytokine IL-10 has been shown to *increase* with the use of corticosteroids.[311-313]

In terms of clinical efficacy, the data regarding use of corticosteroids have been far less consistent. Dietzman and colleagues reported some of the first observational studies on the use of corticosteroids in the setting of human CPB surgery. On the basis of their findings they determined that steroids might lead to decreased vasoconstriction, resulting in improvements in both pulmonary and cardiac function.[314-316] These positive outcomes were soon called into question by the findings of another small study that found that steroid use led to increased blood loss, decreased cardiac function, and an increased requirement for postoperative mechanical ventilation.[317] In the 3 decades since that time, numerous small, randomized trials have been published, but the results have been equally conflicting.[318-326]

These contradictory clinical findings have fueled great controversy on the appropriateness of steroid use in cardiac surgery.[327,328] Proponents point to data that suggest that steroid use is associated with fewer arrhythmias[323] and improved pulmonary function.[322] Limited data indicate that steroids may directly protect the myocardium against ischemic injury as well.[329] Those who advocate against the use of glucocorticoids argue that the existing data do not adequately prove any clinically significant benefit. Because of the lack of proven benefit, and in light of evidence that corticosteroids may prolong mechanical ventilation,[321,330] suppress T-cell function,[331] and decrease glucose tolerance,[322,324,331,332] thereby increasing the risk of wound disruption[333,334] and infection,[103] the potential risk is not justified.

After reviewing the extant data, a joint task force of the American College of Cardiology and American Heart Association recently published guidelines in which they supported the "liberal prophylactic use" of corticosteroids in the setting of surgery with CPB—notably, except for diabetic patients.[5] In the absence of more definitive data, the current authors arrive at a different conclusion. Although the weight of the evidence strongly supports the notion that corticosteroids are effective in ameliorating the proinflammatory response to CPB at a molecular and cellular level, conclusive evidence that corticosteroids lead to clinically significant benefit is lacking. At the same time, the evidence that corticosteroids are harmful is equally insufficient. Until appropriately designed, large, randomized, controlled trials are carried out, expansion of use does not seem warranted at present.

Hemostatic Agents: Aprotinin. As noted earlier, the inflammatory response to CPB includes increased expression and release of a number of serine proteases—including kallikrein, trypsin, plasmin, thrombin, and elastase—which in turn activate multiple coagulation and fibrinolytic cascades. A second major class of drugs used frequently in cardiac surgery is therefore aimed at reducing the intraoperative and postoperative bleeding that occurs as a result of fibrinolytic pathway activation by CPB. Serine protease inhibitors dominate this group, and aprotinin is by far the best studied and most used of this class of drugs. Discovered in the 1930s, aprotinin inhibits trypsin, plasmin, and tissue kallikrein by forming reversible enzyme-inhibitor complexes at the active serine site of the enzyme.[335,336] In addition to reducing fibrinolysis, aprotinin attenuates the inflammatory response by inhibiting cell transmigration and degranulation into soft tissues.[337-341]

Aprotinin has been under investigation in the setting of CPB for more than 40 years,[342] but it did not begin to gain popular acceptance until after 1987, when Royston and colleagues published results of a study of 22 patients undergoing repeat CABG.[343] They reported that high-dose aprotinin led to significantly reduced bleeding (mean blood loss was

286 mL in patients treated with aprotinin compared with 1509 in the 11 control patients, $P < .001$) and decreased the need for blood transfusions by a factor of eight.[343] Prior work had shown that aprotinin inhibits plasmin at a concentration of 125 kallikrein inhibitor units (KIU)/mL, and kallikrein at 250 KIU/mL.[344-346] Unlike in previous clinical investigations of aprotinin, the level of drug administered in the Royston study was sufficient to inhibit kallikrein. Dosing of the drug was divided into three components: a loading dose of 280 mg (2 million KIU), 280 mg in the CPB pump prime (2 million KIU), and an infusion of 70 mg/hr (500,000 KIU) throughout the surgery. This administration schedule subsequently became referred to as the Hammersmith dose, high-dose, or full-dose regimen. A number of lower-dose regimens have been studied[347-350]; most common among these lower dosages has been one half the full-dose regimen.[351,352] Over the past 20 years, use of either the half-dose or full-dose aprotinin regimen has been repeatedly demonstrated in multiple randomized studies to decrease both blood loss and the need for transfusion of blood and blood products.[347,352-356] Recently, aprotinin has been shown to be effective even for treating patients on antiplatelet agents secondary to unstable angina, who are at very high risk of perioperative bleeding.[357]

Despite the overwhelming evidence that aprotinin reduces bleeding and inflammation, clinical outcomes have until recently been less convincing. Because of aprotinin's procoagulant properties, specific concerns have been raised about the theoretical risk of increased thrombus formation, which could potentially lead to decreased graft patency and increased myocardial infarction or stroke. Alderman and colleagues reported an increased probability of vein graft occlusion associated with aprotinin use[358]; however, these authors commented that the poorer outcome with aprotinin was most likely the result of multiple differences in risk factors between their patient populations receiving aprotinin or placebo. The same group subsequently published data indicating that aprotinin had no effect on internal mammary artery graft patency.[140] A number of other small studies designed specifically to assess graft-closure rates have not demonstrated a significant effect.[359-365]

Several early studies showed a nonsignificant increase in myocardial infarction rate in patients who received aprotinin,[347,354] and two very recent studies have reported an increased risk of MI, renal dysfunction, and stroke associated with the use of aprotinin.[366,367] These observational studies involved large numbers of patients treated at a number of institutions and thus may accurately reflect the effects of aprotinin as it is used in common practice. However, despite sophisticated statistical methods to control possible confounding, the lack of randomization is a significant limitation. In contrast to these reports, a recent comprehensive analysis of randomized trials involving aprotinin suggests that aprotinin is not associated with increased MI risk in CABG patients.[368] Interestingly, in the majority of randomized trials in which a difference was observed, aprotinin use has been shown to decrease the risk of stroke,[355,369,370] although this protection may be dosage dependent.[371]

Since the publication of Royston's pivotal study in 1987, more than 50 controlled trials of aprotinin have been conducted. A comprehensive examination of this data is beyond the scope of the present chapter, but a recent meta-analysis by Sedrakyan and colleagues[368] provides an excellent survey of the available literature. Their 2004 report identified 35 randomized, controlled trials of aprotinin use in CABG-only patients conducted between 1988 and 2001. The vast majority[29] of the trials were double-blinded. Full-dose aprotinin was used in 29 trials; both full-dose and low-dose aprotinin were used in six trials. The studies enrolled 3879 patients. Their analysis confirmed that aprotinin reduces transfusion requirements (relative risk [RR], 0.61; 95% confidence interval [CI], 0.58-0.66) relative to placebo, with a 39% risk reduction. Aprotinin therapy had no effect on the risk of mortality (RR, 0.96; 95% CI, 0.65-1.40), myocardial infarction (RR, 0.85; 95% CI, 0.63-1.14), or renal failure (RR, 1.01; 95% CI, 0.55-1.83), but it was associated with a reduced risk of stroke (RR, 0.53; 95% CI, 0.31-0.90) and a trend toward reduced atrial fibrillation (RR, 0.90; 95% CI, 0.78-1.03). Although the evidence in this study strongly supports the routine use of aprotinin, an important caveat is that these data were derived exclusively from studies of CABG-only patients, and therefore they may not apply to non-CABG cardiac surgery patients.

Other Hemostatic Agents. Several other drugs are used to decrease bleeding associated with CPB in the effort to mitigate transfusion-related morbidity. These agents include the lysine analogs tranexamic acid and ε-aminocaproic acid, which reduce bleeding by inhibiting the conversion of plasminogen to plasmin (the serine protease responsible for breaking down fibrinogen); and desmopressin, a vasopressin analog that induces release of the contents of endothelial cell–associated Weibel-Palade bodies, including von Willebrand factor and associated coagulation factor VIII, leading to potentiation of primary hemostasis.[372-377] Several meta-analyses suggest that tranexamic acid and ε-aminocaproic acid may be similarly effective in preventing perioperative bleeding and the risk of transfusion in cardiac surgery patients; desmopressin does not seem to provide as much benefit.[378-380] Data concerning the clinical outcomes associated with the use of these drugs are insufficient to allow conclusive recommendations to be made regarding their use.

Recombinant factor VIIa, which may produce its hemostatic effects by activating platelets in the absence of tissue factor to activate factors IX and X and thus enhance thrombin generation[381] or by directly interacting with tissue factor at the site of injury to initiate thrombin generation,[382] has only recently been introduced to cardiac surgery. Currently, this drug is being used primarily as a measure of last resort to treat uncontrollable hemorrhage, rather than as routine therapy.[383-388]

Although aprotinin is the only one of these drugs that currently has a U.S. Food and Drug Administration (FDA) indication to prevent blood loss and transfusion during CABG surgery, all of these agents are currently used in various centers at the discretion of the operating surgeon. As cardiac surgery patients become increasingly complex and higher risk, the need for multiple pharmacologic options to decrease bleeding will only grow.[389]

Anticomplement Agents. Another class of anti-inflammatory drugs used in the setting of cardiac surgery with CPB is the complement inhibitors. The complement system forms a central component of the inflammatory response to CPB, and the numerous proteins involved in both the classical and alternate pathways present a wealth of potential therapeutic targets. A significant number of the drugs in this category—including such examples as cobra venom factor, C1 esterase inhibitor, complement activation blocker-2 (CAB-2), properdin antibody, factor D antibody, C8 antibody, and Compstatin—remain experimental or have undergone only minimal testing in the clinical setting and therefore are not discussed here. Several soluble complement inhibitors have undergone large randomized trials and show the potential for clinical use, namely soluble complement receptor type 1 (sCR-1) and the C5 complement inhibitor pexelizumab.

Soluble complement receptor-1 inhibits the C3 and C5 convertases, thereby preventing the generation of C3a, C5a, and C5b-9 (the membrane attack complex) and effectively blocking both the classical and alternate pathways. sCR-1 has been shown in a rat model of I/R injury to inhibit neutrophil activation, prevent postischemic myocardial contractile dysfunction, and reduce myocardial infarct size by 44%. Similar results were obtained in a porcine model of I/R injury, in which sCR-1 led to significantly less complement activation than nontreated hearts, less myocardial acidosis, improved ventricular function, and smaller infarct size (24.6% ± 2.0% versus 41% ± 1.3%, respectively; $P < .0001$).[390,391] In a randomized multicenter, prospective, placebo-controlled, double-blind study involving 564 high-risk patients, sCR-1 administered as a single 30-minute infusion prior to median sternotomy significantly inhibited complement activity in the immediate post-CPB period, and this inhibition persisted for 72 hours. Unfortunately, this anti-inflammatory effect did not result in an improvement in the primary endpoint of the study, which was the composite events of death, MI, prolonged (>24 hour) IABP support, and prolonged (>24 hour) intubation.[392] However, when only men were considered, sCR-1 did significantly decrease the incidence of mortality and MI.

Because generalized blockade of the complement system may increase the likelihood of infection,[393] efforts have been made to produce more selective inhibition of the various complement pathways. The terminal complement inhibitor pexelizumab is a recombinant, humanized antibody fragment that binds the human C5 protein.[394,395] Pexelizumab has been shown to block C5 cleavage, thereby preventing the generation of the proinflammatory complement components C5a and C5b-9. In experimental models, the drug was shown to decrease neutrophil and platelet activation, and to significantly inhibit cell apoptosis, necrosis, and polymorphonuclear neutrophil infiltration.[396,397] Importantly, this drug preserves the immunoprotective effects of C3b, which is central to bacterial opsonization and phagocytosis as well as immune complex solubilization and clearance.[397] A phase II study of pexelizumab involving 35 patients undergoing primary, nonemergent CABG demonstrated dosage-dependent inhibition of the generation of C5b-9, reduced leukocyte activation, decreased creatine kinase-MB release, diminished postoperative blood loss, and improved postoperative neurocognitive function.[398]

The PRIMO-CABG trial, a randomized, double-blind, placebo-controlled study, examined more than 3000 patients undergoing CABG with or without valve surgery at 205 hospitals in Europe and North America.[399] Patients were randomly assigned to receive pexelizumab ($n = 1553$) or placebo ($n = 1546$) 10 minutes before undergoing the procedure. The primary endpoint of the study, the incidence of death or MI in the CABG-only subpopulation through day 30 ($n = 2746$), was reduced by 18%. Although this figure did not reach statistical significance, in the larger intent-to-treat population, which included a broad spectrum of patients with diverse baseline risk factors, pexelizumab did statistically significantly reduce the 30-day incidence of death or MI by 18% ($P = .03$). Protection in both groups was maintained at 180 days. The authors concluded that pexelizumab is a safe drug that represents a novel approach for CABG surgery, with the potential for both early and sustained beneficial effects on morbidity and mortality.[399]

Antioxidants. The generation of reactive oxygen species is a major component of the I/R response to cardiac surgery.[400-402] Oxygen radicals are primarily produced by activated neutrophils and may exert their deleterious effects by the peroxidation of membrane lipids and the oxidation of protective proteins. The body's innate antioxidant defenses, including α-tocopherol (vitamin E) and ascorbic acid (vitamin C), are critical in preventing free radical–mediated damage. Indeed, studies have shown an inverse epidemiologic correlation between plasma vitamin E levels and mortality due to ischemic heart disease.[403] CPB induces simultaneous increases in both reactive oxygen species and the body's own antioxidant defense mechanisms; however, these endogenously produced free-radical scavengers may not be able to compensate fully,[404] leading to subsequent tissue destruction. For this reason, a number of investigators have attempted to determine whether administration of exogenous antioxidants is beneficial in CPB.

In animal models, supplementation of vitamin E and vitamin C has been demonstrated to decrease the molecular damage caused by reactive oxygen species[405-408]; the free-radical scavengers superoxide dismutase (SOD) and catalase resulted in significantly better recovery of left ventricular function after reperfusion; and SOD and allopurinol have been shown to reduce significantly the extent of myocardial necrosis that developed after reversible coronary arterial branch occlusion.[409] The same biochemical protection provided by antioxidants has been seen in humans undergoing cardiac surgery[410]; however, in a number of small trials, clinically relevant effects have been minor,[408,411,412] nonexistent,[407] or even potentially harmful.[413]

Alternative Approaches to Myocardial Protection

Previously in this chapter, we discussed protective strategies that are focused either on direct protection of the myocardium or on ameliorating the inflammatory response and I/R injury that are caused by cardiopulmonary bypass. In these final paragraphs, we shall examine two protective strategies that do not easily fit into either of those categories.

Bypassing CPB: Off-pump CABG

Contrary to popular belief, myocardial revascularization without the use of CPB is not a new idea. Indeed, many of the landmark events in the early years of cardiothoracic surgery, including the first CABG, were performed without the aid of the bypass circuit. Although this technique fell out of favor in the late 1960s with the rise of CPB and cardioplegia, the development of new stabilizing devices and the use of a left anterior thoracotomy rather than median sternotomy contributed to their reintroduction into clinical practice in the early 1990s,[414-416] in large part because both off-pump CABG (OPCAB) and minimally invasive direct CABG (MIDCAB) offer the theoretical advantage of eliminating CPB-associated morbidity altogether. With the exception of the short duration of regional myocardial ischemia created when the anastomoses are being performed, blood flow to the beating heart is uninterrupted, thereby minimizing ischemic injury. In addition to avoiding the deleterious effects of CPB, OPCAB has other supposed advantages, including decreased surgical trauma, quicker recovery time, and shorter hospital stays.

A number of studies have attempted to compare the inflammatory response of OPCAB to standard CABG (CABG with CPB). The majority of reported studies are small and nonrandomized, but most have demonstrated that OPCAB is associated with decreased markers of inflammation when compared to standard CABG. For example, leukocyte, neutrophil, and monocyte activation are greater with the use of CPB.[417] Complement levels (C3a, C5a), TNF-α, and IL-1, -6, -8, and -10 are all increased with CPB.[417-426] An important confounding factor in most of these studies is that surgical access (i.e., median sternotomy in standard CABG versus anterolateral thoracotomy for OPCAB) has been demonstrated to play an important role in cytokine release[423,424,427]; indeed, some authors believe that the different surgical approaches may have a greater effect on the inflammatory response than does the use of CPB.[428] In addition, many of the early studies comparing OPCAB to standard CABG did not incorporate the newer drugs and technical modifications (described earlier) that have been specifically designed to ameliorate the effects of CPB. Thus, for example, study protocols that have incorporated normothermia, aprotinin, heparin-bonded circuits, complement inhibitors, and elimination of cardiotomy suction blood from the CPB circuit have yielded results that suggest that surgical trauma, rather than CPB, may prove to be a more significant driver of inflammation than CPB.[418,425,426,429] In low-risk patients, differences in markers of inflammation may be indistinguishable.[425]

A final consideration regarding the role of OPCAB in minimizing inflammation is that although global myocardial ischemia may be avoided, regional myocardial ischemia continues to occur. When the anastomoses are complete and blood flow is restored, all the same factors are in play in terms of I/R injury. The preservation of regional myocardial perfusion by using coronary shunts may preserve left ventricular function[430-432] and prevent severe hemodynamic consequences,[433] but the ability of shunts to prevent I/R injury has not been adequately examined. Thus, although ischemic myocardial damage may be lessened by OPCAB,[434,435] it is not eliminated,[436] nor is I/R injury.

Measuring the clinical impact of OPCAB as compared with standard CABG is equally challenging. No definitive trial has been performed, and meta-analyses are hampered by the fact that in most of the early comparative studies, the degree of revascularization was frequently less with OPCAB than with standard CABG. In others, patient selection bias yielded substantially different study populations. Yet another limitation is that OPCAB has a steep learning curve; thus, outcomes may be significantly influenced by surgeon experience. The American Heart Association Council on Cardiovascular Surgery has recently published an excellent summary of most of the major trials conducted to date that have attempted to compare clinical outcomes of OPCAB with standard CABG.[437] The authors concluded that definitive answers do not yet exist and will not be obtained until a large-scale prospective randomized trial is performed. Still, they arrived at several generalizations, including the observation that the perioperative inflammatory response and degree of I/R injury after OPCAB appears to be less than that associated with standard CABG, as measured by the volume of blood loss, need for transfusion, myocardial enzyme release, and neurocognitive and renal dysfunction. They confirmed that standard CABG generally allows a greater degree of revascularization than OPCAB. With regard to the most important clinical measures—length of hospital stay, mortality, and long-term cardiac outcome—the procedures appear to be equivalent. In the final analysis, these authors commented that both OPCAB and standard CABG result in excellent outcomes, and neither should be considered inferior to the other.[437]

Myocardial Conditioning

As investigation into the molecular machinery of ischemia-reperfusion injury enters its fourth decade, we understand that adaptive, protective cellular mechanisms exist. Much current research is aimed at understanding the key receptors, transduction pathways, and molecular mediators involved so that we may develop methods to modify gene expression in order to shift cellular machinery toward a protective phenotype. The phenomenon of myocardial conditioning is reputed to provide the most powerful protection against ischemic injury yet demonstrated.

Preconditioning. In 1986, Murry and colleagues reported their somewhat paradoxical findings that brief, non-sustained periods of ischemia and reperfusion could actually diminish the effects of a subsequent prolonged ischemic-reperfusion event.[438] This phenomenon, termed *ischemic preconditioning* (IPC), leads not only to smaller infarct size[438] but also to fewer I/R-induced arrhythmias,[439] improved post-ischemic contractile recovery,[440] reduced ventricular remodeling,[441] and improved survival. Later research established that the protection afforded by preconditioning occurs in two phases, with an early period of protection beginning within minutes of the preconditioning event and lasting several hours ("classical" or "early" preconditioning),[442] and a later period of protection beginning approximately 24 hours after

the preconditioning regimen and lasting as long as 3 to 4 days ("delayed preconditioning").[443,444]

Since the initial description by Murry using a canine model, the beneficial effects of IPC have been demonstrated experimentally in multiple species,[445-450] including humans.[451-454] In addition to myocardial ischemia, other physiologic and pharmacologic stimuli have been shown to trigger preconditioning, including remote ischemia,[455] rapid atrial pacing,[456] heat shock,[443] adenosine,[457] opioids,[458] volatile anesthetics,[459,460] endotoxin,[461] and many others. Extensive research has significantly advanced our understanding of the molecular mechanisms underlying both IPC and I/R.[462]

Unfortunately, efforts to translate these promising laboratory findings into clinical therapies have proven disappointing, as recently highlighted by a Working Group of the National Heart, Lung, and Blood Institute.[463] One of the difficulties in translating the gains made in our basic science understanding of the preconditioning phenomenon into clinical practice is that the onset of the ischemic event (e.g., in the case of acute coronary syndromes) is often unpredictable. Although certain at-risk patients may one day benefit from pharmacologic strategies aimed at harnessing the protective power of delayed preconditioning, early preconditioning-focused strategies will be less applicable in these unforeseeable events. On the other hand, cardiac surgery and transplantation are two examples of instances in which the nature and timing of the I/R event are predictable and controllable, and thus surgical I/R is very amenable to strategies aimed at exploiting the resistance to injury provided by early preconditioning.[451,452,464,465]

Unfortunately, despite the wealth of supporting laboratory data, results in humans in the clinical setting have been mixed.[466-468] Thus, 2 decades after its description, preconditioning remains a promising but as yet unproven clinical strategy.

Postconditioning. The beneficial effects of modified reperfusion have been known for many years[469,470] and have been demonstrated in the clinical setting.[471] In 2003, Zhao, Vinten-Johansen, and colleagues at Emory published the first study describing a variation of controlled reperfusion they entitled postconditioning.[472] Using an open-chest canine model, they demonstrated that by briefly interrupting reperfusion in a repetitive fashion at the onset of coronary reflow, infarct size was greatly diminished. These intriguing findings have since been achieved in other animal models, with a degree of protection comparable to that seen with preconditioning.[473,474] In addition to decreasing infarct size, protection against life-threatening arrhythmias has also been shown.[475]

Although the mechanisms of postconditioning protection are undefined, possibilities include an attenuation of injury caused by reactive oxygen species,[472] the prevention of cardiomyocyte hypercontracture,[476] a reduction in ischemia-induced swelling,[477] and activation and "cross-talk" of various "cell survival" pathways.[474,478,479] Some of the key mediators involved in preconditioning have been studied in postconditioning protocols. In addition to ischemia, anesthetics,[480] adenosine,[481,482] bradykinin,[483] and insulin[484] are protective when given immediately before or at the time of reperfusion. Important effectors include mitochondrial KATP channels,[474] the mitochondrial permeability transition pore,[485] and PI3K-Akt.[480,482,486]

Although still in its infancy, the field of postconditioning has tremendous appeal because of its potential therapeutic impact.[472] As noted earlier, one of the great difficulties in applying preconditioning strategies in the clinical setting is that the ischemic event is frequently unpredictable. In postconditioning, by contrast, any proposed intervention comes at the time of reperfusion, the manner and timing of which is under the control of the physician. Furthermore, in cases of planned I/R (e.g., CABG or organ transplantation), a combination of preconditioning and postconditioning strategies may yield protection superior to either alone.[474]

■ REFERENCES

1. Gibbon JH Jr: Application of a mechanical heart and lung apparatus to cardiac surgery. Minn Med 1954;37:171-185.
2. Gibbon JH Jr: The development of the heart-lung apparatus. Am J Surg 1978;135:608-619.
3. Miller BJ, Gibbon JH, Fineberg C: An improved mechanical heart and lung apparatus: Its use during open cardiotomy in experimental animals. Med Clin North Am 1953;1:1603-1624.
4. Edmunds LH: Cardiopulmonary bypass after 50 years. N Engl J Med 2004;351:1603-1606.
5. Eagle KA, Guyton RA, Davidoff R, et al: ACC/AHA 2004 guideline update for coronary artery bypass graft surgery: A report of the American College of Cardiology/American Heart Association Task Force on Practice Guidelines (Committee to Update the 1999 Guidelines for Coronary Artery Bypass Graft Surgery). Circulation 2004;110:e340-437.
6. Gaillard D, Bical O, Paumier D, Trivin F: A review of myocardial normothermia: Its theoretical basis and the potential clinical benefits in cardiac surgery. Cardiovasc Surg 2000;8:198-203.
7. Aldea GS: Invited commentary. Ann Thorac Surg 2005;79:2038-2039.
8. Evidence-based medicine: A new approach to teaching the practice of medicine. Evidence-Based Medicine Working Group. JAMA 1992;268:2420-2425.
9. Tobler HG, Sethi GK, Grover FL, et al: Variations in processes and structures of cardiac surgery practice. Med Care 1995;33(10 Suppl):OS43-58.
10. Karthik S, Grayson AD, Oo AY, Fabri BM: A survey of current myocardial protection practices during coronary artery bypass grafting. Ann R Coll Surg Engl 2004;86:413-415.
11. Bartels C, Gerdes A, Babin-Ebell J, et al: Cardiopulmonary bypass: Evidence or experience based? J Thorac Cardiovasc Surg 2002;124:20-27.
12. Dawson JT, Hall RJ, Hallman GL, Cooley DA: Mortality in patients undergoing coronary artery bypass surgery after myocardial infarction. Am J Cardiol 1974;33:483-486.
13. Hill JD, Kerth WJ, Kelly JJ, et al: Emergency aortocoronary bypass for impending or extending myocardial infarction. Circulation 1971;43(5 Suppl):I105-110.
14. Sustaita H, Chatterjee K, Matloff JM, et al: Emergency bypass surgery in impending and complicated acute myocardial infarction. Arch Surg 1972;105:30-35.
15. Every NR, Maynard C, Cochran RP, et al: Characteristics, management, and outcome of patients with acute myocardial infarction treated with bypass surgery. Myocardial Infarction Triage and Intervention Investigators. Circulation 1996;94(9 Suppl):II81-186.
16. Guyton RA, Arcidi JM Jr, Langford DA, et al: Emergency coronary bypass for cardiogenic shock. Circulation 1987;76(5 Pt 2):V22-27.
17. Gersh BJ, Chesebro JH, Braunwald E, et al: Coronary artery bypass graft surgery after thrombolytic therapy in the Thrombolysis in Myocardial Infarction Trial, Phase II (TIMI II). J Am Coll Cardiol 1995;25:395-402.
18. Magovern JA, Sakert T, Magovern GJ, et al: A model that predicts morbidity and mortality after coronary artery bypass graft surgery. J Am Coll Cardiol 1996;28:1147-1153.
19. Hochman JS, Sleeper LA, Webb JG, et al: Early revascularization in acute myocardial infarction complicated by cardiogenic shock. SHOCK Investigators. Should we emergently revascularize occluded coronaries for cardiogenic shock? N Engl J Med 1999;341:625-634.
20. Kaul TK, Fields BL, Riggins SL, et al: Coronary artery bypass grafting within 30 days of an acute myocardial infarction. Ann Thorac Surg 1995;59:1169-1176.
21. Zaroff JG, diTommaso DG, Barron HV: A risk model derived from the National Registry of Myocardial Infarction 2 database for predicting mortality after coronary artery bypass grafting during acute myocardial infarction. Am J Cardiol 2002;90:1-4.
22. Boden WE, O'Rourke RA, Crawford MH, et al: Outcomes in patients with acute non-Q-wave myocardial infarction randomly assigned to an invasive as compared with a conservative management strategy. Veterans Affairs Non-Q-Wave Infarction Strategies in Hospital (VANQWISH) Trial Investigators. N Engl J Med 1998;338:1785-1792.
23. Tu JV, Sykora K, Naylor CD: Assessing the outcomes of coronary artery bypass graft surgery: How many risk factors are enough? Steering Committee of the Cardiac Care Network of Ontario. J Am Coll Cardiol 1997;30:1317-1323.
24. Braxton JH, Hammond GL, Letsou GV, et al: Optimal timing of coronary artery bypass graft surgery after acute myocardial infarction. Circulation 1995;92(9 Suppl):II66-68.
25. Lee DC, Oz MC, Weinberg AD, et al: Optimal timing of revascularization: Transmural versus nontransmural acute myocardial infarction. Ann Thorac Surg 2001;71:1197-1202; discussion 1202-1204.
26. Lee DC, Oz MC, Weinberg AD, Ting W: Appropriate timing of surgical intervention after transmural acute myocardial infarction. J Thorac Cardiovasc Surg 2003;125:115-119; discussion 119-120.
27. Tuman KJ, Roizen MF: Outcome assessment and pulmonary artery catheterization: Why does the debate continue? Anesth Analg 1997;84:1-4.
28. Dalen JE: PA catheter-guided therapy does not benefit critically ill patients. Am J Med 2005;118:449-451.
29. Gore JM, Goldberg RJ, Spodick DH, Alpert JS, Dalen JE: A community-wide assessment of the use of pulmonary artery catheters in patients with acute myocardial infarction. Chest 1987;92:721-727.
30. Zion MM, Balkin J, Rosenmann D, et al: Use of pulmonary artery catheters in patients with acute myocardial infarction: Analysis of experience in 5,841 patients in the SPRINT Registry. SPRINT Study Group. Chest 1990;98:1331-1335.
31. Tuman KJ, McCarthy RJ, Spiess BD, et al: Effect of pulmonary artery catheterization on outcome in patients undergoing coronary artery surgery. Anesthesiology 1989;70:199-206.
32. Pearson KS, Gomez MN, Moyers JR, et al: A cost/benefit analysis of randomized invasive monitoring for patients undergoing cardiac surgery. Anesth Analg 1989;69:336-341.
33. Connors AF Jr, Speroff T, Dawson NV, et al: The effectiveness of right heart catheterization in the initial care of critically ill patients. SUPPORT Investigators. JAMA 1996;276:889-897.
34. Dalen JE, Bone RC: Is it time to pull the pulmonary artery catheter? JAMA 1996;276:916-918.
35. Kaplan JA, Wells PH: Early diagnosis of myocardial ischemia using the pulmonary arterial catheter. Anesth Analg 1981;60:789-793.
36. Sanchez R, Wee M: Perioperative myocardial ischemia: Early diagnosis using the pulmonary artery catheter. J Cardiothorac Vasc Anesth 1991;5:604-607.
37. Kefalides PT: U.S. mortality trends tell us how we're doing. Ann Intern Med 1998;129:170-172.
38. Ramsey SD, Saint S, Sullivan SD, et al: Clinical and economic effects of pulmonary artery catheterization in nonemergent coronary artery bypass graft surgery. J Cardiothorac Vasc Anesth 2000;14:113-118.
39. Schwann TA, Zacharias A, Riordan CJ, et al: Safe, highly selective use of pulmonary artery catheters in coronary artery bypass grafting:

An objective patient selection method. Ann Thorac Surg 2002;73:1394-1401; discussion 1401-1402.

40. Chaney MA: Pro: Transesophageal echocardiography should be routinely used in all patients undergoing cardiac surgery. Society of Cardiovascular Anesthesiologists Newsletter 2000;October.

41. Bergquist BD, Bellows WH, Leung JM: Transesophageal echocardiography in myocardial revascularization: II. Influence on intraoperative decision making. Anesth Analg 1996;82:1139-1145.

42. Savage RM, Lytle BW, Aronson S, et al: Intraoperative echocardiography is indicated in high-risk coronary artery bypass grafting. Ann Thorac Surg 1997;64:368-373; discussion 373-374.

43. Mishra M, Chauhan R, Sharma KK, et al: Real-time intraoperative transesophageal echocardiography: How useful? Experience of 5,016 cases. J Cardiothorac Vasc Anesth 1998;12:625-632.

44. Bergquist BD, Leung JM, Bellows WH: Transesophageal echocardiography in myocardial revascularization: I. Accuracy of intraoperative real-time interpretation. Anesth Analg 1996;82:1132-1138.

45. Fee M: Con: Transesophageal echocardiography should be routinely used in all patients undergoing cardiac surgery. Society of Cardiovascular Anesthesiologists Newsletter 2000;October.

46. Weinger MB, Herndon OW, Gaba DM: The effect of electronic record keeping and transesophageal echocardiography on task distribution, workload, and vigilance during cardiac anesthesia. Anesthesiology 1997;87:144-155; discussion 29A-30A.

47. Hall RI: Anaesthesia for coronary artery surgery: A plea for a goal-directed approach. Can J Anaesth 1993;40:1178-1194.

48. Kneeshaw JD, Arrowsmith JE: Anesthetic techniques. In Gardner TJ, Spray TL (eds): Operative Cardiac Surgery, ed 5. London, Arnold, 2004, pp 3-14.

49. Riess ML, Stowe DF, Warltier DC: Cardiac pharmacological preconditioning with volatile anesthetics: From bench to bedside? Am J Physiol Heart Circ Physiol 2004;286:H1603-1607.

50. Weber NC, Preckel B, Schlack W: The effect of anaesthetics on the myocardium: New insights into myocardial protection. Eur J Anaesthesiol 2005;22:647-657.

51. Barrington MJ, Kluger R, Watson R, et al: Epidural anesthesia for coronary artery bypass surgery compared with general anesthesia alone does not reduce biochemical markers of myocardial damage. Anesth Analg 2005;100:921-928.

52. Kendall JB, Russell GN, Scawn ND, et al: A prospective, randomised, single-blind pilot study to determine the effect of anaesthetic technique on troponin T release after off-pump coronary artery surgery. Anaesthesia 2004;59:545-549.

53. Loick HM, Schmidt C, Van Aken H, et al: High thoracic epidural anesthesia, but not clonidine, attenuates the perioperative stress response via sympatholysis and reduces the release of troponin T in patients undergoing coronary artery bypass grafting. Anesth Analg 1999;88:701-709.

54. Oransky I: Wilfred Gordon Bigelow. Lancet 2005;365:1616.

55. Bigelow WG, Lindsay WK, Greenwood WF: Hypothermia: Its possible role in cardiac surgery: An investigation of factors governing survival in dogs at low body temperatures. Ann Surg 1950;132:849-866.

56. Bigelow WG: Application of hypothermia to cardiac surgery. Minn Med 1954;37:181-185.

57. Bigelow WG, Mustard WT, Evans JG: Some physiologic concepts of hypothermia and their applications to cardiac surgery. J Thorac Surg 1954;28:463-480.

58. Shumway NE, Lower RR, Stofer RC: Selective hypothermia of the heart in anoxic cardiac arrest. Surg Gynecol Obstet 1959;109:750-754.

59. Griepp RB, Stinson EB, Shumway NE: Profound local hypothermia for myocardial protection during open-heart surgery. J Thorac Cardiovasc Surg 1973;66:731-741.

60. Sealy WC: Hypothermia: Its possible role in cardiac surgery. Ann Thorac Surg 1989;47:788-791.

61. Conte JV: Heart preservation. In Franco KL, Verrier ED (eds): Advanced Therapy in Cardiac Surgery, ed 2. Hamilton, Ontario, BC Decker, 2003, pp 560-569.

62. Lichtenstein SV, Ashe KA, el Dalati H, et al: Warm heart surgery. J Thorac Cardiovasc Surg 1991;101:269-274.

63. Salerno TA, Houck JP, Barrozo CA, et al: Retrograde continuous warm blood cardioplegia: A new concept in myocardial protection. Ann Thorac Surg 1991;51:245-247.

64. Randomised trial of normothermic versus hypothermic coronary bypass surgery. The Warm Heart Investigators. Lancet 1994;343:559-563.

65. Magovern GJ Jr, Flaherty JT, Gott VL, et al: Failure of blood cardioplegia to protect myocardium at lower temperatures. Circulation 1982;66(2 Pt 2):I60-67.

66. Bufkin BL, Mellitt RJ, Gott JP, et al: Aerobic blood cardioplegia for revascularization of acute infarct: Effects of delivery temperature. Ann Thorac Surg 1994;58:953-960.

67. Hayashida N, Weisel RD, Shirai T, et al: Tepid antegrade and retrograde cardioplegia. Ann Thorac Surg 1995;59:723-729.

68. Kaukoranta P, Lepojarvi M, Nissinen J, et al: Normothermic versus mild hypothermic retrograde blood cardioplegia: A prospective, randomized study. Ann Thorac Surg 1995;60:1087-1093.

69. Arom KV, Emery RW, Northrup WF 3rd: Warm heart surgery: A prospective comparison between normothermic and tepid temperature. J Card Surg 1995;10:221-226.

70. Fiore AC, Swartz MT, Nevett R, et al: Intermittent antegrade tepid versus cold blood cardioplegia in elective myocardial revascularization. Ann Thorac Surg 1998;65:1559-1564; discussion 1564-1565.

71. Luciani N, Martinelli L, Gaudino M, et al: Tepid systemic perfusion and intermittent isothermic blood cardioplegia in coronary surgery. J Cardiovasc Surg (Torino) 1998;39:599-607.

72. Elwatidy AM, Fadalah MA, Bukhari EA, et al: Antegrade crystalloid cardioplegia vs antegrade/retrograde cold and tepid blood cardioplegia in CABG. Ann Thorac Surg 1999;68:447-453.

73. De Paulis R, Penta De Peppo A, Colagrande L, et al: Troponin I release after CABG surgery using two different strategies of myocardial protection and systemic perfusion. J Cardiovasc Surg (Torino) 2002;43:153-159.

74. Falcoz PE, Kaili D, Chocron S, et al: Warm and tepid cardioplegia: Do they provide equal myocardial protection? Ann Thorac Surg 2002;74:2156-2160; discussion 2160.

75. Tan TE, Ahmed S, Paterson HS: Intermittent tepid blood cardioplegia improves clinical outcome. Asian Cardiovasc Thorac Ann 2003;11:116-121.

76. Khuri SF: pH-guided Myocardial Management: Evolution and Clinical Application, ed 1. Ann Arbor, Mich, Terumo Cardiovascular Systems Corporation, 2003.

77. Koop A, Piper HM: Protection of energy status of hypoxic cardiomyocytes by mild acidosis. J Mol Cell Cardiol 1992;24:55-65.

78. Nayler WG, Ferrari R, Poole-Wilson PA, Yepez CE: A protective effect of a mild acidosis on hypoxic heart muscle. J Mol Cell Cardiol 1979;11:1053-1071.

79. Webster KA, Discher DJ, Kaiser S, et al: Hypoxia-activated apoptosis of cardiac myocytes requires reoxygenation or a pH shift and is independent of p53. J Clin Invest 1999;104:239-252.

80. Thatte HS, Rhee JH, Zagarins SE, et al: Acidosis-induced apoptosis in human and porcine heart. Ann Thorac Surg 2004;77:1376-1383.

81. Khuri SF, Healey NA, Hossain M, et al: Intraoperative regional myocardial acidosis and reduction in long-term survival after cardiac surgery. J Thorac Cardiovasc Surg 2005;129:372-381.

82. Kumbhani DJ, Healey NA, Birjiniuk V, et al: Intraoperative regional myocardial acidosis predicts the need for inotropic support in cardiac surgery. Am J Surg 2004;188:474-480.

83. Graffigna AC, Nollo G, Pederzolli C, et al: Continuous monitoring of myocardial acid-base status during intermittent warm blood cardioplegia. Eur J Cardiothorac Surg 2002;21:995-1001.

84. Walters FJ, Wilson GJ, Steward DJ, et al: Intramyocardial pH as an index of myocardial metabolism during cardiac surgery. J Thorac Cardiovasc Surg 1979;78:319-330.

85. Trowbridge CC, Vasquez M, Stammers AH, et al: The effects of continuous blood gas monitoring during cardiopulmonary bypass: A prospective, randomized study—Part II. J Extra Corpor Technol 2000;32:129-137.

86. Kumbhani DJ, Healey NA, Biswas KS, et al: Adverse 30-day outcomes after cardiac surgery: Predictive role of intraoperative myocardial acidosis. Ann Thorac Surg 2005;80:1751-1757.

87. Kannel WB, McGee DL: Diabetes and cardiovascular risk factors: The Framingham study. Circulation 1979;59:8-13.
88. Salomon NW, Page US, Okies JE, et al: Diabetes mellitus and coronary artery bypass: Short-term risk and long-term prognosis. J Thorac Cardiovasc Surg 1983;85:264-271.
89. Morris JJ, Smith LR, Jones RH, et al: Influence of diabetes and mammary artery grafting on survival after coronary bypass. Circulation 1991;84(5 Suppl):III275-284.
90. Weintraub WS, Wenger NK, Jones EL, et al: Changing clinical characteristics of coronary surgery patients: Differences between men and women. Circulation 1993;88(5 Pt 2):II79-86.
91. Szabo Z, Hakanson E, Svedjeholm R: Early postoperative outcome and medium-term survival in 540 diabetic and 2239 nondiabetic patients undergoing coronary artery bypass grafting. Ann Thorac Surg 2002;74:712-719.
92. Carson JL, Scholz PM, Chen AY, et al: Diabetes mellitus increases short-term mortality and morbidity in patients undergoing coronary artery bypass graft surgery. J Am Coll Cardiol 2002;40:418-423.
93. Garcia MJ, McNamara PM, Gordon T, Kannel WB: Morbidity and mortality in diabetics in the Framingham population: Sixteen year follow-up study. Diabetes 1974;23:105-111.
94. Lawrie GM, Morris GC Jr, Glaeser DH: Influence of diabetes mellitus on the results of coronary bypass surgery: Follow-up of 212 diabetic patients ten to 15 years after surgery. JAMA 1986;256:2967-2971.
95. Adler DS, Goldman L, O'Neil A, et al: Long-term survival of more than 2,000 patients after coronary artery bypass grafting. Am J Cardiol 1986;58:195-202.
96. Thourani VH, Weintraub WS, Stein B, et al: Influence of diabetes mellitus on early and late outcome after coronary artery bypass grafting. Ann Thorac Surg 1999;67:1045-1052.
97. Cosgrove DM, Loop FD, Lytle BW, et al: Determinants of 10-year survival after primary myocardial revascularization. Ann Surg 1985;202:480-490.
98. Kersten JR, Montgomery MW, Ghassemi T, et al: Diabetes and hyperglycemia impair activation of mitochondrial K(ATP) channels. Am J Physiol Heart Circ Physiol 2001;280:H1744-1750.
99. Kehl F, Krolikowski JG, Mraovic B, et al: Hyperglycemia prevents isoflurane-induced preconditioning against myocardial infarction. Anesthesiology 2002;96:183-188.
100. Murkin JM: Pro: Tight intraoperative glucose control improves outcome in cardiovascular surgery. J Cardiothorac Vasc Anesth 2000;14:475-478.
101. Jacoby RM, Nesto RW: Acute myocardial infarction in the diabetic patient: Pathophysiology, clinical course and prognosis. J Am Coll Cardiol 1992;20:736-744.
102. Chaney MA, Nikolov MP, Blakeman BP, Bakhos M: Attempting to maintain normoglycemia during cardiopulmonary bypass with insulin may initiate postoperative hypoglycemia. Anesth Analg 1999;89:1091-1095.
103. Zerr KJ, Furnary AP, Grunkemeier GL, et al: Glucose control lowers the risk of wound infection in diabetics after open heart operations. Ann Thorac Surg 1997;63:356-361.
104. Furnary AP, Zerr KJ, Grunkemeier GL, Starr A: Continuous intravenous insulin infusion reduces the incidence of deep sternal wound infection in diabetic patients after cardiac surgical procedures. Ann Thorac Surg 1999;67:352-360; discussion 360-362.
105. Furnary AP, Gao G, Grunkemeier GL, et al: Continuous insulin infusion reduces mortality in patients with diabetes undergoing coronary artery bypass grafting. J Thorac Cardiovasc Surg 2003;125:1007-1021.
106. Lorenz RA, Lorenz RM, Codd JE: Perioperative blood glucose control during adult coronary artery bypass surgery. AORN J 2005;81:126-144, 147-150; quiz 151-154.
107. van den Berghe G, Wouters P, Weekers F, et al: Intensive insulin therapy in the critically ill patients. N Engl J Med 2001;345:1359-1367.
108. Consensus conference: Fresh-frozen plasma: Indications and risks. JAMA 1985;253:551-553.
109. Consensus conference: Platelet transfusion therapy. JAMA 1987;257:1777-1780.
110. Consensus conference: Perioperative red blood cell transfusion. JAMA 1988;260:2700-2703.
111. Spiess BD: Transfusion and outcome in heart surgery. Ann Thorac Surg 2002;74:986-987.
112. Ovrum E, Am Holen E, Tangen G: Consistent non-pharmacologic blood conservation in primary and reoperative coronary artery bypass grafting. Eur J Cardiothorac Surg 1995;9:30-35.
113. Stover EP, Siegel LC, Parks R, et al: Variability in transfusion practice for coronary artery bypass surgery persists despite national consensus guidelines: A 24-institution study. Institutions of the Multicenter Study of Perioperative Ischemia Research Group. Anesthesiology 1998;88:327-333.
114. Stover EP, Siegel LC, Body SC, et al: Institutional variability in red blood cell conservation practices for coronary artery bypass graft surgery. Institutions of the MultiCenter Study of Perioperative Ischemia Research Group. J Cardiothorac Vasc Anesth 2000;14:171-176.
115. Hasley PB, Lave JR, Hanusa BH, et al: Variation in the use of red blood cell transfusions: A study of four common medical and surgical conditions. Med Care 1995;33:1145-1160.
116. Hebert PC, Wells G, Martin C, et al: A Canadian survey of transfusion practices in critically ill patients. Transfusion Requirements in Critical Care Investigators and the Canadian Critical Care Trials Group. Crit Care Med 1998;26:482-487.
117. Jan KM, Chien S: Effect of hematocrit variations on coronary hemodynamics and oxygen utilization. Am J Physiol 1977;233:H106-113.
118. Rao SV, Jollis JG, Harrington RA, et al: Relationship of blood transfusion and clinical outcomes in patients with acute coronary syndromes. JAMA 2004;292:1555-1562.
119. Hebert PC, Wells G, Blajchman MA, et al: A multicenter, randomized, controlled clinical trial of transfusion requirements in critical care. Transfusion Requirements in Critical Care Investigators, Canadian Critical Care Trials Group. N Engl J Med 1999;340:409-417.
120. Engoren MC, Habib RH, Zacharias A, et al: Effect of blood transfusion on long-term survival after cardiac operation. Ann Thorac Surg 2002;74:1180-1186.
121. Cosgrove DM, Loop FD, Lytle BW, et al: Determinants of blood utilization during myocardial revascularization. Ann Thorac Surg 1985;40:380-384.
122. Spiess BD, Ley C, Body SC, et al: Hematocrit value on intensive care unit entry influences the frequency of Q-wave myocardial infarction after coronary artery bypass grafting. The Institutions of the Multicenter Study of Perioperative Ischemia (McSPI) Research Group. J Thorac Cardiovasc Surg 1998;116:460-467.
123. Klass O, Mehlhorn U, Zilkens K, et al: Impact of hematocrit value after coronary artery surgery on perioperative myocardial infarction rate. Thorac Cardiovasc Surg 2002;50:259-265.
124. Habib RH, Zacharias A, Schwann TA, et al: Adverse effects of low hematocrit during cardiopulmonary bypass in the adult: Should current practice be changed? J Thorac Cardiovasc Surg 2003;125:1438-1450.
125. DeFoe GR, Ross CS, Olmstead EM, et al: Lowest hematocrit on bypass and adverse outcomes associated with coronary artery bypass grafting. Northern New England Cardiovascular Disease Study Group. Ann Thorac Surg 2001;71:769-776.
126. Fransen E, Maessen J, Dentener M, et al: Impact of blood transfusions on inflammatory mediator release in patients undergoing cardiac surgery. Chest 1999;116:1233-1239.
127. Zallen G, Moore EE, Ciesla DJ, et al: Stored red blood cells selectively activate human neutrophils to release IL-8 and secretory PLA2. Shock 2000;13:29-33.
128. Blumberg N, Triulzi DJ, Heal JM: Transfusion-induced immunomodulation and its clinical consequences. Transfus Med Rev 1990;4(4 Suppl 1):24-35.
129. Triulzi DJ, Vanek K, Ryan DH, Blumberg N: A clinical and immunologic study of blood transfusion and postoperative bacterial infection in spinal surgery. Transfusion 1992;32:517-524.
130. Goodnough LT: Risks of blood transfusion. Anesthesiol Clin North Am 2005;23:241-252, v.
131. Dellinger EP, Anaya DA: Infectious and immunologic consequences of blood transfusion. Crit Care 2004;8(Suppl 2):S18-23.
132. Blumberg N: Deleterious clinical effects of transfusion immunomodulation: Proven beyond a reasonable doubt. Transfusion 2005;45(2 Suppl):33S-39; discussion 39S-40.

133. Hebert PC, Fergusson D, Blajchman MA, et al: Clinical outcomes following institution of the Canadian universal leukoreduction program for red blood cell transfusions. JAMA 2003;289:1941-1949.
134. Sharma AD, Slaughter TF, Clements FM, et al: Association of leukocyte-depleted blood transfusions with infectious complications after cardiac surgery. Surg Infect (Larchmt) 2002;3:127-133.
135. Furnary AP, YingXing, Gately HL, et al: Pre-storage leukoreduction of transfused packed red blood cells improves mid-term survival following cardiac surgery. In 85th Annual Meeting of the American Association for Thoracic Surgery. San Francisco, April 2005.
136. Nugent W: Collaborative practice: A personal journey. Ann Thorac Surg 2001;71:765.
137. Spiess BD: Blood transfusion for cardiopulmonary bypass: The need to answer a basic question. J Cardiothorac Vasc Anesth 2002;16:535-538.
138. Rosenfeldt FL: Myocardial preservation 1987: What is the state of the art? Aust N Z J Surg 1987;57:349-353.
139. Melrose DG, Dreyer B, Bentall HH, Baker JB: Elective cardiac arrest. Lancet 1955;269:21-22.
140. Baker JB, Bentall HH, Dreyer B, Melrose DG: Arrest of isolated heart with potassium citrate. Lancet 1957;273:555-559.
141. Helmsworth JA, Kaplan S, Clark LC Jr, et al: Myocardial injury associated with asystole induced with potassium citrate. Ann Surg 1959;149:200-206.
142. Bretschneider HJ: [Survival time and recuperative time of the heart in normothermia and hypothermia.]. Verh Dtsch Ges Kreislaufforsch 1964;30:11-34.
143. Reidemeister JC, Heberer G, Bretschneider HJ: Induced cardiac arrest by sodium and calcium depletion and application of procaine. Int Surg 1967;47:535-540.
144. Kirsch U, Rodewald G, Kalmar P: Induced ischemic arrest: Clinical experience with cardioplegia in open-heart surgery. J Thorac Cardiovasc Surg 1972;63:121-130.
145. Hearse DJ, Stewart DA, Braimbridge MV: Cellular protection during myocardial ischemia: The development and characterization of a procedure for the induction of reversible ischemic arrest. Circulation 1976;54:193-202.
146. Gay WA Jr, Ebert PA: Functional, metabolic, and morphologic effects of potassium-induced cardioplegia. Surgery 1973;74:284-290.
147. Todd GJ, Tyers GF: Potassium-induced arrest of the heart: Effect of low potassium concentration. Surg Forum 1975;26:255-256.
148. Tyers GF, Manley NJ, Williams EH, et al: Preliminary clinical experience with isotonic hypothermic potassium-induced arrest. J Thorac Cardiovasc Surg 1977;74:674-681.
149. Roe BB, Hutchinson JC, Fishman NH, et al: Myocardial protection with cold, ischemic, potassium-induced cardioplegia. J Thorac Cardiovasc Surg 1977;73:366-374.
150. Bleese N, Doring V, Kalmar P, et al: Clinical application of cardioplegia in aortic cross-clamping periods longer than 150 minutes. Thorac Cardiovasc Surg 1979;27:390-392.
151. Guyton RA, Dorsey LM, Craver JM, et al: Improved myocardial recovery after cardioplegic arrest with an oxygenated crystalloid solution. J Thorac Cardiovasc Surg 1985;89:877-887.
152. Barner HB, Laks H, Codd JE, et al: Cold blood as the vehicle for potassium cardioplegia. Ann Thorac Surg 1979;28:509-521.
153. Follette DM, Fey KH, Steed DL, et al: Reducing reperfusion injury with hypocalcemic, hyperkalemic, alkalotic blood during reoxygenation. Surg Forum 1978;29:284-286.
154. Buckberg GD, Dyson CW, Emerson RC: Techniques for administering blood cardioplegia. In Engelman RM, Levitsky S (eds): Textbook of Clinical Cardioplegia. Mount Kisco, NY, Futura, 1982, pp 305-316.
155. Laks H, Barner HB, Kaiser G: Cold blood cardioplegia. J Thorac Cardiovasc Surg 1979;77:319-322.
156. Fremes SE, Christakis GT, Weisel RD, et al: A clinical trial of blood and crystalloid cardioplegia. J Thorac Cardiovasc Surg 1984;88(5 Pt 1):726-741.
157. Codd JE, Barner HB, Pennington DG, et al: Intraoperative myocardial protection: A comparison of blood and asanguineous cardioplegia. Ann Thorac Surg 1985;39:125-133.
158. Tomasco B, Cappiello A, Fiorilli R, et al: Surgical revascularization for acute coronary insufficiency: Analysis of risk factors for hospital mortality. Ann Thorac Surg 1997;64:678-683.
159. Ibrahim MF, Venn GE, Young CP, Chambers DJ: A clinical comparative study between crystalloid and blood-based St Thomas' hospital cardioplegic solution. Eur J Cardiothorac Surg 1999;15:75-83.
160. Flack JE 3rd, Cook JR, May SJ, et al: Does cardioplegia type affect outcome and survival in patients with advanced left ventricular dysfunction? Results from the CABG Patch Trial. Circulation 2000;102(19 Suppl 3):III84-89.
161. Robinson LA, Schwarz GD, Goddard DB, et al: Myocardial protection for acquired heart disease surgery: Results of a national survey. Ann Thorac Surg 1995;59:361-372.
162. Christakis GT, Lichtenstein SV, Buth KJ, et al: The influence of risk on the results of warm heart surgery: A substudy of a randomized trial. Eur J Cardiothorac Surg 1997;11:515-520.
163. Gundry SR, Kirsh MM: A comparison of retrograde cardioplegia versus antegrade cardioplegia in the presence of coronary artery obstruction. Ann Thorac Surg 1984;38:124-127.
164. Partington MT, Acar C, Buckberg GD, et al: Studies of retrograde cardioplegia: I. Capillary blood flow distribution to myocardium supplied by open and occluded arteries. J Thorac Cardiovasc Surg 1989;97:605-612.
165. Partington MT, Acar C, Buckberg GD, Julia PL: Studies of retrograde cardioplegia: II. Advantages of antegrade/retrograde cardioplegia to optimize distribution in jeopardized myocardium. J Thorac Cardiovasc Surg 1989;97:613-622.
166. Aldea GS, Hou D, Fonger JD, Shemin RJ: Inhomogeneous and complementary antegrade and retrograde delivery of cardioplegic solution in the absence of coronary artery obstruction. J Thorac Cardiovasc Surg 1994;107:499-504.
167. Aronson S, Lee BK, Liddicoat JR, et al: Assessment of retrograde cardioplegia distribution using contrast echocardiography. Ann Thorac Surg 1991;52:810-814.
168. Caldarone CA, Krukenkamp IB, Misare BD, Levitsky S: Perfusion deficits with retrograde warm blood cardioplegia. Ann Thorac Surg 1994;57:403-406.
169. Borger MA, Wei KS, Weisel RD, et al: Myocardial perfusion during warm antegrade and retrograde cardioplegia: A contrast echo study. Ann Thorac Surg 1999;68:955-961.
170. Menasche P, Subayi JB, Piwnica A: Retrograde coronary sinus cardioplegia for aortic valve operations: A clinical report on 500 patients. Ann Thorac Surg 1990;49:556-563; discussion 563-564.
171. Menasche P, Subayi JB, Veyssie L, et al: Efficacy of coronary sinus cardioplegia in patients with complete coronary artery occlusions. Ann Thorac Surg 1991;51:418-423.
172. Hayashida N, Ikonomidis JS, Weisel RD, et al: Adequate distribution of warm cardioplegic solution. J Thorac Cardiovasc Surg 1995;110:800-812.
173. Kaul TK, Agnihotri AK, Fields BL, et al: Coronary artery bypass grafting in patients with an ejection fraction of twenty percent or less. J Thorac Cardiovasc Surg 1996;111:1001-1012.
174. Franke U, Wahlers T, Cohnert TU, et al: Retrograde versus antegrade crystalloid cardioplegia in coronary surgery: Value of troponin-I measurement. Ann Thorac Surg 2001;71:249-253.
175. Borger MA, Rao V, Weisel RD, et al: Reoperative coronary bypass surgery: Effect of patent grafts and retrograde cardioplegia. J Thorac Cardiovasc Surg 2001;121:83-90.
176. Sodi-Pallares D, Ponce de Leon J, Bisteni A, Medrano GA: Potassium, glucose, and insulin in myocardial infarction. Lancet 1969;1:1315-1316.
177. Heng MK, Norris RM, Peter T, et al: The effect of glucose-insulin-potassium on experimental myocardial infarction in the dog. Cardiovasc Res 1978;12:429-435.
178. Lazar HL, Zhang X, Rivers S, et al: Limiting ischemic myocardial damage using glucose-insulin-potassium solutions. Ann Thorac Surg 1995;60:411-416.
179. Whitlow PL, Rogers WJ, Smith LR, et al: Enhancement of left ventricular function by glucose-insulin-potassium infusion in acute myocardial infarction. Am J Cardiol 1982;49:811-820.
180. Lazar HL, Philippides G, Fitzgerald C, et al: Glucose-insulin-potassium solutions enhance recovery after urgent coronary artery

bypass grafting. J Thorac Cardiovasc Surg 1997;113:354-360; discussion 360-362.

181. Lazar HL, Chipkin S, Philippides G, et al: Glucose-insulin-potassium solutions improve outcomes in diabetics who have coronary artery operations. Ann Thorac Surg 2000;70:145-150.

182. Rao V, Borger MA, Weisel RD, et al: Insulin cardioplegia for elective coronary bypass surgery. J Thorac Cardiovasc Surg 2000;119: 1176-1184.

183. Potassium, glucose, and insulin treatment for acute myocardial infarction. Lancet 1968;2:1355-1360.

184. Rao V, Christakis GT, Weisel RD, et al: The insulin cardioplegia trial: Myocardial protection for urgent coronary artery bypass grafting. J Thorac Cardiovasc Surg 2002;123:928-935.

185. Sweeney MS, Frazier OH: Device-supported myocardial revascularization: Safe help for sick hearts. Ann Thorac Surg 1992;54: 1065-1070.

186. Mehlhorn U, Sauer H, Kuhn-Regnier F, et al: Myocardial beta-blockade as an alternative to cardioplegic arrest during coronary artery surgery. Cardiovasc Surg 1999;7:549-557.

187. Kuhn-Regnier F, Natour E, Dhein S, et al: Beta-blockade versus Buckberg blood-cardioplegia in coronary bypass operation. Eur J Cardiothorac Surg 1999;15:67-74.

188. Hekmat K, Clemens RM, Mehlhorn U, et al: Emergency coronary artery surgery after failed PTCA: Myocardial protection with continuous coronary perfusion of beta-blocker-enriched blood. Thorac Cardiovasc Surg 1998;46:333-338.

189. Tassani P, Barankay A, Haas F, et al: Cardiac surgery with deep hypothermic circulatory arrest produces less systemic inflammatory response than low-flow cardiopulmonary bypass in newborns. J Thorac Cardiovasc Surg 2002;123:648-654.

190. Korbmacher B, Simic O, Schulte HD, et al: Intermittent aortic cross-clamping for coronary artery bypass grafting: A review of a safe, fast, simple, and successful technique. J Cardiovasc Surg (Torino) 2004;45:535-543.

191. Chambers DJ, Hearse DJ: Developments in cardioprotection: "Polarized" arrest as an alternative to "depolarized" arrest. Ann Thorac Surg 1999;68:1960-1966.

192. Morris CD, Budde JM, Velez DA, et al: Electroplegia: An alternative to blood cardioplegia for arresting the heart during conventional (on-pump) cardiac operation. Ann Thorac Surg 2001;72: 679-687.

193. Bessho R, Chambers DJ: Experimental study of intermittent cross-clamping with fibrillation and myocardial protection: Reduced injury from shorter cumulative ischemia or intrinsic protective effect? J Thorac Cardiovasc Surg 2000;120:528-537.

194. Liu Z, Valencia O, Treasure T, Murday AJ: Cold blood cardioplegia or intermittent cross-clamping in coronary artery bypass grafting? Ann Thorac Surg 1998;66:462-465.

195. Alhan HC, Karabulut H, Tosun R, et al: Intermittent aortic cross-clamping and cold crystalloid cardioplegia for low-risk coronary patients. Ann Thorac Surg 1996;61:834-839.

196. Rubens FD: Cardiopulmonary bypass: Technique and pathophysiology. In Sellke FW, del Nido PJ, Swanson SJ (eds): Sabiston & Spencer Surgery of the Chest, ed 7. Philadelphia, Elsevier, 2005, pp 1061-1080.

197. Paparella D, Yau TM, Young E: Cardiopulmonary bypass induced inflammation: Pathophysiology and treatment. An update. Eur J Cardiothorac Surg 2002;21:232-244.

198. Drew CE, Keen G, Benazon DB: Profound hypothermia. Lancet 1959;1:745-747.

199. Drew CE, Anderson IM: Profound hypothermia in cardiac surgery: Report of three cases. Lancet 1959;1:748-750.

200. Berglin E, Sandin O, Winstedt P, William-Olsson G: Extracorporeal circulation without an oxygenator in coronary bypass grafting. J Thorac Cardiovasc Surg 1986;92:306-308.

201. Wesolowski SA, Welch CS: Experimental maintenance of the circulation by mechanical pumps. Surgery 1952;31:769-793.

202. Mendler N, Heimisch W, Schad H: Pulmonary function after biventricular bypass for autologous lung oxygenation. Eur J Cardiothorac Surg 2000;17:325-330.

203. Glenville B, Ross D: Coronary artery surgery with patient's lungs as oxygenator. Lancet 1986;2:1005-1006.

204. Richter JA, Meisner H, Tassani P, et al: Drew-Anderson technique attenuates systemic inflammatory response syndrome and improves respiratory function after coronary artery bypass grafting. Ann Thorac Surg 2000;69:77-83.

205. Massoudy P, Zahler S, Tassani P, et al: Reduction of pro-inflammatory cytokine levels and cellular adhesion in CABG procedures with separated pulmonary and systemic extracorporeal circulation without an oxygenator. Eur J Cardiothorac Surg 2000;17:729-736.

206. Royston D: The inflammatory response and extracorporeal circulation. J Cardiothorac Vasc Anesth 1997;11:341-354.

207. Edmunds LH Jr: Inflammatory response to cardiopulmonary bypass. Ann Thorac Surg 1998;66(5 Suppl):S12-16; discussion S25-28.

208. Boyle EM Jr, Pohlman TH, Johnson MC, Verrier ED: Endothelial cell injury in cardiovascular surgery: The systemic inflammatory response. Ann Thorac Surg 1997;63:277-284.

209. Wan S, LeClerc JL, Vincent JL: Inflammatory response to cardiopulmonary bypass: Mechanisms involved and possible therapeutic strategies. Chest 1997;112:676-692.

210. Menasche PA, Edmunds LH Jr: Inflammatory response. In Cohn LH, Edmunds LH Jr (eds): Cardiac Surgery in the Adult, ed 2. New York, McGraw Hill, 2003, pp 361-388.

211. Murphy GJ, Angelini GD: Side effects of cardiopulmonary bypass: What is the reality? J Card Surg 2004;19:481-488.

212. Miller BE, Levy JH: The inflammatory response to cardiopulmonary bypass. J Cardiothorac Vasc Anesth 1997;11:355-366.

213. Krishnadasan B, Morgan EN, Boyle ED, Verrier ED: Mechanisms of myocardial injury after cardiac surgery. J Cardiothorac Vasc Anesth 2000;14(3 Suppl 1):6-10; discussion 37-38.

214. Boyle EM Jr, Morgan EN, Kovacich JC, et al: Microvascular responses to cardiopulmonary bypass. J Cardiothorac Vasc Anesth 1999;13(4 Suppl 1):30-35; discussion 36-37.

215. Boyle EM Jr, Pohlman TH, Cornejo CJ, Verrier ED: Endothelial cell injury in cardiovascular surgery: Ischemia-reperfusion. Ann Thorac Surg 1996;62:1868-1875.

216. Boyle EM Jr, Verrier ED, Spiess BD: Endothelial cell injury in cardiovascular surgery: The procoagulant response. Ann Thorac Surg 1996;62:1549-1557.

217. Sellke FW, Boyle EM Jr, Verrier ED: Endothelial cell injury in cardiovascular surgery: The pathophysiology of vasomotor dysfunction. Ann Thorac Surg 1996;62:1222-1228.

218. Verrier ED, Boyle EM Jr: Endothelial cell injury in cardiovascular surgery. Ann Thorac Surg 1996;62:915-922.

219. Park JL, Lucchesi BR: Mechanisms of myocardial reperfusion injury. Ann Thorac Surg 1999;68:1905-1912.

220. Kukreja RC, Janin Y: Reperfusion injury: Basic concepts and protection strategies. J Thromb Thrombolysis 1997;4:7-24.

221. Ambrosio G, Tritto I: Reperfusion injury: Experimental evidence and clinical implications. Am Heart J 1999;138(2 Pt 2):S69-75.

222. Carden DL, Granger DN: Pathophysiology of ischaemia-reperfusion injury. J Pathol 2000;190:255-266.

223. Anaya-Prado R, Toledo-Pereyra LH, Lentsch AB, Ward PA: Ischemia/reperfusion injury. J Surg Res 2002;105:248-258.

224. Piper HM, Meuter K, Schafer C: Cellular mechanisms of ischemia-reperfusion injury. Ann Thorac Surg 2003;75:S644-648.

225. Braunwald E, Kloner RA: Myocardial reperfusion: A double-edged sword? J Clin Invest 1985;76:1713-1719.

226. Maroko PR, Kjekshus JK, Sobel BE, et al: Factors influencing infarct size following experimental coronary artery occlusions. Circulation 1971;43:67-82.

227. Reimer KA, Jennings RB: The "wavefront phenomenon" of myocardial ischemic cell death: II. Transmural progression of necrosis within the framework of ischemic bed size (myocardium at risk) and collateral flow. Lab Invest 1979;40:633-644.

228. Bolli R: Basic and clinical aspects of myocardial stunning. Prog Cardiovasc Dis 1998;40:477-516.

229. Heyndrickx GR, Millard RW, McRitchie RJ, et al: Regional myocardial functional and electrophysiological alterations after brief coronary artery occlusion in conscious dogs. J Clin Invest 1975;56: 978-985.

230. Gottlieb RA, Burleson KO, Kloner RA, et al: Reperfusion injury induces apoptosis in rabbit cardiomyocytes. J Clin Invest 1994;94: 1621-1628.

231. Kitsis RN, Mann DL: Apoptosis and the heart: A decade of progress. J Mol Cell Cardiol 2005;38:1-2.
232. Anversa P, Kajstura J: Myocyte cell death in the diseased heart. Circ Res 1998;82:1231-1233.
233. Rodriguez M, Lucchesi BR, Schaper J: Apoptosis in myocardial infarction. Ann Med 2002;34:470-479.
234. Rodriguez M, Schaper J: Apoptosis: Measurement and technical issues. J Mol Cell Cardiol 2005;38:15-20.
235. Wildhirt SM, Tarnok A: Immune consequences, pathophysiology, and current perspectives of the extracorporeal circulation. Shock 2001; 16(Suppl 1):1-2.
236. Aldea GS: Use of heparin-bonded cardiopulmonary bypass circuits with alternatives to standard anticoagulation. In Franco KL, Verrier ED (eds): Advanced Therapy in Cardiac Surgery, ed 2. Hamilton, Ont, BC Decker, 2003, p 46-54.
237. Gott VL, Whiffen JD, Dutton RC: Heparin bonding on colloidal graphite surfaces. Science 1963;142:1297-1298.
238. Fosse E, Moen O, Johnson E, et al: Reduced complement and granulocyte activation with heparin-coated cardiopulmonary bypass. Ann Thorac Surg 1994;58:472-477.
239. Moen O, Hogasen K, Fosse E, et al: Attenuation of changes in leukocyte surface markers and complement activation with heparin-coated cardiopulmonary bypass. Ann Thorac Surg 1997;63:105-111.
240. Wendel HP, Schulze HJ, Heller W, Hoffmeister HM: Platelet protection in coronary artery surgery: Benefits of heparin-coated circuits and high-dose aprotinin therapy. J Cardiothorac Vasc Anesth 1999;13:388-392.
241. Pekna M, Hagman L, Halden E, et al: Complement activation during cardiopulmonary bypass: Effects of immobilized heparin. Ann Thorac Surg 1994;58:421-424.
242. Gu YJ, van Oeveren W, Akkerman C, et al: Heparin-coated circuits reduce the inflammatory response to cardiopulmonary bypass. Ann Thorac Surg 1993;55:917-922.
243. Videm V, Mollnes TE, Fosse E, et al: Heparin-coated cardiopulmonary bypass equipment: I. Biocompatibility markers and development of complications in a high-risk population. J Thorac Cardiovasc Surg 1999;117:794-802.
244. Wan S, LeClerc JL, Antoine M, et al: Heparin-coated circuits reduce myocardial injury in heart or heart-lung transplantation: A prospective, randomized study. Ann Thorac Surg 1999;68: 1230-1235.
245. Ovrum E, Mollnes TE, Fosse E, et al: High and low heparin dose with heparin-coated cardiopulmonary bypass: Activation of complement and granulocytes. Ann Thorac Surg 1995;60:1755-1761.
246. Gorman RC, Ziats N, Rao AK, et al: Surface-bound heparin fails to reduce thrombin formation during clinical cardiopulmonary bypass. J Thorac Cardiovasc Surg 1996;111:1-11; discussion 11-12.
247. Aldea GS, Lilly K, Gaudiani JM, et al: Heparin-bonded circuits improve clinical outcomes in emergency coronary artery bypass grafting. J Card Surg 1997;12:389-397.
248. Mirow N, Minami K, Kleikamp G, et al: Clinical use of heparin-coated cardiopulmonary bypass in coronary artery bypass grafting. Thorac Cardiovasc Surg 2001;49:131-136.
249. Ovrum E, Tangen G, Tollofsrud S, Ringdal MA: Heparin-coated circuits and reduced systemic anticoagulation applied to 2500 consecutive first-time coronary artery bypass grafting procedures. Ann Thorac Surg 2003;76:1144-1148; discussion 1148.
250. Aldea GS, Soltow LO, Chandler WL, et al: Limitation of thrombin generation, platelet activation, and inflammation by elimination of cardiotomy suction in patients undergoing coronary artery bypass grafting treated with heparin-bonded circuits. J Thorac Cardiovasc Surg 2002;123:742-755.
251. Caguin F, Carter MG: Fat embolization with cardiotomy with the use of cardiopulmonary bypass. J Thorac Cardiovasc Surg 1963;46: 665-672.
252. Ghatak NR, Sinnenberg RJ, deBlois GG: Cerebral fat embolism following cardiac surgery. Stroke 1983;14:619-621.
253. Kincaid EH, Jones TJ, Stump DA, et al: Processing scavenged blood with a cell saver reduces cerebral lipid microembolization. Ann Thorac Surg 2000;70:1296-1300.
254. Jewell AE, Akowuah EF, Suvarna SK, et al: A prospective randomised comparison of cardiotomy suction and cell saver for recycling shed blood during cardiac surgery. Eur J Cardiothorac Surg 2003;23: 633-636.
255. Body SC, Birmingham J, Parks R, et al: Safety and efficacy of shed mediastinal blood transfusion after cardiac surgery: A multicenter observational study. Multicenter Study of Perioperative Ischemia Research Group. J Cardiothorac Vasc Anesth 1999;13:410-416.
256. Nishida H, Aomi S, Tomizawa Y, et al: Comparative study of biocompatibility between the open circuit and closed circuit in cardiopulmonary bypass. Artif Organs 1999;23:547-551.
257. Schonberger JP, Everts PA, Hoffmann JJ: Systemic blood activation with open and closed venous reservoirs. Ann Thorac Surg 1995;59:1549-1555.
258. Lindholm L, Westerberg M, Bengtsson A, et al: A closed perfusion system with heparin coating and centrifugal pump improves cardiopulmonary bypass biocompatibility in elderly patients. Ann Thorac Surg 2004;78:2131-2138; discussion 2138.
259. Brown Mahoney C, Donnelly JE: Impact of closed versus open venous reservoirs on patient outcomes in isolated coronary artery bypass graft surgery. Perfusion 2000;15:467-472.
260. Wheeldon DR, Bethune DW, Gill RD: Vortex pumping for routine cardiac surgery: A comparative study. Perfusion 1990;5:135-143.
261. Klein M, Dauben HP, Schulte HD, Gams E: Centrifugal pumping during routine open heart surgery improves clinical outcome. Artif Organs 1998;22:326-336.
262. Moen O, Fosse E, Braten J, et al: Roller and centrifugal pumps compared in vitro with regard to haemolysis, granulocyte and complement activation. Perfusion 1994;9:109-117.
263. Baufreton C, Intrator L, Jansen PG, et al: Inflammatory response to cardiopulmonary bypass using roller or centrifugal pumps. Ann Thorac Surg 1999;67:972-977.
264. Ashraf S, Butler J, Tian Y, et al: Inflammatory mediators in adults undergoing cardiopulmonary bypass: Comparison of centrifugal and roller pumps. Ann Thorac Surg 1998;65:480-484.
265. Klein M, Mahoney CB, Probst C, et al: Blood product use during routine open heart surgery: The impact of the centrifugal pump. Artif Organs 2001;25:300-305.
266. Jakob HG, Hafner G, Thelemann C, et al: Routine extracorporeal circulation with a centrifugal or roller pump. ASAIO Trans 1991;37: M487-489.
267. Scott DA, Silbert BS, Blyth C, et al: Blood loss in elective coronary artery surgery: A comparison of centrifugal versus roller pump heads during cardiopulmonary bypass. J Cardiothorac Vasc Anesth 2001;15:322-325.
268. Wesolowski SA, Welch CS: A pump mechanism for artificial maintenance of the circulation. Surg Forum 1950;92:226-233.
269. Son HS, Sun K, Fang YH, et al: The effects of pulsatile versus non-pulsatile extracorporeal circulation on the pattern of coronary artery blood flow during cardiac arrest. Int J Artif Organs 2005;28: 609-616.
270. Orime Y, Shiono M, Hata H, et al: Cytokine and endothelial damage in pulsatile and nonpulsatile cardiopulmonary bypass. Artif Organs 1999;23:508-512.
271. Watarida S, Mori A, Onoe M, et al: A clinical study on the effects of pulsatile cardiopulmonary bypass on the blood endotoxin levels. J Thorac Cardiovasc Surg 1994;108:620-625.
272. Taylor KM, Bain WH, Davidson KG, Turner MA: Comparative clinical study of pulsatile and non-pulsatile perfusion in 350 consecutive patients. Thorax 1982;37:324-330.
273. Zumbro GL Jr, Shearer G, Fishback ME, Galloway RF: A prospective evaluation of the pulsatile assist device. Ann Thorac Surg 1979;28:269-273.
274. Allen GS, Murray KD, Olsen DB: The importance of pulsatile and nonpulsatile flow in the design of blood pumps. Artif Organs 1997;21:922-928.
275. Song X, Throckmorton AL, Untaroiu A, et al: Axial flow blood pumps. ASAIO J 2003;49:355-364.
276. Thalmann M, Schima H, Wieselthaler G, Wolner E: Physiology of continuous blood flow in recipients of rotary cardiac assist devices. J Heart Lung Transplant 2005;24:237-245.
277. Alexiou C, Tang AT, Sheppard SV, et al: A prospective randomized study to evaluate the effect of leukodepletion on the rate of alveolar

production of exhaled nitric oxide during cardiopulmonary bypass. Ann Thorac Surg 2004;78:2139-2145; discussion 2145.

278. Baksaas ST, Flom-Halvorsen HI, Ovrum E, et al: Leucocyte filtration during cardiopulmonary reperfusion in coronary artery bypass surgery. Perfusion 1999;14:107-117.

279. Di Salvo C, Louca LL, Pattichis K, et al: Does activated neutrophil depletion on bypass by leukocyte filtration reduce myocardial damage? A preliminary report. J Cardiovasc Surg (Torino) 1996;37(6 Suppl 1):93-100.

280. Chiba Y, Morioka K, Muraoka R, et al: Effects of depletion of leukocytes and platelets on cardiac dysfunction after cardiopulmonary bypass. Ann Thorac Surg 1998;65:107-113; discussion 113-114.

281. Baksaas ST, Videm V, Mollnes TE, et al: Effects on complement, granulocytes and platelets of a leukocyte-depletion filter during in vitro extracorporeal circulation. Scand Cardiovasc J 1997;31:73-77.

282. Pala MG, Paolini G, Paroni R, et al: Myocardial protection with and without leukocyte depletion: A comparative study on the oxidative stress. Eur J Cardiothorac Surg 1995;9:701-706.

283. Gu YJ, de Vries AJ, Boonstra PW, van Oeveren W: Leukocyte depletion results in improved lung function and reduced inflammatory response after cardiac surgery. J Thorac Cardiovasc Surg 1996;112:494-500.

284. Efstathiou A, Vlachveis M, Tsonis G, et al: Does leukodepletion during elective cardiac surgery really influence the overall clinical outcome? J Cardiovasc Surg (Torino) 2003;44:197-204.

285. Grunenfelder J, Zund G, Schoeberlein A, et al: Modified ultrafiltration lowers adhesion molecule and cytokine levels after cardiopulmonary bypass without clinical relevance in adults. Eur J Cardiothorac Surg 2000;17:77-83.

286. Gu YJ, de Vries AJ, Vos P, et al: Leukocyte depletion during cardiac operation: A new approach through the venous bypass circuit. Ann Thorac Surg 1999;67:604-609.

287. Browning PG, Pullan M, Jackson M, Rashid A: Leucocyte-depleted cardioplegia does not reduce reperfusion injury in hypothermic coronary artery bypass surgery. Perfusion 1999;14:371-377.

288. Mair P, Hoermann C, Mair J, et al: Effects of a leucocyte depleting arterial line filter on perioperative proteolytic enzyme and oxygen free radical release in patients undergoing aortocoronary bypass surgery. Acta Anaesthesiol Scand 1999;43:452-457.

289. Johnson D, Thomson D, Mycyk T, et al: Depletion of neutrophils by filter during aortocoronary bypass surgery transiently improves postoperative cardiorespiratory status. Chest 1995;107:1253-1259.

290. Palatianos GM, Balentine G, Papadakis EG, et al: Neutrophil depletion reduces myocardial reperfusion morbidity. Ann Thorac Surg 2004;77:956-961.

291. Olivencia-Yurvati AH, Ferrara CA, Tierney N, et al: Strategic leukocyte depletion reduces pulmonary microvascular pressure and improves pulmonary status post-cardiopulmonary bypass. Perfusion 2003;18(Suppl 1):23-31.

292. Hayashi Y, Sawa Y, Nishimura M, et al: Clinical evaluation of leukocyte-depleted blood cardioplegia for pediatric open heart operation. Ann Thorac Surg 2000;69:1914-1919.

293. Journois D, Pouard P, Greeley WJ, et al: Hemofiltration during cardiopulmonary bypass in pediatric cardiac surgery: Effects on hemostasis, cytokines, and complement components. Anesthesiology 1994;81:1181-1189; discussion 26A-27A.

294. Roth M, Kraus B, Scheffold T, et al: The effect of leukocyte-depleted blood cardioplegia in patients with severe left ventricular dysfunction: A randomized, double-blind study. J Thorac Cardiovasc Surg 2000;120:642-650.

295. Sawa Y, Matsuda H: Myocardial protection with leukocyte depletion in cardiac surgery. Semin Thorac Cardiovasc Surg 2001;13:73-81.

296. Hiramatsu Y, Koishizawa T, Matsuzaki K, et al: Leukocyte-depleted blood cardioplegia reduces cardiac troponin T release in patients undergoing coronary artery bypass grafting. Jpn J Thorac Cardiovasc Surg 2000;48:625-631.

297. Sawa Y, Matsuda H, Shimazaki Y, et al: Evaluation of leukocyte-depleted terminal blood cardioplegic solution in patients undergoing elective and emergency coronary artery bypass grafting. J Thorac Cardiovasc Surg 1994;108:1125-1131.

298. Hall RI, Smith MS, Rocker G: The systemic inflammatory response to cardiopulmonary bypass: Pathophysiological, therapeutic, and pharmacological considerations. Anesth Analg 1997;85:766-782.

299. Chong AJ, Hampton CR, Pohlman TH, Verrier ED: Anti-inflammatory strategies in cardiac surgery. In Franco KL, Verrier ED (eds): Advanced Therapy in Cardiac Surgery, ed 2. Hamilton, Ont, BC Decker, 2003, p 55-73.

300. Diego RP, Mihalakakos PJ, Hexum TD, Hill GE: Methylprednisolone and full-dose aprotinin reduce reperfusion injury after cardiopulmonary bypass. J Cardiothorac Vasc Anesth 1997;11:29-31.

301. Jorens PG, De Jongh R, De Backer W, et al: Interleukin-8 production in patients undergoing cardiopulmonary bypass: The influence of pretreatment with methylprednisolone. Am Rev Respir Dis 1993;148(4 Pt 1):890-895.

302. Teoh KH, Bradley CA, Gauldie J, Burrows H: Steroid inhibition of cytokine-mediated vasodilation after warm heart surgery. Circulation 1995;92(9 Suppl):II347-353.

303. Engelman RM, Rousou JA, Flack JE 3rd, et al: Influence of steroids on complement and cytokine generation after cardiopulmonary bypass. Ann Thorac Surg 1995;60:801-804.

304. Cavarocchi NC, Pluth JR, Schaff HV, et al: Complement activation during cardiopulmonary bypass: Comparison of bubble and membrane oxygenators. J Thorac Cardiovasc Surg 1986;91:252-258.

305. Jansen NJ, van Oeveren W, van den Broek L, et al: Inhibition by dexamethasone of the reperfusion phenomena in cardiopulmonary bypass. J Thorac Cardiovasc Surg 1991;102:515-525.

306. Wan S, DeSmet JM, Antoine M, et al: Steroid administration in heart and heart-lung transplantation: Is the timing adequate? Ann Thorac Surg 1996;61:674-678.

307. Hill GE, Alonso A, Spurzem JR, et al: Aprotinin and methylprednisolone equally blunt cardiopulmonary bypass-induced inflammation in humans. J Thorac Cardiovasc Surg 1995;110:1658-1662.

308. Hill GE, Alonso A, Thiele GM, Robbins RA: Glucocorticoids blunt neutrophil CD11b surface glycoprotein upregulation during cardiopulmonary bypass in humans. Anesth Analg 1994;79:23-27.

309. Jansen NJ, van Oeveren W, van Vliet M, et al: The role of different types of corticosteroids on the inflammatory mediators in cardiopulmonary bypass. Eur J Cardiothorac Surg 1991;5:211-217.

310. Dernek S, Tunerir B, Sevin B, et al: The effects of methylprednisolone on complement, immunoglobulins and pulmonary neutrophil sequestration during cardiopulmonary bypass. Cardiovasc Surg 1999;7:414-418.

311. Kawamura T, Inada K, Nara N, et al: Influence of methylprednisolone on cytokine balance during cardiac surgery. Crit Care Med 1999;27:545-548.

312. Wan S, LeClerc JL, Schmartz D, et al: Hepatic release of interleukin-10 during cardiopulmonary bypass in steroid-pretreated patients. Am Heart J 1997;133:335-339.

313. Tabardel Y, Duchateau J, Schmartz D, et al: Corticosteroids increase blood interleukin-10 levels during cardiopulmonary bypass in men. Surgery 1996;119:76-80.

314. Dietzman RH, Ersek RA, Lillehei CW, et al: Low output syndrome: Recognition and treatment. J Thorac Cardiovasc Surg 1969;57:138-150.

315. Dietzman RH, Casteda AR, Lillehei CW, et al: Corticosteroids as effective vasodilators in the treatment of low output syndrome. Chest 1970;57:440-453.

316. Dietzman RH, Lunseth JB, Goott B, Berger EC: The use of methylprednisolone during cardiopulmonary bypass: A review of 427 cases. J Thorac Cardiovasc Surg 1975;69:870-873.

317. Coffin LH, Shinozaki T, DeMeules JE, et al: Ineffectiveness of methylprednisolone in the treatment of pulmonary dysfunction after cardiopulmonary bypass. Am J Surg 1975;130:555-559.

318. Morton JR, Hiebert CA, Lutes CA, White RL: Effect of methylprednisolone on myocardial preservation during coronary artery surgery. Am J Surg 1976;131:419-422.

319. Fecht DC, Magovern GJ, Park SB, et al: Beneficial effects of methylprednisolone in patients on cardiopulmonary bypass. Circ Shock 1978;5:415-422.

320. Toledo-Pereyra LH, Lin CY, Kundler H, Replogle RL: Steroids in heart surgery: A clinical double-blind and randomized study. Am Surg 1980;46:155-160.

321. Chaney MA, Nikolov MP, Blakeman B, et al: Pulmonary effects of methylprednisolone in patients undergoing coronary artery bypass grafting and early tracheal extubation. Anesth Analg 1998;87:27-33.

322. Tassani P, Richter JA, Barankay A, et al: Does high-dose methylprednisolone in aprotinin-treated patients attenuate the systemic inflammatory response during coronary artery bypass grafting procedures? J Cardiothorac Vasc Anesth 1999;13:165-172.

323. Yared JP, Starr NJ, Torres FK, et al: Effects of single dose, postinduction dexamethasone on recovery after cardiac surgery. Ann Thorac Surg 2000;69:1420-1424.

324. Chaney MA, Durazo-Arvizu RA, Nikolov MP, et al: Methylprednisolone does not benefit patients undergoing coronary artery bypass grafting and early tracheal extubation. J Thorac Cardiovasc Surg 2001;121:561-569.

325. Fillinger MP, Rassias AJ, Guyre PM, et al: Glucocorticoid effects on the inflammatory and clinical responses to cardiac surgery. J Cardiothorac Vasc Anesth 2002;16:163-169.

326. Kilger E, Weis F, Briegel J, et al: Stress doses of hydrocortisone reduce severe systemic inflammatory response syndrome and improve early outcome in a risk group of patients after cardiac surgery. Crit Care Med 2003;31:1068-1074.

327. Whitlock RP, Rubens FD, Young E, Teoh KH: Pro: Steroids should be used for cardiopulmonary bypass. J Cardiothorac Vasc Anesth 2005;19:250-254.

328. Sulzer CF, Mackensen GB, Grocott HP: Con: Methylprednisolone is not indicated for patients during cardiopulmonary bypass. J Cardiothorac Vasc Anesth 2005;19:255-258.

329. Checchia PA, Backer CL, Bronicki RA, et al: Dexamethasone reduces postoperative troponin levels in children undergoing cardiopulmonary bypass. Crit Care Med 2003;31:1742-1745.

330. Chaney MA, Nikolov MP, Blakeman BP, et al: Hemodynamic effects of methylprednisolone in patients undergoing cardiac operation and early extubation. Ann Thorac Surg 1999;67:1006-1011.

331. Mayumi H, Zhang QW, Nakashima A, et al: Synergistic immunosuppression caused by high-dose methylprednisolone and cardiopulmonary bypass. Ann Thorac Surg 1997;63:129-137.

332. London MJ, Grunwald GK, Shroyer AL, Grover FL: Association of fast-track cardiac management and low-dose to moderate-dose glucocorticoid administration with perioperative hyperglycemia. J Cardiothorac Vasc Anesth 2000;14:631-638.

333. Dostal GH, Gamelli RL: The differential effect of corticosteroids on wound disruption strength in mice. Arch Surg 1990;125:636-640.

334. Durmus M, Karaaslan E, Ozturk E, et al: The effects of single-dose dexamethasone on wound healing in rats. Anesth Analg 2003;97:1377-1380.

335. Rich JB: The efficacy and safety of aprotinin use in cardiac surgery. Ann Thorac Surg 1998;66(5 Suppl):S6-11; discussion S25-28.

336. Poullis M, Manning R, Laffan M, et al: The antithrombotic effect of aprotinin: Actions mediated via the protease-activated receptor 1. J Thorac Cardiovasc Surg 2000;120:370-378.

337. Hess PJ Jr: Systemic inflammatory response to coronary artery bypass graft surgery. Am J Health Syst Pharm 2005;62(18 Suppl 4):S6-9.

338. Engles L: Review and application of serine protease inhibition in coronary artery bypass graft surgery. Am J Health Syst Pharm 2005;62(18 Suppl 4):S9-14.

339. Asimakopoulos G, Thompson R, Nourshargh S, et al: An anti-inflammatory property of aprotinin detected at the level of leukocyte extravasation. J Thorac Cardiovasc Surg 2000;120:361-369.

340. Landis RC, Asimakopoulos G, Poullis M, et al: The antithrombotic and antiinflammatory mechanisms of action of aprotinin. Ann Thorac Surg 2001;72:2169-2175.

341. Wachtfogel YT, Kucich U, Hack CE, et al: Aprotinin inhibits the contact, neutrophil, and platelet activation systems during simulated extracorporeal perfusion. J Thorac Cardiovasc Surg 1993;106:1-9; discussion 9-10.

342. Katz W, Mammen EF, Thal AP: Inhibition of fibrinolysis during extracorporeal circulation. Surg Forum 1965;16:63-64.

343. Royston D, Bidstrup BP, Taylor KM, Sapsford RN: Effect of aprotinin on need for blood transfusion after repeat open-heart surgery. Lancet 1987;2:1289-1291.

344. Blomback B, Blomback M, Olsson P: Action of a proteolytic enzyme inhibitor on blood coagulation in vitro. Thromb Diath Haemorrh 1967;18:190-197.

345. Philipp E: Calculations and hypothetical considerations on the inhibition of plasmin and plasma kallikrein by Trasylol. In Davidson JF, Rowan RM, Samama MM, Desnoyers PC (eds): Progress in Chemical Fibrinolysis and Thrombolysis. New York, Raven Press, 1978, pp 291-295.

346. Fritz H, Wunderer G: Biochemistry and applications of aprotinin, the kallikrein inhibitor from bovine organs. Arzneimittelforschung 1983;33:479-494.

347. Cosgrove DM 3rd, Heric B, Lytle BW, et al: Aprotinin therapy for reoperative myocardial revascularization: A placebo-controlled study. Ann Thorac Surg 1992;54:1031-1036; discussion 1036-1038.

348. Carrel T, Bauer E, Laske A, et al: Low-dose aprotinin also allows reduction of blood loss after cardiopulmonary bypass. J Thorac Cardiovasc Surg 1991;102:801-802.

349. Covino E, Pepino P, Iorio D, et al: Low dose aprotinin as blood saver in open heart surgery. Eur J Cardiothorac Surg 1991;5:414-417; discussion 418.

350. Kawasuji M, Ueyama K, Sakakibara N, et al: Effect of low-dose aprotinin on coagulation and fibrinolysis in cardiopulmonary bypass. Ann Thorac Surg 1993;55:1205-1209.

351. Liu B, Belboul A, Radberg G, et al: Effect of reduced aprotinin dosage on blood loss and use of blood products in patients undergoing cardiopulmonary bypass. Scand J Thorac Cardiovasc Surg 1993;27:149-155.

352. Liu B, Tengborn L, Larson G, et al: Half-dose aprotinin preserves hemostatic function in patients undergoing bypass operations. Ann Thorac Surg 1995;59:1534-1540.

353. Bidstrup BP, Royston D, Sapsford RN, Taylor KM: Reduction in blood loss and blood use after cardiopulmonary bypass with high dose aprotinin (Trasylol). J Thorac Cardiovasc Surg 1989;97:364-372.

354. Lemmer JH Jr, Dilling EW, Morton JR, et al: Aprotinin for primary coronary artery bypass grafting: A multicenter trial of three dose regimens. Ann Thorac Surg 1996;62:1659-1667; discussion 1667-1668.

355. Levy JH, Pifarre R, Schaff HV, et al: A multicenter, double-blind, placebo-controlled trial of aprotinin for reducing blood loss and the requirement for donor-blood transfusion in patients undergoing repeat coronary artery bypass grafting. Circulation 1995;92:2236-2244.

356. Dietrich W, Barankay A, Hahnel C, Richter JA: High-dose aprotinin in cardiac surgery: Three years' experience in 1,784 patients. J Cardiothorac Vasc Anesth 1992;6:324-327.

357. van der Linden J, Lindvall G, Sartipy U: Aprotinin decreases postoperative bleeding and number of transfusions in patients on clopidogrel undergoing coronary artery bypass graft surgery: A double-blind, placebo-controlled, randomized clinical trial. Circulation 2005;112(9 Suppl):I276-280.

358. Alderman EL, Levy JH, Rich JB, et al: Analyses of coronary graft patency after aprotinin use: Results from the International Multicenter Aprotinin Graft Patency Experience (IMAGE) trial. J Thorac Cardiovasc Surg 1998;116:716-730.

359. Bidstrup BP, Underwood SR, Sapsford RN, Streets EM: Effect of aprotinin (Trasylol) on aorta-coronary bypass graft patency. J Thorac Cardiovasc Surg 1993;105:147-152; discussion 153.

360. Kalangos A, Tayyareci G, Pretre R, et al: Influence of aprotinin on early graft thrombosis in patients undergoing myocardial revascularization. Eur J Cardiothorac Surg 1994;8:651-656.

361. Havel M, Grabenwoger F, Schneider J, et al: Aprotinin does not decrease early graft patency after coronary artery bypass grafting despite reducing postoperative bleeding and use of donated blood. J Thorac Cardiovasc Surg 1994;107:807-810.

362. Lemmer JH Jr, Stanford W, Bonney SL, et al: Aprotinin for coronary bypass operations: Efficacy, safety, and influence on early saphenous vein graft patency—A multicenter, randomized, double-blind, placebo-controlled study. J Thorac Cardiovasc Surg 1994;107:543-551; discussion 551-553.

363. Lass M, Welz A, Kochs M, et al: Aprotinin in elective primary bypass surgery: Graft patency and clinical efficacy. Eur J Cardiothorac Surg 1995;9:206-210.

364. Lass M, Simic O, Ostermeyer J: Re-graft patency and clinical efficacy of aprotinin in elective bypass surgery. Cardiovasc Surg 1997;5:604-607.

365. Hayashida N, Isomura T, Sato T, et al: Effects of minimal-dose aprotinin on coronary artery bypass grafting. J Thorac Cardiovasc Surg 1997;114:261-269.

366. Mangano DT, Tudor IC, Dietzel C: The risk associated with aprotinin in cardiac surgery. N Engl J Med 2006;354:353-365.

367. Karkouti K, Beattie WS, Dattilo KM, et al: A propensity score case-control comparison of aprotinin and tranexamic acid in high-transfusion-risk cardiac surgery. Transfusion 2006;46:327-338.

368. Sedrakyan A, Treasure T, Elefteriades JA: Effect of aprotinin on clinical outcomes in coronary artery bypass graft surgery: A systematic review and meta-analysis of randomized clinical trials. J Thorac Cardiovasc Surg 2004;128:442-448.

369. Murkin JM: Attenuation of neurologic injury during cardiac surgery. Ann Thorac Surg 2001;72:S1838-1844.

370. Frumento RJ, O'Malley CM, Bennett-Guerrero E: Stroke after cardiac surgery: A retrospective analysis of the effect of aprotinin dosing regimens. Ann Thorac Surg 2003;75:479-483; discussion 483-484.

371. Smith PK, Muhlbaier LH: Aprotinin: Safe and effective only with the full-dose regimen. Ann Thorac Surg 1996;62:1575-1577.

372. Vander Salm TJ, Kaur S, Lancey RA, et al: Reduction of bleeding after heart operations through the prophylactic use of epsilon-aminocaproic acid. J Thorac Cardiovasc Surg 1996;112:1098-1107.

373. Daily PO, Lamphere JA, Dembitsky WP, et al: Effect of prophylactic epsilon-aminocaproic acid on blood loss and transfusion requirements in patients undergoing first-time coronary artery bypass grafting: A randomized, prospective, double-blind study. J Thorac Cardiovasc Surg 1994;108:99-106; discussion 106-108.

374. Pinosky ML, Kennedy DJ, Fishman RL, et al: Tranexamic acid reduces bleeding after cardiopulmonary bypass when compared to epsilon aminocaproic acid and placebo. J Card Surg 1997;12:330-338.

375. Greilich PE, Brouse CF, Whitten CW, et al: Antifibrinolytic therapy during cardiopulmonary bypass reduces proinflammatory cytokine levels: A randomized, double-blind, placebo-controlled study of epsilon-aminocaproic acid and aprotinin. J Thorac Cardiovasc Surg 2003;126:1498-1503.

376. Hardy JF, Belisle S, Dupont C, et al: Prophylactic tranexamic acid and epsilon-aminocaproic acid for primary myocardial revascularization. Ann Thorac Surg 1998;65:371-376.

377. Ozkisacik E, Islamoglu F, Posacioglu H, et al: Desmopressin usage in elective cardiac surgery. J Cardiovasc Surg (Torino) 2001;42:741-747.

378. Fremes SE, Wong BI, Lee E, et al: Metaanalysis of prophylactic drug treatment in the prevention of postoperative bleeding. Ann Thorac Surg 1994;58:1580-1588.

379. Laupacis A, Fergusson D: Drugs to minimize perioperative blood loss in cardiac surgery: Meta-analyses using perioperative blood transfusion as the outcome. The International Study of Peri-operative Transfusion (ISPOT) Investigators. Anesth Analg 1997;85:1258-1267.

380. Levi M, Cromheecke ME, de Jonge E, et al: Pharmacological strategies to decrease excessive blood loss in cardiac surgery: A meta-analysis of clinically relevant endpoints. Lancet 1999;354:1940-1947.

381. Monroe DM, Hoffman M, Allen GA, Roberts HR: The factor VII-platelet interplay: Effectiveness of recombinant factor VIIa in the treatment of bleeding in severe thrombocytopathia. Semin Thromb Hemost 2000;26:373-377.

382. ten Cate H, Bauer KA, Levi M, et al: The activation of factor X and prothrombin by recombinant factor VIIa in vivo is mediated by tissue factor. J Clin Invest 1993;92:1207-1212.

383. Aldouri M: The use of recombinant factor VIIa in controlling surgical bleeding in non-haemophiliac patients. Pathophysiol Haemost Thromb 2002;32(Suppl 1):41-46.

384. Halkos ME, Levy JH, Chen E, et al: Early experience with activated recombinant factor VII for intractable hemorrhage after cardiovascular surgery. Ann Thorac Surg 2005;79:1303-1306.

385. Karkouti K, Beattie WS, Wijeysundera DN, et al: Recombinant factor VIIa for intractable blood loss after cardiac surgery: A propensity score-matched case-control analysis. Transfusion 2005;45:26-34.

386. Raivio P, Suojaranta-Ylinen R, Kuitunen AH: Recombinant factor VIIa in the treatment of postoperative hemorrhage after cardiac surgery. Ann Thorac Surg 2005;80:66-71.

387. von Heymann C, Schoenfeld H, Sander M, et al: Clopidogrel-related refractory bleeding after coronary artery bypass graft surgery: A rationale for the use of coagulation factor concentrates? Heart Surg Forum 2005;8:E39-41.

388. Vanek T, Straka Z, Hrabak J, et al: Use of recombinant activated factor VII in cardiac surgery for an effective treatment of severe intractable bleeding. Jpn Heart J 2004;45:855-860.

389. Levy JH: Overview of clinical efficacy and safety of pharmacologic strategies for blood conservation. Am J Health Syst Pharm 2005;62(18 Suppl 4):S15-19.

390. Lazar HL, Hamasaki T, Bao Y, et al: Soluble complement receptor type I limits damage during revascularization of ischemic myocardium. Ann Thorac Surg 1998;65:973-977.

391. Lazar HL, Bao Y, Gaudiani J, et al: Total complement inhibition: An effective strategy to limit ischemic injury during coronary revascularization on cardiopulmonary bypass. Circulation 1999;100:1438-1442.

392. Lazar HL, Bokesch PM, van Lenta F, et al: Soluble human complement receptor 1 limits ischemic damage in cardiac surgery patients at high risk requiring cardiopulmonary bypass. Circulation 2004;110(11 Suppl 1):II274-279.

393. Swift AJ, Collins TS, Bugelski P, Winkelstein JA: Soluble human complement receptor type 1 inhibits complement-mediated host defense. Clin Diagn Lab Immunol 1994;1:585-589.

394. Thomas TC, Rollins SA, Rother RP, et al: Inhibition of complement activity by humanized anti-C5 antibody and single-chain Fv. Mol Immunol 1996;33:1389-1401.

395. Fleisig AJ, Verrier ED: Pexelizumab: A C5 complement inhibitor for use in both acute myocardial infarction and cardiac surgery with cardiopulmonary bypass. Expert Opin Biol Ther 2005;5:833-839.

396. Rinder CS, Rinder HM, Smith BR, et al: Blockade of C5a and C5b-9 generation inhibits leukocyte and platelet activation during extracorporeal circulation. J Clin Invest 1995;96:1564-1572.

397. Vakeva AP, Agah A, Rollins SA, et al: Myocardial infarction and apoptosis after myocardial ischemia and reperfusion: Role of the terminal complement components and inhibition by anti-C5 therapy. Circulation 1998;97:2259-2267.

398. Fitch JC, Rollins S, Matis L, et al: Pharmacology and biological efficacy of a recombinant, humanized, single-chain antibody C5 complement inhibitor in patients undergoing coronary artery bypass graft surgery with cardiopulmonary bypass. Circulation 1999;100:2499-2506.

399. Verrier ED, Shernan SK, Taylor KM, et al: Terminal complement blockade with pexelizumab during coronary artery bypass graft surgery requiring cardiopulmonary bypass: A randomized trial. JAMA 2004;291:2319-2327.

400. Granger DN, Hollwarth ME, Parks DA: Ischemia-reperfusion injury: Role of oxygen-derived free radicals. Acta Physiol Scand Suppl 1986;548:47-63.

401. Sussman MS, Bulkley GB: Oxygen-derived free radicals in reperfusion injury. Methods Enzymol 1990;186:711-723.

402. Starkopf J, Zilmer K, Vihalemm T, et al: Time course of oxidative stress during open-heart surgery. Scand J Thorac Cardiovasc Surg 1995;29:181-186.

403. Nagel E, Meyer zu Vilsendorf A, Bartels M, Pichlmayr R: Antioxidative vitamins in prevention of ischemia/reperfusion injury. Int J Vitam Nutr Res 1997;67:298-306.

404. Luyten CR, van Overveld FJ, De Backer LA, et al: Antioxidant defence during cardiopulmonary bypass surgery. Eur J Cardiothorac Surg 2005;27:611-616.

405. Klein HH, Pich S, Lindert S, et al: Combined treatment with vitamins E and C in experimental myocardial infarction in pigs. Am Heart J 1989;118:667-673.

406. Massey KD, Burton KP: Alpha-Tocopherol attenuates myocardial membrane-related alterations resulting from ischemia and reperfusion. Am J Physiol 1989;256(4 Pt 2):H1192-1199.

407. Westhuyzen J, Cochrane AD, Tesar PJ, et al: Effect of preoperative supplementation with alpha-tocopherol and ascorbic acid on

myocardial injury in patients undergoing cardiac operations. J Thorac Cardiovasc Surg 1997;113:942-948.

408. Oktar GL, Sinci V, Kalaycioglu S, et al: Biochemical and hemodynamic effects of ascorbic acid and alpha-tocopherol in coronary artery surgery. Scand J Clin Lab Invest 2001;61:621-629.

409. Gardner TJ, Stewart JR, Casale AS, et al: Reduction of myocardial ischemic injury with oxygen-derived free radical scavengers. Surgery 1983;94:423-427.

410. Sucu N, Cinel I, Unlu A, et al: N-acetylcysteine for preventing pump-induced oxidoinflammatory response during cardiopulmonary bypass. Surg Today 2004;34:237-242.

411. Yau TM, Weisel RD, Mickle DA, et al: Vitamin E for coronary bypass operations: A prospective, double-blind, randomized trial. J Thorac Cardiovasc Surg 1994;108:302-310.

412. Pesonen EJ, Vento AE, Ramo J, et al: Nitecapone reduces cardiac neutrophil accumulation in clinical open heart surgery. Anesthesiology 1999;91:355-361.

413. Butterworth J, Legault C, Stump DA, et al: A randomized, blinded trial of the antioxidant pegorgotein: No reduction in neuropsychological deficits, inotropic drug support, or myocardial ischemia after coronary artery bypass surgery. J Cardiothorac Vasc Anesth 1999;13:690-694.

414. Stanbridge RD, Symons GV, Banwell PE: Minimal-access surgery for coronary artery revascularisation. Lancet 1995;346:837.

415. Calafiore AM, Giammarco GD, Teodori G, et al: Left anterior descending coronary artery grafting via left anterior small thoracotomy without cardiopulmonary bypass. Ann Thorac Surg 1996;61:1658-1663; discussion 1664-1665.

416. Subramanian VA: Less invasive arterial CABG on a beating heart. Ann Thorac Surg 1997;63(6 Suppl):S68-71.

417. Ascione R, Lloyd CT, Underwood MJ, et al: Inflammatory response after coronary revascularization with or without cardiopulmonary bypass. Ann Thorac Surg 2000;69:1198-1204.

418. Diegeler A, Tarnok A, Rauch T, et al: Changes of leukocyte subsets in coronary artery bypass surgery: Cardiopulmonary bypass versus "off-pump" techniques. Thorac Cardiovasc Surg 1998;46:327-332.

419. Matata BM, Sosnowski AW, Galinanes M: Off-pump bypass graft operation significantly reduces oxidative stress and inflammation. Ann Thorac Surg 2000;69:785-791.

420. Schulze C, Conrad N, Schutz A, et al: Reduced expression of systemic proinflammatory cytokines after off-pump versus conventional coronary artery bypass grafting. Thorac Cardiovasc Surg 2000;48:364-369.

421. Chello M, Mastroroberto P, Quirino A, et al: Inhibition of neutrophil apoptosis after coronary bypass operation with cardiopulmonary bypass. Ann Thorac Surg 2002;73:123-129; discussion 129-130.

422. Wan S, Marchant A, DeSmet JM, et al: Human cytokine responses to cardiac transplantation and coronary artery bypass grafting. J Thorac Cardiovasc Surg 1996;111:469-477.

423. Struber M, Cremer JT, Gohrbandt B, et al: Human cytokine responses to coronary artery bypass grafting with and without cardiopulmonary bypass. Ann Thorac Surg 1999;68:1330-1335.

424. Corbi P, Rahmati M, Delwail A, et al: Circulating soluble gp130, soluble IL-6R, and IL-6 in patients undergoing cardiac surgery, with or without extracorporeal circulation. Eur J Cardiothorac Surg 2000;18:98-103.

425. Czerny M, Baumer H, Kilo J, et al: Inflammatory response and myocardial injury following coronary artery bypass grafting with or without cardiopulmonary bypass. Eur J Cardiothorac Surg 2000;17:737-742.

426. Gulielmos V, Menschikowski M, Dill H, et al: Interleukin-1, interleukin-6 and myocardial enzyme response after coronary artery bypass grafting: A prospective randomized comparison of the conventional and three minimally invasive surgical techniques. Eur J Cardiothorac Surg 2000;18:594-601.

427. Gu YJ, Mariani MA, Boonstra PW, et al: Complement activation in coronary artery bypass grafting patients without cardiopulmonary bypass: The role of tissue injury by surgical incision. Chest 1999;116:892-898.

428. Biglioli P, Cannata A, Alamanni F, et al: Biological effects of off-pump vs. on-pump coronary artery surgery: Focus on inflammation, hemostasis and oxidative stress. Eur J Cardiothorac Surg 2003;24:260-269.

429. Lazar HL, Bao Y, Rivers S: Does off-pump revascularization reduce coronary endothelial dysfunction? J Card Surg 2004;19:440-443.

430. Dapunt OE, Raji MR, Jeschkeit S, et al: Intracoronary shunt insertion prevents myocardial stunning in a juvenile porcine MIDCAB model absent of coronary artery disease. Eur J Cardiothorac Surg 1999;15:173-178; discussion 178-179.

431. Lucchetti V, Capasso F, Caputo M, et al: Intracoronary shunt prevents left ventricular function impairment during beating heart coronary revascularization. Eur J Cardiothorac Surg 1999;15:255-259.

432. Yeatman M, Caputo M, Narayan P, et al: Intracoronary shunts reduce transient intraoperative myocardial dysfunction during off-pump coronary operations. Ann Thorac Surg 2002;73:1411-1417.

433. Shin H, Koizumi K, Matayoshi T, Yozu R: Active distal coronary perfusion to prevent regional myocardial ischemia in off-pump coronary artery bypass grafting. Ann Thorac Cardiovasc Surg 2004;10:198-201.

434. Krejca M, Skiba J, Szmagala P, et al: Cardiac troponin T release during coronary surgery using intermittent cross-clamp with fibrillation, on-pump and off-pump beating heart. Eur J Cardiothorac Surg 1999;16:337-341.

435. Koh TW, Carr-White GS, DeSouza AC, et al: Intraoperative cardiac troponin T release and lactate metabolism during coronary artery surgery: Comparison of beating heart with conventional coronary artery surgery with cardiopulmonary bypass. Heart 1999;81:495-500.

436. Bonatti J, Hangler H, Hormann C, et al: Myocardial damage after minimally invasive coronary artery bypass grafting on the beating heart. Ann Thorac Surg 1998;66:1093-1096.

437. Sellke FW, DiMaio JM, Caplan LR, et al: Comparing on-pump and off-pump coronary artery bypass grafting: Numerous studies but few conclusions: A scientific statement from the American Heart Association council on cardiovascular surgery and anesthesia in collaboration with the interdisciplinary working group on quality of care and outcomes research. Circulation 2005;111:2858-2864.

438. Murry CE, Jennings RB, Reimer KA: Preconditioning with ischemia: A delay of lethal cell injury in ischemic myocardium. Circulation 1986;74:1124-1136.

439. Vegh A, Komori S, Szekeres L, Parratt JR: Antiarrhythmic effects of preconditioning in anaesthetised dogs and rats. Cardiovasc Res 1992;26:487-495.

440. Takano H, Tang XL, Kodani E, Bolli R: Late preconditioning enhances recovery of myocardial function after infarction in conscious rabbits. Am J Physiol Heart Circ Physiol 2000;279:H2372-2381.

441. Dairaku Y, Miura T, Harada N, et al: Effect of ischemic preconditioning and mitochondrial KATP channel openers on chronic left ventricular remodeling in the ischemic-reperfused rat heart. Circ J 2002;66:411-415.

442. Burckhartt B, Yang XM, Tsuchida A, et al: Acadesine extends the window of protection afforded by ischaemic preconditioning in conscious rabbits. Cardiovasc Res 1995;29:653-657.

443. Marber MS, Latchman DS, Walker JM, Yellon DM: Cardiac stress protein elevation 24 hours after brief ischemia or heat stress is associated with resistance to myocardial infarction. Circulation 1993;88:1264-1272.

444. Sun JZ, Tang XL, Knowlton AA, et al: Late preconditioning against myocardial stunning: An endogenous protective mechanism that confers resistance to postischemic dysfunction 24 h after brief ischemia in conscious pigs. J Clin Invest 1995;95:388-403.

445. Guo Y, Wu WJ, Qiu Y, et al: Demonstration of an early and a late phase of ischemic preconditioning in mice. Am J Physiol 1998;275(4 Pt 2):H1375-1387.

446. Liu Y, Downey JM: Ischemic preconditioning protects against infarction in rat heart. Am J Physiol 1992;263(4 Pt 2):H1107-1112.

447. Pan HL, Chen SR, Scicli GM, Carretero OA: Cardiac interstitial bradykinin release during ischemia is enhanced by ischemic preconditioning. Am J Physiol Heart Circ Physiol 2000;279:H116-121.

448. Cohen MV, Liu GS, Downey JM: Preconditioning causes improved wall motion as well as smaller infarcts after transient coronary occlusion in rabbits. Circulation 1991;84:341-349.

449. Schott RJ, Rohmann S, Braun ER, Schaper W: Ischemic preconditioning reduces infarct size in swine myocardium. Circ Res 1990;66: 1133-1142.

450. Uematsu M, Gaudette GR, Laurikka JO, et al: Adenosine-enhanced ischemic preconditioning decreases infarct in the regional ischemic sheep heart. Ann Thorac Surg 1998;66:382-387.

451. Yellon DM, Alkhulaifi AM, Pugsley WB: Preconditioning the human myocardium. Lancet 1993;342:276-277.

452. Jenkins DP, Pugsley WB, Alkhulaifi AM, et al: Ischaemic preconditioning reduces troponin T release in patients undergoing coronary artery bypass surgery. Heart 1997;77:314-318.

453. Arstall MA, Zhao YZ, Hornberger L, et al: Human ventricular myocytes in vitro exhibit both early and delayed preconditioning responses to simulated ischemia. J Mol Cell Cardiol 1998;30:1019-1025.

454. Wu ZK, Iivainen T, Pehkonen E, et al: Ischemic preconditioning suppresses ventricular tachyarrhythmias after myocardial revascularization. Circulation 2002;106:3091-3096.

455. Birnbaum Y, Hale SL, Kloner RA: Ischemic preconditioning at a distance: Reduction of myocardial infarct size by partial reduction of blood supply combined with rapid stimulation of the gastrocnemius muscle in the rabbit. Circulation 1997;96:1641-1646.

456. Vegh A, Szekeres L, Parratt JR: Transient ischaemia induced by rapid cardiac pacing results in myocardial preconditioning. Cardiovasc Res 1991;25:1051-1053.

457. Liu GS, Thornton J, Van Winkle DM, et al: Protection against infarction afforded by preconditioning is mediated by A1 adenosine receptors in rabbit heart. Circulation 1991;84:350-356.

458. Schultz JE, Rose E, Yao Z, Gross GJ: Evidence for involvement of opioid receptors in ischemic preconditioning in rat hearts. Am J Physiol 1995;268(5 Pt 2):H2157-2161.

459. Kersten JR, Schmeling TJ, Hettrick DA, et al: Mechanism of myocardial protection by isoflurane: Role of adenosine triphosphate-regulated potassium (KATP) channels. Anesthesiology 1996;85: 794-807; discussion 27A.

460. Cope DK, Impastato WK, Cohen MV, Downey JM: Volatile anesthetics protect the ischemic rabbit myocardium from infarction. Anesthesiology 1997;86:699-709.

461. Eising GP, Mao L, Schmid-Schonbein GW, et al: Effects of induced tolerance to bacterial lipopolysaccharide on myocardial infarct size in rats. Cardiovasc Res 1996;31:73-81.

462. Yellon DM, Downey JM: Preconditioning the myocardium: From cellular physiology to clinical cardiology. Physiol Rev 2003;83: 1113-1151.

463. Bolli R, Becker L, Gross G, et al: Myocardial protection at a crossroads: The need for translation into clinical therapy. Circ Res 2004;95:125-134.

464. Illes RW, Swoyer KD: Prospective, randomized clinical study of ischemic preconditioning as an adjunct to intermittent cold blood cardioplegia. Ann Thorac Surg 1998;65:748-752; discussion 752-753.

465. Teoh LK, Grant R, Hulf JA, et al: The effect of preconditioning (ischemic and pharmacological) on myocardial necrosis following coronary artery bypass graft surgery. Cardiovasc Res 2002;53:175-180.

466. Lu EX, Chen SX, Yuan MD, et al: Preconditioning improves myocardial preservation in patients undergoing open heart operations. Ann Thorac Surg 1997;64:1320-1324.

467. Laurikka J, Wu ZK, Iisalo P, et al: Regional ischemic preconditioning enhances myocardial performance in off-pump coronary artery bypass grafting. Chest 2002;121:1183-1189.

468. Penttila HJ, Lepojarvi MV, Kaukoranta PK, et al: Ischemic preconditioning does not improve myocardial preservation during off-pump multivessel coronary operation. Ann Thorac Surg 2003;75:1246-1252; discussion 1252-1253.

469. Vinten-Johansen J, Buckberg GD, Okamoto F, et al: Superiority of surgical versus medical reperfusion after regional ischemia. J Thorac Cardiovasc Surg 1986;92(3 Pt 2):525-534.

470. Okamoto F, Allen BS, Buckberg GD, et al: Reperfusion conditions: Importance of ensuring gentle versus sudden reperfusion during relief of coronary occlusion. J Thorac Cardiovasc Surg 1986;92(3 Pt 2):613-620.

471. Allen BS, Buckberg GD, Fontan FM, et al: Superiority of controlled surgical reperfusion versus percutaneous transluminal coronary angioplasty in acute coronary occlusion. J Thorac Cardiovasc Surg 1993;105:864-879; discussion 879-884.

472. Zhao ZQ, Corvera JS, Halkos ME, et al: Inhibition of myocardial injury by ischemic postconditioning during reperfusion: Comparison with ischemic preconditioning. Am J Physiol Heart Circ Physiol 2003;285:H579-588.

473. Kin H, Zhao ZQ, Sun HY, et al: Postconditioning attenuates myocardial ischemia-reperfusion injury by inhibiting events in the early minutes of reperfusion. Cardiovasc Res 2004;62:74-85.

474. Yang XM, Proctor JB, Cui L, et al: Multiple, brief coronary occlusions during early reperfusion protect rabbit hearts by targeting cell signaling pathways. J Am Coll Cardiol 2004;44:1103-1110.

475. Galagudza M, Kurapeev D, Minasian S, et al: Ischemic postconditioning: Brief ischemia during reperfusion converts persistent ventricular fibrillation into regular rhythm. Eur J Cardiothorac Surg 2004;25: 1006-1010.

476. Piper HM, Abdallah Y, Schafer C: The first minutes of reperfusion: A window of opportunity for cardioprotection. Cardiovasc Res 2004;61:365-371.

477. Diaz RJ, Wilson GJ: Modifying the first minute of reperfusion: Potential for myocardial salvage. Cardiovasc Res 2004;62:4-6.

478. Hausenloy DJ, Yellon DM: New directions for protecting the heart against ischaemia-reperfusion injury: Targeting the Reperfusion Injury Salvage Kinase (RISK)-pathway. Cardiovasc Res 2004;61: 448-460.

479. Hausenloy DJ, Mocanu MM, Yellon DM: Cross-talk between the survival kinases during early reperfusion: Its contribution to ischemic preconditioning. Cardiovasc Res 2004;63:305-312.

480. Chiari PC, Bienengraeber MW, Pagel PS, et al: Isoflurane protects against myocardial infarction during early reperfusion by activation of phosphatidylinositol-3-kinase signal transduction: Evidence for anesthetic-induced postconditioning in rabbits. Anesthesiology 2005;102:102-109.

481. Xu Z, Yang XM, Cohen MV, et al: Limitation of infarct size in rabbit hearts by the novel adenosine receptor agonist AMP 579 administered at reperfusion. J Mol Cell Cardiol 2000;32:2339-2347.

482. Yang XM, Philipp S, Downey JM, Cohen MV: Postconditioning's protection is not dependent on circulating factors or cells but involves adenosine receptors and requires PI3-kinase and guanylyl cyclase activation. Basic Res Cardiol 2005;100:57-63.

483. Bell RM, Yellon DM: Bradykinin limits infarction when administered as an adjunct to reperfusion in mouse heart: The role of PI3K, Akt and eNOS. J Mol Cell Cardiol 2003;35:185-193.

484. Jonassen AK, Sack MN, Mjos OD, Yellon DM: Myocardial protection by insulin at reperfusion requires early administration and is mediated via Akt and p70s6 kinase cell-survival signaling. Circ Res 2001;89: 1191-1198.

485. Argaud L, Gateau-Roesch O, Raisky O, et al: Postconditioning inhibits mitochondrial permeability transition. Circulation 2005;111: 194-197.

486. Tsang A, Hausenloy DJ, Mocanu MM, Yellon DM: Postconditioning: A form of "modified reperfusion" protects the myocardium by activating the phosphatidylinositol 3-kinase-Akt pathway. Circ Res 2004;95: 230-232.

13 Prevention of Ischemic Injury in Noncardiac Surgery

Don Poldermans

Each year in Western countries, about 4% to 10% of the population is scheduled for noncardiac surgery.[1] Patients undergoing major noncardiac surgery are at significant risk of cardiovascular morbidity and mortality as a result of underlying symptomatic or asymptomatic coronary artery disease (CAD).[1,2] Although the overall perioperative event rate has declined over the past 30 years, 30-day cardiovascular mortality remains as high as 3% to 5%.[1] Myocardial infarction (MI) is the most frequent fatal complication in this respect, accounting for 10% to 40% of postoperative fatalities.

Although the pathophysiology of a perioperative MI is not entirely clear, there is evidence that coronary plaque rupture, leading to thrombus formation and subsequent vessel occlusion, is an important causative mechanism behind such complications, as it is for myocardial infarctions occurring in the nonoperative setting.[3-5] The incidence of plaque rupture, with superimposed thrombosis, is increased by the stress response to major surgery. The perioperative surgical stress response includes a catecholamine surge with associated hemodynamic stress, vasospasm, reduced fibrinolytic activity, platelet activation, and consequent hypercoagulability.[6] In patients with severe CAD, perioperative MI also may be caused by a sustained myocardial supply–demand oxygen imbalance resulting from prolonged tachycardia and increased myocardial contractility.[7] The association of perioperative MI with prolonged, severe, perioperative myocardial ischemia, and the frequency of nontransmural or circumferential subendocardial infarction in the operative setting support this mechanism.[3] Finally, hemodynamic stress and multivessel coronary disease would tend to exacerbate the extent of infarction caused by primary plaque rupture. Studies evaluating the pathophysiology of perioperative MI using noninvasive tests, coronary angiography, and autopsy results showed that coronary plaque rupture occurred in approximately 50% of all fatal cases, and that a sustained mismatch of oxygen supply and demand was responsible for the remaining.[7]

Various approaches for the prevention of devastating perioperative cardiac complications have been proposed, including those aiming at a restoration of the supply–demand mismatch using medical therapy (beta-blockers, alpha-blockers, nitrates, and calcium antagonists), coronary revascularization, anticoagulants, and inhibitors of 3-hydroxy-3-methylglutaryl coenzyme A (statins), which may prevent plaque instability and thrombosis.[1,8,9]

■ BETA-BLOCKERS

In the late 1980s, indications for beta-blockers were hypertension and coronary artery disease, and heart failure and peripheral atherosclerotic disease were considered to be relative contraindications. However, after recent studies, beta-blockers were successfully introduced in patients with stable heart-failure disease and patients undergoing noncardiac, high-risk surgery.[10]

Proposed Mechanisms

The mechanisms by which beta-blockers exert their cardioprotective effect are multifactorial. They reduce heart rate and contractility and, subsequently, myocardial oxygen demand; they induce a shift from free fatty acids as the main cardiac energy substrate toward glucose, resulting in an improved energy efficiency and outcome; and they possess antiarrhythmic and anti-inflammatory effects as well as antirenin and antiangiotensin properties.[10,11]

The onset of the cardioprotective effect has important implications for perioperative management. The effects on heart rate, contractility, and energy substrate shift occur almost instantly. However, the effect on inflammatory response may be observed only after a prolonged period of beta-blocker use.[11] In a randomized study of 200 surgical patients at risk for CAD, Mangano and colleagues found no difference in the incidence of perioperative cardiac events among beta-blocker users, but there was a reduced incidence of late fatal cardiac events.[12] The benefits of beta-blocker use were not immediately apparent but rather evolved over the first 6 to 8 months after initiation of beta-blocker therapy. It could be possible that immediately after initiation of therapy, not all pleiotropic effects are achieved, and that the benefits of beta-blockers become evident only after weeks of treatment.

In addition to the timing of treatment, dosage adjustments for heart rate control are important. In a study by Raby and associates of 150 patients, ischemia was observed prior to vascular surgery using ambulatory electrocardiographic (ECG) monitoring in 26 patients.[13] The heart rate was noted at which ischemia occurred (ischemic threshold). The 26 patients were randomized either to tight heart rate control (i.e., 20% less than the ischemic threshold but >60 beats/min [bpm]) or to normal, nonadjusted beta-blocker therapy. Of 13 patients with heart rates controlled to below the ischemic threshold, one (7.7%) had postoperative ischemia, whereas

12 out of 13 (92%) patients with less tight control had post-operative ischemia. These results suggest that timing followed by titration of beta-blocker dosage is mandatory.

Clinical Evidence

Although beta-blockers are widely prescribed during noncardiac surgery, the evidence for their perioperative use is mainly based on only two small randomized prospective clinical trials and several observational studies. The first trial evaluated the effect of atenolol in high-risk patients undergoing noncardiac surgery.[12,14] In this study, 200 patients with risk factors for known ischemic heart disease were randomized for atenolol (50 or 100 mg) or placebo prior to surgery. Atenolol therapy was not associated with an improved in-hospital outcome (cardiac death or myocardial infarction); however, continuous three-lead Holter monitoring showed a 50% reduction of myocardial ischemia in the atenolol treated group during the first 48 hours after surgery. In a selected high-risk population of 112 vascular surgery patients, the second trial showed a 10-fold reduced incidence of perioperative cardiac death and myocardial infarction, compared with patients without beta-blockers (3.4% versus 34%).[14] The high incidence of perioperative cardiac events was explained by the patient selection: from a population of 1351 patients, the 112 who were included had evidence of stress-induced myocardial ischemia during dobutamine echocardiography.

These promising results were confirmed by a meta-analysis of both retrospective and prospective studies evaluating the incidence of perioperative ischemic episodes in 1092 patients in 15 studies (Fig. 13-1).[15] All studies reported on at least one of three endpoints: perioperative myocardial ischemia, perioperative nonfatal MI, or cardiac mortality. In these studies, 551 beta-blocker users and 541 nonusers were included. There were no significant differences in clinical baseline characteristics. Twelve studies (410 beta-blocker users versus 407 nonusers) reported on myocardial ischemia. Beta-blocker therapy was associated with a 65% relative risk (RR) reduction in perioperative myocardial ischemia ($P < .001$). All studies reported on the incidence of MI. Beta-blocker therapy was associated with a 56% RR reduction ($P = .04$). Also, beta-blocker therapy was associated

with a significant RR reduction of 67% ($P = .002$) in the composite endpoint of cardiac death and nonfatal MI.

A recent large retrospective study performed by Lindenauer and coworkers evaluated the effects from 664,000 surgical procedures and confirmed the benefit of beta-blockers in those patients with increased risk.[16] Patients were evaluated according to the Revised Cardiac Risk Index, in which one point is assigned for each of the following risk factors: high-risk surgery, ischemic heart disease (i.e., angina pectoris and myocardial infarction), cerebrovascular disease, renal dysfunction, and diabetes mellitus. A 0.88, 0.71, and 0.58 risk reduction was observed among those with two, three, or greater than three risk factors on perioperative beta-blocker therapy. However, in patients without risk factors, beta-blockers were associated with a 43% increase of death and a 13% increase among patients with only one risk factor.

These promising results in high-risk patients were not supported by two recent trials evaluating the effect of beta-blockers in low-risk vascular surgery patients and diabetics.[17,18] In the POBBLE trial, low-risk patients (those with a history of ischemic heart disease) were excluded, and those scheduled for vascular surgery were randomized for metoprolol ($n = 55$) or placebo ($n = 48$). Metoprolol, either 25 mg or 50 mg, depending on the patient's weight, was started the day before surgery. Holter monitoring and repeated troponin measurements were performed during the hospital stay. No difference was observed in the incidence of perioperative cardiovascular events, which were 15 (34%) versus 17 (32%) in patients on placebo versus metoprolol, respectively. The only difference was observed in the length of hospital stay, which was significantly shorter in those taking metoprolol, 10 versus 12 days.[17]

The more recently presented Diabetic Postoperative Mortality and Morbidity (DIPOM) trial evaluated the cardioprotective effect of a fixed dosage of metoprolol begun on the evening before major noncardiac surgery and continued postoperatively (mean, 4.6 days) in 921 diabetics. Results demonstrated no difference in 30-day morbidity and mortality.[18] According to the American College of Cardiology/American Heart Association (ACC/AHA) guidelines, diabetes is considered an intermediate cardiac risk factor. High-risk surgery in this study was defined by an operation time of more than

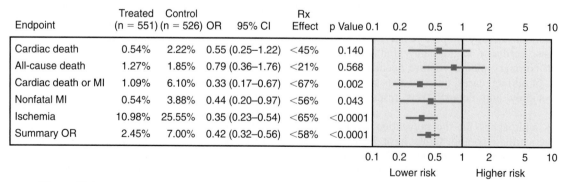

Endpoint	Treated (n = 551)	Control (n = 526)	OR 95% CI	Rx Effect	p Value	0.1 0.2 0.5 1 2 5 10
Cardiac death	0.54%	2.22%	0.55 (0.25–1.22)	<45%	0.140	
All-cause death	1.27%	1.85%	0.79 (0.36–1.76)	<21%	0.568	
Cardiac death or MI	1.09%	6.10%	0.33 (0.17–0.67)	<67%	0.002	
Nonfatal MI	0.54%	3.88%	0.44 (0.20–0.97)	<56%	0.043	
Ischemia	10.98%	25.55%	0.35 (0.23–0.54)	<65%	<0.0001	
Summary OR	2.45%	7.00%	0.42 (0.32–0.56)	<58%	<0.0001	

0.1   0.2   0.5   1   2   5   10
Lower risk   Higher risk

Figure 13-1 ■ Comparison of perioperative and near-term outcomes in patients treated with beta-blocker therapy versus no drug or placebo. Ischemic event data were available from 11 of 15 studies ($n = 410$ treated and $n = 407$ controls). CI, confidence interval; MI, myocardial ischemia; OR, odds ratio; Rx, treatment.

1 hour. These inclusion criteria are different from those in previous studies, in which only high-risk surgical procedures were enrolled. The composite endpoint of all-cause mortality, acute MI, unstable angina, or congestive heart failure was 99 of 462 (21%) in the metoprolol group, versus 93 of 459 (20%) in the placebo group (RR, 1.06; 95% confidence interval [CI] 0.80-1.41; $P = .66$). This design study was similar to that of Mangano, who also failed to show an effect on perioperative cardiac events; both studies started beta-blockers 1 day before surgery during a short perioperative period, and the dosage was not adjusted for heart rate response.

How should we interpret these conflicting beta-blocker results? Potential factors that might influence study outcomes include differences in dosing and variations in the individual responses to β-adrenoceptor blockade. To exert the most beneficial effect, dosage adjustments for heart rate control are important. The study by Raby and coworkers[13] (see Proposed Mechanisms, earlier) showed that the effect of dosing with subsequent reduction of myocardial oxygen demand is mandatory for proper comparison of published trials (Table 13-1).

Also, the individual responses to beta-blockers, because of genotype polymorphism, may vary. In a population of 735 patients with an acute coronary syndrome, 597 patients were on chronic beta-blocker therapy at hospital discharge. The long-term beneficial effect of beta-blockers differed among beta-2-adrenoceptor genotype variants.[19] Patients with the beta-2-adrenoceptor gene locus ADRB2 79 CG experienced 16% mortality during 3-year follow-up, compared with 6% among patients with the GG genotypes.

Available Beta-Blockers

There is no evidence indicating an advantage to any one particular beta-blocker, provided it is beta-1 selective, as emerges from a meta-analysis that reanalyzed five randomized trials in which different molecules were utilized: a class effect is the physiologic mechanism at the basis of prognostic improvement.[20] Beta-blocking agents are characterized not only by their cardioselectivity but also by their liposolubility and intrinsic mimetic sympathetic activity. In regard to the level of lipophilia or hydrophilia, the most validated drugs (atenolol, bisoprolol) in the studies on reduction of perioperative complications have different features. Atenolol is one of the most hydrophilic beta-blockers (together with sotalol and nadolol), and thus it is less linked to proteins, it has less tissue diffusion (it does not pass the hematoencephalic barrier), and it has less variable plasma levels than bisoprolol. Bisoprolol is a lipophilic preparation (like metoprolol) with a greater proteinic link (thus theoretically more subject to interactions with other highly protein-linked drugs), a greater tissue diffusion (including in the central nervous system), a prevalently hepatic metabolism, and more variable plasma levels. However, despite these differences between beta-blockers, no differences were observed with respect to efficacy and side effects.

Beta-blockers with intrinsic mimetic sympathetic activity (ISA) partially activate beta-receptors in the absence of catecholamines and thus have a smaller bradycardic effect (pindolol-acebutolol). For this reason—heart rate reduction

being the precise aim of the treatment—they should probably not be considered first choice in these patients, even if there is no direct clinical evidence to support this, as these molecules have not been investigated in noncardiac surgery.

Safety Endpoints

The most widely reported side effects of beta-blockers are dyspnea and intermittent claudication. These occur particularly in patients using nonselective beta-blockers, because blocking the beta-2-adrenergic receptors in the bronchial smooth muscles can cause bronchospasm in patients with asthma or chronic obstructive bronchitis, or worsening of peripheral circulation in patients with peripheral atherosclerotic disease. In a meta-analysis including 1092 patients, the following safety endpoints were reported: bradycardia, hypotension, atrioventricular (AV) block, pulmonary edema, intermittent claudication, and dyspnea.[15] Nine trials reported bradycardia as a safety endpoint. In these 350 treated patients and 346 control patients, beta-blocker use was associated with a significant 4.3-fold increased risk of bradycardia ($P = .006$). Patients on beta-blocker therapy did not have a significantly increased risk for hypotension (14.1% versus 10.7%, $P = .73$). Other side effects were reported in fewer trials: AV block was reported in only one study (27 treated and 30 controls); pulmonary edema in two studies (93 treated and 89 controls); and bronchospasm in two studies (85 treated and 87 controls). None of these three safety endpoints were statistically associated with beta-blocker use. However, overall beta-blocker therapy was associated with a 1.5-fold risk for the combined safety endpoints ($P = .005$).

Importantly, chronic pulmonary obstructive disease, which is prominent in older adult patients, is considered a relative contraindication for beta-blockers. However, the rates of pulmonary adverse events were similar in treated and untreated patients, a finding that is confirmed in recent publications on cardioselective beta-blockers.

Recommendations

- Although no study has assessed the optimal run-in period for perioperative beta-blocker use, it is preferable that treatment begin 30 days before surgery. Possible additional effects of beta-blockers, such as anti-inflammatory actions, may take a prolonged run-in period.
- The aim is to obtain a resting heart rate of 60 bpm; for this reason, some authors prefer shorter-acting agents (e.g., metoprolol) for a faster titration up to the induction of anesthesia.
- Treatment should not be interrupted during the perioperative period, and beta-blockers being administered orally before surgery might be temporarily substituted with intravenous formulations.
- The ACC/AHA guidelines consider the use of beta-blockers in patients previously treated for angina, symptomatic arrhythmias, or hypertension as an indication of class I (class is discussed in reference 49), and also in patients referred to vascular surgery with signs of ischemia inducible from the noninvasive tests. Class IIa is indicated by beta-blocker use in patients with diagnosed but untreated arterial hypertension, known coronary disease, or a major

13-1   Randomized Controlled Trials of the Effectiveness of Perioperative Beta-Blockade

Study	Year	Type of Noncardiac Surgical Procedure	Cardiac Inclusion Criteria	Beta-blocker Therapy (no. of Analyzed Patients)	Control Therapy (no. of Analyzed Patients)	Preoperative Drug Dosage	Postoperative Drug Dosage	Duration of Treatment
Bayliff et al.[53]	1999	Thoracic	None described	Propranolol (49)	Placebo (50)	10 mg PO	40 mg/day PO	5 days
Bohm et al.[54]	2003	General	NYHA class III or IV	Bisoprolol (64)	Placebo (64)	2.5-10 mg/day PO	2.5-10 mg/day PO	Chronic
Coleman et al.[55]	1980	General	None described	Metoprolol (27)	Placebo (15)	2 or 4 mg IV	—	Premedication
Cucchiara et al.[56]	1986	Vascular	None described	Esmolol (36)	Placebo (37)	500 µg/kg/min for 4 min 300 µg/kg/min for 8 min	—	Premedication
Davies et al.[57]	1992	Vascular	None described	Atenolol (20)	Placebo (20)	50 mg PO	—	Premedication
Jakobsen et al.[58]	1997	Thoracic	None described	Metoprolol (18)	Placebo (17)	100 mg PO	—	4 to 10 days
Magnusson et al.[59]	1986	ENT	None described	Metoprolol (11)	No drug (13)	200 µg/kg IV	—	Premedication
Magnusson et al.[60]	1986	General	None described	Metoprolol (13)	No drug (14)	200 mg/day 15 mg IV preoperative	—	14-34 days + premedication
Poldermans et al.[14]	1999	Vascular	Ischemia during DSE	Bisoprolol (59)	No drug (53)	5-10 mg/day PO	5-10 mg/day PO or metoprolol IV	37 days
Raby et al.[13]	1999	Vascular	Preoperative ischemia	Esmolol (15)	Placebo (11)	—	—	2 days
Rosenberg et al.[61]	1996	General	None described	Metoprolol (19)	Placebo (19)	100 mg PO	—	Premedication
Stone et al.[62]	1988	General	Hypertension	Atenolol (44)	No drug (39)	50 mg PO	—	Premedication
Urban et al.[63]	2000	Orthopedic	Probable IHD	Esmolol/metoprolol (52)	No drug (55)	—	250 mg/hr IV, 50 mg/day PO	2 days
Wallace et al.[64]	1998	General	CAD	Atenolol (101)	Placebo (99)	5-10 mg IV	10-20 mg/day IV or 50-100 mg/day PO	7 days
Zaugg et al.[65]	1999	General	CAD	Atenolol (23)	No drug (20)	5-10 mg IV	10-20 mg IV	3 days

CAD, coronary artery disease; DSE, dobutamine stress echocardiography; ENT, ear, nose, and throat; IHD, ischemic heart disease; NYHA, New York Heart Association.

risk factor for coronary disease (e.g., history of congestive heart failure, prior myocardial infarction, diabetes, heart failure, age >70 years, or poor functional status) especially if undergoing higher-risk surgery (e.g., vascular, thoracic, or major abdominal procedures).[2]

- Beta-blockers have become the first choice in patients with left ventricular dysfunction. However, in this population, use of the drug calls for attention in the initial phase, and no studies are available to assess the effect on patients with heart failure immediately prior to noncardiac surgery; thus, it is generally more prudent not to initiate treatment immediately prior to surgery.

Summary

For patients with stable CAD who are scheduled for low-risk surgery, a low rate of adverse events is anticipated, and beta-blocker therapy does not bring tangible benefits. These patients can undergo surgery without the need for beta-blocker therapy.

For patients with stable CAD who are scheduled for intermediate-risk surgery, beta-blocker therapy is useful and further cardiac evaluations are not required. Therapy should be continued after surgery as long-term prognosis improves.

When patients have CAD or risk factors for CAD and are scheduled for high-risk surgery, their status guides further management. Patients without CAD or cardiac risk for CAD are referred for surgery with beta-blocker therapy without further preoperative testing. Those with CAD or one or more risk factors for CAD are referred for additional noninvasive testing to evaluate the CAD. Patients with one- or two-vessel disease are sent for surgery using beta-blockers. In those with three-vessel disease, left-main disease, or CAD in combination with a reduced left ventricular function, the optimal strategy is not yet defined. The protective effect of beta-blockade is probably insufficient, and coronary revascularization should be considered prior to surgery. If that surgery cannot be postponed, beta-blockers in combination with minimally invasive surgery may be the best option, followed by aggressive postoperative treatment for myocardial ischemia.

■ STATINS: 3-HYDROXY-3-METHYLGLUTARYL COENZYME A REDUCTASE INHIBITORS

Statins (3-hydroxy-3-methylglutaryl coenzyme A reductase inhibitors) are highly effective drugs for reducing low-density lipoprotein (LDL) cholesterol levels. Numerous clinical trials have clearly demonstrated that statin use is associated with a substantial reduction in the risk for cardiovascular morbidity and mortality in patients with or at risk for coronary heart disease.[21-24] Recently, studies have shown that perioperative statin use was associated with an improved postoperative cardiac outcome in patients with or at risk for CAD.[25-28]

Proposed Mechanisms

Apart from being potent LDL-lowering agents, statins have also been shown to attenuate coronary artery plaque inflammation and influence plaque stability, in addition to having antithrombogenic, antiproliferative, and leukocyte-adhesion–inhibiting effects.[22] Coronary plaques at high risk of rupture are known as vulnerable plaques. The prevalence of vulnerable plaques is high even in seemingly stable patients. However, it is impossible to predict whether structurally vulnerable plaques may become unstable in weeks, months, or years after their detection.[29] Surgery imposes an extra myocardial workload, resulting in mechanical stress, stress-induced inflammation, and possibly coronary spasms. This can cause vulnerable plaques to become unstable, leading to the cascade of plaque rupture, thrombus formation, myocardial ischemia, and eventually MI. The pleiotropic and anti-inflammatory effects of statins may stabilize unstable coronary artery plaques, thereby reducing myocardial ischemia and subsequent myocardial necrosis in the perioperative setting.

Factors leading to unstable coronary plaques are multiple and complex. However, in general, the risk of plaque rupture is related to two factors: the intrinsic individual plaque characteristics and an extrinsic force triggering plaque disruption.[30] Intrinsic factors include, for example, plaque morphology. Although it has been proven that statins are capable of positively altering plaque composition,[21] they do not alter these intrinsic factors within a few weeks. Therefore, the perioperative prescription of statins seems less suitable for the prevention of adverse perioperative cardiovascular events by this mechanism. However, the extrinsic factors (e.g., inflammation) might be altered by statins within a few hours to days.

Naghavi and colleagues,[31] in their extensive review on vulnerable plaques, reported that inflammation is one of the major criteria in the definition of vulnerable plaques. It is generally well accepted that inflammation is of imminent importance in the whole process. Therefore, most research has been focused on inflammation of coronary plaques as the ultimate trigger for vulnerable plaque rupture. This interest in inflammatory components has been justified in several population-based studies in which a positive relationship between inflammation markers and the occurrence of cardiovascular events was found.[24] As the histopathologic assessment of inflammation within atheromas is not feasible, serologic inflammatory markers are accepted as a substitute in research and clinical practice. These serum inflammation markers include, among many others, C-reactive protein (which is regulated by tumor necrosis factor [TNF]-α, interleukin [IL]-1b, and IL-6) and serum amyloid A.

Clinical Evidence

Several recent studies have addressed the beneficial effect of statin use in patients undergoing noncardiac surgery, including vascular surgery (Fig. 13-2). In a case-control study among 2816 patients who underwent major vascular surgery, statin use was associated with a significant fourfold reduction in all-cause mortality (adjusted odds ratio [OR], 0.22; 95% CI, 0.10-0.47) compared with patients with no statin use.[25] The beneficial effect of statin use was consistent in subgroups of patients according to the type of vascular surgery, cardiac risk factors, and cardioprotective medication use, including aspirin and beta-blockers. The first blinded, placebo-controlled, randomized trial in which the influence of statin

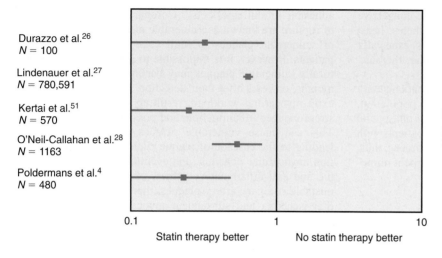

Figure 13-2 ■ The effects of statin use in patients undergoing noncardiac surgery, including vascular surgery.

use on perioperative cardiovascular complications was investigated has been reported by Durazzo and colleagues.[26] In their study, this research group randomly assigned 100 patients to treatment with either 20 mg atorvastatin or placebo. Patients received treatment for 45 days at least 2 weeks before surgery. One month after surgery, patients with elevated cholesterol levels were advised to continue or start statin therapy. The outcome of this trial was the endpoint of cardiovascular events, defined as cardiac death, nonfatal MI, stroke, or unstable angina pectoris. Patients were followed for up to 6 months after the surgical procedure. Of 100 patients, 90 (44 statin users and 46 nonusers) underwent elective vascular surgery. The 6-month incidence of cardiovascular events was reduced 3.1-fold in statin users compared with nonusers ($P = .022$).

Finally, Lindenauer and coworkers[27] and O'Neil-Callahan and associates[28] also confirmed the beneficial effects of statins on the basis of the results of their large-scale retrospective studies. The Lindenauer group's retrospective cohort study was based on the hospital discharge and pharmacy records of over 780,000 patients in 329 hospitals throughout the United States. All patients underwent elective major surgical procedures and survived at least the first 2 postoperative days. In total, 70,159 of these patients were identified as statin users. After correction for numerous baseline differences, statin users had a 1.4-fold reduced risk of in-hospital mortality. Subsequently, Lindenauer concluded that perioperative statin use might result in a reduced risk of death after major surgical procedures.[27]

The O'Neil-Callahan group collected data of 997 patients who underwent noncardiac vascular surgery and found that patients who were statin users had a substantially lower perioperative cardiac complication rate than patients without statin use (OR, 0.52; 95% CI, 0.35-0.77).[28] The protective effect of statin use was similar across different risk group categories and persisted after accounting for the likelihood of statin use in patients with hypercholesterolemia. Although these studies hold promising results for the reduction of perioperative cardiac complications, especially for high-risk patients with multiple cardiac risk factors or with significant

CAD, future clinical trials are required to confirm the efficacy, timing, and safety of perioperative statin use.

Available Statins

Initial reports of perioperative statin use were based on simvastatin, and these were followed by reports of fluvastatin, pravastatin, atorvastatin, and rosuvastatin. All statins reduce low-density lipoprotein cholesterol, but the reduction varies between statins. Data from follow-up studies have shown that more intensive lipid lowering with potent or high-dose statins offers additional benefits after coronary revascularization and during long-term follow-up.

Safety Aspects

A major concern of perioperative statin therapy has been the risk of statin-induced myopathy, rhabdomyolysis, and proteinuria. Perioperatively, factors increasing the risk of statin-induced myopathy are numerous—for example, the impairment of renal function after major surgery and multiple drug use during an anesthesia.[32,33] Furthermore, the use of analgesic agents and postoperative pain may mask signs of myopathy. Failure to detect statin-induced myopathy may then lead to continuous statin use and the subsequent development of rhabdomyolysis and acute renal failure. Probably on the basis of these assumptions, the guidelines of the ACC/AHA/National Heart, Lung, and Blood Institute suggest that there is an increased risk of such rhabdomyolysis during the perioperative period.[33] However, no studies have been published that support this fear, except for some case reports.[34,35] In a retrospective study of 1000 consecutive patients undergoing vascular surgery (238 on statins), no case of rhabdomyolysis or of a significantly higher creatine kinase level in statin users was observed.[32] Considering that the risk of cardiovascular complications is far greater than the risk of statin-induced myopathy and rhabdomyolysis, the potential benefits of perioperative statin use seem to outweigh the potential hazards. However, this should be confirmed in blinded, randomized trials. Recently, tubular proteinuria was observed as a possible side effect of statins, although it should be taken into account that the target population of statin users are patients who have frequent proteinuria as a result of generalized atherosclerosis.[36]

Recommendations

- Perioperative statin use is associated with an improved postoperative outcome in high-risk patients in a limited number of studies, without signs of an increased incidence of side effects. The evidence level is class I. Continuation of statins in high-risk patients after surgery is associated with an improved long-term survival.
- The effect of statins was not related to the preoperative cholesterol levels and type of statin. Therefore, aggressive LDL-cholesterol–lowering treatment prior to surgery might not be indicated, and the dosage might be adjusted after surgery to improve long-term outcome.
- The optimal dosage and run-in period is not yet defined. Side effects are difficult to assess clinically in the perioperative period. Repeated measurements prior to surgery and in the perioperative period of creatine kinase levels, creatinine, and liver function are mandatory to identify early (asymptomatic) side effects. High-dose statin therapy to obtain low LDL-cholesterol levels might be associated with an increased incidence of side effects, especially for those statins metabolized by cytochrome 4A3, a common metabolic pathway for drugs administrated during surgery, and is probably not indicated, as pleiotropic effects are important.
- No intravenous formula exists for statins. Interruption of perioperative therapy in those patients who cannot take medication orally has not been associated with a flare-up of perioperative cardiac events. Statins with a prolonged half-life or in the formulation of a slow-release tablet are preferred.

Summary

Statins should be started prior to surgery in high-risk patients. Evidence from one retrospective study and several large retrospective studies provides class I evidence.

Statins improve postoperative outcome regardless of the type of statin and the achieved LDL-cholesterol level. As side effects might occur more frequently in potent statin regimens, and as these are difficult to assess in the perioperative period, fluvastatin slow-release formulations, simvastatin, and low-dose atorvastatin or rosuvastatin are preferred. Studies provide class IIa evidence.[49]

■ ALPHA-2-ADRENERGIC AGONISTS

The beneficial effect of alpha-2-adrenergic agonists, including clonidine, dexmedetomidine, and mivazerol, during the perioperative period have been studied by several investigators. These drugs exert beneficial cardiovascular effects by reducing central sympathetic nervous system activity, resulting in the attenuation of perioperative catecholamine surges and hemodynamic abnormalities.[37,38] Although potentially promising, earlier small-scale studies failed to demonstrate that clonidine, an alpha-2 agonist, may reduce the incidence of cardiac death and myocardial infarction compared with placebo use.[39,40] When data from some of these studies were

analyzed in a meta-analysis by Nishina and colleagues, the results showed that clonidine use was associated with a reduction in the incidence of perioperative ischemia.[41] Nevertheless, this study was underpowered (358 noncardiac surgical patients in two studies) and effects were reported only on ischemia. In two more recent meta-analyses, the beneficial effect of perioperative alpha-2-agonist use was shown for the reduction of myocardial ischemia and perioperative cardiovascular complications.[8,42] However, as in the study of Nishina, the results of these two meta-analyses were driven mainly by the European Mivazerol Trial, the only large-scale study available to date.[43] The results of the European Mivazerol Trial by Oliver and associates showed no overall effect of mivazerol on the prespecified combined endpoint of cardiac death and myocardial infarction in the total study population of 2854 patients. Only in a post hoc analysis was it revealed that in 904 patients who underwent high-risk major vascular surgery, mivazerol use was associated with a significantly lower incidence of cardiac death and myocardial infarction. These results were confirmed in a study by Wallace and coworkers.[44] In a prospective randomized trial with 190 patients with or at risk for CAD, prophylactic administration of clonidine started the night before surgery and continued until day 4 after surgery reduced perioperative myocardial ischemia. In patients randomized for clonidine, the incidence of ischemia, assessed by a continuous 12-lead ECG recording, was significantly reduced intraoperatively: 14% in the treated group versus 31% in the placebo group during the day of surgery and the first 3 postoperative days ($P = .01$). Clonidine also reduced "hard events" (i.e., cardiac death and myocardial infarction), and both 30-day and long-term mortality were reduced after prophylactic clonidine. This trial convincingly demonstrated the efficacy of these drugs in the reduction of cardiac complications in patients at increased cardiac risk.

Recommendations

- Alpha-2-adrenergic agonists have been shown to have a cardioprotective effect in high-risk surgery patients, with a class Ia level of evidence. They can be considered as an alternative therapy in patients with contraindications for perioperative beta-blockers (level of evidence, class IV).

■ NITRATES

Nitrates are the most frequently used drugs in cases of myocardial ischemia. Nitroglycerin leads to reduction in myocardial oxygen demand by decreasing left ventricular preload and end-diastolic wall tension. This drug also increases coronary collateral perfusion, and as a donor for nitric oxide, it may have direct cardioprotective properties. However, studies of the prophylactic use of intravenous nitroglycerin failed to find any difference in the incidence of intraoperative and perioperative myocardial ischemia between patients receiving nitroglycerin and those receiving placebo.[45,46] A potentially harmful effect might be a vagal withdrawal caused by peripheral vasodilatation, with subsequent cardiac stimulation (or overstimulation) and induction of myocardial ischemia.

Recommendations

- Perioperative nitrate use is not associated with a reduced incidence of cardiac events (level of evidence, class I).

■ CALCIUM CHANNEL BLOCKERS

Calcium channel blockers can be useful to reverse myocardial ischemia caused by coronary artery vasospasm. They also have a variety of cardiovascular effects, especially on heart rate. Use of nifedipine and nicardipine leads to an increased heart rate as the result of a reduction in peripheral arterial tone. In contrast, diltiazem reduces heart rate, and thus it can be useful for the prevention of myocardial ischemia. Nevertheless, use of calcium channel blockers has thus far not been found to be significantly associated with the prevention of myocardial ischemia during noncardiac surgery.[47]

■ PREVENTIVE CORONARY REVASCULARIZATION

When patients with CAD are considered for elective noncardiac surgery, coronary revascularization prior to surgery to improve both perioperative outcome and long-term survival seems to be a logical approach. However, the role of coronary revascularization in candidates for noncardiac surgery has been quite controversial in the past decade. The lack of randomized trials has led to confusion in evaluating the benefits and risks associated with preventive revascularization. Also, the postponement of the index procedure itself with possible worsening of the patient's condition should be taken into account. In support of aggressive treatment before vascular surgery, retrospective data indicate that revascularization improves long-term outcome.[48] However, in the cohort of patients with peripheral vascular disease in the Coronary Artery Surgery Study, a long-term survival benefit was seen only in patients who needed bypass surgery independently of their major noncardiac operation.[48] The latest ACC/AHA guidelines suggest that coronary revascularization before noncardiac surgery should be recommended only in patients with acute coronary syndromes or evidence of high risk on noninvasive tests for ischemia.[49]

Coronary Artery Revascularization Prophylaxis Study

The results of the recently published Coronary Artery Revascularization Prophylaxis (CARP) trial show that preoperative coronary revascularization does not reduce perioperative MI or increase long-term survival in a large group of patients at high risk.[50] The ineffectiveness of preoperative revascularization was partially explained by improved medical therapy—in particular, by the widespread perioperative use of beta-blockers in approximately 90% of the control group.

Indeed, blockade of beta-adrenergic receptors has been associated with a reduced risk of the surrogate endpoint of perioperative myocardial ischemia. However, most of the trials conducted so far have lacked the statistical power to evaluate the protective effect of beta-blockers on the incidence of serious cardiac events such as MI and cardiac death.

Recent findings of the CARP trial support the beneficial effects of beta-blockers and have clarified the role of revascularization in stable patients. Among 5859 patients scheduled for elective vascular surgery (for expanding abdominal aortic aneurysm or severe symptoms of arterial occlusive disease involving the legs) in 18 Veterans Affairs medical centers, a selection was made of those considered at increased risk of cardiac events (on the basis of clinical risk factors or ischemia on an invasive stress imaging study) with evidence of severe coronary stenosis (at least 70%) at coronarography. Anatomic criteria of exclusion included greater than 50% stenosis of the left main coronary artery, left ventricular ejection fraction less than 20%, and severe stenosis of the aorta. The 510 patients selected were randomized to optimal medical therapy with, or optimal medical therapy without, surgical coronary revascularization (more than 80% were on beta-blocker therapy in both groups). The local investigator decided which revascularization procedure to use, whether percutaneous coronary intervention (59%) or coronary artery bypass graft (CABG) (41%). The mean time between randomization and vascular surgery was 54 days for the patients with surgical revascularization, compared with 18 days for the patients treated with the percutaneous procedure. No differences in mortality in the long-term outcome (median follow-up of 2.7 years) were found: 22% in the revascularization group versus 23% in the nonrevascularization group (relative risk, 0.98; 95% CI, 0.70-1.37; $P = .92$). Although the primary endpoint was late mortality, even the findings at 30 days did not show any difference in terms of mortality or postoperative MI (defined by elevated troponin levels, 12% versus 14%), nor did prophylactic revascularization result in a reduction in the length of hospital stay.

On the basis of this multicenter randomized study, it can be concluded that for stable patients, even with known coronary disease, coronary revascularization to reduce the risk of noncardiac surgery is not recommended.

■ CONCLUSIONS

Optimized medical therapy remains the best option for reducing perioperative complications for the majority of patients. The use of effective cardioprotective medication such as beta-blockers and statins can effectively reduce the cardiac complication rate in the majority of those patients undergoing elective high-risk surgery (Fig. 13-3).[51] However, there is always a small group of patients with multiple clinical markers of increased cardiac risk and with extensive myocardial ischemia on preoperative noninvasive testing, for whom cardioprotective medication use may not be sufficient to adequately prevent the occurrence of perioperative cardiac complications.[52] For this small group of patients, the need for further cardiac evaluation and management should at present be based on the ACC/AHA guidelines for perioperative cardiovascular risk evaluation in noncardiac surgery (Box 13-1).[49] These guidelines suggest that coronary angiography and subsequent coronary revascularization should only be considered if there is a clearly defined need, independent of

Assign scores as indicated for each characteristic according to type of vascular procedure, medical history, and long-term medication use.

Characteristics	Scores
Vascular surgery procedures	_____
Medical history	_____
Long-term medication	_____
Total risk score	_____

Vascular Surgical Procedures

	Scores
High risk	
Acute abdominal aortic aneurysm rupture	+43
High-intermediate risk	+26
Thoracoabdominal surgery	
Abdominal aortic surgery	
Low-intermediate risk	+15
Infrainguinal bypass	
Low risk	0
Carotid endarterectomy	

Medical History

	Scores
Cardiovascular morbidity	
Ischemic heart disease	+13
Congestive heart failure	+14
History of cerebrovascular event	+10
Hypertension	+7
Renal dysfunction	+16
Chronic pulmonary disease	+7
Long-term medication	
Beta-Blocker use	+15
Statin use	+10

Calculate the total score by summing the individual scores from the given characteristics and, using the total risk score, read the corresponding estimated probability of perioperative all-cause mortality.

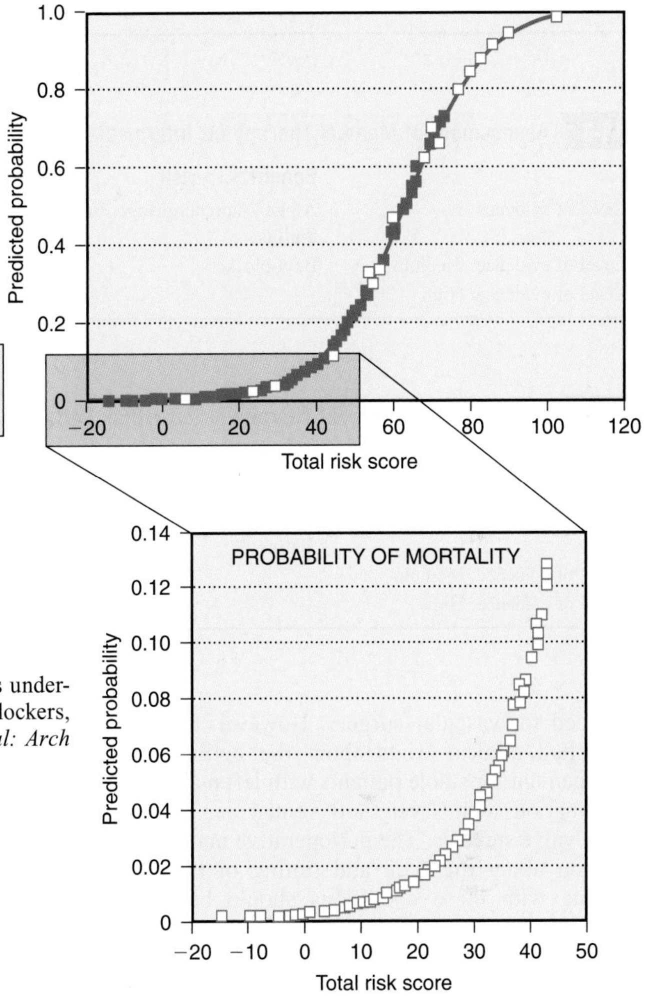

Figure 13-3 ■ Estimated perioperative cardiac event rate in patients undergoing vascular surgery corrected for underlying risk factors, beta-blockers, and statin use. *(Redrawn from Kertai MD, Boersma E, Klein J, et al: Arch Intern Med 2005;165:898-904, with permission.)*

13-1 **Classification of Surgical Procedures According to ACC/AHA Guidelines**

High-Risk Procedures (Reported Cardiac Risk Often >5%)

- Emergent major operations
- Aortic and major vascular surgery
- Peripheral vascular surgery
- Anticipated prolonged surgical procedures

Intermediate-Risk Procedures (Reported Cardiac Risk Generally <5%)

- Carotid endarterectomy
- Head and neck surgery
- Intraperitoneal and intrathoracic surgery
- Orthopedic surgery
- Prostate surgery

Low-Risk Procedures (Reported Cardiac Risk Generally <1%)

- Endoscopic procedures
- Superficial procedures
- Cataract surgery
- Breast surgery

ACC/AHA, American College of Cardiology/American Heart Association.
From Poldermans D, Bax JJ, Kertai MD, et al: Circulation 2003;107:1848-1851.

13-2 Assessment of Medical Therapy for High-Risk Patients Undergoing Surgery

	Benefit >>> Risk	Benefit > Risk	Benefit ≥ Risk	Risk ≥ Benefit
Level of evidence: Low	—	—	Calcium channel blockers Nitrates	—
Level of evidence: Medium	Alpha-2-adrenergic agonists	—	—	—
Level of evidence: High	Beta-blockers Statins	—	—	—

13-3 Assessment of Medical Therapy for Intermediate-Risk Patients Undergoing Surgery

	Benefit >>> risk	Benefit > Risk	Benefit ≥ Risk	Risk ≥ Benefit
Level of evidence: Low	Alpha-2-adrenergic agonists Statins	—	Calcium channel blockers Nitrates	—
Level of evidence: Medium	Beta-blockers	—	—	—
Level of evidence: High	—	—	—	—

13-4 Assessment of Medical Therapy for Low-Risk Patients Undergoing Surgery

	Benefit >>> risk	Benefit > Risk	Benefit ≥ Risk	Risk ≥ Benefit
Level of evidence: Low	Alpha-2-adrenergic agonists Beta-blockers Statins	—	Calcium channel blockers Nitrates	—
Level of evidence: Medium	—	—	—	—
Level of evidence: High	—	—	—	—

the need for vascular surgery. However, there is a lack of controlled clinical trials about the optimal perioperative management for stable patients with left main CAD, CAD in combination with severe left ventricular dysfunction, and aortic valve stenosis. The perioperative management and the decision about the type and timing of the procedure for patients with these conditions should be determined by weighing the risks and benefits of extensive perioperative evaluation and treatment (Tables 13-2 to 13-4).

■ REFERENCES

1. Mangano DT: Perioperative cardiac morbidity. Anesthesiology 1990;72:153-184.
2. Hertzer NR, Beven EG, Young JR, et al: Coronary artery disease in peripheral vascular patients: A classification of 1000 coronary angiograms and results of surgical management. Ann Surg 1984;199: 223-233.
3. Dawood MM, Gupta DK, Southern J, et al: Pathology of fatal perioperative myocardial infarction: Implications regarding pathophysiology and prevention. Int J Cardiol 1996;57:37-44.
4. Poldermans D, Boersma E, Bax JJ, et al: Correlation of location of acute myocardial infarct after noncardiac vascular surgery with preoperative dobutamine echocardiographic findings. Am J Cardiol 2001;88: 1413-1414.
5. Cohen MC, Aretz TH: Histological analysis of coronary artery lesions in fatal postoperative myocardial infarction. Cardiovasc Pathol 1999;8:133-139.
6. Riles TS, Fisher FS, Schaefer S, et al: Plasma catecholamine concentrations during abdominal aortic aneurysm surgery: The link to perioperative myocardial ischemia. Ann Vasc Surg 1993;7:213-219.
7. Fleisher LA, Eagle KA: Lowering cardiac risk in noncardiac surgery N Engl J Med 2001;345:1677-1682.
8. Stevens RD, Burri H, Tramer MR: Pharmacologic myocardial protection in patients undergoing noncardiac surgery: A quantitative systematic review. Anesth Analg 2003;97:623-633.
9. Lindenauer PK, Fitzgerald J, Hoople N, Benjamin EM: The potential preventability of postoperative myocardial infarction: Underuse of perioperative beta-adrenergic blockade. Arch Intern Med 2004;164: 762-766.
10. Cruickshank JM: Beta blockers continue to surprise us. Eur Heart J 2000;21:354-364.
11. Yeager MP, Fillinger MP, Hettleman BD, Hartman GS: Perioperative beta-blockade and late cardiac outcomes: A complementary hypothesis. J Cardiothorac Vasc Anesth 2005;19:237-241.
12. Mangano DT, Layug EL, Wallace A, Tateo I: Effect of atenolol on mortality and cardiovascular morbidity after noncardiac surgery. Multicenter Study of Perioperative Ischemia Research Group. N Engl J Med 1996;335:1713-1720.
13. Raby KE, Brull SJ, Timimi F, et al: The effect of heart rate control on myocardial ischemia among high-risk patients after vascular surgery. Anesth Analg 1999;88:477-482.
14. Poldermans D, Boersma E, Bax JJ, et al: The effect of bisoprolol on perioperative mortality and myocardial infarction in high-risk patients undergoing vascular surgery. Dutch Echocardiographic Cardiac Risk Evaluation Applying Stress Echocardiography Study Group. N Engl J Med 1999;341:1789-1794.
15. Schouten O, Shaw LJ, Boersma H, et al: A meta-analysis of the effectiveness of beta-blocker use in different types of noncardiac surgery. Coron Art Dis 2006 (in press).
16. Lindenauer PK, Pekow P, Wang K, et al: Perioperative beta-blocker therapy and mortality after major noncardiac surgery. N Engl J Med 2005;353:349-361.
17. Brady AR, Gibbs JS, Greenhalgh RM, et al, POBBLE trial investigators: Perioperative beta-blockade (POBBLE) for patients undergoing

infrarenal vascular surgery: Results of a randomized double-blind controlled trial. J Vasc Surg 2005;41:602-609.

18. Juul AB, Wetterslev J, Kofoed-Enevoldsen A, et al, DIPOM Trial Group: Randomized, blinded trial on perioperative metoprolol versus placebo for diabetic patients undergoing non-cardiac surgery. Circulation 2005;111:1725-1728.

19. Lanfear DE, Jones PG, Marsh S, et al: Beta2-adrenergic receptor genotype and survival among patients receiving beta-blocker therapy after an acute coronary syndrome. JAMA 2005;294:1526-1533.

20. Auerbach AD, Goldman L: Beta blockers and reduction of cardiac events in non-cardiac surgery: Clinical applications. JAMA 2002;287:1445-1447.

21. Newby LK, Kristinsson A, Bhapkar MV, et al: Early statin initiation and outcomes in patients with acute coronary syndromes. JAMA 2002;287:3087-3095.

22. Vaughan CJ, Murphy MB, Buckley BM: Statins do more than just lower cholesterol. Lancet 1996;348:1079-1082.

23. Libby P, Ridker PM, Maseri A: Inflammation and atherosclerosis. Circulation 2002;105:1135-1143.

24. Ridker PM, Rifai N, Pfeffer MA, et al: Inflammation, pravastatin, and the risk of coronary events after myocardial infarction in patients with average cholesterol levels. Circulation 1998;98:839-844.

25. Poldermans D, Bax JJ, Kertai MD, et al: Statins are associated with a reduced incidence of perioperative mortality in patients undergoing major noncardiac vascular surgery. Circulation 2003;107:1848-1851.

26. Durazzo AES, Machado FS, Ikeoka DT, et al: Reduction in cardiovascular events after vascular surgery with atorvastatin: A randomized trial. J Vasc Surg 2004;39:967-975.

27. Lindenauer PK, Pekow P, Wang K, et al: Lipid-lowering therapy and in-hospital mortality following major noncardiac surgery. JAMA 2004;291:2092-2099.

28. O'Neil-Callahan K, Katsimaglis G, Tepper MR, et al: Statins decrease perioperative cardiac complications in patients undergoing noncardiac vascular surgery: The Statins for Risk Reduction in Surgery (StaRRS) study. J Am Coll Cardiol 2005;45:336-342.

29. Theroux P: Angiographic and clinical progression in unstable angina: From clinical observation to clinical trials. Circulation 1995;91:2295-2298.

30. Goldstein JA, Demetriou D, Grines CL, et al: Multiple complex coronary plaques in patients with acute myocardial infarction. N Engl J Med 2000;343:915-922.

31. Naghavi M, Libby P, Falk E, et al: From vulnerable plaque to vulnerable patient: A call for new definitions and risk assessment strategies: Part II. Circulation 2003;108:1772-1778.

32. Schouten O, Kertai MD, Bax JJ, et al: Safety of perioperative statin use in high-risk patients undergoing major vascular surgery. Am J Cardiol 2005;95:658-660.

33. Pasternak RC, Smith SC, Bairey-Merz CN, et al: ACC/AHA/NHLBI Advisory on the use and safety of statins. J Am Coll Cardiol 2002;40:568-573.

34. Wilhelmi M, Winterhalter M, Fischer S, et al: Massive postoperative rhabdomyolysis following combined CABG/abdominal aortic replacement: A possible association with HMG-CoA reductase inhibitors. Cardiovasc Drugs Ther 2002;16:471-475.

35. Forestier F, Breton Y, Bonnet E, Janvier G: Severe rhabdomyolysis after laparoscopic surgery for adenocarcinoma of the rectum in two patients treated with statins. Anesthesiology 2002;97:1019-1021.

36. Ferdinand KC: Rosuvastatin: A risk-benefit assessment for intensive lipid lowering. Expert Opin Pharmacother 2005;6:1897-1910.

37. Talke P, Li J, Jain U, et al: Effects of perioperative dexmedetomidine infusion in patients undergoing vascular surgery. The Study of Perioperative Ischemia Research Group. Anesthesiology 1995;82:620-633.

38. Perioperative sympatholysis: Beneficial effects of the alpha-2-adrenoceptor agonist mivazerol on hemodynamic stability and myocardial ischemia. McSPI: Europe Research Group. Anesthesiology 1997;86:346-363.

39. Ellis JE, Drijvers G, Pedlow S, et al: Premedication with oral and transdermal clonidine provides safe and efficacious postoperative sympatholysis. Anesth Analg 1994;79:1133-1140.

40. Stuhmeier KD, Mainzer B, Cierpka J, et al: Small, oral dose of clonidine reduces the incidence of intraoperative myocardial ischemia in

patients having vascular surgery. Anesthesiology 1996;85:706-712.

41. Nishina K, Mikawa K, Uesugi T, et al: Efficacy of clonidine for prevention of perioperative myocardial ischemia: A critical appraisal and meta-analysis of the literature. Anesthesiology 2002;96:323-329.

42. Wijeysundera DN, Naik JS, Scott Beattie W: Alpha-2-adrenergic agonists to prevent perioperative cardiovascular complications: A meta-analysis. Am J Med 2003;114:742-752.

43. Oliver MF, Goldman L, Julian DG, Holme I: Effect of mivazerol on perioperative cardiac complications during non-cardiac surgery in patients with coronary heart disease: The European Mivazerol Trial (EMIT). Anesthesiology 1999;91:951-961.

44. Wallace AW, Galindez D, Salahieh A, et al: Effect of clonidine on cardiovascular morbidity and mortality after noncardiac surgery. Anesthesiology 2004;101:284-293.

45. Coriat P, Daloz M, Bousseau D, et al: Prevention of intraoperative myocardial ischemia during noncardiac surgery with intravenous nitroglycerin. Anesthesiology 1984;61:193-196.

46. Dodds TM, Stone JG, Coromilas J, et al: Prophylactic nitroglycerin infusion during noncardiac surgery does not reduce perioperative ischemia. Anesth Analg 1993;76:705-713.

47. Godet G, Coriat P, Baron JF, et al: Prevention of intraoperative myocardial ischemia during noncardiac surgery with intravenous diltiazem: A randomized trial versus placebo. Anesthesiology 1987;66:241-245.

48. Eagle KA, Rihal CS, Mickel MC, et al: Cardiac risk of noncardiac surgery: Influence of coronary disease and type of surgery in 3368 operations. CASS Investigators and University of Michigan Heart Care Program. Coronary Artery Surgery Study. Circulation 1997;96:1882-1887.

49. Eagle KA, Berger PB, Calkins H, et al: ACC/AHA guideline update for perioperative cardiovascular evaluation for noncardiac surgery: Executive summary. A report of the American College of Cardiology/American Heart Association Task Force on Practice Guidelines (Committee to Update the 1996 Guidelines on Perioperative Cardiovascular Evaluation for Noncardiac Surgery). Circulation 2002;105:1257-1267.

50. McFalls EO, Ward HB, Moritz TE, et al: Coronary artery revascularization before elective major vascular surgery. N Engl J Med 2004;351:2995-2804.

51. Kertai MD, Boersma E, Klein J, et al: Optimizing the prediction of perioperative mortality in vascular surgery using a customized probability model. Arch Intern Med 2005;165:898-904.

52. Boersma E, Poldermans D, Bax JJ, et al: Predictors of cardiac events after major vascular surgery: Role of clinical characteristics, dobutamine echocardiography, and beta-blocker therapy. JAMA 2001;285:1865-1873.

53. Bayliff CD, Massel DR, Inculet RI, et al: Propranolol for the prevention of postoperative arrhythmias in general thoracic surgery. Ann Thorac Surg 1999;67(1):182-186.

54. Bohm M, Maack C, Wehrlen-Grandjean M, Erdmann E: Effect of bisoprolol on perioperative complications in chronic heart failure after surgery (Cardiac Insufficiency Bisoprolol Study II (CIBIS II)). Z Kardiol 2003;92(8):668-676.

55. Coleman AJ, Jordan C: Cardiovascular responses to anaesthesia. Influence of beta-adrenoreceptor blockade with metoprolol. Anaesthesia 1980;35(10):972-978.

56. Cucchiara RF, Benefiel DJ, Matteo RS, et al: Evaluation of esmolol in controlling increases in heart rate and blood pressure during endotracheal intubation in patients undergoing carotid endarterectomy. Anesthesiology 1986;65(5):528-531.

57. Davies MJ, Dysart RH, Silbert BS, et al: Prevention of tachycardia with atenolol pretreatment for carotid endarterectomy under cervical plexus blockade. Anaesth Intensive Care 1992;20(2):161-164.

58. Jakobsen CJ, Bille S, Ahlburg P, et al: Preoperative metoprolol improves cardiovascular stability and reduces oxygen consumption after thoracotomy. Acta Anaesthesiol Scand 1997;41(10):1324-1330.

59. Magnusson H, Ponten J, Sonander HG: Methohexitone anaesthesia for microlaryngoscopy: Circulatory modulation with metoprolol and dihydralazine. Br J Anaesth 1986;58(9):976-982.

60. Magnusson J, Thulin T, Werner O, et al: Haemodynamic effects of pretreatment with metoprolol in hypertensive patients undergoing surgery. Br J Anaesth 1986;58(3):251-260.

61. Rosenberg J, Overgaard H, Andersen M, et al: Double blind randomised controlled trial of effect of metoprolol on myocardial ischaemia during endoscopic cholangiopancreatography. BMJ 1996;313(7052):258-261.

62. Stone JG, Foex P, Sear JW, et al: Myocardial ischemia in untreated hypertensive patients: Effect of a single small oral dose of a beta-adrenergic blocking agent. Anesthesiology 1988;68(4):495-500.

63. Urban MK, Markowitz SM, Gorden MA, et al: Postoperative prophylactic administration of beta-adrenergic blockers in patients at risk for myocardial ischemia. Anesth Analg 2000;90(6):1257-1261.

64. Wallace A, Layug B, Tateo I, et al: Prophylactic atenolol reduces postoperative myocardial ischemia. McSPI Research Group. Anesthesiology 1998;88(1):7-17.

65. Zaugg M, Tagliente T, Lucchinetti E, et al: Beneficial effects from beta-adrenergic blockade in elderly patients undergoing noncardiac surgery. Anesthesiology 1999;91(6):1674-1686.

14 Treatment of Perioperative Ischemia, Infarction, and Ventricular Failure in Cardiac Surgery

Brian Lima and Carmelo A. Milano

An increasing number of high-risk patients are undergoing cardiac surgery. Despite this trend, advances in myocardial preservation, anesthesia, and perioperative care have resulted in reduced morbidity and mortality (Fig. 14-1). Positive outcomes require timely recognition and management of perioperative myocardial ischemic injury and ventricular dysfunction. These sentinel events can have disastrous consequences if mismanaged, and they are determinants of short- and long-term outcomes. This chapter discusses the etiologies of myocardial ischemia and ventricular dysfunction, as well as management that includes pharmacologic, catheter-based, and mechanical treatments.

■ PERIOPERATIVE MYOCARDIAL ISCHEMIA AND INFARCTION

Definition

Perioperative myocardial ischemia is difficult to define, as it represents a continuum with clinically irrelevant events at one end of the spectrum and myocardial infarction at the other end. The diagnosis of perioperative myocardial ischemia and/or infarction is challenging in the setting of cardiac surgery, specifically because of the elevation of cardiac enzymes that accompanies even uncomplicated procedures (Fig. 14-2).[1] Similarly, the electrocardiographic (ECG) changes that typify ischemia and infarction in the nonoperative setting may instead reflect postoperative pericardial inflammation or subclinical myocardial injury incurred during routine surgical manipulation. Therefore, accurate determination of ongoing ischemia often requires a systematic, multifaceted approach, including serial evaluation of ECG changes, biochemical markers, echocardiography, and even angiography. Importantly, early detection of perioperative ischemia may prompt therapies to relieve the ischemia and minimize the incidence of subsequent infarction.

The interpretation of ECG changes remains valuable for defining ischemia in the perioperative period. Table 14-1 summarizes various clinical entities that may lead to ST-segment changes in this setting, including myocardial ischemia and infarction.[2] After cardiac surgery, the initial electrocardiogram may be difficult to interpret because of lead placement changes related to surgical dressings, because of cardiac pacing, and because of the common presence of

conduction abnormalities. For example, right bundle branch block and first-degree atrioventricular (AV) block occur very frequently but typically resolve within the first few postoperative hours.[3]

Other ECG abnormalities in cardiac surgery patients are not uncommon findings, as noted in the Bypass Angioplasty Revascularization Investigation (BARI) study, and often portend increased cardiac mortality, especially the development of postprocedural Minnesota code Q-wave abnormalities (Table 14-2).[4] Therefore, most centers perform preprocedural and serial postprocedural electrocardiograms.[5] Electrocardiography alone, however, may lack sufficient sensitivity and specificity for the detection of myocardial ischemia. Transesophageal echocardiography (TEE), which has become a standard component of perioperative monitoring at most centers, provides a very effective adjunct to the diagnosis of myocardial ischemia and infarction. During surgical revascularization, normal wall motion indicates effective revascularization, whereas newly detected regional wall motion abnormalities usually reflect underlying ischemia or infarction.[3] These regional wall motion abnormalities can consist of akinesia or dyskinesia in a ventricular segment that was normokinetic or hypokinetic preoperatively. A study of 351 coronary artery bypass graft (CABG) patients monitored with intraoperative TEE and electrocardiography demonstrated that wall motion abnormalities detected by TEE were more common than ST-segment changes, but there was only a 17% positive concordance between the two modalities.[6] In addition, TEE was found to be twice as predictive as electrocardiography in identifying patients who ultimately met criteria for myocardial infarction.[6] These results indicate that TEE may be a more sensitive method of detecting myocardial ischemia in the perioperative setting and should probably be routinely utilized in cardiac surgery monitoring. An important observation with TEE is that new interventricular septal wall abnormalities appear to be common postprocedurally but do not appear to be associated with irreversible myocardial damage.[7]

Precise diagnostic criteria for defining perioperative myocardial ischemia have not been uniformly adopted, and thus the published incidence varies. A recent study found that 6.4% of patients undergoing CABG (N = 2052) experienced perioperative myocardial ischemia, using the following criteria: (1) an increase in the creatine kinase–to–creatine

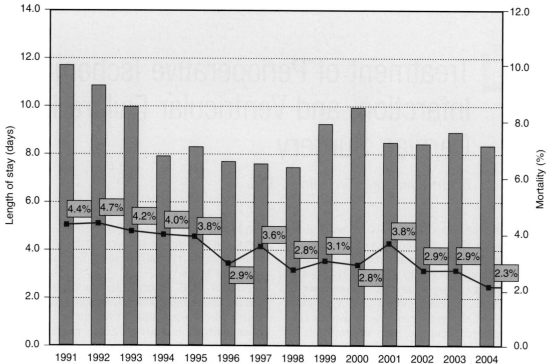

Figure 14-1 ■ Duke cardiac surgery trends in 30-day mortality and length of stay. These data from Duke University Medical Center illustrate improving trends in cardiac surgery perioperative mortality and length of hospitalization.

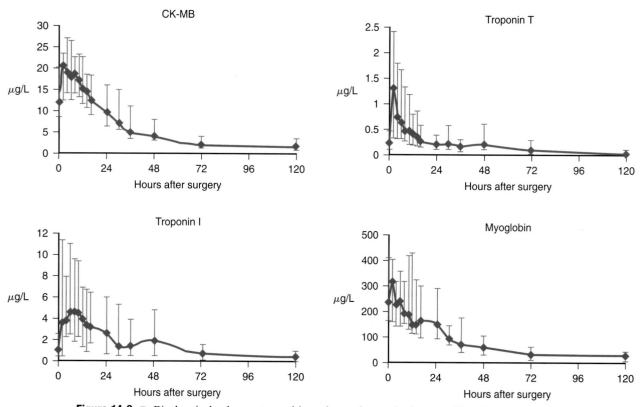

Figure 14-2 ■ Biochemical values measured in patients who received uncomplicated cardiac surgery. CK-MB, creatine kinase–MB isoenzyme. *(Redrawn from Holmvang L, Jurlander B, Rasmussen C, et al: Chest 2002;121:103-111, with permission.)*

14-1 **Conditions That Affect ST-Segment Changes**

Condition	Electrocardiographic Features
Left bundle branch block	Wide QRS complex
	ST-segment deviation
Acute pericarditis	Diffuse ST-segment elevation
	Reciprocal ST-segment depression in lead aVR, not in lead aVL
	Elevation seldom >5 mm
	PR-segment depression
Hyperkalemia	Widened QRS and tall, peaked, tented T waves
	Low-amplitude or absent P waves
	ST-segment usually downsloping
Pulmonary embolism	Changes simulating myocardial infarction, seen often in both inferior and anteroseptal leads
	Classically, right bundle branch block and S1Q3T3 pattern, right axis deviation
Cardioversion	Striking ST-segment elevation, often >10 mm, lasting only minutes immediately after direct-current shock
Myocardial ischemia	Flattened, downsloping ST-segment
	T-wave inversion
Myocardial infarction	ST-segment elevation with a plateau, shoulder, or upsloping
	Reciprocal behavior between aVL and III; progression to Q waves

Adapted from Wang K, Asinger RW, Marriott HJL: N Engl J Med 2003;349: 2128-2135.

14-2 **Incidence of New Electrocardiographic (ECG) Abnormalities among 1427 Patients after Coronary Artery Bypass Graft**

New ECG Abnormality	Incidence n (%)
Major Q wave	65 (4.6)
ST elevation	216 (15.1)
ST depression	220 (15.4)
T-wave abnormality	557 (39.0)
No ECG abnormality	557 (39.0)

From Yokoyama Y, Chaitman BR, Hardison RM, et al: Am J Cardiol 2000;86:819-824.

kinase-MB isoenzyme (CK/CK-MB) ratio of greater than 10%; (2) new onset of elevated ST-segment change of greater than 1 minute's duration and involving a shift from baseline of at least 0.1 mV and a new associated postoperative Q wave; (3) recurrent or sustained ventricular tachyarrhythmia or fibrillation; and (4) hemodynamic deterioration on inotropic support.[8] In a meta-analysis of randomized, controlled trials in patients undergoing cardiac surgery, 20 trials ($n = 1522$ patients) had a 17% overall incidence of ischemic events.[9] Ischemia was defined as ST-segment deviation on the electrocardiogram or new wall motion abnormalities on the transesophageal echocardiogram.

As with myocardial ischemia, there is considerable disagreement on the diagnostic criteria used to define perioperative myocardial infarction (PMI), which again explains discordant reports in the literature of its incidence and prognostic implications. In the same meta-analysis cited earlier, 22 trials of 1853 patients had a 5% overall incidence of PMI.[9] Across the literature, the reported rate of PMI ranges from 5% to 15%. Despite advances in cardiac surgery, this incidence does not appear to be declining.[10] The diagnosis of PMI has classically relied heavily on the development of new and persistent pathologic Q waves on an electrocardiogram, which may not always be truly representative of transmural necrosis.[11] Indeed, in an autopsy study performed on cardiac surgery patients who expired within 1 month after surgery, 23% of patients had significant transmural myocardial necrosis but no pathologic Q waves, and 20% of patients without transmural necrosis exhibited new postprocedural Q waves.[12] Reliance on the presence of Q waves alone to diagnose PMI can dangerously overlook infarctions. In a study of cardiac surgery patients, transthoracic quantitative echocardiography analysis with ECG and radionuclide ventriculography demonstrated non–Q-wave PMI to be three times more common than Q wave PMI, with equally deleterious effects on left ventricular function.[13] A recent study evaluating the clinical significance of a new Q wave after cardiac surgery suggested that patients with this pathologic ECG change, without any concomitant elevation in myocardial enzyme markers or other indicators of PMI, had uneventful outcomes.[14] These findings highlight the critical importance of combining various diagnostic modalities to define PMI.

Although Q waves do not necessarily reflect transmural necrosis, appreciation of these and other ECG changes and their linkage to adverse outcomes cannot be disregarded. New perioperative ST-segment changes (>0.1 mV) have been identified as an independent predictor of PMI, which accounts for up to 40% of preoperative CABG deaths.[15] In the Coronary Artery Surgery Study (CASS, $N = 1340$ patients), 62 patients with a new Q wave postoperatively experienced 9.7% in-hospital mortality, compared with 1.0% in the remaining 1278 patients.[16] In patients who survived to hospital discharge, the presence of new postoperative Q waves did not adversely affect 3-year survival. Among the 1427 CABG patients in the BARI trial, 5-year cardiac mortality was increased with new Q wave development (8.2% versus 3.7% for no new ECG changes; adjusted relative risk, 2.6) (Fig. 14-3).[4] Results from the GUARDIAN study of 2918 high-risk CABG patients further emphasize the negative impact of Q-wave development on survival (Table 14-3).[17] Namay and colleagues reported a 5-year survival rate of 76% in CABG patients ($n = 77$) with new Q waves compared with 90% in the unaffected CABG patients ($n = 1790$).[18]

Along with new postoperative Q-wave development, enzymatic criteria are routinely utilized to define PMI and to enhance the overall sensitivity and specificity of PMI detection.[19] In a study performed on 499 cardiac surgery patients at the Brigham and Women's Hospital, PMI occurred in 5% of patients and was designated by the following criteria: total peak CK greater than 7000 µg/L, CK-MB greater than 30 ng/mL, and new Q waves on electrocardiography.[20] In the GUARDIAN study of 2918 CABG patients, the 6-month mortality associated with a postoperative peak CK-MB of less than 5, of between 5 and 10, of between 10 and 20, and

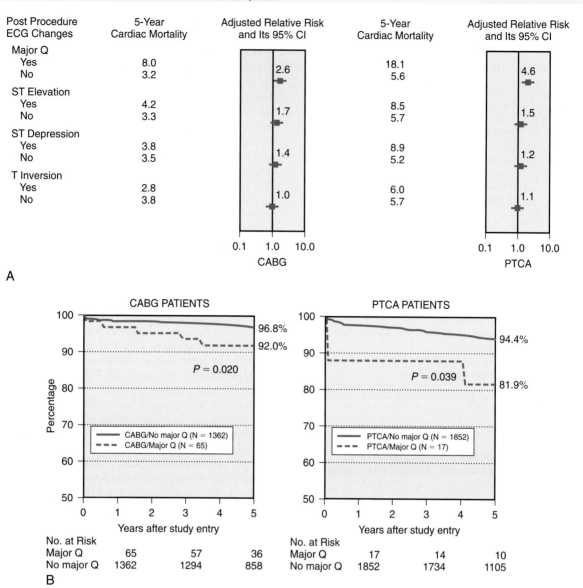

Figure 14-3 ■ **A,** Bypass Angioplasty Revascularization Investigation (BARI) randomized and registry patients' cumulative survival from cardiac mortality. Patients had undergone coronary artery bypass grafting (CABG) or percutaneous transluminal coronary angioplasty (PTCA). The development of major Q waves was associated with significantly increased long-term risk for cardiac mortality in the CABG patients (*P* = .02). **B,** Five-year Kaplan-Meier cardiac mortality and adjusted relative risk for cardiac mortality for any postprocedural electrocardiographic (ECG) changes. Cardiac mortality was significantly increased by the development of new postprocedural major Q waves regardless of the type of coronary revascularization procedure performed. In this analysis, the postprocedural ECG variables were adjusted for study group, treated diabetes, age, prior myocardial infarction, renal dysfunction, congestive heart failure, ejection fraction, body mass index, presence of class C lesions, baseline ST elevation, and baseline ST depression. CI, confidence interval. *(Redrawn from Yokoyama Y, Chaitman BR, Hardison RM, et al: Am J Cardiol 2000;86:819-824, with permission.)*

of greater than 20 times the upper limit of normal (ULN) was 3.4%, 5.8%, 7.8%, and 20.2%, respectively (Fig. 14-4).[17] This highly significant association was conserved even after adjusting for other risk factors. The Cleveland Clinic experience with 3812 CABG patients revealed that a postoperative CK-MB level 10 times ULN was independently predictive of increased mortality at 3 years (Table 14-4 and Fig. 14-5).[21] The Arterial Revascularization Therapies Study (ARTS) prospectively evaluated 496 CABG patients and also demonstrated that increased levels of CK-MB (>5 times ULN) was highly predictive of cardiac death and recurrent myocardial infarction (MI) after the postoperative period (Fig. 14-6).[22]

14-3 **Six-Month Mortality after Coronary Artery Bypass Graft Surgery: Effect of Two-Step Minnesota Code Worsening Electrocardiographic (ECG) Abnormalities**

ECG Abnormality	Frequency (%)	Dead (*n*)	Alive (*n*)	Total (*n*)	Disease Odds	Disease Odds Ratio	95% CI	Incidence (per 100)	Relative Risk	95% CI
None or one step	54.4	74	1194	1268	0.062	1.00*	—	5.84	1.00*	—
2-Step worsening T wave	23.6	18	532	550	0.034	0.55[†]	0.31-0.95	3.27	0.56[†]	0.34-0.93
2-Step worsening ST-segment elevation	14.2	11	320	331	0.034	0.55	0.27-1.09	3.32	0.57	0.31-1.06
2-Step worsening ST-segment depression	2.7	4	59	63	0.068	1.09	0.33-3.24	6.35	1.09	0.41-2.88
2-Step worsening ST-segment elevation and 2-step worsening ST-segment depression	0.4	0	10	10	0.000	0.00	—	0.00	0.00	—
2-Step worsening Q wave	4.7	12	98	110	0.122	1.98	0.98-3.90	10.91	1.87[†]	1.05-3.33

*Reference category.
[†]*P* < .05.
CI, confidence interval.
From Klatte K, Chaitman BR, Theroux P, et al. J Am Coll Cardiol 2001;38:1070-1077.

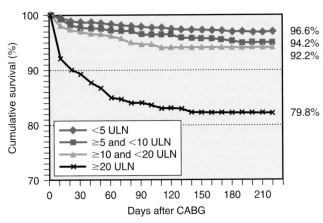

Figure 14-4 ■ Association between survival after coronary artery bypass grafting (CABG) and level of postoperative creatine kinase-MB isoenzyme (CK-MB). All pairwise comparisons between the categories were significant, except for the ≥5 and <10 upper limits of normal (ULN) group versus the ≥10 and <20 ULN group (*P* = .26). (Redrawn from Klatte K, Chaitman BR, Theroux P, et al: J Am Coll Cardiol 2001;38:1070-1077, with permission.)

14-4 **Three-Year Mortality Rates Associated with Elevation of Creatine Kinase (CK)–Isoenzyme MB after Coronary Artery Bypass Graft (CABG) Surgery**

	CABG Patients (*N* = 3812)	
CK-MB Level	**At Risk No. (%)**	**Death (%)**
≤1 × ULN	386 (10)	7.2
1-3 × ULN	1922 (50)	7.7
3-5 × ULN	853 (22)	6.3
5-10 × ULN	427 (11)	7.5
>10 × ULN	224 (6)	20.8
P (trend)	—	<.001

ULN, upper limit of normal.
From Brener SJ, Lytle BW, Schneider JP, et al: J Am Coll Cardiol 2002;40:1961-1967.

The specificity of CK and CK-MB as markers of myocardial injury is limited by the fact that these enzymes are also present in and released from skeletal muscle. Significant skeletal muscle injury and release of large quantities of CK-MB occurs during cardiac surgery.[23] An abundance of experimental evidence has emerged in the literature on the superior sensitivity and specificity of serum troponins as biochemical markers of myocardial damage and predictors of adverse outcomes.[5,7,10,23-32] Cardiac troponin isoforms I and T (cTnI, cTnT) are cardiac-specific proteins involved in regulation of muscle contraction via the tropomyosin complex.[5] No cross-reactivity with skeletal muscle isoforms has been described, and the levels of cardiac troponins do not increase in healthy subjects, even when they are exposed to strenuous muscular activity or after noncardiac operations.[27] The levels of cTnI also appear to be unaltered by renal dysfunction, and its plasma concentration decreases very slowly, allowing for retrospective detection of myocardial damage if necessary.[7,24] Interestingly, troponin levels drawn preoperatively may also enable stratification of patients into subgroups with increased risk for postoperative cardiac complications, notably PMI (Fig. 14-7).[26] Outcomes for these high-risk patients, who

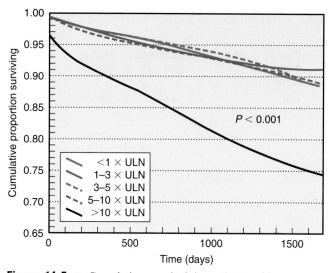

Figure 14-5 ■ Cumulative survival in patients with coronary artery bypass grafting, stratified by postoperative degree of creatine kinase-MB isoform elevation. ULN, upper limit of normal. *(Redrawn from Brener SJ, Lytle BW, Schneider JP, et al: J Am Coll Cardiol 2002;40:1961-1967, with permission.)*

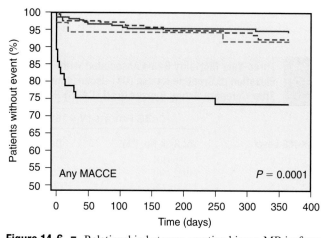

Figure 14-6 ■ Relationship between creatine kinase-MB isoform (CK-MB) levels and major postoperative complications after cardiac surgery. Kaplan-Meier curves illustrate the incidence of major adverse cardiac complications at 1-year follow-up in patients with normal CK-MB levels *(dashed blue line)*, greater than 1 to 3 times normal *(solid blue line)*, ≥3 to 5 times normal *(dashed red line)*, and >5 times normal *(solid black lines)*. MACCE, combined major cardiac death, myocardial infarction, repeat revascularization, and cerebrovascular events. *(Redrawn from Costa MA, Carere RG, Lichtenstein SV, et al: Circulation 2001;104:2689-2693, with permission.)*

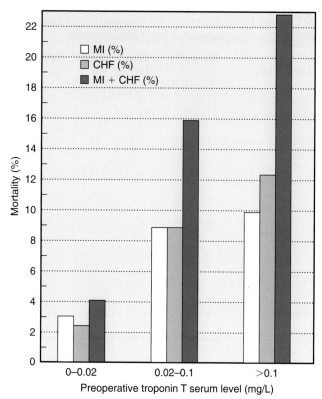

Figure 14-7 ■ Predictive value of preoperative troponin T levels and cardiac events after coronary artery bypass grafting. The positive correlation between circulating troponin T levels before the operation and the rate of postoperative myocardial infarction (MI) ($P = .03$), congestive heart failure (CHF) ($P = .0006$), and combined cardiac events (MI + CHF) ($P = .0001$) was significant. Group 2 was composed of patients with troponin T levels below the discriminator value of 0.02 μg/L. Group 1 patients had elevated troponin T values. They were divided into two subgroups: those with troponin T value between 0.02 μ/L and 0.1 μg/L, and those with values greater than 0.1 μg/L. *(Redrawn from Carrier M, Pelletier LC, Martineau R, et al: J Thorac Cardiovasc Surg 1998;115:1328-1334, with permission.)*

presumably have undetected ongoing myocardial injury, might be improved with a tailored perioperative approach that would include pharmacologic support or an intra-aortic balloon pump (IABP).

A study comparing the efficacies of cTnT and CK-MB in a series of 224 cardiac surgery patients indicated that serum cTnT concentrations greater than 1.58 ng/mL (which

represented the upper quintile) were the most powerful independent predictor of postoperative death or shock within the first 24 hours after surgery.[29] Greenson and colleagues demonstrated that stratification of cardiac surgery patients by peak cTnI levels of less than 40 and greater than 60 ng/mL was exquisitely predictive of intensive care unit length of stay, prolonged mechanical ventilation, new arrhythmia development, and especially cardiac events (Fig. 14-8).[23] Similar results were obtained in a larger series of 502 patients undergoing conventional heart surgery, where the cTnI level proved to be an independent predictor of in-hospital mortality and associated with other major postoperative complications such as PMI, ventricular arrhythmias, low cardiac output, prolonged mechanical ventilation, and acute renal failure requiring dialysis (Table 14-5).[31] The long-term prognostic value of cTnI levels has also been validated, and it is clearly associated with increased mortality, death from cardiac causes, and nonfatal cardiac events within 2 years

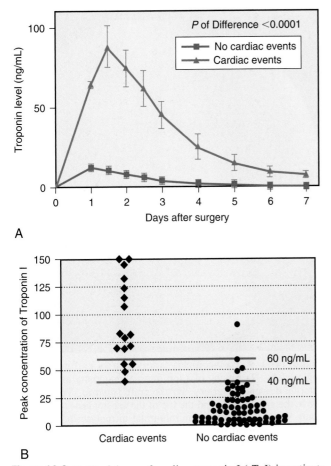

A

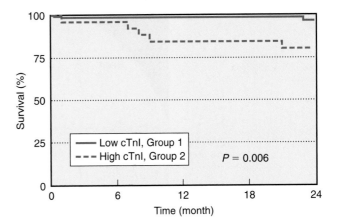

Figure 14-9 ■ Cumulative percentage of surviving patients according to elevation of cardiac troponin I (cTnI). Group 1 (*n* = 174; cTnI < 13 ng/mL, solid red line) and group 2 (*n* = 28; cTnI ≥ 13 ng/mL, dashed red line). Only one patient (in group 1) was lost on follow-up after 1 year. *P* value refers to between-group comparison (log-rank test). *(Redrawn from Fellahi JL, Gue X, Richomme X, et al: Anesthesiology 2003;99:270-274, with permission.)*

B

Figure 14-8 ■ Usefulness of cardiac troponin I (cTnI) in patients undergoing cardiac surgery. **A,** Troponin I levels after cardiac surgery. Levels of troponin I were plotted over time in patients with and without cardiac events. By use of ANOVA, *P* <.0001 between groups. **B,** Cardiac events by peak troponin level. Patients with and without cardiac events are shown with their respective peak cTnI levels. An upper level of 60 ng/mL and a lower level of 40 ng/mL are illustrated. *(Redrawn from Greenson N, Macoviak J, Krishnaswamy P, et al: Am Heart J 2001;141:447-455, with permission.)*

14-5	Cardiac Troponin I (cTnI) Concentrations and Clinical Outcome among 502 Patients	

| | cTnI CONCENTRATION* (ng/mL) | |
Complication	**With Complication (No. of Patients)**	**Without Complication (No. of Patients)**
Q-wave perioperative myocardial infarction	56.5 [43; 175.5][†] (*n* = 7)	4.2 [2.4; 7.6] (*n* = 495)
Ventricular arrhythmias	8.4 [4.2; 28.2][†] (*n* = 17)	4.3 [2.4; 8.0] (*n* = 485)
Low cardiac output	9.5 [4.4; 26.78][†] (*n* = 81)	4.3 [2.4; 7.7] (*n* = 421)
Prolonged (48-hr) mechanical ventilation	56.5 [5.2; 22.3][†] (*n* = 46)	4.5 [2.5; 8.1] (*n* = 456)
Acute renal failure requiring dialysis	18.2 [9.1; 33.5][†] (*n* = 18)	4.6 [2.5; 8.2] (*n* = 484)

*cTnI values are expressed as median [25th; 75th percentiles].
[†]*P* < .0001.
From Lasocki S, Provenchère S, Benessiano J, et al: Anesthesiology 2002;97:405-411.

after CABG (Fig. 14-9).[28] The variable cutoffs of predictive troponin values reported by different studies is concerning and may be attributed to lack of standardization of troponin detection kits by different suppliers.[24]

Etiology

During the preprocedural phase of cardiac surgery, myocardial ischemia usually represents extension of an acute coronary presentation triggered by hypertension, hypotension, hypoxia, tachycardia, bleeding, or surgical manipulation. Causes for postprocedural myocardial ischemic injury include inadequate myocardial protection during surgery, coronary graft failure, native coronary or graft spasm, extension of a preoperative infarction,[33] inadequate revascularization, coronary injury secondary to a valve procedure,[34,35] and distal coronary embolization.[36] These etiologic considerations are notorious predictors of myocardial ischemia, PMI, and other adverse outcomes in cardiac surgery. Predictors of PMI have

been defined and include advanced age, emergent procedure, previous revascularization, longer duration of cardiopulmonary bypass or aortic cross-clamp time, need for inotropic support, prior MI, and preoperative ventricular dysfunction.[20,22,37,38] Awareness of high-risk patients may increase monitoring and enable earlier intervention.

Prior to the widespread implementation of cold potassium cardioplegia and other advancements in myocardial preservation, PMI often resulted from suboptimal myocardial preservation.[37] Consistent with this etiology was the pathologic finding of contraction band necrosis, which indicated intraoperative ischemia and subsequent reperfusion

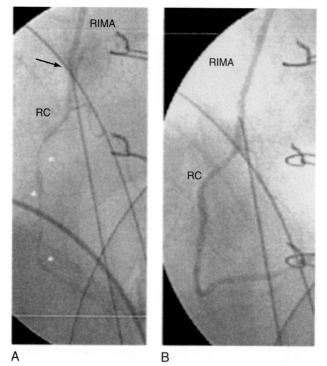

A   B

Figure 14-10 ■ Treatment of right coronary artery (RCA) spasm after coronary artery bypass grafting (CABG). **A,** Coronary artery angiogram showing a diffuse spasm of the RCA beyond the level of the anastomosis *(arrow)* with the right internal mammary artery (RIMA). **B,** RCA spasm resolution after intracoronary infusion of nitroglycerin. *(From Trimboli S, Oppido G, Santini F, Mazzucco A: Eur J Cardiothorac Surg 2003;24:830-833, with permission.)*

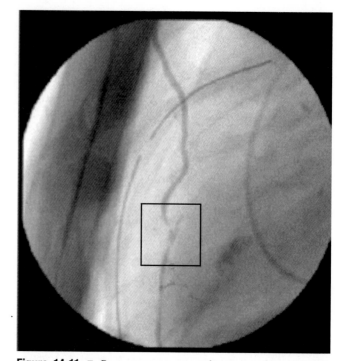

Figure 14-11 ■ Post–coronary artery bypass grafting (CABG) angiography. Narrowing of a left internal mammary artery to left anterior descending artery bypass graft *(square)*. The segment above the anastomosis and the toe of the anastomosis are stenotic. There was no response to intraluminal nitroglycerin. This graft underwent surgical revision. At revision, the upper stenosis was diagnosed to be a spasm, which had been fixed by fibrin glue. The stenosis at the toe was the result of surgical technique. After revision, an open anastomosis and perfect flow were present. *(From Bonatti J, Danzmayr M, Schachner T, Friedrich G: Eur J Cardiothorac Surg 2003;24:647-649, with permission.)*

injury.[12,37] A high percentage of infarctions analyzed from patients in these early studies were in areas supplied by patent grafts, again suggestive of injury mediated by an ischemia-reperfusion phenomenon. Improvements in techniques of myocardial preservation have reduced the incidence of perioperative myocardial ischemia and PMI.[37]

Myocardial preservation techniques have undergone significant evolution during the past decades. The implementation of cold crystalloid cardioplegia was an important early advancement that improved overall outcomes. The introduction of blood cardioplegia led to further improvements in maintaining myocardial energy stores and reducing anaerobic lactate production.[39] Clinically, the advantage of blood cardioplegia is supported in studies that show a reduction in PMI and other morbidity when directly compared with crystalloid cardioplegia.[40] The advent of retrograde delivery of cardioplegia via the coronary sinus was another important advance in myocardial protection, allowing fewer cardioplegic interruptions, perfusion to regions supplied by stenosed arteries, and enhanced cardioplegic delivery to the subendocardial region.[41]

Ischemic injury in the current era may be more frequently the result of technical issues, early graft occlusion, anastomotic stenosis,[42] graft or native coronary spasm (Figs. 14-10 to 14-12),[43-51] poor distal runoff, incomplete revascu-

larization, steal phenomena,[52] or embolization. Graft compression by mediastinal chest drains has even been described as a cause of ischemic injury (Fig. 14-13). Atheromatous embolization in the coronary microcirculation can also occur intraoperatively and lead to PMI. Potential embolic sources include atherosclerotic plaque present in the ascending aorta or major epicardial coronary arteries.[36] In the reoperative setting, mechanical disruption of atheroma in old vein grafts has also been described.[36] Retrograde cardioplegia may be protective in cases of coronary or graft embolization.

PMI caused by coronary spasm occurs with an incidence as high as 1% and involves both grafted and ungrafted vessels.[44-46] Coronary spasm can lead to sudden hemodynamic collapse and is often heralded by acute hypotension. Conventional treatment methods for perioperative hypotension, such as pressor agents, may only exacerbate the vasospastic reaction in this scenario.[44] Similarly, in patients suffering PMI associated with a hyperdynamic state, elevated circulating catecholamine levels create an environment conducive to persistent coronary spasm.[53] Mechanistically, abrupt withdrawal of preoperative calcium channel blockers can lead to rebound vasoconstriction of the native coronary

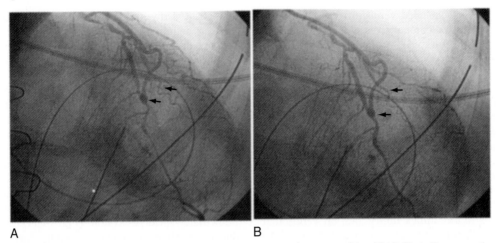

Figure 14-12 ■ Coronary artery spasm after coronary artery bypass grafting (CABG). **A,** Postoperative coronary angiogram showing the left anterior descending artery (LAD) coronary artery spasm just distal to the left internal mammary artery (LIMA) to LAD anastomosis and the first diagonal coronary artery spasm. **B,** Postoperative angiographic control after intracoronary verapamil and nitroglycerin infusion produced relief of the coronary spasm. *(From Caputo M, Nicolini F, Franciosi G, Gallotti R: Eur J Cardiothorac Surg 1999;15:545-548, with permission.)*

Figure 14-13 ■ Angiogram for perioperative myocardial infarction after coronary artery bypass grafting. **A,** The saphenous vein graft to the posterior descending artery was externally compressed by a mediastinal chest tube *(arrow)*. **B,** Obstruction was relieved by removal of tube.

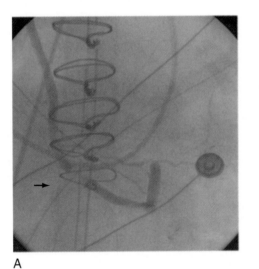
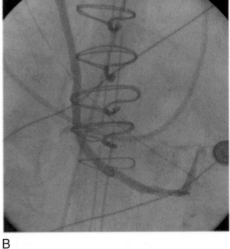

arteries and is an important factor to consider in preoperative planning.[50] Additional factors that may render cardiac surgical patients particularly susceptible to coronary vasospasm include thromboxane release caused by heparin–protamine interactions, cardiopulmonary bypass (CPB), platelet activation, anaphylactic reactions, calcium administration, and increased α-adrenergic tone from vasoconstrictor administration.[54]

Another well-described etiology related to perioperative ischemic injury is the internal mammary artery (IMA) malperfusion syndrome, caused by inadequate myocardial perfusion through the IMA graft.[55] In a series of 2326 CABG patients in which the IMA was utilized, 45 patients (1.9%) with this syndrome were identified.[55] Although the IMA is the proven conduit of choice for myocardial revascularization,[56,57] immediate flow through this arterial graft is gener-

ally less than through a saphenous vein graft and may not adequately meet myocardial demand.[55] Other factors that may precipitate this syndrome include vasospasm, kinking, or overstretching of the IMA; steal phenomena via flow diversion into major intercostal side branches[52]; and residual competitive flow from the native coronary artery.[55] As with radial artery grafts, direct mechanical manipulation of the IMA during harvesting may produce transient endothelial dysfunction and provoke a vasospastic response.[50,54]

A number of large angiographic studies have correlated clinical suspicion of myocardial ischemia or PMI with angiographic evidence of graft failure.[8,58] In a series of 2003 CABG patients, 71 (3.5%) had suspected myocardial ischemia and underwent acute re-angiography (*n* = 59) or an immediate reoperation (*n* = 12) if they were hemodynamically unstable.[58] Angiographic findings in the first group included the following: occluded vein graft(s) (32%), poor distal runoff to the grafted coronary vessel (17%), IMA stenosis (7%), IMA occlusion (5%), vein graft stenoses (5%), and IMA subclavian artery steal (3%).[58] In the immediately reoperated group, 92% of patients had graft occlusions. A more recent study including 2052 CABG patients had similar findings.[8] These studies emphasize that the majority of patients who experience myocardial ischemia or PMI following revascularization have underlying graft failure warranting angiography and either percutaneous or surgical reintervention.

Valvular procedures may lead to technical complications with a specific myocardial ischemia. The proximity of the posterior mitral annulus and the left circumflex coronary artery predisposes to circumflex injury and left ventricular (LV) lateral wall ischemia with mitral reconstruction.[34,35] An analogous situation exists for tricuspid valve surgery and the right coronary artery. Aortic valve procedures may compromise either the left main coronary or the right coronary ostia, and cases of coronary ostial thrombosis with severe ischemia have been reported. Finally, debrided valvular material may also be involved in deleterious coronary embolization.

Management

Intraoperative Preprocedural Phase

The preprocedural phase is a critical period during which appropriate clinical management can prevent myocardial ischemia and PMI. Stabilization of blood pressure and maintenance of normal sinus rhythm should be the goal. A rate–pressure product below 12,000 may minimize perioperative myocardial ischemia.[11] The importance of precise and continuous hemodynamic measurements cannot be overemphasized. It should at least include continuous monitoring of the electrocardiogram, cuff blood pressure, direct arterial pressure, central venous pressure, continuous pulse oximetry, and end-tidal CO_2.[59] Placement of a pulmonary artery (PA) catheter is warranted for high-risk patients, for example, in cases of unstable angina, ventricular hypertrophy, poor ventricular function, and combined valvular and coronary artery disease pathology.[11] The PA catheter enables continuous assessment and maintenance of cardiac filling pressures, cardiac output, and mixed venous oxygen saturation to prevent myocardial ischemia.

Pharmacotherapy with vasodilators such as intravenous nitroglycerin (NTG) may be required preoperatively for patients with unstable angina. The reduction in total ischemic burden may improve prognosis with regard to infarct progression and may prevent deterioration of left ventricular function. Intravenous NTG has also been shown to improve postinduction regional wall motion abnormalities in a prospective study of CABG patients.[60] On the basis of these results, TEE-guided NTG utilization after induction may yield a more optimal baseline echocardiogram.[60] Other important pharmacotherapies to reduce ischemia include intravenous β-blockers, with esmolol as the most titratable agent. β-blockers reduce heart rate, contractility, and blood pressure and thereby greatly reduce overall myocardial work. β-blockers also reduce the incidence of ischemic ventricular

and atrial arrhythmias. Use of intravenous NTG and β-blockers requires careful monitoring and titration, as both agents can induce hypotension; in patients with fixed coronary stenosis, reduced perfusion pressure can result in dangerous ischemia and subsequent myocardial dysfunction.

In patients with cardiogenic shock or medically refractory ischemia, preoperative stabilization with an IABP has been shown to reduce overall surgical mortality and improve outcomes in high-risk coronary patients.[61,62] IABP counterpulsation enhances myocardial perfusion via augmentation of diastolic blood pressure and redistribution of coronary blood flow toward regions of myocardial ischemia.[61] IABP provides partial LV assistance. Proper timing consists of balloon inflation just after aortic valve closure and deflation immediately prior to systole (Fig. 14-14). Balloon inflation during diastole augments coronary perfusion, whereas deflation during systole reduces afterload, decreases cardiac work (myocardial oxygen consumption), and increases stroke volume and cardiac output. Efficacy of IABP support is determined by several factors, including balloon volume, location in the aorta, rate of inflation and deflation, and, most importantly, timing relative to the cardiac cycle.[3] IABP counterpulsation is less effective in the presence of moderate or severe aortic regurgitation. Furthermore, timing may be difficult because of tachycardia or arrhythmias. Aortoiliac or femoral occlusive disease may make placement more difficult and increases the risk for limb ischemia.

Retrospective review of 4756 cases of IABP support at the Massachusetts General Hospital suggests that a 24- to 48-hour period of preoperative IABP support is preferable in unstable or postinfarction angina and enables preoperative recovery of ischemic myocardium.[62] In this study, preoperative IABP placement was associated with a lower mortality (13.6%) than intraoperative (35.7%), or postoperative (35.9%) use.[62] A prospective, randomized study was performed in 60 high-risk CABG patients to evaluate optimal timing for

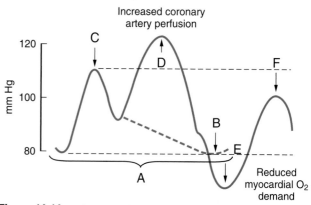

Figure 14-14 ■ Intra-aortic balloon pump (IABP) timing: synchronization with the cardiac cycle. Arterial pressure waveform with correct IABP timing. A, One complete cardiac cycle; B, unassisted aortic end-diastolic pressure; C, unassisted systolic pressure; D, diastolic augmentation; E, reduced aortic end-diastolic pressure; F, reduced assisted systolic pressure. *(Redrawn from Helman DN: In Goldstein DJ, Oz MC [eds]: Cardiac Assist Devices. Armonk, NY, Futura, 2000, p 298, with permission.)*

preoperative IABP placement.[61] In this and other studies, preoperative IABP support led to reduced CPB time, higher postoperative cardiac index, decreased incidence of postoperative low cardiac output, and a diminished period of mechanical ventilation and hospital stay.[61,63] These studies suggest the beneficial impact of preoperative IABP support in high-risk coronary patients. Preoperative risk factors that designated high-risk status in these studies included preoperative left ventricular ejection fraction (LVEF) less than 30%, unstable angina, left main coronary artery stenosis greater than 70%, diffuse coronary artery disease, and reoperative CABG.

Patients with profound preprocedural myocardial ischemia or evolving myocardial infarction probably benefit from a strategy that rapidly establishes CPB. Currently, many surgical revascularizations are performed without CPB, and for others, the initial period of conduit harvest is conducted off CPB. In unstable patients, immediate institution of CPB may dramatically reduce myocardial workload and risk for ischemic injury. Conduit harvest and further surgical preparation can be performed with the heart protected on CPB. In the setting of reoperative cardiac surgery and prior sternotomy, groin dissection and cannulation of the femoral vessels may be the safest and most rapid method to establish CPB. Aggressive utilization of mechanical unloading may help avoid ischemic ventricular arrhythmias and ventricular dysfunction, which may be difficult to reverse once established.

Intraoperative Postprocedural Phase

During the intraoperative postprocedural phase, rigorous attention to ECG pattern, hemodynamic parameters, and TEE findings must be continued. As discussed previously, the collective information obtainable with these modalities can be sensitive and specific for intraoperative myocardial ischemia and PMI. For cases of revascularization, intraoperative ischemic ECG patterns, new regional wall motion abnormalities, or hemodynamic instability requires assessment of the grafts to rule out graft failure as the cause. Assessment of graft integrity and graft patency can be readily accomplished using Doppler flow probes. These probes provide a rapid and highly sensitive method of detecting graft failure, as shown in a recent study of patients undergoing off-pump CABG.[64] In this study, flow probe results were correlated with intraoperative angiographic findings, and Doppler analysis was 100% accurate for confirming graft patency and detecting failed grafts.[64] To qualify as a normal Doppler study, the observed pattern of flow should be predominantly diastolic, with a diastolic flow velocity of greater than 15 cm/sec.[64] Additional flow parameters to consider when evaluating graft integrity include total flow, systolic flow, diastolic-to-total flow ratio, systolic peak flow, diastolic peak flow, systolic-to-diastolic peak flow index, and pulsatility index (PI, defined as difference between systolic peak flow and diastolic flow divided by mean flow).[65] The PI value should be between 1 and 5, where higher values are indicative of a graft problem.[66] When an abnormal Doppler flow study is encountered, consideration should be given to revision of the offending graft. This decision is, however, complex and ultimately relates to the surgeon's confidence in achieving a

better technical result. Small or diffusely diseased target coronary arteries predictably result in grafts with limited flow.

Perhaps one of the most common causes of postprocedural myocardial ischemia is coronary air embolization. This event is important to recognize; the right coronary artery or right coronary graft is specifically affected. Air may actually be seen within the graft, and needle aspiration of the graft can help limit the problem. The left coronary system is more dependent and infrequently involved. Profound right ventricular (RV) dysfunction can follow. TEE may show inferior LV wall myocardial air. Venting of the heart, aorta, or graft is indicated. Often, transiently raising perfusion pressure with an α-adrenergic receptor agonist alleviates the problem, presumably by forcing the obstructing air out of the major coronary arterial branches. Performing procedures under CO_2, which dissolves more readily in blood, may reduce this complication. Importantly, in the absence of continued air embolization, this ischemia should resolve rapidly, and persistent evidence for ischemia warrants consideration of other causes.

Postoperative Phase

The early postoperative phase should include careful hemodynamic and clinical monitoring. Adequate oxygen delivery and systemic blood flow must be ensured: mixed venous oxygen saturation, cardiac output, blood pressure, heart rate, urine output, acid–base status, and pulse should all be carefully monitored. The presence of myocardial ischemia may be indicated by ST-segment changes (via ECG monitoring), ventricular arrhythmia, or hemodynamic collapse. In other cases, more subtle hemodynamic changes or increased inotropic requirement may be the only clues. Many post–cardiac surgery units obtain routine postprocedural 12-lead electrocardiograms and serial serum cardiac enzyme results. Concerns for myocardial ischemia warrant echocardiography to assess LV function and regional wall motion.

Administration of calcium antagonists in the postoperative period may reduce rates of myocardial ischemia, PMI, and long-term mortality.[9,67] These agents enhance the balance between myocardial oxygen supply and demand by mediating negative chronotropy, negative inotropy, afterload reduction, and coronary vasodilation.[9] Recent studies have advocated the use of this therapy to prevent post-CABG graft vasospasm.[50] Native coronary or graft spasm should always be suspected in the setting of postoperative ischemia, and aggressive management with nitroglycerin and a sublingual calcium channel blocker should be instituted.[68] These agents are routinely recommended when radial arterial grafts have been utilized. Unfortunately, postoperative myocardial ischemia may be secondary to hypotension or low cardiac output, limiting the use of calcium channel blockers.

Postoperative ischemia or PMI accompanied by hemodynamic instability necessitates IABP placement and urgent reoperation. In more stable patients with evidence of significant myocardial ischemia, coronary angiography should be strongly considered. Early angiography can identify technical issues and guide further therapy before permanent myocardial damage has occurred.[8,58] Specifically, graft or native artery occlusions or stenoses may be identified, and angioplasty or stenting of the native vessels or new grafts can be safely achieved.[42] Similarly, angiography can identify native coronary or graft vasospasm and enables targeted intraluminal infusion of nitroglycerin or calcium channel blocker (see Figs. 14-10 to 14-12).[43-51] In cases of IMA steal phenomenon, transarterial catheter embolization to obliterate undivided vessels is another effective treatment that is feasible in the angiography suite.[52] Furthermore, specific problems may be identified angiographically that require return to the operating room for surgical revision. Important examples include incomplete revascularization and the IMA malperfusion syndrome, in which placement of an additional saphenous vein graft is widely regarded as the optimal treatment option.[55]

Recent clinical studies have evaluated other alternative pharmacotherapies to prevent ischemia-reperfusion injury and PMI in the setting of cardiac surgery. The Pexelizumab for Reduction in Infarction and Mortality in Coronary Artery Bypass Graft surgery (PRIMO-CABG) study was a randomized, double-blind, placebo-controlled prospective trial evaluating whether pexelizumab, a C5 complement inhibitor, would decrease PMI in CABG patients.[69] Therapy with this agent resulted in a significant reduction in the 30-day incidence of death or MI in 3099 patients undergoing CABG surgery with or without valve surgery.[69] Sodium–hydrogen exchange inhibition with the agent cariporide has also demonstrated promising results.[70] In a study evaluating the CABG cohort of the GUARDIAN trial, therapy with cariporide yielded a modest risk reduction in all-cause mortality and MI that was evident on postoperative day 1 and persisted at 6 months postoperatively.[70]

PERIOPERATIVE VENTRICULAR DYSFUNCTION AND FAILURE

Postoperative ventricular failure with low cardiac output state after cardiac surgery is an important predictor of perioperative mortality and sudden death (Fig. 14-15).[3,71] Even patients with normal preoperative ventricular function exhibit transient dysfunction after uneventful cardiac operations.[54] When ventricular dysfunction is encountered in the perioperative period, treatment should consist of restoring adequate oxygen delivery to prevent end-organ damage and rapid recognition and correction of the underlying cause. In addition, recognition of well-described preoperative risk factors for the development of low cardiac output syndrome may prevent its occurrence via earlier intervention and more aggressive preoperative optimization.[72-74] A retrospective review of 4558 CABG patients identified eight independent predictors of postoperative ventricular dysfunction. These risk factors included preoperative LVEF less than 20%, redo operation, emergency operation, female sex, age greater than 70, left main coronary artery stenosis, recent MI, and extensive three-vessel coronary artery disease.[73] The observed incidence of low cardiac output was 9.1% in this population, with an operative mortality of 16.9%, as opposed to 0.9% in the remaining patients with normal ventricular function.[73] In

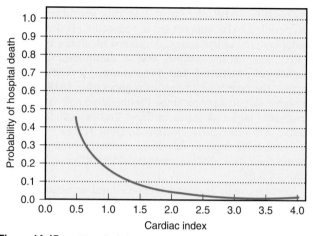

Figure 14-15 ■ Hospital death versus cardiac index. Relationship between postoperative cardiac index (L/min/m²) and probability of death for adults after mitral valve replacement. A sharp rise in hospital mortality is noted among patients with cardiac index less than 2.0. (*Redrawn from Kouchoukos NT: In Davila JC [ed]: Henry Ford Hospital International Symposium on Cardiac Surgery, ed 2. New York, Appleton-Century-Crofts, 1977, with permission.*)

another study of over 20,000 CABG patients, the incidence of low cardiac output syndrome varied from 6% with preoperative LVEF greater than 40%, to 23% in patients with LVEF less than 20%.[74] Importantly, these studies highlight that advances in therapeutic management strategies have led to a decline in mortality rates and perioperative low cardiac output states despite the increasing risk profile of cardiac surgery patients.

Failure to Wean from Cardiopulmonary Bypass

Failure to wean from CPB represents a sentinel intraoperative event in cardiac surgery and warrants independent discussion. An expeditious and properly performed cardiac procedure is the best strategy to avoid this problem. However, the process of successful weaning from CPB is complex and has many prerequisites, not just ventricular function. In general, bradycardia and absence of atrioventricular (AV) synchrony are very detrimental and must be corrected with temporary pacing wires (Figs. 14-16 and 14-17). Atrial fibrillation should be aggressively cardioverted and treated pharmacologically. Frequent premature ventricular contractions (PVCs) should be suppressed with amiodarone or lidocaine. Appropriate preload must be determined relative to preoperative filling pressures, duration of clamp time, and consideration of ventricular stiffness. Appropriate afterload provides critical coronary perfusion pressure and may be compromised by inflammatory responses to prolonged CPB. Perioperative aprotinin and systemic glucocorticoids may limit inflammatory responses and prevent vasodilation. In this setting, agents that promote vasodilation, such as NTG and milrinone, must be stopped. Consideration should include vasopressin or α-adrenergic receptor agonists.

To avoid failure to wean from CPB, a comprehensive checklist of clinical variables should be systematically evaluated prior to initiating weaning efforts. First, intraoperative

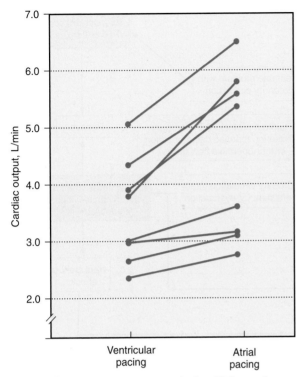

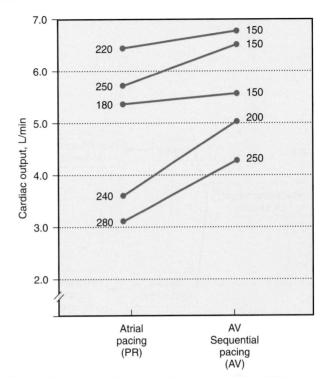

Figure 14-16 ■ Effect of atrioventricular (AV) synchrony on cardiac output after cardiac surgery. Cardiac output with ventricular pacing (without synchronous atrial systole) is compared with cardiac output with atrial pacing. An overall increase in cardiac output of approximately 26% is achieved with A-pacing and restoration of AV synchrony with left ventricular end-diastolic preload augmentation. *(Redrawn from Hartzler GO, Maloney JD, Curtis JJ, Barnhorst DA: Am J Cardiol 1977;40:232, with permission.)*

Figure 14-17 ■ Cardiac output with atrioventricular (AV) sequential versus with atrial pacing: Impact of PR interval duration. A comparison of AV sequential pacing and atrial pacing in patients with a prolonged postoperative PR interval (intrinsic and paced PR intervals are shown in milliseconds to the *left* for atrial pacing and to the *right* for AV sequential pacing). Note the uniform increase in cardiac output despite absolute differences in the shortening of the PR interval that is induced by pacing and overlap between paced PR intervals and intrinsic PR intervals between patients. *(Redrawn from Hartzler GO, Maloney JD, Curtis JJ, Barnhorst DA: Am J Cardiol 1977;40:232, with permission.)*

TEE evaluation of prosthetic valve function and ventricular wall motion, as well as Doppler flow probe analysis of bypass grafts, should be instituted. Any abnormality in body temperature, heart rate and rhythm, preload and perfusion pressures, acid–base status, electrolytes, and hematocrit must be addressed. Hyperkalemia, hypocalcemia, acidosis, hypoxia, and anemia can all profoundly depress ventricular performance and must be rapidly corrected. Surgical correction of mechanical deficiencies may be required to successfully separate from CPB. The status of RV function must also be examined given its important impact on feasibility of CPB weaning and overall outcome.[75] Nitric oxide and inodilators such as milrinone should be considered. Prophylactic initiation of inotropic support in select, high-risk patients may be advocated to enhance the likelihood of successful separation from CPB.[72]

If weaning from CPB is still unsuccessful after these optimizing measures, CPB may need to be reinitiated to allow further recovery of myocardial stunning. Although a period of ventricular rest has proved helpful in many cases, prolonged CPB and repeated failures to wean may result in worsening coagulopathy, emphasizing the importance of a timely decision to institute mechanical support. IABP placement is warranted during this rest period.[76] Refractory ventricular failure in this setting necessitates more advanced mechanical support, including extracorporeal membrane oxygenation (ECMO) or a ventricular assist device (VAD)[77]; these mechanical options should be instituted with even less hesitation if preoperative ventricular dysfunction was present (Fig. 14-18). Complete mechanical support may serve as a bridge to recovery or to transplantation, or as a destination LV assist device (LVAD) therapy. A more detailed discussion of device options for mechanical support, various inotropic agents, and other therapeutic strategies is presented later.

Postoperative Low Cardiac Output State

Assessment

General Assessment

Immediately on arrival to the intensive care unit, the cardiac surgery patient must be thoroughly evaluated in a systematic fashion. Part of this evaluation should encompass the airway and ventilation, body temperature, serum electrolyte levels, acid–base status, hemodynamics, and initial postoperative chest radiograph. Data on the nature of the procedure performed, response of the cardiovascular system to the

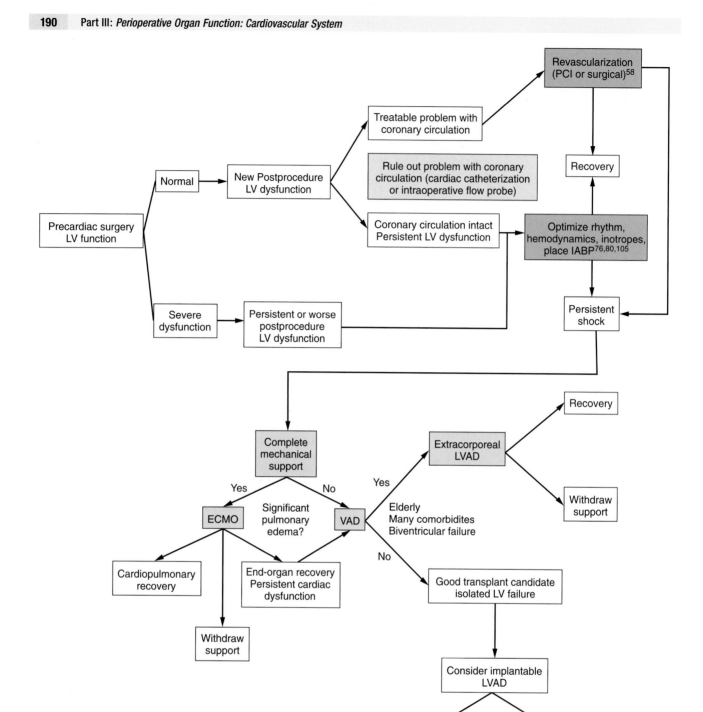

Figure 14-18 ■ Algorithm for management of patients with ventricular failure after cardiac surgery. ECMO, extracorporeal membrane oxygenation; IABP, intra-aortic balloon pump; LV, left ventricular; LVAD, left ventricular assist device; PCI, percutaneous coronary intervention; VAD, ventricular assist device.

procedure, intraoperative complications, current and preoperative medications, and patient comorbidities should be communicated to the intensive care unit (ICU) team. Adequate oxygen delivery (a function of cardiac output, hemoglobin concentration, and arterial oxygen saturation) is the top priority. Therefore, a central feature of the initial evaluation is examination of all physiologic and pathophysiologic parameters that influence the determinants of oxygen delivery and overall global cardiac function (Fig. 14-19).[54] Adequate oxygen delivery and CO_2 elimination can be confirmed via measurements of pulse oximetry, mixed venous oximetry, and arterial gas tensions.

Heart rate is a key determinant of cardiac output, and every effort is made to establish and maintain normal sinus rhythm and adequate rate in the early postoperative period. Arrhythmias may require immediate cardioversion, especially if poorly tolerated from a hemodynamic standpoint. Rhythm disturbances may also be caused by electrolyte or acid–base imbalances, hypothermia, proarrhythmic inotropic agents, or even a malpositioned PA catheter irritating the RV outflow tract.[3] As discussed previously, unexpected ECG changes, such as ST-segment deviation or Q-wave development, may very well reflect myocardial ischemia or PMI, which may also cause arrhythmias.

Despite intraoperative rewarming efforts, residual hypothermia is frequently noted in postoperative cardiac surgery patients, with core temperatures less than 35° C.[54] The characteristic decline in temperature after separation from CPB may be attributed to redistribution of heat within the body or to actual heat loss, particularly if the chest remains open for an extended period after rewarming.[54] Hypothermia impairs cardiac function, causes shivering (which dramatically increases myocardial oxygen demand), aggravates rhythm disturbances, and interferes with coagulation and platelet function, which can contribute to postoperative hemorrhage.[3,54] To limit these deleterious effects, the use of blankets and other auxiliary warming devices should be aggressively implemented.

Recognition of electrolyte and acid–base disturbances is another critical component of the assessment. Typical postoperative electrolyte abnormalities that negatively impact ventricular function include hypokalemia, hypomagnesemia, and hypocalcemia. These electrolyte deficiencies should be aggressively corrected and monitored. Similarly, arterial pH should be checked and often ranges widely in postoperative cardiac surgery patients. Deviations in pH from normal in either direction, regardless of etiology, adversely affect myocardial function and the response to inotropic agents.[78,79]

On arrival to the ICU, an immediate portable chest radiograph should be obtained. The critical items include the position of the endotracheal tube and exclusion of pneumothorax, hemothorax, or lobar collapse (Fig. 14-20). Additionally important features include width of the mediastinal silhouette and correct location of invasive catheters, radiopaque markers, sternal wires, and drainage tubes.[3]

Hemodynamic and Echocardiographic Assessment
A flow-directed PA (Swan-Ganz) catheter enables measurement of ventricular filling pressures, cardiac output, and mixed venous oxygen saturation (MVO_2). These catheters are routinely employed for high-risk cardiac surgery. There

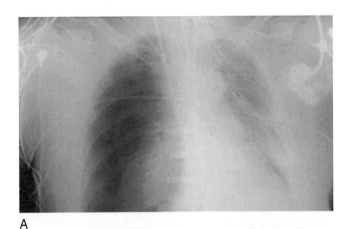

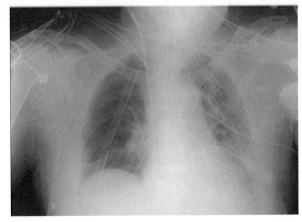

Figure 14-20 ■ Early respiratory distress in a postoperative patient on mechanical ventilation is frequently difficult to assess without emergency chest radiography. A pneumothorax, which can produce intrathoracic tension and hemodynamic compromise, must be differentiated from lobar collapse. A chest radiograph on a patient with respiratory distress early after coronary surgery shows a large right tension pneumothorax (**A**) that is readily reversed with chest tube insertion (**B**).

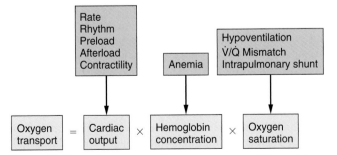

Figure 14-19 ■ Components of oxygen transport. *(Adapted from Levy JH, Michelsen L, Shanewise J, et al: In Kaplan JA, Reich DL, Konstadt SN [eds]: Cardiac Anesthesia, ed 4. Philadelphia, WB Saunders, 1999, pp 1233-1257, with permission.)*

are, however, notable limitations with hemodynamic measurements obtained via PA catheters. For example, cardiac output measurements acquired through thermodilution may be inaccurate in the setting of tricuspid regurgitation. Similarly, positive end-expiratory pressure (PEEP), a common feature of ventilatory management, may artificially elevate filling pressures. Significant mitral valve insufficiency may confound accurate assessment of capillary wedge pressure. Intracardiac shunting may negate the utility of MVO_2 measurements. Finally, malposition or improper setup of the PA catheter can lead to confusing data and inappropriate management. Therefore, although the PA catheter provides critical patient information, the clinical conditions should always be assessed and the limitations of the PA catheters understood.

After cardiac surgery, a cardiac index of at least 2.2 L/min/m² is generally deemed necessary for normal convalescence.[80] Therapeutic manipulation of heart rate and rhythm is critical to optimizing cardiac output and often requires temporary, epicardial, atrial, and ventricular pacing.[81-83] Another fundamental aspect of postoperative management is maintenance of adequate preload. Postoperative cardiac surgery patients generally exhibit relative hypovolemia and labile vascular tone as a result of spontaneous diuresis, ongoing hemorrhage, capillary leak, and vasodilation with rewarming.[84] The end result of these physiologic changes is a diminished preload, as indicated by low pulmonary capillary wedge pressure (PCWP) and central venous pressure (CVP) measurements. Volume expansion can be accomplished with administration of crystalloid or colloid intravenous fluids, or blood products. Optimal preload conditions should be individualized, but a PCWP range of 14 to 18 mm Hg has been proposed.[85] Patients with markedly hypertrophic and noncompliant left ventricles resulting from preoperative aortic stenosis may require significantly higher filling pressures to achieve adequate cardiac output.

Afterload is commonly elevated after cardiac surgery, as indicated by increased blood pressure and systemic vascular resistance (SVR >1200 dynes/sec/cm⁵). The frequency of elevation typically varies with cardiac pathology and operative procedure. The reported incidence ranges between 8% and 12% after valve replacement,[86] and between 8% and 61% after CABG.[87,88] Potential etiologies include decreased baroreceptor sensitivity,[84,89] elevated renin-angiotensin activity,[90,91] elevated catecholamine levels,[88,92,93] and postoperative pain.[94] If cardiac output remains suboptimal despite adequate preload conditions, pharmacologic afterload reduction often improves stroke volume and cardiac output. Importantly, afterload reduction in the setting of inadequate filling can have deleterious consequences, such as compensatory tachycardia or increased infarction size.[95]

Some patients exhibit a vasoplegic syndrome shortly after CPB, with very low SVRs and decreased vascular reactivity.[96] This syndrome, which is further characterized by severe hypotension and increased volume and vasopressor requirements, results from a systemic inflammatory response incited by CPB and may occur even with normal preoperative ventricular function. Given the defective release of baroreflex-mediated arginine vasopressin (AVP) that may

underlie this syndrome, management requires administration of vasoconstrictive agents to normalize afterload.[97]

Assessment of hemodynamics should not occur at a single time point. Early postoperative cardiac surgery patients display rapidly changing hemodynamics, and treatments seldom effect abrupt improvements. Therefore, multiple repeat assessments of hemodynamics are warranted. Trends should be defined and are of greater importance in dictating treatment interventions. Patience in assessing trends may lead to a better understanding of overall physiology.

If postoperative low cardiac output state persists and fails to respond to standard manipulation of heart rate, preload, and afterload, echocardiography may provide supplemental information, such as the status of ventricular filling, the nature of ventricular dysfunction (global, segmental, right or left), and whether there is any evidence of external compression. When abnormal ECG readings or cardiac enzyme levels suggest ischemia or PMI, echocardiography can confirm wall motion abnormalities and guide further therapy. For patients who have undergone valve surgery, low cardiac output state or heart failure symptoms warrant echocardiography to exclude perivalvular leak or disruption of the repair. Specifically for cases of mitral valve repair, systolic anterior motion of the valve and dynamic LV outflow obstruction can occur and is best diagnosed with echocardiography.

Echocardiography can provide valuable additional data to help elucidate the diagnosis of cardiac tamponade.[98] In patients with circumferential pericardial effusion, echocardiography frequently reveals RV diastolic collapse, right atrial collapse, and left atrial collapse, which are useful signs of cardiac tamponade.[99] Recent evidence suggests that early diastolic invagination of the LV free wall and LV diastolic collapse may be a particularly useful echocardiographic finding to aid in the diagnosis of tamponade.[100] Compressive hematomas may selectively affect the superior or inferior vena cava or pulmonary veins, leading to tamponade, and this can often be identified with transthoracic or transesophageal echocardiography.

Cardiac tamponade is caused by accumulation of fluid or clotted blood in the mediastinum, thereby restricting diastolic filling of the ventricles. Studies indicate that it can occur acutely in 3% to 6% of post–cardiac surgery patients.[101-103] The characteristic signs of acute postoperative cardiac tamponade include (1) increased variation in blood pressure with respiration (pulsus paradoxus)[3]; (2) equalization and elevation of CVP, PA diastolic pressure, and left atrial pressure or PCWP[104]; (3) decreased urine output; (4) excessive chest tube drainage or, conversely, sudden cessation of chest tube drainage, when heavy clots obstruct the chest tubes; (5) mediastinal widening on chest radiograph; (6) low cardiac output (late); and (7) hypotension (late). Tamponade is definitively diagnosed and managed with urgent surgical exploration and hematoma evacuation. Temporizing measures include volume loading, inotropic support, and reduction of airway pressure (elimination of PEEP, anesthetic agents, and decreasing tidal volume with increasing ventilatory rate).[3] Although many tests can suggest the diagnosis of cardiac tamponade, there is no single definitive study and the diagnosis remains a clinical judgment. Because this condition is readily treatable, a strategy of aggressive reexploration should be advocated; reexploration in the operating room is definitive and when tamponade is not present, there is little risk to the patient. Persistent treatment of tamponade with transfusion or inotropes can lead to circulatory collapse, cardiac arrest, and precarious wound reopening in an ICU setting. Delayed reexploration is a failure of clinical judgment and can result in loss of the patient.

Management Strategies for Postoperative Low Cardiac Output

Optimization of Cardiac Rate and Rhythm

The first hemodynamic parameters to be addressed in the management of postoperative low cardiac output are heart rate and rhythm. Maintenance of normal sinus rhythm cannot be overemphasized. When sinus rhythm is achieved, the optimal rate for most patients is between 80 and 100 beats/min.[105] AV synchrony provides end-diastolic preload augmentation and can increase cardiac output by 25% (see Fig. 14-16).[106] Heart rate disturbances are common after cardiac surgery and include sinus bradycardia, junctional rhythm, and 1st-, 2nd-, or 3rd-degree heart block. These disturbances are usually temporary and may be secondary to perioperative β-blockade, or to metabolic derangements from cardioplegic arrest.[107,108] Ischemia of the conduction system caused by inadequate myocardial protection, or permanent injury to the conduction system caused by direct surgical trauma are other possible etiologies.[108,109]

Management of heart rate disturbances must be individualized for each patient and commonly incorporates usage of temporary pacing wires placed intraoperatively. If temporary epicardial pacing is not available, alternatives include transvenous or transthoracic pacing, or pharmacologic treatments for bradyarrhythmias (e.g., isoproterenol or atropine).[110] For sinus bradycardia or junctional arrhythmias, simple atrial pacing (range, 90 to 110 beats/min) is appropriate. Conversely, AV nodal blocks are treated with atrioventricular pacing.[111] With this strategy, the optimal AV interval depends

on the chosen heart rate (see Fig. 14-17). It is important to note that normalization of AV synchrony with these strategies leads to a loss of normal ventricular activation sequence and consequent depression of ventricular function by 10% to 15% for a given preload and afterload. Therefore, careful adjustments of heart rate selection must be correlated with cardiac output measurements to determine the optimal settings. Slower heart rate settings may be preferred in patients with dynamic LV outflow obstruction. In these cases, rapid heart rate prevents ventricular filling and accentuates outflow tract obstruction.

Preload and Afterload

Therapeutic measures to optimize preload conditions were discussed previously. Vasodilatory shock, a state of severely depressed afterload, is often effectively managed with arginine vasopressin.[97] However, elevated afterload should be pharmacologically reduced if cardiac output remains suboptimal despite adequate volume loading. The extent to which afterload reduction improves stroke volume is dependent on the end-systolic pressure–volume relationship of each patient. In patients with mitral[112,113] and aortic insufficiency[114], afterload reduction may be more important to enhance forward ejection. NTG and sodium nitroprusside (SNP) are the most frequently utilized pharmacologic agents for afterload reduction. SNP may exacerbate postoperative myocardial ischemia by causing significant intracoronary shunt.[115] Nevertheless, SNP remains the preferred agent for treatment of postoperative hypertension.[112,116,117] NTG is frequently used after CABG surgery because of its favorable effects of improving coronary collateral flow and prevention of coronary spasm.[115,118]

Inotropic State

Postoperative myocardial dysfunction may require inotropic support when measures to optimize heart rate, rhythm, hemoglobin concentration, preload, and afterload have been exhausted. Use of inotropic agents to improve cardiac function must be carefully tempered because of resultant increases in myocardial oxygen consumption. Table 14-6 summarizes

14-6	Pharmacologic Agents for Ventricular Failure after Cardiac Surgery								
		AR Activation			Physiologic Response				
Drug	Dose (μg/kg/min)	α_1	β_1	β_2	SVR	MAP	CO	HR	PAWP
Dopamine	<5	−	++	−	↔	↑	↑	↑	↔
	>5	++	++	−	↑↑	↑↑	↑	↑	↑
Dobutamine	2-20	−	++	+	↓	↑	↑	↑	↓
Epinephrine	<0.05	−	++	+	↓	↑	↑	↑	↓
	>0.05	++	++	+	↑↑	↑↑	↑	↑	↑
Norepinephrine	0.03-1.0	++	+	−	↑↑	↑↑	↔	↑	↑
Phenylephrine	0.6-2.0	++	−	−	↑↑	↑↑	↓	↔	↑
Isoproterenol	0.03-0.15	−	++	++	↓	↔	↑	↑↑	↓
Milrinone	0.3-1.5	—	PDEI	—	↓	↑	↑	↔	↓
Amrinone	5-20	—	PDEI	—	↓	↑	↑	↔	↓
Vasopressin	0.01-0.1*	—	—	—	↑↑	↑↑	↓	↔	↑

*Dosage in U/min.

α_1, Peripheral vasculature; β_1, myocardium; β_2, peripheral vasculature and myocardium; AR, adrenergic receptor activation; CO, cardiac output; HR, heart rate; MAP, mean arterial pressure; PAWP, pulmonary artery wedge pressure; PDEI, phosphodiesterase inhibitor; SVR, systemic vascular resistance.

currently available inotropic agents for pharmacologic support of cardiac function. Inotropic agents are generally administered by continuous infusion through a central venous catheter. The majority of inotropic agents function as β-adrenergic agonists, leading to an increase in intracellular cAMP and calcium concentration.[119] These β-adrenergic agonist agents are also classically associated with proarrhythmic effects and should be used cautiously. Moreover, many inotropes (e.g., dopamine, epinephrine, and norepinephrine) also possess prominent α-adrenergic agonism and at high doses can induce dangerous vasoconstrictive effects, leading to limb, mesenteric, or renal ischemic injury. Nonadrenergic inotropes, such as phosphodiesterase inhibitors (e.g., amrinone, milrinone), can be particularly effective in the management of right heart dysfunction. Combinations of milrinone and β-adrenergic receptor agonists may have synergistic effects on improving myocardial function.

Intra-aortic Balloon Pump

When conventional measures fail to achieve acceptable hemodynamics, mechanical circulatory assist devices should be considered.[120-122] After cardiac surgery, significant ventricular dysfunction requiring mechanical assistance occurs in less than 5% of patients.[77,123] Most of these patients (60% to 90%) can be stabilized with an IABP, and only a small percentage (0.2% to 1%) require more advanced circulatory assist devices such as centrifugal or pneumatic ventricular assist devices.[77,123] The objective for mechanical circulatory assistance in postoperative cardiac surgical patients is to provide adequate circulation and to diminish myocardial work, thus allowing recovery of stunned myocardium.

IABP represents the most frequently employed system for left ventricular mechanical support, with an estimated 100,000 patients being supported annually.[124] The most common design consists of a sheath that is percutaneously placed into the common femoral artery employing a guidewire and a series of dilators. Sheathless introduction has been advocated to reduce vascular complications in smaller patients.[125] The balloon catheter has a central lumen for arterial pressure monitoring and a side lumen for helium gas shuttling; the typical balloon volume is 40 mL, and diameters are 8 to 9.5 F. The balloon catheter is positioned in the descending thoracic aorta, just distal to the left subclavian artery. Appropriate positioning must be confirmed with fluoroscopy or echocardiography.[126] Severe aortoiliac atherosclerotic disease may prevent safe placement by the percutaneous femoral approach. The presence of aneurysmal disease of the aorta or the iliac vessels or the presence of an aortofemoral prosthetic graft increase the risks of femoral placement, but successful IABP placement is still feasible in both of these settings. If femoral placement is not possible, IABP can be placed via the ascending aorta, typically with the balloon placed through a polytetrafluoroethylene (PTFE) or vein graft that is sewn to the aorta. This technique prevents bleeding and enables the device to be well secured. Removal of the IABP from the ascending aorta usually requires that the patient return to the operating room for open removal. Finally, the presence of moderate or severe aortic insufficiency represents a relative contraindication, as aortic counterpulsation is ineffective.

Once IABP is properly positioned, the operator must make several selections on the console. The balloon inflation may be triggered in one of three ways: by the arterial pressure, the R wave of the electrocardiogram, or the pacing spike from an artificial pacemaker. Most commonly, the R wave trigger is most efficient. However, if the patient has frequent arrhythmias, such as PVCs or atrial fibrillation, the arterial pressure may provide a better trigger. The operator also selects whether the balloon counterpulsation will occur with each cardiac cycle (1:1) or with every other or every third cycle (1:2 or 1:3). Generally, 1:1 support is utilized initially, and 1:2 or 1:3 is reserved for when the device is weaned. With frequent arrhythmias or heart rates greater than 120 beats/min, 1:2 support may be more efficient. The most important setting, however, is the timing of balloon inflation and deflation relative to the cardiac cycle. Balloon inflation should begin during early diastole, just beyond the dicrotic notch (closure of the aortic valve). Balloon deflation should end just prior to systole and effect a reduction in diastolic pressure. Proper inflation serves to increase coronary perfusion, and properly timed deflation reduces LV afterload and oxygen consumption (see Fig. 14-14).

Typically, efforts to wean the IABP should proceed cautiously and only after patients are first weaned from significant inotropic support. Patients are frequently treated with significant volume to support hemodynamics and should be aggressively diuresed prior to removal of the device. During weaning of IABP support, MVO$_2$ saturations, cardiac output, and ventricular filling pressures should be carefully monitored. A slight decline in hemodynamics may be anticipated, but significant decreases in cardiac output or mixed venous saturations or large rises in filling pressures indicate that ventricular function is not sufficiently recovered. Development of ventricular or atrial arrhythmias is another indicator that IABP support should not be discontinued.

Postoperative IABP placement does not require immediate anticoagulation. Patients who require postoperative IABP support for more than 48 to 72 hours are generally anticoagulated with heparin, given as a continuous infusion without a bolus dose. Low-molecular-weight dextran has also been used for anticoagulation during the early postoperative period. Failure to anticoagulate patients who have IABP for an extended period may increase the risk for vascular complications. Vascular complications represent the most frequent serious morbidity associated with IABP, occurring in 9% to 36% of cases.[127] These problems range from simple hematoma or false aneurysm to more serious limb ischemia. With femoral IABP, pedal pulses or Doppler signals should be monitored every 2 hours. If pedal Doppler signals cannot be appreciated in the ipsilateral limb, withdrawal of the introducer may occasionally result in return of significant limb perfusion. However, if pedal Doppler signals remain absent, the safest approach is to remove the pump and place a new device in the contralateral femoral artery. If removal of the IABP fails to restore perfusion to the limb, surgical exploration of the femoral artery is warranted with Fogarty catheter embolectomy and arterial repair. If arterial inflow has been lost, femoral–femoral bypass may be performed.

Another well-recognized complication is that of balloon rupture, with a reported rate of 0.5% to 6%.[124] It is heralded by blood in the balloon catheter, and important sequelae include helium gas embolization, infection, and loss of ventricular assistance. The IABP should be removed as soon as possible when this is diagnosed.

Extracorporeal Membrane Oxygenation

ECMO constitutes a temporary method to provide complete cardiac and pulmonary support. Initial experience with ECMO for postcardiotomy cardiogenic shock reported poor survival (25%),[128] but survival has gradually improved to 40% with technical advances in circuit design.[129] A typical ECMO circuit consists of cannulae for drainage and inflow, a centrifugal vortex pump, a membrane oxygenator, and a heat exchanger. The unit is constructed with either a venovenous configuration or, more commonly, a venoarterial configuration; the former provides solely pulmonary support, whereas the latter provides both cardiac and pulmonary support. Cannulation for ECMO may be performed centrally, utilizing the aorta and right atrium for venoarterial support, or peripherally via the femoral artery and vein.

The ECMO circuit has many of the limitations of the centrifugal vortex pumps. Indications for ECMO at our institution consist mainly of primary pulmonary dysfunction—for example, primary graft failure following lung transplant. Other institutions have broadened applications to include cardiogenic shock after cardiac surgery and as a bridge to implantable LVAD.[130-132] In general, patients who do best require only short periods of support (24 to 48 hours). For patients who require longer times, organ recovery is slower and survival is poor. Complications associated with ECMO are common and include leg ischemia, renal failure, hemorrhage, and oxygenator failure.[120] Additional limitations associated with ECMO include inability to unload the left ventricle and the need for a perfusionist to be continuously present throughout its use.[105]

Ventricular Assist Devices

The decision to proceed to VAD support is of critical importance. Because of inexperience with these devices, this decision is often delayed. For example, a patient may be supported on very high doses of epinephrine or norepinephrine (>0.1 µg/kg/min) for many hours with inadequate hemodynamics. In these scenarios, renal or mesenteric injury may occur, or the patient may suffer cardiac arrest. Therefore, a timely decision for VAD support remains an important determinant of positive outcomes. In general, high-dose inotropes and IABP should be attempted first. Most patients show hemodynamic stabilization or gradual improvement. If the patient fails to stabilize or improve within hours, the treatment team should proceed rapidly to VAD. Waiting for more advanced deterioration with oliguria, acidosis, or arrhythmias is a common error, and it prevents successful outcomes.

Choosing the most appropriate type of VAD for the patient with postoperative ventricular failure is complex. Table 14-7 provides a summary of available VADs. The advantages of extracorporeal devices include (1) ease of implantation, (2) capability of being weaned, (3) ease of removal, and (4) the possibility of providing biventricular support (both RV assist device [RVAD] and LVAD). On the other hand, the intracorporeal or implantable LVAD systems (HeartMate and Novacor) have the following advantages: (1) they provide greater mobility and enable discharge from ICU or hospital; (2) they have greater durability and can support patients for months or years; and (3) they are approved as

| **14-7** | **Examples of Mechanical Assistance for Ventricular Failure** |

Device	Pump Design	Indications
Temporary Extracorporeal Support		
Extracorporeal membrane oxygenation	Centrifugal	Cardiopulmonary failure, bridge to recovery
BioMedicus Levitronix CentriMag	Centrifugal	Postcardiotomy ventricular dysfunction, bridge to recovery
Abiomed BVS 5000 Abiomed AB 5000	Pulsatile	Postcardiotomy ventricular dysfunction, bridge to recovery
Thoratec paracorporeal ventricular assist device (VAD)	Pulsatile	Postcardiotomy ventricular dysfunction, bridge to transplantation, bridge to recovery
Implantable Chronic Support		
Thoratec HeartMate Novacor N1000PC	Pulsatile	Bridge to transplantation, destination therapy
Thoratec Intracorporeal VAD	Pulsatile	Bridge to recovery, bridge to transplant
Debakey-VAD HeartMate II Jarvik 2000	Axial flow	Bridge to transplant
Lionheart LVD-2000	Totally implantable pulsatile LVAD	Destination therapy
CardioWest Total Artificial Heart Abiocor	Total artifical heart	Biventricular failure, bridge to transplant, destination therapy

bridges to transplant or destination therapy. Therefore, the extracorporeal devices are more appropriate for patients who are likely to require only short-term support and may experience ventricular recovery. They are also more appropriate for patients who need biventricular support. The implantable device would be the better choice if ventricular recovery is unlikely and the patient is an appropriate candidate for transplantation. Detailed descriptions of specific types of extracorporeal and implantable VADs follow.

One of the first extracorporeal pumps utilized for postoperative support was the centrifugal vortex pump.[133] This device is familiar to cardiac surgeons and perfusionists, as it is commonly utilized in standard CPB circuits. Several commercially centrifugal pumps are available, all of which display pump head velocity (in RPMs) as well as flow. The operator typically is able to increase the RPMs to achieve progressively higher pump flow. In general, the RPMs are set as low as possible to achieve a flow greater than 2.0 L/min/ m^2; this approach limits the hemolysis that can occur at higher RPMs. Ultimately, flow with this system depends on cannula size and placement, preload, and the RPM setting. With this type of support, ventricular filling pressures are monitored and kept within normal physiologic range with infusions of colloid or blood products.

These pumps require early anticoagulation with heparin to prevent thrombus formation in the pump head. The goal of anticoagulation is typically an activated clotting time (ACT) of 180 to 200 seconds, or a partial prothrombin time (PTT) of approximately 80 seconds. Anticoagulation must be balanced against postoperative bleeding and coagulopathy, which are typically a problem in these patients. Most surgeons delay anticoagulation until postoperative bleeding has fallen below 100 mL of chest tube drainage per hour. Centrifugal pumps unfortunately are not designed for long-term support; mechanical failure is frequent and should be anticipated. Seal disruption within the pump head allows fluid accumulation in the magnet chamber and can interfere with pumping.[134] Periodic inspection of the pumps is required, with exchange as needed. Patients supported with centrifugal pumps are typically sedated and mechanically ventilated. These devices do not serve as effective bridges to transplantation, and if prolonged support is required, exchange for an implantable LVAD is needed. Newer designs for centrifugal vortex pumps, such as the Levitronix CentriMag pump, are bearingless and may offer greater durability.

A more popular extracorporeal device for temporary mechanical support is the Abiomed BVS 5000 (Abiomed Cardiovascular, Inc., Danvers, Mass) (Fig. 14-21). The device was approved by the U.S. Food and Drug Administration (FDA) in 1992 for post–cardiac surgery ventricular support.[135] This pump consists of two chambers, an upper chamber that fills passively, employing gravity for venous drainage, and a lower one that is a pneumatically driven pump, isolated by mechanical valves providing unidirectional flow. The console is connected to the pump via pneumatic tubing and can provide right or left ventricular support, or both. The pump relies on gravity drainage and is typically placed at the bedside below the level of the patient and connected to the patient via $\frac{1}{2}$-inch blood-tubing. Unlike the centrifugal

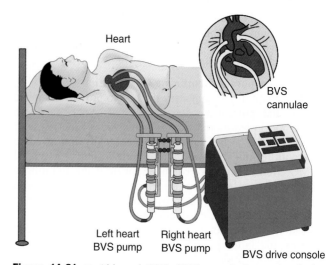

Figure 14-21 ■ Abiomed BVS 5000 ventricular assist device (VAD). A left and right heart assist device is shown at the bedside. The RVAD utilizes right atrial and pulmonary artery cannulation. The LVAD utilizes left atrial and aortic cannulation. The blood pumps are pneumatically driven; pneumatic drivelines connect the pumps to the console. *(From Jett GK: In Goldstein DJ, Oz MC [eds]: Cardiac Assist Devices. Armonk, NY, Futura, 2000, p 236, with permission.)*

pumps, the Abiomed device provides pulsatile perfusion. Furthermore, the Abiomed pump has greater durability, and associated mechanical failure is rare. Limitations include the need for anticoagulation with heparin or Coumadin. After postoperative hemorrhage has stopped, a heparin infusion is begun and gradually titrated to achieve an ACT of 180 to 200 seconds or a PTT of approximately 80 seconds. Thromboembolism, unfortunately, is an important limitation, with thrombus forming commonly on the valve housing. Patients can be extubated and occasionally can ambulate with the device, but full physical rehabilitation is limited by the blood tubing and the sheer size of the console. Most patients supported with this device remain intubated. Decreased device flow is most commonly related to reduced preload, but other conditions, such as cardiac tamponade and malposition of drainage cannula, occasionally manifest as reduced device flow. Relative to centrifugal pumps, the BVS 5000 enables a greater duration of support with improved overall outcomes.[136]

Recently, the Abiomed AB 5000 was introduced for short-term support. It consists of a paracorporeal device that is also pneumatically driven. The AB 5000 pump is compatible with the BVS 5000 cannulae, eliminates extensive blood-tubing, and provides assisted drainage; it is more mobile and less thrombogenic, and it may provide safer long-term support. Both the BVS 5000 and AB 5000 devices have a "weaning" mode that enables controlled reduction of support, so that native ventricular function can be assessed for recovery.

The Thoratec ventricular assist device (Thoratec Laboratories, Corp., Pleasanton, Calif) is another extracorporeal pump that provides left, right, or biventricular support. It consists of four components: a console, an inflow cannula,

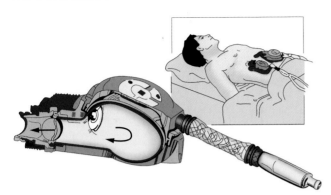

Figure 14-22 ■ Thoratec blood pump (Thoratec Laboratories Corp., Pleasanton, Calif). A patient is shown with a right and left ventricular assist device in place. The cannulae exit in the subcostal region and the pumps lie on the abdomen. The flexible blood sack is isolated by an inflow and outflow valve. The flexible diaphragm separates the blood sack from compressed air used to drive the device. *(Pennington DG: In Goldstein DJ, Oz MC [eds]: Cardiac Assist Devices. Armonk, NY, Futura, 2000, p 252, with permission.)*

an outflow cannula, and the pump. The pump has a flexible blood sack within a rigid outer casing; alternating positive and negative pressure is applied to the outer unit and thereby actuates the flexible blood sack (Fig. 14-22). Two mechanical valves are placed between the cannulae and the pump, enabling unidirectional flow. The Thoratec pump is relatively small and attached directly to the cannulae, which exit the body in the subcostal region. Furthermore, the Thoratec employs active vacuum-assisted drainage and typically lies on the patient's abdomen or flank. The device is termed the PVAD, acknowledging its paracorporeal location; extensive blood-tubing is not part of the design. Given these design advantages, the Thoratec PVAD can serve as a bridge to recovery but may support patients for months serving also as a bridge to transplantation.

The Thoratec device has three modes of operation, but it is operated most frequently in an automatic mode in which the pump ejects when filling is sensed. In this mode, a backup device rate is set; in addition, pneumatic pressures for ejection and vacuum for filling are set by the operator. Finally, the pump should be routinely inspected to ensure complete emptying, as this is important in reducing thromboembolic sequelae.

After the implantation of an extracorporeal VAD device, there are several important patient management goals. First, bleeding must be controlled so that patients may be properly anticoagulated to prevent thromboembolism. The cessation of postoperative bleeding and achieving appropriate anticoagulation is critical to positive outcomes. Initially, these devices should provide complete ventricular unloading, and inotropes should be aggressively weaned off. End-organ function must be monitored and supported: diuresis should be stimulated to clear any pulmonary edema. Patients may require periods of continuous hemodialysis if renal function is severely impaired. Neurologic function is assessed on a daily basis. Echocardiography and weaning efforts may be

initiated as early as 3 days after implantation, but some patients may require weeks of support before ventricular recovery occurs.

Implantable LVADs (see Table 14-7) have received FDA approval as bridges to transplantation. These pumps have an electrically powered, pusher plate design and are implanted in the left upper quadrant under the rectus muscle. Size restraints limit these devices to patients with a body surface area greater than 1.5 m^2.[120] The electrical drive line is tunneled out of the right lower quadrant and is the only component exiting the body. These devices receive drainage from a cannula placed in the LV apex; outflow is via a graft to the ascending aorta. The devices can usually operate in fixed-rate mode or in an automatic mode in which filling triggers activation of the pump.

Implantable LVADs have the major advantage of allowing complete physical recovery. Patients with these devices are extubated, resume ambulation rapidly, and may be successfully discharged to home. Some patients have even returned to work with these devices while they await heart transplantation. Typically, as patients increase their activity, their devices can be powered by light battery packs that can be carried (Fig. 14-23). Finally, the HeartMate (Thoratec Laboratories Corp.) LVAD has the additional advantage of a special textured surface that enables bio-ingrowth with reduced need for anticoagulation. Historically, thromboembolic events affected up to 20% of LVAD patients. However, a multicenter study reported a thromboembolic rate of 0.01 events per patient-month of device use for 223 HeartMate patients, over 531 patient-months.[137,138] HeartMate patients require only aspirin anticoagulation, whch has simplified their management and raised hope that these devices may serve as primary therapies for patients with end-stage heart failure (Fig. 14-24).[139]

Important limitations still exist with implantable LVADs. Postoperative bleeding is typically increased relative to routine cardiac cases. Infection, which can involve the drive line, pocket, or blood-contacting surfaces, represents the most important morbidity. Prophylactic antibiotic and antifungal therapy is recommended until all invasive lines and drains are removed. Importantly, implantable LVADs do not address the difficult problem of right-sided dysfunction, and approximately 5% to 20% of patients require treatment for RV dysfunction, ranging from inotropic support to placement of an extracorporeal RVAD.[75,120]

A common problem with implantable LVADs during the early postoperative period is reduced LVAD flows. The differential diagnosis is important and most commonly includes hypovolemia and cardiac tamponade. Measurements of filling pressures can be helpful, as they are typically elevated with tamponade but reduced with hypovolemia. Other important considerations in the setting of low LVAD flow include tension pneumothorax, RV dysfunction, arrhythmias, and malposition of the device inflow cannula; echocardiography is often helpful in these diagnoses.

In contrast to the current generation of implantable VADs that produce pulsatile cardiac support, a second generation of implantable devices provides continuous flow. These axial flow devices (Fig. 14-25) are smaller, quieter, and

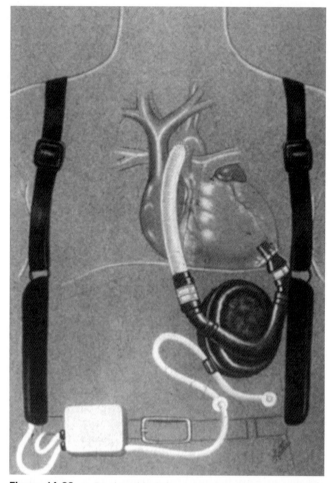

Figure 14-23 ■ Implantable left ventricular (LV) assist device. The Heartmate device (Thermo Cardiosystems Inc., Woburn, Mass) is illustrated. Inflow to the device arises from LV apical cannulation; outflow from the device is via a Dacron graft sewn to the ascending aorta. An electrical driveline exits the patient's abdomen and is attached to a system controller that is in turn attached to two portable battery units. *(Goldstein DJ: In Goldstein DJ, Oz MC [eds]: Cardiac Assist Devices. Armonk, NY, Futura, 2000, p 310, with permission.)*

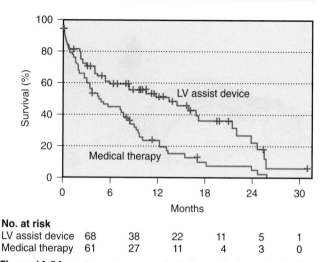

No. at risk

LV assist device	68	38	22	11	5	1
Medical therapy	61	27	11	4	3	0

Figure 14-24 ■ Long-term use of a left ventricular assist device (LVAD) for end-stage heart failure. Improved survival among patients with heart failure randomized to treatment with implantable LVADs or best medical therapies. All patients had advanced heart failure and were not candidates for heart transplantation. *(Redrawn from Rose EA, Gelijns AC, Moskowitz AJ, et al: N Engl J Med 2001;345:1435-1443, with permission.)*

perhaps more power-efficient than pulsatile flow pumps. Trials performed with these pumps suggest these axial flow pumps can provide months of adequate circulatory support and serve as bridges to cardiac transplantation.[140,141] Cardiac output in these devices is dictated by the rotational speed of the pump, which is typically attached to the LV apex with an outflow graft to the ascending or descending aorta.

Perioperative Right Ventricular Dysfunction

Etiology

Perioperative low cardiac output syndromes are usually attributed to LV or biventricular impairment, but occasional patients display isolated RV dysfunction. The incidence of postcardiotomy acute refractory RV failure has a reported range of 0.04% to 0.1%, but RV dysfunction also occurs in 2% to 3% of postoperative heart transplant patients and

nearly 20% to 30% of LVAD recipients.[75] Postoperative RV dysfunction may arise even when preoperative RV function was normal.[142] However, preoperative functional impairment of the RV could be predictive of more severe RV dysfunction postoperatively.[143] In the perioperative setting, abnormalities of RV performance can be related to LV dysfunction, RV ischemia or infarction, inadequate myocardial protection, increased pulmonary vascular resistance (PVR), and altered interventricular balance.[54,75,144] During LVAD support, leftward shift of the interventricular septum occurs as the LV is unloaded. This alteration in interventricular balance leads to significant reductions in RV contractility and afterload which may manifest as RV dysfunction, especially with preexistent or perioperative RV ischemia.[75,145]

Relative to the left, the thin-walled right ventricle has significantly reduced muscular reserve, rendering it more sensitive to increases in afterload (PVR).[54] Reversible increases in PVR during and after CPB have been described[146] and may be attributed to extravascular compression by pulmonary congestion, vasoactive substances released from activated platelets and leukocytes,[147] or obstruction of pulmonary vascular beds by leukocytes or platelet aggregates.[148] Once established, RV dysfunction in the perioperative period has detrimental effects on global cardiac performance and may be self-propagating unless appropriately treated. Specifically, reduced RV stroke volume will decrease LV filling, and RV dilation can induce a leftward shift of the interventricular septum and consequent impaired LV distensibility. The resultant decrease in LV output will exacerbate further the already dysfunctional RV.[54]

Diagnosis

Accurate interpretation of RV function is complex. Hemodynamic parameters suggestive of RV dysfunction include low

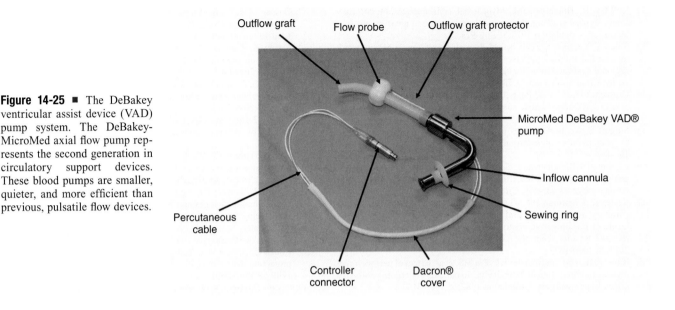

Figure 14-25 ■ The DeBakey ventricular assist device (VAD) pump system. The DeBakey-MicroMed axial flow pump represents the second generation in circulatory support devices. These blood pumps are smaller, quieter, and more efficient than previous, pulsatile flow devices.

cardiac output caused by inadequate LV filling, markedly elevated CVP (>18 mm Hg), and a normal or low PCWP as a result of poor left atrial filling.[75] In cases of severe RV dysfunction, PA pressures are low due to reduced RV work capability. Echocardiographic evaluation is a critical diagnostic tool for determining the status of RV function and identifying potential etiologies of RV impairment. The classic echocardiographic appearance of isolated RV failure is that of a dilated RV with a small, empty, and hypercontractile LV. Echocardiography can quantitate RV function by measurement of RV ejection fraction, provide qualitative assessment of RV size and configuration of the interventricular septum, and detect RV free wall akinesis or dyskinesis, indicative of underlying ischemic injury or infarction.

Management

Treatment of RV dysfunction should begin with optimization of heart rate and rhythm, to maximize the atrial contribution to RV filling. As with the treatment of LV dysfunction, temporary atrial or atrioventricular pacing may be required. Preload, as reflected by the CVP, should be augmented by volume loading provided there are reciprocal increases in cardiac output.[54,75] Efforts to increase RV inotropy through administration of classic agents (e.g., epinephrine, norepinephrine, and dopamine) may paradoxically increase PA vasoconstriction and PVR and thus worsen RV failure. Instead, phosphodiesterase inhibitors (e.g., milrinone, amrinone) are more appropriate pharmacologic treatments because of their positive inotropic effects and capacity to reduce PA pressure and PVR simultaneously. Selective pulmonary vasodilation can be achieved with inhaled nitric oxide to optimize RV function with targeted afterload reduction. Additional effective therapies for pulmonary vasodilation include oral sildenafil[149] and inhaled prostaglandins, such as iloprost.[150] A number of treatable conditions may increase PVR, including hypercapnia, hypoxia, pleural effusion, and pneumonia.

These should be identified and treated. Finally, refractory RV dysfunction may require placement of an RVAD.

■ REFERENCES

1. Holmvang L, Jurlander B, Rasmussen C, et al: Use of biochemical markers of infarction for diagnosing perioperative myocardial infarction and early graft occlusion after coronary artery bypass surgery. Chest 2002;121:103-111.
2. Wang K, Asinger RW, Marriott HJ: ST-segment elevation in conditions other than acute myocardial infarction. N Engl J Med 2003;349:2128-2135.
3. Milano CA, Smith PK: Critical care for the adult cardiac patient. In Sellke FW, Swanson SJ, del Nido PJ (eds): Sabiston & Spencer Surgery of the Chest, ed 7. Philadelphia, Saunders, 2005, pp 1033-1060.
4. Yokoyama Y, Chaitman BR, Hardison RM, et al: Association between new electrocardiographic abnormalities after coronary revascularization and five-year cardiac mortality in BARI randomized and registry patients. Am J Cardiol 2000;86:819-824.
5. Califf RM, Abdelmeguid AE, Kuntz RE, et al: Myonecrosis after revascularization procedures. J Am Coll Cardiol 1998;31:241-251.
6. Comunale ME, Body SC, Ley C, et al: The concordance of intraoperative left ventricular wall-motion abnormalities and electrocardiographic S-T segment changes: Association with outcome after coronary revascularization. Multicenter Study of Perioperative Ischemia (McSPI) Research Group. Anesthesiology 1998;88:945-954.
7. Barron JT: Cardiac troponin I and non-Q-wave myocardial infarction: How useful is it after coronary artery bypass surgery? Crit Care Med 1998;26:1936-1937.
8. Fabricius AM, Gerber W, Hanke M, et al: Early angiographic control of perioperative ischemia after coronary artery bypass grafting. Eur J Cardiothorac Surg 2001;19:853-858.
9. Wijeysundera DN, Beattie WS, Rao V, Karski J: Calcium antagonists reduce cardiovascular complications after cardiac surgery: A meta-analysis. J Am Coll Cardiol 2003;41:1496-1505.
10. Newman MF: Troponin I in cardiac surgery: Marking the future. Am Heart J 2001;141:325-326.
11. Bateman TM, Gray RJ: Perioperative myocardial infarction. In Gray RJ, Matloff JM (eds): Medical Management of the Cardiac Surgical Patient, ed 1. Baltimore, Williams & Wilkins, 1990, pp 178-185.

12. Bulkley B, Hutchins GM: Myocardial consequences of coronary artery bypass grafting: The paradox of necrosis in areas of revascularization. Circulation 1977;56:906-913.

13. Force T, Kemper AJ, Bloomfield P, et al: Non-Q-wave perioperative myocardial infarction: Assessment of the incidence and severity of regional dysfunction with quantitative two-dimensional echocardiography. Circulation 1985;72:781-789.

14. Crescenzi G, Bove T, Pappalardo F, et al: Clinical significance of a new Q wave after cardiac surgery. Eur J Cardiothorac Surg 2004;25:1001-1005.

15. Slogoff S, Keats AS: Does perioperative myocardial ischemia lead to postoperative myocardial infarction? Anesthesiology 1985;62:107-114.

16. Chaitman BR, Alderman EL, Sheffield LT, et al: Use of survival analysis to determine the clinical significance of new Q waves after coronary bypass surgery. Circulation 1983;67:302-309.

17. Klatte K, Chaitman BR, Theroux P, et al: Increased mortality after coronary artery bypass graft surgery is associated with increased levels of postoperative creatine kinase-myocardial band isoenzyme release: Results from the GUARDIAN trial. J Am Coll Cardiol 2001;38:1070-1077.

18. Namay DL, Hammermeister KE, Zia MS, et al: Effect of perioperative myocardial infarction on late survival in patients undergoing coronary artery bypass surgery. Circulation 1982;65:1066-1071.

19. Crescenzi G, Cedrati V, Landoni G, et al: Cardiac biomarker release after CABG with different surgical techniques. J Cardiothorac Vasc Anesth 2004;18:34-37.

20. Greaves SC, Rutherford JD, Aranki SF, et al: Current incidence and determinants of perioperative myocardial infarction in coronary artery surgery. Am Heart J 1996;132:572-578.

21. Brener SJ, Lytle BW, Schneider JP, et al: Association between CK-MB elevation after percutaneous or surgical revascularization and three-year mortality. J Am Coll Cardiol 2002;40:1961-1967.

22. Costa MA, Carere RG, Lichtenstein SV, et al: Incidence, predictors, and significance of abnormal cardiac enzyme rise in patients treated with bypass surgery in the Arterial Revascularization Therapies Study (ARTS). Circulation 2001;104:2689-2693.

23. Greenson N, Macoviak J, Krishnaswamy P, et al: Usefulness of cardiac troponin I in patients undergoing open heart surgery. Am Heart J 2001;141:447-455.

24. Benoit MO, Paris M, Silleran J, et al: Cardiac troponin I: Its contribution to the diagnosis of perioperative myocardial infarction and various complications of cardiac surgery. Crit Care Med 2001;29:1880-1886.

25. Carrier M, Pellerin M, Perrault LP, et al: Troponin levels in patients with myocardial infarction after coronary artery bypass grafting. Ann Thorac Surg 2000;69:435-440.

26. Carrier M, Pelletier LC, Martineau R, et al: In elective coronary artery bypass grafting, preoperative troponin T level predicts the risk of myocardial infarction. J Thorac Cardiovasc Surg 1998;115:1328-1334.

27. Eigel P, van Ingen G, Wagenpfeil S: Predictive value of perioperative cardiac troponin I for adverse outcome in coronary artery bypass surgery. Eur J Cardiothorac Surg 2001;20:544-549.

28. Fellahi JL, Gue X, Richomme X, et al: Short- and long-term prognostic value of postoperative cardiac troponin I concentration in patients undergoing coronary artery bypass grafting. Anesthesiology 2003;99:270-274.

29. Januzzi JL, Lewandrowski K, MacGillivray TE, et al: A comparison of cardiac troponin T and creatine kinase-MB for patient evaluation after cardiac surgery. J Am Coll Cardiol 2002;39:1518-1523.

30. Kathiresan S, Servoss SJ, Newell JB, et al: Cardiac troponin T elevation after coronary artery bypass grafting is associated with increased one-year mortality. Am J Cardiol 2004;94:879-881.

31. Lasocki S, Provenchère S, Benessiano J, et al: Cardiac troponin I is an independent predictor of in-hospital death after adult cardiac surgery. Anesthesiology 2002;97:405-411.

32. Vermes E, Mesguich M, Houel R, et al: Cardiac troponin I release after open heart surgery: A marker of myocardial protection? Ann Thorac Surg 2000;70:2087-2090.

33. Bassan MM, Oatfield R, Hoffman I, et al: New Q waves after aortocoronary bypass surgery: Unmasking of an old infarction. N Engl J Med 1974;290:349-353.

34. Cornu E, Lacroix PH, Christides C, Laskar M: Coronary artery damage during mitral valve replacement. J Cardiovasc Surg (Torino) 1995;36:261-264.

35. Tavilla G, Pacini D: Damage to the circumflex coronary artery during mitral valve repair with sliding leaflet technique. Ann Thorac Surg 1998;66:2091-2093.

36. Keon WJ, Heggtveit HA, Leduc J: Perioperative myocardial infarction caused by atheroembolism. J Thorac Cardiovasc Surg 1982;84:849-855.

37. Force T, Hibberd P, Weeks G, et al: Perioperative myocardial infarction after coronary artery bypass surgery: Clinical significance and approach to risk stratification. Circulation 1990;82:903-912.

38. Jain U, Laflamme CJ, Aggarwal A, et al: Electrocardiographic and hemodynamic changes and their association with myocardial infarction during coronary artery bypass surgery: A multicenter study. Multicenter Study of Perioperative Ischemia (McSPI) Research Group. Anesthesiology 1997;86:576-591.

39. Cohen G, Borger MA, Weisel RD, Rao V: Intraoperative myocardial protection: Current trends and future perspectives. Ann Thorac Surg 1999;68:1995-2001.

40. Loop FD, Higgins TL, Panda R, et al: Myocardial protection during cardiac operations: Decreased morbidity and lower cost with blood cardioplegia and coronary sinus perfusion. J Thorac Cardiovasc Surg 1992;104:608-618.

41. Nicolini F, Beghi C, Muscari C, et al: Myocardial protection in adult cardiac surgery: Current options and future challenges. Eur J Cardiothorac Surg 2003;24:986-993.

42. Piana RN, Adams MR, Orford JL, et al: Rescue percutaneous coronary intervention immediately following coronary artery bypass grafting. Chest 2001;120:1417-1420.

43. Buxton AE, Goldberg S, Harken A, et al: Coronary-artery spasm immediately after myocardial revascularization: Recognition and management. N Engl J Med 1981;304:1249-1253.

44. Lemmer JH Jr, Kirsh MM: Coronary artery spasm following coronary artery surgery. Ann Thorac Surg 1988;46:108-115.

45. Pichard AD, Ambrose J, Mindich B, et al: Coronary artery spasm and perioperative cardiac arrest. J Thorac Cardiovasc Surg 1980;80:249-254.

46. Zeff RH, Iannone LA, Kongtahworn C, et al: Coronary artery spasm following coronary artery revascularization. Ann Thorac Surg 1982;34:196-200.

47. Bonatti J, Danzmayr M, Schachner T, Friedrich G: Intraoperative angiography for quality control in MIDCAB and OPCAB. Eur J Cardiothorac Surg 2003;24:647-649.

48. Caputo M, Nicolini F, Franciosi G, Gallotti R: Coronary artery spasm after coronary artery bypass grafting. Eur J Cardiothorac Surg 1999;15:545-548.

49. Trimboli S, Oppido G, Santini F, Mazzucco A: Coronary artery spasm after off-pump coronary artery by-pass grafting. Eur J Cardiothorac Surg 2003;24:830-833.

50. Sarabu MR, McClung JA, Fass A, Reed GE: Early postoperative spasm in left internal mammary artery bypass grafts. Ann Thorac Surg 1987;44:199-200.

51. Stone GW, Hartzler GO: Spontaneous reversible spasm in an internal mammary artery graft causing acute myocardial infarction. Am J Cardiol 1989;64:822-823.

52. Schmid C, Heublein B, Reichelt S, Borst HG: Steal phenomenon caused by a parallel branch of the internal mammary artery. Ann Thorac Surg 1990;50:463-464.

53. Boudoulas H, Lewis RP, Vasko JS, et al: Left ventricular function and adrenergic hyperactivity before and after saphenous vein bypass. Circulation 1976;53:802-806.

54. Levy JH, Michelsen L, Shanewise J, et al: Postoperative cardiovascular management. In Kaplan JA, Reich DL, Konstadt SN (eds): Cardiac Anesthesia, ed 4. Philadelphia, WB Saunders, 1999, pp 1233-1257.

55. Carrel T, Kujawski T, Zund G, et al: The internal mammary artery malperfusion syndrome: Incidence, treatment and angiographic verification. Eur J Cardiothorac Surg 1995;9:190-195; discussion 196-197.

56. Cameron A, Davis KB, Green G, Schaff HV: Coronary bypass surgery with internal-thoracic-artery grafts: Effects on survival over a 15-year period. N Engl J Med 1996;334:216-219.

57. Loop FD, Lytle BW, Cosgrove DM, et al: Influence of the internal-mammary-artery graft on 10-year survival and other cardiac events. N Engl J Med 1986;314:1-6.

58. Rasmussen C, Thiis JJ, Clemmensen P, et al: Significance and management of early graft failure after coronary artery bypass grafting: Feasibility and results of acute angiography and re-re-vascularization. Eur J Cardiothorac Surg 1997;12:847-852.

59. Pezzella AT, Ferraris VA, Lancey RA: Care of the adult cardiac surgery patient: Part I. Curr Probl Surg 2004;41:458-516.

60. Niimi Y, Morita S, Watanabe T, et al: Effects of nitroglycerin infusion on segmental wall motion abnormalities after anesthetic induction. J Cardiothorac Vasc Anesth 1996;10:734-740.

61. Christenson JT, Simonet F, Badel P, Schmuziger M: Optimal timing of preoperative intraaortic balloon pump support in high-risk coronary patients. Ann Thorac Surg 1999;68:934-939.

62. Torchiana DF, Hirsch G, Buckley MJ, et al: Intraaortic balloon pumping for cardiac support: Trends in practice and outcome, 1968 to 1995. J Thorac Cardiovasc Surg 1997;113:758-764; discussion 764-769.

63. Holman WL, Li Q, Kiefe CI, et al: Prophylactic value of preincision intra-aortic balloon pump: Analysis of a statewide experience. J Thorac Cardiovasc Surg 2000;120:1112-1119.

64. Lin JC, Fisher DL, Szwerc MF, Magovern JA: Evaluation of graft patency during minimally invasive coronary artery bypass grafting with Doppler flow analysis. Ann Thorac Surg 2000;70:1350-1354.

65. Morota T, Duhaylongsod FG, Burfeind WR, Huang CT: Intraoperative evaluation of coronary anastomosis by transit-time ultrasonic flow measurement. Ann Thorac Surg 2002;73:1446-1450.

66. Leong DK, Ashok V, Nishkantha A, et al: Transit-time flow measurement is essential in coronary artery bypass grafting. Ann Thorac Surg 2005;79:854-857; discussion 857-858.

67. Wijeysundera DN, Beattie WS, Rao V, et al: Calcium antagonists are associated with reduced mortality after cardiac surgery: A propensity analysis. J Thorac Cardiovasc Surg 2004;127:755-762.

68. Feldman RL: A review of medical therapy for coronary artery spasm. Circulation 1987;75(6 Pt 2):V96-102.

69. Verrier ED, Shernan SK, Taylor KM, et al: Terminal complement blockade with pexelizumab during coronary artery bypass graft surgery requiring cardiopulmonary bypass: A randomized trial. JAMA 2004;291:2319-2327.

70. Boyce SW, Bartels C, Bolli R, et al: Impact of sodium-hydrogen exchange inhibition by cariporide on death or myocardial infarction in high-risk CABG surgery patients: Results of the CABG surgery cohort of the GUARDIAN study. J Thorac Cardiovasc Surg 2003;126:420-427.

71. Kouchoukos N: Detection and treatment of impaired cardiac performance following cardiac surgery. In Davila JC (ed): Henry Ford Hospital International Symposium on Cardiac Surgery, ed 2. New York, Appleton-Century-Crofts, 1977.

72. McKinlay KH, Schinderle DB, Swaminathan M, et al: Predictors of inotrope use during separation from cardiopulmonary bypass. J Cardiothorac Vasc Anesth 2004;18:404-408.

73. Rao V, Ivanov J, Weisel RD, et al: Predictors of low cardiac output syndrome after coronary artery bypass. J Thorac Cardiovasc Surg 1996;112:38-51.

74. Yau TM, Fedak PW, Weisel RD, et al: Predictors of operative risk for coronary bypass operations in patients with left ventricular dysfunction. J Thorac Cardiovasc Surg 1999;118:1006-1013.

75. Kaul TK, Fields BL: Postoperative acute refractory right ventricular failure: Incidence, pathogenesis, management and prognosis. Cardiovasc Surg 2000;8:1-9.

76. Doyle AR, Dhir AK, Moors AH, Latimer RD: Treatment of perioperative low cardiac output syndrome. Ann Thorac Surg 1995;59(2 Suppl): S3-11.

77. Media N, Blacstone EH: Postcardiotomy mechanical support: Risk factors and outcomes. Ann Thorac Surg 2001;71:S60-66.

78. Cook WA, Webb WR, Unal MO: Myocardial function capacity in response to compensated and uncompensated respiratory alkalosis. Surg Forum 1965;16:186-188.

79. Darby TD, Aldinger EE, Gadsden RH, Thrower WB: Effects of metabolic acidosis on ventricular isometric systolic tension and the response to epinephrine and levarterenol. Circ Res 1960;8: 1242-1253.

80. Kirklin JK, Kirklin JW: Management of the cardiovascular subsystem after cardiac surgery. Ann Thorac Surg 1981;32:311-319.

81. Harris PD, Malm JR, Bowman FO Jr, et al: Epicardial pacing to control arrhythmias following cardiac surgery. Circulation 1968;37(4 Suppl):II178-183.

82. Hodam RP, Starr A: Temporary postoperative epicardial pacing electrodes: Their value and management after open-heart surgery. Ann Thorac Surg 1969;8:506-510.

83. Mills NL, Ochsner JL: Experience with atrial pacemaker wires implanted during cardiac operations. J Thorac Cardiovasc Surg 1973;66:878-886.

84. Hanson EL, Kane PB, Askanazi J, et al: Comparison of patients with coronary artery or valve disease: Intraoperative differences in blood volume and observations of vasomotor response. Ann Thorac Surg 1976;22:343-346.

85. Crexells C, Chatterjee K, Forrester JS, et al: Optimal level of filling pressure in the left side of the heart in acute myocardial infarction. N Engl J Med 1973;289:1263-1266.

86. Estafanous FG, Tarazi RC, Buckley S, Taylor PC: Arterial hypertension in immediate postoperative period after valve replacement. Br Heart J 1978;40:718-724.

87. Estafanous FG, Tarazi RC: Systemic arterial hypertension associated with cardiac surgery. Am J Cardiol 1980;46:685-694.

88. Weinstein GS, Zabetakis PM, Clavel A, et al: The renin-angiotensin system is not responsible for hypertension following coronary artery bypass grafting. Ann Thorac Surg 1987;43:74-77.

89. Fouad FM, Estafanous FG, Bravo EL, et al: Possible role of cardio-aortic reflexes in postcoronary bypass hypertension. Am J Cardiol 1979;44:866-872.

90. Taylor KM, Brannan JJ, Bain WH, et al: Role of angiotensin II in the development of peripheral vasoconstriction during cardiopulmonary bypass. Cardiovasc Res 1979;13:269-273.

91. Taylor KM, Morton IJ, Brown JJ, et al: Hypertension and the renin-angiotensin system following open-heart surgery. J Thorac Cardiovasc Surg 1977;74:840-845.

92. Packer M: Neurohormonal interactions and adaptations in congestive heart failure. Circulation 1988;77:721-730.

93. Whelton PK, Flaherty JT, MacAllister NP, et al: Hypertension following coronary artery bypass surgery: Role of preoperative propranolol therapy. Hypertension 1980;2:291-298.

94. Zelis R, Mansour EJ, Capone RJ, Mason DT: The cardiovascular effects of morphine: The peripheral capacitance and resistance vessels in human subjects. J Clin Invest 1974;54:1247-1258.

95. Redwood DR, Smith ER, Epstein SE: Coronary artery occlusion in the conscious dog: Effects of alterations in heart rate and arterial pressure on the degree of myocardial ischemia. Circulation 1972;46: 323-332.

96. Mekontso-Dessap A, Houel R, Soustelle C, et al: Risk factors for post-cardiopulmonary bypass vasoplegia in patients with preserved left ventricular function. Ann Thorac Surg 2001;71:1428-1432.

97. Morales DL, Gregg D, Helman DN, et al: Arginine vasopressin in the treatment of 50 patients with postcardiotomy vasodilatory shock. Ann Thorac Surg 2000;69:102-106.

98. Chuttani K, Tischler MD, Pandian NG, et al: Diagnosis of cardiac tamponade after cardiac surgery: Relative value of clinical, echocardiographic, and hemodynamic signs. Am Heart J 1994;127(4 Pt 1):913-918.

99. Spodick DH: The normal and diseased pericardium: Current concepts of pericardial physiology, diagnosis and treatment. J Am Coll Cardiol 1983;1:240-251.

100. Chuttani K, Pandian NG, Mohanty PK, et al: Left ventricular diastolic collapse: An echocardiographic sign of regional cardiac tamponade. Circulation 1991;83:1999-2006.

101. Craddock DR, Logan A, Fadali A: Reoperation for haemorrhage following cardiopulmonary by-pass. Br J Surg 1968;55:17-20.

102. Engelman RM, Spencer FC, Reed GE, Tice DA: Cardiac tamponade following open-heart surgery. Circulation 1970;41(5 Suppl):II165-171.

103. Nelson RM, Jenson CB, Smoot WM 3rd: Pericardial tamponade following open-heart surgery. J Thorac Cardiovasc Surg 1969;58:510-516.

104. Weeks KR, Chatterjee K, Block S, et al: Bedside hemodynamic monitoring: Its value in the diagnosis of tamponade complicating cardiac surgery. J Thorac Cardiovasc Surg 1976;71:250-252.

105. Gorman JH 3rd, Gorman RC, Milas BL, Acker MA: Circulatory management of the unstable cardiac patient. Semin Thorac Cardiovasc Surg 2000;12:316-325.

106. Skinner NS Jr, Mitchell JH, Wallace AG, Sarnoff SJ: Hemodynamic effects of altering the timing of atrial systole. Am J Physiol 1963;205:499-503.

107. Ellis RJ, Mavroudis C, Gardner C, et al: Relationship between atrioventricular arrhythmias and the concentration of K^+ ion in cardioplegic solution. J Thorac Cardiovasc Surg 1980;80:517-526.

108. Smith PK, Buhrman WC, Levett JM, et al: Supraventricular conduction abnormalities following cardiac operations: A complication of inadequate atrial preservation. J Thorac Cardiovasc Surg 1983;85:105-115.

109. Smith PK, Buhrman WC, Ferguson TB Jr, et al: Conduction block after cardioplegic arrest: Prevention by augmented atrial hypothermia. Circulation 1983;68(3 Pt 2):II41-48.

110. Zoll PM: Resuscitation of the heart in ventricular standstill by external electric stimulation. N Engl J Med 1952;247:768-771.

111. Hartzler GO, Maloney JD, Curtis JJ, Barnhorst DA: Hemodynamic benefits of atrioventricular sequential pacing after cardiac surgery. Am J Cardiol 1977;40:232-236.

112. Chatterjee K, Parmley WW: The role of vasodilator therapy in heart failure. Prog Cardiovasc Dis 1977;19:301-325.

113. Chatterjee K, Parmley WW, Swan HJ, et al: Beneficial effects of vasodilator agents in severe mitral regurgitation due to dysfunction of subvalvar apparatus. Circulation 1973;48:684-690.

114. Bolen JL, Alderman EL: Hemodynamic consequences of afterload reduction in patients with chronic aortic regurgitation. Circulation 1976;53:879-883.

115. Chiariello M, Gold HK, Leinbach RC, et al: Comparison between the effects of nitroprusside and nitroglycerin on ischemic injury during acute myocardial infarction. Circulation 1976;54:766-773.

116. Bixler TJ, Gardner TJ, Donahoo JS, et al: Improved myocardial performance in postoperative cardiac surgical patients with sodium nitroprusside. Ann Thorac Surg 1978;25:444-448.

117. Franciosa JA, Limas CJ, Guiha NH, et al: Improved left ventricular function during nitroprusside infusion in acute myocardial infarction. Lancet 1972;1:650-654.

118. Goldstein RE, Stinson EB, Scherer JL, et al: Intraoperative coronary collateral function in patients with coronary occlusive disease: Nitroglycerin responsiveness and angiographic correlations. Circulation 1974;49:298-308.

119. Erdmann E: The effectiveness of inotropic agents in isolated cardiac preparations from the human heart. Klin Wochenschr 1988;66:1-6.

120. DiGiorgi P, Kukuy EL, Naka Y, Oz MC: Left ventricular assist devices. In Sellke FW, Swanson SJ, del Nido PJ (eds): Sabiston & Spencer Surgery of the Chest, ed 7. Philadelphia, Saunders, 2005, pp 1613-1629.

121. Emery RW, Joyce LD: Directions in cardiac assistance. J Card Surg 1991;6:400-414.

122. Miller LW: Mechanical assist devices in intensive cardiac care. Am Heart J 1991;121(6 Pt 1):1887-1892.

123. Pennington DG, Joyce LD, Pae WE Jr, Burkholder JA: Circulatory support 1988: Patient selection. Ann Thorac Surg 1989;47:77-81.

124. Bolooki H: Clinical Applications of the Intra-Aortic Balloon Pump, ed 3. Armonk, NY, Futura, 1998.

125. Phillips SJ, Tannenbaum M, Zeff RH, et al: Sheathless insertion of the percutaneous intraaortic balloon pump: An alternate method. Ann Thorac Surg 1992;53:162.

126. Tatar H, Cicek S, Demirkilic U, et al: Exact positioning of intra-aortic balloon catheter. Eur J Cardiothorac Surg 1993;7:52-53; discussion 53.

127. Busch T, Sirbu H, Zenker D, Dalichau H: Vascular complications related to intraaortic balloon counterpulsation: An analysis of ten years' experience. Thorac Cardiovasc Surg 1997;45:55-59.

128. Pennock JL, Pierce WS, Wisman CB, et al: Survival and complications following ventricular assist pumping for cardiogenic shock. Ann Surg 1983;198:469-478.

129. Stolar CJ, Delosh T, Bartlett RH: Extracorporeal Life Support Organization 1993. ASAIO J 1993;39:976-979.

130. Kaplan R, Smedira NG: Extracorporeal membrane oxygenation in adults. In Goldstein D, Oz MC (eds): Cardiac Assist Devices. Armonk, NY, Futura, 2000.

131. Wudel JH, Hlozek CC, Smedira NG, McCarthy PM: Extracorporeal life support as a post left ventricular assist device implant supplement. ASAIO J 1997;43:M441-443.

132. Pagani FD, Lynch W, Swaniker F, et al: Extracorporeal life support to left ventricular assist device bridge to heart transplant: A strategy to optimize survival and resource utilization. Circulation 1999;100(19 Suppl):II206-210.

133. Pae WE Jr, Miller CA, Matthews Y, Pierce WS: Ventricular assist devices for postcardiotomy cardiogenic shock: A combined registry experience. J Thorac Cardiovasc Surg 1992;104:541-552; discussion 552-553.

134. Curtis JJ, Boley TM, Walls JT, et al: Frequency of seal disruption with the Sarns centrifugal pump in postcardiotomy circulatory assist. Artif Organs 1994;18:235-237.

135. Guyton RA, Schonberger JP, Everts PA, et al: Postcardiotomy shock: Clinical evaluation of the BVS 5000 Biventricular Support system. Ann Thorac Surg 1993;56:346-356.

136. Petrofski J, James D, Smigla G, et al: The short-term mechanical ventricular assistance: Advantages of the BVS5000. ASAIO J 2002;48.

137. Goldstein DJ, Oz MC, Rose EA: Implantable left ventricular assist devices. N Engl J Med 1998;339:1522-1533.

138. Slater JP, Rose EA, Levin HR, et al: Low thromboembolic risk without anticoagulation using advanced-design left ventricular assist devices. Ann Thorac Surg 1996;62:1321-1327; discussion 1328.

139. Rose EA, Gelijns AC, Moskowitz AJ, et al: Long-term mechanical left ventricular assistance for end-stage heart failure. N Engl J Med 2001;345:1435-1443.

140. Frazier OH, Myers TJ, Westaby S, Gregoric ID: Clinical experience with an implantable, intracardiac, continuous flow circulatory support device: Physiologic implications and their relationship to patient selection. Ann Thorac Surg 2004;77:133-142.

141. Goldstein DJ: Worldwide experience with the MicroMed DeBakey Ventricular Assist Device as a bridge to transplantation. Circulation 2003;108(Suppl 1):II272-277.

142. Wranne B, Pinto FJ, Hammarstrom E, et al: Abnormal right heart filling after cardiac surgery: Time course and mechanisms. Br Heart J 1991;66:435-442.

143. Fantidis P, Castejon R, Fernandez Ruiz A, et al: Does a critical hemodynamic situation develop from right ventriculotomy and free wall infarct or from small changes in dysfunctional right ventricle afterload? J Cardiovasc Surg (Torino) 1992;33:229-234.

144. Fontes ML, Hines RL: Pharmacologic management of perioperative left and right ventricular dysfunction. In Kaplan JA, Reich DL, Konstadt SN (eds): Cardiac Anesthesia, ed 4. Philadelphia, WB Saunders, 1999, pp 1155-1191.

145. Santamore WP, Austin EH 3rd, Gray L Jr: Overcoming right ventricular failure with left ventricular assist devices. J Heart Lung Transplant 1997;16:1122-1128.

146. Heinonen J, Salmenpera M, Takkunen O: Increased pulmonary artery diastolic-pulmonary wedge pressure gradient after cardiopulmonary bypass. Can Anaesth Soc J 1985;32:165-170.

147. Colman RW: Platelet and neutrophil activation in cardiopulmonary bypass. Ann Thorac Surg 1990;49:32-34.

148. Chenoweth DE, Cooper SW, Hugli TE, et al: Complement activation during cardiopulmonary bypass: Evidence for generation of C3a and C5a anaphylatoxins. N Engl J Med 1981;304:497-503.

149. Trachte AL, Lobato EB, Urdaneta F, et al: Oral sildenafil reduces pulmonary hypertension after cardiac surgery. Ann Thorac Surg 2005;79:194-197; discussion 197.

150. Olschewski H, Rohde B, Behr J, et al: Pharmacodynamics and pharmacokinetics of inhaled iloprost, aerosolized by three different devices, in severe pulmonary hypertension. Chest 2003;124:1294-1304.

15 Perioperative Management of Valvular Heart Disease

Igor Izrailtyan and Joseph P. Mathew

■ PREOPERATIVE ASSESSMENT

Valvular heart disease (VHD) is frequently observed in patients undergoing surgery. With the advent of aggressive statin therapy and widespread use of drug-eluting stents, it is likely that the perioperative management of patients with untreated valvular lesions will present a greater challenge in the next decade than the management of those with severe coronary artery disease. Nevertheless, the association of VHD with other clinical predictors of increased perioperative cardiovascular risk is of prime importance, particularly as it relates to unstable coronary syndromes, decompensated heart failure with left ventricular (LV) dysfunction, and significant arrhythmias.[1] For example, VHD has been reported to be a major predictor of increased perioperative cardiovascular risk, including myocardial infarction, heart failure, and cardiac death.[1] In patients older than 65 years presenting for noncardiac or coronary artery surgery without concomitant valvular surgery, a history of VHD is predictive of lower LV ejection fraction (LVEF) preoperatively.[2] Preoperative symptomatic valvular disease also increases the risk for congestive heart failure (CHF) after elective general surgical procedures,[3] and significant VHD on preoperative physical examination (murmur grade > III) is an independent predictor of supraventricular arrhythmia after noncardiac surgery.[4] Similarly, significant aortic and mitral valvular dysfunction diagnosed by preoperative transthoracic echocardiography is an independent risk factor for perioperative myocardial infarction,[5] and significant aortic stenosis is one of the major factors adversely affecting the clinical outcome after noncardiac surgery.[6,7] Thus, although it is important to preoperatively evaluate the presence, type, and severity of VHD, its natural history and relation to other disease states are key factors in determining the clinical management strategy for the perioperative period.

The physician must know the patient's preoperative history and the results of the physical examination. If a cardiac murmur[8] is present on preoperative evaluation, the anesthesiologist needs to decide whether it represents significant VHD (see later). It may be prudent to delay elective noncardiac surgery if additional diagnostic interventions are needed (Fig. 15-1). For patients who have significant VHD, the relative risks and benefits should be considered of proceeding directly to noncardiac surgery versus delaying it for a diagnostic workup and therapeutic interventions.[9-11] Patients with severe VHD may be more prone to hemodynamic instability during the operation, coupled with longer times for both anesthesia and surgery when compared with patients without VHD.[12] High-risk surgical procedures (emergent major operations, aortic and peripheral vascular surgery, and prolonged surgical procedures associated with large fluid shifts or blood loss) pose a greater risk of hemodynamic instability and increased perioperative morbidity and mortality.[1,6,13,14] Although no randomized trials have been performed to ascertain the best timing of surgical intervention, the indications for evaluation and treatment of valvular lesions prior to elective noncardiac surgery are the same as in the nonoperative setting.[1,10] Thus, symptomatic stenotic lesions often require valve replacement or percutaneous valvotomy prior to noncardiac surgery to decrease cardiac risk,[15] but, in general, regurgitant valve lesions are more likely to be tolerated, as these patients can be stabilized with medical therapy alone.[1]

Although echocardiography usually provides information of greater specificity about the significance of a cardiac murmur, both electrocardiography and chest roentgenography, which are commonly performed preoperatively, can provide clues to the severity of VHD. For example, the presence of ventricular hypertrophy, prior infarction, or active ischemia on the electrocardiogram, or of atrial and pulmonary artery enlargement on the chest roentgenogram, should prompt a more extensive evaluation of the patient. Echocardiography is an important tool for assessing the significance of cardiac murmurs by imaging cardiac structure and function, and the direction and velocity of blood flow through cardiac valves and chambers.[10] Echocardiography is recommended for asymptomatic patients with diastolic murmurs, continuous murmurs, holosystolic murmurs, grade 3 or louder mid-peaking systolic murmurs, or late systolic murmurs, and for patients with murmurs and signs and symptoms of heart failure, myocardial ischemia or infarction, syncope, thromboembolism, infective endocarditis, or other evidence of structural heart disease. However, this recommendation for echocardiography is based on consensus opinion and standard of care alone. If the results of transthoracic echocardiography are inconclusive in defining the diagnosis, other tests, including transesophageal echocardiography (TEE) and cardiac catheterization, should be considered. In determining whether symptoms are present, exercise testing may be helpful, as many patients tend to limit their daily activity.[10,16-19]

Finally, the specific type of surgery and urgency of the operation are important factors in stratifying perioperative

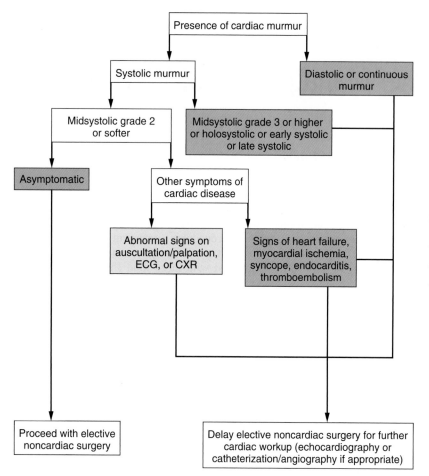

Figure 15-1 ■ Strategy for evaluating cardiac murmurs. CXR, chest radiograph; ECG, electrocardiogram. (*Modified with permission from Bonow RO, Carabello B, de Leon AC, et al: J Am Coll Cardiol 1998;32:1486-1588.* Copyright 1998, The American College of Cardiology Foundation and American Heart Association, Inc.)

risk for VHD surgical patients. High-risk surgical procedures, including emergent major operations, aortic and peripheral vascular surgery, and prolonged surgical procedures associated with large fluid shifts or blood loss, pose a greater threat of hemodynamic instability and portend an increase in perioperative morbidity and mortality.[1,6,13,14]

■ PREOPERATIVE PREPARATION

Antimicrobial Prophylaxis

Surgical procedures may induce bacteremia and thus expose patients to the risk of acquiring infective endocarditis, a potentially lethal disease if not aggressively treated.[20] Valvular abnormalities, particularly those that result in high-velocity jets, can damage the endothelial lining, lead to platelet aggregation and fibrin deposition at those sites, and create a higher risk for bacterial colonization.[10] To date, the efficacy of prophylactic antibiotics is based on laboratory animal models and small clinical series and is not established by large controlled clinical trials.[10,20] Current clinical strategies in endocarditis prevention are based on recommendations from the American Heart Association[21] and are outlined in Boxes 15-1 to 15-3 and Tables 15-1 to 15-3. High-risk patients requiring antimicrobial prophylaxis include surgical patients with prosthetic valves, a previous history of endo-

carditis, complex cyanotic congenital heart disease, or surgically constructed systemic pulmonary shunts. Patients at moderate risk for infection include those with most other congenital cardiac malformations, acquired valvular dysfunction, hypertrophic cardiomyopathy, and mitral valve prolapse with regurgitation or thickened leaflets.[21,22] Antibiotic prophylaxis for at-risk patients (see Box 15-1) is recommended for dental and oral procedures likely to cause bacteremia (see Box 15-2), and for surgical procedures involving the respiratory mucosa and the gastrointestinal and genitourinary tracts (see Box 15-3).[21] The first antimicrobial dose should begin within 1 hour prior to surgical incision.[21,23,24]

Anticoagulation

Some patients with VHD, including those with atrial fibrillation and prosthetic valves, receive anticoagulation therapy, usually with warfarin. A clinician must then weigh the risk of increased bleeding from continued anticoagulation against the increased risk of thromboembolism resulting from a cessation of therapy.[10,25,26] Evidence defining the perioperative management of anticoagulation in this patient population is sparse. For patients with a bileaflet mechanical valve and no other risk factors[27-29] (e.g., atrial fibrillation, previous thromboembolism, hypercoagulable state, older-generation mechanical valves [e.g., Björk-Shiley], LV ejection fraction <30%, or more than one mechanical valve), warfarin should

15-1	**Endocarditis Prophylaxis for Cardiac Conditions**

Endocarditis Prophylaxis Recommended

- High-risk category
  - Prosthetic cardiac valves, including bioprosthetic and homograft valves
  - Previous bacterial endocarditis
  - Complex cyanotic congenital heart disease (e.g., single ventricle states, transposition of the great arteries, tetralogy of Fallot)
  - Surgically constructed systemic pulmonary shunts or conduits
- Moderate-risk category
  - Most congenital cardiac malformations other than the preceding and the following
  - Acquired valvar dysfunction (e.g., rheumatic heart disease)
  - Hypertrophic cardiomyopathy
  - Mitral valve prolapse with valvar regurgitation or thickened leaflets

Endocarditis Prophylaxis Not Recommended

- Negligible-risk category (no greater risk than the general population)
  - Isolated secundum atrial septal defect
  - Surgical repair of atrial septal defect, ventricular septal defect, or patent ductus arteriosus (without residua beyond 6 months)
  - Previous coronary artery bypass graft surgery
  - Mitral valve prolapse without valvar regurgitation[1]
  - Physiologic, functional, or innocent heart murmurs[1]
  - Previous Kawasaki disease without valvar dysfunction
  - Previous rheumatic fever without valvar dysfunction
  - Cardiac pacemakers (intravascular and epicardial) and implanted defibrillators

Reproduced with permission from Dajani AS, Taubert KA, Wilson W, et al: Circulation 1997;96:358-366.

15-2	**Endocarditis Prophylaxis for Dental Procedures**

Endocarditis Prophylaxis Recommended*

- Dental extractions
- Periodontal procedures including surgery, scaling and root planing, probing, and recall maintenance
- Dental implant placement and reimplantation of avulsed teeth
- Endodontic (root canal) instrumentation or surgery only beyond the apex
- Subgingival placement of antibiotic fibers or strips
- Initial placement of orthodontic bands but not brackets
- Intraligamentary local anesthetic injections
- Prophylactic cleaning of teeth or implants when bleeding is anticipated

Endocarditis Prophylaxis Not Recommended

- Restorative dentistry[†] (operative and prosthodontic) with or without retraction cord[‡]
- Local anesthetic injections (nonintraligamentary)
- Intracanal endodontic treatment; post placement and buildup
- Placement of rubber dams
- Postoperative suture removal
- Placement of removable prosthodontic or orthodontic appliances
- Taking of oral impressions
- Fluoride treatments
- Taking of oral radiographs
- Orthodontic appliance adjustments
- Shedding of primary teeth

*Prophylaxis is recommended for patients with high- and moderate-risk cardiac conditions.

[†]This includes restoration of decayed teeth (filling cavities) and replacement of missing teeth.

[‡]Clinical judgment may indicate antibiotic use in selected circumstances that may create significant bleeding.

Reproduced with permission from Dajani AS, Taubert KA, Wilson W, et al: Circulation 1997;96:358-366.

15-3	**Endocarditis Prophylaxis for Nondental Procedures**

Endocarditis Prophylaxis Recommended

- Respiratory tract
  - Tonsillectomy and/or adenoidectomy
  - Surgical operations that involve respiratory mucosa
  - Bronchoscopy with a rigid bronchoscope
- Gastrointestinal tract*
  - Sclerotherapy for esophageal varices
  - Esophageal stricture dilation
  - Endoscopic retrograde cholangiography with biliary obstruction
  - Biliary tract surgery
  - Surgical operations that involve intestinal mucosa
- Genitourinary tract
  - Prostatic surgery
  - Cystoscopy
  - Urethral dilation

Endocarditis Prophylaxis Not Recommended

- Respiratory tract
  - Endotracheal tract
  - Bronchoscopy with a flexible bronchoscope, with or without biopsy[†]
  - Tympanostomy tube insertion

- Gastrointestinal tract
  - Transesophageal echocardiography[†]
  - Endoscopy with or without gastrointestinal biopsy[†]
- Genitourinary tract
  - Vaginal hysterectomy[†]
  - Vaginal delivery[†]
  - Cesarean section
  - In uninfected tissue:
    - Urethral catheterization
    - Uterine dilation and curettage
    - Therapeutic abortion
    - Sterilization procedures
    - Insertion or removal of intrauterine devices
- Other
  - Cardiac catheterization, including balloon angioplasty
  - Implanted cardiac pacemakers, implanted defibrillators, and coronary stents
  - Incision or biopsy of surgically scrubbed skin
  - Circumcision

*Prophylaxis is recommended for high-risk patients; it is optional for medium-risk patients.

[†]Prophylaxis is optional for high-risk patients.

Reproduced with permission from Dajani AS, Taubert KA, Wilson W, et al: Circulation 1997;96:358-366.

15-1 | **Prophylactic Regimens for Dental, Oral, Respiratory Tract, or Esophageal Procedures**

Situation	Agent	Regimen*
Standard general prophylaxis	Amoxicillin	Adults: 2.0 g; children: 50 mg/kg orally 1 hr before procedure
Unable to take oral medications	Ampicillin	Adults: 2.0 g IM or IV; children: 50 mg/kg IM or IV within 30 min before procedure
Allergic to penicillin	Clindamycin or cephalexin[†] or cefadroxil[†] or azithromycin or clarithromycin	Adults: 600 mg; children: 20 mg/kg orally 1 hr before procedure Adults: 2.0 g; children: 50 mg/kg orally 1 hr before procedure Adults: 500 mg; children: 15 mg/kg orally 1 hr before procedure
Allergic to penicillin and unable to take oral medications	Clindamycin or cefazolin[†]	Adults: 600 mg; children: 20 mg/kg IV within 30 min before procedure Adults: 1.0 g; children 25 mg/kg IM or IV within 30 min before procedure

IM, intramuscularly; IV, intravenously.
*Total children's dose should not exceed adult dose.
[†]Cephalosporins should not be used in individuals with immediate-type hypersensitivity reaction (urticaria, angioedema, or anaphylaxis) to penicillins.
Reproduced with permission from Dajani AS, Taubert KA, Wilson W, et al: Circulation 1997;96:358-366.

15-2 | **Prophylactic Regimens for Genitourinary and Gastrointestinal (Excluding Esophageal) Procedures**

Situation	Agent	Regimen*
High-risk patients	Ampicillin plus gentamicin[†]	Adults: ampicillin 2.0 mg IM or IV plus gentamicin 1.5 mg/kg (not to exceed 120 mg) within 30 min of starting procedure; 6 hr later, ampicillin 1 g IM/IV or amoxicillin 1 g orally Children: ampicillin 50 mg/kg IM or IV (not to exceed 2.0 g) plus gentamicin 1.5 mg/kg within 30 min of starting procedure; 6 hr later, ampicillin 25 mg/kg IM/IV or amoxicillin 25 mg/kg orally
	Vancomycin[†] plus gentamicin[†]	Adults: vancomycin 1.0 g IV over 1-2 hr plus gentamicin 1.5 mg/kg IV/IM (not to exceed 120 mg); complete injection/infusion within 30 min of starting procedure
Moderate-risk patients	Amoxicillin or ampicillin	Adults: amoxicillin 2.0 g orally 1 hr before procedure, or ampicillin 2.0 g IM/IV within 30 min of starting procedure Children: amoxicillin 50 mg/kg orally 1 hr before procedure, or ampicillin 50 mg/kg IM/IV within 30 min of starting procedure
Moderate-risk patients allergic to ampicillin/amoxicillin	Vancomycin[†]	Adults: vancomycin 1.0 g IV over 1-2 hr; complete infusion within 30 min of starting procedure Children: vancomycin 20 mg/kg IV over 1-2 hr; complete infusion within 30 min of starting procedure

IM, intramuscularly; IV, intravenously.
*Total children's dose should not exceed adult dose.
[†]No second dose of vancomycin or gentamicin is recommended.
Reproduced with permission from Dajani AS, Taubert KA, Wilson W, et al: Circulation 1997;96:358-366.

be discontinued before the procedure so that the International Normalized Ratio (INR) is less than 1.5 (typically, 24 to 72 hours after discontinuation) and restarted within 24 hours of the procedure.[10,25] For patients at high risk of thrombosis (e.g., those who have mechanical mitral or tricuspid valves, or those with a mechanical aortic valve and any of the previously mentioned risk factors), therapeutic doses of intravenous heparin should be started when the INR falls below 2.0 (typically, 48 hours before surgery) to maintain the activated partial thromboplastin time at 55 to 70 seconds. The heparin should be stopped 4 to 6 hours before the procedure, restarted as early after surgery as possible, and continued until the INR is therapeutic on warfarin therapy. Fresh-frozen plasma may be given to patients with mechanical valves who require interruption of warfarin therapy for emergency noncardiac surgery.

There are theoretical concerns that stopping and restarting warfarin therapy may predispose to a hypercoagulable state because of the suppression of proteins C and S, but it is not clear that the risk of thromboembolism is actually greater despite an increase in the levels of markers defining activation of thrombosis.[30,31] Bridging therapy with subcutaneous low-molecular-weight heparin (LMWH) has been suggested as an alternative to the higher-cost intravenous heparin therapy. In a study of 650 patients, this approach was reported to be feasible, but it was associated with a 3.6% incidence of thromboembolism and a 6.7% incidence of bleeding.[32] Furthermore, concerns over the use of LMWH in patients with mechanical valves persist.[33] With regard to pregnancy, the American College of Chest Physicians recently concluded that it is reasonable to use one of the following three regimens to manage anticoagulation during pregnancy: (1) either LMWH or unfractionated heparin (UFH) between 6 and 12 weeks of gestation and close to term, with warfarin administered at all other times, (2) aggressive dose-adjusted UFH throughout pregnancy, or (3) aggressive dose-adjusted LMWH throughout pregnancy.[26,34]

15-3	Hemodynamic Principles for Perioperative Management of Valvular Heart Disease (VHD)						
VHD	**Cardiac Rhythm**	**HR**	**Contractility**	**Preload**	**SVR**	**PVR**	**Additional Considerations**
AS	Preserve NSR. Treat AF promptly.	Avoid tachycardia. Avoid severe bradycardia. Keep a slower HR (60-80).	Maintain—*may not withstand β-blockade.*	Increase. Avoid rapid fluid infusion.	Avoid sudden, profound decrease (CO is fixed).	Maintain.	Promptly correct hypotension. Consider preinduction external defibrillator placement. Caution with regional anesthesia.
HCM	Maintain NSR. Control tachyarrhythmias promptly.	Keep a slower HR. β-blockers useful.	Decrease. Negative inotropes (e.g., halothane) may be beneficial.	Increase without producing pulmonary edema. Avoid head-up positions.	Avoid decrease.	Maintain.	Consider preoperative baseline and provocative *(nitrates, Valsalva)* TTE. Consider preinduction external defibrillator placement. Caution with regional anesthesia.
MS	Often AF. Control ventricular response *(continue digitalis, β-blockers, Ca-channel blockers).*	Avoid tachycardia. Keep a slower HR (60-80).	Maintain within normal limits.	Maintain without producing pulmonary edema. Avoid rapid fluid infusion. Caution with Trendelenburg position.	Avoid sudden, profound decrease (CO is fixed).	Avoid exacerbation of PHT *(avoid N₂O, hypoxia, hypercarbia, acidosis, hypothermia).*	At premedication, avoid respiratory depression and provide supplemental O₂. Be aware of LA thrombi. PAC: proximal placement to avoid PA rupture, prominent A-wave on PAWP trace; PADP and PAWP overestimate LVEDP. Caution with regional anesthesia. Control pain, ventilation, body temperature postoperatively.
TS	Often in AF. Control ventricular response *(continue digitalis).*	Avoid tachycardia. Keep a slower HR (60-80).	Maintain within normal limits.	Maintain without producing systemic venous congestion.	Avoid sudden and profound decrease.	Maintain.	Consider hepatic dysfunction. Consider hypovolemia, electrolyte wasting from diuretic therapy. PA catheterization may be challenging. Prominent A-wave on CVP trace.
PS	Often AF. Control ventricular response.	Keep a faster HR unless severe RVH.	Maintain. Avoid myocardial depression.	Increase. Avoid rapid fluid infusion.	Maintain.	Keep low to normal range.	Consider hepatic dysfunction. Prominent A-wave often on CVP trace.
AR	Preserve NSR.	Increase HR. Avoid bradycardia.	Inotropic augmentation when appropriate. IABP contraindicated.	Maintain to prevent decrease in CO.	Avoid increase.	Maintain.	Regional anesthesia beneficial. Light premedication. PAC: PADP and PAWP underestimate LVEDP because of mitral valve closure before end-diastole. Prominent V-wave on PCWP trace if acute AR with diastolic MR.

Continued

15-3	**Hemodynamic Principles for Perioperative Management of Valvular Heart Disease (VHD)—cont'd**						
VHD	**Cardiac Rhythm**	**HR**	**Contractility**	**Preload**	**SVR**	**PVR**	**Additional Considerations**
MR	Often AF. Control ventricular response.	Keep a faster HR except for ischemic MR.	Avoid myocardial depression. Use inotropes and inodilators, *IABP* when appropriate.	Maintain without producing pulmonary edema.	Decrease.	Avoid PHT.	At premedication, avoid respiratory depression but provide supplemental O_2. PAC: prominent V-wave on PAWP trace (size does not correlate with MR severity) means PCWP overestimates LVEDP. Regional anesthesia beneficial. Control pain, ventilation, body temperature postoperatively. Avoid hypercarbia, halothane.
MVP	Maintain NSR. Associated with SVT and ventricular arrhythmias.	Keep a slower HR. Avoid anticholinergic agents.	Avoid increase. Avoid positive inotropes and sympathetic discharge.	Avoid decrease.	Avoid decrease. Avoid head-up positions.	Maintain.	
TR	Often AF. Control ventricular response.	Keep a faster HR (>80 bpm).	Avoid myocardial depression. Use inotropes and inodilators when appropriate.	Increase.	Maintain.	Decrease.	Consider hepatic dysfunction. Consider hypovolemia, electrolyte-wasting from diuretic therapy. PAC: prominent V-wave on CVP trace. CO measurement may be inaccurate.
PR	Maintain NSR and AV synchrony to facilitate forward flow.	Keep a faster HR.	Avoid myocardial depression. Use inotropes and inodilators when appropriate.	Increase.	Maintain.	Decrease.	PAC: PADP underestimates PAWP and LVEDP. CO measurement may be inaccurate. Consider propensity to QRS prolongation and monomorphic VT if RV dilation. Consider primary cause of PR (e.g., PHT).

AF, atrial fibrillation; AR, aortic regurgitation; AS, aortic stenosis; AV, atrioventricular; CO, cardiac output; CVP, central venous pressure; HCM, hypertrophic cardiomyopathy; HR, heart rate; IABP, intra-aortic balloon pump; LA, left atrial; LVEDP, left ventricular end-diastolic pressure; MR, mitral regurgitation; MS, mitral stenosis; MVP, mitral valve prolapse; N_2O, nitrous oxide; NSR, normal sinus rhythm; PA, pulmonary artery; PAC, pulmonary artery catheter; PADP, pulmonary artery diastolic pressure; PAWP, pulmonary artery wedge pressure; PHT, pulmonary hypertension; PR, pulmonic regurgitation; PS, pulmonic stenosis; PVR, pulmonary vascular resistance; RVH, right ventricular hypertrophy; SVR, systemic vascular resistance; SVT, supraventricular tachycardia; TR, tricuspid regurgitation; TS, tricuspid stenosis; TTE, transthoracic echocardiography.

Chronic Medications

Patients with severe VHD are often treated with antiarrhythmic, inotropic, or diuretic therapy (or more than one of these) and it is extremely important that these drugs be continued during the perioperative period.[35-37] An inability to administer postoperative oral medications in a timely fashion to heart failure patients could be one reason for the occurrence of postoperative CHF.[37] Similarly, cessation of antiarrhythmic drugs may pose a serious risk for the patient with severe aortic stenosis in whom cardiac output and hemodynamic stability critically depend on normal sinus rhythm.[22] Another consideration in the management of chronic medications is the preoperative assessment for side effects, such as toxicity from digitalis preparations or hypokalemia secondary to diuretic therapy.[36] Finally, therapy aimed at minimizing the perioperative cardiac risk has to be considered. Perioperative beta-blockade has been shown to reduce the risk of cardiac events in patients with a risk of myocardial ischemia who are undergoing noncardiac surgery,[1,12,38-40] but this benefit has to be balanced against the risk of compromising cardiac inotropic function in unstable VHD patients or those with limited contractile reserve. Although randomized trials generally support perioperative use of beta-blockade, it should be noted that very few patients with CHF have been enrolled in these trials. Thus, the safety and efficacy of beta-blockers in heart failure patients undergoing noncardiac surgery is uncertain. Furthermore, recent data have cast some doubt on the efficacy of perioperative beta-blocker therapy in patients with intermediate risk factors.[41,42] There is also growing evidence that alpha-2-agonists and statins reduce the risk of adverse cardiac events in surgical patients[12,43,44]; however, large-scale trials are still needed to further delineate the role of these agents. Finally, although an active inflammatory process contributing to calcific aortic stenosis has recently been recognized,[8,45] a prospective randomized clinical trial[46] concluded that intensive lipid-lowering with statin therapy did not halt the progression of stenosis or induce its regression.

■ INTRAOPERATIVE MANAGEMENT

Pathophysiology of Disease and Physiologic Principles of Management

The current hemodynamic principles of perioperative management of patients with VHD (see Table 15-3) are based on underlying pathophysiology and the natural history of the disease.[8,36,47-53] Discussing all of the pathophysiologic changes that occur with VHD is beyond the scope of this chapter, and interested readers should refer to recent high-quality reviews in the literature.[8,36,47-54] We will focus instead on the basic governing principles that facilitate clinical decision making.

In general, blood flow through a valve is governed by simple hydraulic principles,[49,55] where the valve area, the square root of the pressure gradient across the valve, and the duration of transvalvular flow during a specific phase of the cardiac cycle are the principal determinants of this flow. Lowering or raising these determinant factors will decrease or increase the transvalvular flow accordingly. In stenotic lesions, the anesthetic goal is to support transvalvular flow,

which is partially "fixed" by an obstructive lesion. In regurgitant lesions, the primary goal is to minimize the fraction of regurgitant flow through the abnormal valve and increase the degree of forward flow. Another consideration is that the regurgitant orifice area can change dynamically because of changes in valvular annulus or ventricular dimensions produced by varying loading conditions.[49,56] Thus, the perioperative management of heart rate, preload, and systemic and pulmonary vascular resistance depend on the specific type of valvular abnormality (see Table 15-3).

Nonpharmacologic Management

Nonpharmacologic factors[57,58] may facilitate or interfere with the provision of anesthesia for patients with VHD. For example, the Trendelenburg position may help to support preload in an emergency, but it may also promote pulmonary vascular congestion and decompensation in patients with elevated pulmonary artery pressures (common in severe mitral stenosis) or right heart valvular lesions. Similarly, the upright position can result in pooling of the blood into the lower extremities, causing a decrease in preload, emptying the heart chambers, and reducing the cardiac output settings, which will increase dynamic obstruction to flow in a patient with hypertrophic cardiomyopathy (HCM). Positive-pressure ventilation and positive end-expiratory pressure may also decrease venous return to the right heart and increase pulmonary vascular resistance (PVR).[59] Other important causes of rise in PVR include hypoxia, hypercapnia, acidosis, and hypothermia. Hypothermia also increases the sympathetic drive and represents an additional risk factor for morbid cardiac events.[60] Importantly, preservation of normothermia[61] and administration of supplemental oxygen[62] have been shown to reduce the incidence of surgical infection.

Premedication

Premedication is helpful to prevent anxiety and stress-induced tachycardia. However, in some patients, acutely withdrawing the sympathetic tone may be undesirable. In patients with severe VHD, premedication should be tailored to preserve myocardial function and to avoid significant reduction in preload and systemic vascular resistance (SVR).[50,51] In patients with elevated pulmonary pressures and right heart disease, hypoventilation leading to hypoxemia or hypercapnia should also be avoided.

Type of Anesthesia: General, Regional, or Local with Monitored Sedation

Many anesthetic regimens are used for patients with VHD who are undergoing noncardiac surgery.[51] Today, there is no strong evidence to support that a specific anesthetic technique is associated with better clinical outcomes. Monitored anesthesia care with sedation alone causes less hemodynamic disturbance than a general or neuraxial approach, but it is useful in only a limited number of surgical procedures. The risk of deep venous thrombosis is generally lower with spinal or epidural anesthesia than with general anesthesia.[63] Epidural and spinal anesthesia can, however, produce sympathetic withdrawal and thus decrease SVR as well as preload.[64] Although decreases in afterload may help to maintain forward flow in regurgitant valvular lesions, sudden and profound drops in SVR can be detrimental to patients with stenotic flow obstructions.[51] Unfortunately, the literature lacks the scientific validity provided by randomized clinical trials, and the best available data include only a few case reports in which regional anesthesia was successfully administered to patients with significant stenotic VHD.[65-68] Certain neuraxial techniques, such as continuous spinal and epidural anesthesia, can be tailored to minimize the rapid changes in sympathetic tone.[65] In particular, avoiding the blockade of the sympathetic nerve fibers from T9 to L1 by using lower-level block or with high thoracic epidural analgesia helps to reduce these side effects.[69] Reduction of local anesthetic doses by using them in combination with epidural and intrathecal narcotics also helps to minimize the sympatholytic effects of regional anesthesia.[69]

For patients with normal ventricular function, a balanced general anesthesia with lower concentrations of volatile anesthetics is usually a safe option that minimizes adverse effects on contractility and loading conditions.[36,51] Patients with poor LV function may not be able to tolerate even the lower concentration of volatile gases, and a narcotic-based anesthetic may be the method of choice. Nitrous oxide should be used carefully in patients with mild or moderate pulmonary hypertension, and possibly avoided when significant disease is present, because of the potential of this gas to increase pulmonary artery pressures.[36,51,70,71] Light anesthesia and poor pain control are other factors that may contribute to the increase in sympathoadrenal drive and PVR. The choice of muscle relaxant is related to the specific hemodynamic effects it may cause.[72,73] Regardless of the type of anesthesia, there must be prompt response to sudden hemodynamic changes. Intraoperative fluctuations in mean arterial pressure increase the probability of postoperative heart failure in high-risk patients undergoing elective general surgery.[3] Thus, for patients with severe VHD, cardioactive and vasoactive drips should be readily available.

Monitoring Options

The use of invasive monitoring for patients with VHD is based on the severity of disease, associated cardiac and noncardiac problems, the nature of the surgical procedure, and the practice setting.[36,74,75] Asymptomatic patients without concurrent disease going for minimal-risk surgery require monitoring just as those without VHD do. On the other hand, symptomatic patients undergoing major surgical procedures require invasive monitoring that provides hemodynamic data on a beat-to-beat basis. Such intensive monitoring has been shown to attenuate risk during noncardiac surgery in some patient groups such as those with severe aortic stenosis.[76] Therefore, except for minor surgical procedures (e.g., cataract extraction), direct arterial pressure monitoring should be used for most patients with severe preexisting VHD disease, particularly if there is concomitant LV dysfunction or hemodynamic instability.

Right heart catheterization with a pulmonary artery catheter (PAC) is an important technique to assess the adequacy of circulating blood volume (right ventricular [RV] and LV preload), cardiac output, and mixed venous oxygen-

ation. However, the use of the PAC remains controversial in perioperative medicine.[74,75,77,78] In the recent practice guidelines of the American Society of Anesthesiologists,[75] it is emphasized that with some exceptions, routine pulmonary artery catheterization is generally inappropriate for low- or moderate-risk patients. PAC monitoring is, however, appropriate or necessary in patients undergoing high-risk procedures with large fluid changes or hemodynamic disturbances or with high risk of morbidity and mortality, or in those with severe cardiac disease whose hemodynamic disturbances have a great chance of causing organ dysfunction or death.[75] Additionally, practice settings, particularly catheter use skills and technical support, play an important role in decisions related to PAC use. For patients with VHD, interpretation of PAC data involves understanding that central venous waveforms are altered with significant tricuspid valve lesions, and the pulmonary artery wedge pressures are not reflective of LV end-diastolic pressures in patients with severe mitral disease.[74]

TEE is now widely used during cardiac and noncardiac surgery and in the early postoperative period.[79] Because global and regional heart function, loading conditions, and valvular dysfunction can be effectively monitored by this technique, monitoring with TEE is particularly beneficial for patients with severe VHD[36] and those with a significant risk of hemodynamic disturbances during surgery.[80] There is strong evidence supporting the perioperative use of TEE for evaluating acute, persistent, and life-threatening hemodynamic disturbances in which ventricular function and its determinants are uncertain and have not responded to treatment.[80]

■ POSTOPERATIVE MANAGEMENT

The principles of hemodynamic optimization based on the pathophysiology of specific VHD apply also to the postoperative management of these patients. Both preoperative status[1,3,37] and intraoperative course[3] should be taken into consideration as risk factors for postoperative complications. Patients with severe VHD are prone to develop a number of postoperative problems, including myocardial ischemia, arrhythmias, and heart failure. Continuation of invasive monitoring enables prompt and effective management while the patient is stabilizing after surgery. Effective pain management is of paramount importance so that uncontrolled surges in sympathetic activity are prevented. Alleviation of postoperative pain may also help to decrease perioperative morbidity and mortality.[69,81] Patients who were on beta-blockers preoperatively should have them continued postoperatively to reduce the risk of myocardial ischemia.[82] Antimicrobial agents should be discontinued within 24 hours of the end of surgery.[21,24] Tight blood glucose control, aiming for normoglycemia, reduces the rate of postoperative infections and overall in-hospital mortality among critically ill patients in the surgical intensive care unit.[83-85] Oral anticoagulants should be reinstituted as soon as possible, with initial administration of heparin if necessary.[10,25,26]

■ SPECIFIC VALVULAR LESIONS

The type of valvular lesion should be determined prior to the surgical procedure, because the perioperative management of stenotic lesions differs significantly from that of regurgitant lesions.[22] Each type of VHD imposes a unique set of stresses on the LV and RV, leading to specific hemodynamic profiles and recommendations for anesthetic and therapeutic priorities for each lesion (see Table 15-3).[50] Aortic and mitral lesions are the most common and are discussed in greater detail. Tricuspid and pulmonary lesions are less frequent and therefore less studied in the perioperative environment. Management of tricuspid lesions is generally thought to be similar to the matching lesion in the left heart (i.e., a mitral lesion), but studies are scarce and so are specific guidelines or recommendations.

Aortic Stenosis

Calcific degenerative disease is the most common cause of aortic stenosis (AS) in adults with a normal trileaflet valve.[8,86,87] In those with a congenital bicuspid valve, stenosis usually develops earlier in life. Rheumatic AS is less common and is always accompanied by some degree of mitral valve disease. In patients with aortic stenosis, a hypertrophic process allows the left ventricle to adapt to the pressure overload.[88] The increased wall-thickness with associated diminished LV compliance, however, produces an increase in LV end-diastolic pressure. Therefore, atrial contraction plays an important role in ventricular filling and explains the significant deterioration seen in patients with AS who are tachycardic or who lose the atrial contribution to filling (e.g., atrial fibrillation). Hypertrophy may also reduce coronary blood flow per gram of muscle while increasing the sensitivity to ischemic injury,[89-92] further explaining why this lesion substantially increases risk for patients undergoing noncardiac surgery.[1,6,7,93] Valvotomy or aortic valve replacement prior to noncardiac surgery may be considered for eligible patients with severe AS in order to alleviate the fixed cardiac output that is a hallmark of this lesion.

Mitral Stenosis

Mitral stenosis (MS) is an obstruction to LV inflow that prevents proper opening of the valve during diastolic filling of the left ventricle. Rheumatic carditis is the most common cause of MS, and although MS is seen increasingly rarely because of the decreased incidence of rheumatic disease in the developed world,[94] it remains an important lesion because of the associated perioperative risk.[1] When valve area is reduced, blood can flow into the left ventricle only if it is propelled by a pressure gradient. This transmitral gradient is the characteristic feature of MS that results in elevated left atrial and pulmonary venous pressures and leads eventually to pulmonary edema. As the severity of stenosis increases, cardiac output falls below normal at rest and does not increase with exercise.[95] In patients with chronic MS, pulmonary vascular permeability may decrease significantly, thus diminishing the likelihood of pulmonary edema, but this is often offset by the onset of pulmonary hypertension. For any given orifice size, the transmitral gradient is a function of the square of the transvalvular flow rate and dependent on the diastolic filling period.[55] Thus, perioperative symptoms are often precipitated by stress, infection, or tachycardia.

Aortic Regurgitation

Aortic regurgitant lesions are a very common finding on pulsed Doppler echocardiography, but in the majority of cases, these jets represent a trivial regurgitant volume and are of no clinical significance.[96] Aortic regurgitation (AR) results from multiple abnormalities affecting aortic leaflets or aortic root and annulus.[96,97] The primary pathology includes congenital bicuspid aortic valve, rheumatic heart disease, infective endocarditis, and aortic root diseases. Anoretic drugs have also been recently reported to cause AR.[98] Acute AR, most commonly caused by infective endocarditis, aortic dissection, or blunt chest trauma, results in catastrophic elevation in LV filling pressures and requires emergent surgical replacement of the valve.[97] In chronic AR, compensatory mechanisms include eccentric hypertrophy followed later by concentric hypertrophy and increasing chamber compliance to accommodate a larger diastolic volume.[99] The greater diastolic volume maintains forward stroke volume by ejecting a larger stroke volume, and the hypertrophy helps to maintain normal ejection performance despite an increased afterload.[100,101] Vasodilator therapy reduces the hemodynamic burden in these patients by improving forward stroke volume and reducing the regurgitant volume. Similarly, an increase in heart rate can be beneficial in maintaining cardiac output.

Mitral Regurgitation

Mitral regurgitation (MR) has many causes, the most common being papillary muscle dysfunction, mitral valve prolapse, and dilatation of the mitral valve annulus and left ventricular cavity.[102] Chronic myocardial ischemia can also result in MR secondary to increased leaflet tethering and a reduced closing force of the mitral valve.[56] Acute mitral regurgitation secondary to chordae tendineae rupture or papillary muscle infarction imposes a sudden volume overload on the left atrium and ventricle, resulting in pulmonary edema. Chronic MR also produces eccentric hypertrophy and an increase in LV end-diastolic volume as compensatory mechanisms. The increase in end-diastolic volume restores forward cardiac output, and the increase in left atrial and ventricular size allows accommodation of the regurgitant volume at a lower filling pressure. Afterload reduction is again beneficial in patients with chronic MR associated with LV dilatation and systolic dysfunction.[103] However, there is no indication for vasodilating therapy in asymptomatic patients with MR and preserved LV function.[10,103] As with AR, an increase in heart rate can be beneficial in maintaining cardiac output.

Tricuspid Valve Disease

Tricuspid valve disease is most commonly seen as a congenital abnormality, with Ebstein's anomaly being the most common, wherein failure of leaflet coaptation leads to severe tricuspid regurgitation (TR). Acquired TR is most often secondary to RV dilation and failure resulting from pulmonary

Text continued on p. 216.

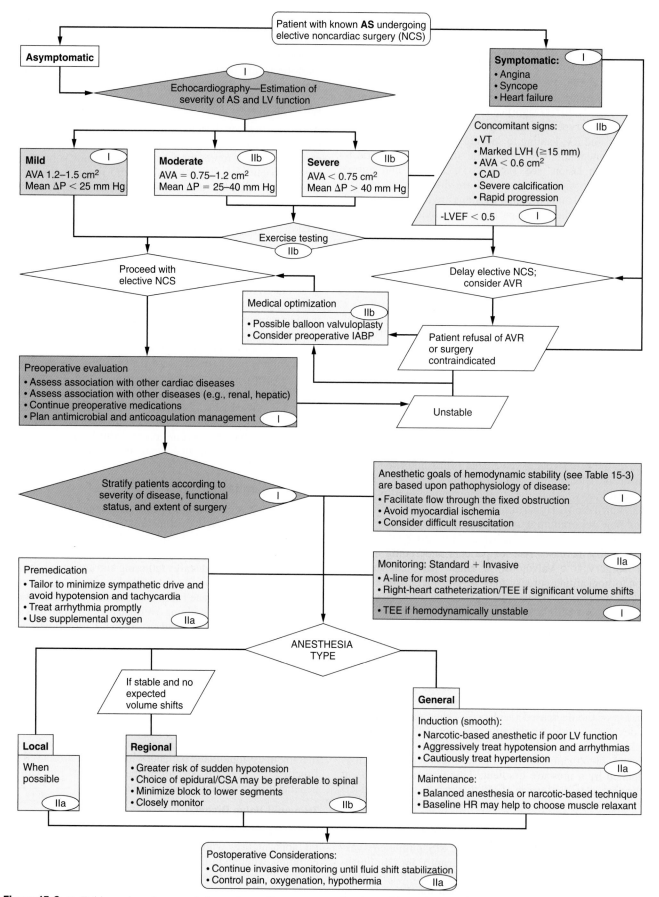

Figure 15-2 ■ Evidence-based approach for perioperative treatment of patient with aortic stenosis (AS). Balloon valvotomy temporarily relieves symptoms but does not prolong survival; 10-year age-corrected rates of survival among patients who underwent aortic valve replacement (AVR) surgery approach the rate in the normal population. Recommendation class (I, IIa, IIb, III) based on ACC/AHA format. AVA, aortic valve area; CAD, coronary artery disease; CSA, continuous spinal anesthesia; HR, heart rate; IABP, intra-aortic balloon pump; LV, left ventricular; LVEF, left ventricular ejection fraction; LVH, left ventricular hypertrophy; NCS, noncardiac surgery; ΔP, pressure gradient; TEE, transesophageal echocardiography; VT, ventricular tachycardia.

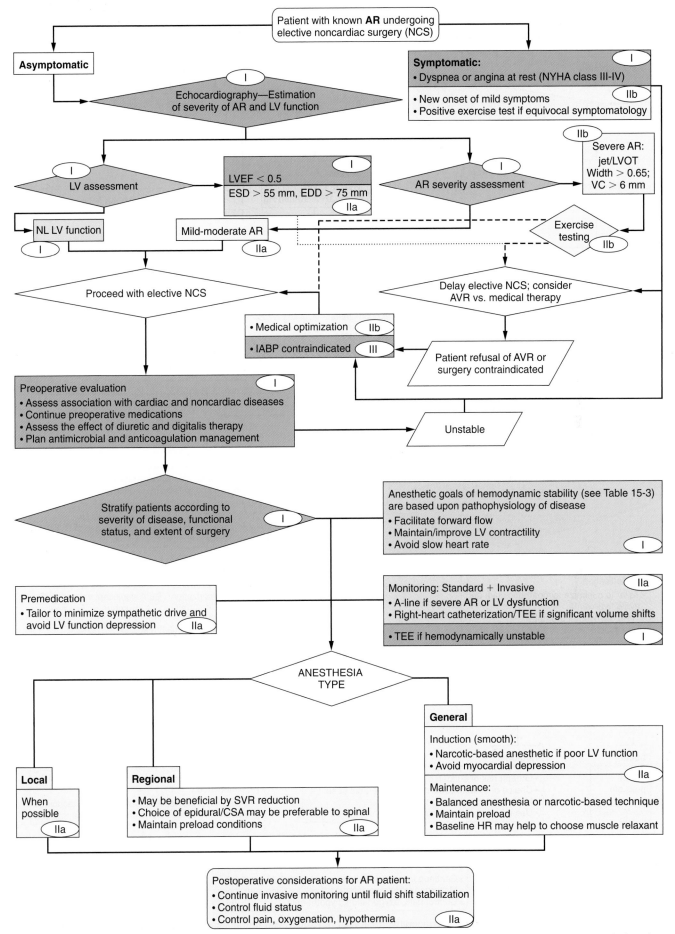

Figure 15-3 ■ Evidence-based approach for perioperative treatment of patient with aortic regurgitation (AR). Recommendation class (I, IIa, IIb, III) based on ACC/AHA format. AVR, aortic-valve replacement; CSA, continuous spinal anesthesia; EDD, end-diastolic dimension; ESD, end-systolic dimension; HR, heart rate; NCS, noncardiac surgery; NL, normal; NYHA, New York Heart Association; LA, left atrial; LV, left ventricular; LVEF, left ventricular ejection fraction; LVOT, left ventricular outflow tract; SVR, systemic vascular resistance; TEE, transesophageal echocardiography; VC, vena contracta.

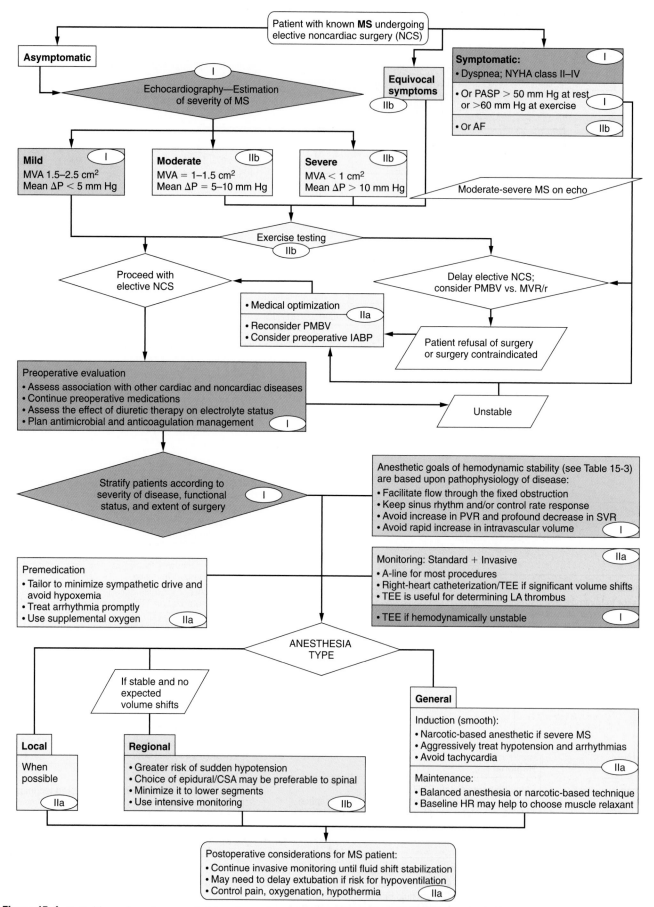

Figure 15-4 ■ Evidence-based approach for perioperative treatment of patient with mitral stenosis (MS). Recommendation class (I, IIa, IIb, III) based on ACC/AHA format. AF, atrial fibrillation; CSA, continuous spinal anesthesia; HR, heart rate; IABP, intra-aortic balloon pump; MVA, mitral valve area; MVR/r, mitral valve replacement/repair; NYHA, New York Heart Association; PASP, pulmonary artery systolic pressure; PMBV, percutaneous mitral balloon valvuloplasty; PVR, peripheral vascular resistance; SVR, systemic vascular resistance; TEE, transesophageal echocardiography.

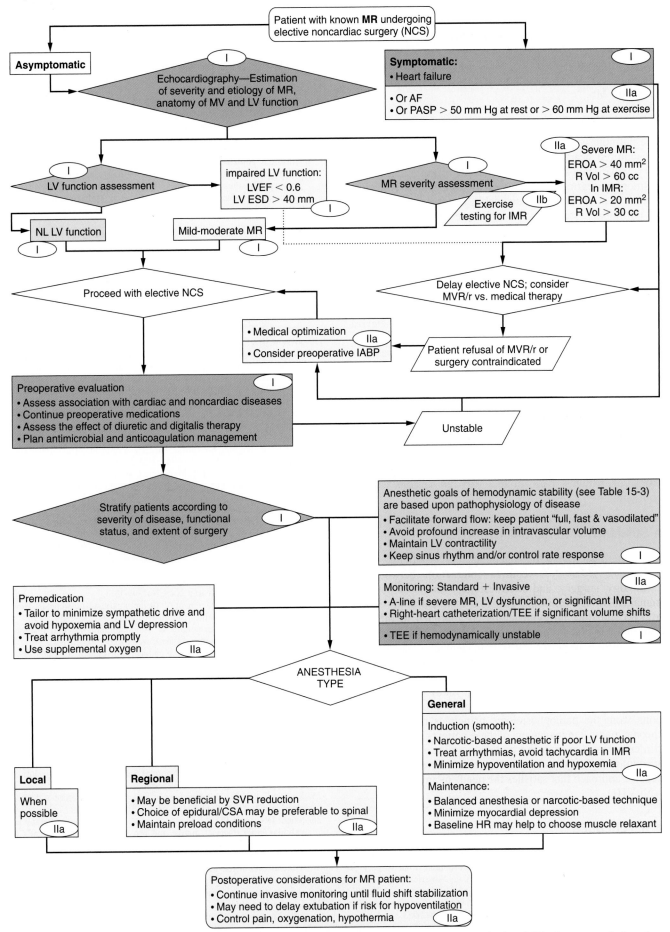

Figure 15-5 ■ Evidence-based approach for perioperative treatment of patient with mitral regurgitation (MR). Recommendation class (I, IIa, IIb, III) based on ACC/AHA format. AF, atrial fibrillation; CSA, continuous spinal anesthesia; EROA, effective regurgitant orifice area; ESD, end-systolic dimension; IABP, intra-aortic balloon pump; IMR, ischemic mitral regurgitation; LV, left ventricular; LVEF, left ventricular ejection fraction; MVR/r, mitral valve replacement/repair; NL, normal; PASP, pulmonary artery systolic pressure; RVol, regurgitant volume; SVR, systemic vascular resistance; TEE, transesophageal echocardiography.

or RV hypertension.[96] Tricuspid stenosis (TS) is most commonly caused by rheumatic disease and is usually associated with MS.[50]

Pulmonic Valve Disease

The pulmonary valve is the least likely valve to be affected by acquired heart disease, and almost all cases of pulmonary valve stenosis are congenital in origin.[10,54] Although pulmonary regurgitation is rare as an isolated congenital lesion, it is an almost unavoidable result of valvuloplasty of pulmonary stenosis or surgical repair of tetralogy of Fallot.[10,54]

Mixed Valvular Lesions

Multivalvular disease occurs in the context of rheumatic heart disease, myxomatous valvular disease, and bacterial endocarditis. The relative contribution of each of these lesions is difficult to assess noninvasively, and cardiac catheterization and angiocardiography are often required.[96] Perioperative management of multivalvular heart disease is based on the severity and hemodynamic significance of each valvular lesion.[50] In mixed single-valve disease (e.g., AR with AS), one lesion usually predominates over the other and the pathophysiology resembles that of the dominant lesion. Similarly, in patients with multiple valve regurgitation (e.g., MR and AR), the best strategy is to determine the dominant lesion and to treat it accordingly. However, it is not always easy to establish which lesion is dominant—the pathophysiology in patients with mixed valvular lesions can be confusing.

■ SUMMARY AND RECOMMENDATIONS

The perioperative management of patients with VHD[10,18,36,47-53,65,80,104-106] requires interaction between the cardiology, surgery, and anesthesiology teams to optimize management and minimize risk to the patient. Figures 15-2 to 15-5 illustrate an evidence-based approach to the most common valvular lesions (AS, AR, MS, and MR). However, when defining the perioperative management of patients with VHD, strong trial-based evidence for most recommendations is lacking—even more so for intraoperative care. Although our knowledge is rapidly expanding, many of the clinical advisories are still based on anecdotal reports or extrapolations from the pathophysiologic principles relevant to the chronic medical management of these patients. Therefore, the clinician has a responsibility to recognize unusual cases, account for specific practice settings, and develop a comprehensive approach that satisfies the needs of any given patient with VHD.

■ REFERENCES

1. Eagle KA, Berger PB, Calkins H, et al: ACC/AHA guideline update for perioperative cardiovascular evaluation for noncardiac surgery: A report of the American College of Cardiology/American Heart Association Task Force on Practice Guidelines (Committee to Update the 1996 Guidelines on Perioperative Cardiovascular Evaluation for Noncardiac Surgery). Am Coll Cardiol 2002;39:542-553.

2. Phillip B, Pastor D, Bellows W, Leung JM: The prevalence of preoperative diastolic filling abnormalities in geriatric surgical patients. Anesth Analg 2003;97:1214-1221.

3. Charlson ME, MacKenzie CR, Gold JP, et al: Risk for postoperative congestive heart failure. Surg Gynecol Obstet 1991;172:95-104.

4. Polanczyk CA, Goldman L, Marcantonio ER, et al: Supraventricular arrhythmia in patients having noncardiac surgery: Clinical correlates and effect on length of stay. Ann Intern Med 1998;129:279-285.

5. Sprung J, Abdelmalak B, Gottlieb A, et al: Analysis of risk factors for myocardial infarction and cardiac mortality after major vascular surgery. Anesthesiology 2000;93:129-140.

6. Goldman L, Caldera DL, Nussbaum SR, et al: Multifactorial index of cardiac risk in noncardiac surgical procedures. N Engl J Med 1977;297:845-850.

7. O'Keefe JH Jr, Shub C, Rettke SR: Risk of noncardiac surgical procedures in patients with aortic stenosis. Mayo Clin Proc 1989;64:400.

8. Bonow RO, Braunwald E: Valvular heart disease. In Zipes DP, Libby P, Bonow RO, Braunwald E (eds): Braunwald's Heart Disease: A Textbook of Cardiovascular Medicine, ed 7. Philadelphia, Saunders, 2005, pp 1553-1632.

9. Park KW: Preoperative cardiac evaluation. Anesthesiol Clin North Am 2004;22:199-208.

10. Bonow RO, Carabello B, Kang C, et al: ACC/AHA 2006 Guidelines for the management of patients with valvular heart disease. A report of the American College of Cardiology/American Heart Association Task Force on Practice Guidelines. Circulation 2006;114:e84-e231.

11. Carabello BA, Crawford FA: Valvular heart disease. N Engl J Med 1997;337:32-41.

12. Kertai MD, Klein J, Bax JJ, Poldermans D: Predicting perioperative cardiac risk. Prog Cardiovasc Dis 2005;47:240-257.

13. Detsky AS, Abrams HB, Forbath N, et al: Cardiac assessment for patients undergoing noncardiac surgery: A multifactorial clinical risk index. Arch Intern Med 1986;146:2131-2134.

14. Lee TH, Marcantonio ER, Mangione CM, et al: Derivation and prospective validation of a simple index for prediction of cardiac risk of major noncardiac surgery. Circulation 1999;100:1043-1049.

15. Torsher LC, Shub C, Rettke SR, Brown DL: Risk of patients with severe aortic stenosis undergoing noncardiac surgery. Am J Cardiol 1998;81:448-452.

16. Amato MC, Moffa PJ, Werner KE, Ramires JA: Treatment decision in asymptomatic aortic valve stenosis: Role of exercise testing. Heart 2001;86:381-386.

17. Das P, Rimington H, Chambers J: Exercise testing to stratify risk in aortic stenosis. Eur Heart J 2005;26:1309-1313.

18. Baumgartner H: Management of asymptomatic aortic stenosis: How helpful is exercise testing? Eur Heart J 2005;26:1252-1254.

19. Botkin N, Seth P, Aurigemma G: Asymptomatic valvular disease: Who benefits from surgery? Curr Cardiol Rep 2005;7:87-93.

20. Moreillon P, Que Y-A: Infective endocarditis. Lancet 2004;363:139.

21. Dajani AS, Taubert KA, Wilson W, et al: Prevention of bacterial endocarditis: Recommendations by the American Heart Association. Circulation 1997;96:358-366.

22. Roizen MF, Fleisher LA: Anesthetic implications of concurrent diseases. In Miller RD (ed): Miller's Anesthesia, ed 6. Philadelphia, Elsevier, 2005, pp 1017-1150.

23. Antimicrobial prophylaxis for surgery. Treat Guidel Med Lett 2004;2:27-32.

24. Bratzler DW, Houck PM: Antimicrobial prophylaxis for surgery: An advisory statement from the National Surgical Infection Prevention Project. Am J Surg 2005;189:395-404.

25. Kearon C, Hirsh J: Management of anticoagulation before and after elective surgery. N Engl J Med 1997;336:1506-1511.

26. Salem DN, Stein PD, Al-Ahmad A, et al: Antithrombotic therapy in valvular heart disease—native and prosthetic: The Seventh ACCP Conference on Antithrombotic and Thrombolytic Therapy. Chest 2004;126(3 Suppl):457S-482S.

27. Moreno-Cabral RJ, McNamara JJ, Mamiya RT, et al: Acute thrombotic obstruction with Björk-Shiley valves: Diagnostic and surgical considerations. J Thorac Cardiovasc Surg 1978;75:321-330.

28. Copans H, Lakier JB, Kinsley RH, et al: Thrombosed Björk-Shiley mitral prostheses. Circulation 1980;61:169-174.

29. Kontos GJ Jr, Schaff HV: Thrombotic occlusion of a prosthetic heart valve: Diagnosis and management. Mayo Clin Proc 1985;60:118-122.

30. Genewein U, Haeberli A, Straub PW, Beer JH: Rebound after cessation of oral anticoagulant therapy: The biochemical evidence. Br J Haematol 1996;92:479-485.

31. Eckman MH, Beshansky JR, Durand-Zaleski I, et al: Anticoagulation for noncardiac procedures in patients with prosthetic heart valves. Does low risk mean high cost? JAMA 1990;263:1513-1521.

32. Kovacs MJ, Kearon C, Rodger M, et al: Single-arm study of bridging therapy with low-molecular-weight heparin for patients at risk of arterial embolism who require temporary interruption of warfarin. Circulation 2004;110:1658-1663.

33. Hirsh J, Fuster V, Ansell J, Halperin JL: American Heart Association/American College of Cardiology Foundation guide to warfarin therapy. J Am Coll Cardiol 2003;41:1633-1652.

34. Bates SM, Greer IA, Hirsh J, Ginsberg JS: Use of antithrombotic agents during pregnancy: The Seventh ACCP Conference on Antithrombotic and Thrombolytic Therapy. Chest 2004;126(3 Suppl):627S-644S.

35. Fleisher LA: Risk of anesthesia. In Miller RD (ed): Miller's Anesthesia, ed 6. Philadelphia, Elsevier, 2005, pp 893-926.

36. Stoelting RK, Diefdorf SF: Valvular heart disease. In Stoelting RK, Diefdorf SF (eds): Anesthesia and Co-Existing Disease, ed 4. New York, Churchill Livingstone, 2002, pp 25-44.

37. Hernandez AF, Newby LK, O'Connor CM: Preoperative evaluation for major noncardiac surgery: Focusing on heart failure. Arch Intern Med 2004;164:1729-1736.

38. Cohn SL, Goldman L: Preoperative risk evaluation and perioperative management of patients with coronary artery disease. Med Clin North Am 2003;87:111-136.

39. Auerbach AD, Goldman L: Beta-Blockers and reduction of cardiac events in noncardiac surgery: Scientific review. JAMA 2002;287:1435-1444.

40. Fleisher LA: Should Beta-adrenergic blocking agents be given routinely in noncardiac surgery? In Fleisher LA (ed): Evidence-Based Practice of Anesthesiology. Philadelphia, Elsevier, 2004, pp 163-167.

41. London MJ, Henderson WG: Perioperative pharmacologic cardioprotection and sodium hydrogen ion exchange inhibitors: One step forward and two steps back? J Cardiothorac Vasc Anesth 2005;19:565-569.

42. Stevens RD, Burri H, Tramer MR: Pharmacologic myocardial protection in patients undergoing noncardiac surgery: A quantitative systematic review. Anesth Analg 2003;97:623-633.

43. Shook DC, Ellis JE: Are alpha-2 agonists effective in reducing perioperative cardiac complications in noncardiac surgery? In Fleisher LA (ed): Evidence-Based Practice of Anesthesiology. Philadelphia, Elsevier, 2004, pp 168-171.

44. Beattie WS: Evidence-based perioperative risk reduction. Can J Anesth 2005;52(suppl 1):R5.

45. Rosenhek R: Statins for aortic stenosis. N Engl J Med 2005;352:2441-2443.

46. Cowell SJ, Newby DE, Prescott RJ, et al: A randomized trial of intensive lipid-lowering therapy in calcific aortic stenosis. N Engl J Med 2005;352:2389-2397.

47. Chen J, Leung JM: Valvular heart disease. In Leung JM (ed): Cardiac and Vascular Anesthesia: The Requisites in Anesthesiology, ed 1. St Louis, Mosby, 2004, pp 86-107.

48. Levin SK, Boyd WC, Rothstein PT, Thomas SJ: Anesthesia for cardiac surgery. In Barash PG, Cullen BF, Stoelting RK (eds): Clinical Anesthesia, ed 4. Philadelphia, Lippincott, Williams & Wilkins, 2001, pp 883-928.

49. Johnston WE: Anesthesia for patient with valvular heart disease. Annual Meeting Refresher Course Lectures, vol 510. Las Vegas, American Society of Anesthesiologists, 2004, pp 1-7.

50. Moore RA, Martin DE: Anesthetic management for valvular heart disease. In Hensley FA Jr, Martin DE (eds): A Practical Approach to Cardiac Anesthesia, ed 3. Philadelphia, Lippincott Williams & Wilkins, 2003, pp 302-335.

51. Ghobashy AM, Barash PG: Valvular heart disease. In Troianos CA (ed): Anesthesia for the Cardiac Patient. St Louis, Mosby, 2002, pp 237-269.

52. Jackson JM, Thomas SJ: Valvular heart disease. In Kaplan JA, Reich DL, Konstadt SN (eds): Cardiac Anesthesia. Philadelphia, WB Saunders, 1999, pp 727-784.

53. Nyhan D, Johns RA: Anesthesia for cardiac surgery procedures. In Miller RD (ed): Miller's Anesthesia, ed 6. Philadelphia, Elsevier, 2005, pp 1941-2004.

54. Warnes CA: The adult with congenital heart disease: Born to be bad? J Am Coll Cardiol 2005;46:1.

55. Gorlin R, Gorlin SG: Hydraulic formula for calculation of the area of the stenotic mitral valve, other cardiac valves, and central circulatory shunts: I. Am Heart J 1951;41:1-29.

56. Pierard LA, Lancellotti P: The role of ischemic mitral regurgitation in the pathogenesis of acute pulmonary edema. N Engl J Med 2004;351:1627-1634.

57. Sessler DI, Akca O: Nonpharmacological prevention of surgical wound infections. Clin Infect Dis 2002;35:1397-1404.

58. Buhre W, Rossaint R: Perioperative management and monitoring in anaesthesia. Lancet 2003;362:1839-1846.

59. Brown M: ICU: Critical care. In Barash PG, Cullen BF, Stoelting RK (eds): Clinical Anesthesia, ed 4. Philadelphia, Lippincott Williams & Wilkins, 2001, pp 1463-1483.

60. Frank SM, Fleisher LA, Breslow MJ, et al: Perioperative maintenance of normothermia reduces the incidence of morbid cardiac events: A randomized clinical trial. JAMA 1997;277:1127-1134.

61. Kurz A, Sessler DI, Lenhardt R: Perioperative normothermia to reduce the incidence of surgical-wound infection and shorten hospitalization. Study of Wound Infection and Temperature Group. N Engl J Med 1996;334:1209-1216.

62. Greif R, Akca O, Horn E-P, Kurz A, Sessler DI: Supplemental perioperative oxygen to reduce the incidence of surgical-wound infection. The Outcomes Research Group. N Engl J Med 2000;342:161-167.

63. Geerts WH, Pineo GF, Heit JA, et al: Prevention of venous thromboembolism: The Seventh ACCP Conference on Antithrombotic and Thrombolytic Therapy. Chest 2004;126(3 Suppl):338S-400S.

64. Brown DL: Spinal, epidural, and caudal anesthesia. In Miller RD (ed): Miller's Anesthesia, ed 6. Philadelphia, Elsevier, 2005, pp 1653-1684.

65. McDonald SB: Is neuraxial blockade contraindicated in the patient with aortic stenosis? Reg Anesth Pain Med 2004;29:496.

66. Pan PH, D'Angelo R: Anesthetic and analgesic management of mitral stenosis during pregnancy. Reg Anesth Pain Med 2004;29:610.

67. Okutomi T, Kikuchi S, Amano K, et al: Continuous spinal analgesia for labor and delivery in a parturient with hypertrophic obstructive cardiomyopathy. Acta Anaesthesiol Scand 2002;46:329-331.

68. Ransom DM, Leicht CH: Continuous spinal analgesia with sufentanil for labor and delivery in a parturient with severe pulmonary stenosis. Anesth Analg 1995;80:418-421.

69. Richman JM, Wu CL: Epidural analgesia for postoperative pain. Anesthesiol Clin North Am 2005;23:125-140.

70. Schulte-Sasse U, Hess W, Tarnow J: Pulmonary vascular responses to nitrous oxide in patients with normal and high pulmonary vascular resistance. Anesthesiology 1982;57:9-13.

71. Konstadt SN, Reich DL, Thys DM: Nitrous oxide does not exacerbate pulmonary hypertension or ventricular dysfunction in patients with mitral valvular disease. Can J Anaesth 1990;37:613-617.

72. Hanson EW, Neerhut RK, Lynch C 3rd: Mitral valve prolapse. Anesthesiology 1996;85:178-195.

73. Larach DR, Hensley FA Jr, Martin DE, et al: Hemodynamic effects of muscle relaxant drugs during anesthetic induction in patients with mitral or aortic valvular heart disease. J Cardiothorac Vasc Anesth 1991;5:126-131.

74. Mark JB, Slaughter TF: Cardiovascular monitoring. In Miller RD (ed): Miller's Anesthesia, ed 6. Philadelphia, Elsevier, 2005, pp 1265-1362.

75. Roizen MF, Berger DL, Gabel RA, et al: Practice guidelines for pulmonary artery catheterization: An updated report by the American Society of Anesthesiologists Task Force on Pulmonary Artery Catheterization. Anesthesiology 2003;99:988-1014.

76. Raymer K, Yang H: Patients with aortic stenosis: Cardiac complications in non-cardiac surgery. Can J Anaesth 1998;45:855-859.

77. Sandham JD, Hull RD, Brant RF, et al: A randomized, controlled trial of the use of pulmonary-artery catheters in high-risk surgical patients. N Engl J Med 2003;348:5-14.

78. Cholley BP, Payen D, Karkouti K, et al: Pulmonary-artery catheters in high-risk surgical patients. N Engl J Med 2003;348:2035-2037.

79. Daniel WG, Mugge A: Transesophageal echocardiography. N Engl J Med 1995;332:1268-1280.

80. Cheitlin MD, Armstrong WF, Aurigemma GP, et al: ACC/AHA/ASE 2003 guideline update for the clinical application of echocardiography: Summary article: A Report of the American College of Cardiology/American Heart Association Task Force on Practice Guidelines (ACC/AHA/ASE Committee to Update the 1997 Guidelines for the Clinical Application of Echocardiography). Circulation 2003;108:1146-1162.

81. Liu S, Carpenter RL, Neal JM: Epidural anesthesia and analgesia: Their role in postoperative outcome. Anesthesiology 1995;82:1474-1506.

82. Taylor RC, Pagliarello G: Prophylactic beta-blockade to prevent myocardial infarction perioperatively in high-risk patients who undergo general surgical procedures. Can J Surg 2003;46:216-222.

83. Van den Berghe G: Insulin therapy for the critically ill patient. Clin Cornerstone 2003;5:56-63.

84. Van den Berghe G, Wouters P, Weekers F, et al: Intensive insulin therapy in the critically ill patients. N Engl J Med 2001;345:1359-1367.

85. Lewis KS, Kane-Gill SL, Bobek MB, Dasta JF: Intensive insulin therapy for critically ill patients. Ann Pharmacother 2004;38:1243-1251.

86. Chambers J: Aortic stenosis. BMJ 2005;330:801-802.

87. Branch KR, O'Brien KD, Otto CM: Aortic valve sclerosis as a marker of active atherosclerosis. Curr Cardiol Rep 2002;4:111-117.

88. Spann JF, Bove AA, Natarajan G, Kreulen T: Ventricular performance, pump function and compensatory mechanisms in patients with aortic stenosis. Circulation 1980;62:576-582.

89. Bache RJ, Vrobel TR, Ring WS, et al: Regional myocardial blood flow during exercise in dogs with chronic left ventricular hypertrophy. Circ Res 1981;48:76-87.

90. Gaasch WH, Zile MR, Hoshino PK, et al: Tolerance of the hypertrophic heart to ischemia: Studies in compensated and failing dog hearts with pressure overload hypertrophy. Circulation 1990;81:1644-1653.

91. Koyanagi S, Eastham CL, Harrison DG, Marcus ML: Increased size of myocardial infarction in dogs with chronic hypertension and left ventricular hypertrophy. Circ Res 1982;50:55-62.

92. Marcus ML, Doty DB, Hiratzka LF, et al: Decreased coronary reserve: A mechanism for angina pectoris in patients with aortic stenosis and normal coronary arteries. N Engl J Med 1982;307:1362-1366.

93. Kertai MD, Bountioukos M, Boersma E, et al: Aortic stenosis: An underestimated risk factor for perioperative complications in patients undergoing noncardiac surgery. Am J Med 2004;116:8-13.

94. Carabello BA: Modern management of mitral stenosis. Circulation 2005;112:432-437.

95. Kasalicky J, Hurych J, Widimsky J, et al: Left heart haemodynamics at rest and during exercise in patients with mitral stenosis. Br Heart J 1968;30:188-195.

96. Bonow RO, Cheitlin MD, Crawford MH, Douglas PS: Task Force 3: Valvular heart disease. J Am Coll Cardiol 2005;45:1334.

97. Bekeredjian R, Grayburn PA: Valvular heart disease: Aortic regurgitation. Circulation 2005;112:125-134.

98. Connolly HM, Crary JL, McGoon MD, et al: Valvular heart disease associated with fenfluramine-phentermine. N Engl J Med 1997;337:581-588.

99. Carabello BA: Aortic regurgitation: A lesion with similarities to both aortic stenosis and mitral regurgitation. Circulation 1990;82:1051-1053.

100. Ricci DR: Afterload mismatch and preload reserve in chronic aortic regurgitation. Circulation 1982;66:826-834.

101. Ross J Jr: Afterload mismatch in aortic and mitral valve disease: Implications for surgical therapy. J Am Coll Cardiol 1985;5:811-826.

102. Otto CM: Evaluation and management of chronic mitral regurgitation. N Engl J Med 2001;345:740-746.

103. Marcotte F, Honos GN, Walling AD, et al: Effect of angiotensin-converting enzyme inhibitor therapy in mitral regurgitation with normal left ventricular function. Can J Cardiol 1997;13:479-485.

104. Thys DM, Abel M, Bollen BA, et al: Practice guidelines for perioperative transesophageal echocardiography: A report by the American Society of Anesthesiologists and the Society of Cardiovascular Anesthesiologists Task Force on Transesophageal Echocardiography. Anesthesiology 1996;84:986-1006.

105. Lung B, Gohlke-Barwolf C, Tornos P, et al: Recommendations on the management of the asymptomatic patient with valvular heart disease. Eur Heart J 2002;23:1252-1266.

106. Carabello BA: Aortic stenosis. N Engl J Med 2002;346:677-682.

16 Prevention and Management of Perioperative Dysrhythmias

Martin Slodzinski

In the past several decades, anesthesiologists, in their role as perioperative consultants, have faced an explosion of information, technology, and therapies in electrophysiologic cardiology. In making perioperative management decisions, they must be cognizant of many developments in arrhythmia management, from development of pacemakers for bradydysrhythmias, to surgery for Wolff-Parkinson-White syndrome from the 1960s and 1980s, to current pharmacologic therapies and technologies such as transvascular ablation and automated internal cardiac defibrillators.

■ EPIDEMIOLOGY

Perioperative arrhythmias are a common source of surgical morbidity, whether from catecholamines (increased with pain and anxiety), structural heart disease, electrolyte imbalances, or myocardial ischemia. Usually well tolerated in the healthy and younger populations, perioperative arrhythmias can be life-threatening in older adults and those with little cardiopulmonary reserve.

Perioperative arrhythmias are common in cardiac surgery. The literature is lacking in documentation of the incidence of supraventricular tachycardia or atrial fibrillation when patients arrive at the operating room. However, 10% to 65% of cardiac surgery patients experience atrial fibrillation during postoperative days 2 and 3.[1] Atrial fibrillation among cardiac surgery patients increases the hospital stay up to 48 hours, with a 1996 cost of $1600 per patient.[2] The cost and morbidity of perioperative arrhythmia is magnified among cardiac surgery patients who were in sinus rhythm preoperatively, because they may develop atrial fibrillation postoperatively and maintain the dysrhythmia for 6 weeks (2% incidence) and 1 year after surgery (1% incidence).[3]

The incidence of perioperative arrhythmia is higher in cardiac surgery, but because the number of older patients with preexisting cardiac disease who undergo noncardiac surgery is so large, new-onset perioperative arrhythmia is an important factor in length of hospital stay and, therefore, the cost of noncardiac surgical procedures. In a study of 4181 patients (>50 years old, in sinus rhythm preoperatively) undergoing non-emergent, noncardiac surgical procedures, almost 8% experienced a perioperative supraventricular arrhythmia that was associated with a one-third increase in the length of stay.[4] The medical risk factors for these patients include male sex, age greater than 70 years, premature atrial complexes on preoperative electrocardiogram (ECG), congestive heart failure, asthma, American Society of Anesthesiology (ASA) class III or IV, and significant vascular disease. Surgical risk factors include prior abdominal aortic aneurysm repair, intrathoracic surgery, intra-abdominal surgery, and vascular surgery.

■ MECHANISMS

The molecular and electrophysiologic mechanisms of clinically significant arrhythmias have yet to be fully elucidated.[5] However, an arrhythmia caused by one mechanism may precipitate an episode of a different arrhythmia caused by a different molecular mechanism. Furthermore, at the clinical level, it is not possible to distinguish a microreentry from a focal change in automaticity. With these limitations in mind, arrhythmogenesis may be classified into four main arrhythmias: sinus node, automaticity, impulse initiation, and reentry (Boxes 16-1 and 16-2).

Sinus tachycardia (>100 beats per minute [bpm]) or sinus bradycardia (<60 bpm) are arrhythmias of normal automaticity, because the molecular mechanism of pacemaker depolarization mirrors the mechanism of normal sinus rate. Fever, anemia, catecholamine surge, and hypotension are a few common precipitating factors of sinus tachycardia. Similarly, sinus bradycardia may result from drug therapy (e.g., beta-adrenergic blockade) or increased vagal tone (e.g., in athletes). Sympathetic dystonias and parasympathetic dystonias are uncommon mechanisms for sinus tachycardia and sinus bradycardia, respectively.

When pacemaker depolarization occurs outside of the location and ionic mechanism of the sinus node, arrhythmia automaticity has occurred. If the sinus node fails to initiate an impulse (e.g., as in sinus pause) or fails to propagate (e.g., as in third-degree heart block), an escape (or ectopic) impulse may be generated. On the other hand, if an ectopic focus generates a repetitive impulse at a rate faster than the normal sinus rate, the ectopic focus may usurp the normal sinus impulse. In general, arrhythmias of automaticity occur when the diastolic resting membrane potential is reduced (e.g., in ischemia, in the presence of digitalis, and perhaps in pulmonary venous origins of cardiac arrhythmias).[6] Regardless of the reason for increased diastolic resting membrane potential, arrhythmias of automaticity occur spontaneously.

Arrhythmias of impulse formation occur when sinus overdrive of latent extra-sinus nodal pacemakers (e.g., in the

16-1	Arrhythmia Mechanisms

- Focal mechanisms
  - Automatic
  - Triggered
- Normal automaticity
  - Sinoatrial node
  - Subsidiary atrial foci
  - Atrioventricular node
  - His-Purkinje system
- Triggered mechanisms occurring from repetitive after-depolarizations
- Reentry
  - Unidirectional block is necessary.
  - Slowed conduction in the alternate pathway exceeds the refractory period of cells at the site of unidirectional block.

From Kaplan JA, Reich DL, Lake CL, Konstadt SN (eds): Kaplan's Cardiac Anesthesia, ed 5. Philadelphia, Elsevier, 2006, p 357, with permission.

16-2	Diagnostic Evaluation of Arrhythmias

- History of palpitations, syncope, and constitutional symptoms
- Physical examination
- 12-lead electrocardiogram
- Echocardiogram
- 24-hour Holter monitoring
- Invasive electrophysiologic testing with multichannel, computerized mapping

From Kaplan JA, Reich DL, Lake CL, Konstadt SN (eds): Kaplan's Cardiac Anesthesia, ed 5. Philadelphia, Elsevier, 2006, p 359, with permission.

16-3	Classification of Arrhythmias

Ventricular Arrhythmias

- Premature ventricular contractions
- Nonsustained ventricular tachycardia
- Repetitive monomorphic ventricular tachycardia
- Sustained ventricular tachycardia
- Polymorphic ventricular tachycardia
- Ventricular fibrillation or ventricular flutter
- Ventricular syndromes
  - Torsades de pointes
  - Long QT syndrome
  - Brugada syndrome
  - Right ventricular tachycardia

Bradyarrhythmias

- Impulse generation failure
- Atrioventricular conduction abnormalities
- Atrioventricular dissociation
- Pacing indications
- Pacemaker-associated arrhythmias

Cardiac Reflexes

- Bezold-Jarisch
- Cushing
- Oculocardiac
- Bainbridge
- Baroreceptor
- Valsalva
- Osborn

atria, pulmonary veins, and coronary sinus[7]) fails. A classic example of this phenomenon is the junctional escape rhythm (at approximately 60 bpm) initiated during sinus bradycardia (<60 bpm). On the other hand, if the extra-sinus nodal pacemaker speeds up, it may usurp the sinus rate (as occurs when premature ventricular contractions develop into ventricular tachycardia).

Arrhythmias of reentry account for a variety of supraventricular and ventricular arrhythmias. Reentry implies a pathologic electrical pathway that results from an anatomic structure (e.g., the Wolff-Parkinson-White [WPW] syndrome) or pathologic dysfunction (e.g., myocardial injury). The magnitude of the reentry loop can vary from the simple reentry loop of the WPW syndrome to the complexity of atrial or ventricular fibrillation. The unrecognized reentrant tachyarrhythmia of WPW may deteriorate into a more complex ventricular tachycardia or fibrillation if the atrioventricular (AV) node is slowed (e.g., as occurs with beta-blockade, adenosine, or calcium channel blockade).

Arrhythmia Evaluation

Evaluation of cardiac arrhythmias requires electrocardiographic analysis of the rhythm in a clinical setting (Box 16-3). The systematic approach to the ECG relies on accurate determination of rate, rhythm, axis, P-wave relationship to QRS, and QRS morphology. In adults, normal sinus rhythm has a rate of 60 to 100 bpm, with sinus bradycardia identified at less than 60 bpm and sinus tachycardia at greater than 100 bpm. A marathon runner may have a physiologic resting heart rate of 40 bpm. At the other end of the clinical spectrum, a patient with an acute coronary syndrome and a heart rate at 40 bpm may not exhibit enough cardiac output. In addition, arrhythmias must be separated into those that cause no symptoms or limited symptoms (e.g., premature ventricular beats) and those that cause sustained or life-threatening symptoms (e.g., supraventricular or ventricular tachycardias, fibrillation, or hemodynamically significant bradycardia).

The 12-lead ECG with a rhythm strip is the most convenient method for the diagnosis of arrhythmia. For most arrhythmias, the relative timing of the P wave to the QRS, their morphologies, and their vectors are sufficient for recognition. A narrow QRS complex (shorter than 0.12 second) indicates a supraventricular arrhythmia. A wide QRS may indicate ventricular origin or a supraventricular origin with a bundle branch block, an aberrant ventricular conduction, or an antegrade accessory pathway. Usually, the standard ECG provides sufficient diagnostic information. An esophageal bipolar lead can be used to record left atrial activity, or an intra-atrial lead can be used to record right atrial activity.

Continuous monitoring of the ECG in outpatients and inpatients may improve diagnostic yield in transient arrhythmias. Patients who report infrequent symptoms that may be caused by a cardiac arrhythmia may be able to activate event recorders. Also, subcutaneous recorders can document very infrequent episodes of arrhythmia.[8]

Stress testing may elucidate arrhythmias, document the exercise relationship to the arrhythmias, and evaluate the efficacy of therapy. In patients with structurally normal hearts without significant coronary artery disease, exercise stress testing may uncover exercise-induced ventricular arrhythmias (e.g., catecholamine-induced polymorphic ventricular tachycardia).[9] These exercise-induced ventricular tachycardias without structural disease respond to beta-blockade but may require implantable defibrillators.

Signal-averaged electrocardiography records low-amplitude signals occurring after termination of the standard electrocardiographic QRS. These low-amplitude signals are caused by delayed activation of parts of the ventricle, and signal averaging removes noise. The resultant signal is used to risk-stratify patients for sudden cardiac death, which is especially useful for older adults who have had a myocardial infarction.[10]

Intracardiac electrocardiography is used when surface electrocardiography is not adequate to assess and treat various forms of supraventricular and ventricular arrhythmias. Multiple catheters map the conducting sequence from the atrium to the ventricle. This electrocardiographic map identifies accessory pathways, reentrant circuits, and sites of origin for tachyarrhythmias.[11] It also guides surgical and nonsurgical ablation therapy.

Arrhythmia Management

Anesthesiologists regularly consider prevention and management of cardiac arrhythmias. Both cardiac and systemic factors in arrhythmia generation are taken into account to determine when to use pharmacologic and nonpharmacologic therapy during the perioperative period. Three factors must be considered in arrhythmia management: structure, triggering factors, and patient suitability and preference for antiarrhythmic therapy.

Structural factors affecting arrhythmias include coronary artery disease, valvular heart disease, and heart failure. In addition to these large-scale structural factors, many molecular structural factors (e.g., ionic channels, receptor mutations, polymorphisms) may predispose patients to arrhythmias.[12] The molecular components of the cardiac rhythm have not been fully elucidated,[5] but recent advances in myocardial repolarization physiology have demonstrated that genetic variation in ionic channels fine-tune the cell to the edge of arrhythmia generation.[12] By administering both cardiac and noncardiac agents (e.g., antihistamines, antimicrobials, phenothiazines, prokinetic agents) anesthesiologists may induce torsades de pointes or QT elongation in certain patients with a genetic predisposition. The relationship between molecular structure and function of ionic channels in arrhythmogenesis remains elusive.

The origin of transient triggering factors in arrhythmogenesis may be cardiac or systemic. These triggering factors include cardiac or neurologic ischemia, volume shifts, electrolyte disturbances, temperature alterations, medications, endocrinopathies, and metabolic abnormalities.[13] The key to management of arrhythmias is an understanding of the inter-

action of triggering factors with underlying molecular and structural anomalies.

Finally, patient suitability and preference for antiarrhythmic therapy must be considered. Because of intolerance of side effects, a patient may refuse or not be suitable for beta-blockade or an implantable defibrillator. The anesthesiologist, surgeon, and cardiologist must balance safety, invasiveness, and efficacy when recommending perioperative antiarrhythmia therapy to a patient. A large spectrum of antiarrhythmia therapy is available, including pharmacologic agents, transvascular ablation, implantable devices, and open surgical ablation. Unfortunately, the lethality and acuity of certain arrhythmias may not relegate the decision to a fully informed consent (Box 16-3).

Supraventricular Tachycardias

Sinus tachycardia (ST) is most commonly an appropriate response to physical or psychological factors. Management is based on control of the exogenous factors (e.g., anemia, thyrotoxicosis, pain, anxiety). Depending on the patient's history and physical examination, perioperative beta-blockade may be beneficial to control the rate of the sinus tachycardia.

In a meta-analysis of 69 studies (out of 3680 reviewed titles), beta-blockers reduced the frequency of ventricular tachycardia (odds ratios [ORs], 0.28 in cardiac surgery, 0.57 in noncardiac surgery), atrial fibrillation/flutter (ORs 0.37 in cardiac surgery, 0.25 in noncardiac surgery), and supraventricular arrhythmia (ORs 0.25 in cardiac surgery, 0.43 in noncardiac surgery). This meta-analysis found that beta-blockers decreased myocardial ischemia but did not impact hospital length of stay, myocardial infarction, or mortality.[14]

Some patients have pharmacologically refractory intermittent or chronic nonparoxysmal inappropriate ST. These pharmacologically resistant patients may require radiofrequency modification or ablation of the sinus node.[15]

Premature atrial contractions (PACs) are ubiquitous in patients with systemic and cardiac disease. PACs are defined by a P wave preceding the next expected sinus impulse with a change in the axis vector of the P wave. Alcohol, tobacco, and caffeine are common exogenous factors in PACs. Like ST, PAC activity may result from physical (e.g., mitral valve prolapse) or psychological (e.g., fear) factors. ST and PACs are linked at the sinus node, where many specialized cells with different intrinsic rates and a nonuniform distribution of autonomic receptors provide the dynamics of heart rate control and PAC activation.[16] PACs usually do not require treatment, but they may be a triggering event for sustained arrhythmias. Beyond the annoying palpitations, repetitive focal PACs and multifocal atrial tachycardia may precipitate atrial flutter and fibrillation.[17] No clinical trials assess the efficacy of beta-blockade in PAC control.

Supraventricular tachycardias (SVTs) include all tachyarrhythmias at or above the bifurcation of the bundle of His. By convention, the atrial rate must be above 100 bpm. The ventricular rate may be slower if conduction through the AV node is incomplete. The QRS duration is usually narrow at less than 0.12 second. In SVTs with bundle branch blocks, aberrant intraventricular conduction, or bypass tracts, the QRS in SVTs may be longer than 0.12 second.[18]

Based on duration, SVTs are separated into three groups: brief paroxysm, persistent, and chronic. Brief paroxysm (onset and offset) SVTs last for minutes to hours and are caused by nodal reentry or WPW syndrome and paroxysm atrial fibrillation or flutter. In contrast, persistent SVTs last for days or weeks (e.g., ST, ectopic atrial tachycardia, or longer episodes of atrial fibrillation or flutter). Finally, the hallmark of chronic SVTs is the inability to revert or convert (with therapy) to a normal rhythm.

The most common SVT is the paroxysmal SVT (PSVT) with AV node reentry. It occurs in 60% of patients with SVT.[19] The hallmark of this arrhythmia is a dual AV nodal pathway. Originally, the dual pathway was thought to exist in the AV node; it is now thought to be the region of the AV node.[20] Because of this dual pathway, P-wave determination is difficult and "pseudo R waves" are seen in V_1 and inferiorly. The rate of PSVT is typically 160 to 190 bpm. In patients with a bundle branch block, it may be difficult to differentiate PSVT from VT.

Management of PSVT depends on the health of the patient. In the healthy patient, intervention is for patient psychological and physical comfort. In patients with cardiac disease, PSVT may be immediately life-threatening. In acute episodes, simple means of reverting include rest, anxiolysis, and vagotonic maneuvers. When pharmacologic intervention is warranted, adenosine is safe and effective at a bolus dose of 6 mg, with a repeated dose of 12 mg.[21] Adenosine, unlike calcium channel blockade, is free of negative inotropic effects. In small dosages, verapamil is effective in 90% of patients with PSVT caused by AV node reentry,[22] but great caution must be used if PSVT with aberrant conduction has a QRS of greater than 0.12 second. If VT is mistakenly diagnosed as PSVT and treated with verapamil, significant hypotension will develop.[23] Because of increased safety and lack of side effects, transvascular radiofrequency ablation has gained wide acceptance in controlling recurrent and persistent PSVT.

PSVT caused by accessory pathways in the atria and ventricles with different conduction properties and refractory periods is the basis of the WPW syndrome. This is the second most common PSVT.[19] The standard ECG is normal during the sinus rhythm because the accessory pathway is unable to conduct in the antegrade direction. Features of the WPW syndrome are the short PR interval, followed by a delta wave at the onset of the QRS.

PSVT in WPW syndrome may manifest from childhood to middle age, with women having an increased likelihood during the stress of pregnancy.[24] Treatment with rest, anxiolysis, and vagal maneuvers is safe with PSVT in WPW syndrome, but verapamil[25] and lidocaine[26] may accelerate the ventricular rate when atrial flutter or fibrillation is also present. Furthermore, digitalis derivatives shorten the refractory period of the accessory pathway and may exacerbate the tachycardia.[27,28] If pharmacologic intervention is not tolerated, as in PSVT with AV node reentry, PSVT with WPW syndrome is amenable to radiofrequency catheter ablation. Atrial flutter or fibrillation in the setting of an accessory

pathway WPW syndrome is dangerous because of the potential of extremely rapid communication down the accessory pathway with resultant rapid ventricular rate and possible deterioration to ventricular fibrillation. Therefore, blocking the AV node may precipitate ventricular fibrillation. Although amiodarone or procainamide may be useful, cardioversion may be the safest urgent therapy.[29]

Multifocal atrial tachycardia (MAT) is diagnosed with a P wave that has three or more different morphologies. This arrhythmia usually has a rate of less than 140 bpm and is most commonly associated with chronic pulmonary disease and metabolic abnormalities.[30] Metoprolol, verapamil, and magnesium have been evaluated in a few studies, but overall, MAT may respond to removal of aggravating factors (pulmonary or metabolic).[31]

Atrial flutter is a regular atrial tachyarrhythmia that is less common than PSVT or atrial fibrillation. Children and young adults who have undergone corrective surgery for tetralogy of Fallot, transposition of vessels, or atrial septal defect are at highest risk for this arrhythmia.[32] The most common AV conduction ratios in atrial flutter are 2:1 and 4:1, generating a ventricular rate of 150 or 75 bpm, respectively. Any narrow complex tachycardia of 150 bpm must lead to the consideration of atrial flutter. Vagal stimulation does not interrupt atrial flutter, but it does distinguish it from other PSVTs. Patients with cardiac disease require rapid rate control with calcium channel blockade or digitalis. If they are hemodynamically unstable, cardioversion is required. If cardioversion is unsuccessful, overdrive pacing may result in conversion to sinus rhythm.[33,34] Radiofrequency ablation is another mechanism to control atrial flutter.[35] In the past, anticoagulation was not recommended for chronic atrial flutter, but now the recommendation is to follow the guidelines established for atrial fibrillation. Anticoagulation of persistent, nonparoxysmal atrial flutter is suggested.[36]

Atrial fibrillation, like other SVTs, can be divided into three groups: paroxysmal (lasting less than 48 hours), persistent (2 days to weeks), and chronic (months to years). Atrial fibrillation is the most common SVT after surgery. Of 916 patients older than 40 years undergoing major noncardiac surgery, the incidence of SVT was 4%, with atrial fibrillation accounting for 63% of these arrhythmias.[37] Atrial fibrillation is even more common after cardiac surgery, with rates of 30% to 40%.[38,39]

Electrophysiologically, atrial fibrillation is grossly disorganized atrial electrical activity that is probably multiple reentrant atrial wavelet circuits interfering with mechanical and electrical synchronization of the atria. Less commonly, atrial fibrillation originates from pulmonary veins.[6] The clinical appearance of atrial fibrillation is an absence of structural cardiac disease, with symptoms ranging from none to many. At the other end of the spectrum, atrial fibrillation may be present in advanced cardiac disease (e.g., valvular disease and cardiomyopathy) or advanced noncardiac disease such as thyrotoxicosis.

Functionally, atrial fibrillation may impair ventricular function in the noncompliant ventricle or in the dilated ventricle with systolic dysfunction. A rapid ventricular rate may induce myocardial ischemia. Cardiac output may be decreased because of decreased filling time. Finally, the long-term risk of thromboembolism and stroke in atrial fibrillation warrants chemical or electrical cardioversion or anticoagulation.

Management of acute atrial fibrillation requires investigation of the underlying causes (structural, hemodynamic, or systemic). If atrial fibrillation occurs without an identified underlying cause, so-called lone atrial fibrillation, the prognosis is very good.[40,41] Long-term antiarrhythmic therapy is rarely needed for the first episode of lone atrial fibrillation, but rate control may be required. For example, in thyrotoxicosis, anticoagulation and rate control are important until the patient is euthyroid and sinus rhythm is restored.[42]

Because the chance of spontaneous conversion of atrial fibrillation to sinus rhythm in the first 24 hours is about 50%, recurrent episodes of paroxysmal atrial fibrillation lasting less than 48 hours are managed by investigation of predisposing factors and rate control (beta-blockers, calcium channel blockers), unless the patient requires the "atrial kick" to maintain cardiac output.[43] Therefore, the decision to intervene in atrial fibrillation requires a balance between hemodynamic tolerance and the tendency of the atrial myocytes to electrically remodel into a form that is resistant to conversion to sinus rhythm.[44] Unless transesophageal echocardiography has confirmed the absence of an atrial thrombus, elective cardioversion should not be attempted until 3 weeks of treatment with anticoagulation therapy[45] has been completed. Management of atrial fibrillation remains controversial[46] with regard to how early to convert atrial fibrillation, the best method for conversion, selection for ablation therapy, and long-term anticoagulation, but for the anesthesiologist, the acuity, hemodynamic situation, and perioperative situation dictate the therapy (Box 16-4). Regardless, perioperative atrial fibrillation increases morbidity, cost, and hospital stay. Whether from atrial stretch during postoperative fluid mobilization or from failure to resume postoperative beta-blockade, postoperative atrial fibrillation occurs in patients predisposed to prolonged hospitalization and other complications. Therefore, without better risk stratification, it is still unclear whether prevention of postoperative atrial fibrillation improves patient outcomes.[38]

16-4	Considerations for the Anesthesiologist before Supraventricular Arrhythmia Surgery and Ablation Procedures

- Be familiar with electrophysiologic study results and associated treatments.
- Place transcutaneous cardioversion or defibrillation pads prior to induction.
- Treat hemodynamically tolerated tachyarrhythmias by slowing conduction across accessory pathway, as opposed to across the atrioventricular node.
- Treat hemodynamically significant tachyarrhythmias with cardioversion.
- Avoid sympathetic stimulation.

From Kaplan JA, Reich DL, Lake CL, Konstadt SN (eds): Kaplan's Cardiac Anesthesia, ed 5. Philadelphia, Elsevier, 2006, p 369, with permission.

Atrioventricular Junctional Rhythms

Originating from the AV node, junctional rhythms may be automatic or reentrant arrhythmias. AV node premature beats, accelerated rhythms, and junctional tachycardias are examples of subordinate pacemakers that may emerge when the sinus rate drops. AV premature beats occur less frequently than premature ventricular and atrial complexes, and usually do not require treatment. When an accelerated junctional rhythm occurs following a sinus bradycardia with enhanced automaticity of the AV node, inferior wall ischemia, hypokalemia, hypoxemia, and digitalis toxicity should be considered. Like AV node premature beats, accelerated AV rates require no specific treatment except treatment of the underlying cause. If needed for maintenance of cardiac output, glycopyrrolate, atropine, or transvenous pacing may increase the sinus rate and allow it to resume its normal function.[47]

AV junctional rhythms may double in rate and become true AV nodal tachycardias.[48] AV junctional tachycardias frequently occur in children after corrective cardiac surgery for congenital defects. Pharmacologic treatment is unpredictable, and ablation therapy is occasionally recommended.[49] Retrospectively, one institution reported favorable results using amiodarone to control AV junctional tachycardia.[50] A rarer permanent junctional reciprocating tachycardia is found in children and may bring on tachycardia-induced heart failure.[51] This uncommon junctional rhythm is caused by a long PR–short PR reentry pattern. In both children and adults, great success with ablation therapy is used to prevent tachycardia cardiomyopathy.[51,52]

Ventricular Tachycardia

The spectrum of ventricular arrhythmias extends from an isolated premature ventricular contraction (PVC) to ventricular tachycardia (VT) to ventricular fibrillation (VF). Ventricular arrhythmias occur distal to the bundle of His. Unifocal PVCs have uniform morphology and are coupled to the preceding sinus beat by a fixed interval. Multifocal PVCs have different morphologies and a coupling to the sinus beat.[53]

VT is identified when three or more PVCs occur in succession. If the VT lasts less than 30 seconds, it is called nonsustained VT; if the VT lasts more than 30 seconds, it is called sustained VT. The risk of PVCs becoming VT is dependent on patient selection, and the occurrence of bigeminy or trigeminy has no prognostic value for the risk of VT beyond the PVC frequency count. In general, the risk of PVC is low in patients after caffeine consumption, with preoperative anxiety, or mitral valve prolapse. The risk of PVCs is higher in patients with idiopathic dilated cardiomyopathy. Beta-blockade and anxiolytics can provide symptomatic relief. Beyond removing inciting factors and symptomatic relief, no data, including data from the Cardiac Arrhythmia Suppression Trial, support PVC suppression.[54]

Nonsustained VT is common after cardiac surgery, especially after aortic valve replacement (incidence, 50%).[55] Nonsustained VT may respond to repletion of post-bypass hypomagnesemia.[56] The CABG Patch Trial found no survival advantage to implantation of a cardiac defibrillator in patients with low ejection fractions at the time of cardiac surgery.[57]

Sustained monomorphic VT is usually a reentrant pathway, best characterized by injury formation after ischemia.[58,59] Lidocaine and procainamide have been the traditional pharmacologic therapies for sustained monomorphic VT.[60] The institution of amiodarone treatment of sustained VT[61] is not without controversy. Amiodarone has a relatively slow onset of its Vaughan Williams class III effect to prolong the myocardial depolarization. In emergency department treatment of acute sustained VT, amiodarone was relatively safe but ineffective for acute termination of sustained monomorphic VT.[62]

Polymorphic ventricular tachycardia requires determination of the QT interval of the sinus rhythm prior to onset. Torsades de pointes is a polymorphic VT that has a prolonged QT. The prolonged QT may be congenital (ionic channelopathy),[63] medication induced,[64] or metabolically induced. Magnesium,[65] cautious potassium repletion, and sinus rate stimulation (atropine, beta agonists, pacing, and implantable defibrillators) are current treatments for hemodynamically stable torsades de pointes.[66]

Clearly, hemodynamically unstable torsades de pointes requires asynchronous direct current countershock. Lidocaine and phenytoin are devoid of potassium channel blocking properties and may be helpful when antiarrhythmic therapy is required. Unlike monomorphic VT, torsades de pointes may benefit from amiodarone.[67]

Sustained monomorphic VT in the perioperative setting has traditionally been treated with lidocaine, yet no human trials support lidocaine in the perioperative setting to promote conversion of sustained monomorphic VT or VF to sinus rhythm. The ALIVE study looked at patients who experienced out-of-hospital fibrillation and found that 22.8% of the amiodarone-treated group survived, compared with 12% of the lidocaine-treated group,[68] but there was no difference in the rate of hospital discharges. Although no controlled trial of amiodarone in the perioperative setting exists, there are numerous reports of perioperative use of amiodarone.[69,70]

Bradyarrhythmias

Severe bradyarrhythmias account for 6.4% of all ASA class III or IV patients in a multicenter study of over 17,000 patients.[71] Whether they occur in the vasovagal obstetric patient (or the patient's partner),[72] or are caused by neostigmine administration[73] or the Bezold-Jarisch reflex,[74] most hemodynamically significant sinus bradycardias and partial or complete heart blocks respond to short-term pharmacologic therapy or transcutaneous or transvenous pacing.[75] The Bezold-Jarisch reflex may be resistant to atropine and direct-acting chronotropic agents (e.g., epinephrine), but controversy over the pathophysiology of the mechanism of the Bezold-Jarisch reflex remains.[74,76] Other bradycardiac reflexes, such as the oculocardiac reflex, merely require removal of the stimulation.[77] No randomized trials are available to evaluate management of perioperative hemodynamically significant bradycardias.

CONCLUSIONS

Perioperative arrhythmias contribute to the significant morbidity in cardiac and noncardiac procedures. Few statistically significant studies have been performed that give anesthesiologists guidance in providing perioperative management of arrhythmias. The available evidence comes from perioperative case studies and series, from nonoperative trials, and from studies of out-of-hospital events. There is a great need for development of rationales for perioperative arrhythmia management.

REFERENCES

1. Maisel WH, Rawn JD, Stevenson WG: Atrial fibrillation after cardiac surgery. Ann Intern Med 2001;135:1061-1073.
2. Mathew JP, Parks R, Savino JS, et al: Atrial fibrillation following coronary artery bypass graft surgery: Predictors, outcomes, and resource utilization. MultiCenter Study of Perioperative Ischemia Research Group. JAMA 1996;276:300-306.
3. Elahi M, Hadjinikolaou L, Galinanes M: Incidence and clinical consequences of atrial fibrillation within 1 year of first-time isolated coronary bypass surgery. Circulation 2003;108(Suppl 1):II207-212.
4. Polanczyk CA, Goldman L, Marcantonio ER, et al: Supraventricular arrhythmia in patients having noncardiac surgery: Clinical correlates and effect on length of stay. Ann Intern Med 1998;129:279-285.
5. Shah M, Akar FG, Tomaselli GF: Molecular basis of arrhythmias. Circulation 2005;112:2517-2529.
6. Chen YJ, Chen SA: Electrophysiology of pulmonary veins. J Cardiovasc Electrophysiol 2006;17:220-224.
7. Katsouras G, Dubuc M, Khairy P: Transcatheter mapping and ablation of arrhythmias in the coronary sinus. Expert Rev Cardiovasc Ther 2006;4:711-720.
8. Marti Almor J, Delclos Urgell J, Bruguera Cortada J: [Atypical sinus node dysfunction: Usefulness of implantable Holter—A case report.] Rev Esp Cardiol 2001;54:1459-1462.
9. Scheinman MM, Lam J: Exercise-induced ventricular arrhythmias in patients with no structural cardiac disease. Annu Rev Med 2006;57:473-484.
10. Iravanian S, Arshad A, Steinberg JS: Role of electrophysiologic studies, signal-averaged electrocardiography, heart rate variability, T-wave alternans, and loop recorders for risk stratification of ventricular arrhythmias. Am J Geriatr Cardiol 2005;14:16-19.
11. Hall MC, Todd DM: Modern management of arrhythmias. Postgrad Med J 2006;82:117-125.
12. Schulze-Bahr E: Arrhythmia predisposition between rare disease paradigms and common ion channel gene variants. J Am Coll Cardiol 2006;48:A67-78.
13. Ellenbogen KA, Chung MK, Asher CR, Wood MA: Postoperative atrial fibrillation. Adv Card Surg 1997;9:109-130.
14. Wiesbauer F, Schlager O, Domanovits H, et al: Perioperative beta-blockers for preventing surgery-related mortality and morbidity: A systematic review and meta-analysis. Anesth Analg 2007;104:27-41.
15. Shen WK: How to manage patients with inappropriate sinus tachycardia. Heart Rhythm 2005;2:1015-1019.
16. Schuessler RB: Abnormal sinus node function in clinical arrhythmias. J Cardiovasc Electrophysiol 2003;14:215-217.
17. Roberts-Thomson KC, Kistler PM, Kalman JM: Focal atrial tachycardia. I: Clinical features, diagnosis, mechanisms, and anatomic location. Pacing Clin Electrophysiol 2006;29:643-652.
18. Kumar UN, Rao RK, Scheinman MM: The 12-lead electrocardiogram in supraventricular tachycardia. Cardiol Clin 2006;24:427-437, ix.
19. Kastor JA: Arrhythmias. 1994, Philadelphia, WB Saunders.
20. Kadish A, Passman R: Mechanisms and management of paroxysmal supraventricular tachycardia. Cardiol Rev 1999;7:254-264.
21. DiMarco JP, Miles W, Akhtar M, et al: Adenosine for paroxysmal supraventricular tachycardia: Dose ranging and comparison with verapamil—Assessment in placebo-controlled, multicenter trials. The

Adenosine for PSVT Study Group. Ann Intern Med 1990;113: 104-110.

22. Rinkenberger RL, Prystowsky EN, Heger JJ, et al: Effects of intravenous and chronic oral verapamil administration in patients with supraventricular tachyarrhythmias. Circulation 1980;62:996-1010.

23. Stewart RB, Bardy GH, Greene HL: Wide complex tachycardia: Misdiagnosis and outcome after emergent therapy. Ann Intern Med 1986; 104:766-771.

24. Lee SH, Chen SA, Wu TJ, et al: Effects of pregnancy on first onset and symptoms of paroxysmal supraventricular tachycardia. Am J Cardiol 1995;76:675-678.

25. McGovern B, Garan H, Ruskin JN: Precipitation of cardiac arrest by verapamil in patients with Wolff-Parkinson-White syndrome. Ann Intern Med 1986;104:791-794.

26. Akhtar M, Gilbert CJ, Shenasa M: Effect of lidocaine on atrioventricular response via the accessory pathway in patients with Wolff-Parkinson-White syndrome. Circulation 1981;63:435-441.

27. Wellens HJ: Effect of drugs in the Wolff-Parkinson-White syndrome. Adv Cardiol 1975;14:233-240.

28. Wellens HJ, Durrer D: Effect of digitalis on atrioventricular conduction and circus-movement tachycardias in patients with Wolff-Parkinson-White syndrome. Circulation 1973;47:1229-1233.

29. Moro Serrano C, Hernandez Madrid A, Lage Silveira J, et al: [Amiodarone in the nineties: To whom and what dosage?] Rev Esp Cardiol 1995;48:272-284.

30. Kastor JA: Multifocal atrial tachycardia. N Engl J Med 1990;322: 1713-1717.

31. McCord J, Borzak S: Multifocal atrial tachycardia. Chest 1998;113: 203-209.

32. Garson A Jr, Moak JP, Friedman RA, et al: Surgical treatment of arrhythmias in children. Cardiol Clin 1989;7:319-329.

33. Lee KW, Yang Y, Scheinman MM: Atrial flutter: A review of its history, mechanisms, clinical features, and current therapy. Curr Probl Cardiol 2005;30:121-167.

34. Mead GE, Flapan AD, Elder AT: Electrical cardioversion for atrial fibrillation and flutter. Cochrane Database Syst Rev 2002: CD002903.

35. Montenero AS, Andrew P: Current treatment options for atrial flutter and results with cryocatheter ablation. Expert Rev Cardiovasc Ther 2006;4:191-202.

36. Scholten MF, Thornton AS, Mekel JM, et al: Anticoagulation in atrial fibrillation and flutter. Europace 2005;7:492-499.

37. Goldman L: Supraventricular tachyarrhythmias in hospitalized adults after surgery: Clinical correlates in patients over 40 years of age after major noncardiac surgery. Chest 1978;73:450-454.

38. Hogue CW Jr, Creswell LL, Gutterman DD, et al: Epidemiology, mechanisms, and risks: American College of Chest Physicians guidelines for the prevention and management of postoperative atrial fibrillation after cardiac surgery. Chest 2005;128(2 Suppl):9S-16S.

39. Favaloro RG, Effler DB, Groves LK, et al: Direct myocardial revascularization with saphenous vein autograft: Clinical experience in 100 cases. Dis Chest 1969;56:279-283.

40. Kopecky SL, Gersh BJ, McGoon MD, et al: The natural history of lone atrial fibrillation: A population-based study over three decades. N Engl J Med 1987;317:669-674.

41. Kopecky SL: Management decisions in lone atrial fibrillation. Hosp Pract (Off Ed) 1992;27:135-138, 143, 147-150.

42. Parmar MS: Thyrotoxic atrial fibrillation. MedGenMed 2005;7:74.

43. Danias PG, Caulfield TA, Weigner MJ, et al: Likelihood of spontaneous conversion of atrial fibrillation to sinus rhythm. J Am Coll Cardiol 1998;31:588-592.

44. Allessie MA, Konings K, Kirchhof CJ, Wijffels M: Electrophysiologic mechanisms of perpetuation of atrial fibrillation. Am J Cardiol 1996; 77:10A-23A.

45. Leung DY, Davidson PM, Cranney GB, Walsh WF: Thromboembolic risks of left atrial thrombus detected by transesophageal echocardiogram. Am J Cardiol 1997;79:626-629.

46. Nattel S, Opie LH: Controversies in atrial fibrillation. Lancet 2006; 367:262-272.

47. Law IH, Von Bergen NH, Gingerich JC, et al: Transcatheter cryothermal ablation of junctional ectopic tachycardia in the normal heart. Heart Rhythm 2006;3:903-907.

48. de Soyza N, Bissett JK, Kane JJ, et al: Association of accelerated idioventricular rhythm and paroxysmal ventricular tachycardia in acute myocardial infarction. Am J Cardiol 1974;34:667-670.

49. Gillette PC: Supraventricular arrhythmias in children. J Am Coll Cardiol 1985;5(6 Suppl):122B-129B.

50. Plumpton K, Justo R, Haas N: Amiodarone for post-operative junctional ectopic tachycardia. Cardiol Young 2005;15:13-18.

51. Vaksmann G, D'Hoinne C, Lucet V, et al: Permanent junctional reciprocating tachycardia in children: A multicentre study on clinical profile and outcome. Heart 2006;92:101-104.

52. Meiltz A, Weber R, Halimi F, et al: Permanent form of junctional reciprocating tachycardia in adults: Peculiar features and results of radiofrequency catheter ablation. Europace 2006;8:21-28.

53. Kessler KM, McAuliffe D, Chakko CS, et al: Multiform ventricular complexes: A transitional arrhythmia form? Am Heart J 1989;118: 441-444.

54. Ruskin JN: The cardiac arrhythmia suppression trial (CAST). N Engl J Med 1989;321:386-388.

55. Michel PL, Mandagout O, Vahanian A, et al: Ventricular arrhythmias in aortic valve disease before and after aortic valve replacement. Acta Cardiol 1992;47:145-156.

56. England MR, Gordon G, Salem M, Chernow B: Magnesium administration and dysrhythmias after cardiac surgery: A placebo-controlled, double-blind, randomized trial. JAMA 1992;268:2395-2402.

57. Bigger JT Jr: Prophylactic use of implanted cardiac defibrillators in patients at high risk for ventricular arrhythmias after coronary-artery bypass graft surgery. Coronary Artery Bypass Graft (CABG) Patch Trial Investigators. N Engl J Med 1997;337:1569-1575.

58. Sugi K, Karagueuzian HS, Fishbein MC, et al: Spontaneous ventricular tachycardia associated with isolated right ventricular infarction, one day after right coronary artery occlusion in the dog: Studies on the site of origin and mechanism. Am Heart J 1985;109:232-244.

59. Lazzara R, Scherlag BJ: Mechanisms of monomorphic ventricular tachycardia in coronary artery disease. J Interv Card Electrophysiol 2003;8:87-92.

60. Gorgels AP, van den Dool A, Hofs A, et al: Comparison of procainamide and lidocaine in terminating sustained monomorphic ventricular tachycardia. Am J Cardiol 1996;78:43-46.

61. Schwab JO, Luderitz B: [Current concepts in diagnosis and treatment of tachyarrhythmias.] Internist (Berl) 2005;46:1021-1031; quiz 1032-1033.

62. Marill KA, deSouza IS, Nishijima DK, et al: Amiodarone is poorly effective for the acute termination of ventricular tachycardia. Ann Emerg Med 2006;47:217-224.

63. Abriel H, Schlapfer J, Keller DI, et al: Molecular and clinical determinants of drug-induced long QT syndrome: An iatrogenic channelopathy. Swiss Med Wkly 2004;134:685-694.

64. Morissette P, Hreiche R, Turgeon J: Drug-induced long QT syndrome and torsades de pointes. Can J Cardiol 2005;21:857-864.

65. Touyz RM: Magnesium in clinical medicine. Front Biosci 2004;9: 1278-1293.

66. Khan IA, Gowda RM: Novel therapeutics for treatment of long-QT syndrome and torsades de pointes. Int J Cardiol 2004;95:1-6.

67. Kathofer S, Thomas D, Karle CA: The novel antiarrhythmic drug dronedarone: Comparison with amiodarone. Cardiovasc Drug Rev 2005;23:217-230.

68. Dorian P, Cass D, Schwartz B, et al: Amiodarone as compared with lidocaine for shock-resistant ventricular fibrillation. N Engl J Med 2002;346:884-890.

69. Yokoyama N, Nishikawa K, Takazawa T, et al: [Ventricular tachycardia induced by the change of position for epidural catheter insertion in a patient with hypertrophic obstructive cardiomyopathy.] Masui 2004; 53:910-913.

70. Installe E, Schoevaerdts JC, Gadisseux P, et al: Intravenous amiodarone in the treatment of various arrhythmias following cardiac operations. J Thorac Cardiovasc Surg 1981;81:302-308.

71. Forrest JB, Rehder K, Cahalan MK, Goldsmith CH: Multicenter study of general anesthesia: III. Predictors of severe perioperative adverse outcomes. Anesthesiology 1992;76:3-15.

72. Tsai PS, Chen CP, Tsai MS: Perioperative vasovagal syncope with focus on obstetric anesthesia. Taiwan J Obstet Gynecol 2006;45: 208-214.

73. Ho KM, Ismail H, Lee KC, Branch R: Use of intrathecal neostigmine as an adjunct to other spinal medications in perioperative and peripartum analgesia: A meta-analysis. Anaesth Intensive Care 2005;33:41-53.

74. Campagna JA, Carter C: Clinical relevance of the Bezold-Jarisch reflex. Anesthesiology 2003;98:1250-1260.

75. Szudi L, Paulovich E, Faluvegi Z, et al: [Perioperative temporary pacemaker therapy.] Orv Hetil 2002;143:401-404.

76. Sia S, Sarro F, Lepri A, Bartoli M: The effect of exogenous epinephrine on the incidence of hypotensive/bradycardic events during shoulder surgery in the sitting position during interscalene block. Anesth Analg 2003;97:583-588.

77. Hunyor AP: Reflexes and the eye. Aust N Z J Ophthalmol 1994;22:155-159; discussion 153.

Renal System

Chapter

17 Preservation of Renal Function

Mark Stafford-Smith

Acute renal impairment, evidenced by the accumulation of nitrogenous waste products (blood urea nitrogen and creatinine) and a rapid decline in glomerular filtration, is a major medical problem, occurring in 5% of all hospital patients and 30% of those admitted to an intensive care unit.[1] Renal injury is particularly common after some surgeries, complicating up to 30% of cardiac, vascular, trauma, and hepatobiliary procedures.[2] The importance of postoperative renal dysfunction lies in its consistent association with increased rates of in-hospital mortality, even after adjustment for other contributing factors.[3-5] Even minor degrees of renal impairment carry with them an increased risk of major complications and mortality, possibly due, at least in part, to the effects of acute renal injury on the normal functioning of many other organ systems.[6-8]

The kidneys are retroperitoneal organs that weigh approximately 150 g each. Although they constitute less than 0.5% of bodyweight, they receive one quarter of the cardiac output, making them the most highly perfused major organs. One of their main roles is to regulate and maintain the volume and composition of body fluids; they filter an amount of water equivalent to a 12-oz can of soda every 3 minutes, returning all but 1%, or approximately 4 mL, to the circulation. The excluded remnant is urine, and the ability to control finely the contents of urine is the basis of whole-body homeostasis. As acknowledged by the renal physiologist, Dr. Homer Smith, "It is no exaggeration to say that the composition of the blood is determined not by what the mouth ingests but by what the kidneys keep; they are the master chemists of our internal environment, which, so to speak, they synthesize in reverse."[9] It is for this reason that acute derangements of renal function, such as occur with postoperative acute renal injury, have ramifications that contrast with the compensated state of chronic renal disorders.

Although some aspects of the pathophysiology of postoperative renal dysfunction are understood, much is still not known about the condition. Components can be loosely grouped into factors affecting kidney vulnerability and factors that contribute to renal insult. Renal vulnerabilities include comorbidities (e.g., diabetes) and are extensively discussed in Chapter 9. However, risk factors explain only a small part of the overall variability in postoperative renal dysfunction.[2,3,10-26] Contributors to insult (e.g., atheroembolism) are also discussed in Chapter 9, and a mechanistic understanding of their involvement is key to the rationale for some of the renal preservation strategies. A burden of perioperative renal vulnerability and insult can therefore be described for each surgical patient. Consideration of the complex interplay among these factors for each patient highlights the need for individualized interventions when a pathophysiology is clear, and the low likelihood that any single intervention will solve this multifactorial problem.

Some practice modifications can significantly influence the likelihood of postoperative renal dysfunction. In contrast, frustration and disappointment have largely accompanied the search for effective renal preservation pharmacotherapies—a concern that has gained attention from members of such research agencies as the U.S. National Institutes of Health[27] and the Cochrane Database of Systematic Reviews.[28] The aim of this chapter is to review existing knowledge supporting or discrediting perioperative renal preservation strategies, including interventions aimed at the critically ill postoperative patient.

■ RENAL PHYSIOLOGY

Medullary Hypoxia

The kidney is inherently at risk for ischemic injury, and the medulla is the most vulnerable kidney region. The medulla receives only 5% of renal blood flow, and medullary perfusion is inefficient: because of the parallel arrangement of entering and exiting vessels, much of the oxygen that enters the medulla is allowed to escape before it is available to tissues. In addition, high demand for oxygen from active transport, particularly from the medullary thick ascending limb (mTAL) of the loop of Henle in the outer medulla, further challenges the adequacy of perfusion. It is, therefore, not surprising that normal oxygen extraction in the medulla is the highest in the body (79%), and normal medullary PO_2 is very low (10 to 20 mm Hg) (Fig. 17-1); this phenomenon is referred to as medullary hypoxia.[29] Paracrine systems (e.g., nitric oxide synthase and the renin-angiotensin system) modulate medullary oxygen delivery by local regulation of microvascular tone and blood flow.[30]

Medullary hypoxia is exacerbated by conditions commonly experienced during the perioperative period, including dehydration and low cardiac output. In these settings, homeostatic reflexes preserve whole-body perfusion at the expense of added risk to the already precarious balance between oxygen supply and demand in the renal medulla. Autoregulatory constriction of the efferent arteriole preserves glomerular filtration but further reduces medullary blood flow. More sluggish medullary blood flow increases oxygen escape from the entering to the exiting vessels. Finally, avid reabsorption of electrolytes by tubular cells increases medullary metabolic requirements. The most at-risk medullary region is adjacent to the cortex in the outer medullary stripe; this is where the first histologic evidence of ischemic renal injury manifests, in the mTAL of the loop of Henle. Urine PO_2 measurement is a sensitive monitor of medullary perfusion[31]; one clinical study found that a drop in urine oxygen levels after cardiac surgery predicted postoperative renal dysfunction.[32]

Ischemic Preconditioning Reflex

In many organs, a brief exposure to ischemia attenuates injury that is caused by subsequent ischemic episodes. This reflex phenomenon, known as ischemic preconditioning, is present in the kidney. Cochrane and colleagues observed in rats that 2 minutes of renal ischemia, or three such episodes separated by 5 minutes of reperfusion, protects the kidney from subsequent prolonged (45-minute) renal ischemia.[33] Interestingly, in this study, more ischemic episodes with reperfusion did not demonstrate renoprotective benefit. Studies by Lee and colleagues indicate that adenosine receptors are involved in mediating the reflex.[34,35] In a rat model, these authors found that adenosine infused just prior to renal ischemia attenuates ischemia-reperfusion injury, an A_1 adenosine receptor agonist–mediated effect. The clinical relevance of this phenomenon is still unclear, and no assessment of its potential as a renoprotective intervention prior to insult has yet been reported in humans (see Agents in the Early Stages of Development as Renal Preservation Therapies, later).

■ MECHANISMS OF SURGERY-RELATED ACUTE RENAL INJURY

The sources of postoperative renal insult are extensively reviewed elsewhere.[6] The two primary mechanisms that contribute to perioperative acute renal injury are ischemia-reperfusion and nephrotoxic effects, and three notable sources of insult (hypoperfusion, inflammation, and atheroembolism) are common to many surgical procedures in which postoperative renal dysfunction is prevalent. Several other, more unusual sources of renal insult may contribute in selected patients (e.g., rhabdomyolysis, drug-related effects).

Ischemia-Reperfusion

Abnormalities of renal perfusion that exceed the autoregulatory reserve of the renal circulation, such as cardiopulmonary

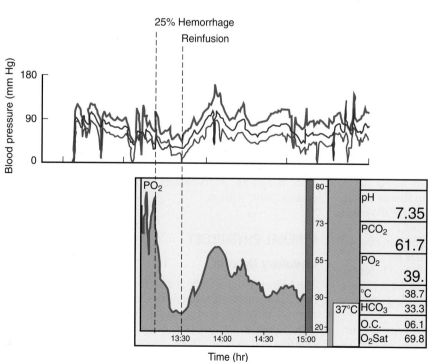

Figure 17-1 ■ An example of renal medullary hypoxia and the adverse effects of hypovolemic shock on medullary perfusion. In a pig model, a renal medullary oxygen sensor demonstrates medullary hypoxemia at baseline. Blood pressure changes are represented during experimental hemorrhage (25% blood volume). Exaggerated medullary hypoxia develops during the period of hypoperfusion. Note the close correlation between perfusion pressure and renal medullary oxygen levels. *(Redrawn from Stafford-Smith M, Grocott HP: Perfusion 2005;20:53-58.)*

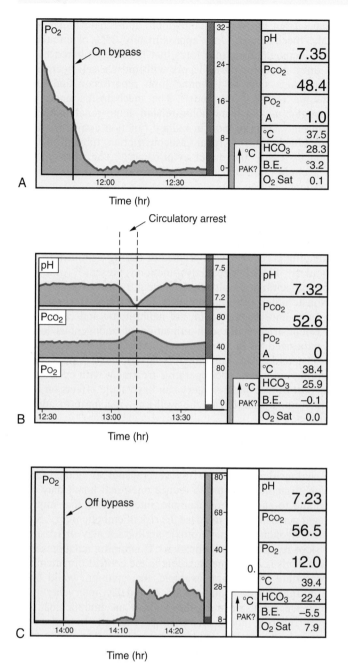

	pH	7.35
	Pco_2	48.4
	Po_2 A	1.0
	°C	37.5
	HCO_3	28.3
	B.E.	°3.2
	O_2 Sat	0.1

	pH	7.32
	Pco_2	52.6
	Po_2 A	0
	°C	38.4
	HCO_3	25.9
	B.E.	−0.1
	O_2 Sat	0.0

	pH	7.23
	Pco_2	56.5
	Po_2	12.0
	°C	39.4
	HCO_3	22.4
	B.E.	−5.5
	O_2 Sat	7.9

Figure 17-2 ■ The effects of cardiopulmonary bypass and circulatory arrest on medullary perfusion. Extreme medullary hypoxia ($Po_2 \times O$) develops in the minutes after initiation of cardiopulmonary bypass **(A).** However, at the onset of circulatory arrest **(B),** this is accompanied by a fall in pH and a rising CO_2 level. Measurable oxygen levels return several minutes after separation from cardiopulmonary bypass **(C).** *(Redrawn from Stafford-Smith M, Grocott HP: Perfusion 2005;20:53-58.)*

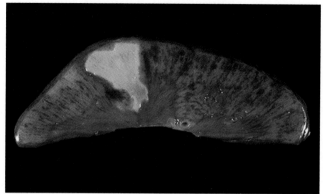

Figure 17-3 ■ A gross kidney specimen demonstrates the wedge-shaped pattern typical of a renal infarct. The organization of the renal vasculature means that embolic arterial obstruction is poorly compensated for by collateral flow. *(From Florida State University College of Medicine and available at www-medlib.med.utah.edu/ WebPath/CINJHTML/CINJ015.html.)*

bypass (Fig. 17-2),[29] are believed to be a major source of perioperative ischemia-reperfusion injury. Other conditions, including low output states, hypovolemic shock (see Fig. 17-1), vasoconstrictor use, and circulatory arrest (see Fig. 17-2B), all may contribute to the renal ischemic burden of specific surgical procedures.[12,17,21] As described earlier, the normally low medullary Po_2 (10 to 20 mm Hg) makes this tissue particularly vulnerable to hypoperfusion.[36] Key to regulation of renal blood flow and modulation of microvascular function and oxygen delivery in the renal medulla are paracrine systems, including the renin-angiotensin system and nitric oxide synthase.[30] Autonomic influences are also important, with the alpha-1-adrenergic receptor–mediated vasoconstriction and alpha-2-adrenergic receptor–mediated vasodilation contributing to modulation of renal perfusion.

Inflammatory

Surgery with disruption of tissues and the potential for endotoxemia is a consistent trigger for the generation of proinflammatory cytokines (e.g., tumor necrosis factor-α [TNFα] and interleukin-6 [IL-6]) and an inflammatory response, both systemically and locally in the kidney.[37,38] Preexisting infection may further predispose surgical patients to postoperative renal dysfunction.[39] Other postoperative factors, such as infectious and septic complications, transfusion, and interventions such as cardiopulmonary bypass, contribute to the generation of cytokines that have major effects on the renal microcirculation and may lead to tubular injury.[40]

Embolic

Showers of emboli are common during certain surgical procedures. Although some types of emboli do not appear to have an important role in postoperative renal dysfunction (e.g., air), others are significant contributors to renal injury. Collateral flow is poorly developed in the kidney, and embolic occlusion of renal vessels usually leads to segmental necrosis of the affected tissue (Fig. 17-3). Atheroembolism is common during some surgical procedures, particularly those involving operative aortic manipulation, and is highly associated with postoperative renal dysfunction.[41] The strong association of intra-aortic balloon counterpulsation with acute renal injury is also thought to be related to the dislodgement of aortic plaque.[42] All degrees of renal injury can result from atheroembolism, ranging from the obstruction of major renal vessels from large fragments of plaque,[43] to the occlusion of multiple small renal vessels by cholesterol microcrystals.[44] Thromboembolism and infectious emboli from endocarditis (Fig. 17-4) may also contribute to renal insult. During cardiac surgery, bone marrow lipid droplets may be returned to the circulation as part of blood salvage and perturb blood flow in renal vessels[45]; however, the significance of these droplets as contributors to postoperative renal dysfunction is unclear.

Pigment (Hemoglobin and Myoglobin)

Hemoglobinuria occurs when intravascular hemolysis releases sufficient hemoglobin to exceed the adsorptive

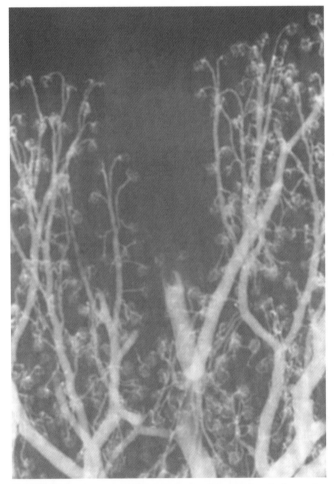

Figure 17-4 ■ Angiography (×30) demonstrates embolic occlusion of an interlobular artery in a patient with subacute bacterial endocarditis. Note the total obstruction, and the complete absence of collateral flow. *(From Bookstein JJ, Clark RL (eds): Renal Microvascular Disease: Angiographic-Microangiographic Correlates. Boston, Little, Brown, 1980.)*

capacity of circulating haptoglobin and renal tubular reuptake mechanisms. Only approximately 25% of circulating free hemoglobin is in a form that is readily filtered by the kidney. Myoglobinuria occurs with muscle cell necrosis in conditions such as ischemic limb reperfusion and major trauma (crush syndrome).[46] The mechanisms underlying myoglobin- and hemoglobin-related acute renal injury are similar.[47] Deterioration in kidney function comes from the combined effects of renal vasoconstriction, tubular obstruction by casts, and direct cytotoxicity.[48] The nitric oxide–scavenging potential of these pigments contributes to renal vasoconstriction.

Nephrotoxins

Several well-known nephrotoxins are relevant to the perioperative period. Contrast-related renal injury is common when imaging is required just prior to or during a procedure, particularly if baseline renal dysfunction is present.[49] Aminoglycoside antibiotics also have potent nephrotoxic effects.[50] Nonsteroidal anti-inflammatory drugs (NSAIDs), such as aspirin and indomethacin, are nephrotoxic and cause renal vasoconstriction through inhibition of endogenous locally synthesized vasodilator prostaglandins (see Steroids, Aspirin, Nonsteroidal Anti-inflammatory Drugs, and Cyclooxygenase Inhibitors, later).[51] Perioperative treatment with cyclosporin as part of transplant surgery can have acute effects on renal function in addition to the well-known long-term adverse effects.[52]

Conflicting Renal Protection Strategies: Mechanism-Directed Renal Preservation

Renal insult often comes from several sources, and preservation strategies directed to reduce one renal insult may contribute to another. For example, interventions that improve renal perfusion may increase the risk of embolic injury. Similarly, avoidance of nephrotoxic antibiotics may increase the risk of septic renal complications. Combining renal preservation goals is sometimes possible in the context of patient and procedure. In the first example, one solution would be to minimize aortic manipulation and delay interventions to increase perfusion until the peak of an embolic load has occurred (i.e., aortic cross-clamp removal). In the second example, an option would be to select a less nephrotoxic antibiotic with similar antibacterial coverage.

■ TIMING OF INTERVENTIONS RELATIVE TO A RENAL INSULT/INJURY

Broadly, perioperative renal preservation studies can be grouped into those in which an intervention is aimed at prevention and those in which renal injury is established or ongoing.

Prophylaxis and Preemption

Renal preservation strategies with the goal of avoiding, preventing, or attenuating renal insult before it occurs include the use of preoperative risk stratification to influence procedure selection, procedure modifications, changes in practice guidelines, and pharmacologic renal protection. Examples include preoperative genetic screening to identify subgroups at high renal risk, stent grafting versus open surgical procedures to treat aortic aneurysmal disease, fluid hydration before contrast dye exposure, and epiaortic scanning to guide aortic manipulation and minimize plaque disruption.

Established Renal Injury

Some renal preservation strategies are aimed at patients with established postoperative renal dysfunction, often defined by a measure of filtration impairment (e.g., a 25% rise in serum creatinine compared with baseline). Most studies in this setting do not differentiate patients no longer sustaining renal injury from those in whom renal insult is ongoing, despite the important differences between these states. The rationales for these interventions are diverse, including the avoidance of further renal insult, attenuation of reflexive components of acute renal injury (e.g., vasoconstriction), and hastening the recovery of tubular function.[53,54] A large number of interventions have failed to show benefit in treating established renal injury, although maintenance of normal serum glucose values with insulin therapy has been useful.

Renal Failure Requiring Dialysis

New-onset postoperative dialysis patients can be broadly divided into two subgroups: (1) those with baseline impairment of renal function severe enough that even a small added perioperative insult is sufficient to cause renal failure, and (2) those who sustained a devastating perioperative renal insult but who had normal baseline renal function. The two patient groups can be differentiated by their preexisting comorbidities, anticipated in-hospital course, and long-term prognosis.[55] Patients with baseline renal impairment have a low in-hospital mortality rate that only slightly exceeds that of patients not requiring dialysis. In contrast, dialysis requirement after a more complicated operation in a patient with normal baseline renal function is typically associated with a devastating renal injury and high in-hospital mortality. Intuitively, each patient subgroup might benefit more from one or another of the preemptive renoprotective strategies; however, once dialysis is required, they are often grouped together for the purpose of study.[56] Studies involve variations in dialysis technique, pharmacologic aids that may reduce or eliminate the need for dialysis, and interventions that may hasten tubular recovery. The molecular biology of tubular regeneration is becoming much better understood, including interventions that may be considered in the future for renoprotection (e.g., stem cells). However, agents that are designed to promote renal regeneration rather than protection are beyond the scope of this chapter and will not be discussed.

■ DEFINITIONS OF PERIOPERATIVE RENAL PRESERVATION

The best evidence of effective renal preservation includes two outcomes: fewer postoperative patients requiring renal replacement therapy and reduced mortality (Table 17-1). For example, optimal management of hyperglycemia in critically ill patients reduces the incidence of dialysis and improves survival (see Insulin, later).[57] Unfortunately, most studies are too small, and the outcomes of mortality or dialysis rates are too infrequent to adequately compare rates between groups as an outcome of interest.

Commonly, renal preservation is evaluated using secondary measures or surrogate endpoints as markers for dialysis and death. Secondary measures most commonly reflect change in postoperative renal filtration rather than renal failure; peak filtration impairment is compared with a predefined critical threshold or with baseline renal function. Although most serum creatinine–derived markers of renal filtration impairment have been associated with postoperative mortality, there is little consensus on a gold standard[58]; one review evaluated 28 controlled perioperative studies, and no two reports used the same criteria for acute renal dysfunction or acute renal failure.[2] Twenty-four-hour urine collection to determine creatinine clearance is useful in stable patients in the intensive care unit (ICU), but 2-hour creatinine clearance measures may be a good and more convenient surrogate.[59] Perioperatively, serum creatinine values combined with other data can provide an estimate of creatinine clearance.[60] The rapid fluid shifts and dynamic changes in renal function that surround the surgical period often make precise measurement of renal glomerular filtration rate at this time impractical. Although controversial, many believe that serum creatinine–derived markers are at least as accurate as more invasive tests in this setting.[61-63] Many studies present several markers of renal function to confirm an effect.[64]

Some consensus definitions for significant renal dysfunction have been published. For example, the Society of Thoracic Surgeons Database definition of acute or worsening perioperative renal failure includes a twofold rise from baseline creatinine level to a serum value of at least 2.1 mg/dL or a new requirement for dialysis.[65] Although no fixed definition of contrast-induced nephropathy exists, many definitions are similar to the one described by Barrett and Parfrey requiring an increase in the serum creatinine of more than 25% or more than 0.5 mg/dL (44 μmol/L) within 48 hours after the administration of the contrast agent.[66] Cystatin C, a cysteine proteinase inhibitor produced by all nucleated cells at a constant rate, is a substance that accumulates in the circulation with renal impairment and can be used as a marker of glomerular filtration. Recent reports indicate that cystatin C may have advantages over serum creatinine as a secondary marker of renal function.[67,68]

Some very sensitive indicators of renal injury exist. The clinical relevance of urinary markers reflecting tubular cell enzyme leakage or changes in tubular functions are not known. Tubular cell enzyme leakage can provide information on the segmental location and ultrastructural origin of injury. For example, the a and p isomers of glutathione S-transferase (GST) are both cytosolic enzymes deriving from the proximal and distal tubular cells, respectively. N-Acetyl-β-D-glucosaminidase (NAG) is predominantly a proximal tubular lysosomal enzyme. Brush border enzymuria (e.g., γ-glutamyl transpeptidase [γGT], alkaline phosphatase [AP], and ala-[leu-gly]-aminopeptidase) identifies brush border injury. Recently, a transcriptome-wide interrogation for renal genes that are induced very early after renal ischemia identified neutrophil gelatinase-associated lipocalin (NGAL) as a

17-1   Measures of Outcomes Reported in Renal Preservation Studies

Level of Evidence*	Commonly Reported Measures of Acute Renal Dysfunction in Perioperative Study	Emerging and Potentially Useful Markers
Level A	• Postoperative mortality • New-onset postoperative dialysis	—
Level B	• STS definition of acute renal failure (see Definitions of Renal Preservation, in text)	• Cystatin C
	Serum Creatinine • Peak postoperative serum creatinine • Maximum change in serum creatinine • Preoperative to peak postoperative fractional (%) change in serum creatinine	

	Inulin Clearance
	Iohexol Clearance
	Creatinine Clearance
	   Measures
	     24-hr urine collection
	     2-hr urine collection
	   Estimates
	     Cockcroft-Gault equation[60]
	     MDRD equation[307]
	• Lowest postoperative measured or estimated clearance
	• Greatest change in measured or estimated clearance
	• Preoperative to lowest postoperative fractional (%) change in clearance	

Level C	• Urine output
	• Blood urea nitrogen (BUN)
	• Tubular cell enzyme leakage (urine)
	   αGST (proximal tubule: cytosol)
	   πGST (distal tubule: cytosol)
	   NAG (proximal tubule: lysosomal)
	   γGT (brush border)
	   AP (brush border)
	   ala-(leu-gly)-aminopeptidase (brush border)
	• Tubular proteinuria (urine: proximal tubule)
	   α_1-Microglobulin
	   β_2-Microglobulin
	   Albumin
	   Retinol-binding protein
	   Lysozyme
	   Ribonuclease
	   Immunoglobulin G
	   Transferrin
	   Ceruloplasmin
	   Light chains (lambda and kappa types)
	   Total protein levels
		• Urinary NGAL (detected at 3 hr, peak at 24 hr, returned to baseline at 72 hr)
		• Urinary SSAT (peak at 12 hr, returned to baseline at 48 hr)
		• Urinary NEP (detected at 3 hr)
		• Urine PO_2
		• Urine cytokine markers
		   ICAM-1
		   AM-1
		   KIM-1
		   P-selectin
		   E-selectin
		   E-selectin
		   MCP-1
		   cyr 61

*Markers of renal preservation can be grouped as follows:
  Level A: Markers that are acceptable as primary evidence of renal preservation.
  Level B: Markers of perioperative renal function that are not sufficient evidence of renal preservation but are known to correlate with level A outcomes, and are supportive evidence for renoprotective properties.
  Level C: Markers that reflect subtle changes in renal function that are of interest but of unknown relevance as evidence of acute renal injury.
  Compared with conventional procedure.
  AP, alkaline phosphatase; cyr, cysteine-rich protein; γGT, γ-glutamyl transpeptidase; GST, glutathione *S*-transferase; ICAM, intercellular adhesion molecule; KIM, kidney injury molecule; MCP, monocyte chemoattractant protein; MDRD, Modification of Diet in Renal Disease Study Group; NAG, *N*-acetyl-β-D-glucosaminidase; NEP, neutral endopeptidase; NGAL, neutrophil gelatinase-associated lipocalcin; SSAT, spermidine/spermine *N*-1-acetyl-transferase; STS, Society of Thoracic Surgeons; VCAM, vascular cell adhesion molecule.

protein generated by ischemic renal tubular cells.[69] NGAL is found in the urine of cardiac surgery patients within 6 hours of surgery, and elevated levels are highly predictive of postoperative acute renal failure.[70] Although this substance demonstrates promise as an early marker of acute renal injury, its validity as a marker for renal preservation studies has not been evaluated. Tubular proteinuria results from the impair-

ments of reuptake of small filtered proteins by the megalin-mediated transport system in the proximal tubule. Markers of tubular proteinuria include urine alpha-1- and beta-2-microglobulin, albumin, retinol-binding protein, lysozyme, ribonuclease, IgG, transferrin, ceruloplasmin, light chains (lambda and kappa types), and total protein levels. Notably, tubular proteinuria is a poor marker of renal tubular function

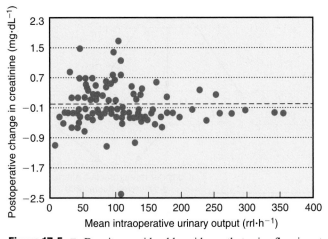

Figure 17-5 ■ Despite considerable evidence that urine flow is not a meaningful assessment of perioperative renal dysfunction, urine output is often reported in renal preservation studies, and it is often monitored to assess kidney function by clinicians. Data from a study comparing postoperative urine output and postoperative rises in serum creatinine after aortic surgery highlight that lack of association of urine output with renal complications. *(Redrawn from Alpert RA, Roizen MF, Hamilton WK, et al: Surgery 1984;95:707-711.)*

in the setting of antifibrinolytic therapy (see Selection of Antifibrinolytic Agent, later). Overall, although studies using these markers generate findings of scientific interest, their utility in assessing the clinical relevance of a renal protective intervention is limited.

Urine output remains the most controversial of outcomes for renal preservation studies. Alpert and colleagues documented urinary output in 137 aortic surgery patients who were given crystalloid solution, mannitol, furosemide, or nothing when urinary flow dropped below 0.125 mL/kg/hr.[71] These authors found no correlation between intraoperative mean urinary output or lowest hourly urinary output and change from preoperative to peak postoperative levels of serum creatinine (Fig. 17-5). The findings of this study are consistent with data from other studies that indicate that urine output is not a useful marker of renal function or preservation. Blood urea nitrogen (BUN) also remains in wide use today, despite its being a poor measure of renal function because of such factors as highly variable rates of endogenous production and significant changes in tubular reabsorption with some conditions (e.g., dehydration). BUN possesses few of the characteristics of an ideal marker for glomerular function.

■ REVIEW OF RENAL PRESERVATION OUTCOME STUDIES

Standard clinical management decisions affect renal outcome (Fig. 17-6), and preoperative renal risk stratification (see Chapter 9) may reduce renal injury by influencing procedure selection.[3,10-15,17-26,72] Finally, pharmacologic interventions have been studied for their ability to protect the kidney during the perioperative period. These factors are reviewed next.

Procedure Planning

Recent surgical innovations have embraced the philosophy that less invasive procedures requiring smaller incisions and less physiologic disturbance can safely achieve surgical goals and may reduce postoperative organ dysfunction and improve overall outcome. Examples include the use of stent-graft technology, videoscopic-assisted procedures, avoidance or modification of cardiopulmonary bypass, and reduced aortic manipulation. Although some innovations appear to confer renal benefit, this is not the case for all minimally invasive procedures.

Modifications of coronary artery bypass surgery have been studied extensively.[73-83] Preliminary reports comparing beating-heart off-pump coronary artery bypass (OPCAB) surgery with standard on-pump coronary artery bypass graft (CABG) procedures identified reductions in subtle markers of renal injury with the off-pump procedure.[84] Three randomized acute renal injury trials compared on- and off-pump procedures, but these studies were small and inconclusive.[73-75] Several large retrospective studies have compared renal outcome after off- and on-pump procedures using a variety of statistical approaches, including multivariable analysis,[76,77] propensity scores,[79,80] case-matching,[78] risk stratification,[82] and meta-analysis of retrospective studies.[81] A major limitation of most of these studies is the baseline differences in renal risk factors between OPCAB and CABG procedure groups, and they have drawn conflicting conclusions. Although the two multivariable analyses that accounted for known renal risk factors identified no difference in renal risk between the two procedures,[76,77] other studies using alternative statistical approaches have favored off-pump over CABG surgery.[78-82] Recently, Cheng and colleagues performed a meta-analysis of randomized studies comparing OPCAB and CABG surgery for all major outcomes.[83] In this review of more than 1400 patients from 10 trials, there was no reduction in the 30-day incidence of renal failure with OPCAB surgery. In their report, these authors particularly highlighted concerns regarding confounding in retrospective OPCAB versus CABG analyses.

A single retrospective report by Chukwuemeka and colleagues[85] has compared postoperative renal impairment in OPCAB and CABG patients with baseline renal dysfunction. The authors used a propensity score analysis to adjust for group differences, comparing 146 off-pump with 438 on-pump procedures, and concluded that even in this high-risk group, off-pump procedures did not confer renal protection.

Clamp occlusion and cannulation of the ascending aorta are actions that can disrupt atheromatous plaque and cause embolization. Measures of atherosclerosis of the ascending aorta and intraoperative arterial emboli counts are strong independent predictors of renal dysfunction after CABG surgery.[41,86] The Symmetry aortic connector system (St. Jude Medical Inc., St. Paul, Minn) is a technology developed to implant saphenous vein coronary bypass grafts onto the aortic wall with less manipulation of the aorta, with the hope that this may reduce embolization and organ dysfunction.[87,88] In a retrospective multivariable analysis of consecutive CABG surgeries, Fischer and colleagues compared renal

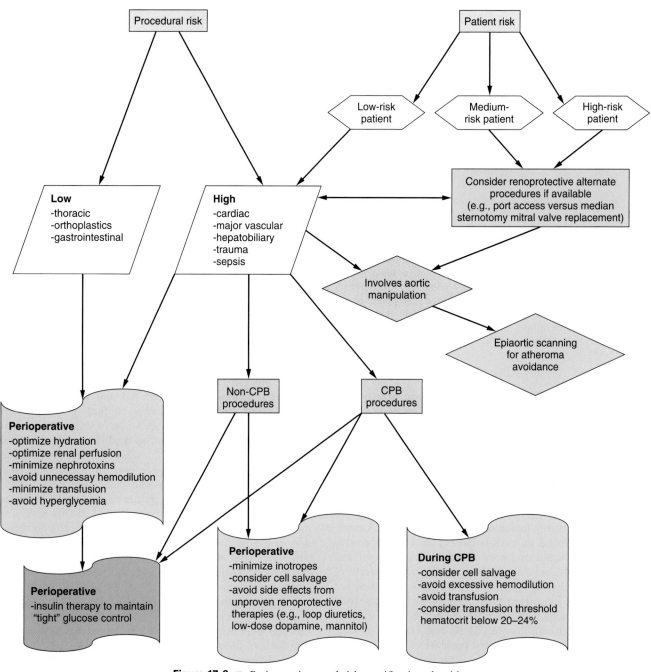

Figure 17-6 ■ Perioperative renal risk stratification algorithm.

dysfunction after 124 OPCAB procedures using Symmetry devices, with 313 standard OPCAB and 2863 standard CABG procedures, and they observed no differences in postoperative renal dysfunction.[77,89]

Collectively, OPCAB studies indicate that surgery with avoidance of cardiopulmonary bypass (CPB) and currently available methods to reduce aortic manipulation do not confer renoprotection. Therefore, renal risk should not be an important factor in selecting the type of coronary artery bypass procedure for a patient.

Catheter-based CPB systems that permit cardiac surgery without median sternotomy may confer renoprotection. Minimally invasive cardiopulmonary bypass systems, such as the EndoCPB or EndoDirect systems (Heartport., Inc, Redwood City, Calif), permit surgical access to the heart through a mini-thoracotomy incision, or port, and have been adopted by some surgeons to facilitate a less invasive approach to mitral and tricuspid valve surgeries. In a nonrandomized retrospective study of 297 port access, minimally invasive, and open mitral valve surgeries, McCreath and colleagues observed approximately a 50% smaller peak rise in creatinine after port access than with the median sternotomy procedures (18.5% versus 35.4%, $P = .01$).[90]

Aortic stent-graft technology is rapidly changing the treatment of thoracic and abdominal aortic disease. In a nonrandomized prospective study involving 279 patients undergoing elective abdominal aortic aneurysm repair by stent-graft placement or open surgery, Greenberg and colleagues noted that stent-graft patients were significantly less likely to meet a criterion for renal dysfunction before hospital discharge (creatinine rise >30%, or creatinine >2.0 mg/dL; 5/198 versus 8/79, $P = .01$); however, only one patient in each group required dialysis postoperatively, and at 30 days, 6 months, and 12 months postoperatively there was no difference between the groups with regard to measures of renal function.[91]

Modifiable Nonpharmacologic Clinical Factors

Preoperative Management

Contrast-induced nephropathy accounts for 10% of all in-hospital acute renal injury. In a group of 27 patients, Garwood and colleagues found that urine markers of tubular injury were elevated in patients presenting for CABG surgery within 5 days of cardiac catheterization.[92] Provenchère and colleagues found radiocontrast agent administration less than 48 hours before surgery to be an independent predictor of postoperative renal dysfunction in a prospective study of 649 cardiac surgery patients.[93] Avoiding elective surgery immediately after contrast administration and permitting recovery of contrast-associated nephropathy before surgery would seem prudent. Patients with baseline renal dysfunction undergoing interventional cardiology procedures have less risk of contrast nephropathy when use of low-osmolar contrast media is accompanied by aggressive prestudy hydration.[49] Hydration for intraoperative contrast studies and the use of low-ionic contrast media are practice changes that are supported by existing literature.

Decisions about the administration of chronic medications are part of preoperative management of perioperative renal risk. Angiotensin-converting enzyme (ACE) inhibitors and angiotensin I receptor blockers delay progression of *chronic* renal disease,[94] but these agents may precipitate acute renal deterioration in situations where angiotensin is critical to the regulation of renal filtration, such as renal artery stenosis or volume depletion.[95,96] In a prospective study of 249 patients undergoing aortic surgery, Cittanova and colleagues noted an association between chronic ACE inhibitor therapy and postoperative renal impairment.[97] However, in a retrospective analysis of 1800 cardiac surgery patients, Weightman and colleagues did not find preoperative ACE inhibitors to be predictive of mortality.[98] In a retrospective cohort study, Charlson and colleagues found preoperative diuretic therapy to be an independent risk factor for postoperative complications in a group of 248 patients undergoing CABG surgery.[99]

There are no clear guidelines regarding renal risk on the merits of giving or withholding chronic drug therapies.

Intraoperative Management

Intravenous Fluid Selection

Intravenous fluid choices have been found to be an attributive risk in some studies of postoperative renal dysfunction. The use of hydroxyethyl starch (HES) preparations for volume expansion is associated with renal dysfunction in surgical and critically ill patients in several retrospective reports.[100-103] In a randomized study of 129 patients with severe sepsis or septic shock who received either 6% HES or 3% gelatin, peak serum creatinine and the frequency of acute renal failure and oliguria was higher in the HES group.[104] In the same study, a multivariable analysis also identified the use of HES as a predictor of acute renal failure independent of other renal risk factors. In contrast, in a study of 40 older adult cardiac surgery patients randomized to receive either 6% HES or gelatin, Boldt and colleagues found no evidence of increased renal risk.[105] A similar study involving 30 major abdominal surgery patients from the same institution came to a similar conclusion.[106] Recent studies have focused on the contents of the solutions supporting the HES preparations and their potential to influence the development of metabolic hyperchloremic acidosis and variations in renal outcome.

Metabolic hyperchloremic acidosis is an acid–base abnormality frequently observed in postoperative patients that results from the use of saline or saline-based colloid solutions. In a randomized blinded trial, 47 older adult patients undergoing major surgery received 6% HES suspended in either a balanced salt solution (Hextend, BioTime, Inc., Berkeley, Calif) or 0.9% sodium chloride (HESPAN, B. Braun Medical, Inc., Irvine, Calif). Two thirds of patients receiving the sodium chloride but none receiving the balanced salt-based solution developed hyperchloremic metabolic acidosis ($P < .0001$).[107] In addition, gastric tonometry identified a larger increase in the CO_2 gap in the saline group ($P = .04$), suggesting poorer splanchnic (and renal) perfusion. There has been speculation that this metabolic abnormality may be a clinically relevant modifier of perioperative renal vulnerability.[108] Elevated chloride levels and acidosis can have adverse effects on renal homeostasis, including reduced renal blood flow and glomerular filtration rate, increased afferent arteriolar tone, and altered renin release.[109,110] The avoidance of saline and the development of metabolic hyperchloremic acidosis may prove to be an important modifier of renal risk. However, an appropriate clinical trial to address this question has not yet been reported.

The efficacy of sodium bicarbonate for prophylaxis against acute renal injury has not been evaluated in the perioperative period but does appear effective for contrast-induced nephropathy. In animal models of acute ischemic renal failure, pretreatment with sodium bicarbonate is more protective than sodium chloride.[111] Merten and colleagues randomized 119 angiography patients to receive either 154 mEq/L of sodium chloride or sodium bicarbonate, as a bolus of 3 mL/kg per hour for 1 hour before iopamidol contrast, followed by an infusion of 1 mL/kg per hour for 6 hours after the procedure.[112] Contrast-induced nephropathy occurred in eight patients (13.6%) infused with sodium chloride but in only one (1.7%) of those receiving sodium bicarbonate

($P = .02$). Whether renal benefit resulted from receiving sodium bicarbonate or from avoiding sodium chloride was not explored in this study.

Cardiopulmonary Bypass Management

Although CPB represents only a small portion of the total perioperative period, research suggests that significant renal risk is associated with this part of cardiac, major vascular, and other related procedures. Animal studies indicate that oxygen supply-and-demand inequalities are exaggerated and that medullary hypoxia is extreme during CPB, with effects that last well beyond separation from circulatory support (see Fig. 17-2).[29] In humans, changes known to occur at the initiation of CPB include greater reduction in renal than in systemic perfusion, loss of renal blood flow autoregulation, and stress hormone and inflammatory responses known to be harmful to the kidney.[113-115] These effects may explain why the duration of CPB independently predicts post–cardiac surgery renal impairment.[3,13,21,22] Many clinical decisions related to CPB management have been studied, and some may influence the occurrence of postoperative acute renal injury.

Modifiers of Renal Oxygen Delivery. Organ perfusion and oxygen delivery are primary goals of CPB. However, the relationship between standard CPB management guidelines and renal complications is only partly understood. Renal blood flow during CPB is not autoregulated and varies with pump flow rates and blood pressure.[113] However, CPB hypotension is not equivalent to hypotension with hemorrhagic shock or low cardiac output states, because low pressure during CPB is rarely associated with low flow. Fischer and colleagues retrospectively compared CPB flow rates and perfusion pressures in a case-control analysis of three groups of patients with normal baseline renal function who postoperatively either required dialysis ($n = 44$), sustained a renal injury without requiring dialysis ($n = 51$), or had no renal impairment ($n = 48$).[116] These authors noted that, on average, greater renal injury was associated with longer bypass durations, lower flows, and longer periods with CPB pressure less than 60 mm Hg. A serious limitation of this study is the potential for confounding CPB variables and known renal risk factors. In contrast, several large retrospective studies that accounted for known risk factors in evaluating perfusion management did not link low CPB blood pressure (with maintained flow) with postoperative acute renal injury.[10,26,117,118]

Renal blood flow is affected by renal artery stenosis. In a retrospective study of 798 aortocoronary bypass patients whose cardiac catheterization procedures routinely included renal angiogram, Conlon and colleagues found that 18.7% of patients had at least 50% stenosis of one renal artery (nine patients had >95% renal artery stenosis bilaterally).[119] However, in a multivariable logistic regression analysis, there was no association of the presence or severity of renal artery stenosis with postoperative acute renal injury.

Hemodilution is another controversial issue in CPB management. When a crystalloid or colloid solution is used to prime the extracorporeal circuit, the initiation of CPB is associated with an acute drop in oxygen-carrying capacity.

Animal studies indicate that moderate hemodilution reduces the risk of kidney injury during CPB through improved regional blood flow and reduction of blood viscosity.[120,121] Extreme CPB hemodilution (hematocrit <20%) is often tolerated as part of current CPB management protocols; however, this practice has recently been linked to adverse outcomes.[122-124] Several large retrospective studies have linked lowest hematocrit levels during CPB with postoperative acute renal injury and failure.[64,125-127] Ironically, one alternative to tolerating extreme CPB hemodilution—transfusion—has also been considered risky.[125,127]

In a retrospective study of 1404 CABG surgery patients, Swaminathan and colleagues found that the lowest CPB hematocrits (in the range of 22% to 24%) were significantly associated with acute kidney damage, a risk that increased as a patient's body weight increased.[125] These authors also observed a strong independent relationship between perioperative transfusion and renal impairment. Habib and colleagues[64] evaluated renal outcome in a cohort of 1780 CABG surgery patients with regard to the lowest hematocrit during CPB, transfusion management, and CPB duration. These authors looked for a threshold detrimental CPB hematocrit and found a nearly sigmoid-shaped "elbow" effect below 24% with increased postoperative renal dysfunction. A more modest effect was observed, also at 24%, when transfused patients were excluded. Finally, the same relationship was exaggerated with extended bypass duration. In another retrospective study, Karkouti and colleagues evaluated the incidence of dialysis relative to nadir CPB hematocrit in 9080 CABG surgery patients. These authors noted a nadir CPB hematocrit of less than 21% to be detrimental (compared with 21% to 25%), with a 2.3-fold increased risk of dialysis.[126] Interestingly, these authors also noted an increased risk for dialysis with high hematocrits (>25%). Although these findings strongly support the avoidance of extreme hemodilution during CPB, they are not helpful in developing guidelines for optimal transfusion practice.

One randomized controlled CPB study involving both normovolemic hemodilution and transfusion evaluated postoperative renal function with an active "target hematocrit" management protocol. Barbeito and colleagues randomized 107 aortocoronary bypass patients to protocols achieving high (>27%) or low (15% to 17%) hematocrit values during CPB; an additional standard practice group of 56 patients was included whose management involved no predefined target CPB hematocrit (median nadir hematocrit, 23%).[128] These authors found no difference in postoperative acute renal injury between groups, concluding that variation in target CPB hematocrit does not have a major effect on postoperative acute renal injury; however, they acknowledged that efficient blood conservation measures that reduce both hemodilution and transfusion (e.g., minimizing CPB pump prime) may well be effective renoprotective strategies.

A second issue in considering transfusion is the age of the blood. Current storage techniques generally provide a 42-day shelf life from the day of donation. In a retrospective multivariable analysis of 6525 CABG surgery patients who received blood, DeSimone and colleagues noted an independent association of older blood with both increased mortality ($P < .0001$) and postoperative acute renal injury ($P = .03$).[129] This same study found no renal or mortality benefit from leukocyte depletion of erythrocytes. In a smaller study, Basran and colleagues evaluated the age of blood in 298 redo-CABG surgery patients and noted a univariate association of older blood with the occurrence of acute renal injury; however, these authors acknowledged their inability to account for potential confounding effects.[130]

In summary, optimal hematocrit management during CPB is currently difficult to define, but it is fair to say that transfusion during CPB appears to contribute to postoperative renal dysfunction and should be considered only after all sources of hemodilution have been minimized.

Modifiers of Renal Oxygen Demand. Profound hypothermia reduces the metabolism and is essential to renal preservation during kidney transplant surgery. It would seem logical, therefore, that hypothermia during CPB would also be renoprotective.[131] However, three prospective randomized studies have not confirmed renal protection from mild CPB hypothermia.[132-134] In the largest study to date, involving 298 aortocoronary bypass patients randomized to hypothermic (28°C to 30°C) or normothermic (35.5°C to 36.5°C) CPB, Swaminathan and colleagues observed no link between normothermic bypass and increased postoperative renal dysfunction.[134]

Hyperglycemia increases renal O_2 demands through the energy-consuming process of glucose reuptake in the proximal tubule.[135] A possible explanation for the absence of renoprotection with CPB hypothermia is that the reduced effectiveness of insulin at cold temperatures may contribute to bypass-related hyperglycemia. Elevations of preoperative and pre-CPB serum glucose in cardiac surgery patients are associated with increased postoperative renal injury, independent of preoperative history of diabetes (see Insulin, later).[13,125]

Avoidance of Ascending Aortic Atheroembolism. Embolic arterial obstruction is poorly compensated for by collateral flow in the kidney, partly because of the organization of renal vasculature[136]; ischemic regions of cortex and medulla from vessel occlusion typically generate wedge-shaped infarcts (see Figs. 17-3 and 17-4). Cardiovascular surgical procedures involving atherosclerotic vessels are known to have high particulate emboli rates (57% to 77%).[137,138] Emboli release is predictable for certain procedures; for example, during cardiac surgery, aortic unclamping is a common time for showers of emboli.[139]

Although some technologies have been introduced to reduce embolization by limiting aortic manipulation or trapping emboli, no strong evidence indicates that these have resulted in benefits. In a multicenter trial of 1289 patients randomized to the use of the Embol-X intra-aortic filtration system (Embol-X, Mountain View, Calif) (Fig. 17-7), a net deployed just prior to aortic cross-clamp release during cardiac surgery to catch emboli, Banbury and colleagues found no difference in a composite outcome of ischemic events; however, in a post hoc comparison of increased-risk patients, filter use was associated with reduced renal complications (17/124 [14%] versus 28/117 [24%], $P = .04$).[140]

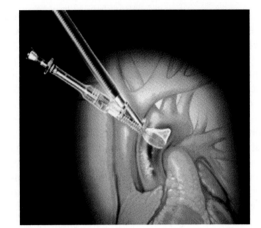

Figure 17-7 ■ The Embol-X intra-aortic filtration system (Embol-X, Mountain View, Calif). (*From Banbury MK, Kouchoukos NT, Allen KB, et al: Ann Thorac Surg 2003;76:508-515.* Copyright 2003, with permission from the *Society of Thoracic Surgeons.*)

A retrospective study of the Symmetry aortic connector device, a method for attaching saphenous vein grafts to the aorta during OPCAB surgery with less aortic manipulation, found no renal benefit relative to standard off-pump or on-pump coronary bypass surgery (see Procedure Planning, earlier).[89]

Selection of Antifibrinolytic Agent. Intraoperative use of serine protease inhibitors (e.g., aprotinin) or lysine analog antifibrinolytic agents (e.g., tranexamic acid, epsilon-aminocaproic acid) is associated with reduced bleeding and transfusion,[141,142] but questions have been raised regarding the renal safety of these agents.[143] Both groups of drugs are filtered by the kidney and saturate brush border binding sites of the low-molecular-weight protein transport system in the proximal renal tubule.[144,145] Saturation by these agents prevents the transport system from processing other small proteins, which pass on into the urine, causing tubular proteinuria, which is presumed to be benign. This phenomenon has confused study of the safety of antifibrinolytic agents, because in other settings, impaired protein reuptake is used as evidence of subtle renal injury.[145] Unreliable markers when antifibrinolytic agents are being used include urine α_1- and β_2-microglobulin, albumin, retinol-binding protein, lysozyme, ribonuclease, IgG, transferrin, ceruloplasmin, light chains (lambda and kappa types), and total protein levels (see Table 17-1). Cardiac surgery studies that use tubular proteinuria as a marker of renal injury without accounting for antifibrinolytic use should be cautiously interpreted for this reason.

Several studies have looked for clinical effects of antifibrinolytic agents on postoperative renal outcome. A meta-analysis of 3003 CABG surgery patients from 17 double-blind, randomized, controlled trials who received either aprotinin or placebo found no difference in mortality or the incidence of renal failure (aprotinin, 1.48%; placebo, 1.28%; relative risk, 1.01; 95% confidence interval, 0.55-1.83).[141] Interestingly, in a retrospective analysis of 1209 cardiac surgery patients with normal baseline renal function, Kincaid and colleagues found that the combination of intraoperative aprotinin with the preoperative ACE inhibitor was predictive of acute renal failure (>0.5 mg/dL postoperative creatinine rise), whereas either of these agents alone was not.[127] A single retrospective study of 1334 aortocoronary bypass patients found no change in the incidence of postoperative acute renal dysfunction during the introduction of epsilon-aminocaproic acid at one institution.[146]

Selection of Vasoactive Agents

In addition to the indirect hemodynamic, humoral, and autonomic effects that typically influence intraoperative renal blood flow,[147,148] use of vasoactive agents may have important additional direct effects on kidney perfusion. Several retrospective studies have identified the use of inotropic agents as a predictor of post–cardiac surgery nephropathy, independent of other markers of poor perfusion[12,17,21]; however, the differences between vasoactive agents have not been studied.

Adrenergic receptor–mediated drug effects are a mainstay in the armamentarium of agents available to the anesthesiologist. In animal models, long-lasting severe renal vasoconstriction and reductions in glomerular filtration result from brief high-dose infusions of norepinephrine.[149,150] In similar experiments, alpha-1-mediated catecholamine effects also raise the minimum pressure at which autoregulation of renal perfusion occurs by 21 to 30 mm Hg.[151] These consequences of norepinephrine appear to be relevant to human physiology[152] and may partially explain the clinical observation that renal blood flow at typical CPB perfusion pressures is not autoregulated.[113] However, in animal models of sepsis, norepinephrine increases both global and medullary renal blood flow.[153] The potential for renoprotection from alpha-1-adrenergic antagonists, such as phenoxybenzamine and phentolamine, has not been examined. Although perioperative β-adrenergic blockade has been associated with improved outcomes, a prospective study of 99 CABG surgery patients randomized to receive pre-CPB placebo or intravenous metoprolol in dosages of 10, 20, or 30 mg did not find a renoprotective benefit from intraoperative beta-blocker therapy.[154] Other catecholamine-mediated renal effects include vasodilation through low-dose dopaminergic and alpha-2-adrenergic agonist effects (see Dopamine, and Alpha-2-Adrenergic Agonist Agents, later).

Arginine vasopressin (also called antidiuretic hormone), a peptide secreted by the posterior pituitary that is increasingly being used to treat vasodilatory hypotension, has widespread effects mediated by V_1 and V_2 receptors.[155,156] Low-dose vasopressin activates baroreceptor reflexes, which explains why this agent is clinically useful when baroreceptor reflexes are impaired such as during septic shock. Higher doses activate vascular smooth muscle V_{1a} receptors that mediate direct vasoconstrictor effects and increase systemic vascular resistance. In animal models of septic shock, vasopressin increases perfusion pressure while preserving renal blood flow.[157] Vasopressin has not been evaluated in the perioperative period. In a case series of 50 patients with severe septic shock who were given vasopressin, Holmes and colleagues[155] noted a 79% increase in urine output, an effect that lasted for at least 48 hours after the infusion was initiated. Although these authors suggested a renal benefit from vasopressin, no assessment of changes in renal filtration was undertaken in this study, and 85% of the patients died. In a small double-blind trial, 24 patients with septic shock were randomized to a 4-hour infusion of either norepinephrine or low-dose vasopressin, and open-label norepinephrine was available to both groups to maintain blood pressure.[158] Urine output increased substantially in the vasopressin group but was unchanged in the norepinephrine group. Similarly, creatinine clearance was increased by 75% in the vasopressin group but did not change in the norepinephrine group (Fig. 17-8) (*P* < .05). The authors concluded that in patients with severe septic shock, short-term vasopressin infusion improved renal function and spared conventional vasopressor use. Some speculate that vasopressin may be a useful renoprotective agent and a preferable selection over conventional catecholamines for the treatment of vasodilatory shock.[155] Although vasopressin demonstrates favorable preliminary evidence, randomized trials are essential to evaluate this agent as a perioperative therapy.

Other vasoconstrictor agents have been less studied for their relationship to postoperative renal impairment. A small study randomized 20 patients who were taking preoperative ACE inhibitor agents to receive either phenylephrine or angiotensin II for the control of systemic vascular resistance during and for 24 hours after cardiac surgery.[159] These authors observed no postoperative renal impairment and concluded that angiotensin II is a safe alternative to phenylephrine in these patients.

Milrinone and enoximone are phosphodiesterase III inhibitors with positive inotropic and vasodilatory effects. Although no studies have compared these agents with other vasoactive drugs, a small number of studies have addressed their renal effects and provide conflicting conclusions. In an animal model, milrinone exacerbates endotoxin-induced renal failure,[160] and anecdotal cases of renal dysfunction and failure in humans have been associated with the use of milrinone.[161,162] In a randomized study of 40 CABG surgery patients receiving enoximone or placebo, Boldt and colleagues noted a significant rise in urinary alpha-1-microglobulin in controls, compared with the enoximone group.[162] In a similar study of 42 CABG surgery patients, Boldt and colleagues observed a postoperative rise in urinary *N*-acetyl-β-D-glucosaminidase in control patients compared with those receiving enoximone combined with an infusion of the beta-adrenergic blocker esmolol.[163] Currently, the data are insufficient to characterize the renal effects of phosphodiesterase III inhibitors.

Postoperative Management

Many issues related to postoperative renoprotection resemble those of the intraoperative period (e.g., intravenous fluid and inotrope selection). In addition, some of the pharmacologic interventions evaluated for renoprotection are continued for an extended period as part of postoperative care. Notably, the renoprotective benefits of insulin have been most convincingly demonstrated in the postoperative period (see Insulin, later).

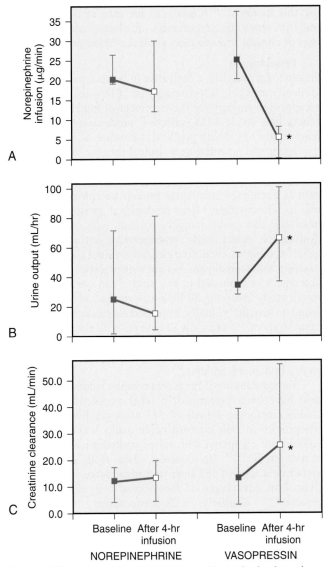

Figure 17-8 ■ In a study of 24 patients with septic shock randomized to a 4-hour infusion of either norepinephrine or low-dose vasopressin, open-label norepinephrine was available to maintain blood pressure. Findings included reduced need for conventional vasopressor use **(A)** ($P < .001$), more than a doubling in urine output **(B)** ($P < .001$), and a 75% increase in creatinine clearance **(C)** ($P < .01$) in the vasopressin group. *Error bars* indicate the range from the 25th to 75th percentile. *(Adapted from Patel BM, Chittock DR, Russell JA, Walley KR: Anesthesiology 2002;96:576-582.)*

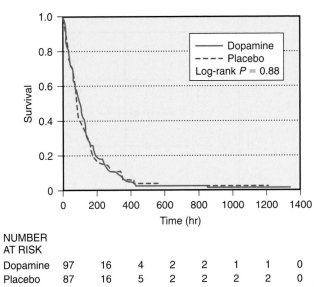

Figure 17-9 ■ Kaplan-Meier curve of time to recovery of normal renal function in 328 critically ill patients with mild renal dysfunction randomized to receive either low-dose dopamine or placebo. *(Redrawn from Bellomo R, Chapman M, Finfer S, et al: Lancet 2000;356:2139-2143. Copyright 2000, with permission from Elsevier.)*

Pharmacologic Interventions

DA₁ Agonist Agents

Dopamine

The controversial issues surrounding dopamine and renal preservation highlight the importance of careful evaluation of a therapy before widespread adoption occurs. Dopamine infusion at rates less than 5 µg/kg/min selectively stimulates mesenteric dopamine-1 (DA₁) receptors, causing increased renal blood flow, decreased renal vascular resistance, natriuresis, and diuresis. Although animal studies 40 years ago promoted the renoprotective potential of dopamine,[165] numerous randomized studies in many different surgical and nonsurgical settings have not substantiated this claim (Fig. 17-9).[166] Meta-analyses of randomized trials have also failed to support dopamine as a renoprotective agent (Fig. 17-10).[167-169] In a recent meta-analysis of 61 trials including 3359 patients randomized to low-dose dopamine versus control, Friedrich and colleagues found no benefit regarding mortality, dialysis, or adverse events.[170] Interestingly, on day 1 after dopamine initiation, these authors noted statistically significant but *clinically insignificant* effects that disappeared by days 2 and 3, including a 24% increase in urine output, a 4% reduction in serum creatinine, and a 6% increase in creatinine clearance. These authors concluded that low-dose dopamine provides small, brief improvements in renal physiology but with no evidence of clinical benefits to patients with or at risk for acute renal failure.

Despite an overwhelming number of negative clinical trials, the use of dopamine for renoprotection remains controversial.[171,172] A growing number of strongly worded editorials and reviews discourages the use of dopamine for renoprotection. Articles entitled "Bad Medicine: Low-Dose

The disposition and management of patients may influence the likelihood of postoperative renal dysfunction. In a large 4-year database analysis, fast-track recovery protocols introduced at three of 30 cardiac surgery centers were associated with an increased incidence of moderate and severe renal failure in patients at high renal risk[164]; when high-risk patients were returned from the fast-track to standard recovery protocols, rates of renal failure returned to normal levels.

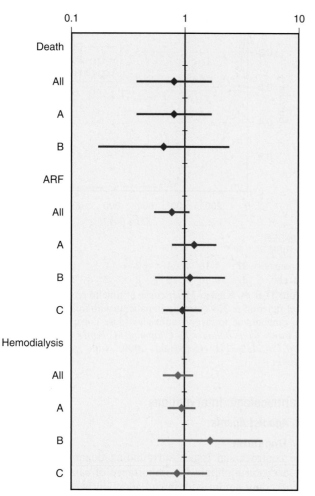

Figure 17-10 ■ Forrest plot showing relative risks *(diamonds)* and 95% confidence intervals *(lines)* of acute renal failure, need for dialysis, and mortality in a meta-analysis of 58 studies published between 1996 and 2000, including 2149 patients randomized to receive either low-dose dopamine or placebo, and for subgroups A, B, and C. Subgroup A excluded studies using radiocontrast dye (661 patients, 14 studies). Subgroup B was limited to heart disease (271 patients, 4 studies). Subgroup C excluded statistical outliers in terms of either control group event rate or the effect size for each outcome as determined by analysis of variance. ARF, acute renal failure. (*Redrawn from Kellum JA, Decker J: Crit Care Med 2001;29:1526-1531.* Copyright 2001, American Medical Association. All rights reserved.)

Dopamine in the ICU"[173] and "Renal-Dose Dopamine: From Hypothesis to Paradigm to Dogma to Myth and, Finally, Superstition?"[174] are not subtle in displaying the opinions of their authors. These articles highlight the numerous negative studies and list undesirable consequences of low-dose dopamine, including worsened splanchnic oxygenation, impaired gastrointestinal function, impaired endocrine and immunologic system function, blunting of ventilatory drive, and increased risk of post–cardiac surgery atrial fibrillation.[173,175] However, dopamine use to treat renal dysfunction or oliguria is still prevalent; for example, 18 of 19 pediatric and neonatal ICUs in The Netherlands and 17 of 24 New Zealand ICUs use this therapy.[169,176] Clearly, in the case of dopamine and renal preservation, practitioners are slow to apply the findings of clinical trials to their evidence-based practice.

Fenoldopam

Fenoldopam mesylate, a derivative of benzazepine, is the first clinically available selective agonist of DA_1 receptors and is an approved therapy for the treatment of hypertension.[177,178] Much like its less-DA_1-selective predecessor, dopamine, fenoldopam has shown preclinical promise as a renoprotective agent and potential as a clinical therapy.[179] Preliminary case series in humans suggested renal benefit.[180] However, the three randomized controlled studies evaluating fenoldopam as a renoprotective agent provide no consensus regarding its effectiveness. One randomized prospective study involving 160 cardiac surgery patients with baseline renal dysfunction noted lower postoperative serum creatinine values and higher creatinine clearance values compared with baseline with fenoldopam, but not with placebo; no long-term outcome was evaluated in this study.[181] In contrast, a more recent study involving 80 high-risk cardiac surgery patients found no benefit.[182] Finally, a prospective randomized double-blind study of 155 critically ill patients with established renal injury (including post–cardiac surgery patients) found no benefit and even discussed possible increased adverse outcomes in diabetic patients.[183,184]

Some randomized renal preservation studies of fenoldopam have been performed in other populations. In three studies, including a total of 533 angiography patients, no renoprotection from contrast nephropathy was evident with fenoldopam compared with saline prehydration alone or N-acetylcysteine.[185-187] In contrast, data from two studies, including a total of 183 liver transplant surgeries, identified short-term advantages of fenoldopam over dopamine and placebo.[188,189] Similarly, in 28 aortic surgery patients, Halpenny and colleagues found a decline in creatinine clearance with aortic cross-clamp application and higher postoperative day 1 serum creatinine values in patients receiving placebo, but not in the fenoldopam group.[190] Overall, current studies provide insufficient data to draw conclusions on the clinical potential of fenoldopam as a renal preservation therapy.

Dopexamine

Dopexamine hydrochloride is a DA_1 receptor and beta-2-adrenoceptor agonist with renal vasodilatory, natriuretic, and diuretic effects that has shown promise in animal studies as a renoprotective agent.[191,192] A notable property of dopexamine is that its metabolism is significantly reduced in the presence of impaired liver function.[193] In a study of 44 CABG surgery patients randomized to three different infusion dosages of dopexamine or placebo, Berendes and colleagues noted improved systemic oxygen delivery, increased postoperative creatinine clearance, and reductions in markers of perioperative inflammatory response with dopexamine.[194] In contrast, in a study of CABG surgery patients with normal ($n = 24$) or impaired ($n = 24$) baseline renal function randomized to dopexamine or placebo, Dehne and colleagues found no evidence of renal protection.[195] In a randomized comparison of dopexamine with dopamine in 24 liver transplant patients, Gray and colleagues found a trend toward better renal function with dopamine but no overall outcome difference between the two therapies.[196] A systematic review of 21 randomized controlled trials involving dopamine by Renton and colleagues concluded that existing evidence is inconsistent and insufficient to recommend dopamine for renoprotection for either high-risk surgical or critically ill patients.[197]

Diuretic Agents

Diuretic agents increase urine generation by reducing reuptake of tubular contents. This can be achieved by numerous mechanisms, including blocking tubular solute reuptake through active transport mechanisms (e.g., loop diuretics), by altering the tubular osmotic gradient to favor solute remaining in the tubule (e.g., mannitol), or by affecting the hormonal signaling to the tubule to increase urine generation (e.g., atrial natriuretic peptide [ANP]). In general, the rationale underlying renoprotection from diuretic agents relates to the decreased likelihood of tubular obstruction by casts, with increased solute flow through injured renal tubules, thus retaining tubular patency and avoiding oliguria or anuria and the need for dialysis. Importantly, despite the clinician's satisfaction at seeing the urine bag fill, the increased urine volume from diuretics does not ensure improved renal function (see Fig. 17-5).[71] Of note, some diuretic agents have added properties that contribute to the rationale for their renoprotective potential (e.g., loop diuretics—reduced tubular oxygen consumption, antioxidant effect). The classes of diuretics are discussed next.

Loop Diuretics

Loop diuretics, also called loop inhibitors because of their mechanism of action, and including furosemide, ethacrynic acid, and bumetanide, inhibit active solute reabsorption in the mTAL of the loop of Henle, causing more solute to remain in the renal tubule and increasing urine generation. Furosemide also induces renal cortical vasodilation. In animal models, administration of furosemide raises oxygen levels in the renal medulla[198] and protects renal tubules from damage after ischemia-reperfusion or nephrotoxic insult.[199-201]

Numerous retrospective renal preservation studies have associated no renal benefit and even harm with loop diuretic use in surgical and critically ill patients.[202-204] In a retrospective multivariable analysis of 50 cardiac surgery patients with normal baseline renal function, furosemide during surgery (dose normalized to body surface area) was highly predictive of postoperative renal dysfunction.[205] In a retrospective study that evaluated 552 critically ill patients with acute renal failure at the time of nephrology consultation, diuretics were given to 59% of patients and were highly associated with an increased risk of death and nonrecovery of renal function (Fig. 17-11).[206] In contrast, Uchino and colleagues recently published a prospective analysis in which 1743 patients with a diagnosis of acute renal failure and/or receiving renal replacement therapy were evaluated for the relationship of diuretic use with mortality[207]; approximately 70% received diuretics (98.3%, furosemide). In this study, multivariable analyses failed to demonstrate a relationship between diuretic use and death.

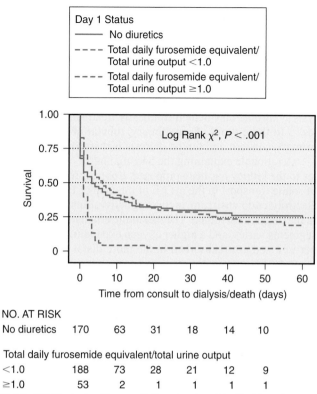

NO. AT RISK

No diuretics	170	63	31	18	14	10

Total daily furosemide equivalent/total urine output

<1.0	188	73	28	21	12	9
≥1.0	53	2	1	1	1	1

Figure 17-11 ■ Avoidance of diuretics in critically ill patients at the time of nephrology consultation is associated with improved avoidance of dialysis and survival. Patients receiving diuretics were grouped by diuretic responsiveness, with responsiveness defined by an index of furosemide dose equivalent per milliliter per day of urine output; a ratio of less than 1.0 on day 1 was a priori selected to reflect diuretic responsiveness. *(Redrawn from Mehta R, Pascual M, Soroko S, et al: JAMA 2002;288:2547-2553.)*

Several randomized trials have investigated the renoprotective effects of loop diuretics. In a randomized study of 121 patients undergoing major thoracoabdominal or vascular surgery procedures, Hager and colleagues found no renoprotective benefit of an extended postoperative furosemide infusion compared with placebo.[202] Notably, another double-blind, randomized, controlled trial comparing infusions of low-dose dopamine, furosemide, and placebo in 126 cardiac surgery patients found a twofold greater postoperative rise in serum creatinine in the group receiving furosemide than in the dopamine and placebo groups.[208] In addition, more patients receiving furosemide in this study reached a threshold for acute renal injury. These authors concluded that furosemide was detrimental to renal function. Finally, in a prospective three-group study of 78 angiography patients with chronic renal dysfunction, randomized to prehydration alone or with furosemide or mannitol, Solomon and colleagues found a higher rate of contrast nephropathy in the mannitol group (11% versus 28%) and the highest rate in the furosemide group (40%; P = .05).[209] These authors concluded that 0.45% saline provided better protection against contrast nephropathy than hydration plus mannitol or furosemide. In sum, the evidence does not support the use of loop diuretics as perioperative renoprotective agents and suggests these agents may have nephrotoxic effects.

Notably, although loop diuretics have not demonstrated renoprotective benefit in studies of cardiac surgery and critically ill patients, disorders with myoglobinuric or hemoglobinuric renal injury or other urinary excreted toxins or drugs (e.g., lithium, theophylline, salicylates) and cases of tumor lysis syndrome may benefit from early treatment with diuretics.[210] In these types of renal injury, tubular obstruction is a primary concern and forced diuresis is therapeutic.

A rationale explaining the potential harm of loop diuretics to the kidney has been proposed. Loop diuretic inhibition of solute transport in the mTAL of the loop of Henle delivers electrolytes downstream, increasing active transport demands in the distal renal tubule. The metabolic efficiency of nephron segments varies, and a higher oxygen expenditure is required per unit sodium reabsorbed in the more distal nephron segments.[211] Thus, loop diuretics may spare injury to the loop of Henle at the expense of subjecting the metabolically less efficient distal renal tubule to added oxygen demand. Confirming the increased distal tubular demands from loop diuretic use are rat studies showing that chronic administration of furosemide results in hypertrophied distal tubular cells with increased numbers of mitochondria.[212] Thus, it is possible that loop diuretics displace injury from the loop of Henle to more distal tubular locations.

Mannitol

Mannitol is an osmotic diuretic with renoprotective potential in animal models[213-216] and effects that include augmentation of renal blood flow[217,218] and increased glomerular filtration rate.[213,215] However, in an animal model of thoracic aortic clamping, mannitol does not provide evidence of improved renal function after de-clamping.[219] In humans, mannitol is commonly used to prime the CPB circuit during cardiac surgery procedures.[220,221] Although several studies have confirmed increased urine output in cardiac surgical patients during the period after mannitol administration,[222,223] very few have carefully assessed postoperative renal dysfunction in these patients. Ip-Yam and colleagues found no benefit of mannitol (0.5 g/kg) during CPB in a randomized study of 23 patients.[132] Carcoana and coworkers also found no benefit of mannitol (1 g/kg) in another randomized study of 100 CABG surgery patients.[180] A third study involving 30 suprarenal and infrarenal aortic surgeries with cross-clamping also found no benefit of mannitol.[224] Finally, Solomon and colleagues found hydration alone (0.45% saline) to be better protection from contrast nephropathy than hydration plus mannitol therapy.[209]

In addition to the lack of beneficial effects on the kidney, inappropriately high dosing of mannitol has nephrotoxic potential, particularly in patients with renal insufficiency.[225] For example, in a randomized study comparing mannitol with placebo in 30 patients with obstructive jaundice, patients receiving mannitol were more likely to have a fall in creatinine clearance.[226] In the absence of large randomized clinical trials, there is insufficient evidence to support the perioperative use of mannitol for renal preservation, except when a significant benefit of forced diuresis is suspected.

Natriuretic Peptides

The natriuretic peptides are hormones that interact with a specific signal transmission system involved in the regulation of volume homeostasis. In response to volume expansion, the release of these hormones is associated with receptor-mediated vasodilation and natriuresis. Assay of B-type natriuretic peptide (BNP) levels has become a diagnostic tool for congestive heart failure. Three natriuretic peptides have been evaluated in human trials: atrial natriuretic peptide (ANP, anaritide), urodilatin (ularitide), and BNP (nesiritide); however, several other less-studied natriuretic peptides also exist.[227]

ANP is normally synthesized by the atria in response to atrial wall tension; anaritide is the human recombinant form of ANP. ANP increases glomerular filtration and urinary output by constricting efferent while dilating afferent arterioles, and it is associated with attenuation of renal cellular injury in animal models of acute renal injury.[228] Unfortunately, human trials of ANP as a renoprotective agent have not been conclusive. In a multicenter randomized double-blind, placebo-controlled clinical trial of ANP as a 24-hour intravenous infusion (0.2 µg/kg/min) in 504 critically ill patients with established acute renal injury, the primary endpoint of improved dialysis-free survival after 21 days was not achieved (47% versus 43%, placebo versus ANP group, $P = .35$).[229] A secondary analysis revealed that dialysis-free survival was higher in the ANP group for oliguric patients (8% versus 27%, $P = .008$). Conversely, in nonoliguric patients, dialysis-free survival was higher in the placebo group (59% versus 48%, $P = .03$). Some have speculated that the disparity of outcomes in this study is caused by the vasodilating properties of ANP; hypotension was more frequent in the nonoliguric patients and may have overwhelmed any renoprotective benefit. However, a similar study designed to reproduce the favorable findings from the first study in 222 critically ill patients with established oliguric renal dysfunction did not find any benefit.[230]

Urodilatin, also known as renal natriuretic peptide, differs from ANP only by the addition of four amino acids to the N-terminus end of the peptide, but it has more potent natriuretic properties. Three small randomized trials indicate renoprotective benefit from this agent in patients with established renal dysfunction, including reduced duration of hemofiltration and frequency of hemodialysis following heart transplant ($n = 24$) and reduced incidence of dialysis after cardiac ($n = 14$) and liver transplant ($n = 9$) surgery.[231-233] However, interpretation of these data is complicated by very high (up to 86% in the control group) dialysis rates. A larger randomized, double-blind trial including 176 critically ill patients with oliguric acute renal failure did not demonstrate a benefit from any of four different urodilatin dosage regimens compared with placebo.[234]

BNP is normally synthesized by the left and right ventricles in response to ventricular dilatation; nesiritide is the human recombinant form of BNP. Nesiritide has potent vasodilating properties and is approved by the U.S. Food and Drug Administration as a treatment for acutely decompensated heart failure, in part because of its ability to rapidly reduce ventricular filling pressures, relieve dyspnea, and induce a sustained diuresis. Although there is interest in evaluating this agent in post–cardiac surgery patients with heart failure as a therapy that may have renal benefit,[235] no randomized data are currently available. Of note, recent publications have indicated that BNP treatment may worsen renal function in heart failure patients.[236,237]

Steroids, Aspirin, Nonsteroidal Anti-Inflammatory Drugs, and Cyclooxygenase-2 Inhibitors

The known propensity of corticosteroids to attenuate the inflammatory response and their renoprotective effects in animal models[238] constitute the rationale for the evaluation of these drugs as renoprotective agents. In a small, randomized, placebo-controlled, double-blind trial of 20 patients undergoing cardiac surgery with cardiopulmonary bypass, Loef and associates found no evidence of renoprotection in patients receiving dexamethasone 1 mg/kg before induction of anesthesia and 0.5 mg/kg 8 hours later.[239] In contrast, whereas there is little evidence or rationale for the use of NSAIDs for renoprotection, in a retrospective study of 5065 coronary artery bypass surgery patients, Mangano reported that early (<48-hour) reinstitution of aspirin therapy after surgery was associated with a threefold reduction in mortality (1.3% versus 4.0%, $P < .001$) and a 74% reduction in the incidence of renal failure (0.9% versus 3.4%, $P < .001$).[240] A review by Lee and collagues reported the combined findings from randomized controlled postoperative NSAID analgesia trials that recorded renal function, including more than 1200 patients receiving ketorolac, diclofenac, indomethacin, or placebo.[241] These authors noted a 16-mL/min decline in creatinine clearance and a reduction in potassium clearance in NSAID patients at 24 hours after surgery, but no episodes of acute renal failure requiring dialysis. Lee and colleagues concluded that postoperative NSAID analgesia has only small temporary negative effects on renal function in adults with normal kidneys at baseline, stressing that these findings may not apply to children or to adults with already impaired renal function. Although similar analyses have not been performed for cyclooxygenase (COX)-2-selective NSAIDs, a greater incidence of serious adverse events in patients receiving valdecoxib/parecoxib, including a trend toward more postoperative renal dysfunction, was reported in a randomized, double-blind, placebo-controlled postoperative analgesia trial involving 462 coronary bypass surgery patients[242]; the interim findings from this trial prompted the investigators to terminate the study for safety reasons. A similar randomized trial including 1671 CABG patients or placebo also noted increased adverse outcomes, in particular an increase in cardiovascular events in patients receiving valdecoxib/parecoxib.[243] The incidence of renal failure or dysfunction in this study was insignificantly higher in the valdecoxib/parecoxib groups than in the placebo group (0.5% versus 1.0%, $P = .32$).

Insulin

The burden of added renal glucose reabsorption from hyperglycemia may contribute significantly to perioperative renal stress. Filtered glucose is mainly reabsorbed in the proximal renal tubule via energy-consuming processes, including the phlorizin-sensitive Na^+/glucose cotransporter.[244] In rats, oxygen consumption is 32% greater in the proximal tubules of diabetic than in nondiabetic animals.[245] In a rat renal ischemia-reperfusion model, diabetic kidneys treated with insulin are protected, but untreated or post-insult treated kidneys sustain significant short- and long-term renal injuries.[246]

Clinical studies indicate that meticulous perioperative glucose management may be one of the most important and effective renal preservation strategies. Several large retrospective studies have associated high preoperative or intraoperative serum glucose values with increased post–cardiac surgery mortality and renal dysfunction, even after adjusting for a history of diabetes.[13,125,247,248] Gandhi and colleagues calculated the average of all intraoperative glucose levels for each of 409 cardiac surgery patients[249]; mean glucose was 126 mg/dL at the start of surgery and peaked at 176 mg/dL after CPB. These authors found that mean glucose levels were significantly higher ($P < .01$) in patients who subsequently met the Society of Thoracic Surgeons definition for acute renal failure; patients with or without diabetes shared the same trend. Ouattra and colleagues recorded glucose values and insulin requirements for 200 cardiac surgery procedures in diabetic patients managed with a dose of intermediate-acting insulin on the morning of the surgery and intraoperatively with a fast-acting insulin protocol and glucose measurements every 30 minutes, which maintained a value between 150 and 200 mg/dL.[250] Poor intraoperative glycemic control was defined as four consecutive values of greater than 200 mg/dL despite the insulin therapy according to the protocol, without any decrease until the end of the surgical procedure. Subjects with poor glycemic control were significantly more likely to require dialysis (15% versus 2%; $P < .05$).

Although no perioperative randomized trials in humans have assessed insulin as a renal protective agent, the van den Berghe study included 1548 critically ill patients (>75% of whom were post-major surgery) randomized to intensive or conventional insulin therapy; this study found that improved glucose management resulted in improved survival and better renal outcome.[57] Compared with conventional therapy (target glucose, 180 to 200 mg/dL), intensive insulin therapy (target in ICU, 80 to 110; after ICU, 180 to 200 mg/dL) was associated with lower peak serum creatinine and urea values, a 41% reduction in the need for renal replacement therapy ($P = .007$), and a 34% lower in-hospital mortality rate ($P = .01$) (Fig. 17-12). Analysis indicated that better metabolic control, rather than insulin dose per se, explained the beneficial effects. Notably, beyond glucose control, effects such as improved immune function, suppression of inflammation, better macrophage function, and normalization of dyslipidemia are attributed as clinical benefits of intensive insulin therapy on renal dysfunction, renal failure, and death.[251,252]

Intraoperative strategies to control serum glucose more tightly are being sought. In an interesting study, Visser and colleagues evaluated an infusion regimen of glucose, insulin, and potassium with aggressive serum glucose monitoring, which they termed a "perioperative hyperinsulinemic

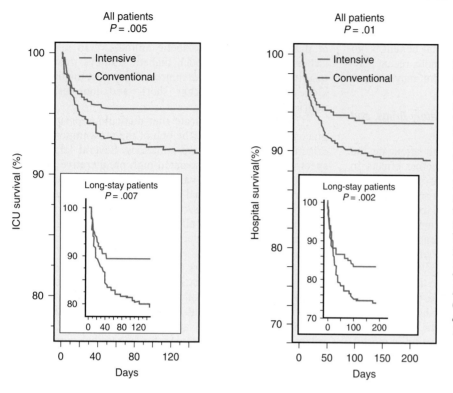

Figure 17-12 ■ The severity of "diabetes of stress" reflects the risk of adverse renal outcome and death. Intensive insulin therapy reduces peak serum creatinine and urea values, the need for renal replacement therapy, and mortality in the intensive care unit (ICU). Kaplan-Meier curves from the van den Berghe study[57] show cumulative survival of 1548 ICU patients (>75% of whom had had major surgery) who received intensive insulin treatment (blood glucose maintained below 110 mg/dL) or conventional insulin treatment (insulin given only when blood glucose exceeded 200 mg/dL, resulting in mean blood glucose levels of 150 to 160 mg/dL) during their ICU or hospital stay. The *upper panels* depict all patients; the *lower panels* depict the subset of long-stay (>5 days) ICU patients. *(Redrawn from van den Berghe G: J Clin Invest 2004;114: 1187-1195.)*

normoglycemic clamp."[253] In this randomized study of 21 nondiabetic CABG surgery patients, these authors noted that compared with standard practice, this proactive approach to serum glucose management was associated with much less perioperative hyperglycemia than is seen with a standard regimen, without the risk of hypoglycemia. In addition, markers of systemic inflammatory response were significantly reduced in the clamp group.

N-*Acetylcysteine*

N-acetylcysteine has antioxidant properties, is a vasodilator, enhances the endogenous glutathione scavenging system, and in animals counteracts renal ischemia and hypoxia. Numerous studies have evaluated its value as a protective agent against contrast nephropathy after radiologic and cardiac angiography procedures. Complicating the interpretation of these studies is recent evidence that *N*-acetylcysteine may have an effect on circulating serum creatinine levels independent of any effects on renal function.[254] Two recent meta-analyses of randomized controlled contrast nephropathy trials of patients receiving *N*-acetylcysteine or placebo concluded that the renoprotective findings were too inconsistent.[255,256] A meta-analysis of studies of patients with baseline renal dysfunction found that *N*-acetylcysteine reduced the risk for contrast nephropathy.[257]

Fewer studies are available that evaluate the role of *N*-acetylcysteine as a renoprotective agent in surgical patients. A study comparing it to mannitol or placebo in 30 abdominal aortic surgery patients suggests benefit.[258] However, a prospective, double-blind, placebo-controlled investigation comparing *N*-acetylcysteine to placebo in 128 cardiac surgery

patients does not demonstrate benefit.[259] In the largest study to date, Burns and colleagues randomized 295 high renal risk CABG surgery patients to receive either four doses of intravenous *N*-acetylcysteine (600 mg) during the perioperative period or placebo.[260] In this quadruple-blinded study, these authors found no evidence of reduced postoperative renal dysfunction, interventions, complications, or mortality.

Alpha-2-Adrenergic Agonist Agents

The normal physiology of the kidney includes a role of adrenergic receptors in modulating vasoconstrictor (alpha-1) and vasodilating (alpha-2) effects. Vasoconstriction contributes to the pathophysiology of acute renal injury, and several studies confirm that clonidine (an alpha-2 agonist) attenuates experimental acute renal injury.[261-265] In animals, clonidine inhibits renin release and causes a water diuresis.[261] A double-blind, randomized, placebo-controlled trial evaluating preoperative clonidine for renal preservation in 48 CABG surgery patients found a significant benefit on the first postoperative day ($P < .05$) but not 3 days after surgery[266]; creatinine clearance was unchanged in treated patients (90 ± 19 preoperative versus 92 ± 17 mL/min) but decreased in those receiving placebo (98 ± 18 preoperative versus 68 ± 19 mL/min postoperative). A second double-blind randomized trial including 156 CABG surgery patients, but not specifically studying renal outcome, supports the finding of higher creatinine clearance values in patients receiving clonidine.[267] In addition, a meta-analysis of 23 randomized studies including 3395 patients receiving perioperative alpha-2 agonists (clonidine, dexmedetomidine, or mivazerol) identified a survival benefit with these agents compared with control.[268] Despite supportive evidence for improved postoperative renal performance and survival benefit with alpha-2 agonists, insufficient data are available to recommend these agents, and currently they are not commonly used for renoprotection.

Calcium Channel Blockers

Three major classes of calcium antagonists exist with varying pharmacologic properties: benzothiazepines (e.g., diltiazem), phenylalkylamines (e.g., verapamil), and dihydropyridines (e.g., nifedipine, nimodipine). Calcium channel blockers decrease renal vascular resistance and increase glomerular filtration[269] and have been reported to exert beneficial effects in experimental models of toxic and ischemic acute renal failure.[270,271] In a three-group study of 35 cardiac surgery patients randomized to 36-hour perioperative diltiazem infusions at 1 mg/kg/min, 2 mg/kg/min, or control, glomerular filtration rate was higher in the high-dose diltiazem group compared with control, but tubular function was not influenced.[272] A similar 24-patient study involving a 24-hour perioperative diltiazem infusion in subjects with elevated baseline serum creatinine found no differences in postoperative serum creatinine levels (days 1, 3, and 5, and 3 weeks).[273] In the same study, iohexol clearance did not differ on day 5 but was higher in the diltiazem group 3 weeks after surgery. Finally, another randomized cardiac surgery study of 20 patients receiving nifedipine (0.24 to 0.59 μg/kg/min) or urapidil (5 mg) to maintain the mean systemic arterial pressure during CPB between 60 and 70 mm Hg found that creatinine clearance and glomerular filtration rate increased after CPB ($P < .001$) and postoperatively ($P < .01$) in the nifedipine group, whereas the two parameters showed small nonsignificant reductions in the urapidil patients.[274] A recent meta-analysis of randomized cardiac surgery studies comparing perioperative use of calcium channel antagonist agents with control or other agents (e.g., nitroglycerin, dopamine) included five reports that documented baseline and postoperative creatinine clearance.[275] These studies involved 161 patients and four agents (diltiazem,[273,276] verapamil,[277] nifedipine,[274,278] and nimodipine[275]). There was no overall effect, but post hoc analysis identified benefit if preoperative creatinine clearance was less than 95 mL/min (13.12 mL/min increase, $P < .001$) but nonsignificant worsening if preoperative creatinine clearance was greater than 95 mL/min (5.03 mL/min decrease, $P = .18$). Separate meta-analyses of postoperative mortality in cardiac and non–cardiac surgery studies did not show a survival benefit of calcium channel blockers.[275,279] The overall inconclusive findings from calcium antagonist blocker trials do not support the use of these agents for renal preservation.

Angiotensin-Converting Enzyme Inhibitor and Angiotensin I Receptor Blocker Agents

The renin-angiotensin system mediates vasoconstriction and contributes to the paracrine regulation of the renal microcirculation. Angiotensin I blocker and ACE inhibitor agents act by decreasing activation of the renin-angiotensin system, and animal studies suggest that these agents may have protective properties in experimental acute renal injury.[280] Although both drug classes are recognized for their ability to slow the progression of chronic renal disease,[281] their role in the clinical prevention of acute renal injury is unclear. Pertinent to the renal effects of these agents is their disconcerting vulnerability to precipitate acute renal deterioration when renin-angiotensin system activation is critical to the regulation of renal filtration, as occurs with renal artery stenosis or volume depletion (see Preoperative Management, earlier).[95,96] These agents can precipitate hemodynamic instability when initiated soon after cardiac surgery.[282] Two retrospective studies have not found perioperative ACE inhibitor therapy to be an independent predictor of renal outcome after cardiac surgery.[77,283] However, in a study of 249 aortic surgery patients, Cittanova and colleagues reported an increased risk of postoperative renal dysfunction in patients receiving chronic ACE inhibitor therapy.[97] Also, in a retrospective review of 23 heart transplant recipients receiving cyclosporine, severe renal dysfunction within 2 weeks of surgery was associated with the use of captopril.[284] In contrast, a clinical trial in 18 CABG surgery patients noted decreases in renal plasma flow and glomerular filtration rate during CPB in a placebo group but not with captopril.[285] A similar study assessing 48 hours of perioperative enalaprilat therapy in 14 CABG surgery patients noted increased renal plasma flow and creatinine clearance after CPB and increased renal plasma flow on postoperative day 7 in the enalaprilat group compared with control.[286] These drugs are being assessed in combination as therapy for chronic renal disease,[287] but their use alone or combined for perioperative renal preservation is largely unexplored.

Agents in the Early Stages of Development as Renal Preservation Therapies

Numerous potentially renoprotective agents have been identified that are in the early stages of development. Some are briefly discussed here.

Adenosine Receptor Agents (Adenosine, Aminophylline, Theophylline)

Paradoxically, a rationale exists for the renoprotective potential of two types of clinically available A_1 receptor agents with opposite effects. A_1 agonists (e.g., adenosine) and A_1 antagonists (e.g., theophylline, aminophylline) have roles in mediating the ischemic preconditioning reflex and inhibition of renal vasoconstriction, respectively (see Ischemic Preconditioning Reflex, earlier). Although testing in rat models supports only the renoprotective potential of adenosine and not A_1 antagonists,[34,35,288] curiously only the latter agents have been tested in humans. In a double-blind, randomized, placebo-controlled trial in 56 CABG surgery patients with normal renal function who received either placebo or a bolus of 4 mg/kg and an infusion of 0.25 mg/kg/hr for up to 4 days postoperatively, the investigators found no evidence of renoprotective benefit from theophylline, although they acknowledged the limitations of such a small study. A second study in 60 coronary angioplasty patients with baseline renal insufficiency receiving hydration starting 2 hours before the procedure with or without aminophylline (4 mg/kg followed by a 0.4-mg/kg/hr infusion) also found no renoprotective benefit.[289]

Endothelin Receptor Antagonists (Bosentan, Tezosentan, Enrasentan TAK-044, SB209670, A-127722)

Endothelin is a potent vasoconstrictor that severely limits renal blood flow and may contribute to the pathophysiology of acute renal failure.[290] Two types of endothelin receptors have been identified: ET_A receptors are located on vascular smooth muscle cells and mediate endothelin-induced vasoconstriction, and ET_B receptors are on endothelial cells and mediate release of nitric oxide and prostacyclin. The development of endothelin receptor antagonists has provided the opportunity to assess the renoprotective potential of this class of drug. Animal studies indicate a protective effect of tezosentan when it is administered either before or, notably, after an ischemic acute renal injury.[291,292] Similarly, tezosentan and TAK-044 improve endotoxin-induced decreases in renal blood flow and indices of glomerular filtration.[293,294] In an animal model of acute liver and renal failure, bosentan given 24 hours after the onset of liver injury prevented the subsequent development of renal failure but had no effect on renal blood flow.[295] Some evidence suggests that renoprotective effects are mediated by ET_A-selective endothelin receptor agents (e.g., A-127722) and not nonselective A/B receptor antagonists (e.g., enrasentan, tezosentan, bosentan, TAK-044, SB209670).[296] In a contrast nephropathy trial involving 158 patients with baseline renal impairment, the nonselective endothelin receptor antagonist SB209670 not only failed to prevent but actually increased the incidence of renal dysfunction.[297]

Erythropoietin

Recombinant human erythropoietin is typically prescribed for anemia associated with cancer chemotherapy or end-stage renal failure. However, this agent also has been shown to have renal protective properties in at least nine studies in animal models of acute ischemic, hypovolemic, endotoxic, and nephrotoxic renal injury.[298] Unfortunately, little is yet known of any renoprotective properties of this agent in humans.

Growth Factors (IGF-I, EGF, HGF)

When the kidney is acutely injured, animal models indicate that growth factors are involved in tubular recovery, such as insulin-like growth factor-I (IGF-I), epidermal growth factor (EGF), and hepatocyte growth factor (HGF). Therefore, providing an exogenous source of these substances has been identified as potential renoprotective strategy. However, human studies do not support the effectiveness of this strategy. In a multicenter, randomized controlled double-blind study of 72 critically ill dialysis patients receiving recombinant human IGF-I or placebo, there was no difference in the rate of recovery of renal function or in mortality.[299] In a second study involving 44 post–renal transplant patients with established renal dysfunction receiving IGF-I or placebo, there was no difference in the return of renal function or subsequent requirement for dialysis.[300]

Omapatrilat

Omapatrilat is a vasopeptidase inhibitor that inhibits the renin-angiotensin-aldosterone system but preserves natri-uretic peptides by simultaneously inhibiting ACE and neutral endopeptidase. In animal studies, this agent reduces glomerular arteriolar resistance with increases in renal blood flow and single nephron plasma flow.[301] Other animal studies show that omapatrilat prevents or reverses nephrotoxic proteinuria and glomerular and arteriolar injury.[301] Although no renal preservation studies have been performed in humans, evaluations of omapatrilat as an antihypertensive therapy in large populations suggest that it has an acceptable safety profile.[302]

Pentoxifylline

Systemic and local inflammatory responses, mediated by inflammatory cytokines (e.g., TNFα), are believed to contribute significantly to perioperative acute renal failure. Pentoxifylline is an inhibitor of TNFα production that has a protective effect in animal models of ischemic and nephrotoxic acute renal failure.[303,304] In a randomized study of 40 older adult CABG surgery patients,[305] Boldt and colleagues noted higher urine alpha-1-microglobulin concentrations and slightly greater serum creatinine values in the untreated control patients, suggesting preserved renal tubular function.

Prostaglandin E₁

Abe and coworkers evaluated urine markers of renal tubular injury in 20 cardiac surgery patients receiving either low-dose prostaglandin E_1 (PGE₁) (0.02 µg/kg/min) or saline during CPB.[306] In this small study, perioperative serum and urine beta-2-microglobulin values were similar between groups, but postoperative urine *N*-acetyl-β-D-glucosaminidase increased more after CPB in the placebo group ($P < .05$). The authors suggest that PGE₁ may have a renoprotective effect.[306]

■ SUMMARY AND FUTURE DIRECTIONS IN RENAL PRESERVATION

Although significant work remains to improve and expand knowledge about perioperative renal protection, there is already much on which to base sound clinical renoprotective practice (Table 17-2). Some of the challenges are to ensure that available information is fully applied. Goals in disseminating available evidence include not just increasing the use of effective strategies but also eliminating ineffective practices. For example, compelling data exist to support meticulous attention to the use of insulin therapy to minimize perioperative hyperglycemia. A growing body of data also supports the avoidance of hemodilution and the minimization of transfusion during cardiopulmonary bypass. In addition, the status quo of the past 20 to 30 years has become unacceptable; few now dispute the lack of benefit from traditional agents such as low-dose dopamine, mannitol, and furosemide, and yet the use of these agents for renoprotection remains prevalent. Continued use of these agents may in fact be deleterious, even distracting the unaware from adopting other effective therapies. The ideal randomized clinical renal preservation trials of the future will avoid the pitfalls of evaluating a substance through numerous small studies that neither strongly support nor refute potential benefit, and will

17-2   Evidence from Studies in Humans for Renal Protective Benefit of Interventions to Protect the Kidney during the Perioperative Period

Level of Evidence	Class I Intervention SHOULD Be Used (Benefit >>> Risk)	Class IIa IT IS REASONABLE to Use the Intervention (Benefit >> Risk)	Class IIb Intervention MAY BE CONSIDERED (Benefit ≥ Risk)	Class III Intervention IS NOT HELPFUL AND MAY BE HARMFUL (Risk ≥ Benefit)
Level A (consistent evidence)	—	—	—	Off-pump CABG* (normal renal function) Low-dose dopamine infusion Loop diuretic therapy Insulin-like growth factor-I
Level B (limited evidence)	Insulin therapy to maintain tight serum glucose control.	Avoid unnecessary hemodilution below 21%-25% hematocrit during CPB. Minimize CPB duration. Restart aspirin within 48 hr of CABG surgery. Alpha-2-adrenergic agonist agents. Avoid unnecessary erythrocyte transfusion.	Avoidance of MHA through use of balanced salt solutions. Avoidance of hydroxyethyl starch solutions for volume expansion. Fenoldopam infusion. Dopexamine infusion. N-Acetylcysteine therapy. Calcium channel blocker therapy. Minimize age (time from donation to administration) of erythrocyte transfusion.	Target-hematocrit CPB management including hemodilution and transfusion. Normothermic CPB.* Avoidance of antifibrinolytic therapy. Mannitol therapy. Steroid therapy. NSAID and COX-2 inhibitor therapy. Beta-blocker therapy. Aminophylline/theophylline therapy. Nonselective ET receptor antagonists. Leukocyte depletion of transfused erythrocytes.
Level C (very limited evidence)	—	Atheroma avoidance during cardiac surgery using epiaortic scanning.	Port access mitral valve surgery.* Stent-graft AAA repair.* Delaying elective surgery after contrast exposure. Withholding preoperative dose of chronic ACE inhibitor. Withholding preoperative dose of chronic loop diuretic. Embol-X intra-aortic filtration system. Vasopressin as preferred vasoconstrictor. Pentoxifylline therapy. PGE$_1$ therapy.	Off-pump CABG* (abnormal renal function). Symmetry aortic connector device.* Maintaining CPB perfusion pressure > 60 mm Hg. ACE inhibitors and AGT1 receptor blocker therapy.

*Compared with conventional procedure.

AAA, abdominal aortic aneurysm; ACE, angiotensin converting enzyme; AGT, angiotensin; CABG, coronary artery bypass surgery; COX, cyclooxygenase; CPB, cardiopulmonary bypass; ET, endothelin; MHA, metabolic hyperchloremic acidosis; NSAID, nonsteroidal anti-inflammatory drug; PGE, prostaglandin E.

be sufficiently large to answer meaningful questions about renal preservation with a yes or a no.

■ REFERENCES

1. Hou SH, Bushinsky DA, Wish JB, et al: Hospital-acquired renal insufficiency: A prospective study. Am J Med 1983;74:243-248.
2. Novis BK, Roizen MF, Aronson S, Thisted RA: Association of preoperative risk factors with postoperative acute renal failure. Anesth Analg 1994;78:143-149.
3. Conlon PJ, Stafford-Smith M, White WD, et al: Acute renal failure following cardiac surgery. Nephrol Dial Transplant 1999;14:1158-1162.
4. Levy EM, Viscoli CM, Horwitz RI: The effect of acute renal failure on mortality: A cohort analysis. JAMA 1996;275:1489-1494.
5. Chertow GM, Levy EM, Hammermeister KE, et al: Independent association between acute renal failure and mortality following cardiac surgery. Am J Med 1998;104:343-348.
6. Stafford-Smith M: Perioperative renal dysfunction: Implications and strategies for protection. In Newman MF (ed): Perioperative Organ Protection. Baltimore, Lippincott Williams & Wilkins, 2003, pp 89-124.
7. Rabb H, Wang Z, Nemoto T, et al: Acute renal failure leads to dysregulation of lung salt and water channels. Kidney Int 2003;63:600-606.
8. Kelly KJ: Distant effects of experimental renal ischemia/reperfusion injury. J Am Soc Nephrol 2003;14:1549-1558.
9. Smith HW: Lectures on the Kidney. Lawrence, Kan, University of Kansas, 1943.
10. Abel RM, Buckley MJ, Austen WG, et al: Etiology, incidence, and prognosis of renal failure following cardiac operations: Results of a

prospective analysis of 500 consecutive patients. J Thorac Cardiovasc Surg 1976;71:323-333.

11. Corwin HL, Sprague SM, DeLaria GA, Norusis MJ: Acute renal failure associated with cardiac operations: A case-control study. J Thorac Cardiovasc Surg 1989;98:1107-1112.

12. Andersson LG, Ekroth R, Bratteby LE, et al: Acute renal failure after coronary surgery: A study of incidence and risk factors in 2009 consecutive patients. Thorac Cardiovasc Surg 1993;41:237-241.

13. Mora-Mangano C, Diamondstone LS, Ramsay JG, et al: Renal dysfunction after myocardial revascularization: Risk factors, adverse outcomes, and hospital resource utilization. The Multicenter Study of Perioperative Ischemia Research Group. Ann Intern Med 1998;128: 194-203.

14. Chertow GM, Lazarus JM, Christiansen CL, et al: Preoperative renal risk stratification. Circulation 1997;95:878-884.

15. Mangos GJ, Brown MA, Chan WY, et al: Acute renal failure following cardiac surgery: Incidence, outcomes and risk factors. Aust N Z J Med 1995;25:284-289.

16. Ostermann ME, Taube D, Morgan CJ, Evans TW: Acute renal failure following cardiopulmonary bypass: A changing picture. Intensive Care Med 2000;26:565-571.

17. Zanardo G, Michielon P, Paccagnella A, et al: Acute renal failure in the patient undergoing cardiac operation. Prevalence, mortality rate, and main risk factors. J Thorac Cardiovasc Surg 1994;107:1489-1495.

18. Yeh T, Brackney E, Hall D, Ellison R: Renal complications of open-heart surgery: Predisposing factors, prevention and management. J Thorac Cardiovasc Surg 1964;47:79-95.

19. Porter GA, Kloster FE, Herr RJ, et al: Renal complications associated with valve replacement surgery. J Thorac Cardiovasc Surg 1967;53: 145-152.

20. McLeish KR, Luft FC, Kleit SA: Factors affecting prognosis in acute renal failure following cardiac operations. Surg Gynecol Obstet 1977;145:28-32.

21. Llopart T, Lombardi R, Forselledo M, Andrade R: Acute renal failure in open heart surgery. Ren Fail 1997;19:319-323.

22. Hilberman M, Myers BD, Carrie BJ, et al: Acute renal failure following cardiac surgery. J Thorac Cardiovasc Surg 1979;77:880-888.

23. Heikkinen L, Harjula A, Merikallio E: Acute renal failure related to open-heart surgery. Ann Chir Gynaecol 1985;74:203-209.

24. Gailiunas P Jr, Chawla R, Lazarus JM, et al: Acute renal failure following cardiac operations. J Thorac Cardiovasc Surg 1980;79: 241-243.

25. Doberneck R, Reiser M, Lillehei C: Acute renal failure after open-heart surgery utilizing extracorporeal circulation and total body perfusion. J Thorac Cardiovasc Surg 1962;43:441-452.

26. Bhat JG, Gluck MC, Lowenstein J, Baldwin DS: Renal failure after open heart surgery. Ann Intern Med 1976;84:677-682.

27. Star R: Why clinical trials fail, and what to do about it. Bethesda, Md, Renal Diagnostics and Therapeutics Unit, U.S. National Institutes of Health. Available at www.isn-online.org/uploadedfiles/ISN/presentations/arf_satellite/STAR.pps.#891,9 (last accessed 10/20/2005).

28. Zacharias M, Gilmore I, Herbison G, et al: Interventions for protecting renal function in the perioperative period. Cochrane Database Syst Rev 2005:CD003590.

29. Stafford-Smith M, Grocott HP: Renal medullary hypoxia during experimental cardiopulmonary bypass: A pilot study. Perfusion 2005;20:53-58.

30. Navar LG, Inscho EW, Majid SA, et al: Paracrine regulation of the renal microcirculation. Physiol Rev 1996;76:425-536.

31. Kainuma M, Kimura N, Shimada Y: Effect of acute changes in renal arterial blood flow on urine oxygen tension in dogs. Crit Care Med 1990;18:309-312.

32. Kainuma M, Yamada M, Miyake T: Continuous urine oxygen tension monitoring in patients undergoing cardiac surgery. J Cardiothorac Vasc Anesth 1996;10:603-608.

33. Cochrane J, Williams BT, Banerjee A, et al: Ischemic preconditioning attenuates functional, metabolic, and morphologic injury from ischemic acute renal failure in the rat. Ren Fail 1999;21:135-145.

34. Lee HT, Emala CW: Protective effects of renal ischemic preconditioning and adenosine pretreatment: Role of A and A receptors. Am J Physiol Renal Physiol 2000;278:F380-387.

35. Lee HT, Gallos G, Nasr SH, Emala CW: A adenosine receptor activation inhibits inflammation, necrosis, and apoptosis after renal ischemia-reperfusion injury in mice. J Am Soc Nephrol 2004;15: 102-111.

36. Brezis M, Rosen S: Hypoxia of the renal medulla: Its implications for disease. N Engl J Med 1995;332:647-655.

37. Cunningham PN, Dyanov HM, Park P, et al: Acute renal failure in endotoxemia is caused by TNF acting directly on TNF receptor-1 in kidney. J Immunol 2002;168:5817-5823.

38. Segerer S, Nelson PJ, Schlondorff D: Chemokines, chemokine receptors, and renal disease: From basic science to pathophysiologic and therapeutic studies. J Am Soc Nephrol 2000;11:152-176.

39. Domart Y, Trouillet JL, Fagon JY, et al: Incidence and morbidity of cytomegaloviral infection in patients with mediastinitis following cardiac surgery. Chest 1990;97:18-22.

40. Heyman SN, Darmon D, Goldfarb M, et al: Endotoxin-induced renal failure: I. A role for altered renal microcirculation. Exp Nephrol 2000;8:266-274.

41. Davila-Roman VG, Kouchoukos NT, Schechtman KB, Barzilai B: Atherosclerosis of the ascending aorta is a predictor of renal dysfunction after cardiac operations. J Thorac Cardiovasc Surg 1999;117: 111-116.

42. Tierney G, Parissis H, Baker M, et al: An experimental study of intra-aortic balloon pumping within the intact human aorta. Eur J Cardiothorac Surg 1997;12:486-493.

43. Tunick PA, Culliford AT, Lamparello PJ, Kronzon I: Atheromatosis of the aortic arch as an occult source of multiple systemic emboli. Ann Intern Med 1991;114:391-392.

44. Smith MC, Ghose MK, Henry AR: The clinical spectrum of renal cholesterol embolization. Am J Med 1981;71:174-180.

45. Deal DD, Jones TJ, Vernon JC, et al: Real time OPS imaging of embolic injury of the renal micro-circulation during cardiopulmonary bypass. Anesth Analg 2001;92:S23.

46. Luft FC, Vinicor F: Recurrent acute renal failure with idiopathic paroxysmal myoglobinuria. JAMA 1975;233:349-351.

47. Corwin HL, Schreiber MJ, Fang LS: Low fractional excretion of sodium: Occurrence with hemoglobinuric- and myoglobinuric-induced acute renal failure. Arch Intern Med 1984;144:981-982.

48. Heyman SN, Rosen S, Fuchs S, et al: Myoglobinuric acute renal failure in the rat: A role for medullary hypoperfusion, hypoxia, and tubular obstruction. J Am Soc Nephrol 1996;7:1066-1074.

49. Porter GA: Contrast-associated nephropathy: Presentation, pathophysiology and management. Miner Electrolyte Metab 1994;20: 232-243.

50. Bennett WM, Luft F, Porter GA: Pathogenesis of renal failure due to aminoglycosides and contrast media used in roentgenography. Am J Med 1980;69:767-774.

51. Baisac J, Henrich W: Nephrotoxicity of nonsteroidal anti-inflammatory drugs. Miner Electrolyte Metab 1994;20:187-192.

52. Olyaei AJ, de Mattos AM, Bennett WM: Immunosuppressant-induced nephropathy: Pathophysiology, incidence and management. Drug Saf 1999;21:471-488.

53. Goligorsky MS: Whispers and shouts in the pathogenesis of acute renal ischaemia. Nephrol Dial Transplant 2005;20:261-266.

54. Myers B, Moran S: Hemodynamically mediated acute renal failure. N Engl J Med 1986;314:97-105.

55. Gaudino M, Luciani N, Giungi S, et al: Different profiles of patients who require dialysis after cardiac surgery. Ann Thorac Surg 2005;79:825-829; author reply 829-830.

56. Stafford-Smith M: Invited commentary. Ann Thorac Surg 2005;79: 829-830.

57. van den Berghe G, Wouters P, Weekers F, et al: Intensive insulin therapy in the critically ill patients. N Engl J Med 2001;345: 1359-1367.

58. Stafford-Smith M, Reddan DN, Phillips-Bute B, et al: Association of perioperative creatinine-derived variables with mortality and other outcomes after coronary bypass surgery. Anesth Analg 2001;92: SCA28.

59. Sladen RN, Endo E, Harrison T: Two-hour versus 22-hour creatinine clearance in critically ill patients. Anesthesiology 1987;67: 1013-1016.

60. Cockcroft DW, Gault MH: Prediction of creatinine clearance from serum creatinine. Nephron 1976;16:31-41.

61. Bloor GK, Welsh KR, Goodall S, Shah MV: Comparison of predicted with measured creatinine clearance in cardiac surgical patients. J Cardiothorac Vasc Anesth 1996;10:899-902.

62. Gowans EM, Fraser CG: Biological variation of serum and urine creatinine and creatinine clearance: Ramifications for interpretation of results and patient care [see comments]. Ann Clin Biochem 1988;25(Pt 3):259-263.

63. Morgan DB, Dillon S, Payne RB: The assessment of glomerular function: Creatinine clearance or plasma creatinine? Postgrad Med J 1978;54:302-310.

64. Habib RH, Zacharias A, Schwann TA, et al: Role of hemodilutional anemia and transfusion during cardiopulmonary bypass in renal injury after coronary revascularization: Implications on operative outcome. Crit Care Med 2005;33:1749-1756.

65. Ferguson TB Jr, Dziuban SW Jr, Edwards FH, et al: The STS National Database: Current changes and challenges for the new millennium. Committee to Establish a National Database in Cardiothoracic Surgery, Society of Thoracic Surgeons. Ann Thorac Surg 2000;69:680-691.

66. Barrett BJ, Parfrey PS: Prevention of nephrotoxicity induced by radiocontrast agents. N Engl J Med 1994;331:1449-1450.

67. Levin A: Cystatin C, serum creatinine, and estimates of kidney function: Searching for better measures of kidney function and cardiovascular risk. Ann Intern Med 2005;142:586-588.

68. Grubb A, Bjork J, Lindstrom V, et al: A cystatin C-based formula without anthropometric variables estimates glomerular filtration rate better than creatinine clearance using the Cockcroft-Gault formula. Scand J Clin Lab Invest 2005;65:153-162.

69. Mishra J, Ma Q, Prada A, et al: Identification of neutrophil gelatinase-associated lipocalin as a novel early urinary biomarker for ischemic renal injury. J Am Soc Nephrol 2003;14:2534-2543.

70. Mishra J, Dent C, Tarabishi R, et al: Neutrophil gelatinase-associated lipocalin (NGAL) as a biomarker for acute renal injury after cardiac surgery. Lancet 2005;365:1231-1238.

71. Alpert RA, Roizen MF, Hamilton WK, et al: Intraoperative urinary output does not predict postoperative renal function in patients undergoing abdominal aortic revascularization. Surgery 1984;95:707-711.

72. Stafford-Smith M, Phillips-Bute B, Reddan DN, et al: The association of postoperative peak and fractional change in serum creatinine with mortality after coronary bypass surgery. Anesthesiology 2000;93:A240.

73. Ascione R, Nason G, Al-Ruzzeh S, et al: Coronary revascularization with or without cardiopulmonary bypass in patients with preoperative nondialysis-dependent renal insufficiency. Ann Thorac Surg 2001;72:2020-2025.

74. Loef BG, Epema AH, Navis G, et al: Off-pump coronary revascularization attenuates transient renal damage compared with on-pump coronary revascularization. Chest 2002;121:1190-1194.

75. Tang AT, Knott J, Nanson J, et al: A prospective randomized study to evaluate the renoprotective action of beating heart coronary surgery in low risk patients. Eur J Cardiothorac Surg 2002;22:118-123.

76. Schwann NM, Horrow JC, Strong MD 3rd, et al: Does off-pump coronary artery bypass reduce the incidence of clinically evident renal dysfunction after multivessel myocardial revascularization? Anesth Analg 2004;99:959-964.

77. Gamoso MG, Phillips-Bute B, Landolfo KP, et al: Off-pump versus on-pump coronary artery bypass surgery and postoperative renal dysfunction. Anesth Analg 2000;91:1080-1084.

78. Hayashida N, Teshima H, Chihara S, et al: Does off-pump coronary artery bypass grafting really preserve renal function? Circ J 2002;66:921-925.

79. Sabik JF, Gillinov AM, Blackstone EH, et al: Does off-pump coronary surgery reduce morbidity and mortality? J Thorac Cardiovasc Surg 2002;124:698-707.

80. Karthik S, Musleh G, Grayson AD, et al: Effect of avoiding cardiopulmonary bypass in non-elective coronary artery bypass surgery: A propensity score analysis. Eur J Cardiothorac Surg 2003;24:66-71.

81. Reston JT, Tregear SJ, Turkelson CM: Meta-analysis of short-term and mid-term outcomes following off-pump coronary artery bypass grafting. Ann Thorac Surg 2003;76:1510-1515.

82. Al-Ruzzeh S, Ambler G, Asimakopoulos G, et al: Off-pump coronary artery bypass (OPCAB) surgery reduces risk-stratified morbidity and mortality: A United Kingdom multi-center comparative analysis of early clinical outcome. Circulation 2003;108(Suppl 1):III-8.

83. Cheng DC, Bainbridge D, Martin JE, Novick RJ: Does off-pump coronary artery bypass reduce mortality, morbidity, and resource utilization when compared with conventional coronary artery bypass? A meta-analysis of randomized trials. Anesthesiology 2005;102:188-203.

84. Ascione R, Lloyd CT, Underwood MJ, et al: On-pump versus off-pump coronary revascularization: Evaluation of renal function. Ann Thorac Surg 1999;68:493-498.

85. Chukwuemeka A, Weisel A, Maganti M, et al: Renal dysfunction in high-risk patients after on-pump and off-pump coronary artery bypass surgery: A propensity score analysis. Ann Thorac Surg 2005;80:2148-2153.

86. Sreeram GM, Grocott HP, White WD, et al: Transcranial Doppler emboli count predicts rise in creatinine after coronary artery bypass graft surgery. J Cardiothorac Vasc Anesth 2004;18:548-551.

87. Scarborough JE, White W, Derilus FE, et al: Combined use of off-pump techniques and a sutureless proximal aortic anastomotic device reduces cerebral microemboli generation during coronary artery bypass grafting. J Thorac Cardiovasc Surg 2003;126:1561-1567.

88. Calafiore AM, Bar-El Y, Vitolla G, et al: Early clinical experience with a new sutureless anastomotic device for proximal anastomosis of the saphenous vein to the aorta. J Thorac Cardiovasc Surg 2001;121:854-858.

89. Fischer SS, Phillips-Bute B, Stafford-Smith M: Does off-pump coronary artery bypass surgery with a connector device reduce postoperative renal dysfunction? Anesth Analg 2004;98:45.

90. McCreath BJ, Swaminathan M, Booth JV, et al: Mitral valve surgery and acute renal injury: Port access versus median sternotomy. Ann Thorac Surg 2003;75:812-819.

91. Greenberg RK, Chuter TA, Lawrence-Brown M, et al: Analysis of renal function after aneurysm repair with a device using suprarenal fixation (Zenith AAA Endovascular Graft) in contrast to open surgical repair. J Vasc Surg 2004;39:1219-1228.

92. Garwood S, Mathew J, Hines R: Renal function and cardiopulmonary bypass: Does time since catheterization impact renal performance? Anesthesiology 1997;87:A90.

93. Provenchère S, Plantefève G, Hufnagel G, et al: Renal dysfunction after cardiac surgery with normothermic cardiopulmonary bypass: Incidence, risk factors, and effect on clinical outcome. Anesth Analg 2003;96:1258-1264.

94. Yusuf S, Lonn E, Bosch J, Gerstein H: Summary of randomized trials of angiotensin converting enzyme inhibitors. Clin Exp Hypertens 1999;21:835-845.

95. Mimran A, Ribstein J: Angiotensin converting enzyme inhibitors and renal function. J Hypertens Suppl 1989;7:S3-9.

96. Kamper AL, Nielsen AH, Baekgaard N, Just S: Renal graft failure after addition of an angiotensin II receptor antagonist to an angiotensin-converting enzyme inhibitor: Unmasking of an unknown iliac artery stenosis. J Renin Angiotensin Aldosterone Syst 2002;3:135-137.

97. Cittanova ML, Zubicki A, Savu C, et al: The chronic inhibition of angiotensin-converting enzyme impairs postoperative renal function. Anesth Analg 2001;93:1111-1115.

98. Weightman WM, Gibbs NM, Sheminant MR, et al: Drug therapy before coronary artery surgery: Nitrates are independent predictors of mortality and beta-adrenergic blockers predict survival. Anesth Analg 1999;88:286-291.

99. Charlson M, Krieger KH, Peterson JC, et al: Predictors and outcomes of cardiac complications following elective coronary bypass grafting. Proc Assoc Am Physicians 1999;111:622-632.

100. Cittanova ML, Leblanc I, Legendre C, et al: Effect of hydroxyethyl-starch in brain-dead kidney donors on renal function in kidney-transplant recipients. Lancet 1996;348:1620-1622.

101. Peron S, Mouthon L, Guettier C, et al: Hydroxyethyl starch-induced renal insufficiency after plasma exchange in a patient with polymyositis and liver cirrhosis. Clin Nephrol 2001;55:408-411.

102. Winkelmayer WC, Glynn RJ, Levin R, Avorn J: Hydroxyethyl starch and change in renal function in patients undergoing coronary artery bypass graft surgery. Kidney Int 2003;64:1046-1049.

103. De Labarthe A, Jacobs F, Blot F, Glotz D: Acute renal failure secondary to hydroxyethylstarch administration in a surgical patient. Am J Med 2001;111:417-418.

104. Schortgen F, Lacherade JC, Bruneel F, et al: Effects of hydroxyethylstarch and gelatin on renal function in severe sepsis: A multicentre randomised study. Lancet 2001;357:911-916.

105. Boldt J, Brenner T, Lang J, et al: Kidney-specific proteins in elderly patients undergoing cardiac surgery with cardiopulmonary bypass. Anesth Analg 2003;97:1582-1589.

106. Kumle B, Boldt J, Piper S, et al: The influence of different intravascular volume replacement regimens on renal function in the elderly. Anesth Analg 1999;89:1124-1130.

107. Wilkes NJ, Woolf R, Mutch M, et al: The effects of balanced versus saline-based hetastarch and crystalloid solutions on acid-base and electrolyte status and gastric mucosal perfusion in elderly surgical patients. Anesth Analg 2001;93:811-816.

108. Parekh N: Hyperchloremic acidosis. Anesth Analg 2002;95:1821.

109. Wilcox C: Regulation of renal blood flow by plasma chloride. J Clin Invest 1983;71:726-735.

110. Hansen PB, Jensen BL, Skott O: Chloride regulates afferent arteriolar contraction in response to depolarization. Hypertension 1998;32:1066-1070.

111. Atkins JL: Effect of sodium bicarbonate preloading on ischemic renal failure. Nephron 1986;44:70-74.

112. Merten GJ, Burgess WP, Gray LV, et al: Prevention of contrast-induced nephropathy with sodium bicarbonate: A randomized controlled trial. JAMA 2004;291:2328-2334.

113. Andersson LG, Bratteby LE, Ekroth R, et al: Renal function during cardiopulmonary bypass: Influence of pump flow and systemic blood pressure. Eur J Cardiothorac Surg 1994;8:597-602.

114. Reves JG, Karp RB, Buttner EE, et al: Neuronal and adrenomedullary catecholamine release in response to cardiopulmonary bypass in man. Circulation 1982;66:49-55.

115. Laffey J, Boylan J, Cheng D: The systemic inflammatory response to cardiac surgery: Implications for the anesthesiologist. Anesthesiology 2002;97:215-252.

116. Fischer UM, Weissenberger WK, Warters RD, et al: Impact of cardiopulmonary bypass management on postcardiac surgery renal function. Perfusion 2002;17:401-406.

117. Urzua J, Troncoso S, Bugedo G, et al: Renal function and cardiopulmonary bypass: Effect of perfusion pressure. J Cardiothorac Vasc Anesth 1992;6:299-303.

118. Swaminathan M, Knauth K, Phillips-Bute B, et al: Lowest CPB hematocrit is inversely associated with creatinine rise after coronary bypass surgery. Anesth Analg 2002;94:S70.

119. Conlon PJ, Crowley J, Stack R, et al: Renal artery stenosis is not associated with the development of acute renal failure following coronary artery bypass grafting. Ren Fail 2005;27:81-86.

120. Shah D, Corson J, Karmody A, Leather R: Effects of isovolemic hemodilution on abdominal aortic aneurysmectomy in high risk patients. Ann Vasc Surg 1986;1:50-54.

121. Messmer K: Hemodilution. Surg Clin North Am 1975;55:659-678.

122. DeFoe G, Ross C, Olmstead E, et al: Lowest hematocrit on bypass and adverse outcomes associated with coronary artery bypass grafting. Ann Thorac Surg 2001;71:769-776.

123. Fang WC, Helm RE, Krieger KH, et al: Impact of minimum hematocrit during cardiopulmonary bypass on mortality in patients undergoing coronary artery surgery. Circulation 1997;96(9 Suppl):II-194-199.

124. Ranucci M, Pavesi M, Mazza E, et al: Risk factors for renal dysfunction after coronary surgery: The role of cardiopulmonary bypass technique. Perfusion 1994;9:319-326.

125. Swaminathan M, Phillips-Bute BG, Conlon PJ, et al: The association of lowest hematocrit during cardiopulmonary bypass with acute renal injury after coronary bypass surgery. Ann Thorac Surg 2003;76:784-791.

126. Karkouti K, Beattie WS, Wijeysundera DN, et al: Hemodilution during cardiopulmonary bypass is an independent risk factor for acute renal failure in adult cardiac surgery. J Thorac Cardiovasc Surg 2005;129:391-400.

127. Kincaid EH, Ashburn DA, Hoyle JR, et al: Does the combination of aprotinin and angiotensin-converting enzyme inhibitor cause renal failure after cardiac surgery? Ann Thorac Surg 2005;80:1388-1393.

128. Barbeito A, Phillips-Bute B, Mathew JP, et al: Hemodilution and acute renal injury: The relationship of three different target CPB hematocrit strategies with post-cardiac surgery renal dysfunction. Anesth Analg 2005;100:SCA18.

129. DeSimone NA, Phillips-Bute B, Hill SE, et al: The association of aging red blood cell and platelet transfusions with mortality after aortocoronary bypass surgery. Anesth Analg 2005;100:SCA7.

130. Basran S, Frumento R, Cohen A, et al: Association between length of storage of erythrocytes and postoperative acute renal dysfunction in patients undergoing reoperative cardiac surgery. Can J Anaesth 2005;52:A21.

131. Lieberthal W, Rennke H, Sandock K, et al: Ischemia in the isolated erythrocyte-perfused rat kidney: Protective effect of hypothermia. Ren Physiol Biochem 1988;11:60-69.

132. Ip-Yam PC, Murphy S, Baines M, et al: Renal function and proteinuria after cardiopulmonary bypass: The effects of temperature and mannitol. Anesth Analg 1994;78:842-847.

133. Regragui IA, Izzat MB, Birdi I, et al: Cardiopulmonary bypass perfusion temperature does not influence perioperative renal function. Ann Thorac Surg 1995;60:160-164.

134. Swaminathan M, East C, Phillips-Bute B, et al: Report of a substudy on warm versus cold cardiopulmonary bypass: Changes in creatinine clearance. Ann Thorac Surg 2001;72:1603-1609.

135. Korner A, Eklof AC, Celsi G, Aperia A: Increased renal metabolism in diabetes: Mechanism and functional implications. Diabetes 1994;43:629-633.

136. Bookstein JJ, Clark RL (eds): Renal Microvascular Disease: Angiographic-Microangiographic Correlates. Boston, Little, Brown, 1980.

137. Thurlbeck W, Castleman B: Atheromatous emboli to the kidneys after aortic surgery. N Engl J Med 1957;257:442-447.

138. Reichenspurner H, Navia JA, Berry G, et al: Particulate emboli capture by an intra-aortic filter device during cardiac surgery. J Thorac Cardiovasc Surg 2000;119:233-241.

139. Barbut D, Yao FS, Lo YW, et al: Determination of size of aortic emboli and embolic load during coronary artery bypass grafting. Ann Thorac Surg 1997;63:1262-1267.

140. Banbury MK, Kouchoukos NT, Allen KB, et al: Emboli capture using the Embol-X intraaortic filter in cardiac surgery: A multicentered randomized trial of 1,289 patients. Ann Thorac Surg 2003;76:508-515; discussion 515.

141. Sedrakyan A, Treasure T, Elefteriades JA: Effect of aprotinin on clinical outcomes in coronary artery bypass graft surgery: A systematic review and meta-analysis of randomized clinical trials. J Thorac Cardiovasc Surg 2004;128:442-448.

142. Fremes SE, Wong BI, Lee E, et al: Metaanalysis of prophylactic drug treatment in the prevention of postoperative bleeding. Ann Thorac Surg 1994;58:1580-1588.

143. Royston D: Aprotinin versus lysine analogues: The debate continues. Ann Thorac Surg 1998;65(4 Suppl):S9-19; discussion S27-28.

144. Rustom R, Maltby P, Grime JS, et al: Effects of lysine infusion on the renal metabolism of aprotinin (Trasylol) in man. Clin Sci (Colch) 1992;83:295-299.

145. Stafford-Smith M: Antifibrinolytic agents make alpha1- and beta2-microglobulinuria poor markers of post cardiac surgery renal dysfunction. Anesthesiology 1999;90:928-929.

146. Stafford-Smith M, Phillips-Bute B, Reddan DN, et al: The association of epsilon-aminocaproic acid with postoperative decrease in creatinine clearance in 1502 coronary bypass patients. Anesth Analg 2000;91:1085-1090.

147. Burchardi H, Kaczmarczyk G: The effect of anaesthesia on renal function. Eur J Anaesthesiol 1994;11:163-168.

148. Sladen RN, Landry D: Renal blood flow regulation, autoregulation, and vasomotor nephropathy. Anesthesiol Clin North Am 2000;18:791-807, ix.

149. Taguma Y, Sasaki Y, Kyogoku Y, et al: Morphological changes in an early phase of norepinephrine-induced acute renal failure in unilaterally nephrectomized dogs. J Lab Clin Med 1980;96:616-632.

150. Baehler RW, Williams RH, Work J, et al: Studies on the natural history of the norepinephrine model of acute renal failure in the dog. Nephron 1980;26:266-273.

151. Persson PB, Ehmke H, Nafz B, Kirchheim HR: Resetting of renal autoregulation in conscious dogs: Angiotensin II and alpha1-adrenoceptors. Pflugers Arch 1990;417:42-47.

152. Hollenberg NK, Meyerovitz M, Harrington DP, Sandor T: Influence of norepinephrine and angiotensin II on vasomotion of renal blood supply in humans. Am J Physiol 1987;252(5 Pt 2):H941-944.

153. Di Giantomasso D, Morimatsu H, May CN, Bellomo R: Intrarenal blood flow distribution in hyperdynamic septic shock: Effect of norepinephrine. Crit Care Med 2003;31:2509-2513.

154. Gardunio C, Funk B, Phillips-Bute B, et al: Beta-adrenergic receptor blockade does not influence postoperative renal dysfunction in cardiac surgical patients. Anesth Analg 1999;88:SCA90.

155. Holmes CL, Walley KR, Chittock DR, et al: The effects of vasopressin on hemodynamics and renal function in severe septic shock: A case series. Intensive Care Med 2001;27:1416-1421.

156. Holmes CL: Is low-dose vasopressin the new reno-protective agent? Crit Care Med 2004;32:1972-1974.

157. Albert M, Losser MR, Hayon D, et al: Systemic and renal macro- and microcirculatory responses to arginine vasopressin in endotoxic rabbits. Crit Care Med 2004;32:1891-1898.

158. Patel BM, Chittock DR, Russell JA, Walley KR: Beneficial effects of short-term vasopressin infusion during severe septic shock. Anesthesiology 2002;96:576-582.

159. Bennett SR, McKeown J, Drew P, Griffin S: Angiotensin in cardiac surgery: Efficacy in patients on angiotensin converting enzyme inhibitors. Eur J Heart Fail 2001;3:587-592.

160. Jonassen TE, Graebe M, Promeneur D, et al: Lipopolysaccharide-induced acute renal failure in conscious rats: Effects of specific phosphodiesterase type 3 and 4 inhibition. J Pharmacol Exp Ther 2002;303:364-374.

161. Saab G, Mindel G, Ewald G, Vijayan A: Acute renal failure secondary to milrinone in a patient with cardiac amyloidosis. Am J Kidney Dis 2002;40:E7.

162. Boldt J, Brosch C, Suttner S, et al: Prophylactic use of the phosphodiesterase III inhibitor enoximone in elderly cardiac surgery patients: Effect on hemodynamics, inflammation, and markers of organ function. Intensive Care Med 2002;28:1462-1469.

163. Boldt J, Brosch C, Lehmann A, et al: The prophylactic use of the beta-blocker esmolol in combination with phosphodiesterase III inhibitor enoximone in elderly cardiac surgery patients. Anesth Analg 2004;99:1009-1017.

164. Page US, Washburn T: Using tracking data to find complications that physicians miss: The case of renal failure in cardiac surgery. Jt Comm J Qual Improv 1997;23:511-520.

165. McNay JL, McDonald RH Jr, Goldberg LI: Direct renal vasodilatation produced by dopamine in the dog. Circ Res 1965;16:510-517.

166. Bellomo R, Chapman M, Finfer S, et al: Low-dose dopamine in patients with early renal dysfunction: A placebo-controlled randomised trial. Australian and New Zealand Intensive Care Society (ANZICS) Clinical Trials Group. Lancet 2000;356:2139-2143.

167. Marik PE: Low-dose dopamine: A systematic review. Intensive Care Med 2002;28:877-883.

168. Kellum JA, Decker J: Use of dopamine in acute renal failure: A meta-analysis. Crit Care Med 2001;29:1526-1531.

169. Prins I, Plotz FB, Uiterwaal CS, van Vught HJ: Low-dose dopamine in neonatal and pediatric intensive care: A systematic review. Intensive Care Med 2001;27:206-210.

170. Friedrich JO, Adhikari N, Herridge MS, Beyene J: Meta-analysis: Low-dose dopamine increases urine output but does not prevent renal dysfunction or death. Ann Intern Med 2005;142:510-524.

171. Carcoana OV, Hines RL: Is renal dose dopamine protective or therapeutic? Yes. Crit Care Clin 1996;12:677-685.

172. Cottee DB, Saul WP: Is renal dose dopamine protective or therapeutic? No. Crit Care Clin 1996;12:687-695.

173. Holmes CL, Walley KR: Bad medicine: Low-dose dopamine in the ICU. Chest 2003;123:1266-1275.

174. Jones D, Bellomo R: Renal-dose dopamine: From hypothesis to paradigm to dogma to myth and, finally, superstition? J Intensive Care Med 2005;20:199-211.

175. Argalious M, Motta P, Khandwala F, et al: "Renal dose" dopamine is associated with the risk of new-onset atrial fibrillation after cardiac surgery. Crit Care Med 2005;33:1327-1332.

176. McHugh GJ: Current usage of dopamine in New Zealand intensive care units. Anaesth Intensive Care 2001;29:623-626.

177. Tumlin JA, Dunbar LM, Oparil S, et al: Fenoldopam, a dopamine agonist, for hypertensive emergency: A multicenter randomized trial. Fenoldopam Study Group. Acad Emerg Med 2000;7:653-662.

178. Panacek EA, Bednarczyk EM, Dunbar LM, et al: Randomized, prospective trial of fenoldopam vs sodium nitroprusside in the treatment of acute severe hypertension. Fenoldopam Study Group. Acad Emerg Med 1995;2:959-965.

179. Shorten GD: Fenoldopam: Potential clinical applications in heart surgery. Rev Esp Anestesiol Reanim 2001;48:487-491.

180. Carcoana OV, Mathew JP, Davis E, et al: Mannitol and dopamine in patients undergoing cardiopulmonary bypass: A randomized clinical trial. Anesth Analg 2003;97:1222-1229.

181. Caimmi PP, Pagani L, Micalizzi E, et al: Fenoldopam for renal protection in patients undergoing cardiopulmonary bypass. J Cardiothorac Vasc Anesth 2003;17:491-494.

182. Bove T, Landoni G, Grazia Calabro M, et al: Renoprotective action of fenoldopam in high-risk patients undergoing cardiac surgery: A prospective, double-blind, randomized clinical trial. Circulation 2005;111:3230-3235.

183. Tumlin J, Finckle K, Murray P, Shaw A: Dopamine receptor 1 agonists in early acute tubular necrosis: A prospective, randomized, double blind, placebo-controlled trial of fenoldopam mesylate. J Am Soc Nephrol 2003;14:PUB001.

184. Tumlin JA, Finkel KW, Murray PT, et al: Fenoldopam mesylate in early acute tubular necrosis: A randomized, double-blind, placebo-controlled clinical trial. Am J Kidney Dis 2005;46:26-34.

185. Ng TM, Shurmur SW, Silver M, et al: Comparison of N-acetylcysteine and fenoldopam for preventing contrast-induced nephropathy (CAFCIN). Int J Cardiol 2006;109:322-328.

186. Stone GW, McCullough PA, Tumlin JA, et al: Fenoldopam mesylate for the prevention of contrast-induced nephropathy: A randomized controlled trial. JAMA 2003;290:2284-2291.

187. Allaqaband S, Tumuluri R, Malik AM, et al: Prospective randomized study of N-acetylcysteine, fenoldopam, and saline for prevention of radiocontrast-induced nephropathy. Catheter Cardiovasc Interv 2002;57:279-283.

188. Della Rocca G, Pompei L, Costa MG, et al: Fenoldopam mesylate and renal function in patients undergoing liver transplantation: A randomized, controlled pilot trial. Anesth Analg 2004;99:1604-1609.

189. Biancofiore G, Della Rocca G, Bindi L, et al: Use of fenoldopam to control renal dysfunction early after liver transplantation. Liver Transpl 2004;10:986-992.

190. Halpenny M, Rushe C, Breen P, et al: The effects of fenoldopam on renal function in patients undergoing elective aortic surgery. Eur J Anaesthesiol 2002;19:32-39.

191. Chintala MS, Lokhandwala MF, Jandhyala BS: Protective effects of dopexamine hydrochloride in renal failure after acute haemorrhage in anaesthetized dogs. J Auton Pharmacol 1990;10(Suppl 1):S95-102.

192. Gomez-Garre DN, Lopez-Farre A, Eleno N, Lopez-Novoa JM: Comparative effects of dopexamine and dopamine on glycerol-induced acute renal failure in rats. Ren Fail 1996;18:59-68.

193. Burns A, Gray PA, Bodenham AR, Park GR: Dopexamine: Studies in the general intensive care unit and after liver transplantation. J Auton Pharmacol 1990;10(Suppl 1):S109-114.

194. Berendes E, Mollhoff T, Van Aken H, et al: Effects of dopexamine on creatinine clearance, systemic inflammation, and splanchnic oxygenation in patients undergoing coronary artery bypass grafting. Anesth Analg 1997;84:950-957.

195. Dehne MG, Klein TF, Muhling J, et al: Impairment of renal function after cardiopulmonary bypass is not influenced by dopexamine. Ren Fail 2001;23:217-230.

196. Gray PA, Bodenham AR, Park GR: A comparison of dopexamine and dopamine to prevent renal impairment in patients undergoing orthotopic liver transplantation [erratum in Anaesthesia 1992;47:92]. Anaesthesia 1991;46:638-641.

197. Renton MC, Snowden CP: Dopexamine and its role in the protection of hepatosplanchnic and renal perfusion in high-risk surgical and critically ill patients. Br J Anaesth 2005;94:459-467.

198. Brezis M, Agmon Y, Epstein FH: Determinants of intrarenal oxygenation: I. Effects of diuretics. Am J Physiol 1994;267(6 Pt 2):F1059-1062.

199. Liss P: Effects of contrast media on renal microcirculation and oxygen tension: An experimental study in the rat. Acta Radiol Suppl 1997;409:1-29.

200. Lindner A, Cutler R, Goodman W: Synergism of dopamine plus furosemide in preventing acute renal failure in the dog. Kidney Int 1979;16:158-166.

201. Heyman SN, Rosen S, Epstein FH, et al: Loop diuretics reduce hypoxic damage to proximal tubules of the isolated perfused rat kidney. Kidney Int 1994;45:981-985.

202. Hager B, Betschart M, Krapf R: Effect of postoperative intravenous loop diuretic on renal function after major surgery. Schweiz Med Wochenschr 1996;126:666-673.

203. Shilliday IR, Quinn KJ, Allison ME: Loop diuretics in the management of acute renal failure: A prospective, double-blind, placebo-controlled, randomized study. Nephrol Dial Transplant 1997;12:2592-2596.

204. Nuutinen L, Hollmen A: The effect of prophylactic use of furosemide on renal function during open heart surgery. Ann Chir Gynaecol 1976;65:258-266.

205. Lombardi R, Ferreiro A, Servetto C: Renal function after cardiac surgery: Adverse effect of furosemide. Ren Fail 2003;25:775-786.

206. Mehta R, Pascual M, Soroko S, et al: Diuretics, mortality, and nonrecovery of renal function in acute renal failure. JAMA 2002;288:2547-2553.

207. Uchino S, Doig GS, Bellomo R, et al: Diuretics and mortality in acute renal failure. Crit Care Med 2004;32:1669-1677.

208. Lassnigg A, Donner E, Grubhofer G, et al: Lack of renoprotective effects of dopamine and furosemide during cardiac surgery. J Am Soc Nephrol 2000;11:97-104.

209. Solomon R, Werner C, Mann D, et al: Effects of saline, mannitol, and furosemide to prevent acute decreases in renal function induced by radiocontrast agents. N Engl J Med 1994;331:1416-1420.

210. Albright RC Jr: Acute renal failure: A practical update. Mayo Clin Proc 2001;76:67-74.

211. Blantz RC, Weir MR: Are the oxygen costs of kidney function highly regulated? Curr Opin Nephrol Hypertens 2004;13:67-71.

212. Ellison DH, Velazquez H, Wright FS: Adaptation of the distal convoluted tubule of the rat: Structural and functional effects of dietary salt intake and chronic diuretic infusion. J Clin Invest 1989;83:113-126.

213. Johnston PA, Bernard DB, Perrin NS, Levinsky NG: Prostaglandins mediate the vasodilatory effect of mannitol in the hypoperfused rat kidney. J Clin Invest 1981;68:127-133.

214. Velasquez MT, Notargiacomo AV, Cohn JN: Comparative effects of saline and mannitol on renal cortical blood flow and volume in the dog. Am J Physiol 1973;224:322-327.

215. Morris CR, Alexander EA, Bruns FJ, Levinsky NG: Restoration and maintenance of glomerular filtration by mannitol during hypoperfusion of the kidney. J Clin Invest 1972;51:1555-1564.

216. Temes SP, Lilien OM, Chamberlain W: A direct vasoconstrictor effect of mannitol on the renal artery. Surg Gynecol Obstet 1975;141:223-226.

217. Stahl WM: Effect of mannitol on the kidney: Changes in intrarenal hemodynamics. N Engl J Med 1965;272:382-386.

218. Braun WE, Lilienfield LS: Renal hemodynamic effects of hypertonic mannitol infusions. Proc Soc Exp Biol Med 1963;114:1-6.

219. Pass LJ, Eberhart RC, Brown JC, et al: The effect of mannitol and dopamine on the renal response to thoracic aortic cross-clamping. J Thorac Cardiovasc Surg 1988;95:608-612.

220. Hett DA, Smith DC: A survey of priming solutions used for cardiopulmonary bypass. Perfusion 1994;9:19-22.

221. Sade RM, Stroud MR, Crawford FA Jr, et al: A prospective randomized study of hydroxyethyl starch, albumin, and lactated Ringer's solution as priming fluid for cardiopulmonary bypass. J Thorac Cardiovasc Surg 1985;89:713-722.

222. Fisher AR, Jones P, Barlow P, et al: The influence of mannitol on renal function during and after open-heart surgery. Perfusion 1998;13:181-186.

223. Nishimura O, Tokutsu S, Sakurai T, et al: Effects of hypertonic mannitol on renal function in open heart surgery. Jpn Heart J 1983;24:245-257.

224. Myers BD, Miller DC, Mehigan JT, et al: Nature of the renal injury following total renal ischemia in man. J Clin Invest 1984;73:329-341.

225. Visweswaran P, Massin EK, Dubose TD Jr: Mannitol-induced acute renal failure. J Am Soc Nephrol 1997;8:1028-1033.

226. Gubern JM, Sancho JJ, Simo J, Sitges-Serra A: A randomized trial on the effect of mannitol on postoperative renal function in patients with obstructive jaundice. Surgery 1988;103:39-44.

227. Joffy S, Rosner MH: Natriuretic peptides in ESRD. Am J Kidney Dis 2005;46:1-10.

228. Deegan PM, Ryan MP, Basinger MA, et al: Protection from cisplatin nephrotoxicity by A68828, an atrial natriuretic peptide. Ren Fail 1995;17:117-123.

229. Allgren RL, Marbury TC, Rahman SN, et al: Anaritide in acute tubular necrosis. Auriculin Anaritide Acute Renal Failure Study Group [see comments]. N Engl J Med 1997;336:828-834.

230. Lewis J, Salem MM, Chertow GM, et al: Atrial natriuretic factor in oliguric acute renal failure. Anaritide Acute Renal Failure Study Group. Am J Kidney Dis 2000;36:767-774.

231. Meyer M, Wiebe K, Wahlers T, et al: Urodilatin (INN: ularitide) as a new drug for the therapy of acute renal failure following cardiac surgery. Clin Exp Pharmacol Physiol 1997;24:374-376.

232. Brenner P, Meyer M, Reichenspurner H, et al: Significance of prophylactic urodilatin (INN: ularitide) infusion for the prevention of acute renal failure in patients after heart transplantation. Eur J Med Res 1995;1:137-143.

233. Kuse ER, Meyer M, Constantin R, et al: Urodilatin (INN: ularitide): A new peptide in the treatment of acute kidney failure following liver transplantation. Anaesthesist 1996;45:351-358.

234. Meyer M, Pfarr E, Schirmer G, et al: Therapeutic use of the natriuretic peptide ularitide in acute renal failure. Ren Fail 1999;21:85-100.

235. Samuels LE, Holmes EC, Lee L: Nesiritide as an adjunctive therapy in adult patients with heart failure undergoing high-risk cardiac surgery. J Thorac Cardiovasc Surg 2004;128:627-629.

236. Sackner-Bernstein JD, Skopicki HA, Aaronson KD: Risk of worsening renal function with nesiritide in patients with acutely decompensated heart failure. Circulation 2005;111:1487-1491.

237. Teerlink JR, Massie BM: Nesiritide and worsening of renal function: The emperor's new clothes? Circulation 2005;111:1459-1461.

238. Tsao CM, Ho ST, Chen A, et al: Low-dose dexamethasone ameliorates circulatory failure and renal dysfunction in conscious rats with endotoxemia. Shock 2004;21:484-491.

239. Loef BG, Henning RH, Epema AH, et al: Effect of dexamethasone on perioperative renal function impairment during cardiac surgery with cardiopulmonary bypass. Br J Anaesth 2004;93:793-798.

240. Mangano DT: Aspirin and mortality from coronary bypass surgery. N Engl J Med 2002;347:1309-1317.

241. Lee A, Cooper MC, Craig JC, et al: Effects of nonsteroidal anti-inflammatory drugs on postoperative renal function in adults with normal renal function. Cochrane Database Syst Rev 2004:CD002765.

242. Ott E, Nussmeier NA, Duke PC, et al: Efficacy and safety of the cyclooxygenase 2 inhibitors parecoxib and valdecoxib in patients undergoing coronary artery bypass surgery. J Thorac Cardiovasc Surg 2003;125:1481-1492.

243. Nussmeier NA, Whelton AA, Brown MT, et al: Complications of the COX-2 inhibitors parecoxib and valdecoxib after cardiac surgery. N Engl J Med 2005;352:1081-1091.

244. Gullans SR: Metabolic basis of solute transport. In Brenner BM (ed): Brenner & Rector's The Kidney, ed 6. Philadelphia, Saunders, 2000, pp 215-246.

245. Baines A, Ho P: Glucose stimulates O_2 consumption, NOS, and Na/H exchange in diabetic rat proximal tubules. Am J Physiol Renal Physiol 2002;283:F286-293.

246. Melin J, Hellberg O, Larsson E, et al: Protective effect of insulin on ischemic renal injury in diabetes mellitus. Kidney Int 2002;61:1383-1392.

247. Anderson RE, Klerdal K, Ivert T, et al: Are even impaired fasting blood glucose levels preoperatively associated with increased mortality after CABG surgery? Eur Heart J 2005;26:1513-1518.

248. Doenst T, Wijeysundera D, Karkouti K, et al: Hyperglycemia during cardiopulmonary bypass is an independent risk factor for mortality in patients undergoing cardiac surgery. J Thorac Cardiovasc Surg 2005; 130:1144.

249. Gandhi GY, Nuttall GA, Abel MD, et al: Intraoperative hyperglycemia and perioperative outcomes in cardiac surgery patients. Mayo Clin Proc 2005;80:862-866.

250. Ouattara A, Lecomte P, Le Manach Y, et al: Poor intraoperative blood glucose control is associated with a worsened hospital outcome after cardiac surgery in diabetic patients. Anesthesiology 2005;103:687-694.

251. Van den Berghe GH: Role of intravenous insulin therapy in critically ill patients. Endocr Pract 2004;10(Suppl 2):17-20.

252. Van den Berghe G: How does blood glucose control with insulin save lives in intensive care? J Clin Invest 2004;114:1187-1195.

253. Visser L, Zuurbier CJ, Hoek FJ, et al: Glucose, insulin and potassium applied as perioperative hyperinsulinaemic normoglycaemic clamp: Effects on inflammatory response during coronary artery surgery. Br J Anaesth 2005;95:448-457.

254. Hoffmann U, Fischereder M, Kruger B, et al: The value of N-acetylcysteine in the prevention of radiocontrast agent-induced nephropathy seems questionable. J Am Soc Nephrol 2004;15:407-410.

255. Kshirsagar AV, Poole C, Mottl A, et al: N-acetylcysteine for the prevention of radiocontrast induced nephropathy: A meta-analysis of prospective controlled trials. J Am Soc Nephrol 2004;15:761-769.

256. Pannu N, Manns B, Lee HH, Tonelli M: Systematic review of the impact of N-acetylcysteine on contrast nephropathy. Kidney Int 2004;65:1366-1374.

257. Alonso A, Lau J, Jaber BL, et al: Prevention of radiocontrast nephropathy with N-acetylcysteine in patients with chronic kidney disease: A meta-analysis of randomized, controlled trials. Am J Kidney Dis 2004;43:1-9.

258. Kretzschmar M, Klein U, Palutke M, Schirrmeister W: Reduction of ischemia-reperfusion syndrome after abdominal aortic aneurysmectomy by N-acetylcysteine but not mannitol. Acta Anaesthesiol Scand 1996;40:657-664.

259. Cote G, Denault A, Belisle S, et al: N-acetylcysteine in the preservation of renal function in patients undergoing cardiac surgery. ASA Annual Meeting Abstracts 2003;99(3A):A420.

260. Burns KE, Chu MW, Novick RJ, et al: Perioperative N-acetylcysteine to prevent renal dysfunction in high-risk patients undergoing CABG surgery: A randomized controlled trial. JAMA 2005;294:342-350.

261. Solez K, Ideura T, Silvia CB, et al: Clonidine after renal ischemia to lessen acute renal failure and microvascular damage. Kidney Int 1980;18:309-322.

262. Ideura T, Solez K, Heptinstall RH: The effect of clonidine on tubular obstruction in postischemic acute renal failure in the rabbit demonstrated by microradiography and microdissection. Am J Pathol 1980;98:123-150.

263. Eknoyan G, Dobyan DC, Senekjian HO, Bulger RE: Protective effect of oral clonidine in the prophylaxis and therapy of mercuric chloride: Induced acute renal failure in the rat. J Lab Clin Med 1983;102:699-713.

264. Eknoyan G, Bulger RE, Dobyan DC: Mercuric chloride-induced acute renal failure in the rat: I. Correlation of functional and morphologic changes and their modification by clonidine. Lab Invest 1982;46:613-620.

265. Zou AP, Cowley AW Jr: Alpha-adrenergic receptor-mediated increase in NO production buffers renal medullary vasoconstriction. Am J Physiol Regul Integr Comp Physiol 2000;279:R769-777.

266. Kulka PJ, Tryba M, Zenz M: Preoperative alpha2-adrenergic receptor agonists prevent the deterioration of renal function after cardiac surgery: Results of a randomized, controlled trial. Crit Care Med 1996;24:947-952.

267. Myles PS, Hunt JO, Holdgaard HO, et al: Clonidine and cardiac surgery: Haemodynamic and metabolic effects, myocardial ischaemia and recovery. Anaesth Intensive Care 1999;27:137-147.

268. Wijeysundera DN, Naik JS, Beattie WS: Alpha-2 adrenergic agonists to prevent perioperative cardiovascular complications: A meta-analysis. Am J Med 2003;114:742-752.

269. Fisher M, Grotta J: New uses for calcium channel blockers: Therapeutic implications. Drugs 1993;46:961-975.

270. Schramm L, Heidbreder E, Kartenbender K, et al: Effects of urodilatin and diltiazem on renal function in ischemic acute renal failure in the rat. Am J Nephrol 1995;15:418-426.

271. Schramm L, Heidbreder E, Lukes M, et al: Endotoxin-induced acute renal failure in the rat: Effects of urodilatin and diltiazem on renal function. Clin Nephrol 1996;46:117-124.

272. Zanardo G, Michielon P, Rosi P, et al: Effects of a continuous diltiazem infusion on renal function during cardiac surgery. J Cardiothorac Vasc Anesth 1993;7:711-716.

273. Bergman AS, Odar-Cederlof I, Westman L, et al: Diltiazem infusion for renal protection in cardiac surgical patients with preexisting renal dysfunction. J Cardiothorac Vasc Anesth 2002;16:294-299.

274. Bertolissi M, Antonucci F, De Monte A, et al: Effects on renal function of a continuous infusion of nifedipine during cardiopulmonary bypass. J Cardiothorac Vasc Anesth 1996;10:238-242.

275. Wijeysundera DN, Beattie WS, Rao V, Karski J: Calcium antagonists reduce cardiovascular complications after cardiac surgery: A meta-analysis. J Am Coll Cardiol 2003;41:1496-1505.

276. Amano J, Suzuki A, Sunamori M, Tofukuji M: Effect of calcium antagonist diltiazem on renal function in open heart surgery. Chest 1995;107:1260-1265.

277. Donmez A, Ergun F, Kayhan Z, et al: Verapamil and nimodipine do not improve renal function during cardiopulmonary bypass. Acta Anaesthesiol Ital 1998;49:173-177.

278. Petry A, Wulf H, Blomer U, Wawersik J: Nifedipine versus nitroglycerin in aortocoronary bypass surgery: The effect on hemodynamics, kidney function and homologous blood requirement. Anaesthesist 1992;41:39-46.

279. Wijeysundera DN, Beattie WS: Calcium channel blockers for reducing cardiac morbidity after noncardiac surgery: A meta-analysis. Anesth Analg 2003;97:634-641.

280. Welch WJ, Wilcox CS: AT1 receptor antagonist combats oxidative stress and restores nitric oxide signaling in the SHR. Kidney Int 2001;59:1257-1263.

281. Kitagawa S, Komatsu Y, Futatsuyama M, et al: Renoprotection of ACE inhibitor and angiotensin II receptor blocker for the patients with severe renal insufficiency. Nephrology 2003;8(Suppl):A26-27.

282. Manche A, Galea J, Busuttil W: Tolerance to ACE inhibitors after cardiac surgery. Eur J Cardiothorac Surg 1999;15:55-60.

283. Rady MY, Ryan T: The effects of preoperative therapy with angiotensin-converting enzyme inhibitors on clinical outcome after cardiovascular surgery. Chest 1998;114:487-494.

284. Macris MP, Ford EG, Van Buren CT, Frazier OH: Predictors of severe renal dysfunction after heart transplantation and intravenous cyclosporine therapy. J Heart Transplant 1989;8:444-448; discussion 449.

285. Colson P, Ribstein J, Mimran A, et al: Effect of angiotensin converting enzyme inhibition on blood pressure and renal function during open heart surgery. Anesthesiology 1990;72:23-27.

286. Ryckwaert F, Colson P, Ribstein J, et al: Haemodynamic and renal effects of intravenous enalaprilat during coronary artery bypass graft surgery in patients with ischaemic heart dysfunction. Br J Anaesth 2001;86:169-175.

287. Rutkowski P, Tylicki L, Renke M, et al: Low-dose dual blockade of the renin-angiotensin system in patients with primary glomerulonephritis. Am J Kidney Dis 2004;43:260-268.

288. Modlinger PS, Welch WJ: Adenosine A1 receptor antagonists and the kidney. Curr Opin Nephrol Hypertens 2003;12:497-502.

289. Abizaid AS, Clark CE, Mintz GS, et al: Effects of dopamine and aminophylline on contrast-induced acute renal failure after coronary angioplasty in patients with preexisting renal insufficiency. Am J Cardiol 1999;83:260-263, A5.

290. Benigni A: Defining the role of endothelins in renal pathophysiology on the basis of selective and unselective endothelin receptor antagonist studies. Curr Opin Nephrol Hypertens 1995;4:349-353.

291. Wilhelm SM, Stowe NT, Robinson AV, Schulak JA: The use of the endothelin receptor antagonist, tezosentan, before or after renal ischemia protects renal function. Transplantation 2001;71:211-216.

292. Knoll T, Schult S, Birck R, et al: Therapeutic administration of an endothelin-A receptor antagonist after acute ischemic renal failure dose-dependently improves recovery of renal function. J Cardiovasc Pharmacol 2001;37:483-488.

293. Mitaka C, Hirata Y, Yokoyama K, et al: Improvement of renal dysfunction in dogs with endotoxemia by a nonselective endothelin receptor antagonist. Crit Care Med 1999;27:146-153.

294. Chin A, Radhakrishnan J, Fornell L, John E: Effects of tezosentan, a dual endothelin receptor antagonist, on the cardiovascular and renal systems of neonatal piglets during endotoxic shock. J Pediatr Surg 2002;37:482-487.

295. Anand R, Harry D, Holt S, et al: Endothelin is an important determinant of renal function in a rat model of acute liver and renal failure. Gut 2002;50:111-117.

296. Forbes JM, Hewitson TD, Becker GJ, Jones CL: Simultaneous blockade of endothelin A and B receptors in ischemic acute renal failure is detrimental to long-term kidney function. Kidney Int 2001;59: 1333-1341.

297. Wang A, Holcslaw T, Bashore TM, et al: Exacerbation of radiocontrast nephrotoxicity by endothelin receptor antagonism. Kidney Int 2000;57:1675-1680.

298. Chatterjee PK: Pleiotropic renal actions of erythropoietin. Lancet 2005;365:1890-1892.

299. Hirschberg R, Kopple J, Lipsett P, et al: Multicenter clinical trial of recombinant human insulin-like growth factor I in patients with acute renal failure. Kidney Int 1999;55:2423-2432.

300. Hladunewich MA, Corrigan G, Derby GC, et al: A randomized, placebo-controlled trial of IGF-1 for delayed graft function: A human model to study postischemic ARF. Kidney Int 2003;64:593-602.

301. Zhou X, Ono H, Ono Y, Frohlich ED: Renoprotective effects of omapatrilat are mediated partially by bradykinin. Am J Nephrol 2003;23:214-221.

302. Kostis JB, Packer M, Black HR, et al: Omapatrilat and enalapril in patients with hypertension: The Omapatrilat Cardiovascular Treatment vs. Enalapril (OCTAVE) trial. Am J Hypertens 2004;17: 103-111.

303. Kim YK, Yoo JH, Woo JS, et al: Effect of pentoxifylline on ischemic acute renal failure in rabbits. Ren Fail 2001;23:757-772.

304. Kim YK, Choi TR, Kwon CH, et al: Beneficial effect of pentoxifylline on cisplatin-induced acute renal failure in rabbits. Ren Fail 2003;25: 909-922.

305. Boldt J, Brosch C, Piper SN, et al: Influence of prophylactic use of pentoxifylline on postoperative organ function in elderly cardiac surgery patients. Crit Care Med 2001;29:952-958.

306. Abe K, Fujino Y, Sakakibara T: The effect of prostaglandin E_1 during cardiopulmonary bypass on renal function after cardiac surgery. Eur J Clin Pharmacol 1993;45:217-220.

307. Levey AS, Bosch JP, Lewis JB, et al: A more accurate method to estimate glomerular filtration rate from serum creatinine: A new prediction equation. Modification of Diet in Renal Disease Study Group. Ann Intern Med 1999;130:461-470.

Chapter

18 Treatment of Acute Oliguria

Ramesh Verhataraman and John A. Kellum

Oliguria is a one of the most common clinical problems encountered by patients perioperatively. The prevalence of the problem has been difficult to establish because of a wide variety of definitions used in the literature. Some studies have estimated that up to 18% of intensive care unit (ICU) patients with intact renal function exhibit episodes of oliguria.[1] Furthermore, 69% of ICU patients who develop acute renal failure (ARF) are oliguric.[2] Early recognition, evaluation, and treatment of oliguria can often halt the progression to ARF. Overall, ARF in the ICU has a poor prognosis (mortality rates range from 30% to 70%), and oliguric ARF is associated with a worse outcome than nonoliguric ARF. Preventing ARF by effective management of oliguria has the potential to significantly alter outcome, and there is now clear evidence that ARF is associated with excess mortality even in the absence of the need for renal replacement therapy (RRT).[3-5] Thus, it is essential to understand the physiologic derangements leading to this exceedingly common problem. The goal of this chapter is to provide both a physiologic background and a practical clinical approach to evaluate and treat oliguria.

Although numerous definitions for oliguria exist, most use a urine output of less than 200 to 500 mL in 24 hours to denote oliguria, whereas urine output of less than 50 to 100 mL/day is generally termed anuria. To standardize the use of the term across different studies and populations, the Acute Dialysis Quality Initiative (ADQI) recently adopted a definition of oliguria as urine output less than 0.3 mL/kg/hr for at least 24 hours (see www.ADQI.net). However, early clinical recognition of oliguria requires a more rapid assessment than can be achieved with a 24-hour measurement. Thus, oliguria should be suspected when the urine flow rate is less than 0.5 mL/kg/hr for 2 consecutive hours.

■ ETIOLOGY

Urine output is a function of the glomerular filtration rate (GFR) and of tubular secretion and reabsorption. GFR is directly dependent on renal perfusion. Therefore, oliguria generally indicates either a dramatic reduction in GFR or a mechanical obstruction to urine flow (Box 18-1).

Prerenal Oliguria

When the cause of oliguria is primarily impaired renal perfusion, it is termed prerenal oliguria. Renal perfusion is a function of circulating volume, cardiac output, mean arterial pressure, and renal vascular resistance. Hence, prerenal oliguria commonly occurs as the result of an absolute or a relative decrease in circulating volume. An absolute decrease in circulating volume can be caused by hemorrhage of fluid

sequestration after surgery. A relative decrease in circulating volume can be caused by an increase in the capacitance of the vasculature that results from vasodilatation (e.g., as a result of sepsis). Decreased renal perfusion and oliguria are commonly a manifestation of impaired cardiac output (e.g., cardiogenic shock, cardiac tamponade). Finally, other less common causes of decreased renal perfusion and oliguria include structural causes, such as thromboembolism, dissection, inflammation (vasculitis, especially scleroderma), affecting either the intrarenal or extrarenal circulation. Renal atheroemboli (usually caused by cholesterol emboli) usually affect older patients with a diffuse erosive atherosclerotic disease. This condition is most often seen after manipulation of the aorta or other large arteries during arteriography, angioplasty, or surgery.[6] This condition may also occur spontaneously or after treatment with heparin, warfarin, or thrombolytic agents.

Rarely, decreased renal perfusion may occur as a result of an outflow problem such as renal vein thrombosis or abdominal compartment syndrome (ACS). ACS is a rare but serious and reversible cause of oliguria and ARF that is often overlooked. It is defined as organ dysfunction that results from an increase in intra-abdominal pressure. ACS can be seen in a wide variety of medical and surgical conditions, most often after major abdominal operations requiring administration of a large volume of fluid (e.g., ruptured abdominal aortic aneurysm repair), emergent laparotomies with tight abdominal wall closures, and abdominal-wall burns with edema. ACS leads to acute oliguria and ARF mainly via increasing renal outflow pressure, and thus it indirectly reduces renal perfusion. Other possible mechanisms for ARF include direct parenchymal compression and renin-mediated arterial vasoconstriction. However, emerging evidence suggests that the rise in renal venous pressure, rather than the direct effect of parenchymal compression, is the primary mechanism of renal dysfunction. Generally, these changes occur in direct response to the increase in intra-abdominal pressure, with oliguria developing at a pressure of greater than 15 mm Hg, and anuria at a pressure of greater than 30 mm Hg.[7,8]

Intrarenal Oliguria

The most common cause of intrarenal oliguria in the ICU is acute tubular necrosis (ATN), which is usually caused by an ischemic or nephrotoxic insult. Although ischemic ATN is often a result of untreated prerenal factors, nephrotoxic ATN occurs as a consequence of the direct nephrotoxicity of agents such as antibiotics, heavy metals, solvents, contrast agents, and crystals (uric acid or oxalate). Uncommonly, drugs (e.g.,

18-1	**Causes of Oliguria**

Prerenal Oliguria

1. Decreased renal perfusion
   a. Decreased intravascular volume: bleeding, gastrointestinal losses, third-spacing
   b. Decreased cardiac output: cardiogenic shock, cardiac tamponade
   c. Decreased renal perfusion pressure: sepsis, drugs
2. Increased renal outflow pressure: abdominal compartment syndrome

Intrarenal Oliguria

1. Ischemic acute tubular necrosis: hypotension, untreated prerenal oliguria
2. Nephrotoxic acute tubular necrosis: drugs (vancomycin, aminoglycosides), contrast media, rhabdomyolysis
3. Acute interstitial nephritis: nafcillin, furosemide

Postrenal Oliguria

1. Urinary obstruction: bilateral renal calculus, prostate enlargement, Foley catheter obstruction

nafcillin, sulfamethoxazole-trimethoprim, furosemide) can cause an acute interstitial nephritis leading to intrarenal oliguria and ARF.

Postrenal Oliguria

Oliguria secondary to mechanical obstruction distal to the kidneys is termed postrenal oliguria. This problem can result from tubular-ureteral obstruction (caused by stones, papillary sloughing, crystals, or pigment), urethral or bladder neck obstruction (secondary to prostatic enlargement), or simply a malpositioned or obstructed urinary catheter. Rarely, urine volume can be increased in cases of partial obstruction due to pressure-mediated impairment of urine concentration.

■ EVALUATION OF PATIENTS WITH OLIGURIA

Oliguria is an early manifestation of either impaired renal function or reduced renal perfusion. If the underlying cause of oliguria is not corrected, ARF usually results. However, merely reversing oliguria, particularly by administering diuretic agents, does not improve outcome and may even worsen injury. Thus, it is essential to determine the cause of the oliguria and correct it rapidly. Empiric treatment or "shotgun" therapy with both fluid and diuretics (which can be said to fix the chart while neglecting the patient) is no substitute for making a diagnosis and prescribing specific therapy.

Instead, an early evaluation of a patient with oliguria includes focused history taking, chart review, and clinical examination. Supplementary urine testing, including examining the urinary sediment and measuring urinary electrolytes, may assist in the diagnosis. However, it is important to be alert to the possibility that oliguria may be postrenal, as identification and correction of this cause can be rapidly rewarding and avoids wasting time with ineffectual testing and interventions. Hence, it is worthwhile to rule out urinary

obstruction as a cause of oliguria prior to embarking on any further workup.

Postrenal Oliguria

In the non-ICU setting, a prior history of prostatic hypertrophy, recent spinal anesthesia, bladder discomfort, and renal colic may provide some clues to the presence of distal obstruction. History of trauma and blood at the urethral meatus along with perineal ecchymoses and a "high-riding" prostate can suggest the diagnosis of urethral disruption. A rapid increase in serum blood urea nitrogen (BUN) concentration and creatinine concentration (especially a doubling every 24 hours) also suggests a diagnosis of urinary obstruction. The urine sediment in postrenal failure is often bland without casts or sediments. Renal ultrasonography is usually the test of choice to exclude urinary tract obstruction.[9] This test is noninvasive, and it can be performed at the bedside. It carries the advantage of avoiding the potential allergic and toxic complications of radiocontrast media. However, under some circumstances, renal ultrasound may not yield good results. For example, in early obstruction or in obstruction associated with severe dehydration, hydronephrosis may not be seen on the initial ultrasound, although it may appear on a subsequent study. Computed tomographic scanning should be considered if the ultrasound results are equivocal or if the kidneys are not well visualized, or if the cause of the obstruction cannot be identified. In the ICU setting, distal obstruction appearing as oliguria is commonly caused by obstruction of the urinary catheter (especially in male patients). Hence, in patients with new-onset oliguria, the urinary catheter must be flushed or changed to rule out obstruction. Early diagnosis of urinary tract obstruction is important, as many cases can be corrected and a delay in therapy can lead to renal injury.

Prerenal versus Intrarenal Oliguria

History

In 50% to 90% of oliguric patients the cause is prerenal, and initial interventions should be conducted presuming this to be the case. A careful, targeted chart review and clinical examination can help differentiate prerenal from intrarenal causes of oliguria. Evidence of ongoing bleeding, perioperative fluid losses or deficits (e.g., gastric/ileostomy losses or vomiting), or extravascular fluid sequestration can lead to intravascular volume depletion and point to a prerenal cause. Cardiac examination should be performed and an electrocardiogram obtained to look for changes consistent with myocardial infarction and impaired cardiac output as a cause of oliguria. Fever, increased white cell count, and a wide pulse pressure indicate sepsis-induced vasodilatation, leading to impaired renal perfusion and relative hypovolemia. A history of perioperative contrast administration for imaging, of intraoperative hypotension, or of administration of nephrotoxic agents can suggest an intrarenal cause of oliguria in an adequately volume-resuscitated patient.

Clinical Parameters

Traditional indicators of hydration status and tissue perfusion, such as systemic blood pressure, heart rate, capillary refill, jugular-venous pulsation, and peripheral edema can provide guidance for making appropriate interventions. In the ICU, hemodynamic monitoring (measurements of central venous pressure [CVP], pulmonary artery occlusion pressure [PAOP], or mixed venous oxygen saturation) can provide important clues for differentiating prerenal from intrarenal oliguria. Mixed venous oxygen saturation is an indirect indication of cardiac output. Recently, Rivers and colleagues showed that this parameter is a valuable guide to targeted early resuscitation in patients with sepsis.[10]

However, many of these traditional measures may be unreliable in the critically ill patient. The jugular-venous pulsation is not an accurate surrogate for right ventricular filling pressures in the presence of positive-pressure ventilation and positive end-expiratory pressure (PEEP). Similarly, peripheral edema is often caused by hypoalbuminemia and decreased oncotic pressure in critically ill patients. Thus, patients may exhibit total-body water overload and yet be intravascularly volume depleted. In addition, blood pressure and heart rate are affected by numerous physiologic and treatment variables in the ICU and are unreliable measures of volume status. In the ICU, increased CVP or PAOP does not ensure adequate preload. The presence of a cardiac index greater than 3.0 L/min/m² generally suggests *adequate* preload, but it may not reflect *optimal* preload. Echocardiography may provide useful information to judge fluid optimization, and an arterial pulse pressure variation of greater than 13% in a patient who is not breathing spontaneously and who is on positive-pressure ventilation is highly predictive of fluid responsiveness (reflecting the likelihood that a fluid challenge will increase cardiac output). However, a fluid challenge (of 250 to 500 mL) is necessary to determine if further increases in preload will augment cardiac output.

Finally, ACS should be suspected in any patient with a tensely distended abdomen, progressive oliguria, and an increased airway pressure (transmitted across the diaphragm). The mainstay of the diagnosis is measurement of intra-abdominal pressure. The most common measure of intra-abdominal pressure is by bladder pressure, which is easily accessible. Sterile saline (50 o 100 mL) is infused into the bladder through an indwelling catheter, and the intravesical pressure is measured using a pressure transducer. Bladder pressure has been shown to correlate well with intra-abdominal pressure over a wide range of pressures. Decompression of the abdomen with laparotomy, sometimes requiring that the abdomen be left open for a time, is the only definitive treatment for ACS.

Laboratory Parameters

Although the yield may be low, examining the urine sediment may provide some important insight into the cause of oliguria. Although hyaline and fine granular casts are common in prerenal disease, acute tubular necrosis is usually associated with coarse granular casts and tubular epithelial casts. However, the discriminating ability of these findings is limited. The main usefulness of examining the urine sediment is for detecting red cell casts, which indicate glomerular disease (rare in the ICU setting). Urine eosinophilia, if

18-1	Urine Indices Useful for Distinguishing Prerenal from Intrarenal Oliguria	
	Prerenal	**Renal**
Osmolality of urine (mOsm/kg)	>500	<400
Urine Na (mmol/L or mEq/L)	<20	>40
FE_{Na} (%)*	<1	>2
FE_{urea} (%)†	<35	>35

*[(Urine Na ÷ serum Na)/(Urine creatinine ÷ serum creatinine)] × 100.
†(Urine$_{urea}$ ÷ serum$_{urea}$)/(Urine$_{cr}$ ÷ serum$_{cr}$) × 100.
FE_{Na}, fractional excretion of sodium; FE_{urea}, fractional excretion of urea.

present, although nonspecific, may point to the diagnosis of acute interstitial nephritis or atheroembolic etiology of oliguria.

Urine sodium and urea concentrations can be of value in differentiating prerenal from intrarenal causes of oliguria (Table 18-1). However, a fractional excretion of sodium (FE_{Na}) is more accurate, and a value of less than 1% has traditionally been used as a marker for a prerenal cause of oliguria, whereas a value of greater than 1% generally suggests an intrarenal cause. Importantly, conditions such as rhabdomyolysis, contrast nephropathy, and sepsis are all causes of intrarenal ARF in which FE_{Na} can be low.[11] Furthermore, these indices are unreliable once the patient has received diuretic or natriuretic agents (including dopamine and mannitol) and may also be confounded by endogenous osmolar substances such as glucose or urea. In patients who have received diuretics, fractional excretion of urea (FE_{urea}) may be useful to differentiate prerenal from intrarenal causes of oliguria. The FE_{urea} is 50% to 65% in normal subjects and usually below 35% in those with prerenal disease. A recent study concluded that low FE_{urea} (≤35%) was a more sensitive and specific index than FE_{Na} in differentiating ARF caused by prerenal azotemia from ARF caused by ATN, especially if diuretics were administered.[12]

■ TREATMENT

A good rule is, Don't just do something; stand there. Telephone orders from the on-call room for fluids and then for diuretics, or for both at the same time, are far too common an occurrence in modern ICUs, and such practices are inherently dangerous. Oliguria is a clinical sign, not a diagnosis. There is no therapy for oliguria; there are only treatments for conditions that cause it. Augmenting urine output with forced dieresis only masks the problem. Always evaluate first and treat the underlying cause of oliguria, not the urine output.

Prerenal Oliguria

The mainstay of treatment of prerenal oliguria is rapid restoration of renal perfusion. The precipitating factors must be identified and corrected early, and supportive measures such as avoidance of nephrotoxic agents must be taken, along with efforts to restore renal perfusion. Renal perfusion can be restored by aggressive correction of hypotension and hypovolemia. Autoregulatory mechanisms that maintain GFR despite fluctuations in mean arterial pressure (MAP) are disrupted in patients with sepsis or other causes of ischemic

ATN. Hence, in these patients, renal perfusion is directly related to systemic arterial pressure. Therefore, rapid correction of hypotension with fluid resuscitation and often with vasoactive drugs is required. Similarly, in patients with chronic hypertension and renal vascular disease, the autoregulation curves are shifted to the right and therefore a higher MAP may be required to ensure adequate renal perfusion. Vasoactive drugs should be initiated only after ensuring adequate intravascular volume. In critically ill patients, vasoactive drugs may be initiated concurrently with volume expansion. Vasoactive drugs, once initiated, should be titrated to maintain adequate renal perfusion pressures. The ideal blood pressure to aim for in patients with oliguria must be individualized on the basis of factors such as premorbid blood pressure or presence of vascular disease. Hemodynamic monitoring devices may provide important information to guide assessment of intravascular volume status and may enable a more streamlined, goal-directed approach to therapy (Fig. 18-1). Some patients may have impaired cardiac contractility despite adequate intravascular volume. These patients may require treatment with an inotrope to improve renal perfusion. Finally, if ACS is diagnosed, prompt opera-

tive decompression of the abdominal cavity with maintenance of an open abdomen through use of temporary abdominal wall closure techniques should be considered to improve renal perfusion.

Low-dose dopamine (<5 μg/kg/min) has been used for decades as therapy to augment renal perfusion in patients with oliguric renal failure. Dopamine increases urine output also because it is a natriuretic agent mediated by inhibition of Na^+,K^+-ATPase at the tubular epithelial cell level[13] and not merely by increasing renal perfusion. There is abundant evidence that low-dose dopamine does not afford any renal protection in oliguria. One multicenter randomized controlled trial and two comprehensive meta-analyses of dopamine in critically ill patients have shown that dopamine does not prevent the onset of ARF, decrease mortality, or reduce the need for dialysis.[14-16]

Fenoldopam mesylate, a dopamine-1 receptor agonist, has been shown, like dopamine, to increase renal blood flow in animal studies and small clinical trials, and, hence, has been evaluated to improve renal perfusion and prevent ARF. A recent placebo-controlled, multicenter trial randomized 315 patients with baseline creatinine clearance less than

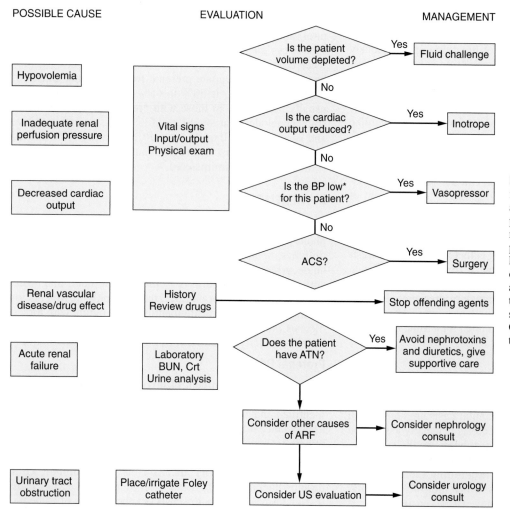

Figure 18-1 ■ An algorithm for the treatment of a patient with acute oliguria. *Note that blood pressure may be within normal range but still be low for a given patient if there is a history of hypertension. ACS, abdominal compartment syndrome; ARF, acute renal failure; ATN, acute tubular necrosis; BP, blood pressure; BUN, blood urea nitrogen; Crt, serum creatinine concentration; US, ultrasound.

60 mL/min to fenoldopam mesylate or placebo[17] and found no difference between the groups in the incidence of contrast nephropathy. Furthermore, fenoldopam mesylate has been shown to cause hypotension and therefore can predispose patients to ARF by reducing renal perfusion pressure.[18] On the basis of these data, we strongly recommend against the use of dopamine and fenoldopam to augment renal perfusion in patients with oliguria.

Intrarenal Oliguria

Continued maintenance of adequate intravascular volume, maintenance of an adequate MAP, and avoidance of nephrotoxic agents are the only interventions shown to impact outcome once intrarenal oliguria (i.e., ARF) occurs. The use of diuretic agents in oliguric renal failure is widespread despite the convincing lack of evidence supporting efficacy. Traditionally, diuretics have been used in the early phases of oliguria in an attempt to convert oliguric ARF to nonoliguric ARF. Presumably, the absence of oliguria makes it easier to regulate volume status, and given that nonoliguric renal failure generally has a better prognosis, clinicians frequently use diuretics in this setting. Many small trials have evaluated the efficacy of loop diuretics in preventing ARF and have provided inconsistent results. One systematic review compared fluids alone with diuretics in people at risk for ARF from various causes. This study failed to show any benefit from diuretics with regard to incidence of ARF, the need for dialysis, or mortality.[19] More recently, two large observational studies have been published. The first was a cohort study (th PICARD study) of patients with ARF in the ICU, in which patients were characterized by the use of diuretics on or before the day of renal consultation.[20] In this study, with adjustments for relevant covariates and propensity scores, diuretic use was associated with significantly increased risk for death or nonrecovery of renal function (odds ratio [OR], 1.77; 95% confidence interval, 1.14-2.76). Although this association does not establish a causal link between diuretic use and harm in the setting of oliguric ARF, it does suggest that this therapy does not afford any benefit to the kidney. Subsequently, a recent multinational observational study of 1743 patients evaluated the effect of loop diuretics on clinical outcomes.[21] The study investigators created three multivariate models to assess the relationship between diuretics and mortality and found that diuretic use was not significantly associated with increased mortality in any of the three models (OR for death was about 1.2 in all three models). However, no benefit was seen, either. On the basis of the current evidence, we suggest that diuretics should be avoided when possible. In other words, diuretics are *never* a treatment for oliguria but may be necessary to manage volume overload.

The natriuretic peptides are another class of drugs used to improve urine output in oliguric patients. These peptides cause natriuresis by both inhibiting tubular sodium reabsorption and improving GFR. In one large randomized controlled trial, 504 patients with early renal dysfunction were randomized to placebo or to 24-hour infusion of anaritide at a dose of 200 ng/kg/min.[22] In this study, there were no differences between the groups in the dialysis-free survival at 21 days

(primary endpoint), need for dialysis, or mortality. However, prospectively defined subgroup analysis suggested that oliguric patients (<400 mL urine/day) had improved dialysis-free survival ($P = .008$) in comparison with the placebo group. Nonoliguric patients had worse dialysis-free survival with anaritide than without it ($P = .03$). This worsening in outcome in nonoliguric patients was thought to be caused by the hypotensive effects of anaritide (46% incidence of hypotension in anaritide group versus 18% in the placebo group). On the basis of these findings, a subsequent randomized controlled trial was performed on patients with oliguric ARF using the same dose of anaritide.[23] This study was terminated after an interim analysis showed no benefit with anaritide. However, more patients in the anaritide group developed significant hypotension (systolic blood pressures <90 mm Hg) than in the placebo group during the drug infusion (95% versus 55%, respectively; $P < .001$).

However, a recent randomized controlled trial studied 61 patients with normal preoperative renal function who had cardiac surgery requiring bypass. When the patients' serum creatinine increased by 50% from baseline, they were randomized to small doses of human recombinant atrial natriuretic peptide (rh-ANP) (50 ng/kg/min) administered by continuous intravenous infusion, or to placebo.[24] In this study, 21% of the patients in the rh-ANP group required dialysis by 21 days compared with 47% of the patients in the placebo group. This small study differed significantly from the previous negative studies in that the patient group was more homogeneous, a smaller dose of natriuretic peptide was used, and the infusion duration was longer. However, this study also has several limitations, including small patient population and baseline differences between the two groups. Hence, larger studies using this dose in cardiac surgical patients are necessary prior to routine use of this drug for prevention of ARF.

A class of drugs similar to ANP is the human B-type natriuretic peptides (hBNP). Nesiritide, the first member of this new drug class, is manufactured using recombinant DNA technology. It is approved by the U.S. Food and Drug Administration for use in patients with advanced congestive heart failure. Nesiritide, like anaritide, induces natriuresis by inhibiting the tubular reabsorption of sodium. It is being used in patients with congestive heart failure both to improve cardiac output and to improve renal function. However, studies have shown that nesiritide can adversely affect outcomes by causing hypotension and impairing renal function. On the basis of this evidence, a recent expert panel that was convened at the request of the company marketing nesiritide reviewed the existing literature. The panel concluded that "use of nesiritide was associated with a dose-dependent increase in serum creatinine indicating renal dysfunction at doses described in the package insert (0.01 to 0.03 µg/kg/min), including the dose recommended for initiation of treatment (0.01 µg/kg/min)." The panel also recommended that nesiritide should not be used to improve renal function or enhance diuresis. In summary, although most natriuretic peptides augment urine output, they cause significant hypotension, thereby worsening renal function. Hence, these peptides should not be used for the purpose of improving renal function or enhancing diuresis.

Finally, oliguric patients with fluid overload should be considered for early dialysis. Although there is little dispute about the necessity of renal replacement therapy for the treatment of fluid overload refractory to diuretic therapy, there is no consensus on the degree of azotemia or duration of renal failure warranting initiation of therapy in the absence of this absolute indication. Intuitively, the earlier an intervention is provided, the better the outcome will be. One retrospective study, which used serum BUN concentration as a surrogate for timing the initiation of dialysis in patients with ARF, showed that patients who were dialyzed earlier in the disease course (mean BUN concentration, 42.6 mg/dL) had a better survival (39% versus 20%) than those in whom dialysis was initiated later (mean BUN concentration, 94.5 mg/dL).[25]

However, a study by Bouman and associates ($N = 106$)[26] does not support this finding. In this study, patients were randomized to three groups: early high-volume hemofiltration ($n = 35$; 72 to 96 L/24 hr), early low-volume hemofiltration ($n = 35$; 24 to 36 L/24 hr), and late low-volume hemofiltration ($n = 36$; 24 to 36 L/24 hr). Survival at 28 days and recovery of renal function were not improved using early initiation of hemofiltration. This study was limited in that it was clearly underpowered to detect any differences in outcome. However, available evidence does not allow recommendation of the optimal timing of the initiation of renal replacement therapy.

Postrenal Oliguria

The definitive treatment for postrenal oliguria is to relieve the obstruction. This might be as simple as flushing or changing the Foley catheter. Other patients require more invasive procedures, such as a percutaneous nephrostomy or a suprapubic decompression of the bladder.

■ CONCLUSION

Oliguria is one of the most common clinical problems encountered by physicians caring for perioperative patients. Any delay in its recognition and treatment can lead to the progression to ARF, which in turn carries significant morbidity and mortality. Hence, the presence of oliguria should alert the clinician to undertake a diligent search for any correctable underlying causes. The mainstay of treatment is to ensure adequate renal perfusion through optimization of cardiac output and volume status and avoidance of nephrotoxins. Dopamine and dopamine-1 receptor agonist such as fenoldopam mesylate do not have any role in augmenting renal perfusion and should not be used for this purpose. Diuretics and natriuretic peptides, although they can convert oliguric ARF to nonoliguric ARF, may worsen the outcome of acute renal failure. Diuretics may be required to treat fluid overload, but they are not treatments for oliguria. Early renal replacement therapy should be considered in patients with oliguria secondary to acute renal failure.

■ REFERENCES

1. Zaloga GP, Hughes SS: Oliguria in patients with normal renal function. Anesthesiology 1990;72:598-602.
2. Brivet FG, Kleinknecht DJ, Loirat P, Landais PJ: Acute renal failure in intensive care units: Causes, outcome, and prognostic factors of hospital mortality—A prospective, multicenter study. French Study Group on Acute Renal Failure. Crit Care Med 1996;24:192-198.
3. Chertow GM, Levy EM, Hammermeister KE, et al: Independent association between acute renal failure and mortality following cardiac surgery. Am J Med 1998;104:343-348.
4. Hoste EA, Clermont G, Kersten A: Clinical evaluation of the new RIFLE criteria for acute renal failure. Crit Care 2004;8(Suppl 1):P162.
5. Levy EM, Viscoli CM, Horwitz RI: The effect of acute renal failure on mortality: A cohort analysis. JAMA 1996;275:1489-1494.
6. Thadhani RI, Camargo CA Jr, Xavier RJ, et al: Atheroembolic renal failure after invasive procedures: Natural history based on 52 histologically proven cases. Medicine (Baltimore) 1995;74:350-358.
7. Bailey J, Shapiro MJ: Abdominal compartment syndrome. Crit Care 2000;4:23-29.
8. Richards WO, Scovill W, Shin B, Reed W: Acute renal failure associated with increased intra-abdominal pressure. Ann Surg 1983;197:183-187.
9. Webb JA: The role of ultrasonography in the diagnosis of intrinsic renal disease. Clin Radiol 1994;49:589-591.
10. Rivers E, Nguyen B, Havstad S, et al: Early goal-directed therapy in the treatment of severe sepsis and septic shock. N Engl J Med 2001;345:1368-1377.
11. Brosius FC, Lau K: Low fractional excretion of sodium in acute renal failure: Role of timing of the test and ischemia. Am J Nephrol 1986;6:450-457.
12. Carvounis CP, Nisar S, Guro-Razuman S: Significance of the fractional excretion of urea in the differential diagnosis of acute renal failure. Kidney Int 2002;62:2223-2229.
13. Seri I, Kone BC, Gullans SR, et al: Locally formed dopamine inhibits Na^+-K^+-ATPase activity in rat renal cortical tubule cells. Am J Physiol 1988;255:666-673.
14. Bellomo R, Chapman M, Finfer S, et al: Low-dose dopamine in patients with early renal dysfunction: A placebo-controlled randomised trial. Australian and New Zealand Intensive Care Society (ANZICS) Clinical Trials Group. Lancet 2000;356:2139-2143.
15. Kellum JA, Decker JM: Use of dopamine in acute renal failure: A meta-analysis. Crit Care Med 2001;29:1526-1531.
16. Marik PE: Low-dose dopamine: A systematic review. Intensive Care Med 2002;28:877-883.
17. Stone GW, McCullough PA, Tumlin JA, et al: Fenoldopam mesylate for the prevention of contrast-induced nephropathy: A randomized controlled trial. JAMA 2003;290:2284-2291.
18. Mathur VS, Swan SK, Lambrecht LJ, et al: The effects of fenoldopam, a selective dopamine receptor agonist, on systemic and renal hemodynamics in normotensive subjects. Crit Care Med 1999;27:1832-1837.
19. Kellum JA: The use of diuretics and dopamine in acute renal failure: A systematic review of the evidence. Critical Care 1997;1:53-59.
20. Mehta RL, Pascual MT, Soroko S, Chertow GM: Diuretics, mortality, and nonrecovery of renal function in acute renal failure. JAMA 2002;288:2547-2553.
21. Uchino S, Doig GS, Bellomo R, et al: Diuretics and mortality in acute renal failure. Crit Care Med 2004;32:1669-1677.
22. Allgren RL, Marbury TC, Rahman SN, et al: Anaritide in acute tubular necrosis. Auriculin Anaritide Acute Renal Failure Study Group. N Engl J Med 1997;336:828-834.
23. Lewis J, Salem MM, Chertow GM, et al: Atrial natriuretic factor in oliguric acute renal failure. Anaritide Acute Renal Failure Study Group. Am J Kidney Dis 2000;36:767-774.
24. Sward K, Valsson F, Odencrants P, et al: Recombinant human atrial natriuretic peptide in ischemic acute renal failure: A randomized placebo-controlled trial. Crit Care Med 2004;32:1310-1315.
25. Gettings LG, Reynolds HN, Scalea T: Outcome in post-traumatic acute renal failure when continuous renal replacement therapy is applied early vs. late. Intensive Care Med 1999;25:805-813.
26. Bouman CS, Oudeman-van Straaten HM, Tijssen JGP: Effects of early high-volume continuous venovenous hemofiltration on survival and recovery of renal function in intensive care patients with acute renal failure: A prospective randomized trial. Crit Care Med 2002;30:2205-2211.

19 Perioperative Management of Renal Failure and Renal Transplant

Per-Olof Jarnberg

Chronic renal disease (CRD) is a pathophysiologic process with a multitude of etiologies, resulting in progressive loss of nephron number and function, which leads to end-stage renal disease (ESRD) with increasing frequency. ESRD ultimately leads to the need for renal replacement therapy—that is, dialysis or transplantation. The diseases most commonly responsible for ESRD are diabetes mellitus (42.8%), hypertension (25.9%), glomerulonephritis (9.0%), and cystic kidney disease (2.3%). Other causes account for the remaining 20%.[1]

Currently, there is a 12% incidence of CRD in the U.S. adult population, and the number of persons with kidney failure who are treated with dialysis and transplantation is projected to increase from 340,000 in 1999 to 651,000 in 2010.[2,3] A widely accepted international classification divides CRD into a number of stages (Table 19-1).[3] The major outcomes of CRD, regardless of cause, include progression to kidney failure, complications of decreased kidney function, and development or worsening of cardiovascular disease. There is evidence that some of these adverse outcomes can be prevented or delayed by early detection and treatment.[4] Unfortunately, CRD is underdiagnosed and undertreated, resulting in lost opportunities for prevention.[5] Recent publications stress the importance of advanced glycation end products, found in patients with both type 1 and type 2 diabetes, for the progression of atherosclerosis and renal disease.[6,7]

Patients with CRD, particularly those with chronic renal failure (CRF) and ESRD, present a number of challenges to the anesthesiologist. For instance, preexisting renal function impairment is a strong risk factor for deterioration of renal function and development of acute renal failure (ARF) in the perioperative period.[8,9] ARF is independently associated with early mortality after cardiac surgery,[8] particularly if the need for dialysis develops. In a study by Conlon and colleagues, mortality for coronary artery bypass graft (CABG) patients who received some form of dialysis was 28%, as opposed to 1.8% in those patients whose ARF did not require renal replacement therapy.[10] The mortality rate for ARF as a complication of nonrenal system failure in the intensive care unit (ICU) setting and requiring dialysis is 50% to 70%, a level that has remained virtually unchanged for the past 3 decades.[11,12] A recent review of perioperative renal protection strategies concluded that existing pharmacologic and other interventions had a limited efficacy in preventing the development or worsening of ARF.[13] The most important elements in preserving renal function were identified as perioperative optimization of hemodynamics and intravascular volume, and avoidance or cautious use of nephrotoxins. Supported pharmacologic interventions were mannitol and calcium antagonists for improvement of outcome in renal transplantation recipients. Also supported were acetylcysteine and probably fenoldopam for prevention of radiocontrast-induced nephropathy. Other considerations are the timing of surgery in relation to diagnostic procedures that require intravenous administration of contrast agents or bowel preparation, as well as the mode and timing of administration of nephrotoxic antibiotics.[14,15]

Impact of Sex on Progression of Nondiabetic Renal Disease

In recent years, evidence has increased that male sex is associated with a more rapid rate of progression of nondiabetic chronic renal disease.[16,17] Neugarten and colleagues performed a meta-analysis of 68 studies containing a total of 11,345 patients and examined the effect of sex on the progression of nondiabetic chronic renal disease (of mixed etiologies), IgA nephropathy, idiopathic membranous nephropathy, and autosomal-dominant polycystic kidney disease.[18] The results strongly indicate that male sex is associated with a more rapid rate of progression and a worse renal outcome in patients with chronic renal disease. A better understanding of the sex-related cellular and molecular renoprotective mechanisms may lead to the development of clinically useful treatment strategies.

■ PATHOPHYSIOLOGY OF CHRONIC RENAL FAILURE

Azotemia is the term for the accumulation of the byproducts of protein and amino acid metabolism. *Uremia* refers to the more advanced stages of renal insufficiency when the complex multiorgan system disturbances become clinically manifest. Uremia is a clinical syndrome, and no single symptom, sign, or laboratory test can reliably identify it. It is generally believed that uremic symptoms correlate only in an approximate and inconsistent way with concentrations of urea in the blood. However, symptoms such as anorexia, fatigue, malaise, vomiting, and headache have generally been ascribed to increased blood urea levels. They represent the basic pathophysiologic disorder of uremia—that is, defective ion transport across cell membranes, resulting in intracellular sodium and water accumulation.[19]

19-1	**Stages of Chronic Renal Disease**	

Stage	Description	Glomerular Filtration Rate (GFR) (mL/min/1.73 m²)
1	Kidney damage with normal or increased GFR	>90
2	Kidney damage with mildly decreased GFR	60-89
3	Moderately decreased GFR	30-95
4	Severely decreased GFR	15-29
5	Kidney failure	<15 or dialysis

Additional uremic toxins include guanido compounds, urates and hippurates, polyamines, myoinositol, phenols, benzoates, and indoles. Other nitrogenous compounds with a molecular mass of 500 to 12,000 Da, so-called middle molecules, are also retained in CRD and contribute to morbidity and mortality of uremic patients.[20]

These toxins impair a number of metabolic and endocrine functions, resulting in anemia; malnutrition; impaired metabolism of carbohydrates, fats, and proteins; defective utilization of energy; and metabolic bone disease (Box 19-1). Plasma levels of a number of polypeptide hormones such as parathyroid hormone (PTH), insulin, glucagon, luteinizing hormone, and prolactin also rise with the development of renal failure.[20] Renal production of erythropoietin (EPO) and vitamin D_3 (1,25-dihydroxycholecalciferol) is impaired. Chronic dialysis can reduce the incidence and severity of those disturbances. However, dialysis is not a complete remedy—some disturbances fail to respond fully and others continue to worsen.

Fluid and Electrolyte Balance

Sodium and Water Homeostasis
In most patients with stable CRD, the body's content of sodium and water is modestly increased. Patients with ESRD have impaired mechanisms for conserving sodium ions, making them prone to volume depletion when extrarenal losses of fluid occur (for instance by diarrhea, vomiting, and sweating), and may thus rapidly become hypovolemic. This may lead to rapid further deterioration of residual renal function, resulting in overt uremia. On the other hand, anuric or oliguric patients are extremely sensitive to excessive sodium and water intake, which rapidly results in hypervolemia, with ensuing hypertension and pulmonary edema.

Potassium Balance
Patients with CRD may present with a wide range of serum potassium levels. Hyperkalemia is more common than hypokalemia, but both are associated with cardiac morbidity. Acute hyperkalemia causes suppression of electrical conduction in the heart and may result in asystolic cardiac arrest. Telltale electrocardiographic (ECG) signs are prolonged PR interval, widened QRS complex, and tall peaked T waves. However, asystole may occur without prior ECG signs.

The ratio of intracellular to extracellular potassium concentration determines the excitability of the cell. Normally, the ratio is 40:1 (160 and 4 mmol/L, respectively). The clini-

19-1	**Clinical Abnormalities in Patients with Chronic Renal Failure**

Fluid and Electrolyte Disturbances
- Hypervolemia, hypovolemia
- Hypernatremia, hyponatremia
- Hyperkalemia, hypokalemia
- Hyperphosphatemia
- Hypocalcemia
- Metabolic acidosis

Cardiovascular Disturbances
- Hypertension
- Coronary artery disease
- Generalized atherosclerosis
- Vascular calcifications
- Congestive heart failure
- Pericarditis

Hematologic and Immunologic Disturbances
- Anemia
- Bleeding diathesis
- Increased susceptibility to infection

Gastrointestinal Disturbances
- Gastritis
- Peptic ulcer
- Bleeding
- Nausea and vomiting
- Delayed gastric emptying

Nutritional and Metabolic Disturbances
- Carbohydrate intolerance
- Hypertriglyceridemia
- Protein-energy malnutrition
- Hypoalbuminemia

Neurologic Disturbances
- Encephalopathy
- Peripheral neuropathy
- Autonomic neuropathy
- Fatigue
- Lethargy
- Impaired mentation
- Neuromuscular irritability
  - Hiccups
  - Muscle cramps and fasciculations

cal and ECG manifestations of hyperkalemia and hypokalemia depend on the speed of change in potassium flux rather than on the serum potassium level itself. Some patients with CRF tolerate stable potassium levels of 6 to 6.5 mmol/L without showing any conduction disturbances. However, if potassium levels increase to greater than that, these patients may rapidly show signs of hyperkalemia. See Box 19-2 for causes that can induce hyperkalemia in patients with CRF.

A preoperative potassium level of 6 mmol/L or greater should be corrected before the start of anesthesia unless there is a dire emergency. Treatment alternatives for lowering potassium level consist of normalizing pH if acidosis is present, and intravenous administration of insulin or glucose and/or a beta-2-adrenergic agonist, all of which work by shifting potassium into the cells. Dialysis or administration

19-2	**Causes of Hyperkalemia in Patients with Chronic Renal Failure**

- Acute acidosis
- Rhabdomyolysis (trauma, major surgery)
- Increased catabolism, sepsis
- Nonsteroidal anti-inflammatory drugs
- Angiotensin-converting enzyme inhibitors
- Potassium-sparing diuretics
- Beta-blockers
- Nephrotoxic drugs (cyclosporine, aminoglycosides)
- Radiocontrast material

of sodium polystyrene sulfonate, either orally or as an enema, removes potassium ions.

Hypokalemia is uncommon in patients with CRD. It usually reflects reduced dietary intake in conjunction with excessive diuretic therapy or gastrointestinal (GI) losses. More rarely, it is associated with primary renal potassium wasting, as seen in Fanconi's syndrome, Bartter's syndrome, and renal tubular acidosis. Acute hypokalemia increases excitability and lowers the arrhythmia threshold. Both supraventricular and ventricular arrhythmias may occur. These may be refractory to normal antiarrhythmic treatment until the serum potassium concentration is normalized.

Magnesium Balance
Magnesium is handled in much the same way as potassium by the kidney. Hypermagnesemia may be induced by intake of magnesium-based antacids or by inadequate dialysis. It may cause muscle weakness and potentiate nondepolarizing muscle relaxants.

Hypomagnesemia renders the heart liable to the development of both supraventricular and ventricular arrhythmias.

Phosphate–Calcium Balance
Decreased glomerular filtration rate leads to reduced phosphate excretion. The retained phosphate has a direct stimulating effect on PTH synthesis. Retained phosphate also indirectly causes increased secretion of PTH through lowering of the level of ionized calcium and by suppression of calcitriol production. Reduced calcitriol leads to reduced Ca^{2+} absorption from the GI tract, causing hypocalcemia, which in its turn stimulates PTH secretion. Taken together, hyperphosphatemia, hypocalcemia, and reduced calcitriol synthesis all promote the production of PTH and the proliferation of parathyroid cells, resulting in secondary hyperparathyroidism. Increased PTH levels lead to high bone resorption and turnover, resulting in abnormal osteoid production and formation of cysts, decreasing bone strength, and increasing risk for fracture.

In addition to abnormalities in bone metabolism, abnormal calcium–phosphate product may lead to calciphylaxis (i.e., extraosseous calcification of soft tissue and blood vessels). Patients with CRD often have highly elevated coronary artery calcification scores, which most likely represents a major factor in the predisposition to occlusive coronary artery disease found in this population.

Metabolic Acidosis
Patients with CRF develop a chronic anion-gap metabolic acidosis, resulting from a decreased ability to excrete acid and a reciprocal decrease in plasma bicarbonate. The metabolic acidosis is usually mild and can most often be corrected by treating the patients with a daily dose of 20 to 30 mmol of $NaHCO_3$ or sodium citrate. However, the buffer base is usually so diminished that a superimposed moderate respiratory acidosis, frequently seen in the immediate postoperative period, may quickly result in acidemia and significant hyperkalemia.

Cardiovascular Disease

Cardiovascular disease (CVD), in the form of hypertension, coronary artery disease (CAD), and congestive heart failure, is the most common cause of morbidity and mortality in patients with CRD and accounts for greater than 50% of the mortality in this group.[21] For patients with ESRD who are treated with dialysis, CVD mortality is 10 to 30 times higher than for patients in the general population.[22] The etiology of CVD in patients with ESRD is multifactorial, stemming from preexisting conditions (diabetes and hypertension), uremia (toxins, hyperlipidemia, and hyperhomocysteinemia), and dialysis-related conditions (dialysis membrane reactions and hemodynamic instability episodes).

Hypertension
Hypertension is the most common cardiovascular problem in patients with CRD. It is associated with further impairment of renal function and progression of CVD. There is ample evidence from studies that a positive correlation exists between the level of blood pressure and the rate of progression of kidney disease.[22] When hypertensive heart disease becomes established, patients present with arrhythmias, CAD, or heart failure, or a combination of these.

Long-term hemodialysis through arteriovenous (AV) fistulas is associated with a 40% incidence of development of pulmonary hypertension. The reason for this is unclear, and a corresponding development in patients undergoing peritoneal dialysis has not been demonstrated.[23] Pulmonary pressures normalize in the majority of patients after kidney transplantation.[23] The creation of AV fistulas may also lead to increased cardiac output, which further increases the cardiac workload. Congestive heart failure, which has a prevalence of 40% among hemodialysis and peritoneal dialysis patients, is an independent predictor of death.[22] CAD and left ventricular hypertrophy constitute risk factors for the development of congestive heart failure.[22]

Coronary Artery Disease
CAD has a prevalence of almost 40% in patients with ESRD.[22] This increased prevalence of CAD among patients with CRD derives from both classic and CRD-related risk factors. The former factors include hypertension, volume overload, dyslipidemia, and hyperhomocysteinemia. The CRD-related risk factors include anemia, hyperphosphatemia, hyperparathyroidism, and low-grade inflammation, which is worsened by dialysis. The inflammatory state elicits a rise in acute-phase proteins such as C-reactive protein and interleukin-6, which contribute to coronary occlusive disease and are predictors

of CVD risk.[24] The acute-phase C-reactive protein is chronically increased in up to 66% of dialysis patients.[25] This protein is considered a marker of a microinflammatory state, and it is a significant predictor of cardiovascular mortality in both the general population and among patients with ESRD.[25,26] Although many subjects with ESRD and CAD have typical exertional angina symptoms, up to 40% of patients have silent ischemia as documented by Holter monitoring.[27] This situation is further complicated by the fact that exercise tolerance testing, which is recommended by some authors, is often impossible because of physical limitations in this patient population. The sensitivity and specificity of stress tests are both low and inconsistent between studies and may not allow prediction of perioperative risk.[28-30]

Uremic pericarditis is well controlled by renal replacement therapy and rarely encountered today. When encountered, it is more commonly observed in underdialyzed patients than in predialysis ESRD patients. Pericarditis may be accompanied by the accumulation of pericardial fluid that is readily detected by echocardiography, and that sometimes leads to cardiac tamponade. Pericardial fluid in uremic pericarditis is more often hemorrhagic than in viral pericarditis.

Hematologic Abnormalities

Anemia

Chronic renal failure induces a normochromic, normocytic anemia, mainly caused by depressed EPO production by the diseased kidneys. Additional causes include iron and folate deficiency, chronic blood loss, hemolysis, and chronic inflammation. The availability of recombinant human EPO has reduced the need for blood transfusions and has improved quality of life as judged by reduced fatigue, improved cardiac function and exercise tolerance, increased sense of well-being, and improved survival.[31] Recently, an EPO analog, darbepoetin alpha, has been introduced for treatment of anemia in patients with CRF. It possesses greater biologic activity and a longer half-life than regular EPO, which allow prolongation of the dose intervals, which in turn improves patient comfort.

Uremic Bleeding Diathesis

Patients with CRF often have a prolonged bleeding time. The origin is multifactorial and includes decreased activity of platelet factor III, abnormal platelet aggregation, abnormal interaction between platelets and vessel walls, and defective release of von Willebrand factor. Patients with CRF are therefore at risk for surgical bleeding, GI tract bleeding, intracranial hemorrhage, and hemorrhagic pericardial effusion.

The bleeding tendency is improved by dialysis, which is the principal treatment, but infusion of desmopressin, cryoprecipitate, and conjugated estrogens may be of value for temporary treatment.[32]

Gastrointestinal Abnormalities

Gastritis, peptic ulcer disease, and mucosal ulcerations, which can occur at any level of the GI tract, are common in uremic patients. Symptoms include abdominal pain, hiccups, nausea, vomiting, and bleeding. Bleeding may be exacerbated by uremic hemostasis defects and use of heparin during hemodialysis. Central nervous system effects of uremia contribute to worsening of hiccups, nausea, and vomiting. Patients with ESRD are therefore at increased risk for regurgitation and aspiration at induction of and emergence from anesthesia.

Nutritional and Metabolic Disturbances

Patients with CRD have impaired glucose and fat metabolism, and they are prone to hyperglycemia and hypertriglyceridemia because of increased peripheral insulin resistance and decreased lipoprotein lipase activity. This contributes to the high incidence of CAD in patients with CRD. These patients are often on a protein-restricted diet to reduce nausea and vomiting, which, in combination with deficient caloric intake or utilization, makes them susceptible to malnutrition. Hypoalbuminemia and decreased colloid oncotic pressure tend to promote interstitial fluid accumulation. In the lungs, this leads to decreased functional residual capacity and ventilatory reserve, increasing the risk for postoperative pulmonary complications.

Neurologic Disturbances

Central, peripheral, and autonomic nervous system neuropathies are common in patients with CRD. Retained nitrogenous metabolites and disturbed calcium homeostasis all contribute to the various manifestations of central neuropathy. Early signs and symptoms include disturbances in memory, concentration, and sleep. Later neuromuscular irritability with hiccups and cramps and muscle fasciculations become evident. Full-blown encephalopathy with myoclonus, seizures, and coma may develop, often precipitated by major surgery or GI bleeding. Uremic encephalopathy is associated with slow delta waves on the electroencephalogram, and magnetic resonance imaging may reveal increased signal intensity in a characteristic pattern in the occipital and parietal lobes.[33] The treatment is dialysis.

Peripheral neuropathy is very common in patients with ESRD. Manifestations include loss of vibration sense, and asymmetric and symmetric neural deficits. Another common deficit is the "glove and stocking" sensory distribution, with pain or sensory loss affecting distal nerves.

The presence of peripheral neuropathy should always trigger an awareness of the possible coexistence of autonomic neuropathy. Important consequences of autonomic dysfunction include silent myocardial ischemia, orthostatic hypotension, impaired circulatory responses to anesthetic and surgical stress, and impaired gastric emptying, which increases the risk for aspiration.

Immunologic Dysfunction

The combination of uremia, anemia, and poor nutritional status induces a state of decreased resistance to infections in patients with ESRD. It is based both on leukocyte dysfunction (depressed chemotaxis, phagocytosis and bactericidal activity) and on immunosuppression (e.g., reduced interleukin-2 production and hypogammaglobulinemia) and is associated with increased mortality.[32] Infections are particularly common, both localized at shunt and peritoneal catheter sites,

19-3	Drugs Chiefly Dependent on Renal Excretion

- Gallamine, metocurine
- Penicillins, cephalosporins, aminoglycosides, vancomycin
- Digoxin

19-2	Drugs with Active Metabolites Dependent on Renal Excretion

Drug	Metabolite	Effect
Morphine	Morphine-6-glucuronide	Analgesic
Meperidine	Normeperidine	Neuroexcitatory
Diazepam	Oxazepam	Sedative
Midazolam	1-Hydroxy-midazolam	Sedative
Pancuronium	3-Hydroxy-pancuronium	Relaxant
Procainamide	N-Acetylprocainamide	Neurotoxic

19-4	Drugs Partially Dependent on Renal Excretion

- Atropine, glycopyrrolate
- Neostigmine, pyridostigmine, edrophonium
- Pancuronium, vecuronium
- Amrinone, milrinone
- Phenobarbital

and disseminated in the form of sepsis. Additional infection risks stem from the impaired wound healing seen in these patients, which results in slow-healing or nonhealing wounds after surgery and a tendency for bedsore development.

■ PHARMACOLOGY IN CHRONIC RENAL FAILURE

The pharmacodynamics and pharmacokinetics of certain drugs may be affected by CRD, which may alter excretion and disposition of drugs, the latter through changes in plasma protein binding and hepatic metabolism.

Elimination of water-soluble, highly ionized drugs is highly dependent on renal excretion. Therefore, depending on the severity of renal failure, excretion of such drugs may be markedly impaired. Digoxin and certain antibiotics and muscle relaxants belong in this group (Box 19-3). Drugs that are partially dependent on renal elimination (e.g., atropine, glycopyrrolate, neostigmine, pancuronium, and vecuronium) may show significant prolongation of action (Box 19-4).

Thiopental and benzodiazepines, frequently used in anesthesia practice, are highly protein bound and increase their unbound free fraction in the presence of uremic conditions (hypoalbuminemia and acidemia), and they may demonstrate exaggerated clinical effects. Depending on the timing and effectiveness of dialysis, volume of distribution for drugs may be increased as well as the plasma volume, which tends to prolong elimination half-life and also counteracts the effects of the increased free fraction of protein-bound drugs.

Many drugs are lipid soluble and depend on hepatic metabolism and/or glucuronization to generate water-soluble compounds that can be excreted by the kidneys. If these compounds maintain some or all of the parent drug's pharmacologic activity, their clinical effects may be quite prolonged (Table 19-2). Another risk is that such accumulated metabolites may have toxic effects when their concentrations increase (Table 19-2).

CRF is often a debilitating condition. Many patients have reduced muscle mass and other characteristics, with the result that pharmacodynamic effects are altered. It is there-

fore prudent, when the clinical situation allows, to titrate drugs to effect rather than to administer "normal" doses of drug.

Choice of Anesthetic Technique

General Considerations

Patients with CRF who present for surgery pose a multitude of challenges to the anesthesiologist. The comorbidities these patients often exhibit affect their whole perioperative course. The following are some of the key factors to which the anesthesiologist should pay particular attention.

At the preoperative visit, the history taking should focus on the cause of CRF and manifestations of systemic disease, keeping in mind that myocardial ischemia may be silent in diabetic patients. The autonomic neuropathy in such patients may also impair circulatory responses to anesthesia and surgery. Bleeding, encephalopathy, and neuropathy are other possible and important complications of CRF that should be ascertained. Whether the patient is anuric or has urine production has significant impact on the planning of fluid management.

Patients on dialysis are not in a homeostatic state. Information on the type of dialysis, frequency, and most recent treatment is important. In most nonurgent surgery patients, the ideal timing of hemodialysis is the day before surgery. This avoids immediate dialysis-related complications, such as rebound heparinization, hypovolemia, hypokalemia, and dysequilibrium syndrome. Ideally, patients should be normovolemic and their potassium should be no higher than 6 mmol/L on the day of surgery. A blood urea nitrogen (BUN) value below 100 mg/L usually keeps coagulopathy and encephalopathy under control. However, this BUN level neither guarantees normal platelet function nor improves immunity and the impaired wound healing that often occur postoperatively.

Individuals with a prior history of perioperative uremic bleeding should be treated before surgery. In addition to dialysis, cryoprecipitate and/or intravenous or intranasal administration of desmopressin, 0.3 μg/kg, should be considered.[34]

There is increasing evidence that perioperative use of beta-blockers improves outcome in seriously ill patients. Lindenauer and colleagues[35] recently published a study involving 782,969 patients undergoing major noncardiac surgery, of whom 122,338 received beta-blockers during their hospital stay. Of these patients, 14% of patients had a Revised Cardiac Risk Index (RCRI) score of 0, and 44% had a score of 4 and higher. The RCRI score was calculated by assigning one point for each of the following risk factors: high-risk surgery, ischemic heart disease, cerebrovascular disease, renal insufficiency, and diabetes mellitus.[36] The relationship between perioperative beta-blockade and the risk for death varied directly with cardiac risk. In patients with an RCRI score of 0 or 1, treatment was associated with no benefit, whereas among patients with a score of 2, 3, or 4 and higher, the adjusted odds ratios were 0.88, 0.71, and 0.58, respectively. The authors list several limitations of their study. Its retrospective nature prevented randomization of treatment and limited the ability to control for differences between patients. The study was restricted to the period of hospitalization and the authors were unable to report on the use of beta-blockers before admission or after discharge, as well as 30-day and 1-year mortality. Despite these limitations, the data are still compelling, and starting beta-blockade before anesthesia induction in high-risk patients who lack contraindications seems indicated. This view was supported in an editorial accompanying the article.[37]

General Anesthesia

General anesthesia is the most common choice for surgical procedures, although regional anesthesia is successfully used in many cases (see later). Before induction of anesthesia, the patient's volume status should be evaluated. If the patient has had recent dialysis (within 12 hours), consider fluid loading with 250 to 500 mL normal saline prior to induction. Gastric emptying is delayed in uremic patients, and they should always be treated as having risk for aspiration. Therefore, use of cricoid pressure is recommended, regardless of whether the induction type is conventional or rapid sequence.

Induction Agents

Thiopental has an increased free fraction in patients who have CRD and hypoalbuminemia, and it is recommended that the induction dose be decreased in these patients.[38] Etomidate also has an increased free fraction, which does not seem to be of clinical importance.[39] Propofol's pharmacokinetic and pharmacodynamic properties are unchanged in patients with CRD. Its safe use in patients with renal failure has been documented.[40] Ketamine is less extensively protein bound than thiopental, and its free fraction is unaffected by renal failure. However, ketamine has the potential of causing impressive increases in blood pressure if it is used in hypertensive patients with CRD,[41] and its use should be limited to emergency anesthetic induction.

Muscle Relaxants

Succinylcholine is often used because it facilitates rapid-sequence anesthetic induction. An intubating dose of succinylcholine (1 mg/kg) increases the serum potassium level by 0.5 to 1 mmol/L within 3 to 5 minutes after administration. Use of succinylcholine in patients with CRF should be restricted to those patients whose potassium concentration is 5.5 mmol/L or less.[42] Vecuronium, rocuronium, and cisatracurium are suitable alternatives to succinylcholine. Of these three drugs, rocuronium has the fastest onset of action. The duration of action of vecuronium and rocuronium may be prolonged in patients with CRF, whereas cisatracurium

undergoes Hoffman elimination in blood and tissue, a process that is totally independent of renal function.[43,44] The long-acting muscle relaxant pancuronium should be avoided because of its high degree of renal elimination. For all nondepolarizing muscle relaxants, except cisatracurium, the reported recovery times from neuromuscular blockade are variable, and careful monitoring of the degree of neuromuscular blockade is recommended.

Opioids

The use of morphine and meperidine is of concern in patients with CRF. Both have metabolites that are dependent on renal elimination. Normeperidine, the active metabolite of meperidine, accumulates in patients with renal failure after repeated doses or continuous infusion and may cause seizures.[45] About 10% of morphine is metabolized to morphine-6-glucuronide, which is a very potent sedative and dependent on excretion by the kidney. This metabolite may accumulate to 10 to 15 times its normal concentration in cerebrospinal fluid in patients with CRF.[46] The pharmacokinetic and pharmacodynamic profiles of alfentanil, fentanyl, remifentanil, and sufentanil are not significantly influenced by renal failure.[47,48] They can therefore be used with little or no modification of their dosage.

Inhaled Anesthetics

Elimination of inhaled anesthetics is independent of renal function. Of the modern inhaled anesthetics, desflurane and isoflurane have no nephrotoxic properties, but there are some concerns with sevoflurane. Sevoflurane is defluorinated during its metabolism to approximately the same extent as enflurane. Initial studies reported plasma levels of fluoride, in connection with sevoflurane anesthesia, comparable to those seen after enflurane administration.[49] More recent studies found that plasma fluoride concentrations often rise to greater than $50\,\mu M$.[50,51] Because of sevoflurane's low blood–gas solubility, only limited stores build up during anesthesia, and as a result, fluoride levels fall very quickly after termination of anesthesia. No renal function impairment has been reported in patients with normal renal function.

The safety of sevoflurane in patients with impaired renal function has been widely studied.[52-54] The consensus from these studies is that sevoflurane has little potential to cause fluoride-induced nephrotoxicity.

Sevoflurane undergoes degradation in carbon dioxide absorbers using soda or barium hydroxide lime. The chief degradation product is fluoromethyl-2,2-difluoro-1(trifluoromethyl) vinylether, also known as compound A. Compound A concentrations in the anesthesia circuit correlate directly with sevoflurane concentrations and absorbent temperature, and inversely with fresh gas inflow rate.[55] Compound A is nephrotoxic in rats at thresholds estimated at 180 ppm/hr.[56,57] Renal toxicity is characterized histologically by corticomedullary necrosis and biochemically by proteinuria, glucosuria, and enzymuria (N-acetyl-D-glucosamine [NAG] and alpha-glutathione-S-transferase [alpha-GST]), with increased serum creatinine and BUN concentrations occurring with severe toxicity.[56-59]

In humans, there seems to be a dose-dependent association between compound A exposure and the appearance of urinary biomarkers such as albumin, glucose, and enzymes (NAG and alpha-GST). These findings appear in studies where the compound A exposure exceeds 160 ppm/hr,[60-62] but they are absent in studies with lower compound A exposure.[63-65] In all studies associated with higher exposure of compound A, the urinary markers have been transient, lasting 3 to 5 days, with total normalization within 1 week. There was no correlation between serum creatinine and the urinary markers. Since its introduction in the United States in 1995, sevoflurane has been administered to tens of millions of patients without a single report of nephrotoxicity.[66]

The concerns around the degradation of sevoflurane can be avoided by using a calcium hydroxide–based absorbent (Amsorb), which does not degrade sevoflurane.[67]

Total Intravenous Anesthesia

Total intravenous anesthesia (TIVA) based on propofol and remifentanil, and using cisatracurium as the muscle relaxant, is a good alternative to inhaled agents, as the pharmacologic properties of these intravenous drugs are not affected by renal failure.

Regional Anesthesia

Regional anesthetic techniques are used successfully in patients with CRF. There are concerns about uremic bleeding diathesis. Prolonged bleeding time (>15 min) is a contraindication to central neuraxial anesthesia. In these patients, it is also best to avoid using the axillary artery puncture technique while administering an arm block. However, a normal platelet count and coagulation parameters is no guarantee against bleeding and hematoma development, because the platelets may be dysfunctional. There are reports of both spinal and epidural hematoma development after use of regional anesthesia in patients with CRF.[68,69] Patients who have CRF and autonomic neuropathy, and who receive epidural or spinal anesthesia, have increased risk for developing significant hypotension caused by exaggerated sympathetic blockade. Patients with CRF have increased risk for catheter site infection, which should be factored into the choice of anesthetic technique.

Brachial plexus and axillary blocks are used in many centers to provide anesthesia for insertion or revision of AV shunts. This is often an excellent anesthetic choice in patients with suitable psychological disposition.

■ INTRAOPERATIVE CONSIDERATIONS

Monitoring

Standard monitoring of patients with CRF should include five-lead ECG, noninvasive blood pressure, pulse oximetry, end-tidal CO_2 and other gases, peripheral nerve stimulator, temperature, and, if applicable, urine output. Preexisting renal function impairment is a major risk factor for further perioperative deterioration of renal function. The maintenance of effective intravascular volume and normal hemodynamics is very important for preventing renal hypoperfusion.[70]

Central venous pressure monitoring is therefore recommended in most patients with advanced renal failure undergoing major surgical procedures, and invasive peripheral arterial pressure monitoring should be considered. The benefits of direct arterial pressure monitoring should be weighed against the risks of arterial damage, making the site unsuitable if future AV shunt placements should become necessary. The use of a pulmonary artery catheter is rarely required, but it may be indicated for patients with severe CAD, left ventricular dysfunction, major valvular disease, or significant pulmonary hypertension. In cases of unexplained refractory hypotension, transesophageal echocardiography, instead of the PA catheter, is preferable for differentiating between hypovolemia and decreased myocardial contractility.

Aseptic Technique

Patients on chronic hemodialysis have a high incidence of hepatitis C because of frequent transfusions and exposure to dialysis equipment contaminated with the hepatitis C virus (HCV). Approximately 10% of hemodialysis patients in the United States have an anti-HCV response.[71,72] Therefore, all patients on hemodialysis should be treated as potentially infected.

Patients with CRF have decreased resistance to infection and are therefore prone to infections perioperatively. Intravenous catheter infections are particularly common. Strict sterile techniques should be used for invasive procedures. Recent studies of general ICU patients have shown that the use of the maximal sterile barrier technique has resulted in a marked decrease in the incidence of both catheter-related bloodstream infections and catheter colonization (local infections associated with central venous catheter insertion). This technique requires the person inserting the catheter to wear a head cap, face mask, and sterile gown and gloves, and to use a full-size sterile drape around the insertion site.[73,74]

Positioning

Patients with CRD often present with both neuropathies and poor nutritional status because of uremia. As a consequence, they are very vulnerable to the development of new nerve deficits or the worsening of existing nerve deficits during surgery, as they have very little endogenous padding for protection. In addition to the standard positioning considerations, extreme diligence should be paid to protecting pressure points with extra padding. If an AV fistula is present in the arm, a rigid cushioned protector is helpful.

■ KIDNEY TRANSPLANTATION

Transplantation of a human kidney is the preferred treatment for advanced CRF. It provides better survival and quality of life than hemodialysis.[75,76] The 5-year survival rate after successful transplantation is 70%, whereas patients with CRF who are treated with dialysis have an increased mortality of 30% to 50%.[76] Although it could be argued that healthier patients are more likely to be referred for transplantation, better-controlled analyses have shown a significantly reduced mortality risk for kidney transplantation recipients when compared with acceptable transplantation candidates waiting on dialysis.[75] Transplantation patients often show significant improvement or even full resolution of some cardiovascular comorbidities associated with ESRD.[77] Regardless of whether the treatment modality is dialysis or transplantation, the major causes of death are, in order, heart disease, sepsis, and stroke.[78] The number of patients listed for deceased donor kidney (DDK) transplantation (this currently preferred term replaces the term *cadaver donor kidney*) continues to grow disproportionately to the number of kidney transplantations performed annually. There are more than five times as many patients with ESRD on the waiting list for DDK transplantations than the number of yearly DDK donations, which has remained constant at between 8000 and 9000 over the past few years. The success of transplantation is negatively affected by the duration of pretransplantation dialysis dependence.[79] Reliable early transplantation can be achieved only with living related-donor kidneys. The advantages of living related-donor renal transplantation compared with DDK transplantation are better probabilities of graft survival, less recipient morbidity, planned timing of the operation, and partial alleviation of the insufficient supply of deceased donor kidneys.

The number of living donor kidney transplants more than doubled (from 2535 to 6236) during the decade from 1992 to 2002, with the largest increase in transplants being from offspring to their parents and from spouses and other genetically unrelated donors. The 5-year graft survival rates among recipients transplanted between 1998 and 2002 were 78.5% and 77.5% for spouse and other unrelated donor grafts, respectively, and these rates were comparable to the 80.7% rate for one-haplotype-matched sibling transplants.[80] The 5-year survival rate for DDKs between 1998 and 2002 was 69.9%.[80]

Recipient Selection

There are few absolute contraindications to renal transplantation. A comprehensive pretransplantation evaluation of the recipient is still important and usually takes place well in advance of the renal transplantation operation and the start of immunosuppression. The aims of the process are to establish the primary cause of kidney failure and its risk for recurrence in the kidney graft, and to rule out active invasive infection, active malignancy, a high probability of operative mortality, noncompliance, and an anatomy unsuitable for technical success.[81]

Transplantation Immunology

The term *allograft* describes organs used for transplantation from nonidentical twin donors of the same species. The two histocompatibility systems of greatest importance in renal transplantation are the cell surface markers of the major histocompatibility complex (MHC) and the ABO blood group.[82] The donor and recipient must be ABO compatible because A and B antigens are present on endothelial cells, and most individuals have antibodies to the red blood cell antigen they lack. Class I MHC antigens (subtypes A, B, and C), also called human leukocyte antigens (HLA), are present on the

surface membranes of all nucleated cells. Class II MHC antigens (subtypes DR, DQ, and DB) are found on B and T lymphocytes, monocytes, macrophages, dendritic cells, and some endothelial cells, and are the primary target for helper T cells.[83] Antibodies against ABO blood group antigens and HLA class I or class II antigens can cause hyperacute rejection if they are present in the recipient at the time of transplantation. Such antibodies bind to vascular endothelium and cause activation of the complement cascade, as well as direct endothelial damage, platelet aggregation, and the formation of microvascular thrombi, with the potential for ischemic necrosis of the transplanted organ. Antibodies against ABO are naturally found in humans. HLA antibodies are produced after prior blood transfusions, multiple pregnancies, or rejection of a prior HLA-incompatible transplant. The presence in the recipient of circulating cytotoxic antibodies against the MHC antigens of a specific donor is checked by pretransplantation cross-matching techniques. A positive complement-dependent T-cell lymphocytotoxicity cross-match is considered a contraindication for renal transplantation.

Because of the inheritance patterns of the HLA antigens, each potential kidney graft recipient is a half-match (or is haploidentical with parents and children) and has a 25% probability of HLA identity, a 50% probability of haploidentity, and a 25% probability of a total HLA mismatch with a sibling. When first-degree relatives are donors, graft survival rates at 1 year are 5% to 7% higher than those of deceased donor grafts. Longer-term graft survival rates still favor the partially matched family donor over a randomly selected DDK (Table 19-3).[80]

Immunosuppressant drugs have been developed to control the immune response and avoid allograft rejection. They all have more or less severe side effects. To minimize side effects, almost all antirejection regimens combine lower dosages of several different drugs. Commonly used drugs include a glucocorticoid in combination with drugs such as cyclosporine or tacrolimus (calcineurin inhibitors), azathioprine or mycophenolate mofetil (purine antagonists), and sometimes antilymphocyte antibody preparations (OKT3, thymoglobulin, basiliximab, and daclizumab), which deplete T cells or interfere with their recruitment.

Preoperative Considerations

The preoperative considerations for renal transplant patients are the same as for patients with advanced CRF and were

19-3	Influence of Histocompatibility on Kidney Transplantation Graft Survival	
Donor	**1-Yr Survival (%)**	**3-Yr Survival (%)**
HLA-identical sibling	96	93
One-haplotype sibling	94	73
Living unrelated	93	86
Deceased donor	89	76

HLA, human leukocyte antigen.

covered earlier in this chapter. The most important considerations are the presence and severity of significant comorbidities (cardiac disease, hypertension, and diabetes), hemostasis abnormalities, fluid and electrolyte status, peripheral and autonomic neuropathies, latest dialysis and possible dialysis-related problems (hypovolemia or hypervolemia, systemic anticoagulation), and, if this is a deceased donor transplantation, the patient's NPO (nil per os) status. The use of perioperative beta-blockade should be considered if there are no contraindications.

Anesthesia Management

Anesthesia management follows the guidelines described earlier for patients with advanced CRF. Adequate venous access is important because there is a potential for significant blood loss. At the author's institution, we routinely insert a central venous catheter, under strict aseptic technique, in addition to a peripheral line. Thiopental or etomidate, depending on the patient's status, is preferred for induction; succinylcholine or rocuronium, depending on the patient's potassium level, is preferred for rapid-sequence induction; and isoflurane is preferred for anesthetic maintenance. Cisatracurium is used for maintenance of muscle blockade as guided by a peripheral nerve stimulator, and fentanyl and hydromorphone are used as analgesics. Transplant recipients receive perioperative drug therapy, in addition to the anesthetics, per protocol. The transplant surgeon provides a list of drugs to administer and the dosage and timing thereof. The list usually covers pre-incision antibiotics, immunosuppressive regimen, albumin, mannitol, and furosemide.

Diabetes and Blood Glucose Control

Diabetes mellitus is increasing at an alarming rate. More than 150 million people currently have diabetes and twice that number are at high risk of developing it in the coming 5 to 10 years.[84] Hyperglycemia is generally accepted to be a major cause of diabetic microvascular complications, and it may also play an important role in the development of macrovascular changes.[85] Knowledge of the mechanisms by which high levels of blood sugar contribute to blindness, cardiovascular disease, and kidney failure remains limited.[86]

Among the irreversible changes that occur as a result of hyperglycemia is the formation of advanced glycation end-products (AGEs) through a reaction between sugars and the free amino groups on proteins, lipids, and nucleic acids. AGEs have a wide range of chemical, cellular, and tissue effects through changes in charge, solubility, and conformation that characterize molecular aging. AGEs also interact with specific receptors (RAGEs) and binding proteins (MSRs) to influence the expression of growth factors and cytokines, thereby regulating the growth and proliferation of the various renal cell types. It seems that many of the pathogenic changes that occur in diabetic nephropathy may be induced by AGEs. Drugs that either inhibit the formation of AGE or break AGE-induced cross-links have been shown to be renoprotective in experimental models of diabetic nephropathy.[87,88] AGEs are able to stimulate directly the production of extracellular matrix and inhibit its degradation. Recent studies have suggested that

angiotensin-converting enzyme (ACE) inhibitors are able to reduce the accumulation of AGEs in diabetes.[89] It is likely that therapies that inhibit the formation of AGEs will form an important part of future therapy in patients with diabetes.[89]

Glycemic management and its influence on outcomes for diabetic and critically ill patients has become an area of great interest during the past decade. The benefits of insulin were first described in the setting of acute myocardial infarction. Long-term outcome was improved by keeping the blood glucose level at less than 215 mg/dL in diabetic patients who had suffered an acute myocardial infarction.[90] Hyperglycemia associated with insulin resistance is common in both diabetic and nondiabetic critically ill patients, and it was postulated that pronounced hyperglycemia might contribute to morbidity and mortality in such patients.[91] In a widely cited study by Van den Berghe and colleagues,[92] 1548 critically ill patients were randomly assigned to receive either intensive or conventional insulin therapy. Intensive therapy was aimed at keeping the blood glucose level between 80 and 110 mg/dL. Conventional therapy was started only if the blood sugar exceeded 215 mg/dL and was then aimed at maintaining blood glucose between 180 and 200 mg/dL. Intensive insulin therapy reduced mortality by 42.5% and also reduced morbidity. The rate of sepsis was decreased by 46%, acute renal failure by 41%, transfusions by 50%, and critical illness polyneuropathy by 44%.[92] Stimulated by these studies, a burgeoning interest has developed in the effect of intraoperative glycemic control on morbidity and mortality. Studies of diabetic patients undergoing CABG have shown that tight glycemic control improves perioperative outcomes, enhances survival, and decreases the incidence of ischemic events and wound complications.[93,94] There are currently no published studies addressing the issue of intraoperative glycemic control and perioperative outcome in diabetic patients undergoing kidney transplantation.

Kidney Viability in Transplant Surgery

Living Kidney Donor

Living donors contribute more than 25% of renal allografts in the United States. Donor nephrectomy is a unique surgery because donor as well as recipient outcomes are required to assess the success of donor surgery. An ideal donor nephrectomy should fulfill the criteria of minimal warm ischemia time, adequate length of damage-free renal vessels, adequate length of well-vascularized ureter, atraumatic organ removal, and a low donor and recipient morbidity. Laparoscopic donor nephrectomy has gained widespread popularity in recent years. The operation is performed under general anesthesia. The renal vein, artery, and ureter are exposed and dissected. An incision is made in the lower midline to facilitate extraction. After systemic heparinization, the ureter, renal artery, and vein are divided, and the kidney is extracted with the help of a plastic specimen-retrieval bag. The kidney is immediately immersed in ice slush and taken out of the operating room for perfusion with preservative solution.

The advantages offered by the laparoscopic technique, as opposed to open nephrectomy, include decreased hospital stay, decreased postoperative pain, improved donor cosmetic outcome, and earlier return to work. Disadvantages include longer surgery time and longer warm ischemia time, which result in longer time for the transplanted kidney to achieve nadir serum creatinine postoperatively. However, long-term outcome does not seem to be negatively influenced by laparoscopic organ procurement.[95,96]

Deceased Donor Kidney

Most kidney recipients lack a suitable or willing living related donor and require a DDK. Factors affecting kidney viability include the donor having primary renal disease, a history of cardiac arrest or prolonged hypotension before harvesting, advanced age (>60 years), the use of vasopressor drugs, the presence of oliguria before harvesting, and the duration of warm and cold ischemia time.[97]

Ischemia time starts with the clamping of the renal vessels in the donor, and it ends with completion of the vascular anastomosis in the recipient. Minimizing ischemia time, particularly the warm ischemia period, is very important, as acute tubular necrosis increases with its duration.

Warm ischemia time starts when the donor vessels are clamped, and it is interrupted when the kidney is perfused with cold preservation solution. Warm ischemia resumes when the kidney is placed in the recipient and ends when the kidney is revascularized and perfusion starts. During cold ischemia, the kidney is usually stored at 4°C. Ideally, the duration of cold ischemia should not exceed 24 hours.

Kidney Preservation

The procured kidney's cellular energy requirements are significantly reduced by hypothermia. This is achieved by surface cooling, followed by hypothermic pulsatile perfusion or flushing with an ice-cold solution.[98,99] The kidney is then put in cold storage. The flush solution is made slightly hyperosmolar with impermanent solutes such as mannitol, lactobionate, raffinose, or hydroxyethyl starch, to prevent endothelial swelling and prevent the "no-reflow" phenomenon. A review of 35,057 DDK transplants demonstrated no significant difference in 3-year graft survival between kidneys preserved by pulsatile machine perfusion and those preserved by simple cold storage.[100]

The two solutions developed by Euro-Collins in 1969 and the newer University of Wisconsin (UW) solution developed in the late 1980s[101] are widely used to preserve kidneys. The UW solution can also be used to preserve other solid organs, and it appears to offer some other advantages over the Euro-Collins solution. A prospective randomized study of 695 DDKs preserved with either UW or Euro-Collins solution and subjected to cold storage up to 24 hours showed that the UW solution resulted in a significantly more rapid reduction in the postoperative serum creatinine level, a significantly lower postoperative dialysis rate, and a 6% higher 1-year graft survival than the Euro-Collins solution.[102] However, the UW solution has limitations, as evidenced by the high failure rate for kidneys subjected to cold storage for more than 24 hours regardless of which of the two preservation solutions are used.[103]

The unavoidable detrimental effects of events surrounding DDK retrieval and preservation, particularly ones resulting from cold storage ischemia, are shown by the 6% better 1-year graft survival in living unrelated donor kidney transplants, compared with primary deceased donor kidney transplants.[104]

Experimental Techniques to Increase Viability

Ischemic Preconditioning. The phenomenon of ischemic preconditioning (IPC), in which short periods of ischemia are followed by reperfusion and this temporarily increases the resistance to further ischemic damage, was first described in the canine heart,[105] and it has subsequently been documented in the kidney.[106] The question of whether IPC would be able to protect the transplanted kidney from the injuries of cold storage and reperfusion, when the renal circulation is restored in the recipient, has been addressed in a couple of recent studies. Torras and colleagues used a rodent model and found a positive IPC effect on kidneys transplanted after 5 hours of cold storage.[107] Using a dog model, Kosieradzki and coworkers were unable to document any effect of IPC on the preservation injury observed after transplantation of kidneys cold-stored for 24 hours.[108] Their conclusion was that IPC had no significantly measurable effect in hypothermic ischemic-reperfusion injury in large animals. The clinical usefulness of IPC under renal ischemia conditions in humans has yet to be determined.

Cold Storage. Recent experimental studies have suggested that two strategies—fortifying the cold storage solution with deferoxamine and preconditioning the kidneys with hemeoxygenase-1 (HO-1)—may prove to be clinically viable to limit cold ischemic injury.

Deferoxamine is an antioxidant. Its renoprotective effect was tested in a rat kidney transplant model, which used 18 hours of cold storage before transplantation and reperfusion of the kidney. Deferoxamine-treated kidneys had 75% better function compared with untreated kidneys, as judged by serum creatinine levels. Deferoxamine treatment was also associated with a significant reduction of renal necrotic and apoptotic injuries.[109]

Stress protein HO-1 is a microsomal enzyme that degrades heme proteins. Overexpression of HO-1 in renal tubular cells, either through gene transfer or induction with hemin, protects these cells against cold storage injury.[110] The renoprotective effects of HO-1 have been supported by in vivo findings in kidney and liver transplantation models.[111] The inducibility of the HO-1 isoenzyme is modulated by a (GT)n dinucleotide polymorphism in the HO-1 gene promoter.[112] Short (class S) GT repeats were found to be associated with highly significant upregulation of HO-1.[112] In a recent study of 101 DDK recipients, 50 patients had received a kidney from a donor with at least one class S allele. These recipients had significantly lower 1-year serum creatinine levels ($P < .01$), compared with the 51 recipients of a non–class S allele donor kidney.[113]

Dopamine is able to induce expression of HO-1 in endothelial cells.[114] In a retrospective study of 254 consecutive DDK recipients, 158 of the donors had received dopamine immediately before their kidneys were harvested, and the remaining 96 had not. Dopamine-treated donor kidneys were associated with both significantly lower 1-day serum creatinine values than untreated kidneys, and also with superior long-term graft survival ($P < .001$).[115] Further studies are required to test the usefulness of HO-1 preconditioning and of adding deferoxamine to the storage solution in the clinical transplant setting.

Intraoperative Management of Kidney Recipients

Deceased donor renal allografts with excellent immediate graft function (IGF), defined as a serum creatinine (Cr) level of less than 3 mg/dL on postoperative day 5, have good long-term outcomes. Recipients with slow graft function (SGF), defined as a Cr level of greater than 3 mg/dL on postoperative day 5 but no need for dialysis, have an increased risk for acute rejection (AR). In the absence of AR, 5-year graft survival of SGF recipients does not differ from that of IGF recipients.[116,117] The impact of delayed graft function (DGF), defined by the need for dialysis in the first week after transplant, is controversial. DGF is associated with a higher incidence of AR than either IGF or SGF recipients.[117] Reports on the outcome for DGF recipients, with no AR, disagree on the impact of DGF. Some authors conclude that DGF is associated with decreased long-term survival when compared with IGF recipients,[104,118] but others have been unable to find any influence of DGF on long-term outcome.[119,120]

We will now examine the supporting evidence for some intraoperative interventions that have been suggested to improve the likelihood of immediate graft function.

Hemodynamics and Intravascular Volume

The intraoperative maintenance of effective intravascular volume and normal hemodynamics is of outmost importance for the prevention of renal hypoperfusion during major surgery.[121] Maintaining a mean pulmonary artery pressure of 20 mm Hg has been shown to reduce the occurrence of postoperative transplant acute renal failure.[122] Maintaining a central venous pressure of 10 to 15 mm Hg has been recommended as a good compromise between optimizing intravascular volume and minimizing the risk of fluid overload.[97] Aggressive intravascular volume expansion has been proposed to enable the use of intraoperative verapamil without inducing hypotensive complications.[123]

Albumin
Colloid plasma volume expansion in living donor-related graft recipients is associated with immediate onset of urine output in more than 90% of patients.[124] Intraoperative plasma volume expansion with albumin also improved outcome in DDK recipients.[125,126] Albumin may have other beneficial effects in addition to plasma volume expansion.[127]

Diuretics
Furosemide. Furosemide blocks the chloride pump in the thick ascending loop of Henle. The decrease in tubular oxygen consumption associated with the reduced workload may confer resistance against ischemic injury. On the basis of such deliberations, furosemide is often included in intraoperative pharmacologic treatment of transplant recipients.

Any certain improvement of kidney transplant outcome has not been documented.[128,129]

Mannitol. Mannitol is an osmotic diuretic. Postulated beneficial effects of mannitol therapy include increased intravascular volume with improvements of preload and cardiac output, increased renal blood flow secondary to release of atrial natriuretic peptide and intrarenal vasodilating prostanoids, increased urinary output, facilitating the flushing out of debris from the tubules and decreased endothelial cell swelling, and promoting increased intrarenal blood flow.[130] Mannitol is a known free radical scavenger, with a possible attenuating effect on reperfusion injury.[131] During DDK renal transplant surgery, mannitol administration before clamp release is associated with a significant reduction in post-transplant ARF.[132]

Calcium Channel Antagonists

Calcium channel blockers have the potential to protect the kidney from the adverse effects of an ischemia-induced rise in intracellular calcium. Detrimental effects of increased intracellular calcium levels include reduced ATP production by uncoupling of mitochondrial oxidative phosphorylation, activation of phospholipases (causing membrane enzyme dysfunction and membrane damage), and free radical generation.[133-135]

A systematic review of perioperative use of calcium channel blockers in kidney transplant recipients in the Cochrane Database yielded nine randomized controlled studies with a total of 445 patients, where calcium channel blockers were given in the peritransplant period.[136] The conclusion was that treatment with calcium channel blockers in the peritransplant period was associated with a significant decrease of post-transplant ARF and delayed graft function. However, the review authors qualified their conclusion: "The result should be treated with caution due to the heterogeneity of the trials, which made comparison of studies and pooling of data difficult."[136]

Dopamine

The use of low-dose dopamine (DA), defined as an infusion of 0.5 to 3.0 µg/kg/min, to prevent or treat renal dysfunction has become a widely accepted clinical practice. This is based on dopamine's ability to increase renal blood flow and glomerular filtration rate, and to induce sodium diuresis. The latter, achieved by inhibition of renal tubular Na^+,K^+-ATPase activity, leads to a decrease in tubular oxygen consumption.[137] These seemingly beneficial effects are well documented in animal models and in human studies. Support for the use of DA to protect renal function was found in some early studies. However, these studies included small numbers of patients and lacked blinding and randomization. Later randomized studies in larger populations of patients undergoing cardiac, vascular, and liver transplant or biliary surgery have failed to demonstrate any efficacy of DA in preventing ARF or improving outcome.[138]

The use of dopamine in the transplant setting can take place both in the DDK setting before procurement or in the recipient in the peritransplant period. The use of dopamine in the donor is, as already discussed, associated with significantly lower 1-day serum creatinine values than untreated kidneys, and also with superior long-term graft survival ($P < .001$).[115] Studies using dopamine in the range of 2 to 3 µg/kg/min perioperatively during DDK transplantation failed to demonstrate any renal protection.[139,140]

Immunosuppressants

The management of immunosuppressants used for renal transplantation, both in the peritransplant period and long term, is very complex and has profound implications for outcome. This topic is too extensive for the scope of this chapter.

However, one drug, murine monoclonal antibody (OKT3), does improve graft survival. However, it has the potential for immediate intraoperative complications in the form of tachycardia and sudden pulmonary edema, induced by the sudden release of cytokines from activated T cells.[141] Prophylactic use of steroids, slow infusion rate, preoperative dialysis, and careful fluid management, guided by central venous pressure, are helpful in preventing the side effects of OKT3.[142]

■ SUMMARY

Organ viability associated with renal transplantation is a very complex issue. The successful kidney transplantation involves the management of the donor, the allograft, and the recipient. Both short- and long-term patient outcomes are influenced by management of perioperative fluid, hemodynamics, and

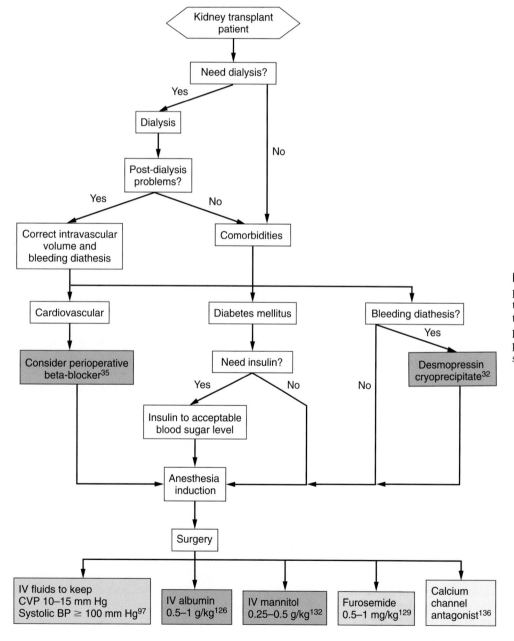

Figure 19-1 ■ Flow chart for preoperative and intraoperative treatment of the kidney transplant recipient. BP, blood pressure; CVP, central venous pressure. For references cited, see reference list.

drugs. The anesthesiologist plays an important role in the perioperative setting by vigilantly monitoring hemodynamics and optimizing intravascular volume to maximize kidney perfusion, thereby contributing to the overall success of renal transplantation (Fig. 19-1).

■ REFERENCES

1. National Kidney Foundation: K/DOQI clinical practice guidelines for chronic kidney disease: Evaluation, classification, and stratification. Am J Kidney Dis 2002;39(2 Suppl 1):S1-266.
2. Coresh J, Byrd-Holt D, Astor BC, et al: Chronic kidney disease awareness, prevalence, and trends among U.S. adults, 1999 to 2000. J Am Soc Nephrol 2005;16:180-188.
3. Levey AS, Coresh J, Balk E, et al: National Kidney Foundation practice guidelines for chronic kidney disease: Evaluation, classification, and stratification. Ann Intern Med 2003;139:137-147.
4. Remuzzi G, Ruggenenti P, Perico N: Chronic renal diseases: Renoprotective benefits of renin-angiotensin system inhibition. Ann Intern Med 2002;136:604-615.
5. Coresh J, Wei GL, McQuillan G, et al: Prevalence of high blood pressure and elevated serum creatinine level in the United States: Findings from the third National Health and Nutrition Examination Survey (1988-1994). Arch Intern Med 2001;161:1207-1216.
6. Heidland A, Sebekova K, Schinzel R: Advanced glycation end products and the progressive course of renal disease. Am J Kidney Dis 2001;38(4 Suppl 1):S100-106.
7. Jandeleit-Dahm KA, Lassila M, Allen TJ: Advanced glycation end products in diabetes-associated atherosclerosis and renal disease: Interventional studies. Ann N Y Acad Sci 2005;1043:759-766.
8. Chertow GM, Lazarus JM, Christiansen CL, et al: Preoperative renal risk stratification. Circulation 1997;95:878-884.
9. Anderson RJ, O'Brien M, MaWhinney S, et al: Renal failure predisposes patients to adverse outcome after coronary artery bypass surgery. VA Cooperative Study #5. Kidney Int 1999;55:1057-1062.
10. Conlon PJ, Stafford-Smith M, White WD, et al: Acute renal failure following cardiac surgery. Nephrol Dial Transplant 1999;14:1158-1162.
11. Metnitz PG, Krenn CG, Steltzer H, et al: Effect of acute renal failure requiring renal replacement therapy on outcome in critically ill patients. Crit Care Med 2002;30:2051-2058.
12. Mehta RL, Chertow GM: Acute renal failure definitions and classification: Time for change? J Am Soc Nephrol 2003;14:2178-2187.
13. Jarnberg PO: Renal protection strategies in the perioperative period. Best Pract Res Clin Anaesthesiol 2004;18:645-660.
14. Prins JM, Buller HR, Kuijper EJ, et al: Once versus thrice daily gentamicin in patients with serious infections. Lancet 1993;341:335-339.
15. Davidman M, Olson P, Kohen J, et al: Iatrogenic renal disease. Arch Intern Med 1991;151:1809-1812.
16. Silbiger SR, Neugarten J: The impact of gender on the progression of chronic renal disease. Am J Kidney Dis 1995;25:515-533.
17. Dubey RK, Jackson EK: Estrogen-induced cardiorenal protection: Potential cellular, biochemical, and molecular mechanisms. Am J Physiol Renal Physiol 2001;280:F365-388.
18. Neugarten J, Acharya A, Silbiger SR: Effect of gender on the progression of nondiabetic renal disease: A meta-analysis. J Am Soc Nephrol 2000;11:319-329.
19. Mujais SK, Sabatini S, Kurtzman NA: Pathophysiology of the uremic syndrome. In Brenner BM, Rector FC (eds): The Kidney, ed 3. Philadelphia, WB Saunders, 1986, pp 1587-1630.
20. Skorecki K, Green J, Brenner BM: Chronic renal failure. In Kasper DL, Braunwald E, Fauci A, et al (eds): Harrison's Principles of Internal Medicine, ed 16. New York, McGraw Hill, 2005, pp 1653-1662.
21. Sarnak MJ, Levey AS, Schoolwerth AC, et al: Kidney disease as a risk factor for development of cardiovascular disease: A statement from the American Heart Association Councils on Kidney in Cardiovascular Disease, High Blood Pressure Research, Clinical Cardiology, and Epidemiology and Prevention. Circulation 2003;108:2154-2169.
22. Foley RN, Parfrey PS, Sarnak MJ: Clinical epidemiology of cardiovascular disease in chronic renal disease. Am J Kidney Dis 1998;32(5 Suppl 3):S112-119.
23. Yigla M, Nakhoul F, Sabag A, et al: Pulmonary hypertension in patients with end-stage renal disease. Chest 2003;123:1577-1582.
24. Date H, Imamura T, Sumi T, et al: Effects of interleukin-6 produced in coronary circulation on production of C-reactive protein and coronary microvascular resistance. Am J Cardiol 2005;95:849-852.
25. Arici M, Walls J: End-stage renal disease, atherosclerosis, and cardiovascular mortality: Is C-reactive protein the missing link? Kidney Int 2001;59:407-414.
26. Lagrand WK, Visser CA, Hermens WT, et al: C-reactive protein as a cardiovascular risk factor: More than an epiphenomenon? Circulation 1999;100:96-102.
27. Conlon PJ, Krucoff MW, Minda S, et al: Incidence and long-term significance of transient ST segment deviation in hemodialysis patients. Clin Nephrol 1998;49:236-239.
28. Steinman TI, Becker BN, Frost AE, et al: Guidelines for the referral and management of patients eligible for solid organ transplantation. Transplantation 2001;71:1189-1204.
29. Kasiske BL, Cangro CB, Hariharan S, et al: The evaluation of renal transplantation candidates: Clinical practice guidelines. Am J Transplant 2001;(1 Suppl 2):3-95.
30. Holley JL, Fenton RA, Arthur RS: Thallium stress testing does not predict cardiovascular risk in diabetic patients with end-stage renal disease undergoing cadaveric renal transplantation. Am J Med 1991;90:563-570.
31. Eknoyan G: The importance of early treatment of the anaemia of chronic kidney disease. Nephrol Dial Transplant 2001;(16 Suppl 5):45-49.
32. Zachee P, Vermylen J, Boogaerts MA: Hematologic aspects of end-stage renal failure. Ann Hematol 1994;69:33-40.
33. Schmidt M, Sitter T, Lederer SR, et al: Reversible MRI changes in a patient with uremic encephalopathy. J Nephrol 2001;14:424-427.
34. Mannucci PM, Remuzzi G, Pusineri F, et al: Deamino-8-D-arginine vasopressin shortens the bleeding time in uremia. N Engl J Med 1983;308:8-12.
35. Lindenauer PK, Pekow P, Wang K, et al: Perioperative beta-blocker therapy and mortality after major noncardiac surgery. N Engl J Med 2005;353:349-361.
36. Lee TH, Marcantonio ER, Mangione CM, et al: Derivation and prospective validation of a simple index for prediction of cardiac risk of major noncardiac surgery. Circulation 1999;100:1043-1049.
37. Poldermans D, Boersma E: Beta-blocker therapy in noncardiac surgery. N Engl J Med 2005;353:412-414.
38. Burch PG, Stanski DR: Decreased protein binding and thiopental kinetics. Clin Pharmacol Ther 1982;32:212-217.
39. Carlos R, Calvo R, Erill S: Plasma protein binding of etomidate in patients with renal failure or hepatic cirrhosis. Clin Pharmacokinet 1979;4:144-148.
40. Kirvela M, Olkkola KT, Rosenberg PH, et al: Pharmacokinetics of propofol and haemodynamic changes during induction of anaesthesia in uraemic patients. Br J Anaesth 1992;68:178-182.
41. Reich DL, Silvay G: Ketamine: An update on the first twenty-five years of clinical experience. Can J Anaesth 1989;36:186-197.
42. Thapa S, Brull SJ: Succinylcholine-induced hyperkalemia in patients with renal failure: An old question revisited. Anesth Analg 2000;91:237-241.
43. Bevan DR, Donati F, Gyasi H, Williams A: Vecuronium in renal failure. Can Anaesth Soc J 1984;31:491-496.
44. Szenohradszky J, Fisher DM, Segredo V, et al: Pharmacokinetics of rocuronium bromide (ORG 9426) in patients with normal renal function or patients undergoing cadaver renal transplantation. Anesthesiology 1992;77:899-904.
45. Szeto HH, Inturrisi CE, Houde R, et al: Accumulation of normeperidine, an active metabolite of meperidine, in patients with renal failure of cancer. Ann Intern Med 1977;86:738-741.
46. D'Honneur G, Gilton A, Sandouk P, et al: Plasma and cerebrospinal fluid concentrations of morphine and morphine glucuronides after oral morphine: The influence of renal failure. Anesthesiology 1994;81:87-93.

47. Chauvin M, Lebrault C, Levron JC, Duvaldestin P: Pharmacokinetics of alfentanil in chronic renal failure. Anesth Analg 1987;66:53-56.

48. Hoke JF, Shlugman D, Dershwitz M, et al: Pharmacokinetics and pharmacodynamics of remifentanil in persons with renal failure compared with healthy volunteers. Anesthesiology 1997;87:533-541.

49. Fujii K, Morio M, Kikuchi H, et al: Pharmacokinetic study on excretion of inorganic fluoride ion, a metabolite of sevoflurane. Hiroshima J Med Sci 1987;36:89-92.

50. Kobayashi Y, Ochiai R, Takeda J, et al: Serum and urinary inorganic fluoride concentrations after prolonged inhalation of sevoflurane in humans. Anesth Analg 1992;74:753-757.

51. Frink EJ Jr, Malan TP Jr, Isner RJ, et al: Renal concentrating function with prolonged sevoflurane or enflurane anesthesia in volunteers. Anesthesiology 1994;80:1019-1025.

52. Conzen PF, Kharasch ED, Czerner SF, et al: Low-flow sevoflurane compared with low-flow isoflurane anesthesia in patients with stable renal insufficiency. Anesthesiology 2002;97:578-584.

53. Conzen PF, Nuscheler M, Melotte A, et al: Renal function and serum fluoride concentrations in patients with stable renal insufficiency after anesthesia with sevoflurane or enflurane. Anesth Analg 1995;81:569-575.

54. Higuchi H, Adachi Y, Wada H, et al: The effects of low-flow sevoflurane and isoflurane anesthesia on renal function in patients with stable moderate renal insufficiency. Anesth Analg 2001;92:650-655.

55. Fang ZX, Eger EI 2nd: Factors affecting the concentration of compound A resulting from the degradation of sevoflurane by soda lime and Baralyme in a standard anesthetic circuit. Anesth Analg 1995;81:564-568.

56. Gonsowski CT, Laster MJ, Eger EI 2nd, et al: Toxicity of compound A in rats: Effect of a 3-hour administration. Anesthesiology 1994;80:556-565.

57. Keller KA, Callan C, Prokocimer P, et al: Inhalation toxicity study of a haloalkene degradant of sevoflurane, compound A (PIFE), in Sprague-Dawley rats. Anesthesiology 1995;83:1220-1232.

58. Morio M, Fujii K, Satoh N, et al: Reaction of sevoflurane and its degradation products with soda lime: Toxicity of the byproducts. Anesthesiology 1992;77:1155-1164.

59. Kharasch ED, Thorning D, Garton K, et al: Role of renal cysteine conjugate beta-lyase in the mechanism of compound A nephrotoxicity in rats. Anesthesiology 1997;86:160-171.

60. Goldberg ME, Cantillo J, Gratz I, et al: Dose of compound A, not sevoflurane, determines changes in the biochemical markers of renal injury in healthy volunteers. Anesth Analg 1999;88:437-445.

61. Higuchi H, Sumita S, Wada H, et al: Effects of sevoflurane and isoflurane on renal function and on possible markers of nephrotoxicity. Anesthesiology 1998;89:307-322.

62. Eger EI 2nd, Gong D, Koblin DD, et al: Dose-related biochemical markers of renal injury after sevoflurane versus desflurane anesthesia in volunteers. Anesth Analg 1997;85:1154-1163.

63. Kharasch ED, Frink EJ Jr, Zager R, et al: Assessment of low-flow sevoflurane and isoflurane effects on renal function using sensitive markers of tubular toxicity. Anesthesiology 1997;86:1238-1253.

64. Bito H, Ikeuchi Y, Ikeda K: Effects of low-flow sevoflurane anesthesia on renal function: Comparison with high-flow sevoflurane anesthesia and low-flow isoflurane anesthesia. Anesthesiology 1997;86:1231-1237.

65. Ebert TJ, Messana LD, Uhrich TD, Staacke TS: Absence of renal and hepatic toxicity after four hours of 1.25 minimum alveolar anesthetic concentration sevoflurane anesthesia in volunteers. Anesth Analg 1998;86:662-667.

66. Bedford RF, Ives HE: The renal safety of sevoflurane. Anesth Analg 2000;90:505-508.

67. Murray JM, Renfrew CW, Bedi A, et al: Amsorb: A new carbon dioxide absorbent for use in anesthetic breathing systems. Anesthesiology 1999;91:1342-1348.

68. Grejda S, Ellis K, Arino P: Paraplegia following spinal anesthesia in a patient with chronic renal failure. Reg Anesth 1989;14:155-157.

69. Basta M, Sloan P: Epidural hematoma following epidural catheter placement in a patient with chronic renal failure. Can J Anaesth 1999;46:271-274.

70. DuBose TD Jr, Warnock DG, Mehta RL, et al: Acute renal failure in the 21st century: Recommendations for management and outcomes assessment. Am J Kidney Dis 1997;29:793-799.

71. Niu MT, Coleman PJ, Alter MJ: Multicenter study of hepatitis C virus infection in chronic hemodialysis patients and hemodialysis center staff members. Am J Kidney Dis 1993;22:568-573.

72. Fabrizi F, Martin P, Dixit V, et al: Quantitative assessment of HCV load in chronic hemodialysis patients: A cross-sectional survey. Nephron 1998;80:428-433.

73. Hu KK, Lipsky BA, Veenstra DL, Saint S: Using maximal sterile barriers to prevent central venous catheter-related infection: A systematic evidence-based review. Am J Infect Control 2004;32:142-146.

74. Berenholtz SM, Pronovost PJ, Lipsett PA, et al: Eliminating catheter-related bloodstream infections in the intensive care unit. Crit Care Med 2004;32:2014-2020.

75. Schnuelle P, Lorenz D, Trede M, Van der Woude FJ: Impact of renal cadaveric transplantation on survival in end-stage renal failure: Evidence for reduced mortality risk compared with hemodialysis during long-term follow-up. J Am Soc Nephrol 1998;9:2135-2141.

76. Wolfe RA, Ashby VB, Milford EL, et al: Comparison of mortality in all patients on dialysis, patients on dialysis awaiting transplantation, and recipients of a first cadaveric transplant. N Engl J Med 1999;341:1725-1730.

77. Ferreira SR, Moises VA, Tavares A, Pacheco-Silva A: Cardiovascular effects of successful renal transplantation: A 1-year sequential study of left ventricular morphology and function, and 24-hour blood pressure profile. Transplantation 2002;74:1580-1587.

78. Excerpts from the 2000 U.S. Renal Data System Annual Data Report: Atlas of End-Stage Renal Disease in the United States. Am J Kidney Dis 2000;36(Suppl):S1-S279.

79. Meier-Kriesche HU, Port FK, Ojo AO, et al: Effect of waiting time on renal transplant outcome. Kidney Int 2000;58:1311-1317.

80. Cecka JM: The OPTN/UNOS Renal Transplant Registry 2003. Clin Transpl 2003:1-12.

81. Barry JM: Current status of renal transplantation: Patient evaluations and outcomes. Urol Clin North Am 2001;28:677-686.

82. VanBuskirk AM, Pidwell DJ, Adams PW, Orosz CG: Transplantation immunology. JAMA 1997;278:1993-1999.

83. Bach FH, Sachs DH: Current concepts: Immunology—Transplantation immunology. N Engl J Med 1987;317:489-492.

84. Zimmet P, Alberti KG, Shaw J: Global and societal implications of the diabetes epidemic. Nature 2001;414:782-787.

85. Hanssen KF: Blood glucose control and microvascular and macrovascular complications in diabetes. Diabetes 1997;46(Suppl 2):S101-103.

86. Brownlee M: Biochemistry and molecular cell biology of diabetic complications. Nature 2001;414:813-820.

87. Soulis T, Cooper ME, Sastra S, et al: Relative contributions of advanced glycation and nitric oxide synthase inhibition to aminoguanidine-mediated renoprotection in diabetic rats. Diabetologia 1997;40:1141-1151.

88. Cooper ME, Thallas V, Forbes J, et al: The cross-link breaker, *N*-phenacylthiazolium bromide prevents vascular advanced glycation end-product accumulation. Diabetologia 2000;43:660-664.

89. Miyata T, van Ypersele de Strihou C, Ueda Y, et al: Angiotensin II receptor antagonists and angiotensin-converting enzyme inhibitors lower in vitro the formation of advanced glycation end products: Biochemical mechanisms. J Am Soc Nephrol 2002;13:2478-2487.

90. Malmberg K, Norhammar A, Wedel H, Ryden L: Glycometabolic state at admission: Important risk marker of mortality in conventionally treated patients with diabetes mellitus and acute myocardial infarction: Long-term results from the Diabetes and Insulin-Glucose Infusion in Acute Myocardial Infarction (DIGAMI) study. Circulation 1999;99:2626-2632.

91. Wolfe RR, Herndon DN, Jahoor F, et al: Effect of severe burn injury on substrate cycling by glucose and fatty acids. N Engl J Med 1987;317:403-408.

92. Van den Berghe G, Wouters P, Weekers F, et al: Intensive insulin therapy in the critically ill patients. N Engl J Med 2001;345:1359-1367.

93. Lazar HL, Chipkin SR, Fitzgerald CA, et al: Tight glycemic control in diabetic coronary artery bypass graft patients improves perioperative outcomes and decreases recurrent ischemic events. Circulation 2004;109:1497-1502.

94. Furnary AP, Gao G, Grunkemeier GL, et al: Continuous insulin infusion reduces mortality in patients with diabetes undergoing coronary artery bypass grafting. J Thorac Cardiovasc Surg 2003;125:1007-1021.

95. Buzdon MM, Cho E, Jacobs SC, et al: Warm ischemia time does not correlate with recipient graft function in laparoscopic donor nephrectomy. Surg Endosc 2003;17:746-749.

96. Koffron A, Herman C, Gross O, et al: Laparoscopic donor nephrectomy: Analysis of donor and recipient outcomes. Transplant Proc 2001;33:1111.

97. Caldwell JE, Cook DR: Kidney transplantation. In Cook DR, Davis PJ (eds): Anesthetic Principles of Organ Transplantation. New York, Raven Press, 1994.

98. Belzer FO, Ashby BS, Dunphy JE: 24-Hour and 72-hour preservation of canine kidneys. Lancet 1967;2:536-538.

99. Collins GM, Bravo-Shugarman M, Terasaki PI: Kidney preservation for transportation: Initial perfusion and 30 hours' ice storage. Lancet 1969;2:1219-1222.

100. Gjertson DW: Multifactorial analysis of renal transplants reported to the United Network for Organ Sharing Registry: A 1994 update. Clin Transpl 1994;519-539.

101. Belzer FO, Southard JH: Principles of solid-organ preservation by cold storage. Transplantation 1988;45:673-676.

102. Ploeg RJ, van Bockel JH, Langendijk PT, et al: Effect of preservation solution on results of cadaveric kidney transplantation. The European Multicentre Study Group. Lancet 1992;340:129-137.

103. Salahudeen AK, Haider N, May W: Cold ischemia and the reduced long-term survival of cadaveric renal allografts. Kidney Int 2004;65:713-718.

104. Cecka JM: The UNOS Scientific Renal Transplant Registry—2000. Clin Transpl 2000:1-18.

105. Murry CE, Jennings RB, Reimer KA: Preconditioning with ischemia: A delay of lethal cell injury in ischemic myocardium. Circulation 1986;74:1124-1136.

106. Hawaleshka A, Jacobsohn E: Ischaemic preconditioning: Mechanisms and potential clinical applications. Can J Anaesth 1998;45:670-682.

107. Torras J, Herrero-Fresneda I, Lloberas N, et al: Promising effects of ischemic preconditioning in renal transplantation. Kidney Int 2002;61:2218-2227.

108. Kosieradzki M, Ametani M, Southard JH, Mangino MJ: Is ischemic preconditioning of the kidney clinically relevant? Surgery 2003;133:81-90.

109. Huang H, He Z, Roberts LJ 2nd, Salahudeen AK: Deferoxamine reduces cold-ischemic renal injury in a syngeneic kidney transplant model. Am J Transplant 2003;3:1531-1537.

110. Salahudeen AA, Jenkins JK, Huang H, et al: Overexpression of heme oxygenase protects renal tubular cells against cold storage injury: Studies using hemin induction and HO-1 gene transfer. Transplantation 2001;72:1498-1504.

111. Katori M, Busuttil RW, Kupiec-Weglinski JW: Heme oxygenase-1 system in organ transplantation. Transplantation 2002;74:905-912.

112. Yamada N, Yamaya M, Okinaga S, et al: Microsatellite polymorphism in the heme oxygenase-1 gene promoter is associated with susceptibility to emphysema. Am J Hum Genet 2000;66:187-195.

113. Exner M, Bohmig GA, Schillinger M, et al: Donor heme oxygenase-1 genotype is associated with renal allograft function. Transplantation 2004;77:538-542.

114. Berger SP, Hunger M, Yard BA, et al: Dopamine induces the expression of heme oxygenase-1 by human endothelial cells in vitro. Kidney Int 2000;58:2314-2319.

115. Schnuelle P, Yard BA, Braun C, et al: Impact of donor dopamine on immediate graft function after kidney transplantation. Am J Transplant 2004;4:419-426.

116. Ferguson CJ, Hillis AN, Williams JD, et al: Calcium-channel blockers and other factors influencing delayed function in renal allografts. Nephrol Dial Transplant 1990;5:816-820.

117. Humar A, Johnson EM, Payne WD, et al: Effect of initial slow graft function on renal allograft rejection and survival. Clin Transplant 1997;11:623-627.

118. Dawidson I, Rooth P, Lu C, et al: Verapamil improves the outcome after cadaver renal transplantation. J Am Soc Nephrol 1991;2:983-990.

119. Troppmann C, Gillingham KJ, Gruessner RW, et al: Delayed graft function in the absence of rejection has no long-term impact: A study of cadaver kidney recipients with good graft function at 1 year after transplantation. Transplantation 1996;61:1331-1337.

120. Boom H, Mallat MJ, de Fijter JW, et al: Delayed graft function influences renal function, but not survival. Kidney Int 2000;58:859-866.

121. Alpert RA, Roizen MF, Hamilton WK, et al: Intraoperative urinary output does not predict postoperative renal function in patients undergoing abdominal aortic revascularization. Surgery 1984;95:707-711.

122. Carlier M, Squifflet JP, Pirson Y, et al: Maximal hydration during anesthesia increases pulmonary arterial pressures and improves early function of human renal transplants. Transplantation 1982;34:201-204.

123. Dawidson IJ, Ar'Rajab A: Perioperative fluid and drug therapy during cadaver kidney transplantation. Clin Transpl 1992:267-284.

124. Dawidson I, Berglin E, Brynger H, Reisch J: Intravascular volumes and colloid dynamics in relation to fluid management in living related kidney donors and recipients. Crit Care Med 1987;15:631-636.

125. Willms CD, Dawidson IJ, Dickerman R, et al: Intraoperative blood volume expansion induces primary function after renal transplantation: A study of 96 paired cadaver kidneys. Transplant Proc 1991;23(1 Pt 2):1338-1339.

126. Dawidson IJ, Sandor ZF, Coorpender L, et al: Intraoperative albumin administration affects the outcome of cadaver renal transplantation. Transplantation 1992;53:774-782.

127. Emerson TE Jr: Unique features of albumin: A brief review. Crit Care Med 1989;17:690-694.

128. Lachance SL, Barry JM: Effect of furosemide on dialysis requirement following cadaveric kidney transplantation. J Urol 1985;133:950-951.

129. Shilliday I, Allison ME: Diuretics in acute renal failure. Ren Fail 1994;16:3-17.

130. Better OS, Rubinstein I, Winaver JM, Knochel JP: Mannitol therapy revisited (1940-1997). Kidney Int 1997;52:886-894.

131. Magovern GJ Jr, Bolling SF, Casale AS, et al: The mechanism of mannitol in reducing ischemic injury: Hyperosmolarity or hydroxyl scavenger? Circulation 1984;70(3 Pt 2):I91-95.

132. van Valenberg PL, Hoitsma AJ, Tiggeler RG, et al: Mannitol as an indispensable constituent of an intraoperative hydration protocol for the prevention of acute renal failure after renal cadaveric transplantation. Transplantation 1987;44:784-788.

133. Wilson DR, Arnold PE, Burke TJ, Schrier RW: Mitochondrial calcium accumulation and respiration in ischemic acute renal failure in the rat. Kidney Int 1984;25:519-526.

134. Matthys E, Patel Y, Kreisberg J, et al: Lipid alterations induced by renal ischemia: Pathogenic factor in membrane damage. Kidney Int 1984;26:153-161.

135. McCord JM: Oxygen-derived free radicals in postischemic tissue injury. N Engl J Med 1985;312:159-163.

136. Shilliday IR, Sherif M: Calcium channel blockers for preventing acute tubular necrosis in kidney transplant recipients. Cochrane Database Syst Rev 2005;CD003421.

137. Seri I, Kone BC, Gullans SR, et al: Locally formed dopamine inhibits Na$^+$-K$^+$-ATPase activity in rat renal cortical tubule cells. Am J Physiol 1988;255(4 Pt 2):F666-673.

138. Weldon BC, Monk TG: The patient at risk for acute renal failure: Recognition, prevention, and preoperative optimization. Anesthesiol Clin North America 2000;18:705-717.

139. Kadieva VS, Friedman L, Margolius LP, et al: The effect of dopamine on graft function in patients undergoing renal transplantation. Anesth Analg 1993;76:362-365.

140. Sandberg J, Tyden G, Groth CG: Low-dose dopamine infusion following cadaveric renal transplantation: No effect on the incidence of ATN. Transplant Proc 1992;24:357.

141. Robinson ST: Administration of OKT3 in the operating room. Transplant Proc 1993;25(2 Suppl 1):41-42.

142. Shield CF 3rd, Beilman G: Safety of OKT3 use in the operating room. Transplant Proc 1993;25(2 Suppl 1):43-44.

Pulmonary System

Chapter

20 Prevention and Treatment of Pulmonary Dysfunction

Christine A. Doyle and Ronald G. Pearl

Pulmonary complications are as likely as cardiac complications to cause perioperative mortality and to prolong hospitalization. These complications may be more severe and more predictive of long-term (2 years or more) mortality.[1] Patients who have chronic obstructive pulmonary disease (COPD) have a 6% to 28% risk of pulmonary complications, and smokers have a 1.4- to 4.3-fold increase. Asthmatics, however, have an increased risk only if they have active disease (e.g., with active wheezing or a peak flow rate below 80% of their personal best).[1]

Management decisions to prevent and treat pulmonary dysfunction increasingly rely on evidence-based medicine. For each patient, the physician integrates pathophysiology, clinician experience, and research to create useful practice guidelines.[2] However, evidence is dynamic and must be continually reviewed as new information is developed, and clinicians must decide whether the evidence applies to each patient. It may take multiple studies and many years to change the standard of care, whether it was evidence based or not.[2,3] Wilkinson notes that the average delay for incorporating new scientific information into the clinical arena is 17 years.[4]

Clinical practice guidelines have been developed to facilitate best-practice treatment for many acute and chronic conditions. However, such guidelines typically deal with only one disease and often do not take comorbidities into account.[5] Most studies define their patient population very specifically, so the results may not apply to the majority of patients in a typical practice. Boyd and colleagues selected 9 of the 15 most common chronic diseases treated in outpatients, collected each of the current guidelines for these diseases, and combined the different recommendations.[5] They identified several conflicts (potential adverse effects on other diseases, drug–drug interactions, and food–drug interactions) and noted that none of the guidelines discussed short-term versus long-term goals and effects on quality of life. None addressed patients with more than three concurrent diseases, but nearly half of Medicare beneficiaries have at least three conditions, and over 20% have five or more. Physicians need to reconcile guidelines with local conditions, resources, and capabilities.[6] Guidelines are not meant to replace clinical judgment but to give an organizational framework for patient management.

■ PREOPERATIVE ASSESSMENT AND RISK FACTORS

Underlying Pulmonary Disease

Many patients have chronic lung disease combined with cardiovascular disease. Even after correction for smoking, there appears to be an association between these two disease processes. Inflammatory responses in the lungs may increase cardiovascular risk through increased autonomic instability (arrhythmias), increased inflammatory cytokines (thrombosis), or increased number of leukocytes (plaque rupture). Furthermore, the increased work of breathing and pulmonary hypertension associated with severe lung disease increases stress on the heart.[7] More than a third of all patients with a diagnosis of COPD are likely to die of a cardiovascular event.[8]

Chronic Obstructive Pulmonary Disease

Chronic obstructive pulmonary disease, the only major fatal disease with an increasing death rate,[7] is characterized by airflow limitation that is not fully reversible. The airflow limitation is usually progressive and is associated with an abnormal inflammatory response of the lungs to noxious particles or gases.[9] Although COPD primarily affects the lungs, it also produces significant systemic consequences[10] and thus is a heterogeneous disease with variable presentations.[11]

20-1	Classification of the Severity of Chronic Obstructive Pulmonary Disease (COPD)	
Stage	**Severity**	**Characteristics**
0	At risk	Normal spirometry
		Chronic symptoms*
I	Mild COPD	FEV_1/FVC <70%
		$FEV_1 \geq 80\%$ predicted
		With or without chronic symptoms*
II	Moderate COPD	FEV_1/FVC <70%
		FEV_1 <80% but $\geq 30\%$ predicted
		IIA: $FEV_1 \geq 50\%$ predicted
		IIB: FEV_1 <50% predicted
		With or without chronic symptoms*
III	Severe COPD	FEV_1/FVC <70%
		FEV_1 <30% predicted,
		Or presence of respiratory failure,†
		Or clinical signs of right heart failure

*Chronic symptoms include cough and sputum production.
†PaO_2 <60 mm Hg while breathing air at sea level.
FEV_1, forced expiratory volume in 1 second; FVC, forced vital capacity.
Adapted from Pauwels RA, Buist AS, Calverley PM, et al; GOLD Scientific Committee: Am J Respir Crit Care Med 2001;163:1256-1276.

20-2	Grading Exacerbations of Chronic Obstructive Pulmonary Disease	
Type	**Severity**	**Symptoms**
Type 1	Severe	Dyspnea, cough, and sputum production
Type 2	Moderate	Any two of the above
Type 3	Mild	Any one of the above

In "Global Strategy for the Diagnosis, Management, and Prevention of Chronic Obstructive Pulmonary Disease" (the GOLD paper),[9] the American Thoracic Society proposed diagnostic criteria for COPD. A post-bronchodilator forced expiratory volume in 1 second (FEV_1) of less than 80% of the predicted value, in combination with an FEV_1 or forced vital capacity (FVC) of less than 70% confirms the presence of airflow limitation that is not fully reversible. As seen in Table 20-1, the disease is stratified into mild, moderate, and severe, based on the reduction in FEV_1 from the predicted value. Patients with class IIB disease are more likely to present with exacerbations. All stages are characterized by chronic inflammation throughout the airways, parenchyma, and pulmonary vasculature. Inflammation is an important part of the disease process, particularly in smokers. However, in subsets of patients, the primary problem is inflammatory changes caused by underlying biochemical defects, such as alpha-1-antitrypsin deficiency[7] or cystic fibrosis.

Chronic bronchitis is a clinical diagnosis based on a chronic productive cough lasting at least 3 months in each of 2 successive years when other causes have been excluded. Emphysema is defined pathologically, with permanent enlargement of airspaces distal to terminal bronchioles, destruction of alveolar walls, and no obvious fibrosis.[10]

Exacerbation of disease is defined by episodic increases in dyspnea, cough, and sputum production.[12] No model satisfactorily predicts exacerbations for all patients. Exacerbations can be graded on the basis of the number of symptoms present (Table 20-2). Exacerbations of COPD are associated with approximately 120,000 deaths per year.[13] Atypical bacteria such as chlamydia (e.g., *Chlamydia pneumoniae*) are responsible for less than 10% of exacerbations of COPD.[14] Viruses such as influenza, parainfluenza, and rhinoviruses are often responsible.

The functional status of the patient with COPD should be assessed, as there may be significant compensation at rest. Patients should be questioned about work limitations and ability to perform activities of daily living. Expiratory flow limitations and hyperinflation in exercise have been implicated as major causes of dyspnea, reduced diaphragm force output, and reduced exercise performance in patients with varying types of increased airway resistance.[15] A normal resting $PaCO_2$ may be present despite extensive ventilation–perfusion ($\dot{V}/\dot{Q}$) inhomogeneity in patients with COPD; supplemental oxygen may uncouple the compensatory mechanisms (hypoxic vasoconstriction and increased central drive) and thus give a better estimate of extent of disease.[16]

Asthma

Asthma occurs in 5% to 7% of the U.S. population, and the incidence is increasing. It is defined by the American Thoracic Society (ATS) as reversible obstructive airways disease, with an FEV_1 of 15% or less of the predicted value plus an improvement of at least 15% with inhalation of a beta-2-adrenergic selective bronchodilator or with other treatment such as corticosteroids.[17] Asking patients whether they have ever had asthma diagnosed by a physician or have had wheezing during the previous 12 months has good sensitivity and specificity for the diagnosis.[18] Asthmatics who require surgery have a 10% complication rate if their preoperative American Society of Anesthesiologists (ASA) physical status (PS) is class 2; the complication rate is 28% with PS class 3, and 46% with PS class 4.[19]

Outpatient treatment of chronic asthma is predominantly directed at the chronic inflammation, whereas treatment of acute asthma is directed primarily at bronchospasm, mucus plugging, $\dot{V}/\dot{Q}$ mismatch, and hypoxemia.[19] Patients who have "resistant" asthma and do not respond to inhaled corticosteroids with or without long-acting bronchodilators should be evaluated to ensure the correct diagnosis, to identify previously unrecognized systemic disease, to identify potential triggers (e.g., occupational exposures), to assess compliance with the prescribed treatment regimen, and to assess for psychosocial problems.[20] A pre-bronchodilator FEV_1 of less than 70% of the predicted value despite high-dose inhaled steroids and long-acting beta-agonist therapy suggests resistance to treatment.

Restrictive Lung Disease

Restrictive lung disease is defined by a symmetric decrease in FEV_1 and FVC, with a reduction in the total lung capacity (TLC). There may also be a concomitant obstructive component, reducing FEV_1 even further.[21] Acute symptoms include tachypnea, tachycardia, and hypoxemia. In general, there is increased load on the inspiratory pump at the same time as there is decreased pressure-generating capacity of the respiratory muscles.[22] Extrinsic causes of restrictive lung diseases include kyphoscoliosis, chest trauma, and muscular dystrophies; intrinsic causes include sarcoidosis, pulmonary fibrosis, alveolar proteinosis, acute pulmonary edema, and acute respiratory distress syndrome or acute lung injury.

Smoking

Nearly one quarter of adults in the United States smoke.[23] The pharmacologic effects of nicotine and carbon monoxide, combined with the particulate components of smoke, produce a proinflammatory[23] and a hypercoagulable state,[24] which contributes to the pathophysiology of COPD and atherosclerosis (Table 20-3).

Physiologic changes from cigarette smoke include nicotine-mediated hemodynamic effects and decreased tissue oxygen delivery resulting from increased carboxyhemoglobin (decreasing oxyhemoglobin concentrations) and a corresponding leftward shift in the oxygen dissociation curve. Nicotine causes increased myocardial work by increasing both heart rate (by 10 to 15 bpm) and blood pressure (by 5 to 10 mm Hg) resulting from increased sympathetic tone.[24,25] Nicotine also vasoconstricts the epicardial and resistance vessels in the heart. The proinflammatory effects of cigarette smoke include increased numbers and activation of macrophages and neutrophils.[24,26] Serum lipids are increased, with increased lipolysis and increased plasma free fatty acids. Increased mucus volume and decreased mucociliary clearance are caused by goblet cell hyperplasia and epithelial abnormalities of the airways.[24] In combination with increased oxidant injury, this contributes to the fibrosis of the airway wall and destruction of alveolar attachments typical of COPD.[26]

Smoking promotes atherosclerosis as a result of inflammation, endothelial injury, oxidant injury, and adverse effects on lipids. Smoking also produces a hypercoagulable state, with increased factor VII levels, platelet aggregation (decreasing platelet life span), and fibrinogen.[24] Although platelets are activated (as measured by increased levels of thromboxane A_2), nicotine alone does not affect platelets.[25] Hypercoagulability leading to acute thrombosis in areas of myocardial atherosclerosis is the cause of most acute myocardial infarctions.

Smoking results in acute and chronic abnormalities of pulmonary function, with a 15% incidence of symptomatic COPD and an additional 50% incidence of chronic bronchitis

20-3	**Effects of Cigarette Smoke**	
Acute Effects on Physiology	**Contributions to Pathophysiology**	**Chronic Effects on Pharmacology**
↑ Sympathetic tone	Atherosclerosis	Nicotine receptor function
Lung inflammation	↓ Mucociliary clearance	Drug metabolism
↓ Tissue P_{O_2}	Endothelial dysfunction	

↑, Increased; ↓, decreased.

without obstruction. Smoking increases intraoperative airway events such as cough and laryngospasm during induction of anesthesia. Smoking also markedly increases the incidence of postoperative respiratory events, including respiratory failure, pneumonia, and unanticipated admission to the intensive care unit (ICU).[23,27] It results in an increased need for postoperative respiratory or aerosol therapy. Finally, it adversely affects wound healing because of the small-vessel vasoconstriction and decreased tissue oxygen delivery described earlier. Patients with a recent history of smoking should be considered for nicotine replacement therapy to prevent physiologic and psychological nicotine withdrawal in the perioperative period.[23] Smoking cessation for a short period before surgery can decrease carboxyhemoglobin levels, but abstinence for a period of several weeks is required to decrease the increased airway reactivity.

Pulmonary Infectious Diseases

Lower respiratory tract infections are the main cause of the deaths caused by infectious diseases in the United States, and pneumonia is the sixth most common cause of death overall. Community-acquired pneumonia (CAP) has a mortality rate of about 2% if outpatient treatment is adequate; mortality increases to 14% if the patient requires hospitalization. About 45,000 cases of CAP occur each year. Hospital-acquired or nosocomial pneumonia is more common, with 300,000 cases per year and a mortality rate ranging from 33% to 50%.

For patients with CAP, a prognostic scoring tool, such as the Pneumonia Patient Outcomes Research Team (PORT) Severity Index, which uses demographic factors, coexisting conditions, physical findings, and laboratory data, can be used to determine the initial site of treatment.[28] In patients with CAP, an etiologic agent is not identified in up to 50% of cases.[29] When a bacterial agent is identified, *Streptococcus pneumoniae* is responsible for two thirds of the cases. *Mycoplasma pneumoniae* is a common organism for outpatient cases. Multiple guidelines for treatment of CAP have been developed by organizations. In general, monotherapy with a macrolide or doxycycline is appropriate in patients without comorbidities (e.g., COPD, diabetes mellitus, congestive heart failure, chronic renal insufficiency, end-stage renal disease) who have not had antibiotic therapy in the past 3 months, but a fluoroquinolone or a combination of antibiotics should be used in other patients. The use of high dosages for shorter durations may increase efficacy and decrease the development of antibiotic resistance. For patients who have had CAP, surgery should be delayed until they are asymptomatic (or symptoms have returned to baseline). Patients with hospital-acquired pneumonia are frequently infected with multidrug-resistant bacterial pathogens and require broad-spectrum antibiotic therapy.[13]

Interactions between Pulmonary Dysfunction and Cardiac Disease

The beta-adrenergic system relies on a negative feedback mechanism. Downregulation (reduction in density of receptors) and desensitization (decreased affinity of available receptors) occur rapidly in the presence of continued adrenergic stimulation. Paradoxically, then, inhaled beta-agonist use may be beneficial in the short term, but continued use is detrimental to both cardiac and pulmonary function.[30,31] Meta-analysis shows that at the onset of beta-blockade, there is a modest (7%) decrease in FEV_1 without symptomatic change; use of beta-agonists after this point will generate a 5% increase in FEV_1.[30] With chronic beta-blockade, the improved response to inhaled beta-agonists is maintained. Withdrawal of chronic beta-blockade (e.g., by allowing nothing by mouth) can lead to a transient fourfold increase in the risk of myocardial infarction. Initiating inhaled beta-agonists in patients with known cardiovascular disease has a sevenfold increased risk of acute myocardial infarction. Chronic beta-agonist use in patients with cardiovascular disease has a dose-dependent risk of increased myocardial infarction and angina, with patients requiring three to five metered-dose inhalers (MDIs) in a 90-day period increasing their risk by 50%, and those using six or more MDIs in a 90-day period nearly doubling their risk. When patients use a beta-blocker and a beta-agonist concomitantly, risk of myocardial infarction is increased threefold if they use six or more MDIs in 90 days, whereas those who use less beta-agonist have an essentially unchanged risk from baseline.

Perioperative beta-blockade using atenolol resulted in a 50% reduction in the incidence of myocardial ischemia within the first 48 hours of surgery.[32,33] An episode of myocardial ischemia in the perioperative period was associated with an increased risk of death within the next 2 years. The use of perioperative beta-blockade with a beta-1-selective agent does not increase the incidence of bronchospasm.

Patients with pulmonary dysfunction have an increased incidence of supraventricular arrhythmias, both because of the pulmonary disease and because of the adverse effects of bronchodilators.[34] COPD alters autonomic tone, and both inhaled beta-adrenergic agonists and anticholinergic agents can produce tachycardia and arrhythmias. The most common arrhythmias are atrial fibrillation, atrial flutter, multifocal atrial tachycardia, and supraventricular tachycardia without discernible P waves. In patients undergoing noncardiac surgery, supraventricular arrhythmias primarily occur within the first 3 days of surgery, and the incidence is doubled in patients with asthma.[35] Patients with supraventricular arrhythmias have an increased incidence of perioperative morbidity.

Patients with pulmonary disease frequently have significant pulmonary artery hypertension, defined as a resting mean pulmonary artery systolic pressure greater than 25 mm Hg as assessed by pulmonary artery catheterization or Doppler echocardiography. Pulmonary hypertension may lead to the development of cor pulmonale, with right ventricular dysfunction, elevated right atrial pressure, and decreased cardiac output. Management of pulmonary hypertension has been described elsewhere. Patients with pulmonary disease and pulmonary hypertension may require evaluation for acute or chronic pulmonary thromboembolic disease.

Gastroesophageal Reflux Disease

Gastroesophageal reflux disease (GERD) is present in 20% to 30% of patients with lung disease, and it may be seen in up to 70% to 80% of patients with asthma.[17,36] Most of these patients are asymptomatic. Bronchoconstriction may produce or exacerbate GERD by decreasing intrathoracic pressure.[37] Furthermore, the beta-agonists used to treat asthma decrease lower esophageal sphincter tone in a dose-dependent manner.[38] Patients who have adult-onset asthma, nocturnal asthma, or steroid-resistant asthma and are nonsmokers should be considered at risk for GERD.[39]

Although GERD is frequently associated with asthma, it is less frequent in patients with COPD. Typically, the prevalence is less than 20% in those with class I and IIA disease (see Table 20-1); there is an increasing prevalence if FEV_1 is less than 50%.[40] Baseline use of antacids and antireflux medications (either over the counter or by prescription) is twice as high in COPD patients as in controls. However, there are no significant changes in pulmonary function tests (PFTs) with or without GERD.

Obesity and Obstructive Sleep Apnea

Patients with obesity may have significant pulmonary dysfunction, including the obesity hypoventilation (Pickwickian) syndrome, normally associated with a body mass index (BMI) of 40. In addition to associated diseases such as diabetes mellitus and hypertension, patients with obesity hypoventilation syndrome may also have obstructive sleep apnea (OSA).[41] Patients with obesity hypoventilation syndrome always have resting hypercapnia, whereas patients with OSA alone may have a normal $PaCO_2$. Obesity itself impairs pulmonary function by decreasing pulmonary compliance and decreasing airway caliber, and it is associated with an increased incidence of intraoperative and postoperative pulmonary complications.[27]

OSA may be central and/or obstructive in origin. Symptoms commonly include snoring, daytime somnolence, and fatigue. Its severity can be assessed by measures such as the Epworth sleepiness scale and the Berlin questionnaire, but it is frequently undiagnosed and may be first recognized in the perioperative period, particularly in patients who have received opioids for analgesia and sedation.[19,42] OSA may be more prominent in edentulous patients when their dentures are removed.[43]

Allergies

Latex allergies are becoming more common, possibly because of increased use of latex products (gloves, in particular). Patients who have a history of atopy, including patients with asthma, have an increased risk of latex sensitivity. The typical response may include bronchospasm and cardiovascular collapse within 30 to 40 minutes of exposure, although delays of up to 6 hours have been reported.[44] Lebenbom-Mansour and colleagues assessed an outpatient surgical population to determine the incidence of latex allergy.[45] IgE antibodies were present in 6.7% of the patients. Patients filled out an extensive historical questionnaire, and, although both specificity and positive predictive value were low, factors that were associated with increased risk of latex sensitivity included asthma, spinal cord abnormalities, food allergies (especially kiwi fruit), and prior allergic symptoms when exposed to latex.

■ PULMONARY FUNCTION TESTING

The role of pulmonary function testing in predicting postoperative pulmonary complications is more extensively discussed in Chapter 10. Spirometry is generally indicated in patients who smoke or have COPD, or who have unexplained symptoms that may be pulmonary in origin.[1]

Measurement of FEV_1 is the best single standardized pulmonary function test currently available. The ratio of FEV_1 to FVC is diagnostic and distinguishes between COPD and asthma (irreversible versus reversible airflow obstruction).[46] Assessment of preoperative FEV_1 may underestimate potential complications, and predicted postoperative FEV_1 (ppoFEV$_1$) along with predicted postoperative diffusing capacity of the lung for carbon monoxide (ppoDLCO) may be a more useful measurement in those patients undergoing lung surgery.[47]

Flow-volume loops are particularly useful for distinguishing between respiratory and cardiac causes of shortness of breath, obstructive versus restrictive lung diseases, and reversible versus nonreversible lung diseases.[48] The positive predictive value of the flow loop in restrictive disease is approximately 40%, but the negative predictive value is 2.4%, so a normal FVC makes restrictive lung disease a very unlikely diagnosis. A diminished FVC and restrictive pattern on flow loop indicates a need for specific measurement of TLC.[49] Expiratory flow limitations are seen in approximately one quarter of all patients with COPD, typically in those patients with the lowest FEV_1 and FEV_1-to-FVC ratio. In patients with restrictive lung disease and obesity, such flow limitations are not seen or are transiently seen and overcome.[50]

A peak flow meter can be a useful tool given its ease of use and portability. Serial measurements of peak flow (which is analogous to FEV_1 but not identical to it) can be used not only to follow the course of respiratory abnormalities but also to help to make a diagnosis. For example, a patient whose peak flow routinely drops in the mid morning (a "morning dipper") may have an occupational exposure, whereas a "night dipper" may have sleep apnea or GERD.

Edentulous patients may show changes in PFTs. Spirometry in patients with and without dentures can show significant differences. If tested without dentures, patients with normal lungs and interstitial lung disease demonstrate a decrease in volumes and flow rates, but not those patients with COPD. It is hypothesized that the relative collapse of the retropharyngeal space is analogous to pursed-lip breathing.[43]

Arterial blood gas (ABG) analysis is frequently performed in conjunction with PFTs. It may help estimate the severity of COPD, particularly of an exacerbation. Hypoxia demonstrates the need for supplemental oxygen therapy, whereas hypercapnia and acidosis help assess the need for mechanical ventilation or other supplemental modalities such as bilevel positive airway pressure (BiPAP). An elevated serum bicarbonate level may suggest chronic respiratory failure; the venous bicarbonate level may be used for this purpose.

Chest radiography is one of the most commonly performed tests in the United States, but its value is limited. The primary question to be asked when obtaining a perioperative radiograph is how it will alter treatment in terms of additional tests, optimization of pulmonary function, alterations in anesthetic and surgical management, or via demonstration of increased perioperative risk.[51] Mendelson and colleagues reported that 19% of routine preoperative chest radiographs were abnormal, and the test altered postoperative management in 9%.[52] Silvestri and coworkers reported a similar incidence of abnormal preoperative chest radiographs (18%), and indicated that anesthetic management was changed for 5% of patients.[53] It is likely that half or more of the abnormal chest radiographs show previously noted findings; this likelihood increases with patient age. Many patients (from 5% to 25%) demonstrate pulmonary congestion on chest radiography.[54] It is important to distinguish between a chest radiograph from an asymptomatic patient and one from a symptomatic patient. Patients with exacerbations of COPD should have a chest radiograph obtained, as one in five of these patients do have infiltrates or other abnormalities that will change medical and surgical management.[10] The likelihood of an abnormal chest radiograph increases with age (>60 years), ASA physical status (≥ 3), respiratory disease, and two or more comorbidities.[53]

Exercise testing is perhaps the best measure for both cardiac and pulmonary function, as it assesses both oxygen uptake and cardiopulmonary reserve. Contraindications include unstable angina or myocardial infarction within the past month. Hypertension may be a relative contraindication. All patients should have immediate access to emergency services, including antianginal medications, oxygen, and a crash cart, along with the personnel to manage such a situation.

The 6-minute walk test assesses submaximal exercise tolerance as patients walk as far as they can over 6 minutes on a flat, firm surface. It does not diagnose causes of dyspnea or mechanisms of exercise limitation. The test is easily reproducible and requires only a 100-foot-long pathway and a watch. The shuttle-walking test uses a signal on an audiotape to direct the pace as the patient walks back and forth on a 10-m course. The test is concluded when the patient can no longer reach the turn-around point within the required time. As with exercise-treadmill testing, this test is symptom limited and it correlates with peak oxygen uptake. Stair climbing is a low-tech method to assess cardiac and pulmonary function. Girish and colleagues studied patients preoperatively, having them climb up to seven flights of stairs.[55] Those unable to climb one flight had an 89% complication rate, and as a whole, those with complications climbed fewer stairs, had a lower FVC and FEV_1, spent longer times in the ICU, and had a longer length of stay in the hospital.[47,55] Inability to climb at least two flights of stairs was associated with a positive predictive value of 80%, although sensitivity was only 38%; ability to climb five or more flights had a negative predictive value of 95% and a specificity of 32%.

However, stairs climbed did not accurately predict mortality. Oxygen desaturation during exercise is a predictor of prolonged hospital stay and respiratory failure. This test identified 50% of those who died, all of whom had an FEV_1 of 1.5 L or greater. However, the sensitivity of the test is low.[56]

■ PREOPERATIVE OPTIMIZATION

Medications

Differences in drug response among patients led to the challenge of optimizing a medication regimen for individuals. This variability is multifactorial and includes environmental, genetic, and disease determinants.[4] Historical information about a patient's response to other medications should be included when formulating a perioperative plan. It is important to distinguish between medications prescribed and those actually used by the patient.[57] All medications should be continued preoperatively and resumed postoperatively. Medications should be given intraoperatively as indicated by the duration of procedure and the clinical assessment.[47]

The mainstay of medical management for pulmonary disease is inhaled beta-agonist therapy (Table 20-4). These drugs are currently divided into long-acting and short-acting medications, and they are used for maintenance and acute management, respectively. The currently available long-acting beta-agonists are salmeterol and formoterol. Both are used twice a day for maintenance. The short-acting beta-agonists are albuterol (also known as salbutamol), fenoterol, and terbutaline. Beta-agonists may have adverse effects. Higher dosages decrease lower esophageal tone, which may

play a role in aspiration events.[38] Cardiac side effects may be significant. Beta-agonists cause both positive inotropic and chronotropic effects. Tachycardia is both a marker of sympathetic stimulation and a direct contributor to increased myocardial work. A single dose of a beta-agonist will increase heart rate by 10 to 15 beats per minute and decrease serum potassium by 0.36 mmol/dL (by pushing potassium intracellularly). This may contribute to a higher risk of sinus tachycardia, ventricular tachycardia, syncope, atrial fibrillation, congestive heart failure, heart attack, cardiac arrest, and sudden death.[3] The rapid desensitization (within minutes) and downregulation (within hours) and the equally rapid reversal of these can contribute to tolerance to beta-agonists and to the maximal side effects seen with each use if the dosing regimen is spaced out. The development of tolerance may explain the increased risk of fatal and near-fatal asthma attacks in long-term users.[30] The currently available intravenous (IV) beta-adrenergic agonists are either nonselective (epinephrine, isoproterenol) or lose their selectivity with IV or subcutaneous use (terbutaline). This can limit their utility in exacerbations.

Steroids are useful for the prevention and minimization of inflammatory changes in the pulmonary tree. Most steroids used chronically are administered in an inhaled form, which limits many of the side effects associated with systemic administration. Systemic steroids often cause hyperglycemia, which is not seen with inhaled steroids. The currently available inhaled steroids (Table 20-5) include fluti-

20-4	**Inhaled Beta-Adrenergic Agonists**		
Drug	**Delivery Device**	**Adult Dosages**	**Mechanism**
Albuterol 5% (Proventil, Ventolin, others)	Neb	0.3 mL q6-8h	$\beta2 > \beta1$
	MDI	90 µg/puff, 2 puffs q6-8h	
	DPI	200 µg/capsules, q4-6h	
Epinephrine (Adrenalin, Vaponefrine)	Neb	0.25-0.5 mL qid	α- and β-agonist
	MDI	0.2 mg/puff, qid	
	IV		
Formoterol (Foradil)	DPI	12 µg q12h	$\beta2 > \beta1$
Isoetharine 1% (Bronkosol)	Neb	0.25-0.50 mL q2-4h	
Isoproterenol 0.5% (Isuprel)	Neb	0.25-0.5 mL q2-4h	Nonselective β-agonist
	MDI	131 µg/puff, 2 puffs qid	
	IV		
Levalbuterol (Xopenex)	Neb	0.625 mg q6-8h *or* 1.25 mg q6-8h	$\beta2 > \beta1$
Metaproterenol 5% (Alupent)	Neb	0.3 mL tid-qid	$\beta2 > \beta1$
	MDI	650 µg/puff, 2-3 puffs tid-qid	
Pirbuterol (Maxair)	MDI	200 µg/puff	$\beta2 > \beta1$
Racemic epinephrine	Neb	0.25-0.5 mL qid	$\beta2 > \beta1$
Salmeterol (Serevent)	MDI	21 µg/puff, 2 puffs bid	$\beta2 > \beta1$
	DPI	48 µg/capsules, bid	
Terbutaline 0.1% (Brethine, Bricanyl)	MDI	200 µg/puff, 2 puffs q2-6h	$\beta2 > \beta1$
	SQ		
	PO		

bid, twice a day; DPI, dry powder inhaler; IV, intravenous; MDI, metered-dose inhaler; Neb, nebulizer; PO, by mouth; q, once every; qid, four times a day; SQ, subcutaneously; tid, three times a day.

20-5	**Inhaled Steroids**	
Drug	**Delivery Device**	**Dosage**
Beclomethasone (Vanceril, others)	MDI	42 µg/puff, 2 puffs q6h 48 µg/puff, 2 puffs q6h
Budesonide (Pulmicort)	DPI	200 µg/capsule, 1-2 capsules bid
Flunisolide (Aero-Bid)	MDI	250 µg/puff, 2 puffs bid
Fluticasone (Flovent)	MDI	44, 110, 220 µg/puff, 2 puffs bid
	DPI	500, 100, 250 mg/disk, 1 disk bid
Triamcinolone (Astrocort, Azmacort, others)	MDI	100 µg/puff, 2-4 puffs q6h
Dexamethasone	Neb	1 mg q6h

bid, twice a day; DPI, dry powder inhaler; MDI, metered-dose inhaler; Neb, nebulizer; q6h, every 6 hours.

20-6	**Inhaled Anticholinergic Bronchodilators**		
Drug	**Delivery Device**	**Dosage**	**Mechanism**
Atropine 2% or 5%	Neb	2.5 mg q6-8h	Cholinergic blocker; decreases cAMP
Ipratropium 0.03% (Atrovent)	Neb MDI	0.5 mg tid or qid 18 µg/puff, 2 puffs tid-qid	Competitive muscarinic blocker
Tiotropium (Spiriva)	DPI	18 µg/puff, q day	Competitive muscarinic blocker

DPI, dry powder inhaler; MDI, metered-dose inhaler; Neb, nebulizer; q, once every; qid, four times a day; tid, three times a day.

casone, beclomethasone, budesonide, and triamcinolone. Dosing is usually twice a day. The inhaled steroids are not indicated for exacerbations of COPD. Systemic steroids are known to increase the FEV_1 the most within the first 24 hours, less so on days 2 and 3, and then insignificantly after that.[10]

Anticholinergic bronchodilators (Table 20-6), such as ipratropium and tiotropium, are competitive muscarinic acetylcholine receptor antagonists. Both have quaternary nitrogens, so they are poorly absorbed orally. If given via inhalation, the systemic side effects are negligible. Potency decreases from bronchial smooth muscle to cardiac to urinary bladder muscle if given intravenously. Because their onset of action is slower than that of beta-agonists (30 to 60 minutes), they are not indicated as first-line single-agent treatment. Ipratropium is a relatively short-acting agent, typically administered three to four times a day, whereas tiotropium is a long-acting agent administered once a day. Ipratropium is also found in a combination formulation with albuterol, which can be used via nebulizer or MDI.

The inhaled beta-agonists are available in combination with either an inhaled anticholinergic or an inhaled steroid (Table 20-7).

20-7	**Inhaled Combination Therapy**	
Drug	**Delivery Device**	**Dosage**
Duoneb (albuterol & ipratropium)	Neb MDI	Ipratropium 0.5 mg/albuterol 3 mg
Advair (fluticasone & salmeterol)	DPI	Fluticasone 100 µg/salmeterol 50 µg Fluticasone 250 µg/salmeterol 50 µg Fluticasone 500 µg/salmeterol 50 µg

DPI, dry powder inhaler; MDI, metered-dose inhaler; Neb, nebulizer.

The methylxanthines (theophylline, theobromine, and caffeine) have several actions, including smooth muscle relaxation (especially bronchial muscle), central nervous system stimulation, cardiac muscle stimulation, and diuresis, which are all seen in patients using this class of drugs. Although caffeine is considered the most potent of the methylxanthines, theophylline is a more profound and potentially more dangerous central nervous system stimulant. Side effects involve the nervous system, cardiac system, and gastrointestinal tract. Theophylline (and its salt aminophylline, for IV use) has a narrow therapeutic window, and seizures may occur as the initial sign of toxicity. Adenosine receptor blockade is considered the most important mechanism of action of both theophylline and caffeine.[58] Theophylline antagonizes A_1 and A_2 receptors more effectively than A_3 receptors, and it appears that the A_2B receptor indirectly activates sensitized mast cells via the release of histamine and leukotrienes.[59] The mechanism of methylxanthine action also includes weak and nonspecific competitive phosphodiesterase inhibition, which increases the concentration of cAMP in the target tissues.[58,59] Recent research has indicated that theophylline also has anti-inflammatory effects at low dosages (i.e., at concentrations less than 10 mg/L). This is believed to be mediated by increased histone deacetylase activity, and it is associated with the increased efficacy of concomitantly administered corticosteroids.[59]

Methylxanthines are metabolized in the liver by cytochrome P-450 demethylation or oxidation, so there may be significant drug–drug interactions with ciprofloxacin, erythromycin, allopurinol, and cimetidine. Smoking also slows liver metabolism, as do liver disease, congestive heart failure, and cor pulmonale. Theophylline is ineffective if inhaled. Given these limitations, theophylline is now considered to be a second- or third-line choice in patients with pulmonary disease.

Cromolyn and nedocromil inhibit the release of histamine, leukotrienes, and other autacoids from mast cells (sensitized or not) in the lungs (Table 20-8). Thus, they are useful for prevention of both extrinsic and allergic asthma. Both block the acute reaction (release of preformed histamine) and the delayed reaction (secondary inflammation). Neither is absorbed well orally, and thus they are used only via inhalation. Although a single dose before antigenic challenge is

20-8   **Additional Drugs Used for Reactive Airways Disease**

Drug	Delivery Device	Dosage	Mechanism
Cromolyn (Intal)	Neb	20 mg q6h	Suppresses mast cell response; inhibits both early- and late-phase bronchoconstriction
	MDI	2 puffs qid	
Nedocromil (Tilade)	MDI	1.75 mg/puff, 2 puffs q6-12h	
Montelukast (Singulair)	PO	10 mg daily	Leukotriene-D4 receptor blocker
Zileuton (Zyflo)	PO	600 mg qid	5-Lipoxygenase inhibitor
Zafirlukast (Accolate)	PO	20 mg bid	Leukotriene-C4 receptor blocker

bid, twice a day; MDI, metered-dose inhaler; Neb, nebulizer; PO, by mouth; q, once every; qid, four times a day.

20-9   **Inhaled Drug Delivery Devices**

Device	Advantages	Disadvantages
Small-volume jet nebulizer	Patient coordination not required High dose possible Can be used with supplemental oxygen	Lack of portability Pressurized gas source required Lengthy treatment time Not all medication available in solution form Device preparation required Expensive compressor required
Ultrasonic nebulizer	Patient coordination not required High dose possible Small dead volume Newer designs small and portable Quiet Faster delivery than jet nebulizer	Expensive Requires electrical power source Contamination possible Device preparation required before treatment
Pressurized metered dose inhaler (MDI)	Portable and compact Short treatment time No drug preparation required No contamination possible High dose reproducibility	Requires coordination of breathing and actuation High pharyngeal deposition Limited dose Potential for abuse
Dry powder inhaler (DPI)	Breath-actuated Less patient coordination required Portable and compact Short treatment time No propellant	Requires moderate to high inspiratory flow Cannot be used with ventilator High pharyngeal deposition
Spacer or holding chamber	Less patient coordination required Decreased pharyngeal deposition	Less portable and more expensive than MDI alone More complex Dose may be decreased if used improperly

Modified from Dolovich MB, Ahrens RC, Hess DR, et al; American College of Chest Physicians; American College of Asthma, Allergy, and Immunology: Chest 2005;127:335-371.

useful, long-term prophylaxis of 4 to 12 weeks is optimal to prevent response to allergen exposure.

Leukotriene receptor antagonists available in the United States include montelukast, zafirlukast, and zileuton (see Table 20-8). Like cromolyn, these drugs are used to prevent asthma attacks, and they are not useful once an attack has begun. Zafirlukast blocks the action of leukotriene-C4 (LTC$_4$) on its receptors. It also inhibits CYP2C9 and CYP3A4. Montelukast blocks the action of leukotriene-D4 (LTD$_4$), and does not inhibit the cytochrome system. Zileuton inhibits 5-lipoxygenase, the first enzyme in the synthetic pathway for cysteinyl-leukotrienes.

Cyclic nucleotide phosphodiesterases (PDEs) are a family of enzymes that catalyze the degradation of cAMP and cGMP. PDE-4 is the subset that is a major regulator of cAMP metabolism in proinflammatory and immune cells. However, the PDE-4 inhibitor drugs under study are hampered by a low therapeutic ratio and a propensity to produce side effects similar to those of nonsteroidal anti-inflammatory drugs (NSAIDs). An additional potential toxic effect is arteritis or periarteritis. Dual-specificity inhibitors, targeting PDE-4 and either PDE-1, PDE-3, or PDE-7, may be useful to improve therapeutic response as well as safety, and are under study.[60]

A variety of inhalational delivery devices are available for inhaled drug delivery, each of which has specific risks and benefits (Table 20-9). In general, the devices provide similar outcomes if the patient is using the correct technique for inhalation. Not all drugs are available in all formats, and the side effects may differ depending on the delivery format.

Dose-scale comparisons are used to identify the true difference in drug delivery to the site of action. The brand of the device may make a difference, particularly with the dry powder inhaler (DPI) devices (e.g., the characteristics of the Rotahaler are different from those of the Spinhaler). In addition, different formulations of the same drug may have different aerosolization properties and thus different delivered doses. There appears to be little difference in drug delivery when comparing nebulizers with MDIs that have spacers; however, proving device efficacy can be difficult in patients with COPD because of the limited reversibility associated with the disease.[61] Inpatient treatment offers an opportunity to instruct both patient and family in the proper use of the various delivery devices. It may also provide an opportunity to evaluate prior (outpatient) use and education, and to adjust medication regimens on the basis of the patient's ability to use the various delivery devices.

Mechanical ventilation can severely limit the delivery of medications. Drug is adsorbed onto the circuit, and the adapters required to access the circuit can change delivery efficacy. Unfortunately, there are few data indicating the relevant details with each drug or device. The general rule is to give twice as much as would be given to a nonventilated patient.

Antibiotic Therapy

Antibiotics should be reserved for patients with acute infections (e.g., pneumonia) or severe exacerbations of COPD. Unfortunately, inappropriate use is common and may increase the duration of hospital stay and predispose to development of antibiotic resistance.[13] The Council for Appropriate and Rational Antibiotic Therapy (CARAT), formed to address these issues,[62] established five criteria to help determine the right drug, the right dose, and the right duration: (1) evidence-based studies have been performed; (2) therapeutic benefits have been shown; (3) safety is established; (4) it is the optimal drug for the optimal duration; and (5) the drug is cost effective. Local and regional resistance patterns should be reviewed on a regular basis; these may change empiric drug choices significantly.

The joint statement by the American Thoracic Society and the Infectious Diseases Society of America (see Suggested Readings) emphasizes the initial dichotomy between patients without risk factors for multidrug-resistant (MDR) bacteria and those with such risk factors. Patients without risk factors, and whose disease course is in its early stages, do not need broad-spectrum antibiotics, but those with risk factors do. The key recommendations include grouping health-care–associated pneumonia (HCAP) with hospital-acquired pneumonia (HAP) and ventilator-associated pneumonia (VAP), all of which need broad-spectrum antibiotics until either semiquantitative or quantitative culture data are obtained. An empiric regimen should include agents that are in a class that is different from the class of agents recently administered to the patient. HCAP is defined as occurring in a patient who (1) has been hospitalized 2 or more days within the past 90 days, (2) resides in a nursing facility or long-term-care facility, (3) has received IV antibiotics, chemotherapy, or wound care within the past 30 days, or (4) has attended a hospital or hemodialysis clinic. Recommendations for initial empiric antibiotic therapy based on categorization for risk factors for MDR pathogens, early versus late onset,

and disease severity are shown in Tables 20-10 and 20-11. Dosage regimens are in Table 20-12.

The major classes of antibiotics used for pulmonary infections include the beta-lactams (penicillins and cephalosporins), fluoroquinolones, and macrolides. Each has a different mechanism of action, which must be taken into account when selecting dosage and duration of therapy. Beta-lactams exhibit time-dependent killing, so efficacy relies on multiple

20-10	Initial Empiric Antibiotic Therapy for Hospital-Acquired Pneumonia or Ventilator-Associated Pneumonia in Patients with No Known Risk Factors for Multidrug-Resistant Pathogens, with Early-Onset Disease, and with Any Disease Severity
Potential Pathogens	**Recommended Antibiotic**
Streptococcus pneumoniae	Ceftriaxone
Haemophilus influenzae	or
Methicillin-sensitive *Staphylococcus aureus*	Levofloxacin, moxifloxacin, or ciprofloxacin
Antibiotic-sensitive enteric gram-negative bacilli	or
Escherichia coli	Ampicillin/sulbactam
Klebsiella pneumoniae	or
Enterobacter species	Ertapenem
Proteus species	
Serratia marcescens	

Modified from American Thoracic Society; Infectious Diseases Society of America: Am J Respir Crit Care Med 2005;171:388-416.

20-11	Initial Empiric Therapy for Hospital-Acquired Pneumonia, Ventilator-Associated Pneumonia, and Health-Care–Associated Pneumonia in Patients with Late-Onset Disease or Risk Factors for Multidrug-Resistant Pathogens, and with Any Disease Severity
Potential Pathogens	**Combination Antibiotic Therapy**
Pathogens listed in Table 20-10, and multidrug-resistant pathogens	Antipseudomonal cephalosporin (cefepime, ceftazidime)
Pseudomonas aeruginosa	or
Klebsiella pneumoniae (ESBL[+])*	Antipseudomonal carbapenems (imipenem or meropenem)
Acinetobacter species*	or
Methicillin-resistant *Staphylococcus aureus* (MRSA)	β-Lactam/β-lactamase inhibitor (piperacillin-tazobactam)
*Legionella pneumophila**	plus
	Antipseudomonal fluoroquinolone[†] (ciprofloxacin or levofloxacin)
	or
	Aminoglycoside (amikacin, gentamicin, or tobramycin)
	plus
	Linezolid or vancomycin[†]

*If an extended-spectrum beta-lactamase (ESBL)[+] strain, such as *K. pneumoniae*, or an *Acinetobacter* species is suspected, a carbapenem is a reliable choice. If *L. pneumophila* is suspected, the combination antibiotic regimen should include a macrolide (e.g., azithromycin), or a fluoroquinolone (e.g., ciprofloxacin or levofloxacin) should be used rather than an aminoglycoside.
[†]When MRSA risk factors are present or there is a high incidence locally.
Modified from American Thoracic Society; Infectious Diseases Society of America: Am J Respir Crit Care Med 2005;171:388-416.

20-12	**Initial Intravenous, Adult Doses of Antibiotics for Empiric Therapy of Hospital-Acquired Pneumonia**

Antibiotic	Dosage*
Antipseudomonal cephalosporin	
Cefepime	1-2 g every 8-12 hr
Ceftazidime	2 g every 8 hr
Carbapenems	
Imipenem	500 mg every 6 hr or 1 g every 8 hr
Meropenem	1 g every 8 hr
β-Lactam/β-lactamase inhibitor	
Piperacillin-tazobactam	4.5 g every 6 hr
Aminoglycosides	
Gentamicin	7 mg/kg/day[†]
Tobramycin	7 mg/kg/day[†]
Amikacin	20 mg/kg/day[†]
Antipseudomonal quinolones	
Levofloxacin	750 mg every day
Ciprofloxacin	400 mg every 8 hr
Vancomycin	15 mg/kg every 12 hr[‡]
Linezolid	600 mg every 12 hr

*Dosages are based on normal renal and hepatic function.
[†]Trough levels for gentamicin and tobramycin should be less than 1 µg/mL, and for amikacin they should be less than 4-5 µg/mL.
[‡]Trough levels for vancomycin should be 15-20 µg/mL.
Modified from American Thoracic Society; Infectious Diseases Society of America: Am J Respir Crit Care Med 2005;171:388-416.

doses.[14] In contrast, fluoroquinolones exhibit concentration-dependent killing, so higher dosages with short courses work well. This shorter course may decrease selection pressure.[13] Macrolides reversibly bind to the ribosomal subunit to inhibit protein synthesis; efficacy relies on both adequate concentration and duration.

Combination therapy may result in additive adverse-event profiles and increased drug–drug interactions.[13]

Other Drugs

One of the most common other classes of drugs that patients with pulmonary disease may benefit from is beta-blockers. Beta-blockade must be cardioselective. The current cardioselective beta-blockers have a 20-fold increased affinity for the beta-1-receptor[8] and include acebutolol, atenolol, betaxolol, bisoprolol, esmolol, and metoprolol. The original studies listing asthma and COPD as contraindications for beta-blockade used isoproterenol, a nonselective drug, at dosages ranging from 240 to 1600 mg/day.[30]

If patients use an inhaled beta-agonist and no beta-blocker, there is an increased risk of acute coronary syndrome. If they use both agents, there is no increased risk unless they use more than six refills of the inhaled beta-agonist in 90 days (i.e., unless the situation is poorly controlled or the drug improperly used).[31]

GERD associated with pulmonary disease is generally managed with proton pump inhibitors at a doubled dosage (e.g., omeprazole, 40 mg/day). This antireflux therapy promptly alleviates the GERD symptoms in most patients, but it typically takes 2 months or more to resolve the pulmonary symptoms. The PFTs of approximately one quarter of patients will improve, but predicting which patients will most benefit from this treatment is not currently successful.[36]

Smoking Cessation

Intercession to stop smoking is the most important intervention for COPD.[6] Repeated discussion (every physician at every encounter) with patients about smoking cessation is important, but it frequently takes a specific event, a "teachable moment," to make these efforts finally bear fruit. The withdrawal symptoms contribute to the high relapse rate and must be addressed as part of the entire smoking cessation plan. A combination of pharmacologic therapy (either nicotine replacement or withdrawal treatment) and behavioral interventions works best to improve the cessation rate. In addition to the pulmonary effects, smoking cessation may be beneficial for other reasons, such as wound healing.

Nicotine-replacement therapy (NRT) can be accomplished with several different products: two forms of patch, a gum, and an inhaler are available. Transdermal nicotine produces lower plasma levels than the gum or inhaler. Both the gum and the inhaler have very rapid delivery via the buccal mucosa and are not recommended for patients with cardiac disease.[24] Overwhelming evidence supports the safety of NRT in patients with concomitant cardiac disease,[23] as these products avoid the other chemicals and particulates found in cigarettes.[24] Smokers who cut back or quit while using nicotine patches have actually had improvements in exercise-induced perfusion defects, which is attributed to the decrease in carboxyhemoglobin concentration rather than the nicotine concentration.[25] The few contraindications include the period after acute myocardial infarction, severe arrhythmias, and unstable or low-threshold angina.[24] Significant decreases in exercise-induced ischemia as assessed by exercise thallium perfusion is noted in ex-smokers on NRT, although there may be exaggerated heart rate responses to stimuli such as intubation.

Other therapies focus on the withdrawal effects of smoking cessation,[24] which include anxiety, depression, dysphoria, intense cravings, and hunger. These symptoms are mediated by decreased levels of dopamine, norepinephrine, and serotonin, all of which are downregulated by routine use of nicotine. Bupropion (Zyban or Wellbutrin) is an antidepressant that has both noradrenergic and dopaminergic activity and is believed to minimize the withdrawal effects. Behavioral counseling can be an effective adjunct. It usually involves a multidisciplinary approach with office visits, group meetings, and phone calls. Patients who participate in some form of behavioral counseling are more likely to still be ex-smokers at 1 year.

Useful abstinence requires 8 to 12 weeks to decrease overall morbidity, but in the first 4 weeks, cessation may actually increase complications.[19,23] Mucociliary clearance improves after about 1 week; mucus production is not quantified but may actually be increased in the short term. Postoperative complications occur in about 50% of patients who currently smoke or have stopped within the last 8 weeks. This rate drops to about 10% to 15% if smoking cessation has been for 12 weeks or longer.[23] The specific risk profile varies depending on the specific complication and the surgical procedure. It takes at least 6 months before the cytokine response to the stress associated with anesthesia and surgery is equal in smokers and ex-smokers,[63] and inflammation may actually be more extensive in ex-smokers who also have COPD than in those without COPD. Cellular inflammation is a negative consequence of smoking, but it is an integral part of the repair process.[26] Although the inflammatory changes begin to reverse after 6 months, it may be 3 years before ex-smokers return to nonsmoker cytokine, macrophage, and plasma cell levels.[64]

Lapperre and colleagues studied the changes in inflammatory mediators in patients with COPD at different times after smoking cessation.[64] Ex-smokers had higher $CD3^+$, $CD4^+$, and plasma cell levels than current smokers with COPD. Patients who had quit smoking for longer than 3.5 years had a decrease of $CD4^+$, $CD8^+$, and mast cells and an increase in plasma cells when compared with both short-term ex-smokers and current smokers. The ongoing inflammation suggests the presence of a persistent stimulus from chronic colonization with viral or bacterial pathogens and self-perpetuating inflammation from an altered balance between endogenous proinflammatory and anti-inflammatory mechanisms.

Additional Therapies for Chronic Obstructive Pulmonary Disease

Patients with chronic pulmonary dysfunction may benefit from multiple nonpharmacologic therapies.[6,65] Patients with COPD commonly have peripheral muscle disuse atrophy and respiratory muscle overuse fatigue.[66] Pulmonary rehabilitation exercise training can improve exercise tolerance, symptoms, and quality of life, and specific inspiratory muscle training may have additional beneficial effects.[67,68] In fact, 15% of the patients enrolled in the National Emphysema Treatment Trial withdrew after mandatory pulmonary rehabilitation because they had significant symptomatic improvement and no longer would consider surgery. However, the ability of exercise training to decrease postoperative pulmonary complications has not been convincingly demonstrated.

■ PREVENTION OF VENTILATOR-ASSOCIATED PNEUMONIA

The development of VAP markedly increases morbidity, mortality, and health-care costs in postoperative patients. Multiple individual interventions such as nursing patients in the semiupright position, not routinely changing ventilator circuits, oral hygiene, daily spontaneous breathing trials, and daily interruption or downtitration of sedation have been demonstrated to decrease the incidence of VAP.[69] Efficacy is markedly increased when several such interventions are combined in a ventilator "bundle" and applied as part of a multidisciplinary approach to VAP prevention.

Strategies to Prevent Postoperative Pulmonary Complications

A recent systematic review examined strategies to prevent postoperative pulmonary complications after noncardiothoracic surgery.[70] The authors concluded that there was strong evidence that lung expansion interventions such as incentive spirometry, deep-breathing exercises, and continuous positive airway pressure decrease pulmonary complications. There was fair evidence that selective (versus routine) use of nasogastric tubes after abdominal surgery and the use of intraoperative short-acting (versus long-acting) neuromuscular blocking (paralyzing) agents decreased the risk of postoperative pulmonary complications. There was evidence that routine total enteral or parenteral nutrition does not decrease risk, but enteral formulations to improve immune status may decrease risk. Finally, there was insufficient or conflicting evidence regarding preoperative smoking cessation, epidural analgesia, and the use of laparoscopic (versus open) surgical techniques.

■ REFERENCES

1. Joehl RJ: Preoperative evaluation: Pulmonary, cardiac, renal dysfunction and comorbidities. Surg Clin North Am 2005;85:1061-1073.
2. Cook DJ: Moving toward evidence-based practice. Respir Care 2003;48:859-868.
3. Salpeter SR, Ormiston TM, Salpeter EE: Cardiovascular effects of beta-agonists in patients with asthma and COPD: A meta-analysis. Chest 2004;125:2309-2321.
4. Wilkinson GR: Drug metabolism and variability among patients in drug response. N Engl J Med 2005;352:2211-2221.
5. Boyd CM, Darer J, Boult C, et al: Clinical practice guidelines and quality of care for older patients with multiple comorbid diseases: Implications for pay for performance. JAMA 2005;294:716-724.
6. Pierson DJ: Translating new understanding into better care for the patient with chronic obstructive pulmonary disease. Respir Care 2004;49:99-109.
7. Rennard SI: Clinical approach to patients with chronic obstructive pulmonary disease and cardiovascular disease. Proc Am Thorac Soc 2005;2:94-100.
8. Andrus MR, Holloway KP, Clark DB: Use of beta-blockers in patients with COPD. Ann Pharmacother 2004;38:142-145.
9. Pauwels RA, Buist AS, Calverley PM, et al; GOLD Scientific Committee: Global strategy for the diagnosis, management, and prevention of chronic obstructive pulmonary disease NHLBI/WHO Global Initiative for Chronic Obstructive Lung Disease (GOLD) Workshop summary. Am J Respir Crit Care Med 2001;163:1256-1276.
10. McCrory DC, Brown C, Gelfand SE, Bach PB: Management of acute exacerbations of COPD: A summary and appraisal of published evidence. Chest 2001;119:1190-1209.
11. Sterk PJ: Let's not forget: The GOLD criteria for COPD are based on post-bronchodilator FEV_1. Eur Respir J 2004;23:497-498.
12. Snow V, Lascher S, Mottur-Pilson C; Joint Expert Panel on COPD of the American College of Chest Physicians and the American College of Physicians–American Society of Internal Medicine: The evidence base for management of acute exacerbations of COPD: Clinical practice guideline: Part 1. Chest 2001;119:1185-1189.
13. Grossman RF, Rotschafer JC, Tan JS: Antimicrobial treatment of lower respiratory tract infections in the hospital setting. Am J Med 2005;118:29S-38S.
14. Martinez FJ, Anzueto A: Appropriate outpatient treatment of acute bacterial exacerbations of chronic bronchitis. Am J Med 2005;118(Suppl 7A):39S-44S.
15. Dempsey JA: Exercise carbon dioxide retention in chronic obstructive pulmonary disease: A case for ventilation/perfusion mismatch combined with hyperinflation. Am J Respir Crit Care Med 2002;166:634-635.
16. O'Donnell DE, D'Arsigny C, Fitzpatrick M, Webb KA: Exercise hypercapnia in advanced chronic obstructive pulmonary disease: The role of lung hyperinflation. Am J Respir Crit Care Med 2002;166:663-668.
17. Liou A, Grubb JR, Schechtman KB, Hamilos DL: Causative and contributive factors to asthma severity and patterns of medication use in patients seeking specialized asthma care. Chest 2003;124:1781-1788.

18. Weissman DN: Epidemiology of asthma: Severity matters. Chest 2002; 121:6-8.

19. Tamul PC, Peruzzi WT: Assessment and management of patients with pulmonary disease. Crit Care Med 2004;32(4 Suppl):S137-145.

20. Heaney LG, Conway E, Kelly C, et al: Predictors of therapy resistant asthma: Outcome of a systematic evaluation protocol. Thorax 2003;58: 561-566.

21. Balfe DL, Lewis M, Mohsenifar Z: Grading the severity of obstruction in the presence of a restrictive ventilatory defect. Chest 2002;122: 1365-1369.

22. Garcia-Rio F, Pino JM, Ruiz A, et al: Accuracy of noninvasive estimates of respiratory muscle effort during spontaneous breathing in restrictive diseases. J Appl Physiol 2003;95:1542-1549.

23. Warner DO: Perioperative abstinence from cigarettes: Physiologic and clinical consequences. Anesthesiology 2006;104:356-367.

24. Ludvig J, Miner B, Eisenberg MJ: Smoking cessation in patients with coronary artery disease. Am Heart J 2005;149:565-572.

25. Benowitz NL, Gourlay SG: Cardiovascular toxicity of nicotiol: Implications for nicotine replacement therapy. J Am Coll Cardiol 1997;29: 1422-1431.

26. Willemse BW, ten Hacken NH, Rutgers B, et al: Effect of 1-year smoking cessation on airway inflammation in COPD and asymptomatic smokers. Eur Respir J 2005;26:835-845.

27. Chung F, Mezei G, Tong D: Pre-existing medical conditions as predictors of adverse events in day-case surgery. Br J Anaesth 1999;83: 262-270.

28. Fine MJ, Auble TE, Yealy DM, et al: A prediction rule to identify low-risk patients with community-acquired pneumonia. N Engl J Med 1997;336:243-250.

29. Segreti J, House HR, Siegel RE: Principles of antibiotic treatment of community-acquired pneumonia in the outpatient setting. Am J Med 2005;118(Suppl 7A):21S-28S.

30. Ormiston TM, Salpeter SR: Beta-blocker use in patients with congestive heart failure and concomitant obstructive airway disease: Moving from myth to evidence-based practice. Heart Fail Monit 2003;4: 45-54.

31. Au DH, Curtis JR, Every NR, et al: Association between inhaled beta-agonists and the risk of unstable angina and myocardial infarction. Chest 2002;121:846-851.

32. Mangano DT, Layug EL, Wallace A, Tateo I: Effect of atenolol on mortality and cardiovascular morbidity after noncardiac surgery. N Engl J Med 1996;335:1713-1721.

33. Wallace A, Layug B, Tateo I, et al: Prophylactic atenolol reduces postoperative myocardial ischemia. McSPI Research Group. Anesthesiology 1998;88:7-17.

34. Seshadri N, Gildea TR, McCarthy K, et al: Association of an abnormal exercise heart rate recovery with pulmonary function abnormalities. Chest 2004;125:1286-1291.

35. Polanczyk CA, Goldman L, Marcantonio ER, et al: Supraventricular arrhythmia in patients having noncardiac surgery: Clinical correlates and effect on length of stay. Ann Intern Med 1998;129:279-285.

36. Kiljander TO, Laitinen JO: The prevalence of gastroesophageal reflux disease in adult asthmatics. Chest 2004;126:1490-1494.

37. Zerbib F, Guisset O, Lamouliatte H, et al: Effects of bronchial obstruction on lower esophageal sphincter motility and gastroesophageal reflux in patients with asthma. Am J Respir Crit Care Med 2002;166: 1206-1211.

38. Crowell MD, Zayat EN, Lacy BE, et al: The effects of an inhaled beta(2)-adrenergic agonist on lower esophageal function: A dose-response study. Chest 2001;120:1184-1189.

39. Jiang SP, Liang RY, Zeng ZY, et al: Effects of antireflux treatment on bronchial hyper-responsiveness and lung function in asthmatic patients with gastroesophageal reflux disease. World J Gastroenterol 2003;9:1123-1125.

40. Mokhlesi B, Morris AL, Huang CF, et al: Increased prevalence of gastroesophageal reflux symptoms in patients with COPD. Chest 2001;119:1043-1048.

41. Kessler R, Chaouat A, Schinkewitch P, et al: The obesity-hypoventilation syndrome revisited: A prospective study of 34 consecutive cases. Chest 2001;120:369-376.

42. Gupta RM, Parvizi J, Hanssen AD, Gay PC: Postoperative complications in patients with obstructive sleep apnea syndrome undergoing hip or knee replacement: A case-control study. Mayo Clin Proc 200;76: 897-905.

43. Bucca CB, Carossa S, Colagrande P, et al: Effect of edentulism on spirometric tests. Am J Respir Crit Care Med 2001;163:1018-1020.

44. Hepner DL: Sudden bronchospasm on intubation: Latex anaphylaxis? J Clin Anesth 2000;12:162-166.

45. Lebenbom-Mansour MH, Oesterle JR, Ownby DR, et al: The incidence of latex sensitivity in ambulatory surgical patients: A correlation of historical factors with positive serum immunoglobulin E levels. Anesth Analg 1997;85:44-49.

46. Celli BR, MacNee W; ATS/ERS Task Force: Standards for the diagnosis and treatment of patients with COPD: A summary of the ATS/ERS position paper. Eur Respir J 2004;23:932-946.

47. Robles AM, Shure D: Optimization of lung function before pulmonary resection: Pulmonologists' perspectives. Thorac Surg Clin 2004;14: 295-304.

48. Pierce R: Spirometry: An essential clinical measurement. Aust Fam Physician 2005;34:535-539.

49. Aaron SD, Dales RE, Cardinal P: How accurate is spirometry at predicting restrictive pulmonary impairment? Chest 1999;115:869-873.

50. Baydur A, Wilkinson L, Mehdian R, et al: Extrathoracic expiratory flow limitation in obesity and obstructive and restrictive disorders: Effects of increasing negative expiratory pressure. Chest 2004;125: 98-105.

51. Joo HS, Wong J, Naik VN, Savoldelli GL: The value of screening preoperative chest x-rays: A systematic review. Can J Anaesth 2005;52: 568-574.

52. Mendelson DS, Khilnani N, Wagner LD, Rabinowitz JG: Preoperative chest radiography: Value as a baseline examination for comparison. Radiology 1987;165:341-343.

53. Silvestri L, Maffessanti M, Gregori D, et al: Usefulness of routine preoperative chest radiography for anaesthetic management: A prospective multicentre pilot study. Eur J Anaesthesiol 1999;16:749-760.

54. Bouillot JL, Fingerhut A, Paquet JC, et al: Are routine preoperative chest radiographs useful in general surgery? A prospective, multicentre study in 3959 patients. Eur J Surg 1996;162:597-604.

55. Girish M, Trayner E Jr, Dammann O, et al: Symptom-limited stair climbing as a predictor of postoperative cardiopulmonary complications after high-risk surgery. Chest 2001;120:1147-1151.

56. Rao V, Todd TR, Kuus A, et al: Exercise oximetry versus spirometry in the assessment of risk prior to lung resection. Ann Thorac Surg 1995;60:603-608.

57. Pont LG, van der Molen T, Denig P, et al: Relationship between guideline treatment and health-related quality of life in asthma. Eur Respir J 2004;23:718-722.

58. Chou T: Wake up and smell the coffee: Caffeine, coffee, and the medical consequences. West J Med 1992;157:544-553.

59. Barnes PJ: Theophylline in chronic obstructive pulmonary disease: New horizons. Proc Am Thorac Soc 2005;2:334-339.

60. Giembycz MA: Life after PDE4: Overcoming adverse events with dual-specificity phosphodiesterase inhibitors. Curr Opin Pharmacol 2005; 5:238-244.

61. Dolovich MB, Ahrens RC, Hess DR, et al; American College of Chest Physicians; American College of Asthma, Allergy, and Immunology: Device selection and outcomes of aerosol therapy: Evidence-based guidelines. Chest 2005;127:335-371.

62. Slama TG, Amin A, Brunton SA, et al: A clinician's guide to the appropriate and accurate use of antibiotics: The Council for Appropriate and Rational Antibiotic Therapy (CARAT) criteria. Am J Med 2005;118(Suppl 7A):1S-6S.

63. Kotani N, Kushikata T, Hashimoto H, et al: Recovery of intraoperative microbicidal and inflammatory functions of alveolar immune cells after a tobacco smoke-free period. Anesthesiology 2001;94:999-1006.

64. Lapperre TS, Postma DS, Gosman MME, et al: GLUCOLD Study Group: Relation between duration of smoking cessation and bronchial inflammation in COPD. Thorax 2006;61:115-121.

65. Currie GP, Douglas JG: ABC of chronic obstructive pulmonary disease: Non-pharmacological management. BMJ 2006;332:1379-1381.

66. MacIntyre NR: Muscle dysfunction associated with chronic obstructive pulmonary disease. Respir Care 2006;51:840-852.

67. Nici L, Donner C, Wouters E, et al: ATS/ERS Pulmonary Rehabilitation Writing Committee. American Thoracic Society/European Respi-

ratory Society statement on pulmonary rehabilitation. Am J Respir Crit Care Med 2006;173:1390-1413.

68. Sanchez Riera H, Montemayor Rubio T, Ortega Ruiz F, et al: Inspiratory muscle training in patients with COPD: Effect on dyspnea, exercise performance, and quality of life. Chest 2001;120:748-756.

69. Craven DE: Preventing ventilator-associated pneumonia in adults: Sowing seeds of change. Chest 2006;130:251-260.

70. Lawrence VA, Cornell JE, Smetana GW: American College of Physicians: Strategies to reduce postoperative pulmonary complications after noncardiothoracic surgery: Systematic review for the American College of Physicians. Ann Intern Med 2006;144:596-608.

■ SUGGESTED READINGS

American Thoracic Society, Infectious Diseases Society of America: Guidelines for the management of adults with hospital-acquired, ventilator-associated, and healthcare-associated pneumonia. Am J Respir Crit Care Med 2005;171:388-416.

Harrison BD: Difficult asthma. Thorax 2003;58:555-556.

Kiljander TO: The role of proton pump inhibitors in the management of gastroesophageal reflux disease-related asthma and chronic cough. Am J Med 2003;115(Suppl 3A):65S-71S.

Rodenbaugh DW, Collins HL, Dicarlo SE: Spirometry: Simulations of obstructive and restrictive lung diseases. Adv Physiol Educ 2002;26: 222-223.

SECTION 4

Central Nervous System

Chapter

21 Carotid and Intracranial Surgery

Frederick W. Lombard, Michael L. James, John C. Keifer, David McDonagh, David Warner, and Cecil O. Borel

◼ ANESTHESIA FOR CAROTID SURGERY

Approximately 700,000 strokes occur annually in the United States, and 20% to 30% are secondary to carotid artery disease.[1] Many strokes are therefore potentially preventable with appropriate carotid intervention. Carotid endarterectomy (CEA) is the most commonly performed peripheral vascular procedure in the United States today.

Indications for Carotid Endarterectomy

Carotid endarterectomy is recommended for symptomatic patients (e.g., with ipsilateral transient ischemic attacks [TIAs] or nonprogressing, nondisabling stroke within the previous 6 months) who have 70% to 99% angiographic stenosis of the internal carotid artery.[2,3] It is reasonable to consider CEA for men with 50% to 69% symptomatic stenosis, especially men older than 75 years, but additional clinical and angiographic variables that might alter the risk-to-benefit ratio should be considered. For symptomatic patients, life expectancy should be at least 5 years and the perioperative stroke or death rate should be less than 6%.

CEA can be considered for patients between the ages of 40 and 75 years who have asymptomatic stenosis of 60% to 99%. Life expectancy should be at least 5 years and the perioperative stroke or death rate should be less than 3%.

Women with symptomatic stenosis of 50% to 69% did not show clear benefit in any of the large trials.[4]

Patients presenting with retinal ischemia (amaurosis fugax or retinal infarction) have a lower risk for subsequent stroke compared with patients with hemispheric events. However, CEA may be beneficial when other risk factors for stroke are also present.[5]

CEA should not be considered for symptomatic patients when stenosis is less than 50%. Symptomatic patients with near occlusion angiographically also do not derive any long-term benefit from CEA.

Preoperative Assessment

Cardiovascular System

Up to 28% of patients presenting for carotid endarterectomy have severe angiographic coronary artery disease,[6] and myocardial infarction is a leading cause of death after CEA. However, the overall incidence of perioperative myocardial infarction is low (0.3% from North American Symptomatic Carotid Endarterectomy Trial [NASCET] data),[7] and extensive preoperative cardiac testing is therefore unnecessary and cost ineffective. Furthermore, because these patients are intensively monitored in the perioperative period, additional preoperative testing has little potential to alter perioperative management. In accordance with the guidelines for perioperative evaluation for noncardiac surgery,[8] patients with major clinical predictors, such as suspected unstable coronary syndrome, may require cardiac catheterization independent of the need for carotid endarterectomy. In the unusual patient requiring coronary revascularization, staged or combined operations may be necessary, depending on the severity of the coronary and carotid disease. Other major clinical predictors such as high-grade valvular lesions, decompensated congested cardiac failure, and significant arrhythmias should be investigated and treated aggressively prior to CEA.

Central Nervous System

Risk factors for stroke resulting from CEA can be divided into preoperative medical, neurologic, and radiographic risk factors. Based on these factors, a risk stratification system was proposed[9] and has been validated as a valuable tool in predicting adverse neurologic outcome after CEA.[10] An adaptation of this risk stratification is presented in Box 21-1.

21-1	**Preoperative Risk Factors for Perioperative Stroke**

Medical Risk Factors

- Female sex[4,118,119]
- Chronic renal insufficiency (creatinine >1.5 mg/dL)[120,121]
- Active coronary artery disease (unstable angina or angina with minimal activity in the past 12 months)[122]
- Diabetes mellitus, on insulin[121]
- Congested cardiac failure
- Severe, poorly controlled hypertension
- Advanced age (>70 yr) with comorbidities
- Obesity
- Chronic obstructive airways disease

Neurologic Risk Factors

- Crescendo transient ischemic attacks (TIAs) (i.e., more than one TIA per day)
- TIA while anticoagulated with heparin
- Multiple completed strokes
- Ischemic symptoms less than 24 hours before the surgical procedure
- Symptom status of the patient: asymptomatic patients and patients with only ocular ischemic events < patients with TIA < patients with stroke

Radiographic Risk Factors

- Occlusion of the contralateral internal carotid artery
- Near occlusion on the operative side
- Lack of angiographic collateral blood flow
- Ipsilateral intracranial stenosis
- Plaque extension more than 3 cm distal to the origin of the internal carotid artery or 5 cm proximal to the common carotid artery
- High bifurcation of the carotid artery
- Thrombus extending from the operative lesion

Perioperative Stroke Risk Stratification

- Group 1: no preoperative risks
- Group 2: angiographic risks only
- Group 3: medical risks with or without angiographic risks
- Group 4: neurologic risks with or without medical or angiographic risks

Adapted from Sundt TM, Sandok BA, Whisnant JP: Mayo Clin Proc 1975;50:301-306.

Anesthetic Management

Physiologic Management

Meticulous maintenance of physiologic stability (in particular, systemic, coronary, and cerebrovascular hemodynamic stability) is the ultimate goal in CEA anesthesia. Beyond avoiding factors that could put the patient at risk for myocardial or cerebral ischemia, at present there is relatively little else the anesthesiologist can do to improve outcome.

As part of the preoperative assessment, a series of blood pressure and heart rate measurements should be obtained from which acceptable ranges for perioperative management can be determined. Blood pressure should be maintained in the high-normal range throughout the procedure and particularly during the period of carotid clamping,

in an attempt to increase collateral flow and to prevent cerebral ischemia.

Hemodynamic fluctuations are common during carotid endarterectomy. Hypotension is more common under general anesthesia, and it often occurs immediately after the induction of anesthesia or after carotid unclamping and cerebral reperfusion.[11] In patients with contralateral internal carotid artery occlusion or severe stenosis, induced hypertension to approximately 10% to 20% above baseline is advocated during the period of carotid clamping when neurophysiologic monitoring is not used. Blood pressure preservation or augmentation can be accomplished by appropriate intravascular hydration, avoiding unnecessarily deep levels of general anesthesia, and vasopressor therapy such as phenylephrine and ephedrine. In the absence of severe left ventricular systolic dysfunction, phenylephrine is preferred over ephedrine because the increase in contractility and heart rate associated with ephedrine therapy increases myocardial oxygen consumption to a greater extent than the increase in wall stress caused by phenylephrine.

Because of the unnecessary increase in myocardial oxygen consumption, blood pressure elevations more than 20% of the baseline and tachycardia should be avoided. Furthermore, such increases in blood pressure might put the patient with a recent stroke at risk for intracerebral hemorrhage. Hypertension should be treated appropriately, taking into account the stage of the operation, the level of anesthesia, and the patient's heart rate. Deepening the anesthetic, beta-blocker therapy, nitroglycerine, and sodium nitroprusside are commonly used. In this situation, agents with a short half-life are preferred.

Bradycardia might occur during surgical manipulation of the carotid sinus or direct stimulation of the vagus nerve during dissection. Prophylactic injection of 1 to 2 mL of a local anesthetic between the internal and external carotid arteries before manipulation of these vessels might attenuate the bradycardia. However, local anesthetic infiltration may increase the incidence of intraoperative and postoperative hypertension. Other than a more gentle surgical approach, specific treatment is usually not needed. Administration of anticholinergic drugs can result in tachycardia, excessive hypertension, and increased myocardial oxygen requirements, so their use should be avoided.

Severe carotid stenosis, in particular during cross-clamping, represents a state of gross regional flow inequality and collateral dependence. The vessels supplying the ischemic areas are already maximally vasodilated, and blood flow could be diverted from these vascular beds to those already adequately perfused by cerebral vasodilators such as carbon dioxide, volatile anesthetic agents, and nitrates (i.e., cerebral steal). The reverse may occur in hypocapnia or as a result of intravenous anesthetic agents such as thiopental and propofol (i.e., inverse steal). On balance, normocarbia is recommended, and low levels of volatile anesthetic agents are acceptable.

Evidence is accumulating to suggest that hyperglycemia is detrimental in cerebral ischemia.[12] Although there are no good outcome studies in humans, it is appropriate to maintain normoglycemia during CEA.

General Anesthesia

General anesthesia offers ideal operating conditions. Provided that close attention is paid to the physiologic variables, and a rapid, controlled emergence from anesthesia is ensured, there is no evidence based on outcome data that favors the use of one anesthetic over another. Although it would seem logical that isoflurane or even barbiturate pretreatment would offer cerebral protection during carotid cross-clamping, no outcome data suggest a reduction in either the incidence or severity of intraoperative stroke during CEA.

Remifentanil infusion (0.05 to 0.2 µg/kg/min) ablates the sympathetic response to surgery, although phenylephrine infusion may be needed to maintain perfusion pressure. For amnesia, a low dose of volatile anesthetic (isoflurane or sevoflurane, usually between 0.3 and 0.5 of the minimum alveolar concentration [MAC]), or less commonly a propofol infusion, is titrated to maintain a bispectral index (BIS) number just below 60. Muscle relaxation is maintained with a nondepolarizing agent. This approach provides hemodynamic stability as well as stable conditions for electroencephalographic (EEG) monitoring. There is no consensus on the importance of the increase in cerebral metabolic rate and cerebral blood flow (CBF) caused by nitrous oxide, but when nitrous oxide is combined with remifentanil in this setting, vasopressor requirements are increased. Furthermore, as nitrous oxide has little to add to this technique, it is usually avoided.

After closure of the deep fascial layers, the volatile anesthetic is discontinued and neuromuscular reversal agents are administered. On skin closure, the remifentanil infusion rate is reduced to 0.02 to 0.04 µg/kg/min, allowing the patient to gently emerge from anesthesia. This approach allows neurologic assessment while the patient is still intubated. Hypertension on emergence usually responds well to labetalol, if required.

Regional Anesthesia

A superficial cervical plexus block, in combination with additional local anesthetic infiltration by the surgeon, can achieve the necessary sensory blockade of the C2 to C4 dermatomes. Deep cervical plexus blockade adds unnecessary risks, such as inadvertent intravascular or intrathecal injections, paralysis of the ipsilateral diaphragm, and local anesthetic toxicity, without reducing the need for intraoperative local anesthetic supplementation.[13] Sedation should be kept to a minimum to allow continuous neurologic assessment, in particular during carotid cross-clamping. Levels of consciousness, speech, and contralateral handgrip are assessed throughout the procedure. Patient refusal, language barriers, and difficult surgical anatomy such as a high carotid bifurcation are contraindications to performing CEA under regional anesthesia.

Postoperative Management

Blood pressure may continue to be labile for several days postoperatively, sometimes requiring continued use of vasoactive drugs. Untreated hypertension in the postoperative period may lead to cerebral hyperperfusion syndrome, myocardial ischemia, and neck hematoma. Hypertension unresponsive to labetalol may require a nicardipine infusion.

In patients with severe carotid stenosis, parts of the intracerebral circulation may have lost the ability to autoregulate blood flow and remain maximally vasodilated in the postoperative period. The sudden increase in cerebral perfusion pressure (CPP) and blood flow may lead to perfusion breakthrough edema. This typically occurs within the first few hours after surgery and may manifest as a severe headache, seizure, or even intracranial hemorrhage. Intracranial hemorrhage after CEA has a high mortality, so blood pressure should be carefully controlled in these patients.

Wound hematoma is one of the most common early postoperative complications, occurring in about 4% of patients.[14] Because of the increased risk of airway obstruction, these patients have to be intubated and surgically explored as soon as possible. Tracheal deviation caused by the hematoma, and pharyngeal edema caused by venous and lymphatic obstruction may complicate mask ventilation and intubation. Furthermore, pharyngeal edema may not resolve immediately after hematoma evacuation, and patients should be extubated with great care if this was present at the time of intubation.

■ ANESTHESIA FOR INTRACRANIAL SURGERY

Anesthesia for intracranial surgery is in many ways similar to general anesthesia for other procedures, but there are several special considerations. The brain is enclosed in a rigid skull and may be intolerant of volume increases, but it is a highly vascular organ and has the potential for massive hemorrhage. Tolerance to interruption of substrate delivery is minimal, and the brain is therefore equipped with a highly developed and responsive ability to autoregulate regional blood flow. Anesthetics and physiologic factors controlled by the anesthesiologist have profound effects on the brain, and it is reasonable to expect an anesthesiologist who is providing care for patients undergoing craniotomy to understand these interactions.

Preoperative Evaluation

Preoperative considerations for neurosurgical patients are similar to those for all surgical patients, with some significant adjuncts. Of first importance is the baseline neurologic evaluation. At emergence from anesthesia, failure to recover baseline neurologic function can be attributed to a number of surgical or anesthetic-related factors of varying degrees of urgency. The anesthesiologist must recognize changes from baseline and participate in the decision-making process. Second, the anesthesiologist must recognize the magnitude of preoperative intracranial pressure (ICP) and intracranial compliance, and the potential for intraoperative intracranial hypertension. Third, the anesthesiologist should be familiar with the location and size of the lesion, as this has a bearing on the surgical approach and patient positioning, the potential for intraoperative hemorrhage, the effects of cerebral edema, and possible postoperative neurologic deficits, including airway protection and arousal difficulties. Finally, the list of current medications is important for a variety of reasons.

During the course of surgery, scheduled doses of antiepileptics, steroids, and antibiotics may be missed, which could result in postoperative complications. High-dose steroid requirements may require intensive insulin regimens to maintain normal serum glucose, and patients receiving antihypertensive therapy may exhibit exaggerated hemodynamic responses to volatile anesthetics.[15,16] A focused history and brief physical should incorporate all these issues and adequately prepare the anesthesiologist for the neurosurgical procedure.

In addition to preoperative evaluation, the anesthesiologist should consider any necessary premedication. As a general rule, long-acting preoperative medications that might result in an alteration of the postoperative neurologic status should be minimized or avoided. It is reasonable to use premedications for prophylaxis against postoperative nausea and vomiting, as this is a common complication.

Anesthesia Induction

Concerns unique to induction of anesthesia for craniotomy are principally related to maintaining cerebral perfusion pressure and preventing intracranial hypertension. To maintain cerebral perfusion in the presence of impaired autoregulation, hypotension or intracranial hypertension must be avoided. Early studies recognized that the induction of anesthesia for craniotomies is associated with major increases in ICP,[17] so techniques evolved to minimize this increase. The sympathetic responses and associated increases in ICP caused by noxious stimuli such as endotracheal intubation, line placement, and surgical stimulation can be effectively blunted with an adequate depth of anesthesia. Complete muscle relaxation should be achieved and maintained to avoid coughing and straining, and the use of opioids and intravenous lidocaine prior to intubation is commonplace. Intravenous anesthetic agents, in addition to reducing the intubation response, also decrease cerebral metabolic rate and therefore CBF, volume, and ICP. Volatile anesthetic agents are potent cerebrovascular vasodilators that overcome the reduction in blood flow caused by metabolic suppression and result in a dose-dependent increase in CBF, blood volume, and ICP. This increase in ICP can be blunted by simultaneous moderate hyperventilation.[18] Unfortunately, data relevant to the effects of various anesthetics on ICP have for the most part come from animal studies and are thus limited for humans. More importantly, clinical outcome data related to anesthetic effects on ICP and craniotomy are limited, and the few human studies available used crude outcome assays. As a result, it is unclear whether the use of anesthesia for ICP control actually improves outcome after craniotomy, and it is difficult to advocate any specific anesthetic or technique for ICP control during induction.

Anesthesia Maintenance

Maintenance of neurosurgical anesthesia, like that of other surgeries, is usually uncomplicated. Most aspects of anesthesia for craniotomy are universal to all general anesthetics. However, two special considerations pertain: attendance to brain bulk and the necessity for rapid emergence. ICP and brain bulk are easily managed by careful positioning of the

head to avoid neck vein compression, by maintaining normocapnia and normotension, by avoiding high dosages of volatile anesthetic, by maintaining full muscle paralysis, and by administering routine osmotic diuretics such as mannitol. Occasionally, problems arise, particularly when the dura is being opened or the procedure involves the posterior fossa. A swollen brain can herniate through the dural defect, prohibiting further dural incision or adequate surgical visualization of the field. The management of acute intracranial hypertension is discussed later.

The other significant difference in the anesthetic technique for craniotomy is the necessity of rapid emergence, which is related to the need to be able to quickly and fully assess the patient for any postoperative neurologic deficit that may have a treatable cause (e.g., hematoma or cerebral edema). If the patient does not return to preoperative neurologic function, then requisite brain imaging and possible empiric treatment can be performed. Therefore, it is imperative that residual anesthetics play no role in altered levels of consciousness or postoperative neurologic deficit. Methods that result in a fully awake, cooperative patient after anesthesia include the use of a low-dose volatile agent augmented by remifentanil infusion.[19] Because of the relatively minimal amount of postoperative pain, this technique allows excellent hemodynamic control through titration of remifentanil dosage during the stimulating portion of the surgery, with rapid awakening at its end. For a totally intravenous technique that produces a predictable and rapid emergence pattern, the low-dose volatile agent can be replaced by a propofol infusion used together with a remifentanil infusion.

Management of Arterial Blood Pressure

In general, normotension is maintained in craniotomy patients. However, at times either low or high blood pressure may be more suitable. Blood pressure management can usually be accomplished by adjusting the anesthetic level. However, anesthetic techniques based largely on high-dose opioid infusion may induce more pronounced vasodilation and hypotension, and alpha agonism via phenylephrine may be used to offset the hypotension caused by the anesthetic. When increased arterial blood pressure may be of benefit (e.g., in a patient with a high ischemic risk), the usual means is through phenylephrine. However, patients who might be in a low cardiac output state may derive more benefit from appropriate intravascular volume therapy and inotropic support in the form of beta-agonism (i.e., dobutamine) or mixed alpha–beta agonism (i.e., norepinephrine). When strict blood pressure maintenance is essential to avoid even minimal amounts of hypertension (e.g., at induction during aneurysm clipping and at emergence from anesthesia), the usual method entails the infusion of a vasodilator—classically nitroprusside, and more recently the calcium channel blocker, nicardipine. Either agent rapidly and effectively treats increased systemic blood pressure, and both agents allow blood pressure to be maintained within a very strict range. The choice of agent depends primarily on the risk for intracranial hypertension. The use of nitroprusside may interfere with brain autoregulation of blood flow and cause increased intracranial pressure via increased blood volume in the arterial vasculature; this concern is not present with the use of nicardipine.[20] When less precise control is acceptable, longer-acting agents such as labetalol or occasionally clonidine may be used.

Management of Ventilation

Alteration of $PaCO_2$, within the range of approximately 20 to 80 mm Hg, causes a parallel change in CBF, which is a surrogate for cerebral blood volume (CBV). Because of the rigid structure of the skull and the relatively unchangeable volume outside the intravascular space, CBV is a direct determinant of ICP. Although CBF is easy to measure, CBV is not (particularly in humans). It is logical, however, that given a constant mean arterial pressure (MAP), $PaCO_2$-induced changes in CBF would correlate with reproducible changes in CBV. Indeed, abundant clinical evidence in patients with ICP monitors shows that reduction of $PaCO_2$ results in a transient reduction in ICP, and vice versa.[21] Historically, large reductions in $PaCO_2$ were common practice. However, use of techniques to measure retrograde jugular venous hemoglobin O_2 saturation in patients with traumatic head injury has repeatedly shown that reduction in $PaCO_2$ can exacerbate cerebral hypoperfusion, presumably as a result of vasoconstriction.[22] As a result, it is no longer advocated that major reductions in $PaCO_2$ be made in patients undergoing craniotomy for space-occupying lesions. Modest reductions in $PaCO_2$ remain valuable, however, to counteract vasodilatory effects of volatile anesthetics.[23] Finally, it is important to measure arterial to end-tidal CO_2 gradients in all neurosurgical patients, because physiologic dead space variability can be unpredictable.

Intraoperative Fluid Management

The intraoperative fluid management for patients undergoing craniotomy is somewhat different from that during anesthesia for other procedures. The induction of hyperosmotic therapy for the treatment of brain edema results in a predictable diuresis. It is essential that euvolemia be maintained, as it has been shown that both hypervolemia and hypovolemia are detrimental in some forms of brain injury[24]: euvolemia promotes improved osmotic diuresis, and hypovolemia results in hypoperfusion, especially if there is a sudden large surgical blood loss. Therefore, preoperative fluid deficit should be replaced, and once hyperosmotic therapy has been instituted, euvolemia should be maintained by replacing urine volume. Because urine output should be replaced with the solution that most closely approximates the goal osmolality of 310 mM/dL, normal saline (with an osmolality of 308 mM/dL) is preferred over hypo-osmolar lactated Ringer's solution. In the setting of major blood loss, fluid management becomes more challenging. Because of osmotic diuresis, urine output cannot be used as a gauge for intravascular volume, and surgical loss should be carefully estimated while observing the patient closely for signs of hypovolemia. Central venous pressure monitoring, if in place, can be valuable in maintaining euvolemia. Coagulopathy should be anticipated and treated early with appropriate products, as indicated by coagulation studies. Controversy over the use of

colloid to replace surgical blood loss continues. Colloids allow smaller infusion volumes during resuscitation and, theoretically, less extravasation into the third-space compartment. However, they are generally more expensive, and there is concern over potential bleeding diathesis with the use of synthetic colloids.[25] Human albumin solutions, which have little effect on coagulation and a very low risk for allergic reactions, might therefore be the preferred colloid in neurosurgery.

Muscle Relaxants

Succinylcholine has received special consideration in the context of craniotomy. There is clear evidence from studies in both experimental animals and humans that succinylcholine can increase ICP when intracranial compliance is poor, although the increase is typically small and transient. Animal evidence supports the idea that fasciculation plays a role in the ICP effects of succinylcholine, and there are data in humans that ICP changes caused by this drug can be prevented by preadministration of a de-fasciculating dose of nondepolarizing relaxants.[26] A probable mechanism is that the massive fasciculation-induced afferent barrage from muscle spindles to the brain causes transient increases in metabolic rate and coupled increases in CBF.[27] As with any decision, the risk-to-benefit ratio must be weighed when deciding whether succinylcholine is the appropriate agent. In controlled settings for nonemergent craniotomy, the ICP effects of succinylcholine can easily be offset by pretreatment with a nondepolarizing agent. At the same time, emergency airway management and the need to minimize hypercapnia and hypoxemia in patients with traumatic brain injury dictate that succinylcholine can be an appropriate adjunct for tracheal intubation.

The majority of patients undergoing craniotomy have been recently exposed to anticonvulsant agents. There is clear evidence that the duration of action of nondepolarizing muscle relaxants is reduced by anticonvulsant medications,[28] and even limited exposure can elicit this change. The mechanism for this remains unclear, but nondepolarizing agents that are metabolized by Hoffman elimination (e.g., atracurium and *cis*-atracurium) are largely resistant to the effects of anticonvulsants.

Management of Emergence

With neurosurgical procedures involving craniotomy, planning for emergence from anesthesia begins with induction. The goals of emergence are a predictable recovery to allow testing of neurologic function in the context of stable hemodynamics and a stable airway. A unique concern is that failure to emerge may be attributable to either anesthesia or surgery, which drastically alters subsequent treatment. If failure to emerge is attributable to surgery, a computerized tomographic (CT) scan is usually obtained to rule out hematoma formation or malignant cerebral edema. In contrast, if residual anesthesia is the issue, the use of opioid antagonists or additional reversal of neuromuscular blockade may be necessary. Therefore, when planning the anesthetic, it is helpful to restrict the use of agents to those that can be monitored for concentration or to those for which sufficient knowledge of pharmacodynamics allows highly probable and predictable clearance or reversal for emergence. It is best to keep the anesthetic simple so that each compound can be independently ruled out as an etiology for failure to emerge.

The magnitude of surgical stimulation after dural opening is minimal, and postoperative pain is often minor. However, one of the strongest intraoperative stimuli occurs at the very end of the procedure—that is, application of the head dressing, which causes sustained motion of the endotracheal tube. This, combined with a decreasing level of anesthesia for the anticipated emergence, can result in loss of control of hemodynamics and difficulty in airway management. A practical approach is to assume that the anesthesiologist needs 5 to 10 minutes after completion of the head dressing to allow a controlled emergence. Thus, neuromuscular blockade is maintained until completion of the head dressing, elimination of volatile anesthetics is complete by the time of head dressing, and anesthesia is maintained by either residual concentration of opioid (e.g., fentanyl or sufentanil) or continued infusion of remifentanil. Additionally, nitrous oxide can be used to supplement the anesthetic. This technique is probably better than using intravenous agents because its concentration can be defined by end-tidal gas analysis, which aids in defining failure to emerge. However, although nitrous oxide is usually well tolerated, the anesthesiologist should be vigilant in monitoring for a clinically apparent expanding pneumocephalus. Furthermore, rapidly cleared intravenous agents such as lidocaine can be of value in sustaining anesthesia for a few additional minutes. Finally, if remifentanil is used, the rate of infusion can remain unchanged until the dressing is complete.[29] It is important, however, to provide transitional analgesia (typically 5 mg morphine or 50 μg fentanyl in adults) before discontinuation of remifentanil.

After the need for a predictable emergence so that a neurologic examination can be performed, the second concern is hypertension. For reasons not yet understood, patients undergoing craniotomy often exhibit extreme hypertension during emergence that is sustained through the early phases of recovery. Because of the implications of intracranial hemorrhage, it is imperative to plan for treatment of hypertension before it manifests. Aside from ensuring adequate analgesia, prophylactic dosages of labetalol are helpful—usually 40 to 60 mg is required to be effective. Additionally, a nicardipine infusion is rapidly and easily titratable and does not contribute to increases in ICP (see Management of Arterial Blood Pressure, earlier). The concern about emergence hypertension is that it may contribute to postoperative hematoma formation, although this has not been proved. It has been shown, however, that many patients who develop postoperative hematomas have had episodes of hypertension during emergence or early recovery.[30] The source of hemorrhage is almost always within the surgical field, and thus the quality of hemostasis is undoubtedly important. However, because the mortality associated with postoperative hematoma formation requiring emergent evacuation is high, it is important to mitigate hypertension during emergence.

Finally, postoperative nausea and vomiting (PONV) is a frequent problem after craniotomy,[31,32] and in addition to being uncomfortable for the patient, it can contribute to postoperative hypertension. Several studies have shown that greater than 50% of patients suffer this complication. Its incidence appears to be independent of anesthetic technique (awake or general) or opioid dose, suggesting that surgery itself is contributory. Women, younger patients, and those undergoing infratentorial craniotomy are at greater risk, but prophylactic antiemetic therapy markedly reduces the magnitude of this problem. Droperidol (0.625 mg) appears to be at least as effective as 4 mg ondansetron without causing detectable sedation.[32] Many patients require multiple agents to ultimately control nausea and emesis. Regardless, some form of prophylaxis is generally warranted in patients undergoing craniotomy.

■ PROCEDURE-SPECIFIC ISSUES

Awake Craniotomy

Although brain scanning modalities (magnetic resonance imaging [MRI] and positron-emission tomography [PET]) can identify the speech-dominant cerebral hemisphere noninvasively, intraoperative mapping of the eloquent cortex is still the most reliable method to ensure preservation of speech function when the speech center is close to the surgical field.[33] Mapping the speech cortex, originally developed to allow maximal resection of epileptic foci in the dominant hemisphere, is equally useful for safely maximizing the extent of other cortical resections near language cortex, especially resections for low-grade gliomas and vascular malformations.[34] Neuroleptanalgesia with intermittent periods of general analgesia has been the technique most often utilized in the past. The development of short-acting titratable anesthetics and narcotics has led to an "asleep-awake-asleep" technique (e.g., spontaneously ventilating general anesthesia with intraoperative wakeup) for use during craniotomy when the eloquent cortex is at risk. The combined use of narcotics and intravenous anesthetics can result in decreased respiratory drive, hypercarbia, and elevated intracranial pressure. Patients with reflux risk, morbid obesity, chronic obstructive airways disease, or a tendency to airway obstruction pose a particular challenge, and these risk factors might even prohibit the use of this technique.

The Wada Test: Determining Whether Speech Mapping Is Required

Because the speech cortex is a unilateral structure, preoperative identification by a Wada test of the hemisphere containing it may be required.[35] The Wada test is advocated as a preliminary to operations in the vicinity of the Sylvan area in left-handed and ambidextrous patients, and also in the right-handed patient if any doubt exists as to which cerebral hemisphere is dominant for speech. The test is performed by intracarotid amytal injection. This results in immediate speech disruption, contralateral hemiparesis, and maintenance of consciousness when the injected carotid supplies the speech-dominant hemisphere. The nondominant hemisphere is identified by speech preservation and contralateral hemiparesis after carotid amytal injection.[35]

Intraoperative Electrophysiologic and Anatomic Components of Speech Mapping

Ojemann and colleagues described the technique of electrical stimulation of the cortex to map for speech.[34] Language function is measured by showing the patient pictures of objects with common names. While the patient names the pictures, cortical sites are stimulated. Three sets of sites have been identified. At one set of sites, repeated errors are evoked; a second set shows only single errors on multiple samples, and the third group shows no effect of stimulation at all. Regions in which repeated errors are evoked seem to be essential for a particular language function because when the cortical resection encroaches on these sites, aphasia commonly occurs. However, regions in which stimulation produces only occasional errors do not seem to be essential for that particular language function, and at least some of these sites can be included in a resection without producing aphasia. Too low a current may not adequately block local cortical function, whereas too large a current is likely to evoke seizures.

Thus, it is essential to determine the after-discharge threshold on electrocorticography (ECoG), and to use a current just below that threshold to identify language cortex with stimulation mapping while decreasing the chance of inducing a generalized seizure. Alteration of the seizure threshold by pharmacologic agents should be minimal, and ideally the seizure threshold should be constant during the period of testing. Intraoperative seizures may be aborted by irrigating the stimulated cortex with iced solution. Alternatively, a small dose of a short-acting sedative (e.g., barbiturate or propofol) may be required.

Comparing Neurolept and General Anesthesia for Awake Cortical Mapping

The practice of neuroleptanalgesia, also called conscioussedation analgesia, for treatment of epileptics at the Montreal Neurologic Institute was outlined by Trop.[36] The technique of neuroleptanalgesia relies on the titration of fentanyl and droperidol to a specific endpoint rather than the administration of a dose based on bodyweight. The goals of the neuroleptanalgesia technique were to enable the patient to tolerate surgical discomfort during prolonged immobility while maintaining verbal responsiveness. Short periods of unconsciousness were induced to complete painful portions of the procedure by increasing doses of fentanyl. The neurolept craniotomy technique is therefore more accurately described as neuroleptanalgesia with intermittent periods of general anesthesia. Loss of consciousness could be accompanied by hypoventilation or airway obstruction, leading to hypoxia, hypercarbia, and elevation of the intracranial pressure. These complications would occasionally necessitate the conversion to general anesthesia.

Although the majority of patients undergoing awake cortical testing can be managed successfully with a conscious sedation technique, a small percentage of patients (2% to 16%) are unable to tolerate the conditions of the surgery and require conversion to general anesthesia. In these patients, gaining control of the airway can be a challenge. Intubation by direct laryngoscopy necessitates rapid uncovering of the drapes and, if applicable, removal of the patient's head from the fixation holder. Emergency blind nasal intubation may be an option, although it is not always fast or successful.[37] Alternative options include the use of a fiberoptic bronchoscope or an intubating laryngeal mask airway (LMA), or the combined use of these two devices. To obviate these airway problems, and to prevent intraoperative hypercarbia, Huncke and coworkers proposed an anesthetic technique that they called asleep-awake-asleep.[37] The strategy includes awake fiberoptic intubation of a sedated patient after local anesthetic topicalization of the airway. To eliminate coughing on the endotracheal tube during intraoperative emergence, the airway is retopicalized by injection of a local anesthetic into a long, thin multi-orifice catheter that has been wrapped around the endotracheal tube prior to intubation. After awake brain mapping, some in this small series of 10 patients were reintubated over a tube changer that was left in place, and others were reintubated with a fiberoptic bronchoscope.

An alternative approach to providing an airway for positive-pressure ventilation is with an LMA.[38] In a series of 32 patients, LMA placement in the lateral position, together with controlled ventilation, was successful in all patients. The author reported excellent brain relaxation as assessed by the neurosurgeon. The anesthetic maintenance included sevoflurane and nitrous oxide. All patients received a bupivacaine scalp block after the placement of the LMA. All patients awoke smoothly and none experienced bucking or coughing on emergence for speech mapping. Exclusion criteria for this study included sleep apnea, a potentially difficult airway, risk of aspiration, and severe claustrophobia.

Although there are potential advantages to routine endotracheal intubation or LMA insertion, no large trials have documented the benefits or the incidence of associated risks. To minimize the coughing and Valsalva associated with airway instrumentation, or at the time of emergence, techniques relying on spontaneous ventilation through a natural or splinted airway continue to evolve. Careful titration of remifentanil and propofol infusions in an asleep-awakeasleep technique produced very good results, with only 2% of cases requiring conversion to general anesthesia during cortical mapping.[39] Airway support was dictated by the patient's ability to maintain airway patency and sufficient respiratory drive, and when required, this was usually established with positive-pressure ventilation through nasal trumpets or LMA. This technique was successful in most cases, with 2% requiring conversion to general anesthesia during cortical testing. Adverse side effects were equivalent to previously reported rates using a neurolept technique. Some degree of hypercarbia (median $PaCO_2$, 50; range, 47 to 55 mm Hg) was seen, and the incidence of apnea was high, underscoring the importance of an available method to offer positive-pressure ventilation.

Table 21-1 summarizes anesthesia techniques for craniotomy with awake intraoperative language testing, and it illustrates that no one method for the anesthetic management

21-1   **Summary of Awake Craniotomy Studies**

Study Authors	Date	Number of Patients	Monitors	Drugs	Technique	Side Effects and Outcome
Trop et al.[36]	1986	2000 (descriptive review)	Noninvasive No Foley	Droperidol 0.15 mg/kg Fentanyl 0.5-0.75 μg/kg Methohexital Local anesthetic: Infiltration used, but type, quantity, and location not specified.	**Neurolept technique** Repeat fentanyl and droperidol to maintain analgesia and adequate ventilation Methohexital used for brief loss of consciousness in painful portions of procedure	70% managed with neuroleptic technique 25% required methohexital (Brevital) in addition 5% required conversion to GA Nausea and vomiting, 12% Seizure, frequency not stated
Archer et al.[123]	1988	354	Noninvasive No Foley Arterial catheter for those converting to GA	Fentanyl 6(1-24) μg/kg Droperidol 10(0-40) mg Methohexital 150(0-890) mg Local anesthetic: dibucaine, 50:50 mix of 0.67% and 0.25% with epinephrine Scalp infiltrated initially, and along middle meningeal artery and dura if needed during opening of the bone flap	**Neurolept technique** Supplemental fentanyl kept to a minimum to maintain normal respiration, conserve airway reflexes, and provide alertness for testing Methohexitone given to majority to stimulate cortical activity Also given for sedation or control of seizures	Seizures, 16% Nausea/vomiting, 8% Excessive sedation, 3% Change to GA,* 2% "Tight" brain, 1.4% Local anesthetic toxicity, 2%
Sartorius et al.[124]	1997	Not stated	Arterial catheter Foley catheter	—	**Neurolept technique** The goal is patient responsiveness to verbal commands with sufficient analgesia to tolerate both local anesthetic infiltration and prolonged relative immobility	—
Silbergeld et al.[125]	1992	9	Not stated	Droperidol, 1.25-2.5 mg Fentanyl, 50-150 μg Propofol bolus, 1-2 mg/kg	**Sedative technique with intermittent GA** Premedicate with droperidol, 1.25-2.5 mg Fentanyl, 50-150 μg Propofol titrated for sedation without apnea "Adequate level of anesthesia is obtained prior to beginning any potentially painful part of the procedure"	Recall of portions of procedure during propofol administration, 33% Duration of recovery and nature of recovery not altered by propofol dosage or duration ECoG not altered by propofol

| 21-1 | **Summary of Awake Craniotomy Studies—cont'd** |

Study Authors	Date	Number of Patients	Monitors	Drugs	Technique	Side Effects and Outcome
Herrick et al.[126]	1997	37	Noninvasive	Propofol PCS: propofol 0.5 mg/kg bolus with a 3-min lockout and basal infusion of 0.5 mg/kg/hr Neurolept: initial bolus droperidol (0.04 mg/kg), fentanyl, 0.7 µg/kg bolus, and fentanyl infusion, 0.7 µg/kg/hr All patients received scalp and meningeal local anesthetic, bolus fentanyl (25 µg), and Dramamine as needed	**Sedative technique vs. neurolept technique** Prospective trial of PCS with propofol vs. neurolept technique	Sedation scores significantly higher (i.e., patients more alert) in the propofol group Recall of intraoperative events not depressed in either group All patients easily aroused throughout procedure Respiratory rate <8 more common in the fentanyl/propofol group Pain associated with tachycardia more common in the neurolept group Intraoperative seizures more common in the neurolept group
Welling and Donegan[127]	1989	4	Arterial catheter in 1 case	Droperidol, 2.5 mg Alfentanil bolus, 5-7.5 µg/kg, repeated Infusion, 0.25-2.0 µg/kg/min	**Neurolept technique** Patient sedated, breathing spontaneously and comfortable Alfentanil infusion maintained at low level during testing	Etomidate used to elicit seizure in one patient "Tight" brain in one patient unresponsive to decreasing alfentanil infusion and auto-hyperventilation Mannitol achieved good result
Gignac et al.[128]	1993	30	Noninvasive BP Nasal prong CO_2	Droperidol, 0.014 mg/kg Dimenhydrinate, 0.25 mg/kg <u>Opioid bolus and infusion:</u> Fentanyl 0.75 µg/kg and 0.01 µg/kg/min Sufentanil 0.075 µg/kg and 0.0015 µg/kg/min Alfentanil 7.5 µg/kg and 0.5 µg/kg/min	**Neurolept technique**	Nasal prong CO_2 >45 mm Hg in 33% Nausea in 50% Conversion to GA, 2/30 Oversedation, 2/30 Desaturation, 3/30 Seizure, 5/30
Huncke[37]	1998	10	Arterial catheters Foley catheter Both inserted after GA induction	Induction: pentothal or propofol Maintenance: N_2O and desflurane, isoflurane, or sevoflurane Propofol Bupivacaine 0.5% for pin sites and scalp incision	**GA with intraoperative wakeup, "asleep-awake-asleep"** Patient self-positioned Awake nasal or oral intubation Hyperventilation Topical lidocaine to trachea prior to intraoperative extubation Reintubation after cortical mapping with bronchoscope or with tube changer	Nosebleed, 2 patients Reintubation attempts >50% of patients

Continued

21-1   Summary of Awake Craniotomy Studies—cont'd

Study Authors	Date	Number of Patients	Monitors	Drugs	Technique	Side Effects and Outcome
Taylor[129]	1999	200	Infrequent use of arterial catheters, CVP, or Foley catheters	Local anesthetic to pin sites Short-acting sedatives propofol, midazolam, and fentanyl (dosage not specified) to keep patient comfortable	—	Exclusion criteria explicitly stated (inability to cooperate because of dysphasia, severe language barrier, mental retardation, emotional instability, decreased level of consciousness) eliminated 105/305 patients. Five mapping-negative patients developed new permanent deficits. Two mapping-positive patients developed new permanent deficits. Patients with intact preoperative mental status had lower a complication rate than those with preoperative deficits. 67% did not stay in ICU postoperatively.
Vlessides[38]	2000	32	Not stated	Bupivacaine scalp block Sevoflurane and nitrous oxide maintenance	**GA with intraoperative wakeup, "asleep-awake-asleep"** LMA placement in lateral position	4/32 patients experiencing grand mal seizure during speech testing were treated with thiopental, and their airways were immediately secured with an LMA
Keifer et al.[39]	2005	98	Arterial catheter Foley catheter	Remifentanil, 0.05 µg/kg/min Propofol, 115 µg/kg/min	**Asleep-awake-asleep** Spontaneous ventilation with natural or "stented" airway Positive-pressure ventilation when indicated by apnea	Successful testing, 98% Disoriented on emergence, 5% Required conversion to GA, 2% Episodic apnea, 66% Hypercarbia, hypertension at placement of Mayfield head frame and at emergence Headache, 16% Nausea, 8%

*Tracheal intubation, lateral position.

CVP, central venous pressure; ECoG, electrocorticography; GA, general anesthesia; ICU, intensive care unit; LMA, laryngeal mask airway; PCS, patient-controlled sedation.

of awake testing during craniotomy is perfect. The choice of technique and the management of intraoperative complications are directed by the patient and the surgical requirements (patient position, duration of surgery, duration of wakefulness, and multiple periods of wakefulness). Close communication (both preoperative and intraoperative) between surgeon, patient, anesthesiologist, and the electrophysiologists is critical. Focus on details of patient comfort, details of patient monitoring, and requirements for patient wakefulness are necessary to increase the rate of successful procedures.

Cerebral Aneurysm Clipping and Coiling Procedures

Rupture of an intracranial aneurysm, the most common cause of subarachnoid hemorrhage (SAH), occurs with a frequency of between six and eight per 100,000 in most populations.[40] SAH is associated with a 32% to 67% case fatality rate, and with long-term dependence in 10% to 20% of survivors because of brain damage.[41] To ablate the aneurysm and prevent rebleeding, aneurysm clipping or endovascular coiling is commonly performed on patients who survive to reach the hospital after aneurysmal subarachnoid bleeding.

21-2	Hunt and Hess' Modified Clinical Grades

Grade	Criteria
Grade 0	Unruptured aneurysm (0%-2%)
Grade I	Asymptomatic or minimal headache and slight nuchal rigidity (0%-2%)
Grade II	Moderate to severe headache, nuchal rigidity, but no neurologic deficit other than cranial nerve (2%-10%)
Grade III	Drowsiness, confusion, or mild deficit (10%-15%)
Grade IV	Stupor, mild to severe hemiparesis, possible early decerebrate rigidity, and vegetative disturbance (60%-70%)
Grade V	Deep coma, decerebrate rigidity, moribund appearance (70%-100%)

From Hunt WE, Hess RM: J Neurosurg 1968;28:14-20.

21-3	World Federation of Neurological Surgeons (WFNS) Grading Scale for Patients with Subarachnoid Hemorrhage

WFNS Grade	Glasgow Coma Score (Sum Score)	Motor Deficit
I	15	Absent
II	14-13, without focal deficit*	Absent
III	14-13, with focal deficit	Present
IV	12-7	Present or absent
V	6-3	Present or absent

*Cranial nerve palsies are not considered a focal deficit.
From Report of World Federation of Neurological Surgeons Committee on a Universal Subarachnoid Hemorrhage Grading Scale. J Neurosurg 1988;68:985-986.

In addition, unique pathophysiologic changes occur after rupture of an intracranial aneurysm that require special anesthetic and intensive care management.

Hypertension, frequently seen with acute SAH, may represent autonomic hyperactivity induced by cerebral ischemia or direct trauma to cerebral autonomic control mechanisms. Sudden or sustained elevations of MAP or reductions of ICP tend to distend the aneurysmal sac and may cause rupture and rebleeding of the aneurysm, the most significant early complication after SAH. On the other hand, prolonged reductions of CPP (MAP – ICP) may produce neurologic ischemia in poorly perfused areas with impaired autoregulation, and may globally increase ICP through ischemic disruption of the blood–brain barrier.[42]

Preoperative Management

Not only does SAH injure the brain at the time of the hemorrhage, but it is frequently followed by further neurologic insults that may occur over a period of weeks. In addition, the complications are by no means limited to the central nervous system, and there is frequent impairment of cardiac and pulmonary function. Finally, there is a complex interaction between neurologic and medical complications.

Neurologic

Headache, the most common clinical symptom of SAH, occurs in 85% to 95% of patients.[43] Many patients present with a brief loss of consciousness followed by various degrees of decreased mental acuity. Other symptoms of SAH include nausea, vomiting, and photophobia. Other signs of neurologic involvement include motor or sensory deficits, visual field deficits, abnormal motor posturing, or loss of various brainstem reflexes.

Two grading scales are commonly used to assess neurologic status after SAH: the modified Hunt and Hess grade[44] (Table 21-2) and the grading scale of the World Federation of Neurological Surgeons[45] (Table 21-3). The scales are useful for identifying a baseline neurologic status from which any acute changes should be assessed. In addition, the scales may correlate with physiologic status. Patients who are Hunt and Hess grades I and II have near normal cerebral autoregulation and ICP. Serious systemic disease or vasospasm, if present, raises the Hunt and Hess grade one level to the next worse grade.

Cardiopulmonary

Electrocardiographic Abnormalities and Cardiac Injury. The stratification of cardiac dysfunction after SAH ranges from isolated electrocardiographic (ECG) abnormalities and myocardial enzyme elevation to pulmonary edema and cardiogenic shock. Injury to the posterior hypothalamus may stimulate the release of norepinephrine from the adrenal medulla and sympathetic cardiac efferents.[46] Norepinephrine, either through direct toxicity or via significant elevation of myocardial afterload, produces ischemic changes in the subendocardium.[47] Pathologic examination of the myocardium after SAH may reveal microscopic subendocardial hemorrhages and myocytolysis.[48] By performing ECG spectral analysis and measuring cardiac enzymes and plasma catecholamines in patients with SAH, it was found that not only sympathetic activity but also vagal activity is enhanced during the acute phase of SAH, thus contributing to the ECG abnormalities and the onset of cardiac injury.[49]

ECG changes accompany 50% to 80% of SAH episodes, occur during the first 48 hours, and normalize over a 6-week period. Most ECG abnormalities appear to be neurogenic rather than cardiogenic.[50,51] Also, the risk of death from cardiac causes is low in patients with SAH and ECG readings consistent with ischemia or myocardial infarction. ECG abnormalities are associated with more severe neurologic injury but are not independently predictive of mortality. Therefore, a dilemma exists as to whether ECG changes suggesting cardiac injury suggest frank myocardial injury and increase the risk of anesthesia and surgery.

The correlation between the ECG abnormalities and cardiac ischemia is not good. However, it appears that cardiac troponin I (cTnI) is a highly sensitive and specific indicator of myocardial dysfunction and injury after aneurysmal SAH.[52] Cardiac dysfunction is usually reversible and should not necessarily preclude these patients from undergoing operative interventions.[53] Nevertheless, serial cardiac enzymes, assessment of ventricular function, or cardiac catheterization may be necessary to establish functional and therapeutic implications associated with the severity of the cardiac injury.

Dysrhythmias. Life-threatening dysrhythmias may occur in patients during the first 48 hours after SAH.[54] Cardiac dysrhythmias include sinus tachycardia, sinus bradycardia, premature supraventricular complexes, supraventricular tachycardia, atrial fibrillation, premature ventricular complexes, ventricular tachycardia, ventricular fibrillation (VF), torsades de pointes, and QT prolongation. The QT interval was significantly prolonged in those cases where torsades de pointes was followed by life-threatening ventricular dysrhythmias.[54] The development of VF is frequently preceded by torsades de pointes. Female sex and hypokalemia are independent risk factors for QT interval prolongation after SAH.[55] An inverse correlation between the serum catecholamines and potassium levels suggests that a catecholamine surge after SAH plays an important role in the pathogenesis of hypokalemia during the acute phase of SAH.

Hypertension. Management of hypertension is a difficult issue, especially if the blood pressure rises above 200/110 mm Hg. The primary reason for treating hypertension is to reduce transmural pressure to prevent hemorrhage or aneurysmal rupture. However, after SAH, the range between the upper and lower limits of the autoregulation of CBF becomes narrower, which makes brain perfusion more dependent on MAP.[56] In fact, intraoperative hypotension could have a significantly adverse effect on the outcome of SAH.[57] Moreover, hypotension is also related to more frequent and severe manifestations of vasospasm. Thus, it seems best to reserve antihypertensive drugs for patients with extreme elevations of blood pressure as well as evidence of rapidly progressive end-organ deterioration, diagnosed from either clinical signs (e.g., new retinopathy, heart failure) or laboratory evidence (e.g., signs of left ventricular failure on chest radiograph, proteinuria, or oliguria with a rapid rise of creatinine level).

Calcium channel blockers have been effective in treating acute hypertension and may have an additional beneficial effect on cerebral vasospasm. (We suggest administration of nicardipine, 1 to 15 mg/hr. A bolus of labetalol [50 to 100 mg] is useful as an adjunct.) Adrenergic blockers have the advantage of not directly affecting CBF[58] and have the theoretical advantage of shifting the autoregulatory curve to the left.[59]

Most of the assessment of the risk of anesthesia and surgery is derived from experience with cerebral aneurysm surgery, not endovascular coiling. Endovascular aneurysmal coiling may have less cardiovascular impact than craniotomy and aneurysm clipping. The timing of endovascular aneurysm coiling must be determined in the context of the disease course, especially with respect to the risk of rebleeding and vasospasm. Significant cardiopulmonary edema, malignant dysrhythmias, or severe heart failure may warrant postponement of surgery until adequate medical management can be achieved.

Anesthetic Management for Aneurysm Clipping

The goals of intraoperative management for cerebral aneurysm surgery include preventing intraoperative aneurysm rupture, minimizing potential neurologic injury, facilitating surgical exposure, and providing optimal conditions for smooth emergence and stable recovery.

Premedication

In patients presenting for aneurysm surgery with decreased levels of consciousness (grades III to V), significant anxiety is unlikely. Sedative premedication is not required in these patients. Grades I and II patients may require only a reassuring preoperative visit. Heavy sedation hinders preoperative neurologic assessment and depresses ventilation. Depression of ventilation may produce hypercarbia and corresponding increases in CBF and ICP. If preoperative sedation is required to prevent potential hemodynamic perturbations associated with anxiety, a small dose of a benzodiazepine is usually sufficient. If the patient is at increased risk for aspiration because of a decreased level of consciousness, prophylactic administration of agents that reduce gastric acidity and volume should be given before induction.

Monitoring

Adequate monitoring should be established prior to maneuvers that are likely to alter CBF, ICP, and transmural aneurysmal pressure. Induction of anesthesia and laryngoscopy are critical events that directly influence intracranial physiology. Intra-arterial blood pressure monitoring is particularly useful as an early detector of hemodynamic alterations. Many clinicians prefer to place an intra-arterial catheter with local anesthesia prior to induction so that blood pressure responses can be assessed continuously. Central venous access is helpful in assessing volume replacement needs prior to aneurysm clipping, and in managing hypervolemic therapy in patients at risk for vasospasm. Rapid titration of vasoactive medications can be best achieved with the use of a central venous catheter. There is a poor correlation between central venous and left ventricular end-diastolic pressure in SAH.[60] Therefore, placement of a pulmonary artery catheter may be more helpful in assessing perioperative volume status and cardiac dysfunction than a central venous catheter.

Intraoperative neurologic monitoring may be helpful in patients undergoing aneurysm surgery. SSEPs detect reversible ischemia during temporary vessel occlusion.[61] Monitoring of somatosensory evoked potential (SSEP) for cerebral ischemia during temporary vessel occlusion is limited by its inability to detect ischemia in the motor cortex, subcortical structures, and sensory regions not topographically represented by the stimulated peripheral nerve. Studies demonstrate relatively high false-positive (38% to 60%) and false-negative (5% to 34%) detection rates.[62,63] Posterior circulation aneurysms appear best suited to brainstem auditory evoked potential monitoring,[64,65] but they may also benefit from SSEP monitoring. Intraoperative EEG monitoring may also be helpful for detection of cerebral ischemia during aneurysm surgery.[64]

The probability of increased ICP during the first 24 to 48 hours after SAH is high. Some groups monitor ICP intraoperatively with intraventricular catheters. This allows intraoperative drainage of cerebrospinal fluid (CSF) to improve operating conditions and management of elevated ICP.

Angiography is a useful diagnostic test when focal neurologic deficits evolve in the intraoperative or perioperative period. Intraoperative cerebral angiography ensures complete obliteration of the aneurysmal neck, and it helps the surgeon recognize clip occlusion of the parent arterial trunk or perforating arterial branches.[66] Repositioning the clip before emergence may decrease the incidence of ischemic complications and reduce the need for reoperation.

Induction

Rupture of an aneurysm during induction is associated with a mortality approaching 75%.[67] Although it seems appropriate to maintain lower blood pressures during induction to prevent abrupt elevations in transmural pressure, significant reductions in cerebral perfusion pressure cause focal and global neurologic deficits in animal models.[68] This is particularly relevant to the patient with SAH who may have impaired autoregulation and vasospasm. Decreases in cerebral perfusion pressure for brief periods during induction are probably less detrimental than sudden elevations in transmural pressure.

To avoid increases in transmural pressure, the sympathetic response to laryngoscopy and intubation must be attenuated, while preventing coughing and straining. Anesthesia is induced in the usual fashion.[69,70] Barbiturates and propofol are similar in their ability to reduce transmural pressure and cerebral metabolism. Narcotics are usually added to the induction sequence to blunt the hemodynamic response to laryngoscopy and intubation. Remifentanil infusion (0.3 to 0.5 μg/kg/min) administered over 3 to 5 minutes before laryngoscopy to deepen anesthesia is extremely effective in attenuating sympathetic responses. Additional propofol (20 to 50 mg), intravenous lidocaine (1.5 to 2.0 mg/kg), esmolol (0.5 mg/kg), or labetalol (10 to 20 mg) administered 90 seconds before laryngoscopy, can further attenuate rises in transmural pressure during intubation.

The indication for rapid sequence induction in the patient with an unclipped cerebral aneurysm is controversial. The incidence of clinically significant aspiration is 0.05% during general anesthesia.[71] The incidence of aneurysm rupture during induction is in the range of 1% to 2%.[72] Therefore, careful consideration should be given to the risks and benefits before choosing a classic rapid sequence technique.

Maintenance

The hemodynamic goals during maintenance are similar to those during induction. Ideally, a maintenance agent allows rapid and reversible titration of blood pressure, protects against cerebral ischemia, minimizes formation of cerebral edema, allows control of intracranial pressure, and provides for rapid emergence. Commonly, anesthesia is maintained with combinations of oxygen, narcotic, isoflurane or sevoflurane, and nondepolarizing muscle relaxant. As with induction, choosing a particular agent is less important than matching anesthetic depth to the level of surgical stimulation. Maintaining stable hemodynamic responses to the varying level of stimulation may be particularly important in preventing aneurysm rupture. Painful stimuli (e.g., pin insertion) should be anticipated and adverse hemodynamic responses prevented by additional anesthesia and/or sympathetic blockers. Local anesthetic infiltration at the Mayfield pin sites prior to application can reduce the hemodynamic response.

Intraoperative fluid administration is governed by the patient's maintenance requirements, urine volume, blood loss, and measured cardiac filling pressures if central venous access has been established. Profound hypovolemia should be avoided in patients with subarachnoid hemorrhage, as it can be associated with cerebral ischemia and perioperative neurologic deficits, especially if there is also vasospasm.[73] Dextrose-containing solutions should be avoided, as an increased incidence of neurologic deficits is associated with hyperglycemia and focal cerebral ischemia in experimental models.[74]

Intraoperative maintenance of adequate CPP is imperative. Although elevations of CPP increase transmural pressure and may predispose to aneurysm rupture, this concern is much less important after the aneurysm has been secured. The acceptable and safe upper limit of blood pressure after the aneurysm has been clipped has not been systematically evaluated. Arterial pressure tends to rise spontaneously when anesthetic levels are decreased after clip placement in volume-replete patients. This rise in pressure may benefit patients, especially those with potential vasospasm, by increasing CPP and CBF. Reasonable outcomes were observed when systolic blood pressures of 160 to 200 mm Hg were maintained after aneurysm clipping in a study of 42 patients with suspected vasospasm.[67] Before aneurysm clipping, the systolic blood pressure was kept between 120 and 150 mm Hg. In some patients, however, the elevation in blood pressure can be considerable and may damage the blood–brain barrier, leading to the formation of vasogenic edema. Systolic pressure above 240 mm Hg, or a mean pressure greater than 150 mm Hg, may warrant pharmacologic reduction to prevent formation of vasogenic edema caused by breakthrough of autoregulation.[74]

Emergence

The primary goals during emergence are to avoid coughing, straining, hypercarbia, and wide fluctuations in blood pressure. All anesthetic drugs should be discontinued, the patient should be well oxygenated, and residual neuromuscular blockade should be reversed. Intravenous administration of 1.5 mg/kg of lidocaine a few minutes prior to extubation may minimize coughing. Blood pressure should be reduced pharmacologically if there is evidence of cardiac ischemia, pulmonary edema, or excessive prolonged blood pressure elevation. In patients with multiple or unclippable aneurysms, blood pressure should be kept within 20% of normal (120 to 160 mm Hg).

SAH grade I or II patients usually do not require postoperative ventilation or airway support. Grade III patients may not be extubated after surgery, depending on their level of consciousness at emergence and their preoperative ventilatory status. Grade IV and V patients often require postoperative ventilation. Patients with surgical clipping of vertebral-basilar aneurysms may require postoperative airway support because of injury to swallowing or airway protective reflexes.

If the patient does not return to preoperative neurologic status, any residual effects of anesthetic agents should be reversed, including neuromuscular blocking agents, narcotics, and sedative agents. After elimination of anesthetic agents as a cause for poor emergence, a thorough diagnostic evaluation should be undertaken. Metabolic causes of poor emergence include hypoxia, hypercarbia, and hyponatremia. Although epileptic seizure activity is usually evident from clinical examination, subclinical status epilepticus is a possible cause of delayed emergence and should be evaluated by diagnostic EEG. A CT scan is imperative to rule out subdural hematoma, hydrocephalus, pneumocephalus, and intracranial hemorrhage. A cerebral angiogram may be helpful in ruling out the possibility of vascular occlusion.

Special Situations

Temporary Vessel Occlusion

Local decreases in transmural pressure can be achieved by occlusion of the aneurysm's feeding vessels with temporary clips. The advantages include more effective reduction of transmural pressure, reduced intraoperative rupture, technically easier clipping, and reduced requirement for controlled hypotension.[75] Considerable controversy exists concerning the techniques and duration of temporary arterial occlusion. The critical threshold for conversion of temporary cerebral ischemia to permanent focal cerebral infarction is unknown. A recent study concluded that 15 to 20 minutes of temporary occlusion is a critical threshold for the development of postoperative cerebral infarctions.[76] In contrast, other series have reported safe time limits of up to 120 minutes.[77] If temporary occlusion involves ischemia to major deep nuclei or the brainstem, temporary clip application times of less than 10 minutes may be more appropriate.[78]

Several risk factors predispose patients to new neurologic deficits after temporary vessel occlusion. These factors include age greater than 61 years, poor neurologic condition before surgery (Hunt and Hess grades III to IV), and distributions of the perforating arteries of the distal basilar and horizontal segment of the middle cerebral artery.[76]

Intraoperative Cerebral Protection

The International Hypothermia Aneurysm Trial (IHAST) is the only randomized prospective trial to address cerebral protection during aneurysm clipping.[79] IHAST did not demonstrate any benefit to mild (33° C) intraoperative hypothermia. No other putative protective strategies have been submitted to prospective randomized trials.

Despite this, some centers use a variety of anesthetic-based techniques. The most common are barbiturates or propofol given to achieve burst suppression.[80] Barbiturates decrease CBF, intracranial pressure, and metabolic rate. Although animal investigations have shown that barbiturates can protect against focal ischemia, the few uncontrolled human series in aneurysm surgery have not demonstrated improvement in morbidity or mortality.[81] In addition, the large dosages required to suppress EEG activity and significantly reduce the cerebral metabolic rate can produce profound cardiovascular depression.[82] Propofol's cerebral hemodynamic profile is similar to that of the barbiturates, and like these drugs, it can cause burst suppression. Animal studies have been equivocal in demonstrating cerebroprotective effects.[83]

Intraoperative Rupture

Aneurysmal rupture may occur during induction of anesthesia or during the operative procedure. The incidence of intraoperative rupture is 2% to 19%.[84] The stage in the operative procedure at which the rupture occurs influences the severity of the outcome. Sudden sustained elevations of blood pressure with or without bradycardia suggest the possibility of aneurysm rupture. Alterations in hemodynamic parameters may be subtle when the patient is anesthetized. One report used transcranial Doppler ultrasound to detect aneurysm rupture immediately after induction[85]; this information was used clinically to manage intracranial hypertension. In most circumstances when aneurysmal rupture is suspected during induction, the surgery is postponed to allow reassessment of the neurologic status and prognosis. Therapy should be instituted to control ICP and maintain cerebral perfusion. Some centers have demonstrated good results with "rescue clipping" of an aneurysm that ruptures at the time of induction.[67]

Rupture occurring during aneurysm dissection usually has a lower mortality than when it occurs during induction. The immediate anesthetic goals after rupture are to maintain adequate systemic perfusion and to facilitate prompt surgical control of bleeding. Bleeding during repair of the aneurysm does not change morbidity if it is quickly controlled.[86] However, if significant amounts of blood enter the subarachnoid space, intraoperative rupture has resulted in marked brain swelling that tends to be refractory to steroids and diuretics. Rapid induction of hypotension to achieve a MAP of 40 to 50 mm Hg may reduce bleeding enough to clip the aneurysm. If this method does not reduce bleeding enough, brief periods of manual compression of the ipsilateral carotid may be considered for an anterior-circulation aneurysm. The induction of hypotension to control bleeding may be associated with a worsened neurologic outcome compared with maintaining cerebral perfusion pressure, and compared with controlling bleeding with the placement of temporary clips.[87]

Cerebral Aneurysm Embolization

Endovascular treatment of intracranial aneurysms was first described in the early 1970s by Fedor Serbinenko.[88] In 1990, Guido Guglielmi was the first to describe the technique of occluding aneurysms from an endovascular approach with electrolytic detachable platinum coils, termed Guglielmi detachable coils (GDCs).[89] As clinical experience with this technique has increased and coil design has improved, coil embolization has been used with increasing frequency even in patients who could be treated by conventional surgical clipping for some ruptured intracranial aneurysms.[90,91]

Recently, in a randomized trial of 2143 patients with acutely ruptured intracranial aneurysm, the International Subarachnoid Aneurysm Trial (ISAT) showed that endovascular treatment reduced relative and absolute risks of dependency or death, compared with neurosurgical clipping, at the 1-year follow up.[92]

Anesthesiologists have several important concerns when providing care to patients undergoing interventional neuroradiology (INR) procedures: (1) maintenance of patient immobility and physiologic stability, (2) manipulating systemic or regional blood flow, (3) managing anticoagulation, (4) treating and managing sudden unexpected complications during the procedure, (5) guiding the medical management of critical care patients during transport to and from the radiology suites, and (6) ensuring rapid recovery from anesthesia and sedation during and immediately after the procedure to facilitate neurologic examination and monitoring.[93,94]

Induction and Maintenance of Anesthesia

The goals of anesthetic management specific to endovascular aneurysm ablation are immobility, cardiorespiratory stability, and rapid emergence from anesthesia. Two coincident radiologic techniques, contrast angiography and real-time fluoroscopy, enable the precise localization of aneurysm and placement of intravascular coils and stents. The images derived from these two methods are superimposed on a single monitoring screen, producing an "interactive road map" of the cerebral vasculature. If there is any movement of the patient's head after obtaining the road map, the position of the intravascular catheter noted on fluoroscopy is inaccurate and may be dangerously misleading. Immobility is therefore essential throughout the procedure to ensure that the angiogram and fluoroscopic image are precisely aligned.

To promote adequate CPP, normotension and normocarbia are maintained. The current methods to determine the adequacy of cerebral perfusion include angiography, transcranial Doppler, electroencephalography, and clinical testing of neurologic function. Many of these modalities require access to the patient's head and are not practical to perform during the coiling procedure. Clinical neurologic testing of an awake patient is the standard for assessing cerebral perfusion. However, the value of this testing may be decreased in the sedated patient. Therefore, if a general anesthetic technique is used, rapid emergence enabling timely and accurate neurologic testing is important to assess outcome.

General Anesthesia versus Sedation

In choosing an anesthetic for intravenous sedation, the primary goals are to alleviate pain, anxiety, and discomfort, and to provide patient immobility. With adequate local anesthetic infiltration, the procedure itself is generally not painful. However, a long period of recumbence can cause significant pain and discomfort. A variety of sedation regimens are available, and the decision is based not only on the primary goals but also on the experience of the practitioner. Common to all intravenous sedation techniques is the potential for upper airway obstruction. Placement of a nasopharyngeal airway may cause troublesome bleeding in anticoagulated patients and is generally avoided. An LMA may be helpful in the rare emergency when a patient with a difficult airway has a neurologic crisis.

The primary reasons to use general anesthesia are to reduce motion artifacts and to improve the quality of images, especially in small children and uncooperative adult patients. Total intravenous anesthesia with remifentanil and propofol is suitable, and it is advantageous when no scavenging is available. Another technique is nitrous oxide combined with a low dose of inhaled agent. Both of these techniques provide rapid wakeup for neurologic assessment. Although Hashimoto and colleagues[93] suggest that N_2O should be avoided because of the possibility of introducing air emboli into the cerebral circulation, no evidence is available to support this opinion.[95]

No data exist to show whether sedation is better than general anesthesia. In large part, the choice of the anesthetic technique depends on institutional preference. However, the tendency is for more centers to opt for general anesthesia with a secure airway, probably because more complicated procedures are performed in increasingly compromised patients.[96]

Management of Procedural Complications

Although the complications of aneurysm embolization were lower than those of surgery in the ISAT trial,[92] complications during INR treatment of cerebral aneurysms can be rapid and life-threatening and require multidisciplinary collaboration. During these procedures, anesthesiologists must be aware of the potential for two very serious complications of aneurysm rupture and thromboembolism.[91]

Aneurysm Rupture

Aneurysm rupture may occur by perforation with the microcatheter or microwire, or during delivery of the GDC coils. Sudden sustained increases in MAP, with or without bradycardia, suggest the possibility of aneurysm rupture. Hemodynamic stability (normotension or mild hypertension), adequate preload and filling, and hemodilution are essential. In patients with signs of persistent intracranial hypertension (Cushing's response), a remifentanil infusion and continuous infusion of nicardipine with or without beta-blocker is preferred. Meanwhile, deepening the anesthetic level with a high-dose barbiturate or propofol bolus followed by infusion therapy may also be indicated. If intracranial bleeding is suspected, the patient can be given intravenous protamine to reverse the systemic heparinization. Emergent placement of a continuous intracranial pressure monitor via ventriculostomy may be necessary.[97] However, with small hemorrhages, management with mannitol and hyperventilation may be all that is needed. The determination must be made whether to continue coiling the aneurysm to seal the bleed, or to bring the patient emergently to the operating room for microsurgical clipping of the aneurysm.

Thrombotic Complications

Thromboembolic and ischemic complications occur at a rate of 1% to 5% depending on the complexity of the aneurysm during and after endovascular procedures. The thrombogenic characteristics of arterial catheters, contrast agents, and implanted devices such as coils and stents are thought to be related to arterial injury.

The anesthesiologist is integrally involved in the careful management of coagulation parameters to prevent and treat thromboembolic complications during and after the procedures. Activated clotting times (ACT) are typically used in the interventional suite to monitor heparin therapy. In patients undergoing complex aneurysm embolizations (e.g., stent-assisted procedures), potent antiplatelet therapy, such as clopidogrel treatment, should be considered prior to the procedure. Abnormal thrombus formation can usually be seen on the angiogram during the procedure, however, occasionally patients emerge from anesthesia with new neurologic deficits. Intra-arterial thrombolytic therapy with tissue plasminogen activator and urokinase has been described.[98] However, if there is abnormal thrombus formation despite heparin therapy, the platelet glycoprotein (GP) IIb/IIIa receptor antagonist abciximab can be used, as it appears to be particularly effective in dissolving thrombus. Nevertheless, the use of abciximab in conjunction with aspirin, clopidogrel, and heparin as an adjunct to INR procedures can result in rapidly progressive intracerebral hemorrhages.[99] Further research is required to develop both prophylactic and treatment strategies to reduce the rate of thromboembolic complications associated with INR procedures and thus improve their overall success.

■ MANAGEMENT OF INTRACRANIAL HYPERTENSION

The management of ICP (target, <20 mm Hg) is a necessary skill for the anesthesiologist. Perioperative ICP management is frequently needed when there is cranial trauma. In this setting, ICP control may have to be attempted empirically on the basis of the clinical neurologic examination, without an actual ICP measurement. Alternatively, therapy may be titrated to a specific ICP if the patient has an intracranial monitor in place. Perioperative ICP control is often an issue in other settings as well. Patients with spontaneous intracranial hemorrhage, aneurysmal subarachnoid hemorrhage, ischemic stroke, or mass lesions may require ICP control when coming to the operating room for neurosurgical or non-neurosurgical intervention. Finally, the need to prevent cerebral herniation through an open craniotomy is a concern in any brain surgery. Interventions to control ICP can also be used to control brain volume, shift, and herniation.

Interventions to control ICP fall into two general categories. First are the interventions primarily aimed at the reduction of intracranial contents, with secondary improvements in ICP. Second are the interventions aimed at the reduction of cerebral metabolic rate ($CMRO_2$), with secondary reductions in CBF, CBV, and ICP.

Reducing Intracranial Contents

Removal of Mass Lesions. All efforts in the preoperative care of the neurologically deteriorating patient with intracranial hypertension are focused on the safe, expedient delivery of the neurosurgical intervention.[100] Removal of intracranial mass lesions provides the most definitive control of ICP.

Head Positioning. The patient's head should be positioned to avoid jugular venous compression so as to facilitate venous drainage from the skull. Similarly, the head should be kept in a nondependent position (usually elevated about 20 degrees) to avoid cerebral venous congestion.

Ventricular CSF Drainage. Drainage of CSF by means of a ventriculostomy is a definitive treatment for intracranial hypertension caused by hydrocephalus, and it is an effective method of reducing ICP in many nonhydrocephalic patients.

In the perioperative setting, care must be taken to maintain the drain at an appropriate height, with close attention to opening and closing. These measures are necessary to avoid both over-drainage and unintended ICP spikes caused by unintended clamping. Lumbar cisternal CSF drainage must be used with extreme caution and is generally contraindicated in any patient with an intracranial mass lesion.

Hyperventilation. Hyperventilation provides a progressive reduction in CBV and ICP as $PaCO_2$ declines.[101,102] Hyperventilation can be quickly implemented once the anesthesiologist has control of the airway (target $PaCO_2$, 25 to 30 mm Hg).[103] Critical reductions in CBF can result, necessitating caution in the administration of this therapy.[104] It is best used as a temporizing measure to control ICP or to reduce brain size. Efforts to restore normocapnia should follow as soon as prudently possible.

Cerebral Perfusion Pressure. Maintenance of cerebral perfusion pressure (CPP = MAP − ICP) is critical for the patient with elevated ICP. Brain injury guidelines (see www2.braintrauma.org/guidelines) recommend a CPP of greater than 60 mm Hg. This was a 2003 update to the original recommendation of 70 mm Hg in 2000.[103] In a patient with intracranial hypertension, a drop in CPP causes a compensatory cerebral vasodilation to maintain CBF, with a subsequent elevation in ICP. The cerebral hypoperfusion is clearly injurious as well. In general, systemic (arterial) hypertension is much safer than hypotension.[105] Hypertension can become injurious beyond the range of cerebral autoregulation, and there is concern about promoting continued intracranial bleeding with hemorrhagic lesions. Current recommendations are to maintain a MAP of less than 130 mm Hg (<110 mm Hg postoperatively).[106] Intra-arterial blood pressure monitoring is highly advantageous when managing ICP.

Hyperosmotic Therapy. Hyperosmotic therapy reduces intracranial contents primarily by removing extravascular water from the brain. Mannitol and hypertonic saline are the hyperosmotic agents in current use. Older methods using other solutes such as urea or glycerol have fallen out of favor. The goal of hyperosmotic therapy is hyperosmolar euvolemia with maintenance of CPP and CBF. Mannitol (20% solution; 1160 mOsm/L) is typically given in bolus doses of 0.25 to 1 g/kg until the ICP target is reached. Dosing beyond a serum osmolality of 320 mOsm/L is generally contraindicated because of concerns about renal toxicity.[107] Clinical trial data comparing mannitol with hypertonic saline are limited, and there is no good evidence to support the use of one over the other.[108] Different formulations of hypertonic saline (2% to 30%) have been used in various clinical studies, and there is no consensus for a specific tonicity.[108] Our preference is for 23.4% NaCl (23% solution; 8008 mOsm/L).[109] This is administered in 30-mL doses via central venous catheter and is often used for ICP refractory to mannitol in our practice. The generally accepted limit on this therapy is a serum osmolality of 320 mOsm/L.

Reducing Cerebral Metabolism

Anesthetic Depth. Adequate anesthetic depth, usually coupled with neuromuscular blockade in the operative setting, is essential to avoid increases in ICP in response to laryngoscopy, bladder catheterization, line placement, or surgical stimulation. Furthermore, anesthetic depth can be increased to achieve a reduction in ICP through a reduction in $CMRO_2$. Burst suppression, as determined by EEG monitoring, is associated with a 50% reduction in $CMRO_2$.[110] Therefore, increasing anesthetic depth decreases both noxious stimulation and ICP (the latter through a reduction in $CMRO_2$). The anesthesiologist must choose the anesthetic agent carefully, as potent inhaled anesthetics, such as isoflurane and sevoflurane, progressively increase the CBF as alveolar concentration (MAC) increases.[111] This may offset the reduction in ICP because of the decrease in $CMRO_2$. Propofol and barbiturates decrease ICP without causing cerebral vasodilation, but, like the inhaled anesthetics, they still decrease the MAP and $CMRO_2$.[112-114] Attention to CPP is critical when reducing ICP with anesthetic agents. The issue of neuroprotection is discussed separately.

Hypothermia. Hypothermia causes approximately a 5% reduction in $CMRO_2$ per degree Celsius[115] and can be used to control ICP in the perioperative setting. The fastest practical way to induce hypothermia is with intravenous boluses of refrigerated saline (4° C, 0.9% NaCl).[116] However, this is an extrapolation from the cardiac arrest literature and has not been studied in a perioperative setting. Neuromuscular blockade is necessary to prevent shivering. Maintenance cooling can be accomplished with surface (liquid or air blankets) or, if available, intravascular methods.[117]

Summary

The anesthesiologist usually chooses a multimodal approach to control intracranial hypertension in the perioperative arena. Ideally, therapy is guided by an ICP monitor, but it often has to be administered empirically in a rapidly decompensating patient. Jugular venous compression should be avoided, and the head of the bed should be elevated to promote venous drainage from the skull. Hyperventilation can be quickly implemented while hyperosmotic therapy is being infused. Anesthetic depth is increased, along with neuromuscular blockade, while maintaining an uncompromised CPP (>60 mm Hg). If needed, systemic hypothermia can be initiated with cold intravenous fluids and maintained with surface cooling. Attention must be paid to restoring normocapnia when other methods of ICP control have been successfully implemented.

■ REFERENCES

1. Timsit SG, Sacco RL, Mohr JP, et al: Early clinical differentiation of cerebral infarction from severe atherosclerotic stenosis and cardioembolism. Stroke 1992;23:486-491.
2. Biller J, Feinberg WM, Castaldo JE, et al: Guidelines for carotid endarterectomy: A statement for healthcare professionals from a special writing group of the Stroke Council, American Heart Association. Stroke 1998;29:554-562.
3. Chaturvedi S, Bruno A, Feasby T, et al: Carotid endarterectomy: An evidence-based review—Report of the Therapeutics and Technology Assessment Subcommittee of the American Academy of Neurology. Neurology 2005;65:794-801.
4. Rothwell PM, Eliasziw M, Gutnikov SA, et al: Endarterectomy for symptomatic carotid stenosis in relation to clinical subgroups and timing of surgery. Lancet 2004;363:915-924.
5. Benavente O, Eliasziw M, Streifler JY, et al: Prognosis after transient monocular blindness associated with carotid-artery stenosis. N Engl J Med 2001;345:1084-1090.
6. Hertzer NR, Young JR, Beven EG, et al: Coronary angiography in 506 patients with extracranial cerebrovascular disease. Arch Intern Med 1985;145:849-852.
7. Beneficial effect of carotid endarterectomy in symptomatic patients with high-grade carotid stenosis. North American Symptomatic Carotid Endarterectomy Trial Collaborators. N Engl J Med 1991;325:445-453.
8. Eagle KA, Brundage BH, Chaitman BR, et al: Guidelines for perioperative cardiovascular evaluation for noncardiac surgery. Report of the American College of Cardiology/American Heart Association Task Force on Practice Guidelines. Committee on Perioperative Cardiovascular Evaluation for Noncardiac Surgery. Circulation 1996;93:1278-1317.
9. Sundt TM, Sandok BA, Whisnant JP: Carotid endarterectomy: Complications and preoperative assessment of risk. Mayo Clin Proc 1975;50:301-306.
10. Sieber FE, Toung TJ, Diringer MN, et al: Preoperative risks predict neurological outcome of carotid endarterectomy related stroke. Neurosurgery 1992;30:847-854.
11. Gibbs BF: Temporary hypotension following endarterectomy for severe carotid stenosis: Should we treat it? Vasc Endovascular Surg 2003;37:33-38.
12. Bruno A, Levine SR, Frankel MR, et al: Admission glucose level and clinical outcomes in the NINDS rt-PA Stroke Trial. Neurology 2002;59:669-674.
13. Stoneham MD, Doyle AR, Knighton JD, et al: Prospective, randomized comparison of deep or superficial cervical plexus block for carotid endarterectomy surgery. Anesthesiology 1998;89:907-912.
14. Munro FJ, Makin AP, Reid J: Airway problems after carotid endarterectomy. Br J Anaesth 1996;76:156-159.
15. Abe K, Iwanaga H, Shimada Y, Yoshiya I: The effect of nicardipine on carotid blood flow velocity, local cerebral blood flow, and carbon dioxide reactivity during cerebral aneurysm surgery. Anesth Analg 1993;76:1227-1233.
16. Felding M, Jakobsen CJ, Cold GE, et al: The effect of metoprolol upon blood pressure, cerebral blood flow and oxygen consumption in patients subjected to craniotomy for cerebral tumours. Acta Anaesthesiol Scand 1995;38:271-275.
17. Jennett WB, McDowall DG, Barker J: The effect of halothane on intracranial pressure in cerebral tumors: Report of two cases. J Neurosurg 1967;26:270-274.
18. Adams RW, Cucchiara RF, Gronert GA, et al: Isoflurane and cerebrospinal fluid pressure in neurosurgical patients. Anesthesiology 1981;54:97-99.
19. Guy J, Hindman BJ, Baker KZ, et al: Comparison of remifentanil and fentanyl in patients undergoing craniotomy for supratentorial space-occupying lesions. Anesthesiology 1997;86:514-524.
20. Combes P, Durand M: Combined effects of nicardipine and hypocapnic alkalosis on cerebral vasomotor activity and intracranial pressure in man. Eur J Clin Pharmacol 1991;41:207-210.
21. Cold GE, Bundgaard H, von Oettingen G, et al: ICP during anaesthesia with sevoflurane: A dose-response study—Effect of hypocapnia. Acta Neurochir Suppl 1998;71:279-281.
22. Gopinath SP, Valadka AB, Uzura M, Robertson CS: Comparison of jugular venous oxygen saturation and brain tissue Po_2 as monitors of cerebral ischemia after head injury. Crit Care Med 1999;27:2337-2345.
23. McCulloch TJ, Boesel TW, Lam AM: The effect of hypocapnia on the autoregulation of cerebral blood flow during administration of isoflurane. Anesth Analg 2005;100:1463-1467.
24. Paczynski RP, Venkatesan R, Diringer MN, et al: Effects of fluid management on edema volume and midline shift in a rat model of ischemic stroke. Stroke 2000;31:1702-1708.
25. Van der Linden P, Ickx BE: The effects of colloid solutions on hemostasis. Can J Anaesth 2006;53:S30-39.

26. Minton MD, Grosslight K, Stirt JA, Bedford RF: Increases in intracranial pressure from succinylcholine: Prevention by prior nondepolarizing blockade. Anesthesiology 1986;65:165-169.

27. Lanier WL, Iaizzo PA, Milde JH: The effects of intravenous succinylcholine on cerebral function and muscle afferent activity following complete ischemia in halothane-anesthetized dogs. Anesthesiology 1990;73:485-490.

28. Ornstein E, Matteo RS, Schwartz A, et al: The effect of phenytoin on the magnitude and duration of neuromuscular block following atracurium or vecuronium. Anesthesiology 1987;67:191-196.

29. Balakrishnan G, Raudzens P, Samra SK, et al: A comparison of remifentanil and fentanyl in patients undergoing surgery for intracranial mass lesions. Anesth Analg 2000;91:163-169.

30. Basali A, Mascha EJ, Kalfas I, Schubert A: Relation between perioperative hypertension and intracranial hemorrhage after craniotomy. Anesthesiology 2000;93:48-54.

31. Fabling JM, Gan TJ, Guy J, et al: Postoperative nausea and vomiting: A retrospective analysis in patients undergoing elective craniotomy. J Neurosurg Anesthesiol 1997;9:308-312.

32. Fabling JM, Gan TJ, El-Moalem HE, et al: A randomized, double-blind comparison of ondansetron, droperidol, and placebo for prevention of postoperative nausea and vomiting after supratentorial craniotomy. Anesth Analg 2000;91:358-361.

33. Vinas FC, Zamorano L, Mueller RA, et al: [^{15}O]-water PET and intraoperative brain mapping: A comparison in the localization of eloquent cortex. Neurol Res 1997;19:601-608.

34. Ojemann G, Ojemann J, Lettich E, Berger M: Cortical language localization in left, dominant hemisphere: An electrical stimulation mapping investigation in 117 patients. J Neurosurg 1989;71:316-326.

35. Wada J, Rasmussen T: Intracarotid injection of sodium amytal for the lateralization of cerebral speech dominance. J Neurosurg 1960;17:266-282.

36. Trop D: Conscious-sedation analgesia during the neurosurgical treatment of epilepsies: Practice at the Montreal Neurological Institute. Int Anesthesiol Clin 1986;24:175-184.

37. Huncke K, Van de Wiele B, Fried I, Rubinstein EH: The asleep-awake-asleep anesthetic technique for intraoperative language mapping. Neurosurgery 1998;42:1312-1317.

38. Vlessides M: LMA use safe, effective during craniotomy for speech mapping (Poster presentation A578 at the 2000 annual meeting of the American Society of Anesthesiologists), by A-TT Nguyen. Anesthesiology News 2000, p 16.

39. Keifer JC, Dentchev D, Little K, et al: A retrospective analysis of a remifentanil/propofol general anesthetic for craniotomy before awake functional brain mapping. Anesth Analg 2005;101:502-508.

40. Linn FH, Rinkel GJ, Algra A, van Gijn J: Incidence of subarachnoid hemorrhage: Role of region, year, and rate of computed tomography—A meta-analysis. Stroke 1996;27:625-629.

41. Hop JW, Rinkel GJ, Algra A, van Gijn J: Case-fatality rates and functional outcome after subarachnoid hemorrhage: A systematic review. Stroke 1997;28:660-664.

42. Richardson AE, Jane JA, Payne PM: The prediction of morbidity and mortality in anterior communicating aneurysms treated by proximal anterior cerebral ligation. J Neurosurg 1966;25:280-283.

43. Jennett B, Bond M: Assessment of outcome after severe brain damage. Lancet 1975;1:480-484.

44. Hunt WE, Hess RM: Surgical risk as related to time of intervention in the repair of intracranial aneurysms. J Neurosurg 1968;28:14-20.

45. Report of World Federation of Neurological Surgeons Committee on a Universal Subarachnoid Hemorrhage Grading Scale [comment]. J Neurosurg 1988;68:985-986.

46. Cruickshank JM, Neil-Dwyer G, Stott AW: Possible role of catecholamines, corticosteroids, and potassium in the production of electrocardiographic abnormalities associated with subarachnoid hemorrhage. Br Heart J 1974;36:697-706.

47. Marion DW, Segal R, Thompson ME: Subarachnoid hemorrhage and the heart. Neurosurgery 1986;18:101-106.

48. Doshi R, Neil-Dwyer G: A clinicopathological study of patients following a subarachnoid hemorrhage. J Neurosurg 1980;52:295-301.

49. Kawahara E, Ikeda S, Miyahara Y, Kohno S: Role of autonomic nervous dysfunction in electrocardiographic abnormalities and cardiac injury in patients with acute subarachnoid hemorrhage. Circ J 2003;67:753-756.

50. Rudehill A, Gordon E, Sundqvist K, et al: A study of ECG abnormalities and myocardial specific enzymes in patients with subarachnoid hemorrhage. Acta Anaesthesiol Scand 1982;26:344-350.

51. Samra SK, Kroll DA: Subarachnoid hemorrhage and intraoperative electrocardiographic changes simulating myocardial ischemia: Anesthesiologist's dilemma. Anesth Analg 1985;64:86-89.

52. Parekh N, Venkatesh B, Cross D, et al: Cardiac troponin I predicts myocardial dysfunction in aneurysmal subarachnoid hemorrhage. J Am Coll Cardiol 2000;36:1328-1335.

53. Deibert E, Barzilai B, Braverman AC, et al: Clinical significance of elevated troponin I levels in patients with nontraumatic subarachnoid hemorrhage. J Neurosurg 2003;98:741-746.

54. Andreoli A, di Pasquale G, Pinelli G, et al: Subarachnoid hemorrhage: Frequency and severity of cardiac arrhythmias—A survey of 70 cases studied in the acute phase. Stroke 1987;18:558-564.

55. Fukui S, Katoh H, Tsuzuki N, et al: Multivariate analysis of risk factors for QT prolongation following subarachnoid hemorrhage. Crit Care 2003;7:R7-12.

56. Kaneko T, Sawada T, Niimi T, et al: Lower limit of blood pressure in treatment of acute hypertensive intracranial hemorrhage (AHCH). J Cereb Blood Flow Metab 1983;3(Suppl 1):S51-52.

57. Chang CC, Kuwana N, Ito S, et al: Cerebral haemodynamics in patients with hydrocephalus after subarachnoid hemorrhage due to ruptured aneurysm. Eur J Nucl Med Mol Imaging 2003;30:123-126.

58. Schroeder T, Schierbeck J, Howardy P, et al: Effect of labetalol on cerebral blood flow and middle cerebral arterial flow velocity in healthy volunteers. Neurol Res 1991;13:10-12.

59. Fitch W, Ferguson GG, Sengupta D, et al: Autoregulation of cerebral blood flow during controlled hypotension in baboons. J Neurol Neurosurg Psychiatry 1976;39:1014-1022.

60. Foley PL, Caner HH, Kassell NF, Lee KS: Reversal of subarachnoid hemorrhage-induced vasoconstriction with an endothelin receptor antagonist. Neurosurgery 1994;34:108-113.

61. Boisvert VP, Gelb AW, Tang C, et al: Brain tolerance to middle cerebral artery occlusion during hypotension in primates. Surg Neurol 1989;31:6-13.

62. Manninen PH, Lam AM, Nantau WE: Monitoring of somatosensory evoked potentials during temporary arterial occlusion in cerebral aneurysm surgery. J Neurosurg Anesth 1990;2:97-104.

63. Pickard JD, Matheson M, Patterson J, Wyper D: Prediction of late ischemic complications after cerebral aneurysm surgery by the intraoperative measurement of cerebral blood flow. J Neurosurg 1980;53:305-308.

64. Little JR, Lesser RP, Lueders H: Electrophysiological monitoring during basilar aneurysm operation. Neurosurg 1987;20:421-427.

65. Lam AM, Keane JF, Manninen PH: Monitoring of brainstem auditory evoked potentials during basilar artery occlusion in man. Br J Anaesth 1985;57:924-928.

66. Martin N, Doberstein C, Bentson J, et al: Intraoperative angiography in cerebrovascular surgery. Clin Neurosurg 1991;37:312-331.

67. Tsementzis SA, Hitchcock ER: Outcome from "rescue clipping" of ruptured intracranial aneurysms during induction anaesthesia and endotracheal intubation. J Neurol Neurosurg Psychiatry 1985;48:160-163.

68. Farrar JK, Gamache FW, Ferguson GG, et al: Effects of profound hypotension on cerebral blood flow during surgery for intracranial aneurysms. J Neurosurg 1981;55:857-864.

69. Payne KA, Murray WB, Oosthvizen JH: Obtunding the sympathetic response to intubation. S Afr Med J 1988;73:584-586.

70. Holldin M, Wahlin A: Effect of succinylcholine on the intraspinal fluid pressure. Acta Anaesthesiol Scand 1959;3:155-161.

71. Olsson GL, Hallen B, Hambraeus-Jonzon K: Aspiration during anaesthesia: A computer-aided study of 185,358 anaesthetics. Acta Anaesthesiol Scand 1986;30:84-92.

72. Hanley DF, Borel CO: Hypervolemic hypertensive therapy for subarachnoid hemorrhage induced vasospasm: Current therapy. In Neurologic Surgery. Philadelphia, BC Deeker, 1988, pp 169-172.

73. Sieber FE, Smith DS, Traystman RJ, Wollman H: Glucose: A reevaluation of its intraoperative use. Anesthesiology 1987;67:72-81.

74. Dernbach PD, Little JR, Jones SC, Ebrahim ZY: Altered cerebral autoregulation and CO_2 reactivity after aneurysmal subarachnoid hemorrhage. Neurosurgery 1988;22:822-826.

75. Charbel FT, Ausman J, Diaz FG, et al: Temporary clipping in aneurysm surgery: Techniques and results. Surg Neurol 1991;36:83-90.

76. Samson D, Batjer HH, Bowman G, et al: A clinical study of the parameters and effects of temporary arterial occlusion in the management of intracranial aneurysms. Neurosurgery 1994;34:22-29.

77. Jabre A, Symon L: Temporary vascular occlusion during aneurysm surgery. Surg Neurol 1987;27:47-63.

78. Rosenorn J, Diemer N: The risk of cerebral damage during graded brain retractor pressure in the rat. J Neurosurg 1985;63:608-611.

79. Todd MM, Hindman BJ, Clarke WR, Torner JC: Mild intraoperative hypothermia during surgery for intracranial aneurysm. N Engl J Med 2005;352:135-145.

80. Spetzler RF, Hadley MN: Protection against cerebral ischemia: The role of barbiturates. Cerebrovasc Brain Metab Rev 1989;1:212-229.

81. Hoff JT, Pitts LH, Spetzler R, Wilson CB: Barbiturates for protection from cerebral ischemia during aneurysm surgery. Acta Neurol Scand 1977;56:158-159.

82. Todd MM, Drummond JC, Hoi SU: Hemodynamic effects of high dose pentobarbital: Studies in elective neurosurgical patients. Neurosurgery 1987;20:559-563.

83. Ridenour TR, Warner DS, Todd MM, Gionet TX: Comparative effects of propofol and halothane on outcome from temporary middle cerebral artery occlusion in the rat. Anesthesiology 1992;76:807-812.

84. Sundt TM, Whisnant JP: Subarachnoid hemorrhage from intracranial aneurysm surgical management and natural history of disease. N Engl J Med 1978;299:116-122.

85. Calvin CE, Lam AM, Byrd S, Newell DW: The diagnosis and management of a perianesthetic cerebral aneurysmal rupture aided with transcranial Doppler ultrasonography. Anesthesiology 1993;78:191-194.

86. Sundt TM, Kobayoshi S, Fode NC, Whisnant JP: Results and complications of surgical management of 809 intracranial aneurysms in 722 cases. J Neurosurg 1982;56:753-765.

87. Giannotta SL, Oppenheimer JH, Levy ML, Zelman V: Management of intraoperative rupture of aneurysms without hypotension. Neurosurgery 1991;28:531-535.

88. Serbinenko FA: Balloon catheterization and occlusion of major cerebral vessels. J Neurosurg 1974;41:125-145.

89. Guglielmi G, Vinuela F, Dion J, Duckwiler G: Electrothrombosis of saccular aneurysms via endovascular approach: Part 2: Preliminary clinical experience [comment]. J Neurosurg 1991;75:8-14.

90. Johnston SC, Wilson CB, Halbach VV, et al: Endovascular and surgical treatment of unruptured cerebral aneurysms: Comparison of risks [comment]. Ann Neurol 2000;48:11-19.

91. Johnston SC, Zhao S, Dudley RA, et al: Treatment of unruptured cerebral aneurysms in California. Stroke 2001;32:597-605.

92. Molyneux A, Kerr R, Stratton I, et al: International Subarachnoid Aneurysm Trial (ISAT) of neurosurgical clipping versus endovascular coiling in 2143 patients with ruptured intracranial aneurysms: A randomised trial [comment]. Lancet 2002;360:1267-1274.

93. Hashimoto T, Gupta DK, Young WL: Interventional neuroradiology: Anesthetic considerations. Anesthesiol Clin North Am 2002;20:347-359, vi.

94. Young WL, Pile-Spellman J: Anesthetic considerations for interventional neuroradiology. Anesthesiology 1994;80:427-456.

95. Condette-Auliac S, Bracard S, Anxionnat R, et al: Vasospasm after subarachnoid hemorrhage: Interest in diffusion-weighted MR imaging. Stroke 2001;32:1818-1824.

96. Lai YC, Manninen PH: Anesthesia for cerebral aneurysms: A comparison between interventional neuroradiology and surgery. Can J Anaesth 2001;48:391-395.

97. Gorji R, Willoughby PH, Cozza C, Thomas PS: Guglielmi detachable coil: Report of intraoperative complications. J Neurosurg Anesthesiol 2001;13:40-42.

98. Hahnel S, Schellinger PD, Gutschalk A, et al: Local intra-arterial fibrinolysis of thromboemboli occurring during neuroendovascular procedures with recombinant tissue plasminogen activator [comment]. Stroke 2003;34:1723-1728.

99. Qureshi AI, Saad M, Zaidat OO, et al: Intracerebral hemorrhages associated with neurointerventional procedures using a combination of antithrombotic agents including abciximab. Stroke 2002;33:1916-1919.

100. Bullock MR, Chesnut R, Ghajar J, et al; Surgical Management of Traumatic Brain Injury Author Group: Surgical management of acute epidural hematomas. Neurosurgery 2006;58:S7-15; discussion Si-iv.

101. Raichle ME, Plum F: Hyperventilation and cerebral blood flow. Stroke 1972;3:566-575.

102. Fortune JB, Feustel PJ, deLuna C, et al: Cerebral blood flow and blood volume in response to O_2 and CO_2 changes in normal humans. J Trauma 1995;39:463-472.

103. The Brain Trauma Foundation, American Association of Neurological Surgeons, Joint Section on Neurotrauma and Critical Care: Methodology. J Neurotrauma 2000;17:561-562.

104. Muizelaar JP, Marmarou A, Ward JD, et al: Adverse effects of prolonged hyperventilation in patients with severe head injury: A randomized clinical trial. J Neurosurg 1991;75:731-739.

105. Bouma GJ, Muizelaar JP: Relationship between cardiac output and cerebral blood flow in patients with intact and with impaired autoregulation. J Neurosurg 1990;73:368-374.

106. Broderick JP, Adams HP Jr, Barsan W, et al: Guidelines for the management of spontaneous intracerebral hemorrhage: A statement for healthcare professionals from a special writing group of the Stroke Council, American Heart Association. Stroke 1999;30:905-915.

107. Mendelow AD, Teasdale GM, Russell T, et al: Effect of mannitol on cerebral blood flow and cerebral perfusion pressure in human head injury. J Neurosurg 1985;63:43-48.

108. White H, Cook D, Venkatesh B: The use of hypertonic saline for treating intracranial hypertension after traumatic brain injury. Anesth Analg 2006;102:1836-1846.

109. Suarez JI, Qureshi AI, Bhardwaj A, et al: Treatment of refractory intracranial hypertension with 23.4% saline [see comment]. Crit Care Med 1998;26:1118-1122.

110. Newman MF, Murkin JM, Roach G, et al: Cerebral physiologic effects of burst suppression doses of propofol during nonpulsatile cardiopulmonary bypass. CNS Subgroup of McSPI. Anesth Analg 1995;81:452-457.

111. Bundgaard H, von Oettingen G, Larsen KM, et al: Effects of sevoflurane on intracranial pressure, cerebral blood flow and cerebral metabolism. A dose-response study in patients subjected to craniotomy for cerebral tumours. Acta Anaesthesiol Scand 1998;42:621-627.

112. Pierce EC Jr, Lambertsen CJ, Deutsch S, et al: Cerebral circulation and metabolism during thiopental anaesthesia and hypoventilation in man. J Clin Invest 1962;41:1664-1671.

113. Nimkoff L, Quinn C, Silver P, Sagy M: The effects of intravenous anesthetics on intracranial pressure and cerebral perfusion pressure in two feline models of brain edema. J Crit Care 1997;12:132-136.

114. Eisenberg HM, Frankowski RF, Contant CF, et al: High-dose barbiturate control of elevated intracranial pressure in patients with severe head injury. J Neurosurg 1988;69:15-23.

115. Yager JY, Asselin J: Effect of mild hypothermia on cerebral energy metabolism during the evolution of hypoxic-ischemic brain damage in the immature rat. Stroke 1996;27:919-925, discussion 926.

116. Bernard S, Buist M, Monteiro O, Smith K: Induced hypothermia using large volume, ice-cold intravenous fluid in comatose survivors of out-of-hospital cardiac arrest: A preliminary report. Resuscitation 2003;56:9-13.

117. Schmutzhard E, Engelhardt K, Beer R, et al: Safety and efficacy of a novel intravascular cooling device to control body temperature in neurologic intensive care patients: A prospective pilot study [see comment]. Crit Care Med 2002;30:2481-2488.

118. Rothwell PM, Warlow CP: Prediction of benefit from carotid endarterectomy in individual patients: A risk-modeling study. European Carotid Surgery Trialists' Collaborative Group. Lancet 1999;353:2105-2110.

119. Barnett HJ, Meldrum HE, Eliasziw M: The appropriate use of carotid endarterectomy. AJ 2002;166:1169-1179.

120. Rigdon EE, Monajjem N, Rhodes RS: Is carotid endarterectomy justified in patients with severe chronic renal insufficiency? Ann Vasc Surg 1997;11:115-119.

121. Stoner MC, Abbott WM, Wong DR, et al: Defining the high-risk patient for carotid endarterectomy: An analysis of the prospective

National Surgical Quality Improvement Program database. J Vasc Surg 2006;43:285-296.

122. Halm EA, Hannan EL, Rojas M, et al: Clinical and operative predictors of outcomes of carotid endarterectomy. J Vasc Surg 2005;42: 420-428.

123. Archer DP, McKenna JM, Morin L, Ravussin P: Conscious-sedation analgesia during craniotomy for intractable epilepsy: A review of 354 consecutive cases. Can J Anaesth 1988;35:338-344.

124. Sartorius CJ, Wright G: Intraoperative brain mapping in a community setting: Technical considerations. Surg Neurol 1997;47:380-388.

125. Silbergeld DL, Mueller WM, Colley PS, et al: Use of propofol (Diprivan) for awake craniotomies: Technical note. Surg Neurol 1992;38: 271-272.

126. Herrick IA, Craen RA, Gelb AW, et al: Propofol sedation during awake craniotomy for seizures: Electrocorticographic and epileptogenic effects. Anesth Analg 1997;84:1280-1284.

127. Welling EC, Donegan J: Neuroleptanalgesia using alfentanil for awake craniotomy. Anesth Analg 1989;68:57-60.

128. Gignac E, Manninen PH, Gelb AW: Comparison of fentanyl, sufentanil and alfentanil during awake craniotomy for epilepsy. Can J Anaesth 1993;40:421-424.

129. Taylor MD, Bernstein M: Awake craniotomy with brain mapping as the routine surgical approach to treating patients with supratentorial intraaxial tumors: A prospective trial of 200 cases. J Neurosurg 1999;90:35-41.

22 Protecting the Central Nervous System during Cardiac Surgery

Hilary P. Grocott

Despite the passage of more than 50 years since the development of cardiopulmonary bypass (CPB) heralded the arrival of modern-day cardiac surgery, complications involving the brain remain a significant concern in the perioperative care of the cardiac surgical patient. Decades of research have led to an evolved understanding of how frequently these complications occur, how they manifest (stroke versus encephalopathy versus neurocognitive dysfunction), what the various risk factors are, and what their purported multifactorial etiologies are.[1,2] On the surface, it might seem that we have largely failed in developing strategies to universally protect the brain, because complications remain common. However, the population now being treated has become progressively sicker and older, and many advances have been made. The development of new strategies is complicated because cardiac surgery is always evolving, with different procedures and a changing population presenting for surgery. The increased number of elderly and sick patients makes cerebral complications all the more relevant in the hierarchy of perioperative considerations. New strategies and techniques must be evaluated for the robustness of their clinical effectiveness. To evaluate protective strategies, criteria have been developed to categorize the levels of evidence. These criteria are summarized in Table 22-1.[3]

A number of strategies, both nonpharmacologic and pharmacologic, have been used to try to protect the brain. The nonpharmacologic can be further classified into manipulations of physiology (e.g., blood pressure, temperature, and glucose management) and the technical or mechanical modifications to the CPB apparatus (e.g., arterial line filtration and management of aortic atherosclerosis). The evidence for these interventional strategies will be discussed.

In the related sub-discipline of cardiac surgery, thoracic aortic operations have been complicated by neurologic injury to the spinal cord. As a result, protecting the spinal cord has been the focus of a decades-long pursuit for answers. And, whereas there is still a surprisingly small amount of information on how to protect the brain, there is even less information to guide us in protecting the spinal cord. This is partly because of the relatively low number of operations involving the thoracic aorta, which is just a fraction of the number involving the heart. As a result, significantly less funding has been focused on how to protect the spinal cord, and fewer patients have been available to participate in clinical evaluations of protective technologies.

Overall, no particular therapy, either for the brain or for the spinal cord, either technological or pharmacologic, is sufficiently well accepted and efficacious to have acquired any regulatory approval, by the U.S. Food and Drug Administration (FDA) or by any foreign regulatory organization, or to have been adopted as a standard of care by allied professional bodies.

■ CEREBRAL INJURY AFTER CARDIAC SURGERY

Incidence and Significance

Injury to the central nervous system (CNS) after CPB results in a variety of clinical entities. Deficits include a spectrum of diagnoses from neurocognitive deficits, occurring in approximately 25% to 80% of patients, to overt stroke, occurring in 1% to 5% of patients.[4-7] Between these are varying degrees of encephalopathy. The results of studies to determine the incidence of these adverse cerebral outcomes differ significantly, partly because of how the neurologic and neurocognitive outcomes are defined and partly because of methodological differences in measuring them. In addition, the assessment of neurologic deficits (particularly with stroke) is sometimes retrospective and sometimes prospective, which accounts for a significant part of the variation in incidence, as does the degree of detail and sensitivity of the neurologic examination performed. Another difference relates to the timing of postoperative testing. For example, cognitive deficits at discharge may be seen in as many as 80% of patients, but this figure decreases to 10% to 35% by 6 or more weeks after coronary artery bypass grafting (CABG), and to 10% to 15% at more than a year after surgery. A recurrence of higher rates of cognitive deficits occurs 5 years after surgery, when as many as 42% of patients have been documented to have deficits.[5]

Although the incidence of cerebral dysfunction, must notably neurocognitive deficit, varies greatly, the significance of these injuries cannot be underestimated. Cerebral injury is a most disturbing outcome of cardiac surgery. To have a patient's cardiac condition treated by a successful operation only to have the patient lose cognitive or physical function from a stroke can be devastating. The personal, family, and financial consequences of extending a patient's life with surgery only to reduce quality of the life and overall functional status are enormous.[7,8] Furthermore, mortality after

Class of Rating

Class I: Interventions are always acceptable, proven safe, and definitely useful.

Class IIa: Interventions are acceptable, safe, and useful. Considered the standard of care; reasonably prudent physicians can choose. Considered the intervention of choice by majority of experts.

Class IIb: Interventions are acceptable, safe, and useful. Considered "within" the standard of care: reasonably prudent physicians can choose. Considered optional or alternative intervention by majority of experts.

Class indeterminate: Interventions can still be used but insufficient evidence to suggest efficacy.

Class III: No evidence of efficacy and/or studies suggesting it.

Criteria

More than one randomized, controlled trial that is considered of excellent quality, with robust and consistently positive results supporting intervention.

A number of studies of good to very good quality with a positive result. Weight of evidence/expert opinion more strongly favors intervention than for class IIb recommendation. Magnitude of benefit higher than class IIb recommendation.

Level of evidence low to intermediate. Only a few studies of fair or poor quality support its use. Weight of evidence/expert opinion less in favor of usefulness/efficacy. Results not always positive.

Evidence found but available studies have one or more shortcomings.
Intervention is promising, but studies fail to address relevant clinical outcomes and are inconsistent, noncompelling, or have inconsistent results.
Positive evidence is completely absent or evidence is strongly suggestive of harm.

Used with permission from Hogue CW Jr, Palin CA, Arrowsmith JE: Anesth Analg 2006;103:21-37.

CABG, which reached relatively low levels (approximately 1% overall) in the past decade, is increasingly being attributed to neurologic injury.[7]

Risk Factors for CNS Injury

Strategies for perioperative brain and spinal cord protection require a thorough understanding of the risk factors, etiology, and pathophysiology of the injury. Risk factors for CNS injury can be considered from several different perspectives. Older studies outlining risk factors considered only stroke, but now studies are consistently reporting the preoperative risk for postcardiac surgery cognitive loss.[9] Preoperative factors such as a poor baseline cognitive state, years of education (with a more advanced education being protective), age, diabetes, and CPB time are frequently described.[9-11]

Nonetheless, stroke is far better characterized from a risk factor perspective. Although studies differ somewhat as to the complete spectrum of risk factors, certain patient characteristics consistently demonstrate an increased risk for stroke after cardiac surgery. In the well-documented Multicenter Study of Perioperative Ischemia (McSPI), the incidence of adverse cerebral outcome after CABG surgery was determined and the risk factors analyzed for more than 2000 patients.[7] Two types of adverse cerebral outcomes were defined: type I (nonfatal stroke, transient ischemic attack [TIA], stupor or coma at time of discharge, or death caused by stroke or hypoxic encephalopathy) and type II (significant new deterioration in intellectual function, confusion, agitation, disorientation, residual memory deficit without evidence of focal injury). Overall, 6.1% patients had an adverse cerebral outcome in the perioperative period. The two types of outcomes occurred in similar numbers (3.1% and 3%, respectively). Statistical analysis identified eight independent predictors of type I outcomes and seven independent predictors of type II outcomes (Table 22-2).

In a subsequent study from the same McSPI database, a stroke risk index using preoperative factors was developed (Fig. 22-1). This risk index allowed preoperative determina-

22-2   **Risk Factors for Adverse Neurologic Outcomes after Cardiac Surgery**

Risk Factor	Type I Outcomes* OR (95% CI)	Type II Outcomes* OR (95% CI)
Proximal aortic atherosclerosis	4.52 (2.52-8.09)	—
History of neurologic disease	3.19 (1.65-6.15)	—
Use of IABP	2.60 (1.21-5.58)	—
Diabetes mellitus	2.59 (1.46-4.60)	—
History of hypertension	2.31 (1.20-4.47)	—
History of pulmonary disease	2.09 (1.14-3.85)	2.37 (1.34-4.18)
History of unstable angina	1.83 (1.03-3.27)	—
Age (per additional decade)	1.75 (1.27-2.43)	2.20 (1.60-3.02)
Admission systolic BP >180 mm Hg	—	3.47 (1.41-8.55)
History of excessive alcohol intake	—	2.64 (1.27-5.47)
History of CABG	—	2.18 (1.14-4.17)
Arrhythmia on day of surgery	—	1.97 (1.12-3.46)
Antihypertensive therapy	—	1.78 (1.02-3.10)

*Adjusted odds ratio (OR) (95% confidence interval [CI]) for type I and type II cerebral outcomes associated with selected risk factors from the McSPI study.

BP, blood pressure; CABG, coronary artery bypass graft surgery; IABP, intraaortic balloon pump.

From Arrowsmith JE, Grocott HP, Reves JG, et al. Br J Anaesth 2000;84:378-393. By permission of Oxford University Press.

tion of the stroke risk based on a weighted combination of preoperative factors that included age, unstable angina, diabetes mellitus, neurologic disease, prior coronary cardiac surgery, vascular disease, and pulmonary disease.[12] In that long study, as in many other analyses,[7,13-16] age appears to be the most overwhelmingly robust predictor of both stroke and

Risk factor	Score
Age	(Age − 25) × 1.43
Unstable angina	14
Diabetes mellitus	17
Neurologic disease	18
Prior CABS	15
Vascular disease	18
Pulmonary disease	15

Figure 22-1 ■ Preoperative stroke risk for patients undergoing coronary artery bypass graft surgery. The individual patient stroke risk can be determined from the corresponding cumulative risk index score in the nomogram. CABS, coronary artery bypass surgery; CNS, central nervous system. *(Adapted from Newman MF, Wolman R, Kanchuger M, et al: Circulation 1996;94:II74-80, and redrawn from Arrowsmith JE, Grocott HP, Reves JG, et al: Br J Anaesth 2000;84:378-393.)*

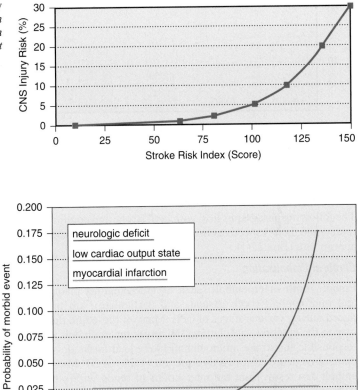

Figure 22-2 ■ The relative effect of age on the probability of neurologic and cardiac morbidity after cardiac surgery. *(Redrawn from Tuman KJ, McCarthy RJ, Najafi H, et al: J Thorac Cardiovasc Surg 1992;104:1510-1517.)*

neurocognitive dysfunction[5] after cardiac surgery.[4] Indeed, Tuman and colleagues described that age has a greater impact on neurologic outcome than it does on perioperative myocardial infarction or low cardiac output states after cardiac surgery (Fig. 22-2).[16]

Atheromatous disease of the aorta is another consistent risk factor for stroke after cardiac surgery. In addition to increasing the risk of atheromatous emboli, the atherosclerotic aorta also indicates a high likelihood of cerebrovascular disease,[17] and patients who have had a prior stroke or TIA are more likely to suffer a perioperative stroke.[18-21] Even in the absence of symptomatic cerebrovascular disease (as would be indicated by a carotid bruit), the risk of stroke increases with the severity of the carotid disease.[22,23]

Atheromatous disease of the ascending aorta, aortic arch, and descending thoracic aorta has been consistently implicated as a risk factor for stroke in cardiac surgical patients.[24-27] The increased use of ultrasonography, both transesophageal echocardiography (TEE) and epiaortic scanning, has added new dimensions to the detection of aortic atheromatous disease and to the understanding of its relationship to stroke risk. The risk of cerebral embolism from aortic atheroma was described early in the history of cardiac surgery[28] and has repeatedly been described in detail since.[7,29-31] Studies have consistently reported higher stroke rates in patients with increasing atheromatous aortic involvement (particularly the ascending and arch segments).[32,33] This risk relationship is outlined in Figure 22-3.

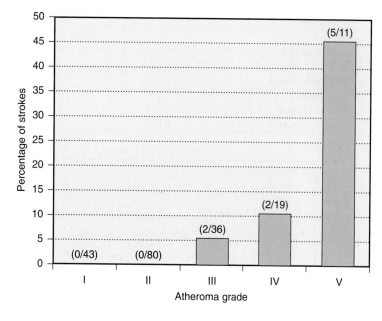

Figure 22-3 ■ Stroke rate 1 week after cardiac surgery as a function of atheroma severity. Atheroma was graded by transesophageal echocardiography as follows: I, normal; II, intimal thickening; III, plaque <5 mm in height; IV, plaque >5 mm in height; V, any plaque with a mobile segment. *(Redrawn with permission from Hartman GS, Yao FS, Brue-fach M 3rd, et al: Anesth Analg 1996;83:701-708.)*

Etiology of Perioperative Brain Injury

The following paragraphs deal with both stroke and cognitive injury, and their respective etiologies are differentiated where appropriate (Box 22-1).

Cerebral Embolization

Emboli, both macroemboli (such as atheromatous plaque) and microemboli (both gaseous and particulate), are produced during various stages of CPB. Many of these find their way to the cerebral vasculature.[34] Whereas macroemboli are responsible for stroke, microemboli likely lead to the development of neurocognitive dysfunction (Table 22-3). Microemboli can result from the interactions of blood within the CPB apparatus (e.g., platelet–fibrin aggregates), and they can be generated in the body by the mobilization of atheromatous material. Entrainment of air from the operative field, and of lipid-laden debris in the salvaged blood aspirated from the chest cavity by cardiotomy suction, are also sources of emboli.[35]

Numerous studies outline the relationship between emboli and cognitive decline after cardiac surgery.[36-38] However, one of the major limitations to understanding this relationship has been the difficulty in discerning between gaseous and particulate microemboli. Typically, Doppler ultrasonography has been used to measure cerebral embolic signals, but most Doppler techniques cannot reliably distinguish between gaseous and particulate emboli.[39] However, some newer techniques are improving this ability using multifrequency technologies.[40,41] Other evidence for cerebral embolic injury comes from Moody and coworkers,[34] who performed histologic analyses on brains from cardiac surgical patients and described the presence of thousands of cerebral emboli in the form of small capillary arteriolar dilations (SCADs).

The impact of aortic atheroma on cognitive decline is incompletely understood. Although it is known from nonsur-

22-1	**Possible Causes of Cognitive Dysfunction after Cardiac Surgery**

- Cerebral microemboli
- Global cerebral hypoperfusion
- Inflammation (systemic and cerebral)
- Cerebral hyperthermia
- Cerebral edema
- Blood–brain barrier dysfunction
- Pharmacologic influences
- Genetics

22-3	**Risk Factors for Adverse Cognitive Outcomes after Cardiac Surgery**

Effect	Odds Ratio (95% Confidence Interval)	P
Prolonged intensive care unit stay (>24 hr)	1.88 (1.27-2.79)	.002
Abnormal left ventricular function	1.53 (1.02-2.30)	.042
Elevated preoperative serum creatinine level	1.01 (1.00-1.03)	.017
Intraoperative/perioperative normothermia	1.15 (1.01-1.31)	.042
Low level of education	1.52 (1.01-2.28)	.042

Used with permission and modified from Boodhwani M, Rubens FD, Wozny D, et al: Circulation 2006;114:I461-466.

gical and cardiac surgery studies that there is a clear relationship between the presence of aortic atheroma and stroke,[24,42-44] the relationship between cognitive outcome and cerebral atheroma is much less uncertain. Studies report different results.[45,46] Whereas some data suggest that the higher the degree of aortic atheroma, the more likely there are to be cerebral emboli,[47] these atheroma may not relate to cognitive decline.[45] Part of the discordance between these findings may be because Doppler technology has a limited ability to discriminate between gaseous and particulate emboli, thus misrepresenting somewhat their relative injurious cerebral embolic loads.[1]

Global Cerebral Hypoperfusion

In the earlier days of cardiac surgery, when profound and often prolonged systemic hypotension was a relatively common event, it was believed that this hypotension would lead to global cerebral hypoperfusion. However, studies of the relationship between mean arterial pressure and cognitive decline after cardiac surgery have not consistently demonstrated any significant relationship.[11,48,49] This is different from stroke, as Hartman and colleagues[31] and Gold and coworkers[50] demonstrated that hypotension was associated with worse neurologic outcome in the presence of a significantly atheromatous aorta.

Hypoperfusion of the brain can occur, however, in patients with otherwise normal blood pressure. The unphysiologic nonpulsatile flow during CPB may cause microvascular hypoperfusion as a result of shunting at the capillary level.[51] In addition, relative hypoperfusion can occur when an otherwise normal blood pressure is accompanied by an elevated central venous pressure (CVP) secondary to cerebral venous engorgement from steep Trendelenburg positioning (such as that seen during off-pump surgery[52]) or from venous cannula malposition.[53]

Temperature Considerations

The data are inconsistent in showing whether *hypothermia* can protect the brain during cardiac surgery. However, *hyperthermia* can have an injurious effect, potentially causing some brain injury patterns. Indeed, hyperthermia can occur during particular periods during and after cardiac surgery. During rewarming from hypothermic CPB, there can be an overshoot in cerebral temperature. This cerebral hyperthermia may be responsible for some of the injury that occurs in the brain,[54] or at least it may counteract some of the protection that may have been afforded by the hypothermia during CPB. (For the role of temperature management in optimizing cerebral outcome after CPB, see Temperature and Neurologic Injury, later.)

During the postoperative period, hyperthermia can contribute to brain injury.[55,56] Grocott and colleagues[55] demonstrated that the peak temperature in the postoperative period (24 hours after cardiac surgery) was associated with worse cognitive decline 6 weeks later. It was not clear, however, whether this hyperthermia caused new injury or whether it exacerbated injury that had already occurred (such as the injury that might be induced by cerebral microembolization or global cerebral hypoperfusion).

This issue highlights a common problem in studies of risk factors or etiologic events—determining whether they are contemporaneous or causal. However, assuming that the brain is injured during CPB, and as experimental brain injury is known to cause hyperthermia (secondary to hypothalamic injury[57]), then the hyperthermia that is demonstrated in the postoperative period may very well be caused by the brain injury. However, if the hyperthermia is caused by the inflammatory response to bypass, this hyperthermia may induce or exacerbate cerebral injury.[58]

Inflammation

Although CPB stimulates a profound inflammatory response via the interaction of blood with the surfaces of the pump-oxygenator,[59] the systemic end-organ effects of this inflammatory response are less clearly defined. Many of the experimental and clinical studies relating CNS organ dysfunction to the inflammatory response have relied on indirect evidence. For example, it is not clear whether a cerebral inflammatory response occurs as a result of CPB in humans, but Hindman and coworkers reported that in animals, cyclooxygenase mRNA was upregulated after CPB, suggesting that on the molecular biological level, CPB induces an overexpression of this proinflammatory gene in the brain.[60] What is not clear was whether this was a primary event (i.e., a direct result of the proinflammatory effects of CPB) or a secondary event, resulting from other injurious effects of CPB (such as microembolization). In settings other than cardiac surgery, inflammation has been demonstrated to directly injure brain (e.g., in sepsis-mediated encephalopathy),[61] but it is also known to occur as a response to various cerebral injuries (e.g., ischemic stroke).[62]

In humans, Mathew and associates demonstrated a relationship between poor cognitive outcome and an impaired immune response to circulating endotoxin (which inevitably translocates from the gut to the bloodstream because of alterations in splanchnic blood flow during CPB).[63] It is known that having a low antibody response to circulating endotoxin is paradoxically associated with an overstimulated inflammatory response.[64] Thus, the relationship between low endotoxin antibodies and poor cognitive outcome may be mediated by an augmented inflammatory response. Other data come from smaller studies directly correlating high systemic cytokine levels with adverse cognitive outcome.[65] Some genetic association studies are also pointing to inflammation as an important pathway to cerebral injury.[66]

Possible Pharmacologic Influences

Although no direct human studies have implicated anesthetics in the etiology of this injury, experimental studies of cognitive outcome in rats exposed to anesthetics have demonstrated that relatively brief (several hours) exposure to isoflurane led to long-term cognitive changes.[67] Studies with other experimental models of necrosis in neonatal brains after exposure to anesthetic agents (isoflurane, midazolam, nitrous oxide)[68] and findings of protein changes in the brain after exposure to anesthetics[69] identify this as an area for further research.

Blood–Brain Barrier Dysfunction

The blood–brain barrier (BBB) aids in maintaining the homeostasis of the extracellular cerebral milieu that protects the brain against fluctuations in ion concentrations, neurotransmitters, growth factors, and other factors that are present in the serum.[70]

The BBB has been incompletely interrogated in the setting of CPB, in part because of an inability to clinically assess BBB function and in part because of a relative lack of animal models of brain dysfunction after CPB. Several studies do provide some information aout BBB integrity during CPB, however, but the data are conflicting. Using carbon-14 aminoisobutyric acid tracer techniques in post-bypass brain homogenates, Gillinov and colleagues[71] were unable to show any changes in BBB dysfunction after 2 hours of CPB in piglets. More recently, however, Bokesch and coworkers[72] were able to demonstrate impairment in the BBB by using a technique that measures the leakage of fluorescent albumin from blood vessels in brain slices after bypass. However, both of these studies looked at a single time point—immediately after CPB—and any temporal changes are not known.

It is difficult to determine whether the changes in BBB integrity, if present at all, are a primary cause of brain dysfunction or simply a result of other initiating events such as ischemia (from cerebral microembolization), a diffuse cerebral inflammatory event, or the cerebral edema that has been seen after bypass.[73]

Genetic Influences

Genetic influences are likely to play a role in modifying the susceptibility to brain injury or in affecting the ability of the brain to recover once injury has occurred. Among the several investigations of genetic influences on cerebral outcome after CPB, the most commonly explored gene variant, or single nucleotide polymorphism (SNP), has been the ε4 allele of the apolipoprotein gene. This gene has been reported to be responsible for increasing the risk of both sporadic and late-onset Alzheimer's disease (as well as complicating outcome after a variety of other brain injuries).[74] Although early reports suggested that this may have an important influence

on cognitive decline,[75] later reports have shed some doubt on the robustness of this effect.[76] A second SNP examined relates to the PLA-II receptor polymorphism. This platelet integrin receptor polymorphism has been shown to be important in the etiology of acute coronary syndromes and other thrombotic disorders.[77,78] A small study in cardiac surgery patients demonstrated that PLA-II–positive patients had worse impairments in the mini-mental status examination than PLA-II negative patients.[79]

Most recently, a large genotyping study[66,80-82] has identified more complex gene and gene-to-gene interactions that may contribute to the susceptibility of the brain to injury. However, the understanding of the role genetics plays is in its infancy.

■ NONPHARMACOLOGIC NEUROPROTECTIVE STRATEGIES

Table 22-4 lists some evidence-based ratings for nonpharmacologic and pharmacologic neuroprotective strategies that can be used during CPB.[3]

Emboli Reduction Techniques

There are many sources of emboli, both particulate and gaseous, during cardiac surgery. Gaseous emboli can be created in the circuit, or augmented if already present, by turbulence-related cavitation, and potentially even by vacuum-assisted venous drainage.[83] The techniques used to reduce the number of emboli presented to the brain include arterial line filters, insufflation of the surgical field with CO_2, and the judicious use of cell salvage techniques to reduce reinfusion of exogenous lipid-containing emboli.

Depending on the procedure being performed, significant quantities of air can be entrained from the surgical field into the heart. Various means have been proposed to deal with these emboli. One way is to reduce their size by flooding the operative field with CO_2, which may be effective because

22-4 Evidence-Based Classes* of Pharmacologic and Nonpharmacologic Neuroprotection during Cardiopulmonary Bypass	
Intervention	**Rating**
Epiaortic ultrasound-guided changes in surgical approach	Class IIb
Modified aortic cannula	Class indeterminate
Cell-saver processing of pericardial aspirate	Class indeterminate
CO_2 wound insufflation	Class indeterminate
Maintaining higher MAP targets (i.e., > the lower target of 50 mm Hg)	Class IIb for patients at high risk for neurologic injury
Nonpulsatile (versus pulsatile) perfusion	Class IIb (class indeterminate for patients at high risk for neurologic injury)
Alpha-stat (versus pH-stat) acid–base management	Class IIb (class indeterminate for patients at high risk for neurologic injury)
Thiopental, propofol, nimodipine, prostacyclin, GM1-ganglioside, pegorgotein, clomethiazole	Class III
Remacemide, lidocaine, aprotinin, pexelizumab	Class indeterminate
Intraoperative glucose control	Class indeterminate
Hypothermia	Class indeterminate

*See Table 22-1 for definitions of classes.
MAP, mean arterial pressure.
Used with permission and modified from Hogue CW Jr, Palin CA, Arrowsmith JE: Anesth Analg 2006;103:21-37.

of its high solubility.[84] However, its ability to specifically reduce cerebral injury has not been rigorously evaluated, although it has been demonstrated to significantly reduce the number of bubbles detectable by TEE in the heart after cardiac surgery.[85] Even with CO_2 in the surgical field, however, significant amounts of air can be entrained.

The impact of perfusionist interventions on cerebral embolic load has also been studied. Borger and colleagues found that following injections (for drug or other interventions) into the venous reservoir, gaseous emboli may be allowed rapid passage through to the arterial outflow.[86] Limiting these perfusionist interventions reduced both emboli generation and neurocognitive impairment.

Although the oxygenator or venous reservoir design attempts to purge the air before it reaches the inflow cannula, the arterial line filter is expected to deal with what is left. However, the capacity of the arterial filter to remove all sources of emboli (gaseous or particulate) has significant limitations, so emboli easily pass into the aortic root. The data supporting the use of arterial filtration are surprisingly weak,[38] considering this is one of the fundamental techniques in the bypass apparatus to reduce organ injury, and the filter has undergone little rigorous evaluation in relevant populations with regard to preventing neurologic injury.

The aortic cannula also affects cerebral emboli production. Placing the cannula into an area of the aorta with an atheromatous lesion may lead to the direct generation of emboli from the "sandblasting" of atherosclerotic material in the aorta. However, using a long aortic cannula, whose tip can lie beyond the origin of the cerebral vessels, has been found to reduce embolic load.[87] Other cannula designs reduce the sandblasting-type jets emanating from the aortic cannula. Some have gained acceptance and others have not. For example, a baffled cannula and cannulae that allow the incorporation of regional brain hypothermia as well as diversion of emboli away from the cerebral vessels have all been used.[88] The uniquely designed and widely available Embol-X cannula has a basket-like extension that can be inserted just prior to cross-clamp removal.[89] However, in a large ($N = 1289$) study, this cannula was unable to reduce the incidence of neurologic injury,[90] perhaps because of the increase in embolic signals that have been reported with its deployment in the aorta.[91] Few other embolus-reducing strategies, besides arterial line filtration and reduction of perfusion interventions,[38,86] have been studied sufficiently to determine their impact on cognitive loss after cardiac surgery.

Particulate emboli, such as the lipid emboli described as SCADs (see Cerebral Embolization, earlier), may be removed by processing the shed blood before returning it to the CPB circuit. Using cell salvage devices to process shed blood prior to returning it to the venous reservoir may minimize the amount of particulate and lipid-laden material that contributes to embolization.[35,92] A significant amount of this material is either small or highly deformable (because of its lipid composition), so it easily passes through standard arterial filters. Although the cell saver may reduce the number of lipid emboli, a potential disadvantage to its excessive use is a reduction in both platelet and coagulation factors through its intrinsic washing processes. Using cell salvage for only

a limited volume of blood (e.g., two cycles) is probably prudent.

Pulsatile Perfusion

Flow generated during CPB by either roller or centrifugal pumps can be either pulsatile or nonpulsatile. Nonpulsatile CPB is the most commonly practiced form of artificial perfusion. It is unclear how this unphysiologic nonpulsatile flow pattern moderates cerebral injury, as it would seem that matching the heart's normal pulsing should be beneficial. One adequately sized ($N = 316$), but not definitive, study provides some guidance: Murkin and coworkers compared the effects of pulsatile and nonpulsatile CPB on neurologic and neuropsychological outcome, and they found no significant benefit to pulsatility.[93] This study, however, probably suffered from one limitation: in all conventional pulsatile systems, for technical reasons, true physiologic pulsatility is almost never accomplished. The variations of sinusoidal pulse waveforms that are generated fail to replicate the hydrodynamics of normal physiologic pulsation. Another study of balloon pump–induced pulsatile perfusion during CPB failed to show any improvement in jugular venous oxygen saturation or regional brain oxygenation.[94]

Most studies to date do not present enough convincing evidence that suggests that routine pulsatile flow during CPB is warranted. More physiologic approaches to pulsatility are needed, such as the biologically variable systems developed by Mutch and colleagues.[51]

Acid–Base Management

Acid–base management is particularly relevant to cardiac surgery, largely because of its close link to temperature manipulations that have always been a major issue during CPB. As hypothermia becomes commonplace, the question of whether to "correct" the pH to the patient's temperature becomes relevant. If the blood gas is adjusted to the temperature (e.g., to hypothermia), then to maintain a normal pH, CO_2 must be added to the CPB system (or less must be removed by the oxygenator). This would result in significant hypercarbia at an uncorrected temperature, with all of its predictable effects on the cerebral circulation. Theoretically, alpha-stat management maintains normal cerebral blood flow (CBF) autoregulation, with the coupling of cerebral metabolism ($CMRO_2$) to CBF allowing adequate oxygen delivery while minimizing the potential for emboli. On the other hand, pH stat management (in which CO_2 is added to the fresh oxygenator gas flow) results in a higher CBF than is needed for the brain's metabolic requirements. This luxury perfusion risks excessive delivery of emboli to the brain. Although early studies[93] were unable to document a difference in neurologic or neuropsychological outcome between the two techniques, more recent studies have shown reductions in cognitive performance when pH-stat management is used, particularly in cases with prolonged CPB times.[95] A notable exception is that presented by deep hypothermic circulatory arrest (DHCA), for which recent outcome data (from pediatric populations) support the utilization of pH-stat management because of its more homogeneous brain cooling before circulatory arrest.[96,97]

Glucose Management

Hyperglycemia commonly occurs during the course of cardiac surgery, partly because cardioplegic solutions containing glucose are administered, but also because of stress response–induced alterations in both insulin secretion and resistance, coupled with hypothermic impairment of insulin utilization, which all combine to increase the overall potential for significant hyperglycemia.[98] In experimental cerebral ischemia, both focal and global, hyperglycemia has been repeatedly demonstrated to impair neurologic outcome.[99-101] There are several mechanisms for this injurious relationship. One relates to the effects hyperglycemia has on the anaerobic conversion of glucose to lactate, which ultimately causes intracellular acidosis and impairs intracellular homeostasis and metabolism.[102] Another injurious mechanism involves an increase in the release of excitotoxic amino acids in response to hyperglycemia in the setting of cerebral ischemia.[100]

Furthermore, some evidence suggests that the presence of hyperglycemia itself may enhance the inflammatory response.[103] Hyperglycemia has been shown to increase perioperative C-reactive protein levels, indicative of a causal relationship to inflammation.[104] As CPB itself has a much enhanced inflammatory response,[105,106] and inflammation may mediate several adverse outcomes, including cerebral outcome, the additional hyperglycemia-mediated inflammation may cause further injury. Cerebral ischemia has the potential to occur during cardiac surgery, which may link adverse cerebral outcome with hyperglycemia during cardiac surgery. If hyperglycemia is injurious to the brain, the threshold for making injuries worse appears to be approximately 180 to 200 mg/dL.[107,108]

Although its effects on cerebral injury are well defined experimentally, there is currently insufficient, though emerging, information on its clinical cerebral effects in the bypass setting. There is, however, a growing amount of data linking hyperglycemia to other adverse endpoints after bypass—most notably, infectious complications. Mediastinitis is a particularly ominous infection that can occur in the post–cardiac surgery period. Although there are multiple risk factors for this potentially devastating infectious complication, hyperglycemia has recently been demonstrated to be associated with a higher incidence of mediastinitis, particularly in patients who are diabetic or obese.[109,110] As a result, efforts have been targeted at reducing hyperglycemia to decrease significant mediastinal infection.

Some of the most compelling data associating hyperglycemia with adverse outcome were recently published by Lazar and associates.[111] These data implicated hyperglycemia not just on adverse short-term outcome but on mortality and morbidity some years after cardiac surgery. The mechanism behind this possible longer-term effect was most likely twofold. It is possible that even short durations of intense hyperglycemia are injurious; however, it is also possible that those patients who exhibit a hyperglycemic response are the ones who are more prone to other seemingly unrelated pathologies that cause premature death, such pathologies that involve an enhanced inflammatory response.

Thus far, however, most studies have been too small (and as a result underpowered) to demonstrate any meaningful associations between adverse cerebral outcome and hyperglycemia during cardiac surgery; this is particularly true for stroke. Metz and Keats found no difference in neurologic outcome between patients undergoing CPB with a glucose prime (blood glucose during CPB of 600 to 800 mg/dL) and those with no glucose prime (a blood glucose level of 200 to 300 mg/dL).[112] However, Hindman, in an accompanying editorial, cautioned against the use of glucose-containing prime for CPB.[113] In another study, by Nussmeier and colleagues, the use of a glucose-containing prime was demonstrated not to be a risk factor for cerebral injury in nondiabetic or diabetic patients having CABG procedures.[114] In a very large retrospective review ($N = 2862$), no association between the intraoperative maximal glucose concentration and major adverse neurologic outcome or in-hospital mortality was found.[115,116] However, this early absence of strong evidence supporting any link between hyperglycemia and adverse cerebral outcome after cardiac surgery may not amount to evidence of absence of any effect.

Recently, for example, our research group reported the results of a large (but still too small to adequately examine any stroke effect) study of 595 patients.[117] In this study, the cognitive function of patients undergoing CABG with CPB was assessed both preoperatively and postoperatively (at 6 weeks). The incidence of cognitive deficit was compared between those with hyperglycemia and those without. The hyperglycemic patients had a cognitive deficit rate of 40%, compared with 29% in the normoglycemic group (odds ratio, 1.85; 95% confidence interval [CI], 1.1-3.0; $P = .0165$). The presence of hyperglycemia increased the risk of cognitive dysfunction by as much as 85%.[117] Butterworth and coworkers[118] also studied a large number of patients ($N = 360$) to determine whether reducing glucose levels could impact favorably on neurologic outcome after cardiac surgery. Following the experimental rationale that neurologic injury commonly occurs during cardiac surgery, along with data supporting an injurious role of hyperglycemia in other settings of cerebral ischemic injury, these authors hypothesized that lowering intraoperative glucose levels could have a beneficial impact. However, they did not find any benefit in the high-dose insulin group. They were, however, as others have been before, unable to adequately regulate glucose levels to below a level that would be considered neurologically neutral (i.e., <140 to 150 mg/dL), which significantly limited the applicability of their "negative" findings. Their data also suggested that insulin itself was not likely to be intrinsically neuroprotective without a concomitant decrease in blood glucose levels.

There are risk/benefit considerations that must be taken into account when considering interventional therapy, even something as relatively routine as insulin therapy. One of the limitations of insulin therapy in this setting is the risk of the significant hypoglycemia that can occur after prolonged periods of aggressive insulin regimens. Chaney and colleagues reported that not only is normoglycemia difficult to attain during cardiac surgery but also large insulin doses administered during surgery increase the risk of hypoglycemia in the period after bypass.[119] High-dose insulin can also result in hypokalemia because it facilitates potassium transmembrane transport mechanisms.

Although adequate glycemic control has been difficult to obtain, moderate success has recently been demonstrated with a novel insulin glucose infusion protocol to better maintain adequate serum glucose levels during surgery. Indeed, Carvalho and coworkers described methodology to successfully target a particular glucose level.[120] Although their study was relatively small ($N = 47$), it demonstrated clear efficacy compared with previous surgery trials[119] and warrants further large-scale evaluation. Using a more aggressive approach than seen in previous studies, they described a hyperinsulinemia normoglycemic clamp technique that, instead of administering insulin in reaction to hyperglycemia, purposely administered high doses of insulin so that exogenous glucose would have to be administered to prevent hypoglycemia. Thus, when patients were exposed to bypass-induced hyperglycemia, the amount of glucose that was being infused was reduced, which resulted in better glucose control. Importantly, they supplemented potassium by continuous infusion and also monitored glucose levels every 5 to 10 minutes. Compared with conventionally treated patients, greater than 95% of patients managed by this clamp technique achieved normoglycemia. The same technique was also reported by Visser and colleagues.[104] In their small study ($N = 21$), hyperglycemia was present in only 15% of patients who were treated with the normoglycemic insulin clamp technique, compared with 80% of control patients. The requirement for frequent (and as a result, difficult to achieve) glucose monitoring is the inherent weakness in this technique.

Significant progress is being made on the glucose monitoring front, however. Recently, a continuous glucose monitor has been approved by the FDA for marketing. This device (Minimed, Medtronic Diabetes, Northridge, Calif) records glucose levels from the subcutaneous interstitial fluid every 5 seconds, averaging and displaying them every 5 minutes. It is this type of rapid glucose measurement that may make intraoperative glucose control easier when employing aggressive insulin or insulin-glucose-potassium strategies. It should also be noted that these types of devices were approved for ambulatory nonsurgical settings, and it is not clear how well they will work in operative settings. They do require the placement of a small needle into the subcutaneous tissue, which may have some disadvantages for heparinized patients. The utility and accuracy of these devices in this setting need further validation, but in principle they hold considerable promise.

■ BLOOD PRESSURE MANAGEMENT DURING CPB

The global cerebral hypoperfusion that follows the unphysiologic flow during CPB was one of the first factors targeted to improve cerebral outcome. The idea that hypotension potentially contributes to cerebral injury originated in the early days of cardiac surgery when significant systemic hypotension (both in degree and duration) was a frequent event. Although it was logical to assume that hypotension would lead to global cerebral hypoperfusion, studies that have examined the relationship between blood pressure and cognitive decline after cardiac surgery have generally failed to show any significant relationship.[11,48,49,121]

Although there does not appear to be a convincing link between blood pressure and cognitive outcome, some data support a link between lower blood pressure during bypass and postoperative stroke. Gold and coworkers[50] and Hartman and colleagues[31] demonstrated a link between hypotension (coupled with the presence of a significantly atheromatous aorta) and an increased risk of stroke (see Fig. 22-3). Gold and coworkers[50] randomized 248 patients to low (50 to 60 mm Hg) or to high (80 to 100 mm Hg) mean arterial pressure (MAP) during CPB. Although a difference was demonstrated in their composite endpoint of adverse cardiac plus neurologic outcome (4.8% high versus 12.9% low, $P = .026$), there was no statistical difference in stroke itself. However, a secondary analysis of the same data subsequently performed by Hartman and coworkers[31] described a very interesting interaction between pressure, aortic atheroma, and stroke: those patients who were at risk of cerebral embolic stroke (from having severely atheromatous aortas) were more likely to manifest a stroke if blood pressure was maintained in the lower range than in the higher range.[31] The relationship is complex and most likely represents an interaction between macroembolism of atheromatous plaque material superimposed on global cerebral hypoperfusion. Collateral perfusion in a region of the brain at risk for ischemia, caused by the presence of either a rear-occlusive obstructive lesion in the cerebral vasculature or a vessel acutely obstructed from an embolus, is highly pressure dependent. Vessel obstruction concomitant with hypotension could lead to irreversible focal cerebral damage (i.e., stroke).

The concept that the unphysiologic flow provided by the CPB apparatus leads to general and cerebral hypothermia is supported experimentally by Mutch and colleagues.[51] Further supportive clinical data come from a magnetic resonance spectroscopy (MRS) study demonstrating that there are MRS characteristics in the post-bypass brain that are consistent with global cerebral ischemia, and that these signatures are associated with cognitive decline, and return to baseline is accompanied by a normalized MRS pattern.[122]

The relationship between pressure during CPB and CBF is pertinent to understanding whether blood pressure can be optimized to prevent neurologic injury. Plochl and coworkers examined the threshold of the autoregulatory curve in dogs, at which lowering blood pressure further would result in inadequate CBF and oxygen delivery during CPB.[123] In that study, the brain becomes perfusion pressure dependent below 50 mm Hg. They also demonstrated that hypothermia did not shift this threshold leftward. Clinically, the available data suggest that in an otherwise normal patient, CBF during nonpulsatile hypothermic CPB using alpha-stat blood gas management is largely independent of MAP as long as that MAP is within or near the autoregulatory range for the patient (i.e., 50 to 100 mm Hg).[124] However, although the autoregulatory curve is traditionally considered a horizontal plateau, this plateau actually has a slightly positive slope. This slightly positive incline, however, is unlikely to have a clinically meaningful effect. For example, Newman and associates demonstrated that under hypothermic conditions, for every 10 mm Hg change in MAP, CBF changes only 0.86 mL/100 g/min.[11] Although this change was greater with normothermia (1.78 mL/100 g/min),[125] these changes represent a relatively small fraction of the normal CBF, which is approximately 50 mL/100 g/min. The effects of underlying hypertension as a comorbidity, however, probably have the effect of shifting rightward the autoregulatory curve. The degree to which this rightward shift occurs, however, is not clear, but it would be reasonable to expect that it is at least 10 mm Hg, suggesting that the lower range of autoregulatory blood flow in chronically hypertensive patients is more likely to be 60 mm Hg than 50 mm Hg.[126]

Although the data associating MAP with neurologic and neurocognitive outcome after CABG surgery are inconclusive, most data suggest that MAP during CPB is not a primary predictor of cognitive decline. However, with increasing age, MAP during CPB may play a role in improving cerebral collateral perfusion to embolized regions, and in those with significant aortic atheroma, it may be prudent to modestly increase blood pressure.

■ TEMPERATURE AND NEUROLOGIC INJURY

Normothermic versus Hypothermic Bypass

Hypothermia has been a fundamental aspect of CPB management. Its widespread use relates to its putative, though far from definitively proven, global organ protective effects. Although hypothermia has a suppressing effect on cerebral metabolism (about a 6% to 7% decline per °C),[127] it most likely has other neuroprotective effects that are mediated by nonmetabolic pathways. Moreover, moderate hypothermia has multimodal effects in the ischemic brain, including blocking the release of glutamate,[128] reducing calcium influx,[129] hastening recovery of protein synthesis,[130] diminishing membrane-bound protein kinase-C activity,[131] reducing of the time to onset of depolarization,[132] reducing the formation of reactive oxygen species (ROS),[133] and suppressing nitric oxide synthase activity.[134] It is most likely the additive effect of these mechanisms that conveys any neuroprotection from hypothermia. Although experimental demonstrations of the neuroprotective benefits of hypothermia are abundant, clinical examples, until recent demonstrations of its efficacy after cardiac arrest, have been few.[135-138]

Some of the most illustrative data outlining the pros and cons of various temperature strategies during CPB have come within the past 15 years. In the late 1980s and early 1990s, warm CPB was revisited because of its putative myocardial salvaging effects when used concomitantly with continuous warm cardioplegia.[139-142] This prompted investigation into possible cerebral effects, as CPB was being carried out at higher temperatures than what were considered conventional, and there was concern that cerebral outcome could be compromised. Several large studies have been undertaken to examine the effects of temperature management on cerebral outcome after cardiac surgery. The Warm Heart Investigators Trial,[139] another trial performed at Emory University,[143] and

a later trial at Duke University,[144] although they had important methodological differences, had very similar neurocognitive outcome results.[145,146] However, the results pertaining to stroke differed remarkably. None of the studies demonstrated any neuroprotective benefit from hypothermia on neurocognitive outcome. The Warm Heart Investigators Trial and the Duke trial showed no difference with respect to stroke. In contrast, the Emory trial demonstrated an apparently injurious effect (as manifested by a worse stroke outcome) of what was most likely mild degrees of hyperthermia during CPB. These divergent results could be partly explained by differences in how temperature was monitored (i.e., nasopharyngeal versus bladder), what the peak and nadir temperatures were, and how normothermia was maintained (actively warmed versus allowing the patient's temperature to passively drift). Most relevant to the issue of stroke was that the Emory investigators actively warmed their patients, which per se is not injurious if precisely carried out, but coupled with the fact that they did not measure nasopharyngeal temperature, made it highly likely that they exposed the brain to hyperthermic temperatures. These data suggest that active warming to maintain temperatures at (or greater than) 37° C may pose an unnecessary risk of stroke.

Avoidance of Hyperthermia

Just as hypothermia, at least experimentally, has protective effects on the brain, *hyperthermia,* in an opposite and disproportionate fashion, has injurious effects.[128] The lack of neuroprotective effects seen in the normothermic versus hypothermic CPB studies referred to previously[139,143,144] might be related to the obligate rewarming that occurs at the end of bypass. Indeed, Grigore and colleagues,[54] studying the effect of different rewarming rates on neurocognitive outcome after CABG, compared conventional "fast" rewarming to slower rewarming and found a lower incidence of neurocognitive dysfunction 6 weeks after cardiac surgery. These slower rewarming rates were accompanied by lower peak cerebral temperatures during rewarming, which was consistent with past observations that rapid rewarming can lead to an overshoot in cerebral temperature and result in inadvertent cerebral hyperthermia.[147] By reducing this rewarming rate, the overshoot in temperature is limited and perhaps prevented, thereby avoiding the negative effects of cerebral hyperthermia. Supporting the concept that limiting rewarming may be neuroprotective was a study by Nathan and associates[148] that demonstrated a neurocognitive benefit for patients who had limited rewarming and were maintained between 34° and 36° C for a prolonged (12-hour) period postoperatively. Indeed, the beneficial effect may actually have been mediated by the avoidance of cerebral hyperthermia during rewarming rather than by the prolonged hypothermia.[148] These rewarming studies, when coupled with the postoperative temperature data suggesting that early postoperative fever is associated with worse neurocognitive decline,[55] suggest that avoiding hyperthermia may be beneficial in this population.

Monitoring Brain Temperature

Fundamental to the issue of temperature management is how to measure temperature when the brain is at particular risk from hyperthermia. When measuring temperature directly within the brain is not practical or possible, a surrogate for brain temperature should be chosen. Two surrogates are nasopharyngeal temperature and tympanic membrane temperature. A more invasive brain temperature surrogate is the measurement of jugular bulb temperature with a thermistor placed retrogradely from the internal jugular vein.[147,149] Use of these sites has shown that significant temperature gradients exist across the body and across the brain during bypass. It is likely that during periods of rapid flux (such as during rewarming[150]), these temperature gradients are maximal, making a noncerebral brain temperature site particularly prone to misrepresenting brain temperature.

■ AORTIC ATHEROMA AND NEUROLOGIC OUTCOMES

Aortic Assessment

Among patients undergoing CABG surgery, cerebral atheroemboli account for the majority of stroke outcomes, with noncalcific plaque likely to be the greatest contributor to these emboli.[151] Unfortunately, noncalcific plaque is least likely to be identified by the intraoperative surgical palpation of the aorta that is performed prior to instrumentation.[152] Advanced age, diabetes mellitus, and vascular disease are all well-known risk factors for perioperative stroke, and are also predictors of advanced aortic atherosclerosis with an attendant risk of systemic atheroemboli.[24,153] Significant atherosclerosis (defined as intimal thickening more than 5 mm in the aortic arch), present in up to 20% of CABG patients, has previously been associated with an increased risk of stroke after CABG.[153,154] Although the use of TEE was first described to intraoperatively image aortic atherosclerosis, epiaortic ultrasound is significantly more sensitive than TEE for identification of atherosclerosis of the ascending aorta and provides complementary information regarding thoracic aortic atherosclerosis. Both ultrasound techniques are clearly superior to palpation.[152,155,156]

The widespread use of TEE and complementary (and preferably routine) epiaortic scanning has had a tremendous impact on our understanding of the risks involved in the patient with a severely atheromatous aorta. There is strong evidence linking stroke to atheroma,[24,42-44] but the link between atheroma and cognitive decline is far less clear.[45] At this point, the data are insufficient to say without doubt that there is a relationship between atheroma and cognitive decline, but regardless of whether atheroma causes cognitive dysfunction, its importance to the etiology of cardiac surgery–associated stroke is enough to warrant specific strategies for its management.

Modification of surgical technique on the basis of results of intraoperative epiaortic ultrasound and TEE in older adult patients undergoing cardiac procedures may prevent atheroembolic complications.[47,153,157,158] Epiaortic ultrasound and TEE may facilitate the reduction of neurologic injury through the identification of areas free from atherosclerosis for aortic cannulation, by avoidance of the ascending aorta entirely in favor of femoral or axillary artery sites, or by use of off-pump techniques.[157-160]

For patients at increased risk of adverse neurologic events who are undergoing CPB, strong consideration should be given to intraoperative TEE or epiaortic ultrasound scanning of the aorta to detect nonpalpable plaque and thus reduce cerebral emboli.[161]

Management of Aortic Atherosclerosis

The aorta is a significant source of injurious emboli during CPB, largely because of atheromatous aortic debris that can embolize to various vascular beds, including the brain. Many strategies can be used to minimize the atheromatous material being liberated from the aortic wall and keep it from embolizing into the cerebral circulation. Although there are considerable data outlining the relationship of aortic atheroma to adverse outcome, there are, as in most areas pertaining to decreasing injury to the brain, relatively limited good data demonstrating clear benefit to any particular procedural or interventional strategy. Ultrasonographic guidance is useful for avoiding atheromatous sections of the ascending aorta, and for making decisions about cannulation, clamping, and anastomosis placement.[46]

Studies of modifications to aortic manipulation when aortic atheromas are detected have rarely been well controlled or blinded. For the most part, a strategy is chosen on the basis of the presence of known atheroma, and then the results of these patients are compared with historical controls. Techniques to potentially limit atheromatous material from being liberated from the aortic wall and embolizing into the cerebral circulation range from the most conservative, such as placing the cannula in an area of the aorta that is relatively devoid of plaque, to the most extreme, such as aortic atherectomy or replacement under DHCA.

For example, various procedural differences have been used to try to avoid adverse neurologic injury. A small study used a combination of epiaortic scanning and atheroma avoidance techniques (with respect to cannulation, clamping, and vein graft anastomosis placement) to attempt to reduce neurocognitive deficits.[46] In that study ($N = 47$), the incidence of cognitive decline was significantly lower when an avoidance technique (guidance by epiaortic scanning) was used than when no epiaortic scanning or guided alteration was used.

Specialized cannulae that reduce the "sandblasting" of the aortic wall have also been described. Embolization of atheromatous plaque can be decreased by using alternative aortic cannulae or different insertion points. Partial-occlusion clamping for proximal vein graft anastomosis can be avoided by using either single-step automated anastomotic devices or other occlusive technologies that do not require clamping, and this can mitigate injury caused by embolization. Furthermore, specialized cannulae that integrate filtering technologies[89] and other means to deflect emboli to more distal sites have been developed and are being studied.[162] None of these variations to minimize aortic manipulations has yet yielded significant neuroprotective results in large prospective randomized trials, but their potential holds promise.

Hammon and coworkers have recently demonstrated that avoiding manipulation of the aorta by using only a single clamp application can significantly reduce cognitive loss.[163] Similar, although underpowered, studies have also reported differences in stroke with the use of minimizing aortic clamping.[164] Technology is advancing rapidly, and proximal (as well as distal) coronary artery anastomotic devices are becoming increasingly available to minimize manipulation of the ascending aorta.

■ PHARMACOLOGIC NEUROPROTECTION

Decades of investigations to find a preventative or therapeutic agent to address neurologic injury after cardiac surgery have yet to uncover a robust pharmacologic agent. This failure is not unique to the cardiac surgical setting, as stroke in the nonsurgical population has few pharmacologic options. For example, thrombolytic therapy (with recombinant tissue plasminogen activator [rtPA] or similar compounds) has benefited relatively few stroke patients, and no other drug options are currently available for these patients. These failures in other stroke settings have not, however, stemmed the flow of investigations in cardiac surgery (Table 22-5). Indeed, CPB has been considered by some in the field of neuroprotection to be an optimal model for the preemptive delivery of a neuroprotective drug. It is a situation where there is a well-defined onset of injury (i.e., at the start of the bypass), and all patients present within a well-defined therapeutic window.

All of the compounds that have been investigated have as their basis a molecular target in the cell that can be defined by understanding the events that occur with the onset of ischemia. The CNS ischemic cascade is triggered and propagated by critical reductions in global or regional CBF to the point at which the demands of cerebral metabolism are no longer met (Fig. 22-4).[165] This cerebral energy failure results in ionic pump failure within the cell membrane, initiating a number of injurious events that are mediated via the influx of sodium, the opening of voltage-dependent calcium gates, the release of stored intracellular calcium, and overall membrane depolarization. Membrane depolarization results in the release of the excitatory amino acids glutamate and aspartate, which, when interacting with N-methyl-D-aspartate (NMDA) or a similar receptor, cause a dramatic increase in intracellular calcium. This increase in cytoplasmic calcium further propels the cascade through the activation of various calcium-dependent enzymes, including endonucleases, nitric oxide synthase, various proteases, protein kinases, and phospholipase. If left unabated, these enzymes result ultimately in cellular death.

Theoretically, many of these events are potentially reversible if reperfusion is quickly reestablished; however, reperfusion itself can initiate other destructive pathways. For example, the reestablishment of oxygen delivery provides substantial substrate for the production of various reactive oxygen species (ROS). In addition to the generation of free

| **22-5** | **Agents Studied as Pharmacologic Neuroprotectants during Cardiac Surgery** |

Drug	Proposed Primary Mechanism	Reference	Patients (N)	Type of Surgery	Main Findings
Thiopental	↓CMRO$_2$	Nussmeier et al.[48]	182	Valvular	Fewer cognitive complications 10 days after surgery.
		Zaiden et al.[167]	300	CABG	No difference in neurologic outcomes between thiopental and placebo.
Propofol	↓CMRO$_2$	Roach et al.[173]	225	Valvular	No difference in cognitive complications.
Remacemide	NMDA receptor antagonist	Arrowsmith et al.[174]	171	CABG	Remacemide led to better performance on 3 of 10 psychometric measures and better global cognitive function.
Aprotinin	Mechanism(s) unknown; maybe due to ↓inflammation or ↓pericardial aspirate	Levy et al.[205]	287	CABG	No strokes in "high" and "low" dose aprotinin groups compared with control ($n = 5$) and "pump" prime only ($n = 1$) groups ($P = .01$).
		Harmon et al.[207]	36	CABG	Cognitive deficits 6 wk after surgery lower in aprotinin than in placebo group (23% versus 55%; $P < .05$).
Lidocaine	Na$^+$ channel blockade; membrane stabilization, or ↓EAA release	Mitchell et al.[185]	55	Valvular	Neurocognitive outcome better 10 days and 10 wk after surgery in lidocaine than in placebo group, but not at 6 mo.
		Wang et al.[186]	42	CABG	Improved neurocognitive function 9 days after surgery with lidocaine compared with placebo.
Pexelizumab	↓C5a and C5b-9	Mathew et al.[203]	800	CABG	Pexelizumab had no effect on global cognition but did lower decline in the visuospatial domain more than placebo.

CABG, coronary artery bypass graft; CMRO$_2$, cerebral metabolic rate for oxygen; EAA, excitatory amino acid; NMDA, N-methyl-D-aspartate.
Used with permission and modified from Hogue CW Jr, Palin CA, Arrowsmith JE: Anesth Analg 2006;103:21-37.

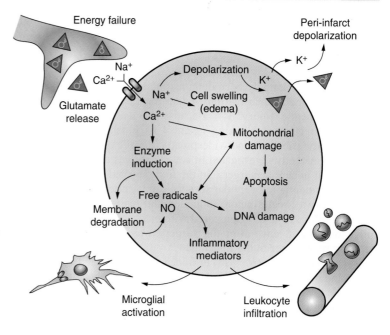

Figure 22-4 ■ Cerebral ischemic cascade. A simplified overview of central nervous system events that occur following energy failure in the ischemic brain. *(Redrawn with permission from Dirnagl U, Iadecola C, Moskowitz M: Trends Neurosci 1999;22:391-397.)*

radicals, reperfusion initiates other damaging extracellular events, including BBB breakdown, endothelial swelling, and localized thrombosis that together culminate in microvascular occlusion and further ischemia. Each of these ischemic cascade pathways represents discreet targets for the institution of neuroprotective therapeutics.

Although dozens of drug trials have been performed,[58,166] the subsequent discussion includes only those drugs that either had some clinical success (even if only in a limited way) or are clinically and widely available but have proven unsuccessful.

Barbiturates

The barbiturate thiopental, one of the first agents investigated as a potential neuroprotective agent, launched a series of investigations in this field. Nussmeier and associates reported administering thiopental (with a dosage aimed at obtaining electroencephalographic [EEG] isoelectricity) prior to cannulation and continuing until separation from CPB, and they found a reduction in neuropsychiatric complications on postoperative day 10 in those receiving thiopental.[48] The mechanism of this beneficial effect was attributed to the suppressive effects of barbiturates on cerebral metabolism. However, a subsequent investigation by Zaidan and associates[167] and a later one by Pascoe and colleagues[168] failed to support a beneficial effect of thiopental on neurologic outcome after cardiac surgery. These negative trials and the prolonged sedation associated with the high drug dosages tempered optimism for barbiturates.

Propofol

Propofol was evaluated as a potential neuroprotectant in the setting of cardiac surgery because its suppressing effect on cerebral metabolism was similar to that of barbiturates, it demonstrated superior pharmacokinetics (i.e., a large volume of distribution and a shorter duration of action), and its effects on CMRO$_2$ and CBF were similar to those of thiopental. It has also been shown to have some antioxidant and calcium-channel antagonist properties,[169] and further support for its investigation was provided by beneficial results from experimental cerebral ischemia studies.[170-172] Roach and colleagues, in a prospective randomized clinical trial, evaluated whether propofol at a dosage sufficient to induce EEG burst-suppression would reduce the incidence or severity of cerebral injury during valvular surgery.[173] However, there was no beneficial effect on cognitive outcome at 2 months in patients randomized to receive propofol.

Remacemide

Because excitotoxicity plays a central role in cerebral ischemic injury, it was an obvious target in the search to prevent cerebral injury after cardiac surgery. One such NMDA antagonist is remacemide. In a well-designed study by Arrowsmith and colleagues, patients scheduled for CABG were given remacemide orally for 4 days preoperatively.[174] A neurocognitive battery was performed 1 week before and 8 weeks after CABG, with a cognitive deficit defined as a decrease in one standard deviation in two or more of the 12 tests within the neurocognitive battery. In addition, an analysis of a global Z score (reflective of overall learning ability) was also evaluated. Although there was no difference between groups with respect to the binary outcome of cognitive deficit ($P = .6$), examination of learning ability showed there was a beneficial cognitive effect to remacemide ($P = .028$). However, despite these positive results, this drug was not further pursued for this indication because of the length of time that it took to perform this single-center trial (a limitation in most single-center trials), initial nonbeneficial preliminary results, and the lengthy period of data analysis and review for publication. This study was instrumental, however, in facilitating other investigations examining other NMDA receptor antagonists during cardiac surgery.[175-178]

Lidocaine

Lidocaine has repeatedly been demonstrated to have neuroprotective properties in various experimental models of cerebral ischemic injury.[179-182] Because of its properties as a sodium channel–blocking agent,[183] its potential anti-inflammatory effects,[184] and widespread clinical experience, it has been recently investigated in several studies as a neuroprotectant in cardiac surgery. In the first reported study of 55 patients undergoing valvular surgery, a lidocaine infusion (1 mg/min) was begun before induction and maintained for 48 hours after surgery.[185] Compared with placebo, neurocognitive outcome 8 days after the surgery was significantly better in patients receiving lidocaine ($P = .025$). The second neuroprotective study ($N = 118$) of lidocaine was reported by Wang and coworkers[186] and similarly demonstrated a benefit. However, the effect was examined on only postoperative day 9, significantly limiting its longer-term applicability. A much larger double-blind randomized trial in cardiac surgery examining cognition at 6 weeks after surgery has failed to replicate these positive findings.[187] Currently, lidocaine cannot be recommended as a clinically effective neuroprotective agent in cardiac surgery.

Beta-Blockers

The use of beta-blockers in patients with cardiac disease has principally been focused on the prevention of adverse myocardial events.[188] However, there is some evidence supporting the use of beta-blockers for noncardiac benefits. In a recent study of neurologic outcomes after cardiac surgery, beta-blockers were demonstrated to be associated with better neurologic outcome.[189] In this nonrandomized retrospective study of nearly 3000 patients, those receiving beta-blocker therapy had a significantly lower incidence of neurologic deficit (stroke and encephalopathy) than those not receiving beta-blockers. Although more rigorous evaluation is needed, there is a plausible basis of this CNS effect. Potential mechanisms by which beta-blockers could be efficacious include the modulation of both cerebrovascular tone and CPB-related inflammatory events.[190,191] More specific potential neuroprotective effects from beta-blockers were demonstrated in a study of carvedilol, known to have not only mixed adrenergic antagonist effects but also antioxidant apoptosis inhibitor properties.[192]

Steroids

Despite a paucity of data on their efficiency, corticosteroids are frequently utilized during CPB. Because of their ability to reduce the inflammatory response, and because inflammation is considered an important factor in propagating ischemia-mediated brain injury, they may indeed have some benefit. Thorough evaluation in this setting, however, has not been performed.[193,194] Furthermore, with the exception of nonthoracic aortic surgery–related spinal cord injury,[195] they have never been demonstrated to possess any significant clinical neuroprotective properties. In fact, in the CRASH

trial ($N = 10,000$), the administration of steroids actually worsened cerebral outcome with an increased relative risk of death (1.18 [95% CI, 1.09-1.27]; $P = .0001$) in those receiving high-dose steroids within 8 hours of closed-head injury.[196,197] It could be speculated that part of their lack of effect may result from the hyperglycemia that generally follows their administration. Hyperglycemia, in animal models and several human studies of cerebral injury, has been associated with worsened neurologic outcome.[107,198]

In the absence of significant supporting data, the argument opposing the routine use of steroids is straightforward. Some of the more concerning data about steroids in cardiac surgery comes from recent well-designed studies associating steroid use to impairments in pulmonary physiology. Many studies have focused on the pathophysiologic mechanism of lung injury after CPB, which appears to be related to the systemic inflammatory response and more specifically represents an inflammatory response of the lungs. It shares similarities with what the American-European Consensus Conference on adult respiratory distress syndrome (ARDS) defined as being a mild form of ARDS or acute lung injury (ALI).[199] The risk and severity of ALI have been linked with the duration of CPB. Steroids were an obvious early and promising therapeutic; however, recent publications have highlighted a perplexing paradox in this regard. That is, steroids decrease inflammation, and inflammation can lead to pulmonary dysfunction, yet steroids actually worsen pulmonary function after CPB.

Chaney and associates, in two separate studies,[119,200] described how the administration of steroids not only led to hyperglycemia, which itself is an unrelated yet difficult problem to treat successfully,[119] but also caused adverse effects relative to post-bypass pulmonary function. Both studies demonstrated either no improvement or worsening in lung compliance, shunt, alveolar-arterial (A-a) oxygen gradient (A-a DO_2), and delays in extubation. These authors speculated that the worsened A-a DO_2 and delayed pulmonary extubation associated with steroid administration was attributable to steroid-induced sodium retention and vasodilation, leading to increased shunt and increased lung water and resulting in pulmonary edema. In a similar recent study, Oliver and colleagues,[201] comparing placebo to either steroids or hemofiltration, noted that the steroid-treated patients had larger increases in postoperative A-a DO_2. Using a preset mechanical ventilation protocol to guide ventilation or weaning, these authors also showed that steroids failed to reduce the time to tracheal extubation (519 ± 293 versus 618 ± 405 min, $P = .21$),[201] confirming the finding of Chaney and associates.[200]

In light of the lack of any demonstrable neurologic benefit, coupled with data suggesting that steroids have an injurious effect in CPB patients, routine use of steroids cannot be recommended in these patients. There is as yet no demonstrable link between this inhibition of inflammation and improved outcome, and the paradox remains.

Pexelizumab

Other targets of the inflammatory cascade, including complement inhibitors, have begun to be investigated.[202] The activation of complement is central to the inflammatory response seen in response to CPB.[106] In a small study ($N = 18$) using a simple assessment of cognitive function, patients receiving an inhibitor to C5 (h5G1.1-scFv; pexelizumab) demonstrated fewer visuospatial deficits at hospital discharge.[203] Further large-scale (phase III) investigations of this compound to more adequately delineate any potential longer-term neuroprotective effects from this drug in this setting have been performed. Mathew and colleagues studied pexelizumab in a 914-patient study aimed at evaluating its effect on both myocardial outcome and mortality.[203] A secondary endpoint of neurocognitive outcome demonstrated that pexelizumab, although it had no effect on global measures of cognition, appeared to have a benefit with respect to the visuospatial domain.

Aprotinin

Aprotinin, first used in the 1950s for the treatment of pancreatitis, is a nonspecific serine protease inhibitor. A widely used drug in cardiac surgery, its current indication is for transfusion and the prevention of blood loss, and although that was the primary reason for its initial clinical use, it has more frequently been used for a perceived neurologic benefit. However, no prospective randomized trials have been conducted to evaluate its potential neuroprotective benefit. Some data do exist, suggesting that it should be evaluated more rigorously.

In a large multicenter trial evaluating the blood loss–reducing effects of aprotinin in patients undergoing primary or redo CABG and valvular surgery, the group receiving a high-dose aprotinin regimen had a lower stroke rate than the group that received placebo ($P = .032$).[204,205] Similarly, Frumento and coworkers retrospectively examined patients at high risk for stroke (due to the presence of significant aortic atheroma); those who received aprotinin had a significantly lower stroke rate.[206] The evidence for a neurocognitive benefit is weak but sufficiently promising to justify further work. In a small study ($N = 36$) examining the effect of aprotinin on cognitive deficit after CABG surgery, the aprotinin group had a reduced incidence of cognitive deficit (58%, aprotinin versus 94% placebo; $P = .01$).[207] However, the excessively high incidence of cognitive deficit in the placebo group, the small size of the study, and methodologic concerns limit the conclusions from that study.[208] Interestingly, animal investigations in the setting of cerebral ischemia failed to show any direct benefit on either functional or neurohistologic outcome after cerebral ischemia.[209] However, there is some evidence of functional benefit after cerebral ischemia superimposed on CPB.[210]

There has been considerable discussion, not necessarily accompanied by evidence-producing study, about the potential mechanism for any aprotinin-derived neuroprotection. Initial interest was based on the possibility that its anti-inflammatory effects might prevent some of the adverse inflammatory sequelae of cerebral ischemia. However, the aprotinin may not have provided a direct neuroprotective effect but instead an indirect effect via modulation of cerebral emboli. Brooker and associates identified the cardiotomy suction as a major source of cerebral emboli during CPB.[35]

By extrapolation, a drug that reduces overall blood loss, and thereby reduces the amount of particulate-containing blood returning from the operative field to the cardiotomy reservoir, might also decrease cerebral emboli (and the resulting neurologic consequences).

Most recently, however, considerable question has been added to the aprotinin picture. Mangano and colleagues reported an actual increase in stroke rate in those receiving aprotinin in a subsequent study that used propensity scoring to adjust for the higher overall risk in patients receiving aprotinin.[211] Further randomized prospective studies will be needed to fully understand the neurologic effects of this drug.

■ OFF-PUMP CARDIAC SURGERY AND BRAIN PROTECTION

Many of the adverse cerebral complications that follow CPB, particularly cognitive loss, have been attributed to the cardiopulmonary bypass itself. However, it has not been shown that elimination of bypass, as seen with off-pump coronary artery bypass (OPCAB), can reduce these complications.[212] Technological advancements (particularly, improved myocardial stabilizing devices, but also in robotics) led to an increase in the use of OPCAB cardiac surgery in the past 5 to 8 years. The increase reached a plateau, and now OPCAB accounts for approximately 20% CABG procedures. Although further exploration with longitudinal prospective randomized clinical trials is needed to find the optimal treatment for coronary disease (with maintenance of long-term graft patency), it is clear that OPCAB and similar operations will always be among the therapeutic options available to patients requiring CABG. Whether they will lead to a reduction in the neurologic complications of cardiac surgery remains unproven in any large-scale studies.

A series of studies have partially addressed the impact of OPCAB surgery on both stroke and neurocognitive outcome.[213] All are too small to offer meaningful information about stroke risk (although most tend toward stroke reduction), but at least two are large enough to provide some meaningful information about cognitive outcome. One of the largest trials comparing OPCAB to conventional CABG surgery was reported by Van Dijk and coworkers, and although the trend is toward a short-term reduction in neurocognitive decline, the trial failed to demonstrate a decrease at 1 year after surgery.[212] The reasons for this are unclear but may reflect the complex pathophysiology of cognitive decline. For example, if inflammatory processes play a role,[214] then OPCAB, which, like conventional CABG surgery, involves sternotomy, heparin administration,[215] and wide hemodynamic swings,[53] may be a significant reason that cognitive dysfunction was still seen. In addition, traditional embolic theories are still at play here, as ascending aortic manipulation, with its ensuing particulate embolization, is still commonly used. In addition, significant hemodynamic compromise due to manipulation of the heart can lead to hypotension that has been associated with significant cerebral desaturation.[216] This type of jugular venous desaturation is similar to that demonstrated by Croughwell and colleagues, who described an association with cognitive decline in patients undergoing conventional on-pump CABG.[217] Even though this was a well-designed and adequate-size study (*N* = 281), it is still probably not large enough to determine subtle differences between the groups, and it is likely that the failure to see a difference at 1 year was related to a consequent lack of statistical power.[52]

Recently, Al-Ruzzeh and coworkers also examined the issue of potential neurocognitive benefits of OPCAB over on-pump CABG.[218] In their study (*N* = 168), patients were given not only a thorough neurocognitive assessment but also an angiographic assessment of their coronary anastomosis. Patients in the OPCAB group showed a reduction in cognitive loss up to 6 months postoperatively, and, importantly, the authors demonstrated that using the off-pump technique did not compromise the quality of the coronary grafting.

The divergent results of the van Dijk and Al-Ruzzeh trials have left unanswered the question of neurocognitive benefit to OPCAB. The results of further large prospective studies will help determine whether off-pump procedures have lower neurologic complications, and to which patient population this procedure should be targeted. At the present time, the data are insufficient to determine whether there is any neurologic benefit to OPCAB surgery.

PROTECTING THE SPINAL CORD DURING THORACIC AORTIC SURGERY

Surgery on the descending thoracic aorta involves numerous risks to the patient. One of the most devastating complications is spinal cord ischemic injury. When the thoracic aorta is cross-clamped during the procedure to allow the placement of an interposition graft, blood flow to the spinal cord may be transiently interrupted; if intercostal arteries are ligated, it is often permanently interrupted. The resulting ischemia can lead to permanent damage to the spinal cord, particularly in the region of the anterior motor neurons. As a result of this ischemic injury, variable degrees of paraparesis occur. The incidence of paraplegia varies from 2% to 21% or more, depending on the individual patient's risk and on the acuity of the problem requiring surgery.[219-221] For example, the risk is higher for acute dissections requiring emergency surgery in a patient with significant vascular disease than for simple coarctation repair in a young patient.

A number of protective strategies have been used to prevent paraplegia in these patients[222-224] (Box 22-2). They include manipulation of spinal cord hydrodynamics (cerebral spinal fluid [CSF] pressure), distal perfusion techniques, and a number of pharmacologic strategies.[225] The relative efficacy of each in protecting the spinal cord will be discussed.

Because relatively few patients present for these procedures (less than a few thousand patients per year), rigorous prospective randomized double-blind trials of these techniques have been difficult to undertake. As a result, the data supporting any particular technique are somewhat scant and often rely on comparisons with historical controls. However, several lines of evidence can be followed to assess their efficacies.

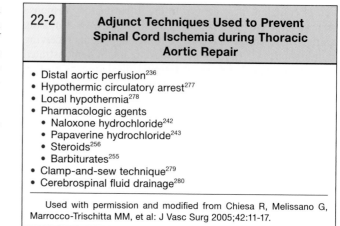

22-2	**Adjunct Techniques Used to Prevent Spinal Cord Ischemia during Thoracic Aortic Repair**

- Distal aortic perfusion[236]
- Hypothermic circulatory arrest[277]
- Local hypothermia[278]
- Pharmacologic agents
  - Naloxone hydrochloride[242]
  - Papaverine hydrochloride[243]
  - Steroids[256]
  - Barbiturates[255]
- Clamp-and-sew technique[279]
- Cerebrospinal fluid drainage[280]

Used with permission and modified from Chiesa R, Melissano G, Marrocco-Trischitta MM, et al: J Vasc Surg 2005;42:11-17.

Distal Perfusion Techniques

Distal perfusion techniques are used to optimize the proximal hemodynamics during the cross-clamp phase and to increase distal perfusion pressure to the arteries that supply nutrients to the spinal cord. Other bypass techniques that have been used include left atrial-to-femoral artery bypass, various shunts,[226] and full femoral-to-femoral CPB.

Following the rationale that distal perfusion techniques provide blood flow to patent arteries distal to the aortic cross-clamp, and that in so doing they provide nutrient blood flow to the spinal cord, a number of techniques have been used to maintain this distal blood flow. Initial attempts at providing distal perfusion included the use of Gott shunts, which provided passive blood flow to the distal aorta.[226] Although used with variable success, these techniques typically resulted in lower distal perfusion pressures than desired. As a result, more active techniques including left atrial–femoral[227-232] and full femoral–femoral artery bypass[233-235] were used. In addition to providing adequate distal perfusion, these bypass techniques also help maintain blood flow to the mesentery and to distal extremities and as a result can prevent some of the metabolic acidosis that can occur in "clamp and sew" situations. When desired, the integration of heat exchangers helps to prevent intraoperative hypothermia, although disadvantages include a potentially prolonged operative time to place them and a requirement for substantial systemic heparinization and the resultant risk of trauma-related bleeding.

One difficulty in evaluating case series that address different distal perfusion techniques is the tendency to use these more complex techniques for more complex and extensive aneurysms. Such aneurysms have a higher rate of spinal cord ischemia, making the association between the distal perfusion techniques and paraplegia one that is very likely neither causative (in the case of worse paraplegia) nor preventive (in the case of significant spinal cord protection). One of the largest series to date was reported by Coselli and colleagues.[236] In this long-term study (387 consecutive patients over a 15-year period), two thoracic aortic aneurysm repair techniques were compared: clamp-and-sew technique versus left heart bypass techniques. Although the study is significantly limited by being retrospective, left heart bypass did not provide any significant reduction in the risk of paraplegia over the clamp-and-sew technique. Indeed, the most important factors associated with the high incidence of paraplegia were advanced age, increased aortic cross-clamp time, acute dissection, and an increasing need for red blood cell transfusion. From this study, it appears that no strong recommendation regarding the use, or, for that matter, the avoidance, of left heart bypass techniques can be made.

Cerebrospinal Fluid Drainage

One of the techniques used extensively in some centers involves draining variable amounts of CSF just prior to and during cross-clamping of the aorta.[237-240] This involves placing a large (14-gauge) epidural needle into the intrathecal space and advancing a 5- to 15-cm catheter into the CSF space. With the subsequent drainage of CSF (to maintain optimal spinal cord perfusion pressure and a CSF pressure of ideally <10 mm Hg), spinal cord perfusion is optimized. This technique has received more rigorous prospective evaluation than any other and yet the data are still not sufficient to suggest that this should be used in all patients. However, this technique may be warranted in some subset of patients. The study of any particular spinal cord protective technique is significantly limited by patient variability and by the low number of patients who present for treatment. Nonetheless, the best information about CSF drainage comes from a study by Coselli and associates.[241] In this prospective trial, 145 patients were randomized to having CSF drainage or no CSF drainage. The operative strategy in these patients included moderate heparinization, permissive mild hypothermia, the use of left heart bypass, and the reattachment of critical intercostal arteries, and the CSF drainage was considered an adjunct to these other techniques. Paraplegia or paraparesis developed in 13% of the control patients but in only 2.6% of the patients in the CSF drainage group ($P = .03$). Overall, the CSF drainage resulted in an 80% reduction in the relative risk of postoperative spinal cord ischemic deficits. On the basis of this study and other reported case series, this continues to be a widely used technique.[242-247]

Hypothermia

Hypothermia has been used to protect the myocardium during cardiac surgery, and it has been used (but with limited supporting data, as previously mentioned) in an attempt to protect the brain during CPB. It has also been used in various forms to protect the spinal cord during thoracic aortic surgery. Varying degrees of hypothermia have been used, from the mild permissive hypothermia of a few degrees, to, at one extreme, deep hypothermic circulatory arrest. In addition, regional cooling techniques have been used, including the administration of cold epidural saline.

Prospective randomized data are generally not available to help determine which, if any, of these techniques should be used. Because this surgery involves exposure of large skin and body-cavity surface area to the environment, some degree of hypothermia is unavoidable, and this type of permissive hypothermia is recommended by several authors.[243,248] Extensive aneurysms have been repaired under DHCA, a

technique recommended by Kouchoukos and associates.[249] However, there are no randomized data evaluating the efficacy of DHCA. With respect to regional hypothermia of the spinal cord, Cambria and colleagues[250] reported a technique involving epidural injection of iced saline. In this study comparing regional hypothermia to historical controls, the rate of ischemia in the regional perfusion was 7%, compared with 18.5% in the historical controls ($P = .003$). Again, because this study was retrospective, it is difficult to make definitive conclusions. Furthermore, and unexpectedly for a technique used to protect the spinal cord, this regional perfusion led to very high CSF pressure, which could itself have significant disadvantages.

Neuroanesthesia Adjuncts

A number of neuroanesthetic adjuncts[251] have been used experimentally, including the induction of mild hyperventilation (to a $PaCO_2$ of 30 to 32 mm Hg), and the intravenous administration of mannitol (2.0 g/kg). No clinical studies have been performed specifically using these regimens, but because of their wide availability and ease of use, they are discussed here. There are physiologic reasons for their possible effectiveness, as follows. One consequence of cross-clamping the thoracic aorta is a tremendous increase in intracranial pressure (ICP) because of the redistribution of vascular volume into the central vascular compartment with a subsequent increase in CVP. Hyperventilation causes a reduction in cerebral blood flow and volume. The intracranial compartment contents become smaller, resulting in a lower ICP. As a result, the CSF pressure is lowered, with a resultant increase in spinal cord perfusion pressure. Similar hemodynamic adjuncts have been used, including the modest use of phlebotomy to try to offset the increase in CVP and to optimize spinal cord perfusion pressure.[252] These techniques have the significant advantage of being noninvasive, as opposed to the placement of a CSF drain, which may increase the risk of central neuraxial hematoma.

Pharmacologic Spinal Cord Protection

Although many pharmacologic approaches have been used in experimental settings of spinal cord ischemia for aortic surgery,[225,253] few have been investigated clinically, and none are sufficiently efficacious to warrant recommendation. Methylprednisolone has been shown to lessen neurologic dysfunction in the setting of direct spinal cord injury,[195,254] but this was not in the setting of thoracic aortic surgery. No similar clinical trials of steroid use in thoracic aorta cross-clamping have been performed.

In the setting of CPB, more than two dozen pharmacologic agents have been studied in clinical trials, but few have been clinically studied for the prevention of spinal cord injury. A number of agents have been used in experimental models (deferoxamine, allopurinol, superoxide dismutase, mimetics, and barbiturates), but none of these has entered the clinical trials arena.[255,256] In addition, NMDA-receptor antagonists such as raluzole[257] and memantine,[258] as well as magnesium sulfates have been evaluated in animals.[259] Several inhibitors of the inflammatory response have also been used including methylprednisolone,[260] as well as the synthetic steroid tirilazad, which is a 21-amino-steroid that has also been used experimentally.[256,261] The anti-inflammatory effects of prostaglandin E_1,[262] as well as activated protein C,[263] have also been examined. Finally, agonism of the adenosine A_2A receptor has also been investigated experimentally with some promising results, but no clinical trial has been forthcoming.[264]

The only drugs that have been trialed clinically have been papaverine hydrochloride[243] and naloxone hydrochloride.[242] In summary, the clinical data are insufficient to recommend any particular pharmacologic strategy for the protection of spinal cord injury.

Endovascular Stent Repair of the Thoracic Aorta

As minimal-access techniques and less invasive approaches continue to flourish in all sectors of cardiac surgery, less invasive approaches to repair the thoracic aorta are also being developed.[265] The devices and techniques of these procedures continue to evolve, and the ability of endovascular approaches to reduce spinal cord ischemia has been evaluated.[222,265-268]

Spinal cord ischemia after endovascular thoracic aortic repair, although less common than after open procedures, remains a significant risk.[265] Overall incidences of spinal cord ischemia with this less invasive approach have been reported from 0% to −12%.[219,221,222,266,269-273] The pathophysiology of spinal cord ischemia after endovascular repair appears unique in that in the absence of aortic cross-clamping, the hemodynamic and consequent CSF hydrodynamic effects, are unlikely to be contributing factors. The exclusion of intercostal arteries originating within or near the aneurysm by the overlying of the endograft appears to play a critical role.[267]

Patients with previous or concomitant abdominal aortic repair appear to be at particularly high risk because the ligation of arteries in that procedure results in a marginal blood supply. In addition, occlusion of the subclavian artery may compromise vertebral artery collateral contributions to the anterior spinal artery. In a case series by Baril and coworkers,[267] of 125 patients who underwent endovascular repair of the thoracic aorta, 14.3% who had had previous abdominal aortic repair developed spinal cord ischemia, compared with 1.0% of the remaining patients. Delayed (>3 days) onset of ischemia was a common finding, more so than in open repairs.[274,275] In a series of 186 patients reported by Criado and coworkers, eight patients (4.3%) developed ischemia, and half of these developed delayed-onset ischemia.[266]

Although reports in the literature are increasing, these case series still represent weak data for drawing any evidenced-based conclusions about spinal cord risk or protection. It is unclear whether spinal cord protection techniques used in open procedures should be applied to closed procedures.

■ REFERENCES

1. Grocott HP, Homi HM, Puskas F: Cognitive dysfunction after cardiac surgery: Revisiting etiology. Semin Cardiothorac Vasc Anesth 2005;9: 123-129.
2. Grocott HP, Arrowsmith JE: Serum S100 protein as a marker of cerebral damage during cardiac surgery. Br J Anaesth 2001;86: 289-290.
3. Hogue CW Jr, Palin CA, Arrowsmith JE: Cardiopulmonary bypass management and neurologic outcomes: An evidence-based appraisal of current practices. Anesth Analg 2006;103:21-37.
4. Wolman RL, Nussmeier NA, Aggarwal A, et al: Cerebral injury after cardiac surgery: Identification of a group at extraordinary risk. Stroke 1999;30:514-522.
5. Newman MF, Kirchner JL, Phillips-Bute B, et al: Longitudinal assessment of neurocognitive function after coronary artery bypass surgery. N Engl J Med 2001;344:395-402.
6. Nussmeier N: Adverse neurologic events: Risks of intracardiac versus extracardiac surgery. J Cardiothorac Vasc Anesth 1996;10: 31-37.
7. Roach GW, Kanchuger M, Mangano CM, et al: Adverse cerebral outcomes after coronary bypass surgery. N Engl J Med 1996;335: 1857-1863.
8. Newman MF, Grocott HP, Mathew JP, et al: Report of the substudy assessing the impact of neurocognitive function on quality of life 5 years after cardiac surgery. Stroke 2001;32:2874-2881.
9. Boodhwani M, Rubens FD, Wozny D, et al: Predictors of early neurocognitive deficits in low-risk patients undergoing on-pump coronary artery bypass surgery. Circulation 2006;114:I461-466.
10. Arrowsmith JE, Grocott HP, Reves JG, et al: Central nervous system complications of cardiac surgery. Br J Anaesth 2000;84: 378-393.
11. Newman MF, Croughwell ND, Blumenthal JA, et al: Effect of aging on cerebral autoregulation during cardiopulmonary bypass: Association with postoperative cognitive dysfunction. Circulation 1994;90: II243-249.
12. Newman MF, Wolman R, Kanchuger M, et al: Circulation 1996;94: II74-80.
13. Cosgrove D, Loop F, Lytle B, et al: Primary myocardial revascularizations. J Thorac Cardiovasc Surg 1984;88:673-684.
14. Gardner TJ, Horneffer PJ, Gott VL, et al: Coronary artery bypass grafting in women: A ten-year perspective. Ann Surg 1985;201: 780-784.
15. Newman M, Kramer D, Croughwell N, et al: Differential age effects of mean arterial pressure and rewarming on cognitive dysfunction after cardiac surgery. Anesth Analg 1995;81:236-242.
16. Tuman KJ, McCarthy RJ, Najafi H, et al: Differential effects of advanced age on neurologic and cardiac risks of coronary artery operations. J Thorac Cardiovasc Surg 1992;104:1510-1517.
17. Amarenco P, Duyckaerts C, Tzourio C, et al: The prevalence of ulcerated plaques in the aortic arch in patients with stroke. N Engl J Med 1992;1992:221-225.
18. Hogue CW Jr, De Wet CJ, Schechtman KB, et al: The importance of prior stroke for the adjusted risk of neurologic injury after cardiac surgery for women and men. Anesthesiology 2003;98:823-829.
19. Martin WR, Hashimoto SA: Stroke in coronary bypass surgery. Can J Neurol Sci 1982;9:21-26.
20. Sotaniemi K: Brain damage and neurological outcome after open-heart surgery. J Neurol Neurosurg Psychiatry 1980;43:127-135.
21. Turnipseed WD, Berkoff HA, Belzer FO: Postoperative stroke in cardiac and peripheral vascular disease. Ann Surg 1980;192: 365-368.
22. Breslau PJ, Fell G, Ivey TD, et al: Carotid arterial disease in patients undergoing coronary artery bypass operations. J Thorac Cardiovasc Surg 1981;82:765-767.
23. Brener BJ, Brief DK, Alpert J, et al: The risk of stroke in patients with asymptomatic carotid stenosis undergoing cardiac surgery: A follow-up study. J Vasc Surg 1987;5:269-279.
24. Blauth CI, Cosgrove DM, Webb BW, et al: Atheroembolism from the ascending aorta: An emerging problem in cardiac surgery. J Thorac Cardiovasc Surg 1992;103:1104-1111; discussion 1111-1102.
25. Blumenthal J, Mahanna E, Madden D, et al: Methodological issues in the assessment of neuropsychologic function after cardiac surgery. Ann Thorac Surg 1995;59:1345-1350.
26. Borowicz L, Goldsborough M, Selenes O, et al: Neuropsychological changes after cardiac surgery: A critical review. J Cardiothorac Vasc Anesth 1996;10:105-112.

27. Branthwaite MA: Neurological damage related to open-heart surgery: A clinical survey. Thorax 1972;27:748-753.

28. Harris LS, Kennedy JH: Atheromatous cerebral embolism: A complication of surgery of the thoracic aorta. Ann Thorac Surg 1967;4: 319-326.

29. Barbut D, Lo YW, Hartman GS, et al: Aortic atheroma is related to outcome but not numbers of emboli during coronary bypass. Ann Thorac Surg 1997;64:454-459.

30. Davila-Roman VG, Barzilai B, Wareing TH, et al: Intraoperative ultrasonographic evaluation of the ascending aorta in 100 consecutive patients undergoing cardiac surgery. Circulation 1991;84:III47-53.

31. Hartman GS, Yao FS, Bruefach M 3rd, et al: Severity of aortic atheromatous disease diagnosed by transesophageal echocardiography predicts stroke and other outcomes associated with coronary artery surgery: A prospective study. Anesth Analg 1996;83:701-708.

32. Katz ES, Tunick PA, Rusinek H, et al: Protruding aortic atheromas predict stroke in elderly patients undergoing cardiopulmonary bypass: Experience with intraoperative transesophageal echocardiography. J Am Coll Cardiol 1992;20:70-77.

33. Cheng MA, Theard MA, Tempelhoff R: Intravenous agents and intraoperative neuroprotection: Beyond barbiturates. Crit Care Clin 1997;13:185-199.

34. Moody DM, Brown WR, Challa VR, et al: Brain microemboli associated with cardiopulmonary bypass: A histologic and magnetic resonance imaging study. Ann Thorac Surg 1995;59:1304-1307.

35. Brooker RF, Brown WR, Moody DM, et al: Cardiotomy suction: A major source of brain lipid emboli during cardiopulmonary bypass. Ann Thorac Surg 1998;65:1651-1655.

36. Stump D, Rogers A, Hammon J, et al: Cerebral emboli and cognitive outcome after cardiac surgery. J Cardiothorac Vasc Anesth 1996;10: 113-119.

37. Stump DA, Kon NA, Rogers AT, et al: Emboli and neuropsychological outcome following cardiopulmonary bypass. Echocardiography 1996;13:555-558.

38. Pugsley W, Klinger L, Paschalis C, et al: Microemboli and cerebral impairment during cardiac surgery. Vasc Surg 1990;24:34-43.

39. Tegeler CH, Babikian VL, Gomez CR: Neurosonology. St Louis, Mosby, 1996.

40. Markus HS, Punter M: Can transcranial Doppler discriminate between solid and gaseous microemboli? Assessment of a dual-frequency transducer system. Stroke 2005;36:1731-1734.

41. Mackinnon AD, Aaslid R, Markus HS: Ambulatory transcranial Doppler cerebral embolic signal detection in symptomatic and asymptomatic carotid stenosis. Stroke 2005;36:1726-1730.

42. Djaiani G, Fedorko L, Borger M, et al: Mild to moderate atheromatous disease of the thoracic aorta and new ischemic brain lesions after conventional coronary artery bypass graft surgery. Stroke 2004;35: e356-358.

43. Davila-Roman VG, Murphy SF, Nickerson NJ, et al: Atherosclerosis of the ascending aorta is an independent predictor of long-term neurologic events and mortality. J Am Coll Cardiol 1999;33:1308-1316.

44. Amarenco P, Cohen A, Tzourio C, et al: Atherosclerotic disease of the aortic arch and the risk of ischemic stroke. N Engl J Med 1994;331:1474-1479.

45. Bar-Yosef S, Anders M, Mackensen GB, et al: Aortic atheroma burden and cognitive dysfunction after coronary artery bypass graft surgery. Ann Thorac Surg 2004;78:1556-1562; discussion 1562-1553.

46. Royse AG, Royse CF, Ajani AE, et al: Reduced neuropsychological dysfunction using epiaortic echocardiography and the exclusive Y graft. Ann Thorac Surg 2000;69:1431-1438.

47. Mackensen GB, Ti LK, Phillips-Bute BG, et al: Cerebral embolization during cardiac surgery: Impact of aortic atheroma burden. Br J Anaesth 2003;91:656-661.

48. Nussmeier N, Arlund A, Slogoff S: Neuropsychiatric complications after cardiopulmonary bypass: Cerebral protection by a barbiturate. Anesthesiology 1986;64:165-170.

49. Newman M, Murkin J, Roach G, et al: Cerebral physiologic effects of burst suppression doses of propofol during nonpulsatile cardiopulmonary bypass. Anesth Analg 1995;81:452-457.

50. Gold JP, Charlson ME, Williams-Russo P, et al: Improvement of outcomes after coronary artery bypass. J Thorac Cardiovasc Surg 1995;110:1302-1314.

51. Mutch W, Lefevre G, Thiessen D, et al: Computer-controlled cardiopulmonary bypass increases jugular venous oxygen saturation during rewarming. Ann Thorac Surg 1998;65:59-65.

52. Mark DB, Newman MF: Protecting the brain in coronary artery bypass graft surgery. JAMA 2002;287:1448-1450.

53. Murkin JM: Hemodynamic changes during cardiac manipulation in off-CPB surgery: Relevance in brain perfusion. Heart Surg Forum 2002;5:221-224.

54. Grigore AM, Grocott HP, Mathew JP, et al: The rewarming rate and increased peak temperature alter neurocognitive outcome after cardiac surgery. Anesth Analg 2002;94:4-10.

55. Grocott HP, Mackensen GB, Grigore AM, et al: Postoperative hyperthermia is associated with cognitive dysfunction after coronary artery bypass graft surgery. Stroke 2002;33:537-541.

56. Thong WY, Strickler AG, Li S, et al: Hyperthermia in the forty-eight hours after cardiopulmonary bypass. Anesth Analg 2002;95: 1489-1495.

57. Gerriets T, Stolz E, Walberer M, et al: Neuroprotective effects of MK-801 in different rat stroke models for permanent middle cerebral artery occlusion: Adverse effects of hypothalamic damage and strategies for its avoidance. Stroke 2003;34:2234-2239.

58. Grocott HP, Stafford-Smith M: Organ protection during cardiopulmonary bypass. In Kaplan JA, Reich DL, Lake CL, et al (eds): Cardiac Anesthesia, ed 5. Philadelphia, Elsevier, 2006, pp 985-1022.

59. Pintar T, Collard CD: The systemic inflammatory response to cardiopulmonary bypass. Anesthesiol Clin North America 2003;21: 453-464.

60. Hindman BJ, Moore SA, Cutkomp J, et al: Brain expression of inducible cyclooxygenase 2 messenger RNA in rats undergoing cardiopulmonary bypass. Anesthesiology 2001;95:1380-1388.

61. Bogdanski R, Blobner M, Becker I, et al: Cerebral histopathology following portal venous infusion of bacteria in a chronic porcine model. Anesthesiology 2000;93:793-804.

62. Chamorro A: Role of inflammation in stroke and atherothrombosis. Cerebrovasc Dis 2004;17(Suppl 3):1-5.

63. Mathew JP, Grocott HP, Phillips-Bute B, et al: Lower endotoxin immunity predicts increased cognitive dysfunction in elderly patients after cardiac surgery. Stroke 2003;34:508-513.

64. Hamilton-Davies C, Barclay GR, Cardigan RA, et al: Relationship between preoperative endotoxin immune status, gut perfusion, and outcome from cardiac valve replacement surgery. Chest 1997;112: 1189-1196.

65. Nakamura K, Ueno T, Yamamoto H, et al: Relationship between cerebral injury and inflammatory responses in patients undergoing cardiac surgery with cardiopulmonary bypass. Cytokine 2005;29: 95-104.

66. Mathew JP, Grocott HP, Podgoreanu MV, et al: Inflammatory and prothrombotic genetic polymorphisms are associated with cognitive decline after CABG surgery. Anesthesiology 2004;101:A274.

67. Culley DJ, Baxter M, Yukhananov R, et al: The memory effects of general anesthesia persist for weeks in young and aged rats. Anesth Analg 2003;96:1004-1009.

68. Jevtovic-Todorovic V, Beals J, Benshoff N, et al: Prolonged exposure to inhalational anesthetic nitrous oxide kills neurons in adult rat brain. Neuroscience 2003;122:609-616.

69. Futterer CD, Maurer MH, Schmitt A, et al: Alterations in rat brain proteins after desflurane anesthesia. Anesthesiology 2004;100: 302-308.

70. Kandel ER, Schwartz JH, Jessell TM: Principles of Neural Science, ed 3. Norwalk, Conn, Appleton and Lange, 1991.

71. Gillinov AM, Davis EA, Curtis WE, et al: Cardiopulmonary bypass and the blood-brain barrier: An experimental study. J Thorac Cardiovasc Surg 1992;104:1110-1115.

72. Bokesch PM, Cavaglia M, Dombrowski S, et al: Cardiopulmonary bypass causes dysfunction of the blood brain barrier. Anesthesiology 2002:A-1282.

73. Harris D, Oatridge A, Dob D, et al: Cerebral swelling after normothermic cardiopulmonary bypass. Anesthesiology 1998;88: 340-345.

74. Saunders A, Strittmatter W, Schmechel D, et al: Association of apolipoprotein E allele epsilon 4 with late-onset familial and sporadic Alzheimer's disease. Neurology 1993;43:1467-1472.

75. Tardiff BE, Newman MF, Saunders AM, et al: Preliminary report of a genetic basis for cognitive decline after cardiac operations. Ann Thorac Surg 1997;64:715-720.

76. Gaynor JW, Gerdes M, Zackai EH, et al: Apolipoprotein E genotype and neurodevelopmental sequelae of infant cardiac surgery. J Thorac Cardiovasc Surg 2003;126:1736-1745.

77. Barakat K, Kennon S, Hitman GA, et al: Interaction between smoking and the glycoprotein IIIa P1(A2) polymorphism in non-ST-elevation acute coronary syndromes. J Am Coll Cardiol 2001;38:1639-1643.

78. Kenny D, Muckian C, Fitzgerald DJ, et al: Platelet glycoprotein Ib alpha receptor polymorphisms and recurrent ischaemic events in acute coronary syndrome patients. J Thromb Thrombolysis 2002;13:13-19.

79. Mathew JP, Rinder CS, Howe JG, et al: Platelet PlA2 polymorphism enhances risk of neurocognitive decline after cardiopulmonary bypass. Multicenter Study of Perioperative Ischemia (McSPI) Research Group. Ann Thorac Surg 2001;71:663-666.

80. Grocott HP, White WD, Morris RW, et al: Genetic polymorphisms and the risk of stroke after cardiac surgery. Stroke 2005;36:1854-1858.

81. Stafford-Smith M, Podgoreanu M, Swaminathan M, et al: Association of genetic polymorphisms with risk of renal injury after coronary bypass graft surgery. Am J Kidney Dis 2005;45:519-530.

82. Welsby IJ, Podgoreanu MV, Phillips-Bute B, et al: Genetic factors contribute to bleeding after cardiac surgery. J Thromb Haemost 2005;3:1206-1212.

83. Lapietra A, Grossi EA, Pua BB, et al: Assisted venous drainage presents the risk of undetected air microembolism. J Thorac Cardiovasc Surg 2000;120:856-862.

84. Webb WR, Harrison LH Jr, Helmcke FR, et al: Carbon dioxide field flooding minimizes residual intracardiac air after open heart operations. Ann Thorac Surg 1997;64:1489-1491.

85. Svenarud P, Persson M, van der Linden J: Effect of CO_2 insufflation on the number and behavior of air microemboli in open-heart surgery: A randomized clinical trial. Circulation 2004;109:1127-1132.

86. Borger MA, Peniston CM, Weisel RD, et al: Neuropsychologic impairment after coronary bypass surgery: Effect of gaseous microemboli during perfusionist interventions. J Thorac Cardiovasc Surg 2001;121:743-749.

87. Borger MA, Taylor RL, Weisel RD, et al: Decreased cerebral emboli during distal aortic arch cannulation: A randomized clinical trial. J Thorac Cardiovasc Surg 1999;118:740-745.

88. Cook DJ, Zehr KJ, Orszulak TA, et al: Profound reduction in brain embolization using an endoaortic baffle during bypass in swine. Ann Thorac Surg 2002;73:198-202.

89. Reichenspurner H, Navia JA, Berry G, et al: Particulate emboli capture by an intra-aortic filter device during cardiac surgery. J Thorac Cardiovasc Surg 2000;119:233-241.

90. Banbury MK, Kouchoukos NT, Allen KB, et al: Emboli capture using the Embol-X intraaortic filter in cardiac surgery: A multicentered randomized trial of 1,289 patients. Ann Thorac Surg 2003;76:508-515; discussion 515.

91. Eifert S, Reichenspurner H, Pfefferkorn T, et al: Neurological and neuropsychological examination and outcome after use of an intraaortic filter device during cardiac surgery. Perfusion 2003;18(Suppl 1):55-60.

92. Aldea GS, Soltow LO, Chandler WL, et al: Limitation of thrombin generation, platelet activation, and inflammation by elimination of cardiotomy suction in patients undergoing coronary artery bypass grafting treated with heparin-bonded circuits. J Thorac Cardiovasc Surg 2002;123:742-755.

93. Murkin J, Martzke J, Buchan A, et al: A randomized study of the influence of perfusion technique and pH management strategy in 316 patients undergoing coronary artery bypass surgery. J Thorac Cardiovasc Surg 1995;110:349-362.

94. Kawahara F, Kadoi Y, Saito S, et al: Balloon pump-induced pulsatile perfusion during cardiopulmonary bypass does not improve brain oxygenation. J Thorac Cardiovasc Surg 1999;118:361-366.

95. Patel RL, Turtle MR, Chambers DJ, et al: Alpha-stat acid-base regulation during cardiopulmonary bypass improves neuropsychologic outcome in patients undergoing coronary artery bypass grafting. J Thorac Cardiovasc Surg 1996;111:1267-1279.

96. Duebener LF, Hagino I, Sakamoto T, et al: Effects of pH management during deep hypothermic bypass on cerebral microcirculation: Alpha-stat versus pH-stat. Circulation 2002;106:I103-108.

97. Laussen PC: Optimal blood gas management during deep hypothermic paediatric cardiac surgery: Alpha-stat is easy, but pH-stat may be preferable. Paediatr Anaesth 2002;12:199-204.

98. Lanier WL: Glucose management during cardiopulmonary bypass: Cardiovascular and neurologic implications. Anesth Analg 1991;72:423-427.

99. Dietrich WD, Alonso O, Busto R: Moderate hyperglycemia worsens acute blood-brain barrier injury after forebrain ischemia in rats. Stroke 1993;24:111-116.

100. Siesjö B: Acidosis and ischemic brain damage. Neurochem Pathol 1988;9:31-88.

101. Warner DS, Gionet TX, Todd MM, et al: Insulin-induced normoglycemia improves ischemic outcome in hyperglycemic rats. Stroke 1992;22:1775-1781.

102. Feerick AE, Johnston WE, Jenkins LW, et al: Hyperglycemia during hypothermic canine cardiopulmonary bypass increases cerebral lactate. Anesthesiology 1995;82:512-520.

103. Kinoshita K, Kraydieh S, Alonso O, et al: Effect of posttraumatic hyperglycemia on contusion volume and neutrophil accumulation after moderate fluid-percussion brain injury in rats. J Neurotrauma 2002;19:681-692.

104. Visser L, Zuurbier CJ, Hoek FJ, et al: Glucose, insulin and potassium applied as perioperative hyperinsulinaemic normoglycaemic clamp: Effects on inflammatory response during coronary artery surgery. Br J Anaesth 2005;95:448-457.

105. Bourbon A, Vionnet M, Leprince P, et al: The effect of methylprednisolone treatment on the cardiopulmonary bypass-induced systemic inflammatory response. Eur J Cardiothorac Surg 2004;26:932-938.

106. Levy JH, Tanaka KA: Inflammatory response to cardiopulmonary bypass. Ann Thorac Surg 2003;75:S715-720.

107. Lam A, Winn H, Cullen B, et al: Hyperglycemia and neurological outcome in patients with head injury. J Neurosurg 1991;75:545-551.

108. Li PA, Shuaib A, Miyashita H, et al: Hyperglycemia enhances extracellular glutamate accumulation in rats subjected to forebrain ischemia. Stroke 2000;31:183-192.

109. Rao N, Schilling D, Rice J, et al: Prevention of postoperative mediastinitis: A clinical process improvement model. J Healthc Qual 2004;26:22-27.

110. Guvener M, Pasaoglu I, Demircin M, et al: Perioperative hyperglycemia is a strong correlate of postoperative infection in type II diabetic patients after coronary artery bypass grafting. Endocr J 2002;49:531-537.

111. Lazar HL, Chipkin SR, Fitzgerald CA, et al: Tight glycemic control in diabetic coronary artery bypass graft patients improves perioperative outcomes and decreases recurrent ischemic events. Circulation 2004;109:1497-1502.

112. Metz S, Keats AS: Benefits of a glucose-containing priming solution for cardiopulmonary bypass. Anesth Analg 1991;72:428-434.

113. Hindman B: Con: Glucose priming solutions should not be used for cardiopulmonary bypass. J Cardiothorac Vasc Anesth 1995;9:605-607.

114. Nussmeier N, Marino M, Cooper J, et al: Use of glucose-containing prime is not a risk factor for cerebral injury or infection in nondiabetic or diabetic patients having CABG procedures. Anesthesiology 1999;91:A122.

115. Hill SE, van Wermeskerken GK, Lardenoye JW, et al: Intraoperative physiologic variables and outcome in cardiac surgery: Part I. In-hospital mortality. Ann Thorac Surg 2000;69:1070-1075; discussion 1075-1076.

116. van Wermeskerken GK, Lardenoye JW, Hill SE, et al: Intraoperative physiologic variables and outcome in cardiac surgery: Part II. Neurologic outcome. Ann Thorac Surg 2000;69:1077-1083.

117. Puskas F, Grocott HP, White WD, et al: Hyperglycemia and increased incidence of cognitive deficit after cardiac surgery. Anesth Analg 2005;100:SCA19.

118. Butterworth J, Wagenknecht LE, Legault C, et al: Attempted control of hyperglycemia during cardiopulmonary bypass fails to improve neurologic or neurobehavioral outcomes in patients without diabetes

mellitus undergoing coronary artery bypass grafting. J Thorac Cardiovasc Surg 2005;130:1319.

119. Chaney MA, Nikolov MP, Blakeman BP, et al: Attempting to maintain normoglycemia during cardiopulmonary bypass with insulin may initiate postoperative hypoglycemia. Anesth Analg 1999;89: 1091-1095.

120. Carvalho G, Moore A, Qizilbash B, et al: Maintenance of normoglycemia during cardiac surgery. Anesth Analg 2004;99:319-324.

121. Green A, White WD, Grocott H, et al: Hypotension during cardiopulmonary bypass is not associated with cognitive decline after CABG: Anesth Analg 2006;102:SCA39.

122. Bendszus M, Reents W, Franke D, et al: Brain damage after coronary artery bypass grafting. Arch Neurol 2002;59:1090-1095.

123. Plochl W, Liam BL, Cook DJ, Orszulak TA: Cerebral response to haemodilution during cardiopulmonary bypass in dogs: The role of nitric oxide synthase. Br J Anaesth 1999;82:237-243.

124. Govier AV, Reves JG, McKay RD, et al: Factors and their influence on regional cerebral blood flow during nonpulsatile cardiopulmonary bypass. Ann Thorac Surg 1984;38:592-600.

125. Newman MF, Croughwell ND, White WD, et al: Effect of perfusion pressure on cerebral blood flow during normothermic cardiopulmonary bypass. Circulation 1996;94:II353-357.

126. Barry DI, Strandgaard S, Graham DI, et al: Cerebral blood flow in rats with renal and spontaneous hypertension: Resetting of the lower limit of autoregulation. J Cereb Blood Flow Metab 1982;2: 347-353.

127. Michenfelder J, Milde J: The relationship among canine brain temperature, metabolism, and function during hypothermia. Anesthesiology 1991;75:130-136.

128. Busto R, Globus M, Dietrich W, et al: Effect of mild hypothermia on ischemia-induced release of neurotransmitters and free fatty acids in rat brain. Stroke 1989;20:904-910.

129. Bickler PE, Buck LT, Hansen BM: Effects of isoflurane and hypothermia on glutamate receptor-mediated calcium influx in brain slices. Anesthesiology 1994;81:1461-1469.

130. Widmann R, Miyazawa T, Hossmann K: Protective effect of hypothermia on hippocampal injury after 30 minutes of forebrain ischemia in rats is mediated by postischemic recovery of protein synthesis. J Neurochem 1993;61:200-209.

131. Busto R, Globus M, Neary J, et al: Regional alterations of protein kinase C activity following transient cerebral ischemia: Effects of intraischemic brain temperature modulation. J Neurochem 1994;63:1095-1103.

132. Nakashima K, Todd MM, Warner DS: The relation between cerebral metabolic rate and ischemic depolarization: A comparison of the effects of hypothermia, pentobarbital, and isoflurane. Anesthesiology 1995;82:1199-1208.

133. Globus M, Busto R, Lin B, et al: Detection of free radical activity during transient global ischemia and recirculation: Effects of intraischemic brain temperature modulation. J Neurochem 1995;65: 1250-1256.

134. Kader A, Frazzini V, Baker C, et al: Effect of mild hypothermia on nitric oxide synthesis during focal cerebral ischemia. Neurosurgery 1994;35:272-277.

135. Bernard SA, Gray TW, Buist MD, et al: Treatment of comatose survivors of out-of-hospital cardiac arrest with induced hypothermia. N Engl J Med 2002;346:557-563.

136. Hypothermia after Cardiac Arrest Study Group: Mild therapeutic hypothermia to improve the neurologic outcome after cardiac arrest. N Engl J Med 2002;346:549-556.

137. Clifton GL, Miller ER, Choi SC, et al: Lack of effect of induction of hypothermia after acute brain injury. N Engl J Med 2001;344: 556-563.

138. Todd MM, Hindman BJ, Clarke WR, et al: Mild intraoperative hypothermia during surgery for intracranial aneurysm. N Engl J Med 2005;352:135-145.

139. The Warm Heart Investigators: Randomized trial of normothermic versus hypothermic coronary bypass surgery. Lancet 1994;343: 559-563.

140. Gaillard D, Bical O, Paumier D, et al: A review of myocardial normothermia: Its theoretical basis and the potential clinical benefits in cardiac surgery. Cardiovasc Surg 2000;8:198-203.

141. Nicolini F, Beghi C, Muscari C, et al: Myocardial protection in adult cardiac surgery: Current options and future challenges. Eur J Cardiothorac Surg 2003;24:986-993.

142. Panos AL, Deslauriers R, Birnbaum PL, et al: Perspectives on myocardial protection: Warm heart surgery. Perfusion 1993;8: 287-291.

143. Martin T, Craver J, Gott J, et al: Prospective, randomized trial of retrograde warm blood cardioplegia: Myocardial benefit and neurologic threat. Ann Thorac Surg 1994;57:298-302.

144. Grigore AM, Mathew J, Grocott HP, et al: Prospective randomized trial of normothermic versus hypothermic cardiopulmonary bypass on cognitive function after coronary artery bypass graft surgery. Anesthesiology 2001;95:1110-1119.

145. Mora CT, Henson MB, Weintraub WS, et al: The effect of temperature management during cardiopulmonary bypass on neurologic and neuropsychologic outcomes in patients undergoing coronary revascularization. J Thorac Cardiovasc Surg 1996;112:514-522.

146. McLean RF, Wong BI, Naylor CD, et al: Cardiopulmonary bypass, temperature, and central nervous system dysfunction. Circulation 1994;90:II250-255.

147. Grocott HP, Newman MF, Croughwell ND, et al: Continuous jugular venous versus nasopharyngeal temperature monitoring during hypothermic cardiopulmonary bypass for cardiac surgery. J Clin Anesth 1997;9:312-316.

148. Nathan HJ, Wells GA, Munson JL, et al: Neuroprotective effect of mild hypothermia in patients undergoing coronary artery surgery with cardiopulmonary bypass: A randomized trial. Circulation 2001;104:I85-191.

149. Cook DJ, Oliver WC Jr, Orszulak TA, et al: A prospective, randomized comparison of cerebral venous oxygen saturation during normothermic and hypothermic cardiopulmonary bypass. J Thorac Cardiovasc Surg 1994;107:1020-1028; discussion 1028-1029.

150. Stone JG, Young WL, Smith CR, et al: Do standard monitoring sites reflect true brain temperature when profound hypothermia is rapidly induced and reversed? Anesthesiology 1995;82:344-351.

151. Likosky DS, Marrin CA, Caplan LR, et al: Determination of etiologic mechanisms of strokes secondary to coronary artery bypass graft surgery. Stroke 2003;34:2830-2834.

152. Davila-Roman VG, Phillips KJ, Daily BB, et al: Intraoperative transesophageal echocardiography and epiaortic ultrasound for assessment of atherosclerosis of the thoracic aorta. J Am Coll Cardiol 1996;28: 942-947.

153. Davila-Roman VG, Barzilai B, Wareing TH, et al: Atherosclerosis of the ascending aorta: Prevalence and role as an independent predictor of cerebrovascular events in cardiac patients. Stroke 1994;25: 2010-2016.

154. Mizuno T, Toyama M, Tabuchi N, et al: Thickened intima of the aortic arch is a risk factor for stroke with coronary artery bypass grafting. Ann Thorac Surg 2000;70:1565-1570.

155. Sylivris S, Calafiore P, Matalanis G, et al: The intraoperative assessment of ascending aortic atheroma: Epiaortic imaging is superior to both transesophageal echocardiography and direct palpation. J Cardiothorac Vasc Anesth 1997;11:704-707.

156. Royse C, Royse A, Blake D, et al: Screening the thoracic aorta for atheroma: A comparison of manual palpation, transesophageal and epiaortic ultrasonography. Ann Thorac Cardiovasc Surg 1998;4: 347-350.

157. Trehan N, Mishra M, Dhole S, et al: Significantly reduced incidence of stroke during coronary artery bypass grafting using transesophageal echocardiography. Eur J Cardiothorac Surg 1997;11:234-242.

158. Gold JP, Torres KE, Maldarelli W, et al: Improving outcomes in coronary surgery: The impact of echo-directed aortic cannulation and perioperative hemodynamic management in 500 patients. Ann Thorac Surg 2004;78:1579-1585.

159. Ribakove G, Katz E, Galloway A, et al: Surgical implications of transesophageal echocardiography to grade the atheromatous aortic arch. Ann Thorac Surg 1992;53:758-763.

160. Baribeau YR, Westbrook BM, Charlesworth DC, et al: Arterial inflow via an axillary artery graft for the severely atheromatous aorta. Ann Thorac Surg 1998;66:33-37.

161. Shann KG, Likosky DS, Murkin JM, et al: An evidence-based review of the practice of cardiopulmonary bypass in adults: A focus on

neurologic injury, glycemic control, hemodilution, and the inflammatory response. J Thorac Cardiovasc Surg 2006;132:283-290.

162. Cook DJ, Orszulak TA, Zehr KJ, et al: Effectiveness of the Cobra aortic catheter for dual-temperature management during adult cardiac surgery. J Thorac Cardiovasc Surg 2003;125:378-384.

163. Hammon JW, Stump DA, Butterworth JF, et al: Single crossclamp improves 6-month cognitive outcome in high-risk coronary bypass patients: The effect of reduced aortic manipulation. J Thorac Cardiovasc Surg 2006;131:114-121.

164. Tsang JC, Morin JF, Tchervenkov CI, et al: Single aortic clamp versus partial occluding clamp technique for cerebral protection during coronary artery bypass: A randomized prospective trial. J Card Surg 2003;18:158-163.

165. Dirnagl U, Iadecola C, Moskowitz M: Pathobiology of ischaemic stroke: An integrated view. Trends Neurosci 1999;22:391-397.

166. Grocott HP, Nussmeier NA: Neuroprotection in cardiac surgery. Anesthesiol Clin North America 2003;21:487-509.

167. Zaidan J, Klochany A, Martin W: Effect of thiopental on neurologic outcome following coronary artery bypass grafting. Anesthesiology 1991;74:406-411.

168. Pascoe E, Hudson R, Anderson B, et al: High-dose thiopentone for open-chamber cardiac surgery: A retrospective review. Can J Anaesth 1996;43:575-579.

169. Zhou W, Fontenot HJ, Liu S, et al: Modulation of cardiac calcium channels by propofol. Anesthesiology 1997;86:670-675.

170. Pittman JE, Sheng HX, Pearlstein R, et al: Comparison of the effects of propofol and pentobarbital on neurologic outcome and cerebral infarct size after temporary focal ischemia in the rat. Anesthesiology 1997;87:1139-1144.

171. Young Y, Menon DK, Tisavipat N, et al: Propofol neuroprotection in a rat model of ischaemia reperfusion injury. Eur J Anaesthesiol 1997;14:320-326.

172. Wang J, Yang X, Camporesi CV, et al: Propofol reduces infarct size and striatal dopamine accumulation following transient middle cerebral artery occlusion: A microdialysis study. Eur J Pharmacol 2002;452:303-308.

173. Roach GW, Newman MF, Murkin JM, et al: Ineffectiveness of burst suppression therapy in mitigating perioperative cerebrovascular dysfunction. Multicenter Study of Perioperative Ischemia (McSPI) Research Group [see comments]. Anesthesiology 1999;90:1255-1264.

174. Arrowsmith JE, Harrison MJG, Newman SP, et al: Neuroprotection of the brain during cardiopulmonary bypass: A randomized trial of remacemide during coronary artery bypass in 171 patients. Stroke 1998;29:2357-2362.

175. Ma D, Yang H, Lynch J, et al: Xenon attenuates cardiopulmonary bypass-induced neurologic and neurocognitive dysfunction in the rat. Anesthesiology 2003;98:690-698.

176. Homi HM, Yokoo N, Ma D, et al: The neuroprotective effect of xenon administration during transient middle cerebral artery occlusion in mice. Anesthesiology 2003;99:876-881.

177. Homi HM, Yokoo N, Venkatakrishnan K, et al: Neuroprotection by antagonism of the N-methyl-D-aspartate receptor NR2B subtype in a rat model of cardiopulmonary bypass. Anesthesiology 2004: A878.

178. Lockwood GG, Franks NP, Downie NA, et al: Feasibility and safety of delivering xenon to patients undergoing coronary artery bypass graft surgery while on cardiopulmonary bypass: Phase I study. Anesthesiology 2006;104:458-465.

179. Lei B, Cottrell JE, Kass IS: Neuroprotective effect of low-dose lidocaine in a rat model of transient focal cerebral ischemia. Anesthesiology 2001;95:445-451.

180. Terada H, Ohta S, Nishikawa T, et al: The effect of intravenous or subarachnoid lidocaine on glutamate accumulation during transient forebrain ischemia in rats. Anesth Analg 1999;89:957-961.

181. Liu K, Adachi N, Yanase H, et al: Lidocaine suppresses the anoxic depolarization and reduces the increase in the intracellular Ca^{2+} concentration in gerbil hippocampal neurons. Anesthesiology 1997;87:1470-1478.

182. Fujitani T, Adachi N, Miyazaki H, et al: Lidocaine protects hippocampal neurons against ischemic damage by preventing increase of extracellular excitatory amino acids: A microdialysis study in Mongolian gerbils. Neurosci Lett 1994;179:91-94.

183. Wendt DJ, Starmer CF, Grant AO: pH dependence of kinetics and steady-state block of cardiac sodium channels by lidocaine. Am J Physiol 1993;264:H1588-1598.

184. de Klaver MJ, Buckingham MG, Rich GF: Lidocaine attenuates cytokine-induced cell injury in endothelial and vascular smooth muscle cells. Anesth Analg 2003;97:465-470.

185. Mitchell SJ, Pellett O, Gorman DF: Cerebral protection by lidocaine during cardiac operations. Ann Thorac Surg 1999;67:1117-1124.

186. Wang D, Wu X, Li J, et al: The effect of lidocaine on early postoperative cognitive dysfunction after coronary artery bypass surgery. Anesth Analg 2002;95:1134-1141.

187. Mathew JP, Grocott HP, Phillips-Bute B, et al: Lidocaine does not prevent cognitive dysfunction after cardiac surgery. Anesth Analg 2004;98:SCA13.

188. Mangano DT, Layug EL, Wallace A, et al: Effect of atenolol on mortality and cardiovascular morbidity after noncardiac surgery. Multicenter Study of Perioperative Ischemia Research Group. N Engl J Med 1996;335:1713-1720.

189. Amory DW, Grigore A, Amory JK, et al: Neuroprotection is associated with beta-adrenergic receptor antagonists during cardiac surgery: Evidence from 2,575 patients. J Cardiothorac Vasc Anesth 2002;16:270-277.

190. Ohtsuka T, Hamada M, Hiasa G, et al: Effect of beta-blockers on circulating levels of inflammatory and anti-inflammatory cytokines in patients with dilated cardiomyopathy. J Am Coll Cardiol 2001;37:412-417.

191. Yang SP, Ho LJ, Cheng SM, et al: Carvedilol differentially regulates cytokine production from activated human peripheral blood mononuclear cells. Cardiovasc Drugs Ther 2004;18:183-188.

192. Savitz SI, Erhardt JA, Anthony JV, et al: The novel beta-blocker, carvedilol, provides neuroprotection in transient focal stroke. J Cereb Blood Flow Metab 2000;20:1197-1204.

193. Clark RK, Lee EV, White RF, et al: Reperfusion following focal stroke hastens inflammation and resolution of ischemic injured tissue. Brain Res Bull 1994;35:387-392.

194. Chopp M, Zhang RL, Chen H, et al: Postischemic administration of an anti-Mac-1 antibody reduces ischemic cell damage after transient middle cerebral artery occlusion in rats. Stroke 1994;25:869-875; discussion 875-866.

195. Bracken MB, Shepard MJ, Collins WF, et al: A randomized, controlled trial of methylprednisolone or naloxone in the treatment of acute spinal-cord injury: Results of the Second National Acute Spinal Cord Injury Study. N Engl J Med 1990;322:1405-1411.

196. Roberts I, Yates D, Sandercock P, et al: Effect of intravenous corticosteroids on death within 14 days in 10,008 adults with clinically significant head injury (MRC CRASH trial): Randomised placebo-controlled trial. Lancet 2004;364:1321-1328.

197. Wass CT, Lanier WL: Glucose modulation of ischemic brain injury: Review and clinical recommendations. Mayo Clin Proc 1996;71:801-812.

198. Li P, Kristian T, Shamloo M, et al: Effects of preischemic hyperglycemia on brain damage incurred by rats subjected to 2.5 or 5 minutes of forebrain ischemia. Stroke 1996;27:1592-1602.

199. Bernard GR, Artigas A, Brigham KL, et al: The American-European Consensus Conference on ARDS: Definitions, mechanisms, relevant outcomes, and clinical trial coordination. Am J Respir Crit Care Med 1994;149:818-824.

200. Chaney MA, Nikolov MP, Blakeman B, et al: Pulmonary effects of methylprednisolone in patients undergoing coronary artery bypass grafting and early tracheal extubation. Anesth Analg 1998;87:27-33.

201. Oliver WC Jr, Nuttall GA, Orszulak TA, et al: Hemofiltration but not steroids results in earlier tracheal extubation following cardiopulmonary bypass: A prospective, randomized double-blind trial. Anesthesiology 2004;101:327-339.

202. Fitch JC, Rollins S, Matis L, et al: Pharmacology and biological efficacy of a recombinant, humanized, single-chain antibody C5 complement inhibitor in patients undergoing coronary artery bypass graft surgery with cardiopulmonary bypass. Circulation 1999;100:2499-2506.

203. Mathew JP, Shernan SK, White WD, et al: Preliminary report of the effects of complement suppression with pexelizumab on neurocogni-

tive decline after coronary artery bypass graft surgery. Stroke 2004;35:2335-2339.

204. Levy J, Ramsay J, Murkin J: Aprotinin reduces the incidence of strokes following cardiac surgery. Circulation 1996;94:I-535.

205. Levy JH, Pifarre R, Schaff HV, et al: A multicenter, double-blind, placebo-controlled trial of aprotinin for reducing blood loss and the requirement for donor-blood transfusion in patients undergoing repeat coronary artery bypass grafting. Circulation 1995;92:2236-2244.

206. Frumento RJ, O'Malley CM, Bennett-Guerrero E: Stroke after cardiac surgery: A retrospective analysis of the effect of aprotinin dosing regimens. Ann Thorac Surg 2003;75:479-483; discussion 483-484.

207. Harmon DC, Ghori KG, Eustace NP, et al: Aprotinin decreases the incidence of cognitive deficit following CABG and cardiopulmonary bypass: A pilot randomized controlled study. [L'aprotinine reduit l'incidence de deficit cognitif a la suite d'un PAC et de la circulation extracorporelle: Une etude pilote randomisee et controlee.] Can J Anaesth 2004;51:1002-1009.

208. Murkin JM: Postoperative cognitive dysfunction: Aprotinin, bleeding and cognitive testing. [Dysfonction cognitive postoperatoire: Aprotinine, hemorragie et epreuves cognitives.] Can J Anaesth 2004;51:957-962.

209. Grocott HP, Sheng H, Miura Y, et al: The effects of aprotinin on outcome from cerebral ischemia in the rat. Anesth Analg 1999;88:1-7.

210. Homi HM, Sheng H, Mackensen GB, et al: Aprotinin does not decrease cerebral infarct volume in an experimental model of stroke during cardiopulmonary bypass. Anesth Analg 2005;100:SCA14.

211. Mangano DT, Tudor IC, Dietzel C: The risk associated with aprotinin in cardiac surgery. N Engl J Med 2006;354:353-365.

212. Van Dijk D, Jansen EW, Hijman R, et al: Cognitive outcome after off-pump and on-pump coronary artery bypass graft surgery: A randomized trial. JAMA 2002;287:1405-1412.

213. Bainbridge D, Martin J, Cheng D: Off pump coronary artery bypass graft surgery versus conventional coronary artery bypass graft surgery: A systematic review of the literature. Semin Cardiothorac Vasc Anesth 2005;9:105-111.

214. Tomic V, Russwurm S, Moller E, et al: Transcriptomic and proteomic patterns of systemic inflammation in on-pump and off-pump coronary artery bypass grafting. Circulation 2005;112:2912-2920.

215. McBride WT, Armstrong MA, McMurray TJ: An investigation of the effects of heparin, low molecular weight heparin, protamine, and fentanyl on the balance of pro- and anti-inflammatory cytokines in in-vitro monocyte cultures. Anaesthesia 1996;51:634-640.

216. Kalkman CJ, Traast H, Zuurmond WW, et al: Differential effects of propofol and nitrous oxide on posterior tibial nerve somatosensory cortical evoked potentials during alfentanil anaesthesia. Br J Anaesth 1991;66:483-489.

217. Croughwell N, Newman M, Blumenthal J, et al: Jugular bulb saturation and cognitive dysfunction after cardiopulmonary bypass. Ann Thorac Surg 1994;58:1702-1708.

218. Al-Ruzzeh S, George S, Bustami M, et al: Effect of off-pump coronary artery bypass surgery on clinical, angiographic, neurocognitive, and quality of life outcomes: Randomised controlled trial. BMJ 2006;332:1365.

219. Bell RE, Taylor PR, Aukett M, et al: Mid-term results for second-generation thoracic stent grafts. Br J Surg 2003;90:811-817.

220. Criado FJ, Clark NS, Barnatan MF: Stent graft repair in the aortic arch and descending thoracic aorta: A 4-year experience. J Vasc Surg 2002;36:1121-1128.

221. Greenberg R, Resch T, Nyman U, et al: Endovascular repair of descending thoracic aortic aneurysms: An early experience with intermediate-term follow-up. J Vasc Surg 2000;31:147-156.

222. Chiesa R, Melissano G, Marrocco-Trischitta MM, et al: Spinal cord ischemia after elective stent-graft repair of the thoracic aorta. J Vasc Surg 2005;42:11-17.

223. Juvonen T, Biancari F, Rimpilainen J, et al: Strategies for spinal cord protection during descending thoracic and thoracoabdominal aortic surgery: Up-to-date experimental and clinical results—A review. Scand Cardiovasc J 2002;36:136-160.

224. Zvara DA: Thoracoabdominal aneurysm surgery and the risk of paraplegia: Contemporary practice and future directions. J Extra Corpor Technol 2002;34:11-17.

225. Reece TB, Kern JA, Tribble CG, et al: The role of pharmacology in spinal cord protection during thoracic aortic reconstruction. Semin Thorac Cardiovasc Surg 2003;15:365-377.

226. Verdant A, Cossette R, Page A, et al: Aneurysms of the descending thoracic aorta: Three hundred sixty-six consecutive cases resected without paraplegia. J Vasc Surg 1995;21:385-390; discussion 390-381.

227. Griepp RB, Ergin MA, Galla JD, et al: Looking for the artery of Adamkiewicz: A quest to minimize paraplegia after operations for aneurysms of the descending thoracic and thoracoabdominal aorta. J Thorac Cardiovasc Surg 1996;112:1202-1213; discussion 1213-1205.

228. Schepens MA, Vermeulen FE, Morshuis WJ, et al: Impact of left heart bypass on the results of thoracoabdominal aortic aneurysm repair. Ann Thorac Surg 1999;67:1963-1967; discussion 1979-1980.

229. Borst HG, Jurmann M, Buhner B, et al: Risk of replacement of descending aorta with a standardized left heart bypass technique. J Thorac Cardiovasc Surg 1994;107:126-132; discussion 132-123.

230. Coselli JS, LeMaire SA, Ledesma DF, et al: Initial experience with the Nikkiso centrifugal pump during thoracoabdominal aortic aneurysm repair. J Vasc Surg 1998;27:378-383.

231. Coselli JS: Thoracoabdominal aortic aneurysms: Experience with 372 patients. J Card Surg 1994;9:638-647.

232. Safi HJ, Miller CC 3rd: Spinal cord protection in descending thoracic and thoracoabdominal aortic repair. Ann Thorac Surg 1999;67:1937-1939; discussion 1953-1938.

233. Bachet J, Guilmet D, Rosier J, et al: Protection of the spinal cord during surgery of thoraco-abdominal aortic aneurysms. Eur J Cardiothorac Surg 1996;10:817-825.

234. Kouchoukos NT, Masetti P, Rokkas CK, et al: Safety and efficacy of hypothermic cardiopulmonary bypass and circulatory arrest for operations on the descending thoracic and thoracoabdominal aorta. Ann Thorac Surg 2001;72:699-707; discussion 707-698.

235. Moriyama Y, Iguro Y, Hisatomi K, et al: Thoracic and thoracoabdominal aneurysm repair under deep hypothermia using subclavian arterial perfusion. Ann Thorac Surg 2001;71:29-32.

236. Coselli JS, LeMaire SA, Conklin LD, Adams GJ: Left heart bypass during descending thoracic aortic aneurysm repair does not reduce the incidence of paraplegia. Ann Thorac Surg 2004;77:1298-1303; discussion 1303.

237. Gravereaux EC, Faries PL, Burks JA, et al: Risk of spinal cord ischemia after endograft repair of thoracic aortic aneurysms. J Vasc Surg 2001;34:997-1003.

238. Tiesenhausen K, Amann W, Koch G, et al: Cerebrospinal fluid drainage to reverse paraplegia after endovascular thoracic aortic aneurysm repair. J Endovasc Ther 2000;7:132-135.

239. Fuchs RJ, Lee WA, Seubert CN, et al: Transient paraplegia after stent grafting of a descending thoracic aortic aneurysm treated with cerebrospinal fluid drainage. J Clin Anesth 2003;15:59-63.

240. Ortiz-Gomez JR, Gonzalez-Solis FJ, Fernandez-Alonso L, et al: Reversal of acute paraplegia with cerebrospinal fluid drainage after endovascular thoracic aortic aneurysm repair. Anesthesiology 2001;95:1288-1289.

241. Coselli JS, Lemaire SA, Koksoy C, et al: Cerebrospinal fluid drainage reduces paraplegia after thoracoabdominal aortic aneurysm repair: Results of a randomized clinical trial. J Vasc Surg 2002;35:631-639.

242. Acher CW, Wynn MM, Hoch JR, et al: Combined use of cerebral spinal fluid drainage and naloxone reduces the risk of paraplegia in thoracoabdominal aneurysm repair. J Vasc Surg 1994;19:236-246; discussion 247-238.

243. Svensson LG, Hess KR, D'Agostino RS, et al: Reduction of neurologic injury after high-risk thoracoabdominal aortic operation. Ann Thorac Surg 1998;66:132-138.

244. Safi HJ, Bartoli S, Hess KR, et al: Neurologic deficit in patients at high risk with thoracoabdominal aortic aneurysms: The role of cerebral spinal fluid drainage and distal aortic perfusion. J Vasc Surg 1994;20:434-444; discussion 444-445.

245. Safi HJ, Hess KR, Randel M, et al: Cerebrospinal fluid drainage and distal aortic perfusion: Reducing neurologic complications in repair of thoracoabdominal aortic aneurysm types I and II. J Vasc Surg 1996;23:223-228; discussion 229.

246. Hollier LH, Money SR, Naslund TC, et al: Risk of spinal cord dysfunction in patients undergoing thoracoabdominal aortic replacement. Am J Surg 1992;164:210-213; discussion 213-214.

247. Crawford ES, Svensson LG, Hess KR, et al: A prospective randomized study of cerebrospinal fluid drainage to prevent paraplegia after high-risk surgery on the thoracoabdominal aorta. J Vasc Surg 1991; 13:36-45; discussion 45-46.

248. Coselli JS, LeMaire SA: Left heart bypass reduces paraplegia rates after thoracoabdominal aortic aneurysm repair. Ann Thorac Surg 1999;67:1931-1934; discussion 1935-1938.

249. Kouchoukos NT, Daily BB, Rokkas CK, et al: Hypothermic bypass and circulatory arrest for operations on the descending thoracic and thoracoabdominal aorta. Ann Thorac Surg 1995;60:67-76; discussion 76-77.

250. Cambria RP, Davison JK, Carter C, et al: Epidural cooling for spinal cord protection during thoracoabdominal aneurysm repair: A five-year experience. J Vasc Surg 2000;31:1093-1102.

251. Mutch WA, Graham MR, Halliday WC, et al: Use of neuroanesthesia adjuncts (hyperventilation and mannitol administration) improves neurological outcome after thoracic aortic cross-clamping in dogs. Stroke 1993;24:1204-1210.

252. Mutch WA, Thomson IR, Teskey JM, et al: Phlebotomy reverses the hemodynamic consequences of thoracic aortic cross-clamping: Relationships between central venous pressure and cerebrospinal fluid pressure. Anesthesiology 1991;74:320-324.

253. Gharagozloo F, Larson J, Dausmann MJ, et al: Spinal cord protection during surgical procedures on the descending thoracic and thoracoabdominal aorta: Review of current techniques. Chest 1996;109: 799-809.

254. A randomized, controlled trial of methylprednisolone or naloxone in the treatment of acute spinal-cord injury [comment on ref. 195]. N Engl J Med 1990;323:1207-1209.

255. Qayumi AK, Janusz MT, Jamieson WR, et al: Pharmacologic interventions for prevention of spinal cord injury caused by aortic cross-clamping. J Thorac Cardiovasc Surg 1992;104:256-261.

256. Fowl RJ, Patterson RB, Gewirtz RJ, et al: Protection against postischemic spinal cord injury using a new 21-aminosteroid. J Surg Res 1990;48:597-600.

257. Lips J, de Haan P, Bodewits P, et al: Neuroprotective effects of riluzole and ketamine during transient spinal cord ischemia in the rabbit. Anesthesiology 2000;93:1303-1311.

258. von Euler M, Li-Li M, Whittemore S, et al: No protective effect of the NMDA antagonist memantine in experimental spinal cord injuries. J Neurotrauma 1997;14:53-61.

259. Simpson JI, Eide TR, Schiff GA, et al: Intrathecal magnesium sulfate protects the spinal cord from ischemic injury during thoracic aortic cross-clamping. Anesthesiology 1994;81:1493-1499; discussion 1426A-1427.

260. Laschinger JC, Cunningham JN Jr, Cooper MM, et al: Prevention of ischemic spinal cord injury following aortic cross-clamping: Use of corticosteroids. Ann Thorac Surg 1984;38:500-507.

261. Francel PC, Long BA, Malik JM, et al: Limiting ischemic spinal cord injury using a free radical scavenger 21-aminosteroid and/or cerebrospinal fluid drainage. J Neurosurg 1993;79:742-751.

262. Grabitz K, Freye E, Prior R, et al: Does prostaglandin E1 and superoxide dismutase prevent ischaemic spinal cord injury after thoracic aortic cross-clamping? Eur J Vasc Surg 1990;4:19-24.

263. Hirose K, Okajima K, Taoka Y, et al: Activated protein C reduces the ischemia/reperfusion-induced spinal cord injury in rats by inhibiting neutrophil activation. Ann Surg 2000;232:272-280.

264. Cassada DC, Tribble CG, Kaza AK, et al: Adenosine analogue reduces spinal cord reperfusion injury in a time-dependent fashion. Surgery 2001;130:230-235.

265. Bortone AS, De Cillis E, D'Agostino D, et al: Endovascular treatment of thoracic aortic disease: Four years of experience. Circulation 2004;110:II262-267.

266. Criado FJ, Abul-Khoudoud OR, Domer GS, et al: Endovascular repair of the thoracic aorta: Lessons learned. Ann Thorac Surg 2005;80:857-863; discussion 863.

267. Baril DT, Carroccio A, Ellozy SH, et al: Endovascular thoracic aortic repair and previous or concomitant abdominal aortic repair: Is the increased risk of spinal cord ischemia real? Ann Vasc Surg 2006;20:188-194.

268. Peterson BG, Eskandari MK, Gleason TG, et al: Utility of left subclavian artery revascularization in association with endoluminal repair of acute and chronic thoracic aortic pathology. J Vasc Surg 2006;43:433-439.

269. Dake MD, Miller DC, Mitchell RS, et al: The "first generation" of endovascular stent-grafts for patients with aneurysms of the descending thoracic aorta. J Thorac Cardiovasc Surg 1998;116:689-703; discussion 703.

270. Ellozy SH, Carroccio A, Minor M, et al: Challenges of endovascular tube graft repair of thoracic aortic aneurysm: Midterm follow-up and lessons learned. J Vasc Surg 2003;38:676-683.

271. Greenberg RK, O'Neill S, Walker E, et al: Endovascular repair of thoracic aortic lesions with the Zenith TX1 and TX2 thoracic grafts: Intermediate-term results. J Vasc Surg 2005;41:589-596.

272. Makaroun MS, Dillavou ED, Kee ST, et al: Endovascular treatment of thoracic aortic aneurysms: Results of the phase II multicenter trial of the GORE TAG thoracic endoprosthesis. J Vasc Surg 2005;41: 1-9.

273. Neuhauser B, Perkmann R, Greiner A, et al: Mid-term results after endovascular repair of the atherosclerotic descending thoracic aortic aneurysm. Eur J Vasc Endovasc Surg 2004;28:146-153.

274. Maniar HS, Sundt TM 3rd, Prasad SM, et al: Delayed paraplegia after thoracic and thoracoabdominal aneurysm repair: A continuing risk. Ann Thorac Surg 2003;75:113-119; discussion 119-120.

275. Azizzadeh A, Huynh TT, Miller CC 3rd, et al: Postoperative risk factors for delayed neurologic deficit after thoracic and thoracoabdominal aortic aneurysm repair: A case-control study. J Vasc Surg 2003;37:750-754.

276. Newman MF, Wolman R, Kanchuger M, et al: Multicenter preoperative stroke risk index for patients undergoing coronary artery bypass graft surgery. Circulation 1996;94:II74-80.

277. Safi HJ, Miller CC 3rd, Subramaniam MH, et al: Thoracic and thoracoabdominal aortic aneurysm repair using cardiopulmonary bypass, profound hypothermia, and circulatory arrest via left side of the chest incision. J Vasc Surg 1998;28:591-598.

278. Cambria RP, Davison JK, Zannetti S, et al: Clinical experience with epidural cooling for spinal cord protection during thoracic and thoracoabdominal aneurysm repair. J Vasc Surg 1997;25:234-241.

279. Biglioli P, Spirito R, Porqueddu M, et al: Quick, simple clamping technique in descending thoracic aortic aneurysm repair. Ann Thorac Surg 1999;67:1038-1043; discussion 1043-1044.

280. Cina CS, Abouzahr L, Arena GO, et al: Cerebrospinal fluid drainage to prevent paraplegia during thoracic and thoracoabdominal aortic aneurysm surgery: A systematic review and meta-analysis. J Vasc Surg 2004;40:36-44.

23 Preservation of Spinal Cord Function

Michael M. McGarvey and Albert T. Cheung

Acute spinal cord injury (SCI) is a devastating medical condition because of the magnitude of permanent disability produced by paraplegia or quadriplegia. It creates enormous problems for the health-care systems treating the injured patient, and even greater challenges for the family and the patient trying to reintegrate into society. The tragic consequences of acute SCI are amplified further because the patient often remains fully cognitive of the disability, and the health-care team recognizes that most injuries are permanent and treatment is unlikely to improve the disability. For these reasons, the primary emphasis for preservation of spinal cord function is prevention of injury. Once injury has occurred, treatment is primarily supportive. Fortunately, understanding the mechanisms and causes of spinal cord injury associated with neuraxial anesthetic techniques may decrease the frequency of this complication. In addition, some progress has been reported for the prevention and treatment of spinal cord ischemia after thoracoabdominal aortic aneurysm repair.

SCI can be classified as ischemic, toxic, or mechanical according to the etiology. The mechanisms leading to permanent disability from structural damage to the spinal cord after the initial injury can be further classified into primary mechanisms and secondary mechanisms. Primary mechanisms of injury include immediate neuronal cell death from infarction, exposure to toxic substances, or direct mechanical forces such as contusion, shear, laceration, distraction, or compression. Primary mechanisms of injury may also be a consequence of direct injury to blood vessels, glial cells, or the vertebral column necessary for spinal cord function. Secondary mechanisms of injury are more complex and are the consequence of biochemical, cellular, and pathophysiologic pathways, initiated by the primary injury, that exacerbate the initial injury. Secondary mechanisms of injury begin immediately after the primary injury and have been attributed to inflammation, apoptosis, intracellular protein synthesis inhibition, glutaminergic dysfunction, electrolyte shifts, neurotransmitter derangements, vascular changes, edema, and loss of energy metabolism.[1] Secondary mechanisms result in the eventual death of an additional population of neuronal or glial cells over the course of days to weeks that survived the primary injury. Finally, spinal cord injuries can be further classified as complete or incomplete based on the absence of function or the presence of partial neurologic function below the level of the injury.

The importance of classifying spinal cord injuries according to etiology and mechanism is that categorization provides potential targets for medical intervention. Incomplete injuries may offer some hope for recovery of additional function. Ischemic injuries may be treated, prevented, or limited by medical interventions directed at improving spinal cord perfusion. The severity of mechanical injuries may be limited by surgical stabilization or decompression. Medical strategies to limit damage caused by secondary mechanisms are often referred to as neuroprotection. The promise of neuroprotection strategies rests on the basis that treatment can be instituted after the primary injury has occurred, and that preserving even a small quantity of functioning neuronal structures can result in marked differences in rehabilitation potential. Unfortunately, evidence supporting the effectiveness of medical treatments directed at secondary mechanisms of injury or neuroprotection remains controversial.

■ TRAUMATIC SPINAL CORD INJURY

Traumatic spinal cord injury has an incidence 15 to 40 spinal injuries per million people worldwide, with approximately 12,000 new cases per year in the United States alone.[1] Approximately 50% of spinal cord injuries occur in patients between ages of 15 and 30 years as the direct result of motor vehicle accidents, occupational injuries, violence, falls, or sports. The 1-year case-fatality rate of spinal cord injuries averages 46%, with 11% of patients dying during their initial hospitalization.[2] The annual cost attributed to spinal cord injuries in the United States in 1990 was estimated to be 4 billion dollars.[3] Greater than 50% of spinal cord injuries occur at the cervical level, and 45% of those injuries are complete lesions with total loss of function below the level of the lesion. The most common cause of death after survival from the initial injury is pulmonary complications. The primary injury in SCI accounts for a majority of neurologic dysfunction that occurs, although the amount of dysfunction occurring from secondary injury may be clinically significant, and the prevention of secondary injury may be critical for long-term outcome.[4]

The approach to preventing secondary injury after traumatic SCI is to stabilize cardiovascular and pulmonary function, immobilize the spine, determine the level and extent of injury, consider pharmacologic neuroprotection, and stabilize the spine surgically. The highest immediate priority for preventing secondary injury in traumatic SCI is resuscitation and medical stabilization of the patient to ensure an adequate airway, oxygenation, ventilation, and blood pressure without worsening the spinal cord injury. Supplemental oxygen should be administered and an airway established with the head and neck immobilized in a neutral position. The treatment of airway compromise in a patient with suspected traumatic SCI is challenging because it is difficult to prevent movement of the cervical spine during emergency maneuvers to establish a patent airway.[5,6] The jaw-thrust maneuver should be tried initially in a patient making respiratory efforts with evidence of airway obstruction. This maneuver is performed by placing the palms of both hands on either side of the head to stabilize the neck and using the first two or three fingers of each hand to lift the mandible forward and outward; it can be combined with the use of an oral or nasopharyngeal airway or used to facilitate mask ventilation (Fig. 23-1).

Ventilation should be assessed, and if it is inadequate, tracheal intubation should be performed with the two-person orotracheal or nasotracheal technique, in which one rescuer performs the tracheal intubation while the other provides manual in-line immobilization of the head and neck in the neutral position.[7] Manual in-line immobilization is performed by cradling the occiput in the palms of the hands and gently applying forces that are equal and opposite in direction to those being applied during laryngoscopy and tracheal intubation in an effort to keep the head and neck in a neutral position. It is important to avoid traction of the neck during manual in-line immobilization because it could cause distraction of the spine at the site of injury.[7] If time permits and equipment is available, tracheal intubation can be performed using fiberoptic bronchoscopic techniques instead of direct laryngoscopy to decrease the risk of spinal movement, but outcome data are lacking to demonstrate the advantage of any specific technique for tracheal intubation.[7,8] If an airway cannot be established by oral or nasotracheal intubation, emergency cricothyroidotomy should be considered.[8] Although failure to immobilize the head and neck may increase neurologic injury by 7- to 10-fold in patients with cervical spine injuries,[9] existing evidence supports the safety of tracheal intubation with manual in-line immobilization.[7]

Blood pressure should be measured and treatment directed to maintain a mean arterial pressure (MAP) in the range of 85 to 90 mm Hg during the first week after traumatic injury.[8] Hypotension associated with traumatic SCI may be caused by hypovolemic or neurogenic shock. The etiology of hypotension should be determined and treated with intravascular volume expansion, vasopressor therapy, or inotropic medications. Expert opinion, observational studies, and published clinical guidelines support treatment of hypoxia and hypotension to lessen secondary ischemic injury and improve outcome after acute traumatic SCI.[4,10,11]

After initial resuscitation of the patient with suspected acute traumatic SCI, the next priority is immobilization of the head, neck, and body until radiographic assessment for spinal fracture can be performed. Optimally, immobilization should be performed concurrently with resuscitation, but there may need to be a compromise if it interferes with efforts to reestablish cardiopulmonary function or treatment of other immediately life-threatening injuries. The entire spine, including the cervical spine, should be immobilized if the site of injury is not known. Clinical indications for immobilization of the spine include trauma from motor vehicle accidents, diving accidents, or acceleration-deceleration injuries that have a high risk of associated spinal cord injury. Indications for immobilization also include physical signs of tenderness along the posterior spine, decreased cervical range of motion, pain with motion, neurologic deficits, deformities, or decreased level of consciousness prohibiting neurologic examination.[7]

The first step in immobilization is manual stabilization of the head without applying traction until the application of an appropriate-size rigid or semi-rigid cervical collar. The patient can then be log-rolled with the spine in a neutral position onto a rigid spine board. The body is positioned on the board with the arms straightened with the palms against the body, and the legs straightened with the ankles secured to each other with padding between them. Straps are applied to the lower extremities, the pelvis, and then the trunk, in that order, to secure the body snugly against the board. Tape is then applied across the forehead and the cervical collar to

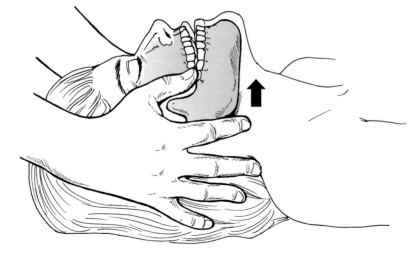

Figure 23-1 ▪ The jaw thrust maneuver to establish an airway. The head and neck are immobilized in a neutral position to prevent injury to the spinal cord in patients with suspected cervical spine injuries.

prevent head and neck movement. Wedges or a lightweight head block provide additional stability to prevent lateral movement of the head and neck. If the patient is placed on a long spinal board in the supine position for the physical examination, forehead padding and a semi-rigid or rigid cervical collar should be considered. If there is obvious deformity of the spine, immobilization should be modified to maintain a neutral position of the deformity. Advanced Trauma Life Support (ATLS) recommends that no effort be made to reduce an obvious deformity, especially in children.[8]

The objective of immobilization is to maintain the spine in a neutral position. Neutral position can be defined as the normal anatomic position of the head and torso when standing and looking straight ahead.[12] Other definitions of the neutral position include maintaining the external auditory meatus in line with the shoulder in the coronal plane[13] or supine without rotating or bending the spinal column.[5] Achieving a neutral cervical spine position in adults requires elevating the occiput approximately 2 cm above the spine board.[12] The occipital elevation distance may need to be greater than 2 cm in patients with truncal obesity. In contrast, achieving a neutral cervical spine position in children on a spine board may require elevating the back and shoulders to accommodate a relatively larger head.[14]

The proper radiographic evaluation of a patient with suspected SCI varies based on the availability of imaging modalities, level of consciousness, and the presence of systemic or neurologic deficit. The first aspect of radiographic clearance of spinal injuries requires immobilization and radiologic evaluation of the patient. In injuries involving the cervical spine, two sets of criteria have been developed to identify low-risk patients. The National Emergency X-Radiography Utilization Study (NEXUS) identified five criteria that must be met to exclude patients from radiologic evaluation: lack of midline cervical tenderness, lack of neurologic deficits, normal consciousness, no intoxication, and lack of significant systemic injuries that affect the ability to adequately examine the patient.[7] This practice demonstrated a high sensitivity (99%) but a low specificity (12%) in a study of 34,069 patients. Only two patients in the NEXUS had clinically significant cervical injuries missed by the screening.[7] The Canadian C-Spine Rule for Radiography (CCSRR) after trauma examined only alert and medically stable patients. The decision to image the cervical spine was based on whether the patient had any high-risk factors (age greater than 65, paresthesias, mechanism of injury) or low-risk factors (simple rear-end motor vehicle collision, sitting position in emergency department, ambulatory at any time since injury, delayed onset of neck pain, or absence of midline C-spine [i.e., cervical spine] tenderness) for injury, followed by the ability to rotate the head actively 45 degrees to the right and left.[15] This study demonstrated 100% sensitivity and 42.5% specificity in 8924 patients. Patients with potential cervical spine injury who meet both the NEXUS and CCSRR criteria can have spinal precautions relaxed and their cervical spines cleared.

In patients with suspected cervical spinal injury based on NEXUS and CCSRR criteria, radiographic evaluation begins with a three-view cervical series (lateral, anteroposterior, and odontoid). When done with adequate technique, three-view cervical spine plain films have a sensitivity for detecting injury approaching 90%.[7] A large percentage of cervical spine films are inadequate because of lack of visualization of the craniocervical and cervical-thoracic junction. The combination of cervical spine radiographs and supplemental computed tomography (CT) through the areas that are poorly visualized increases negative predictive values to 99% (Fig. 23-2). Clearance in the awake and neurologically normal patient is then completed by moving the neck actively and evaluating for pain. In a patient who cannot be evaluated clinically but is at high risk for a cervical fracture, the three-view cervical series, supplemented by high resolution CT imaging, reduces the risk of missing a fracture to less than 1%.[7]

In conscious patients who have normal plain films and cervical CT but neurologic deficits and cervical pain, flexion–extension radiographs should be considered for clearance.[16] In the unconscious patient, several options should be considered in patients with normal plain films and supplemental CT. The first option is close observation with removal of hard collar but maintenance of in-line positioning until the patient is awake and a neurologic examination can be completed. The other options in the unconscious patient are a magnetic resonance imaging (MRI) scan and dynamic fluoroscopy.[16] The benefit of performing MRI in addition to plain radiography and supplemental CT is unclear, as it adds only minimal information on ligamental injury, but it may identify spinal cord injury in patients with neurologic deficits.[7,17]

Guidelines for performing a detailed neurologic assessment for spinal cord injury have been developed by the American Spinal Injury Association (ASIA).[18,19] The neurologic examination includes assessment and rating of the level of consciousness using the Glasgow Coma Scale. Testing for sensation is performed in response to pinprick and light touch over each dermatome, and the most caudal dermatome having normal sensation is documented. Sensory deficits below the suspected level of injury are characterized as present, diminished, or absent. Motor function is examined by testing the strength of flexion and extension in the proximal and distal muscle groups of each extremity. Strength is rated on a six-point scale ranging from 0 to 5, with 0 indicating total paralysis and 5 indicating full strength against resistance. Strength of elbow flexion and extension, wrist extension, finger spread and flexion, hip flexion, leg extension, foot plantar and dorsiflexion, and great toe extension can then be numerically tabulated and compared with a total of 100 possible points for normal strength in all four extremities. This standardized neurologic examination and the ASIA scale can be used to stratify patients according to the severity of neurologic injury, and it has been shown to correlate with clinical outcomes[19,20] (Fig. 23-3). In unconscious patients, motor and sensory function is assessed by eliciting biceps (C5-C6), triceps (C6-C7), patellar (L4), and Achilles (S1) deep tendon reflexes. A rectal examination is performed to test anal sphincter tone (S2-S4) and perianal sensation (S2-S5).

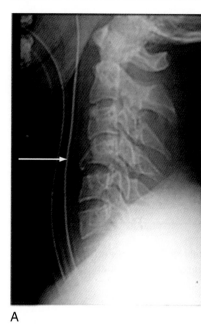

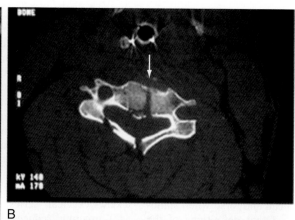

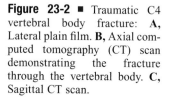

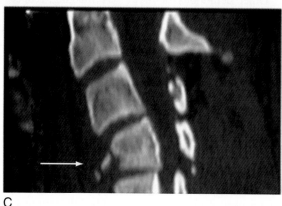

A

B

C

Figure 23-2 ■ Traumatic C4 vertebral body fracture: **A,** Lateral plain film. **B,** Axial computed tomography (CT) scan demonstrating the fracture through the vertebral body. **C,** Sagittal CT scan.

Pharmacologic Therapy

Pharmacologic therapies for treatment of acute spinal cord injury have shown little benefit.[21] The corticosteroid methylprednisolone has been the most extensively tested for SCI. Its mechanism of action is thought to involve decreasing of cord edema, support of energy metabolism, anti-inflammatory properties, membrane stabilization, antioxidant effects, and free-radical scavenging.[22,23] There is controversial class 1 clinical evidence to support its use in SCI.[4] This controversy has arisen over several large clinical trials. The first National Acute Spinal Cord Injury Studies (NASCIS) trial in 1984 randomized 330 patients to either a high or a low dosage of methylprednisolone for 10 days. There was not a placebo arm in NASCIS I. The trial demonstrated a significant increase in wound infections without statistical difference in clinical outcomes in the two dosage groups. The landmark NASCIS II study reported results in 1990 and 1992 for 487 patients who were randomized into this double-blind, controlled, multicenter trial of either naloxone, high-dose methylprednisolone (30 mg/kg bolus followed by a 5.4-mg/kg/hr infusion) or placebo during a 24-hour period after the injury. The NASCIS II trial showed no difference in clinical outcomes, although a secondary analysis demonstrated that patients given methylprednisolone within 8 hours of the injury had a statistically significant improvement in their motor function at 1 year. The NASCIS III trial (1997) randomized 499 patients to tirilazad mesylate (an inhibitor of

lipid peroxidation) and methylprednisolone (30 mg/kg), methylprednisolone only for 24 hours, or methylprednisolone only for 48 hours (30 mg/kg bolus followed by a 5.4-mg/kg/hr infusion). The trial showed no significant improvement in any of the primary outcome measures at 1 year, although secondary analysis demonstrated that patients treated with 48 hours of methylprednisolone between 3 to 8 hours after injury had an improvement in motor function at both 6 weeks and 6 months over patients in the 24-hour treatment group.

The current recommended dosage of methylprednisolone is a 30 mg/kg bolus over 15 minutes followed by a maintenance dose of 5.4 mg over 23 hours if the injury occurred within 3 hours (Table 23-1), or over 48 hours if the injury occurred between 3 to 8 hours before treatment.[8] Although it was not clinically significant, a trend has been noted toward a high complication rate associated with methylprednisolone in the three NASCIS trials. Complications include myopathy, infection, respiratory failure, and sepsis. The current recommendation for the use of methylprednisolone after traumatic SCI is that it is an option for either 24 or 48 hours, but that it should be undertaken only with the understanding that evidence supporting harmful side effects may outweigh any clinical benefit.[21] The use of methylprednisolone in acute SCI is probably no longer the standard of care.[24]

Other pharmaceuticals studied in randomized clinical trials for SCI (GM-1 ganglioside, tirilazad mesylate, naloxone) have not shown a benefit. Future treatments for SCI

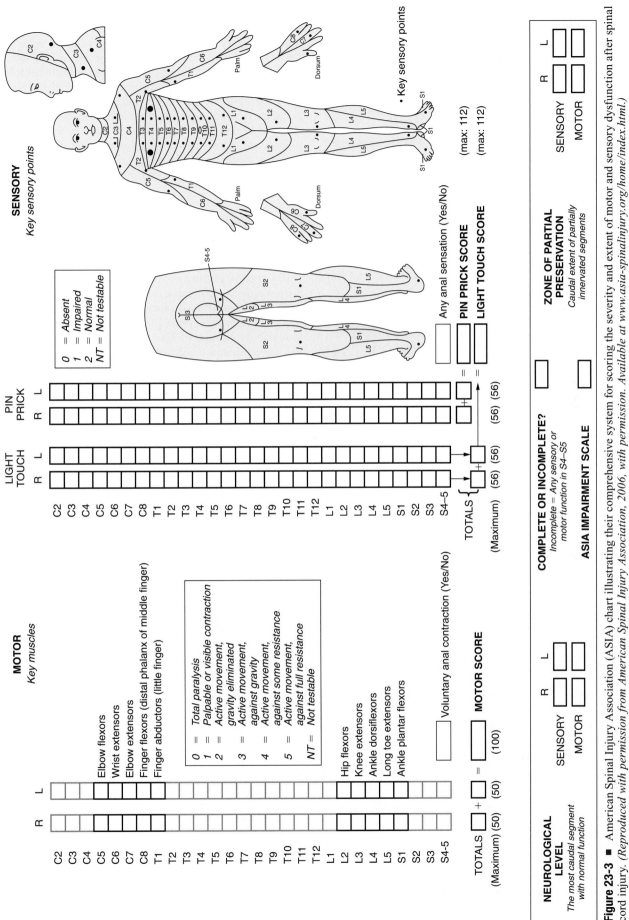

Figure 23-3 ■ American Spinal Injury Association (ASIA) chart illustrating their comprehensive system for scoring the severity and extent of motor and sensory dysfunction after spinal cord injury. (*Reproduced with permission from American Spinal Injury Association, 2006, with permission. Available at www.asia-spinalinjury.org/home/index.html.*)

include transplantation of progenitor or stem cells into injured spinal cord, and pharmacologic treatments including minocycline (regulation of growth factors, anti-inflammatory, inhibition of free radicals, and modulation of apoptosis) and Cethrin-activated macrophage implantation.[4]

Surgery

Surgery for patients who have suffered SCI can be considered for stabilization of an unstable spine, to reduce a deformity, or to decompress neural tissues.[11] Surgical stabilization of unstable spine lesions may prevent primary neurologic injury. Most unstable injuries require anterior and posterior fixation, although some cervical injuries require anterior discectomy and fusion, or posterior fixation alone.[11] The treatment of vertebral fractures is controversial and may benefit from conservative treatment with an orthosis.[11] Although they do not result in an unstable spine, vertebral burst fractures may require surgery because the lesion may result in collapse of the vertebral body with time, causing the loss of anterior height or kyphosis.[11] Surgery to relieve a complete neurologic injury is not indicated, because primary cell death has already occurred and reversal of this deficit would not occur. Incomplete injuries or progressive neurologic injuries are more likely to benefit from decompressive surgery for lesions impinging on the spinal cord. Decompressive surgery should occur as soon as possible, as it may prevent further primary injury and improve tissue perfusion, thus limiting secondary injury.

■ PARAPLEGIA AFTER THORACIC OR THORACOABDOMINAL AORTIC ANEURYSM REPAIR

Despite improvements in surgical and medical care, spinal cord ischemia causing postoperative paraplegia or paraparesis remains a major cause of morbidity and mortality after thoracoabdominal aortic aneurysm (TAAA) repair, isolated thoracic aortic aneurysm (TAA) repair, and even after endovascular stent repair of TAA (Fig. 23-4). This complication has an estimated incidence that ranges between 2.7% and 41%.[25-29] Temporary or permanent interruption of vascular collaterals to the spinal cord from the intercostals or lumbar segmental arteries is believed to be the cause of spinal cord ischemia and subsequent infarction. Infarction may affect the entire spinal cord from the lumbar to the mid-thoracic level, causing dense paraplegia or spare regions of the cord, producing paraparesis or selective motor weakness with preserved sensation.[30] Existing clinical experience suggests that the risk of spinal cord ischemia is related to the extent of disease in the descending aorta and the length of the interposition or endovascular stent graft[31,32] (Fig. 23-5). Risk factors for spinal cord ischemia include Crawford extent I, II, or III TAAA (Fig. 23-6), emergent operations, ruptured aneurysm, acute Stanford type B aortic dissection, and endo-

23-1	Schedule of Methylprednisolone* Administration for Treatment of Acute Spinal Cord Injury				
	BOLUS			**MAINTENANCE**	
Body Surface Area Regimen	**Dosage**	**Rate**		**Dosage**	**Rate**
1.16-1.70 m²	1,938 mg	7,750 mg/hr		8,625 mg	375 mg/hr
1.71-2.35 m²	2,750 mg	11,000 mg/hr		11,500 mg	500 mg/hr
2.36-3.00 m²	3,688 mg	14,750 mg/hr		15,813 mg	688 mg/hr
Bodyweight Regimen					
—		30 mg/kg over 15 min (first hr)		5.4 mg/kg/hr for next 23 hr	

*Methylprednisolone was prepared to a concentration of 62.5 mg/mL and administered intravenously.
From Bracken MB, Shepard MJ, Collins WF, et al: N Engl J Med 1990;322:1405-1411, with permission.

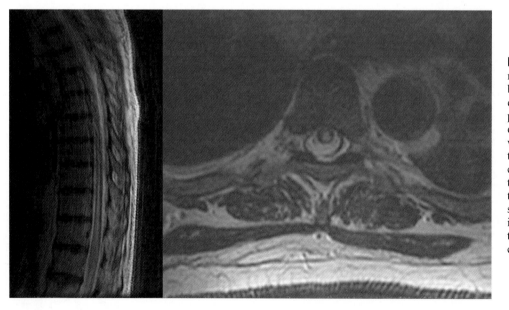

Figure 23-4 ■ Magnetic resonance images of the thoracolumbar spine demonstrating spinal cord infarction in a patient with paraplegia after thoracoabdominal aneurysm repair. T2-weighted sagittal imaging through the center of the spinal cord *(left)* showed central infarction extending from the high thoracic level into the lumbar segments. T2-weighted axial images of the spinal cord at the thoracic level demonstrated central infarction *(right)*.

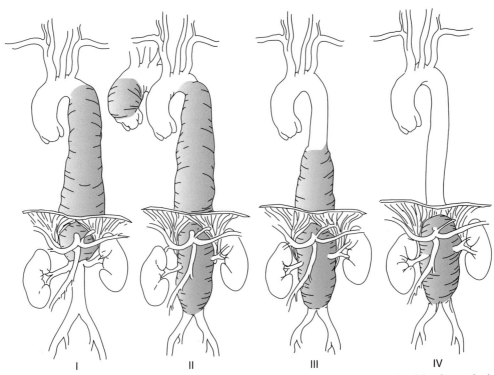

Figure 23-5 ■ Crawford classification of thoracoabdominal aortic aneurysms. The risk of paraplegia after surgery correlates with the extent of disease. *(Modified with permission from Coselli JS: Descending thoracoabdominal aortic aneurysms. In Edmunds LH [ed]: Cardiac Surgery in the Adult. New York, McGraw Hill, 1997, p 1232.)*

Figure 23-6 ■ Proposed classification for isolated descending thoracic aortic aneurysms. The risk of paraplegia from spinal cord ischemia after endovascular stent graft repair correlated with the extent of aortic coverage by the stent graft. The risk of postoperative paraplegia is greatest in patients with prior abdominal aortic aneurysm repair undergoing the extent of coverage of the thoracic aorta shown in **C.** *(Adapted with permission from Estrera AL, Rubenstein FS, Miller CC 3rd, et al: Ann Thorac Surg 2001;72:481-486.)*

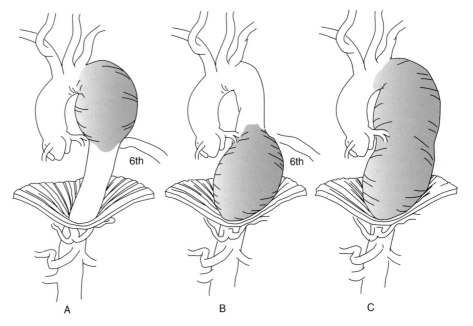

vascular stent graft repair of TAA in patients after prior abdominal aortic aneurysm repair.[26,27,31,32] Permanent paraplegia after TAAA repair has an associated mortality rate ranging from 50% to 100%.

Clinical strategies to prevent and treat spinal cord ischemia consist of surgical techniques to preserve vascular collaterals and maintain spinal cord perfusion during surgery, anesthetic techniques to decrease central nervous system (CNS) metabolic demand and augment spinal cord perfusion, pharmacologic agents to protect against neuronal injury, and monitoring of spinal cord function to permit early intervention (Box 23-1).[33] Except for lumbar cerebrospinal fluid (CSF)

23-1	Management Strategies to Prevent and Treat Spinal Cord Ischemia after Thoracoabdominal Aortic Aneurysm Repair

Surgical Techniques

- Reimplantation of intercostal and lumbar segmental arteries
- Partial left heart bypass to provide distal aortic perfusion
- Staged cross-clamping of aortic segments to decrease ischemic duration
- Deliberate hypothermia or deep hypothermic circulatory arrest
- Maintenance of left vertebral artery flow by revascularization of the left subclavian artery (endovascular stent repair)

Anesthetic Techniques

- Intraoperative somatosensory evoked potential monitoring (SSEP)
- Intraoperative motor evoked potential monitoring (MEP)
- Lumbar cerebrospinal fluid drainage
- Arterial pressure augmentation
- Deliberate mild systemic hypothermia
- Selective cooling of the spinal cord
- Serial neurologic examination
- Pharmacologic neuroprotection agents (e.g., glucocorticoids, naloxone, papaverine, intravenous lidocaine, magnesium, central nervous system depressants)

drainage, none of these techniques has been studied by randomized controlled trials, and clinical efficacy remains unproven (class indeterminate) or must be inferred by clinical series, case reports, rational conjecture, tradition, and routine use in established practices.

The physiologic basis for lumbar CSF drainage is that increased lumbar CSF pressure decreases the net spinal cord perfusion pressure. Decreasing lumbar CSF pressure by draining CSF has the potential to increase perfusion pressure to the spinal cord. The technique can be performed prophylactically before surgery or, in the event of spinal cord ischemia, by percutaneous insertion of a Silastic catheter into the subarachnoid space between lumbar spinal processes. The lumbar CSF pressure is measured by transducer, and CSF is drained into a sealed reservoir to achieve a lumbar CSF pressure of 10 mm Hg.[30,34] Two meta-analyses on the efficacy of lumbar CSF drainage have been published and are based on 372 reports that include three randomized controlled trials involving 289 patients, and five cohort studies involving 505 patients.[35,36] Pooled data from the three randomized trials indicated that lumbar CSF drainage was effective in decreasing the risk of paraplegia, with a pooled odds ratio (OR) of 0.30 ($P = .05$; 95% confidence interval [CI], 0.17-0.54).[16] However, the analysis by the Cochrane Collaborative indicated insufficient evidence to support the efficacy of lumbar CSF drainage alone (OR, 0.57; 95% CI, 0.28-1.17), because one randomized controlled trial was disqualified for administration of intrathecal papaverine in combination with lumbar CSF drainage.[36] Although the Cochrane report concluded that use of lumbar CSF drainage *alone* as protection has not been established from the available evidence, lumbar

CSF drainage was recommended as a component of the multimodality approach for prevention of neurologic injury (class IIa).[36] Although the safety of lumbar CSF drainage appears to be acceptable even in patients subjected to full anticoagulation for extracorporeal circulation,[37] complications associated with the technique include subdural hematoma,[38] intraspinal hematoma,[39] remote cerebellar hemorrhage,[40] infection,[37] and even catheter fracture.[37] The most serious complications appear to be associated with intracranial hypotension from rapid drainage of CSF.[38]

Augmenting the arterial pressure alone or in combination with lumbar CSF drainage is another technique for treating spinal cord ischemia (class IIa).[30,31,41] In general, vasopressor agents are administered to maintain a MAP of 80 mm Hg or greater to ensure a spinal cord perfusion pressure of at least 70 mm Hg. The MAP can be augmented further in increments of 5 mm Hg if spinal cord ischemia persists.[30,31] Inconsistent control of the arterial pressure may also explain in part the controversy surrounding the effectiveness of lumbar CSF drainage, because decreasing CSF pressure alone without controlling the arterial pressure may limit the ability to improve spinal cord perfusion. Hypotension from bleeding or other causes is often associated with the onset of spinal cord ischemia after TAAA repair, but clinical observations also suggest that spinal cord ischemia may contribute to hypotension as a consequence of autonomic dysfunction from neurogenic shock.[30,31,42,43] In this situation, hypotension may represent an early sign of spinal cord ischemia. Immediate treatment of hypotension associated with spinal cord ischemia is necessary to prevent infarction (Figs. 23-7 and 23-8). The benefits of arterial pressure augmentation must be weighed against the risk of bleeding when implementing this technique in the perioperative period.

Early detection of spinal cord ischemia is important and very likely contributes to the effectiveness of treatment.[30,31,41] Inability to detect intraoperative spinal cord ischemia in anesthetized patients may explain in part the lack of success in treating patients with immediate onset paraplegia after TAAA repair. Successes reported in the treatment of delayed postoperative spinal cord ischemia may be attributed to early diagnosis by serial neurologic assessment and immediate interventions to increase spinal cord perfusion.[30,31,41-43] Neurologic assessment of lower extremity motor function can be performed and documented objectively by the nursing staff of the intensive care unit, and any deficit should be considered to be spinal cord ischemia until disproved.

Intraoperative monitoring of somatosensory evoked potentials (SSEPs) or motor evoked potentials (MEPs) may improve the ability to detect and treat spinal cord ischemia during surgery, but clinical experience remains limited (class indeterminate).[44,45] During surgery on the descending thoracic aorta, spinal cord ischemia may be caused by loss of perfusion to the spinal cord due to hypoperfusion, or by loss of collateral blood flow through critical radicular, intercostal, or lumbar arteries, either because of dissection itself, thrombosis, or embolization, or through surgical ligation of these arteries. The clinical objectives for intraoperative monitoring of spinal cord function during these operations are to ensure

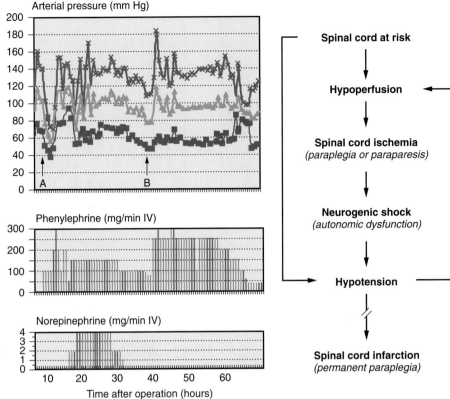

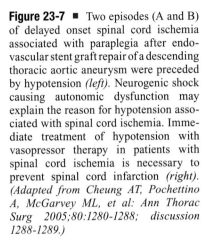

Figure 23-7 ■ Two episodes (A and B) of delayed onset spinal cord ischemia associated with paraplegia after endovascular stent graft repair of a descending thoracic aortic aneurysm were preceded by hypotension *(left)*. Neurogenic shock causing autonomic dysfunction may explain the reason for hypotension associated with spinal cord ischemia. Immediate treatment of hypotension with vasopressor therapy in patients with spinal cord ischemia is necessary to prevent spinal cord infarction *(right)*. *(Adapted from Cheung AT, Pochettino A, McGarvey ML, et al: Ann Thorac Surg 2005;80:1280-1288; discussion 1288-1289.)*

adequate spinal cord perfusion throughout the procedure and to identify critical vessels for reimplantation. The detection of reversible transient spinal cord ischemic changes by intraoperative monitoring may identify patients who may be at risk for delayed postoperative paraplegia. Clinical experience suggests that improved techniques for detecting and preventing intraoperative spinal cord ischemia have decreased the incidence of immediate postoperative paraplegia but have not eliminated the risk of delayed postoperative spinal cord ischemia.[30] SSEP and MEP changes have been shown to correlate with spinal cord ischemia. These techniques may serve as a warning of impending injury in that the loss of neuronal function may precede permanent structural injury. In patients undergoing both acute and chronic type B dissection repair, monitoring SSEP and MEP may be more critical than during atherosclerotic aneurysm repair, because the dissections are associated with a greater number of patent radicular and intercostal arteries than are seen with atherosclerotic aneurysms, thus increasing the risk of paraplegia when these branch vessels are sacrificed.[46,47]

Intraoperative changes in (or loss of) SSEP or MEP signals are not always caused by spinal cord ischemia. A functioning peripheral nerve is required to generate both SSEP and MEP signals, and peripheral nerve ischemia from any cause will affect the associated SSEP or MEP. Vascular malperfusion of a lower extremity can cause loss of peripheral SSEP or MEP in the absence of spinal cord ischemia if blood flow to the limb is significantly compromised. Malperfusion causes a loss of SSEP or MEP from the ischemic limb. Lower extremity malperfusion may be caused by the aortic dissection itself, by atheroembolism, or most commonly by arterial cannulation of the femoral artery for extracorporeal circulation. As is seen in malperfusion, operations performed by cross-clamping the aorta without distal aortic perfusion will cause SSEP and MEP signals from the lower extremities to decay over time after aortic cross-clamping, and loss of SSEP or MEP signals in this situation is a nonspecific indicator for spinal cord ischemia. Acute intraoperative stroke also alters SSEP or MEP. SSEP or MEP changes caused by stroke can be distinguished from changes caused by spinal cord ischemia by comparing signals recorded at different sites along the neural conduction pathway. Stroke is associated with selective loss of cortical signals and typically affects both upper and lower extremity evoked potentials. The various modalities, including the wakeup test, have certain advantages and disadvantages that can be tailored, depending on the patient's operative risk and the type of anesthesia that may be required for the procedure (Table 23-2).

Intraoperative monitoring of SSEP is performed by placing stimulating electrodes on the skin adjacent to peripheral nerves in the arms or legs. Electrical stimulation of the peripheral nerves in the limbs generates action potentials that can be measured from recording electrodes over the lumbar plexus, brachial plexus, spine, brainstem, thalamus and cerebral cortex. The SSEP from the legs may also travel in the more lateral spinocerebellar tracts of the spinal cord. This is important because the anterior spinal artery supplies

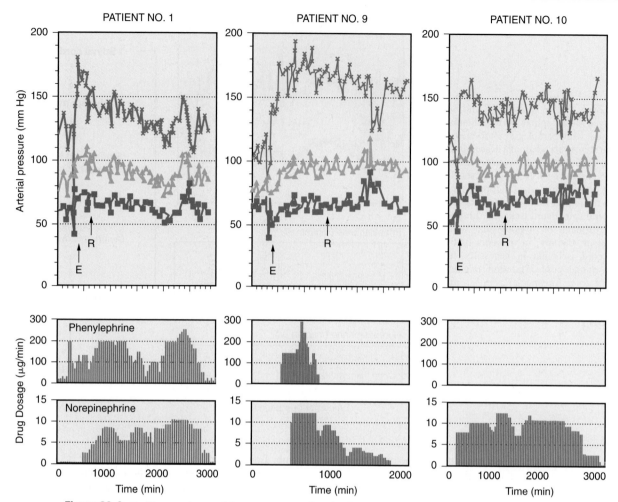

Figure 23-8 ■ Changes in arterial pressure over time in three patients with delayed-onset paraplegia caused by spinal cord ischemia after open thoracoabdominal aortic aneurysm repair. In each case, the onset of paraplegia (E) was preceded by hypotension. Each patient recovered in response to vasopressor therapy combined with lumbar cerebrospinal fluid drainage (R). Recovery of motor function coincided with recovery of arterial pressure, indicating the return of autonomic function. *(Reproduced from Cheung AT, Weiss SJ, McGarvey ML, et al: Ann Thorac Surg 2002;74:413-419; discussion 420-421.)*

23-2	Assessing Spinal Cord Function during Surgery	
Technique	**Advantages**	**Disadvantages**
Wakeup test	Simple to perform	Complete neurologic assessment limited by residual anesthetic agents, patient's ability to move, or surgical restrictions
Somatosensory evoked potential (SSEP)	Signals less affected by general anesthetic agents and agent concentrations	Does not assess motor pathways
		Impaired by high depth of general anesthesia
	Not affected by neuromuscular blocking drugs	May have about a 20-min delay in SSEP changes after spinal cord ischemia
Motor evoked potential (MEP)	Assesses integrity of motor pathways	Attenuated by inhaled anesthetic agents
	Immediate detection of spinal cord ischemia	Neuromuscular blocking drugs cannot be used
	Difficult to achieve reproducible recordings	

the spinocerebellar tracts, and ischemia in the territory of the anterior spinal artery is manifested by changes in the SSEP.[48] A potential limitation of SSEP monitoring is that spinal cord ischemia confined to the anterior spinal cord may cause a selective motor deficit with intact sensation. In this situation, SSEP monitoring may fail to detect spinal cord ischemia. However, clinical experience suggests that isolated motor dysfunction is uncommon. In one clinical series, 90% of patients with spinal cord ischemia after TAAA repair had sensory deficits.[30] An advantage of SSEP monitoring is that it is relatively reliable to perform and easy to interpret. SSEP signals are improved with neuromuscular blockade under general anesthesia. Although high concentrations of inhaled anesthetics, thiopental, or propofol can attenuate cortical SSEP signals, inhaled anesthetics maintained at a concentration of 0.5 MAC provide consistent conditions for monitoring intraoperative SSEP. A specific classification system has been developed to describe the findings of SSEP monitoring during thoracic aneurysm repairs (Table 23-3).[44]

Myogenic and neurogenic MEPs elicited through transcortical electrical stimulation have been advocated for the detection of intraoperative spinal cord ischemia. However, evidence to support the efficacy of MEP for prevention of spinal cord ischemia and infarction remains limited. To monitor MEP, myogenic potentials are produced in extremity muscle groups by delivering multipulse electrical stimulation to the scalp, overlying the motor cortex. The neurogenic MEP is recorded from peripheral nerves after this stimulation. The evoked potentials elicited from this stimulation travel from the motor cortex, through cortical spinal tracts, anterior horn cell, and peripheral nerve, and finally to muscle. An interruption in this pathway will result in loss of the MEP. Monitoring MEP from the legs of patients undergoing TAAA repair would be expected to detect spinal cord ischemia in the lumbar to thoracic myotomes. In theory, monitoring MEP should be more sensitive and specific than SSEP to detect spinal cord ischemia. A small study of 56 patients using both MEP and SSEP monitoring demonstrated that MEP was able to detect more transient changes and persistent changes consistent with spinal cord ischemia than SSEP monitoring.[49] MEP monitoring has been used to identify critical intercostal arteries for reattachment after the acute loss of lower extremity MEP signals during TAAA repair.[45]

Limitations of MEP monitoring include the inability to monitor it in the postoperative period.[45] MEP recording also requires special anesthetic protocols that limit or avoid the use of neuromuscular blocking agents and inhaled anesthetics. General anesthetic regimens involving intravenous infusions of remifentanil, ketamine, propofol, or etomidate are often required to maintain satisfactory MEP signals during surgery.

At present, the morbidity associated with spinal cord ischemia after TAAA, combined with the difficulty of performing randomized controlled trials to test the effectiveness of interventions, justifies the continued use of techniques with acceptable safety in an effort to decrease the incidence of this complication until better evidence becomes available. Algorithms have been developed to attempt to identify and reverse this complication, both intraoperatively and postoperatively, with some success (Fig. 23-9).[30,31]

■ SPINAL CORD INJURY FROM CENTRAL NEURAXIAL ANESTHESIA AND ANALGESIA

Spinal cord injury after central neuraxial anesthesia and analgesia is a well-established but rare complication. Mechanisms purported to cause spinal cord injury as a consequence of epidural or spinal anesthesia include epidural hematoma (resulting in compressive myelopathy), mechanical injury to the spinal cord or nerve roots (via instrumentation), direct

23-3	Classification of Intraoperative Somatosensory Evoked Potential (SSEP) Alterations during Thoracoabdominal Aortic Aneurysm Repair
Type	**Etiology**
Type 1	Distal spinal cord ischemia from aortic cross-clamping
Type 2	Peripheral nerve ischemia from femoral artery occlusion
Type 3	Segmental spinal ischemia from vascular insufficiency
Type 4	Left hemispheric ischemia from left carotid occlusion
Type 5	Global cortical ischemia from hypotension or stroke

Modified with permission from Guerit JM, Witdoeckt C, Verhelst R, et al: Ann Thorac Surg 1999;67:1943-1946; discussion 1953-1958.

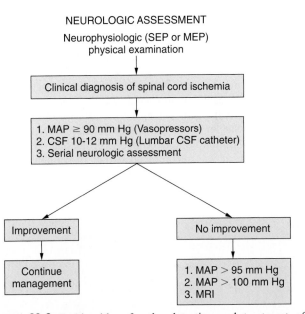

Figure 23-9 ■ Algorithm for the detection and treatment of spinal cord ischemia after surgery on the thoracic and thoracoabdominal aorta. Neurologic deficits detected by intraoperative somatosensory evoked or motor evoked potential monitoring or postoperative deficits detected by neurologic examination are treated by augmenting the arterial pressure with vasopressor therapy and decreasing the cerebrospinal fluid (CSF) pressure by lumbar CSF drainage. MAP, mean arterial pressure; MEP, motor evoked potential; MRI, magnetic resonance imaging; SSEP, somatosensory evoked potential.

injection of medications into the spinal cord or blood vessels (resulting in toxic neurolysis), and infection.[50] The incidence of complications related to central neuraxial anesthesia and analgesia has been estimated to be in the range of 1 per 10,000 to 1 per 100,000 cases.[51,52] Although the majority of neurologic complications attributed to perioperative neuraxial anesthesia and analgesia are more likely the consequence of improper patient positioning, resulting in pressure palsies or surgical trauma,[53] it is important to recognize the potential for complications in patients at risk.

The most frequent neurologic injury associated with neuraxial anesthesia is spinal hematoma, caused by intraspinal or epidural bleeding after instrumentation for intradural or epidural catheter placement. Based on limited reports, risks for spinal epidural hematoma include female sex, age (>75 years), traumatic procedure, history of gastrointestinal bleeding, anticoagulation therapy, and administration of anticoagulants shortly after instrumentation or catheter placement.[54,55] Additional potential risk factors include preexisting coagulopathy, spine deformities, vascular malformations, and tumors in the spinal canal. The increasing use of anticoagulation and antiplatelet therapy has generated increased concern for the risk of hemorrhagic complications associated with neuraxial anesthetic techniques.

For this reason, the American Society of Regional Anesthesia (ASRA) has published a consensus statement that provides recommendations on the safe use of neuraxial anesthetic techniques in patients receiving anticoagulation and antiplatelet therapy.[55] The ASRA guidelines recommend that neuraxial techniques can be performed safely in patients on aspirin, nonsteroidal anti-inflammatory drugs (NSAIDs), subcutaneous (mini-dose) heparin for deep venous thrombosis prophylaxis, or intraoperative heparin for vascular surgical procedures. The ASRA guidelines recommend against the use of neuraxial anesthetic techniques in patients on therapeutic doses of low-molecular-weight heparin (LMWH) (enoxaparin, dalteparin, tinzaparin), warfarin, thrombolytic agents, antiplatelet agents (clopidogrel, ticlopidine), or platelet IIb/IIIa inhibitors (abciximab, eptifibatide, tirofiban). Furthermore, it was recommended that instrumentation of the spine should not be performed within 10 to 12 hours after

the last dose of LMWH, 7 days after clopidogrel, 10 days after thrombolytic therapy, and 14 days after ticlopidine.

Despite adherence to the ASRA recommendations, spinal hematoma causing neurologic injury complicating epidural anesthesia has been reported.[56-60] It is also recognized that hemorrhagic complications associated with epidural anesthesia are present at the time of catheter insertion and the time of removal. Although the therapeutic action of unfractionated heparin therapy can be assessed by measuring the partial thromboplastin time (PTT) or activated coagulation time (ACT), and the therapeutic level of warfarin can be measured by the prothrombin time (PT) or International Normalized Ratio (INR), there are no laboratory assays to assess the effects of LMWH or antiplatelet therapy on coagulation. The ASRA recommendations may not apply to patients on combination therapy, with renal insufficiency, with hepatic dysfunction, or with underlying coagulation defects that result in increased risk of hemorrhagic complications. Patients at risk for hemorrhagic or spinal cord injury associated with neuraxial anesthesia or analgesia should be managed with local anesthetic or narcotic analgesics that do not completely block sensory and motor function, in order to permit neurologic assessment, and they should be monitored for neurologic deficits at least every 2 hours.

Signs and symptoms of spinal epidural hematoma include back pain, lower extremity paresthesia, leg weakness, urinary retention, and bowel dysfunction (Fig. 23-10). The clinical diagnosis of spinal epidural hematoma complicating neuraxial blockade can be difficult because the spectrum of manifestations varies, and signs and symptoms may be attributed to the actions of the local anesthetic block. Persistence or progression of signs and symptoms such as back pain or lower extremity numbness and weakness beyond the expected duration of the local anesthetic block may indicate spinal epidural hematoma with cord compression. MRI scans demonstrating an epidural or paraspinal heme-containing collection causing cord compression or displacement is diagnostic for spinal epidural hematoma. Spontaneous resolution of spinal epidural hematoma without treatment has been reported,[56] but two case series reported that outcomes were best when surgical decompression was performed within 8 to

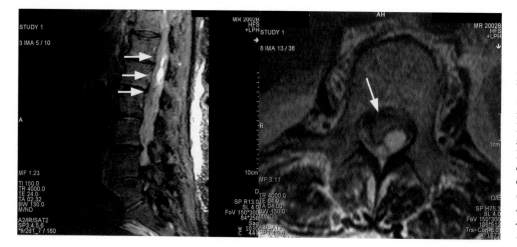

Figure 23-10 ■ Magnetic resonance imaging of the thoracolumbar spine, demonstrating an epidural hematoma in a patient after spinal anesthesia. T2-weighted sagittal imaging showed extension of the epidural hematoma from T12 to L3 *(arrows, left)*. T2-weighted axial imaging at the level of L2 showed anterior compression of the spinal cord from the epidural hematoma *(arrow, right)*. *(Adapted with permission from Litz RJ, Gottschlich B, Stehr SN: Anesthesiology 2004;101:1467-1470.)*

12 hours after the onset of symptoms.[61,62] Recovery of neurologic function after surgical decompression also correlated to the severity of the neurologic deficits before surgery.

Infection complicating neuraxial blockade and causing meningitis, arachnoiditis, or spinal epidural abscess has always been a concern, particularly in patients with sepsis, localized infections, bacterial colonization, or immunosuppression. However, clinical experience suggests that infections related to neuraxial anesthesia are rare, with an incidence ranging from 1 per 1000 to 1 per 10,000 cases.[63] In reported cases, infectious complications have been attributed to performing procedures in patients with sepsis, infections close to the site of instrumentation, traumatic catheter insertion, or indwelling catheters left in for prolonged periods.[37,63] Signs and symptoms of spinal or CNS infection as a consequence of neuraxial techniques include back pain, radiculopathy, paresthesia, paraplegia, bowel or bladder dysfunction, fever, and altered mentation. On the basis of clinical experience, it has been recommended that neuraxial anesthesia can be performed safely in patients with systemic infections or at risk for bacteremia when appropriate antibiotic therapy has been initiated prior to the procedure.[63] Neuraxial anesthesia should be avoided when needle insertion or catheter placement is in a region with a high risk of bacterial contamination.

Cauda equina syndrome with permanent neurologic injury is a recognized complication of continuous spinal anesthesia and has been attributed to the neurotoxic potential of local anesthetic agents.[64] Reports of this complication suggest a mechanism of injury caused by high concentrations of local anesthetic administered into a restricted region within the subarachnoid space. This condition can be achieved by continuous spinal anesthesia with local anesthetic administered through a small-bore (<24-gauge) spinal catheter, repeated injections of local anesthetic into the subarachnoid space, or inadvertent injection of a large dose of local anesthetic into the subarachnoid space originally intended for epidural administration. The local anesthetic agent that cases of cauda equina syndrome are most commonly associated with is lidocaine, but they have also been reported with chloroprocaine. This association is consistent with the finding that lidocaine is more neurotoxic than other local anesthetic agents when tested in a laboratory setting.[65,66] For this reason, it has been recommended that lidocaine should not be administered at a dosage of greater than 60 mg or at a concentration greater than 2.5% when used for subarachnoid injection. The safety of combining vasoconstrictor agents such as epinephrine to prolong the duration of lidocaine subarachnoid blocks has also been questioned, because vasoconstrictor agents have the potential to increase local anesthetic toxicity by promoting ischemia or by limiting the distribution and uptake of the local anesthetic agent.[64]

■ SPINAL CORD INJURY AND SPINE SURGERY

Complete or incomplete paraplegia is a recognized complication of spine surgery. Although the precise incidence of this complication is unknown, a retrospective analysis indicated an estimated rate of 0.6% for the surgical treatment of scoliosis with a high degree of correction, 0.14% for spinal fusion, 0.07% for cervical discectomy, and 0.03% for lumbar discectomy.[67,68] Because of the limited reports in the literature, the precise mechanism of spinal cord injury after orthopedic spine surgery is not completely understood. Proposed mechanisms of spinal cord injury include ischemia, mechanical injury, or more likely a combination of both. Ischemic injury can occur as a consequence of operative injury, sacrifice, or ligation of radicular arteries providing collateral circulation to the anterior spinal artery. Hypotension, low cardiac output states, increased central venous pressure, or "kinking" of arteries supplying the spinal cord as a consequence of realigning the spine all may contribute to ischemic injury. Mechanical injury to the spinal cord may occur as a consequence of traction or transverse forces to the cord during realignment, misplaced implants, or direct injury to the spinal cord during surgical exposure. Compression of the spinal cord from epidural hematoma, bone chips, scar formation, or bone may cause both mechanical injury and vascular insufficiency. The incidence of postoperative epidural hematoma after spine surgery has been estimated to be 0.2% in one series.[69] Risk factors for spinal cord injury after spine surgery include operations for short-curved kyphosis (as opposed to long-curved scoliosis), congenital deformities with spinal cord malformation, preoperative neurologic deficits, and coagulopathy.[67] Risk factors for postoperative epidural hematoma complicating spine operations include age greater than 60 years, preoperative use of NSAIDs, Rh-positive blood type, surgery involving more than five vertebral levels, hemoglobin concentration less than 10 g/dL, estimated blood loss greater than 1 L, or INR greater than 2.0 within the first 48 hours after surgery.[69] Clinical strategies to prevent and detect spinal cord injury during spine operations include intraoperative wakeup testing, SSEP monitoring, MEP monitoring, or a combination of techniques, but the evidence to support the effectiveness of these interventions is indeterminate.

■ ANESTHETIC AND MEDICAL MANAGEMENT OF THE PATIENT WITH EXISTING OR PRIOR SPINAL CORD INJURY

It is not uncommon that a patient with an acute or established spinal cord injury requires anesthetic and surgical care. Even though the neurologic injury may be established and nothing can be done to decrease the severity of injury, spinal cord injuries cause profound physiologic alterations and are associated with a spectrum of systemic problems that require medical attention. Autonomic nervous system dysfunction may cause neurogenic shock, bradycardia, orthostatic hypotension, or autonomic dysreflexia. Altered autonomic nervous system function impairs vascular autoregulation to external temperature changes and to intravascular volume shifts, making the patient more susceptible to hypothermia from exposure and to hypovolemia from blood and fluid losses associated with surgery. The renin-angiotensin-aldosterone system may exert a more important role in blood pressure regulation to compensate for autonomic dysfunction, making the spinal cord–injured patient more susceptible to the antihypertensive actions of angiotensin-converting enzyme (ACE) inhibitors or angiotensin receptor blocking (ARB) drugs. In addition, urinary retention and neurogenic bladder dysfunction as a consequence of spinal cord injury predispose the patient to urinary tract infections and renal insufficiency. Constipation associated with spinal cord injuries may lead to bowel obstruction, malnutrition, or an increased risk of aspiration pneumonia. Motor paralysis affecting the respiratory accessory muscles and abdominal muscles is associated with reduced pulmonary reserve and impaired cough, predisposing the patient to respiratory failure or respiratory infections. Pulmonary function testing can be useful to assess respiratory function and pulmonary reserve in the patient with spinal cord injury. Finally, spinal cord injury causing quadriplegia, paraplegia, or paraparesis is a chronic disease state and is associated with anemia, poor nutritional status, skin breakdown, decubitus ulcers, risk of deep venous thrombosis, and risk of infection.

Neurogenic shock is a complication of acute complete spinal cord injury above the thoracic T6 level. Hypotension attributed to neurogenic shock has also been observed as a consequence of spinal cord ischemia and infarction after TAAA surgery.[30] Neurogenic shock is caused by autonomic nervous system dysfunction with dysfunction of the sympathetic paravertebral ganglia innervated by the thoracic lumbar segments of the spinal cord, in particular, that exert an important role in the maintenance of peripheral vascular tone. In the classic description, neurogenic shock is characterized as a state of hypotension with low systemic vascular resistance and normal or increased cardiac output. Episodes of hypotension from neurogenic shock typically occur in about half of spinal cord injury patients within the first 24 hours after injury.[70] Neurogenic shock generally persists for 1 to 3 weeks after injury. The incidence and severity of neurogenic shock appear to correlate with the level of the injury and the extent of the injury.[71] Patients with paraplegia may have compensatory tachycardia, whereas quadriplegic patients may suffer from bradycardia caused by unopposed vagal tone. The treatment of neurogenic shock is directed at pharmacologic support of blood pressure and circulatory function until autonomic nervous system function is restored or compensatory physiologic mechanisms are able to maintain blood pressure within a physiologic range. Intravenous vasopressor therapy with norepinephrine, phenylephrine, dopamine, epinephrine, or vasopressin, often in high doses, is necessary to treat hypotension and support the arterial pressure. During treatment with vasopressor therapy, it is important to assess intravascular fluid status and treat hypovolemia with volume expansion.

Neurogenic shock should be distinguished from the term *spinal shock,* which is a neurologic phenomenon describing the transient inexcitability of the spinal cord below the level of injury in the acute phase of injury. Spinal shock is characterized by the loss of deep tendon reflexes; motor and sensory function below the level of the lesion and may or may not be associated with neurogenic shock.

Autonomic dysreflexia or hyperreflexia is a complication that occurs in patients with spinal cord injuries that is often precipitated during surgical procedures; it is considered a medical emergency.[72] Its incidence ranges from 19% to 70% in patients with spinal cord injuries.[73] It is more common in patients with complete lesions above the thoracic T6 level and a viable spinal cord below the level of the lesion. Autonomic dysreflexia may occur soon after spinal cord injury or may not manifest for years after injury. Its pathophysiology is exaggerated sympathetic activity triggered in response to a stimulus below the level of the lesion. The "mass reflex" and discharge of adrenergic transmitters occurs because the cord lesion prevents brainstem and higher cortical regulation of autonomic tone. It is possible also that the peripheral vasculature has increased responsiveness to adrenergic agonists.

The primary clinical sign of autonomic dysreflexia is severe hypertension, with systolic blood pressures as high as 200 to 300 mm Hg. Severe vasoconstriction may even render the noninvasive blood pressure monitor and pulse oximeter nonfunctional. The adrenergic discharge may produce signs and symptoms as mild as headache, tinnitus, nausea, nasal congestion, cutaneous flushing, anxiety, blurred vision, piloerection, fever, or ventricular ectopic activity. Severe reactions may cause respiratory distress, loss of consciousness, pulmonary edema, heart failure, cardiac arrhythmias, stroke, encephalopathy, intracranial hemorrhage, or retinal hemorrhages. The episode may be associated with reflex bradycardia and may be followed by hypotension. Known triggers for autonomic dysreflexia include painful stimuli, trauma, instrumentation of the genitourinary tract, bladder distention, vesicoureteral reflux, constipation, bowel obstruction, biliary colic, or exposure to heat or cold.

Autonomic dysreflexia can be prevented in anticipation of a potential triggering event by providing topical, local, regional, or general anesthesia prior to stimulation. Pretreatment with nifedipine or the alpha-adrenergic antagonist terazosin or prazosin to prevent autonomic dysreflexia has also been described.[74,75] The emergency treatment is to remove the offending stimulus and administer antihypertensive agents to control the blood pressure. No single therapeutic agent has been systematically evaluated for the treatment of hypertension caused by autonomic dysreflexia, but commonly used agents include sodium nitroprusside, nitroglycerin, trimethaphan, hydralazine, nifedipine, nicardipine, and labetalol.

■ REFERENCES

1. Sekhon LH, Fehlings MG: Epidemiology, demographics, and pathophysiology of acute spinal cord injury. Spine 2001;26(24 Suppl): S2-12.
2. Kraus JF, Franti CE, Riggins RS, et al: Incidence of traumatic spinal cord lesions. J Chronic Dis 1975;28:471-492.
3. Harvey C, Rothschild BB, Asmann AJ, Stripling T: New estimates of traumatic SCI prevalence: A survey-based approach. Paraplegia 1990; 28:537-544.
4. Hurlbert RJ: Strategies of medical intervention in the management of acute spinal cord injury. Spine 2006;31(11 Suppl):S16-21; discussion S36.
5. Donaldson WF 3rd, Heil BV, Donaldson VP, Silvaggio VJ: The effect of airway maneuvers on the unstable C1-C2 segment: A cadaver study. Spine 1997;22:1215-1218.
6. Brimacombe J, Keller C, Kunzel KH, et al: Cervical spine motion during airway management: A cinefluoroscopic study of the posteriorly destabilized third cervical vertebrae in human cadavers. Anesth Analg 2000;91:1274-1278.

7. Crosby ET: Airway management in adults after cervical spine trauma. Anesthesiology 2006;104:1293-1318.

8. American College of Surgeons Committee on Trauma: Management of spinal cord injury. 1998. Available at www.facs.org/trauma/publications/spinalcord.pdf.

9. Reid DC, Henderson R, Saboe L, Miller JD: Etiology and clinical course of missed spine fractures. J Trauma 1987;27:980-986.

10. Vale FL, Burns J, Jackson AB, Hadley MN: Combined medical and surgical treatment after acute spinal cord injury: Results of a prospective pilot study to assess the merits of aggressive medical resuscitation and blood pressure management. J Neurosurg 1997;87:239-246.

11. Licina P, Nowitzke AM: Approach and considerations regarding the patient with spinal injury. Injury 2005;36(Suppl 2):B2-12.

12. Schriger DL: Immobilizing the cervical spine in trauma: Should we seek an optimal position or an adequate one? Ann Emerg Med 1996;28:351-353.

13. Herzenberg JE, Hensinger RN, Dedrick DK, Phillips WA: Emergency transport and positioning of young children who have an injury of the cervical spine: The standard backboard may be hazardous. J Bone Joint Surg Am 1989;71:15-22.

14. Curran C, Dietrich AM, Bowman MJ, et al: Pediatric cervical-spine immobilization: Achieving neutral position? J Trauma 1995;39:729-732.

15. Stiell IG, Wells GA, Vandemheen KL, et al: The Canadian C-spine rule for radiography in alert and stable trauma patients. JAMA 2001;286:1841-1848.

16. Richards PJ: Cervical spine clearance: A review. Injury 2005;36:248-269; discussion 270.

17. Hogan GJ, Mirvis SE, Shanmuganathan K, Scalea TM: Exclusion of unstable cervical spine injury in obtunded patients with blunt trauma: Is MR imaging needed when multi-detector row CT findings are normal? Radiology 2005;237:106-113.

18. Maynard FM Jr, Bracken MB, Creasey G, et al: International standards for neurological and functional classification of spinal cord injury. American Spinal Injury Association. Spinal Cord 1997;35:266-274.

19. American Spinal Injury Association: Practice guidelines, 2006. Available at www.asia-spinalinjury.org/home/index.html.

20. Stevens RD, Bhardwaj A, Kirsch JR, Mirski MA: Critical care and perioperative management in traumatic spinal cord injury. J Neurosurg Anesthesiol 2003;15:215-229.

21. Pharmacological therapy after acute cervical spinal cord injury. Neurosurgery 2002;50(3 Suppl):S63-72.

22. Dumont RJ, Verma S, Okonkwo DO, et al: Acute spinal cord injury: Part II. Contemporary pharmacotherapy. Clin Neuropharmacol 2001;24:265-279.

23. Bracken MB, Shepard MJ, Collins WF, et al: A randomized, controlled trial of methylprednisolone or naloxone in the treatment of acute spinal-cord injury: Results of the Second National Acute Spinal Cord Injury Study. N Engl J Med 1990;322:1405-1411.

24. Fu ES, Tummala RP: Neuroprotection in brain and spinal cord trauma. Curr Opin Anaesthesiol 2005;18:181-187.

25. Safi HJ, Hess KR, Randel M, et al: Cerebrospinal fluid drainage and distal aortic perfusion: Reducing neurologic complications in repair of thoracoabdominal aortic aneurysm types I and II. J Vasc Surg 1996;23:223-228; discussion 229.

26. Coselli JS, LeMaire SA, Miller CC 3rd, et al: Mortality and paraplegia after thoracoabdominal aortic aneurysm repair: A risk factor analysis. Ann Thorac Surg 2000;69:409-414.

27. Svensson LG, Crawford ES, Hess KR, et al: Experience with 1509 patients undergoing thoracoabdominal aortic operations. J Vasc Surg 1993;17:357-368; discussion 368-370.

28. Sullivan TM, Sundt TM 3rd: Complications of thoracic aortic endografts: Spinal cord ischemia and stroke. J Vasc Surg 2006;43(Suppl A):85A-88.

29. Katzen BT, Dake MD, MacLean AA, Wang DS: Endovascular repair of abdominal and thoracic aortic aneurysms. Circulation 2005;112:1663-1675.

30. Cheung AT, Weiss SJ, McGarvey ML, et al: Interventions for reversing delayed-onset postoperative paraplegia after thoracic aortic reconstruction. Ann Thorac Surg 2002;74:413-419; discussion 420-421.

31. Cheung AT, Pochettino A, McGarvey ML, et al: Strategies to manage paraplegia risk after endovascular stent repair of descending thoracic

aortic aneurysms. Ann Thorac Surg 2005;80:1280-1288; discussion 1288-1289.

32. LeMaire SA, Miller CC 3rd, Conklin LD, et al: Estimating group mortality and paraplegia rates after thoracoabdominal aortic aneurysm repair. Ann Thorac Surg 2003;75:508-513.

33. Gharagozloo F, Larson J, Dausmann MJ, et al: Spinal cord protection during surgical procedures on the descending thoracic and thoracoabdominal aorta: Review of current techniques. Chest 1996;109:799-809.

34. Coselli JS, Lemaire SA, Koksoy C, et al: Cerebrospinal fluid drainage reduces paraplegia after thoracoabdominal aortic aneurysm repair: Results of a randomized clinical trial. J Vasc Surg 2002;35:631-639.

35. Cina CS, Abouzahr L, Arena GO, et al: Cerebrospinal fluid drainage to prevent paraplegia during thoracic and thoracoabdominal aortic aneurysm surgery: A systematic review and meta-analysis. J Vasc Surg 2004;40:36-44.

36. Khan SN, Stansby G: Cerebrospinal fluid drainage for thoracic and thoracoabdominal aortic aneurysm surgery. Cochrane Database Syst Rev 2004:CD003635.

37. Cheung AT, Pochettino A, Guvakov DV, et al: Safety of lumbar drains in thoracic aortic operations performed with extracorporeal circulation. Ann Thorac Surg 2003;76:1190-1196; discussion 1196-1197.

38. Dardik A, Perler BA, Roseborough GS, Williams GM: Subdural hematoma after thoracoabdominal aortic aneurysm repair: An underreported complication of spinal fluid drainage? J Vasc Surg 2002;36:47-50.

39. Weaver KD, Wiseman DB, Farber M, et al: Complications of lumbar drainage after thoracoabdominal aortic aneurysm repair. J Vasc Surg 2001;34:623-627.

40. Leyvi G, Ramachandran S, Wasnick JD, et al: Case 3: 2005 risk and benefits of cerebrospinal fluid drainage during thoracoabdominal aortic aneurysm surgery. J Cardiothorac Vasc Anesth 2005;19:392-399.

41. Ackerman LL, Traynelis VC: Treatment of delayed-onset neurological deficit after aortic surgery with lumbar cerebrospinal fluid drainage. Neurosurgery 2002;51:1414-1421; discussion 1421-1422.

42. Chiesa R, Melissano G, Marrocco-Trischitta MM, et al: Spinal cord ischemia after elective stent-graft repair of the thoracic aorta. J Vasc Surg 2005;42:11-17.

43. Maniar HS, Sundt TM 3rd, Prasad SM, et al: Delayed paraplegia after thoracic and thoracoabdominal aneurysm repair: A continuing risk. Ann Thorac Surg 2003;75:113-119; discussions 119-120.

44. Guerit JM, Witdoeckt C, Verhelst R, et al: Sensitivity, specificity, and surgical impact of somatosensory evoked potentials in descending aorta surgery. Ann Thorac Surg 1999;67:1943-1946; discussion 1953-1958.

45. Jacobs MJ, Elenbaas TW, Schurink GW, et al: Assessment of spinal cord integrity during thoracoabdominal aortic aneurysm repair. Ann Thorac Surg 2002;74:S1864-1866; discussion S1892-1898.

46. Chiappini B, Schepens M, Tan E, et al: Early and late outcomes of acute type A aortic dissection: Analysis of risk factors in 487 consecutive patients. Eur Heart J 2005;26:180-186.

47. Schepens M, Dossche K, Morshuis W, et al: Introduction of adjuncts and their influence on changing results in 402 consecutive thoracoabdominal aortic aneurysm repairs. Eur J Cardiothorac Surg 2004;25:701-707.

48. Cunningham JN Jr, Laschinger JC, Spencer FC: Monitoring of somatosensory evoked potentials during surgical procedures on the thoracoabdominal aorta: IV. Clinical observations and results. J Thorac Cardiovasc Surg 1987;94:275-285.

49. Dong CC, MacDonald DB, Janusz MT: Intraoperative spinal cord monitoring during descending thoracic and thoracoabdominal aneurysm surgery. Ann Thorac Surg 2002;74:S1873-1876; discussion S1892-1898.

50. Jacob AK, Borowiec JC, Long TR, et al: Transient profound neurologic deficit associated with thoracic epidural analgesia in an elderly patient. Anesthesiology 2004;101:1470-1471.

51. Auroy Y, Narchi P, Messiah A, et al: Serious complications related to regional anesthesia: Results of a prospective survey in France. Anesthesiology 1997;87:479-486.

52. Moen V, Dahlgren N, Irestedt L: Severe neurological complications after central neuraxial blockades in Sweden 1990-1999. Anesthesiology 2004;101:950-959.

53. Wedel DJ: Regional anesthesia and pain management: Reviewing the past decade and predicting the future. Anesth Analg 2000;90: 1244-1245.

54. Foo D, Rossier AB: Preoperative neurological status in predicting surgical outcome of spinal epidural hematomas. Surg Neurol 1981; 15:389-401.

55. Horlocker TT, Abel MD, Messick JM Jr, Schroeder DR: Small risk of serious neurologic complications related to lumbar epidural catheter placement in anesthetized patients. Anesth Analg 2003;96:1547-1552.

56. SreeHarsha CK, Rajasekaran S, Dhanasekararaja P: Spontaneous complete recovery of paraplegia caused by epidural hematoma complicating epidural anesthesia: A case report and review of literature. Spinal Cord 2006;44:514-517.

57. Tam NL, Pac-Soo C, Pretorius PM: Epidural haematoma after a combined spinal-epidural anaesthetic in a patient treated with clopidogrel and dalteparin. Br J Anaesth 2006;96:262-265.

58. Litz RJ, Gottschlich B, Stehr SN: Spinal epidural hematoma after spinal anesthesia in a patient treated with clopidogrel and enoxaparin. Anesthesiology 2004;101:1467-1470.

59. Chan L, Bailin MT: Spinal epidural hematoma following central neuraxial blockade and subcutaneous enoxaparin: A case report. J Clin Anesth 2004;16:382-385.

60. Cullen DJ, Bogdanov E, Htut N: Spinal epidural hematoma occurrence in the absence of known risk factors: A case series. J Clin Anesth 2004;16:376-381.

61. Vandermeulen EP, Van Aken H, Vermylen J: Anticoagulants and spinal-epidural anesthesia. Anesth Analg 1994;79:1165-1177.

62. Lawton MT, Porter RW, Heiserman JE, et al: Surgical management of spinal epidural hematoma: Relationship between surgical timing and neurological outcome. J Neurosurg 1995;83:1-7.

63. Wedel DJ, Horlocker TT: Regional anesthesia in the febrile or infected patient. Reg Anesth Pain Med 2006;31:324-333.

64. Drasner K: Local anesthetic neurotoxicity: Clinical injury and strategies that may minimize risk. Reg Anesth Pain Med 2002;27:576-580.

65. Lambert LA, Lambert DH, Strichartz GR: Irreversible conduction block in isolated nerve by high concentrations of local anesthetics. Anesthesiology 1994;80:1082-1093.

66. Bainton CR, Strichartz GR: Concentration dependence of lidocaine-induced irreversible conduction loss in frog nerve. Anesthesiology 1994;81:657-667.

67. Delank KS, Delank HW, Konig DP, et al: Iatrogenic paraplegia in spinal surgery. Arch Orthop Trauma Surg 2005;125:33-41.

68. MacEwen GD, Bunnell WP, Sriram K: Acute neurological complications in the treatment of scoliosis: A report of the Scoliosis Research Society. J Bone Joint Surg Am 1975;57:404-408.

69. Awad JN, Kebaish KM, Donigan J, et al: Analysis of the risk factors for the development of post-operative spinal epidural haematoma. J Bone Joint Surg Br 2005;87:1248-1252.

70. Lehmann KG, Lane JG, Piepmeier JM, Batsford WP: Cardiovascular abnormalities accompanying acute spinal cord injury in humans: Incidence, time course and severity. J Am Coll Cardiol 1987;10: 46-52.

71. Bilello JF, Davis JW, Cunningham MA, et al: Cervical spinal cord injury and the need for cardiovascular intervention. Arch Surg 2003;138:1127-1129.

72. Hambly PR, Martin B: Anaesthesia for chronic spinal cord lesions. Anaesthesia 1998;53:273-289.

73. Lindan R, Joiner E, Freehafer AA, Hazel C: Incidence and clinical features of autonomic dysreflexia in patients with spinal cord injury. Paraplegia 1980;18:285-292.

74. Vaidyanathan S, Soni BM, Sett P, et al: Pathophysiology of autonomic dysreflexia: Long-term treatment with terazosin in adult and paediatric spinal cord injury patients manifesting recurrent dysreflexic episodes. Spinal Cord 1998;36:761-770.

75. Krum H, Louis WJ, Brown DJ, Howes LG: A study of the alpha-1 adrenoceptor blocker prazosin in the prophylactic management of autonomic dysreflexia in high spinal cord injury patients. Clin Auton Res 1992;2:83-88.

24 Perioperative Management of Acute Central Nervous System Injury

W. Andrew Kofke

Neural function is essential to human existence, and loss of any neural element in the course of a critical illness is a major loss for an individual. Neurons or supporting elements may be lost in a small, virtually unnoticeable manner, perhaps seen as a cognitive or behavioral deficit, or, at the other end of the spectrum, widespread selective neuronal loss or tissue infarction may produce more apparent and disabling deficits. Perioperative management must therefore include consideration of neural viability and of the impact of primary diseases and therapeutics on the nervous system.

A patient may present with neurologic dysfunction in numerous perioperative scenarios, often involving ischemia, trauma, or neuroexcitation. As they progressively worsen, each of these at some point typically involves a period of decreased cerebral perfusion pressure (CPP), usually caused by elevated intracranial pressure (ICP), eventually compromising cerebral blood flow sufficiently to produce permanent neuronal loss, infarction, and possibly brain death. A variety of biochemical pathways play a major role. In this chapter, I review the important physiologic factors, ICP considerations, and therapeutic options critical to the perioperative care of the patient with central nervous system (CNS) injury.

■ PHYSIOLOGY OF INTRACRANIAL HYPERTENSION

The brain, spinal cord, cerebrospinal fluid (CSF), and blood are encased in the skull and vertebral canal, thus constituting a nearly incompressible system (Fig. 24-1). In a totally incompressible system, pressure would vary linearly with volume. However, there is capacitance in the system, thought to be provided by the intervertebral spaces and the vasculature. Once this capacitance is exhausted, the ICP increases dramatically with increased intracranial volume (Fig. 24-2). The relationship can be expressed by the following equation:

$$CBF = (MAP - ICP)/CVR,$$

where CBF is cerebral blood flow, MAP is mean arterial pressure, and CVR is cerebrovascular resistance.

The concern arises that increased ICP is necessarily associated with decrements in CBF. However, the effect on CBF of increased ICP is not straightforward, as MAP may increase with ICP elevations,[1] and CVR adjusts with decreasing CPP (increasing cerebral blood volume) to maintain CBF until maximal vasodilatation occurs.[2-5] This is thought to occur at a CPP of less than 50 mm Hg, although considerable

interindividual heterogeneity in this value exists.[6] Thus, increased ICP is often associated with cerebral vasodilatation or with increasing MAP to maintain CBF.

Normal ICP is less than 10 mm Hg. An ICP of greater than 20 mm Hg is generally associated with escalation of ICP-reducing therapy.[7,8] However, this is an epidemiologically derived number. Head trauma studies have indicated that patients with an ICP of greater than 20 mm Hg generally do not do well.[7] However, physiologically, simply elevating ICP to greater than 20 mm Hg is not necessarily associated with decrements in CBF, provided the compensatory mechanisms noted earlier occur.[9]

Nonetheless, increased ICP resulting from mass lesions or obstruction of CSF outflow can exhaust compensatory mechanisms. When this occurs, compromise of CBF does eventually take place. Initially, abnormality arises in distal runoff of the cerebral circulation. As the process continues, compromise of diastolic perfusion arises. With this, the normally continuous (through systole and diastole) cerebral perfusion becomes discontinuous (Fig. 24-3).[10] Further compromise of CPP results in anaerobic metabolism, exacerbation of edema, and, ultimately, intracranial circulatory arrest.[10,11] Thus, when ICP increases it is important to detect it and ascertain whether this lethal sequence of events may be occurring.

Factors That Exacerbate Intracranial Hypertension

The skull and vertebral canal contain the brain and spinal cord, CSF, and blood. Abnormal masses composed of blood (hematoma) or neoplasia may also occupy this space. When the volume of one or more of these compartments enlarges sufficiently to exhaust normal capacitive compensatory mechanisms, ICP begins to rise, leading to the sequence of events associated with increasing ICP as just described.[12,13]

Two Types of Intracranial Hypertension

In a general sense, there are two types of intracranial hypertension, categorized according to CBF as hyperemic or oligemic (Fig. 24-4). Although conceptualized here as a dichotomous process, undoubtedly the real physiology is more of a continuum between the two.

In the normal state, increases in CBF are not associated with increased ICP, as the normal capacitive mechanisms absorb the increased intracranial blood volume. However, in the situation of disordered intracranial compliance, small increases in intracranial volume caused by increased CBF produce increases in ICP. When cerebral blood volume (CBV) increases, intracranial contents increase, thereby increasing ICP in a noncompliant system.[3,14]

This raises an important issue. Elevated ICP has traditionally raised concern because it indicates that cerebral perfusion might be jeopardized. It is, however, unclear whether it is appropriate to be concerned about high ICP inducing intracranial oligemia when the cause of the high ICP is intracranial hyperemia. There have been no detailed examinations of this issue, although some studies have questioned the significance of hyperemic intracranial hypertension.

Short-lived noxious stimuli briefly increase ICP in the setting of decreased intracranial compliance. Recent studies have shown that such situations are associated with hyperemia, strongly suggesting that hyperemic intracranial hypertension is not a dangerous situation.[15] However, it is reasonable to be concerned, at least theoretically, about such hyperemia for three reasons. First, elevated ICP caused by hyperemia in one portion of the brain may increase ICP in other areas of the brain, compromising CBF where regional CBF (rCBF) is

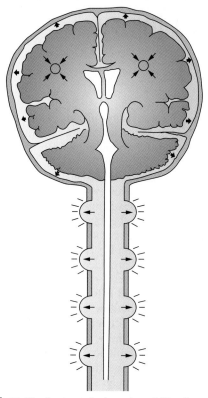

Figure 24-1 ■ The brain, spinal cord, and blood are encased in the skull and vertebral canal, thus constituting a nearly incompressible system. System capacitance is thought to be provided via intervertebral spaces and blood volume. *(Redrawn from Kofke WA, Yanes H, Wechsler L, et al: Neurologic intensive care. In Albin MS [ed]: Textbook of Neuroanesthesia with Neurosurgical and Neuroscience Perspectives. New York, McGraw-Hill, 1997, pp 1247-1347.)*

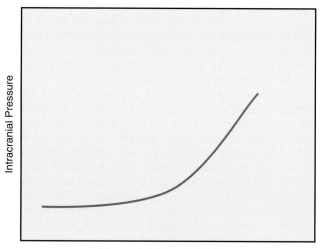

Figure 24-2 ■ Nonlinear relationship between intracranial pressure (ICP) and intracranial volume. At normal ICP, small changes in the volume produce small changes in the pressure. However, as ICP increases, the increases in pressure per unit change in volume become progressively larger and more dramatic.

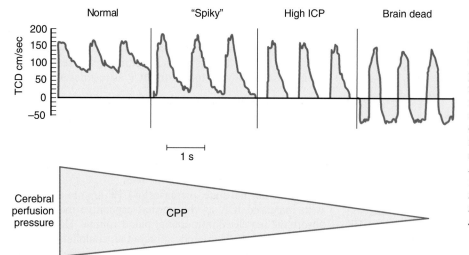

Figure 24-3 ■ Transcranial Doppler (TCD) waveforms after head injury. The progression is from intact CBF and normal-appearing TCD waveform to intracranial pressure (ICP), or hypertension, sufficient to induce intracerebral circulatory arrest. Schematic of decreasing cerebral perfusion pressure (CPP) is shown in the lower panel. *(Redrawn from Hassler W, Steinmetz H, Gawlowski J: Transcranial Doppler ultrasonography in raised intracranial pressure and in intracranial circulatory arrest. J Neurosurg 1988;68:745-751.)*

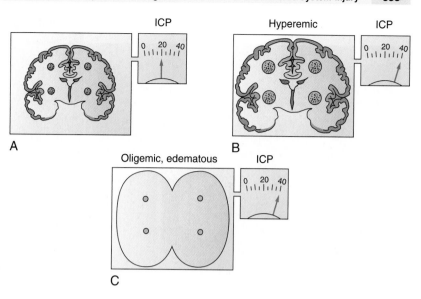

Figure 24-4 ■ Two types of intracranial hypertension. From a baseline condition, intracranial pressure (ICP) can increase in two ways. One is via an increase in cerebral blood volume associated with reflex vasodilation caused by moderate blood pressure decreases or by hyperemia. The second mechanism is via malignant brain edema or other expanding masses that encroach on the vascular bed and produce intracranial ischemia. *(Redrawn from Kofke WA, Yanes H, Wechsler L, et al: Neurologic intensive care. In Albin MS [ed]: Textbook of Neuroanesthesia with Neurosurgical and Neuroscience Perspectives. New York, McGraw-Hill, 1997, pp 1247-1347.)*

marginal. Second, increased pressure in one area of the brain may produce gradients that might lead to a herniation syndrome. The third theoretical concern is that inappropriate hyperemia may predispose the brain to worsened edema or hemorrhage, as occurs with other hyperperfusion syndromes.[14,16] Thus, theoretically, hyperemic intracranial hypertension has the potential to be deleterious, although this has yet to be conclusively demonstrated. For brief periods, as may occur during intubation or limited exposure to other noxious stimuli, it may not be a problem.[17]

In contrast, oligemic intracranial hypertension is associated with compromised cerebral perfusion.[18] This is supported by the high mortality observed in head trauma patients, in whom ICP rises as a result of brain edema after head injury, with decrements in CBF.[7,19] Transcranial Doppler (TCD) and CBF studies on these patients have demonstrated that CBF is low and perfusion is discontinuous during the cardiac cycle (see Fig. 24-3).[10,19] Moreover, jugular venous bulb data indicate that O_2 extraction is markedly increased,[20] suggesting anaerobic metabolism.[19] In this setting, noxious stimuli can further increase the ICP, thus producing the situation of hyperemic or oligemic intracranial hypertension. Presumably, in this setting, the hyperemic rise in ICP acts to further compromise rCBF in areas of brain edema.

■ TREATMENT OF INTRACRANIAL HYPERTENSION

The goals in treating intracranial hypertension are to maintain adequate CPP, oxygenation, and glucose supply (without hyperglycemia). The clinical strategy is to diagnose and treat underlying causes, avoid exacerbating factors, and reduce ICP. Underlying causes include masses (tumors, hematomas), hydrocephalus, cerebral edema, and cerebrovascular dilatation.

Therapy for intracranial hypertension is directed at removing the primary cause. When this is not possible, therapy is aimed at controlling ICP. Controlling ICP is thus supportive, intended to preserve viable neuronal tissue until

the high ICP situation resolves. There are six types of therapy: (1) decrease cerebral blood volume, (2) decrease CSF volume, (3) induce serum hyperosmolarity, (4) resect dead or injured brain tissue or resect viable but less important brain tissue (e.g., anterior temporal lobe), (5) resect non-neural masses or hematomas, and (6) remove the calvarium to permit unopposed outward brain swelling. Recent advances in the use of brain tissue oxygen monitors occasionally affect the manner in which these maneuvers are employed to ensure continued optimal oxygen tension of brain tissue ($P_{br}O_2$).

Cerebral Blood Volume Reduction

Cerebral blood volume can be decreased with hyperventilation and cerebral blood volume–decreasing drugs.

Hyperventilation

Hyperventilation can be used to acutely reduce cerebral blood flow and volume to reduce ICP.[21-25] Under normal conditions, however, CBF returns to its original state within hours,[21,25] so it is unclear why sustained decreases in ICP can be achieved with hyperventilation. In the intubated patient, hyperventilation is performed by increasing tidal volume or rate.

Hyperventilation produces several adverse effects. It introduces a risk of decreasing CBF to a dangerous level (Fig. 24-5).[26] In a recent study in trauma patients, routine hyperventilation was associated with worse neurologic outcome at 3 and 6 months after the injury (Fig. 24-6).[27] The reason for this is uncertain, as it has not been demonstrated that anaerobic metabolism occurs with hyperventilation in this setting. There are several possible explanations: (1) hyperventilation produces alkalemia and increased affinity of oxygen for hemoglobin; (2) it decreases seizure threshold[28]; (3) the potential exists for hyperventilation to produce only a transient effect on, or a paradoxical increase in, ICP (Fig. 24-7); and (4) on discontinuation of hyperventilation, a paradoxical CSF acidosis can occur.[21,25] Although these adverse effects indicate that hyperventilation should not be used as routine

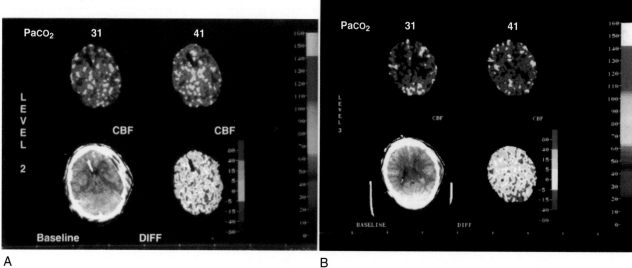

Figure 24-5 ■ Two examples of disparate effects of hyperventilation on cerebral blood flow (CBF). Both figures are stable xenon-enhanced computed tomographic (CT) scans of CBF in patients with head trauma and with and without hyperventilation. CBF scale is indicated on the right in mL/100 g/min and is indicated at the top of each study. CT images are in the *lower portions* and CBF maps are in the *upper portions*. CBF change is noted in the lower right panel with adjacent change scale. **A** was decreased from 41 to 31 mm Hg. The baseline scan *(right)* shows satisfactory flows with some areas of hyperemia, and the hyperventilated scan *(left)* shows CBFs of approximately 30 mL/100 g/min, probably acceptable flows. **B** was decreased from 41 to 31 mm Hg. The baseline CBF *(right)* had only marginally acceptable CBF. The effect of hyperventilation *(left)* was to produce widespread areas of CBF less than 20 mL/100 g/min, probably unacceptable flows.

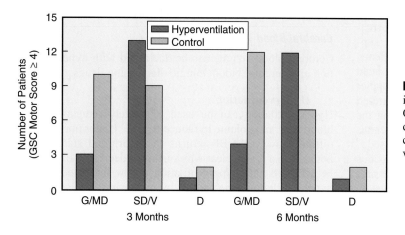

Figure 24-6 ■ Patients with head trauma were randomized to receive hyperventilation or normoventilation. Outcome was worse in hyperventilated patients. D, death; GCS, Glasgow Coma Scale; G/MD, good recovery, moderate disability; SD/V, severe disability or vegetative state.

prophylaxis, it can be an effective means to decrease ICP if the patient has hyperemic intracranial hypertension or an emergent herniation syndrome. The presence of hyperemia can be determined by use of direct brain CBF determination or via jugular bulb oximetry.[29] Brain tissue $P_{br}O_2$ may be helpful but this has not been definitively demonstrated. High ICP associated with a low arteriovenous oxygen difference ($AVDO_2$) across the brain (i.e., 3% to 4% by volume) is thought to indicate that hyperventilation can be safely used. In an emergent situation, even if it is not known whether the high ICP is oligemic or hyperemic, hyperventilation should be administered acutely to keep ICP down or to reverse a herniation syndrome or plateau wave until a more definitive diagnosis can be obtained or therapy performed.

Cerebral Blood Volume–Decreasing Drugs
CBF-decreasing (and therefore CBV-decreasing) drugs that can decrease ICP include barbiturates,[30-32] benzodiazepines,[33] etomidate,[34,35] and propofol.[32,36] As all are CNS depressants, their use indicates acceptance on the part of the clinician to lose the ability to perform a reliable neurologic examination. Unlike hyperventilation, these agents decrease CBF coupled to cerebral metabolic rate (CMR). Therefore, the CBF decreases should not provide a milieu for anaerobic

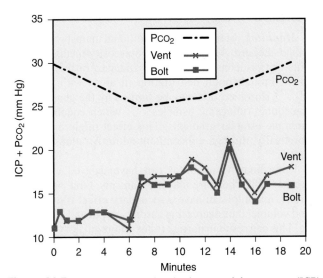

Figure 24-7 ■ Paradoxical rise in intracranial pressure (ICP) induced by mechanical hyperventilation, presumably the result of mechanical pressure effects predominating over hypocarbic cerebral vasoconstriction. It is likely that hyperventilation induced a decrease in blood pressure, which resulted in an opposing reflex increase in cerebral blood volume. Bolt, subarachnoid screw; vent, ventricular catheter. *(Redrawn from Ropper A, Kennedy S: Postoperative neurosurgical care. In Ropper A [ed]: Neurological and Neurosurgical Intensive Care. New York, Raven Press, 1993, pp 185-191.)*

metabolism. Lidocaine also decreases CBF and CMR to decrease ICP, although with a less pronounced decrement in neurologic function.[37,38] The immediate effects of mannitol are thought to be mediated by a reduction in cerebral blood volume,[25] but this is undoubtedly minor and temporary.

Barbiturates. Barbiturates decrease ICP by decreasing CBF, CBV, CMR, and seizure activity.[30-32] Barbiturate therapy usually decreases ICP, its failure to lower ICP is a bad prognostic sign. Ultrashort barbiturates such as thiopental and methohexital can be helpful in the intubated patient for acute increases in ICP. In addition, barbiturates can be used when intracranial hypertension is refractory to other treatments. Moreover, barbiturates have the advantage of decreasing the amount of mannitol needed and thus its side effects. In addition, by blunting shivering, they can facilitate use of hypothermia therapy, and they can be helpful to blunt the rise in ICP secondary to suctioning and other nursing procedures.

Prolonged barbiturate therapy for high ICP has several adverse effects. Because barbiturates blunt the neurologic examination, a growing intracranial mass lesion or other neurologic exacerbation may not be obvious until it causes a further increased ICP or the barbiturate requirement to maintain normal ICP increases. Hypotension and respiratory depression may occur. Blood pressure may need to be pharmacologically supported, and intubation and mechanical ventilation are mandatory. Dysfunction of the alimentary tract may occur, making it difficult to use enteral nutrition. Thermoregulation is disturbed. Hypothermia may occur

inadvertently, and infection may be masked because of the lack of fever. Finally, physical addiction and tolerance may occur with prolonged use, making it difficult to discontinue barbiturate treatment without seizures.

Thiopental can be given at a dosage of 1 to 4 mg/kg, repeated as needed to control ICP. It is subsequently infused as needed. Pentobarbital is given at a loading dose of 3 to 5 mg/kg over 30 to 60 minutes, followed by 1 mg/kg/hr with the infusion adjusted as needed to control ICP. Electroencephalography (EEG) can be used concurrently to assist in titration by defining the upper effective dose (isoelectric EEG). Infusion can be increased until a burst-suppression pattern arises on the electroencephalogram. Increasing the barbiturate dosage beyond that needed to produce burst suppression is unlikely to provide further decreases in ICP, as further decrements in CMR are not thought to occur at dosages beyond that needed for significant burst suppression.[39] Alternatively, serum pentobarbital levels can be monitored, aiming for 30 to 50 µg/mL. Discontinuation of barbiturate therapy can be considered when (1) there is no decrease in ICP with barbiturate loading; (2) after an initially favorable response, intracranial hypertension recurs despite maximal barbiturate therapy; or (3) ICP has remained at less than 15 mm Hg for greater than 24 to 48 hours. In the latter case, barbiturates should be weaned with continued ICP monitoring.

Etomidate. Etomidate decreases ICP by decreasing CBF and CMR.[34,35] It does not have the potent hemodynamic effects of barbiturates, in that it can decrease ICP without decreasing CPP, which occurs with thiopental. It is not suitable for prolonged infusion to control ICP, because it inhibits adrenal corticosteroid synthesis[40] unless steroids are concomitantly administered. Nonetheless, it can be used for brief periods as an adjunct in ICP control, especially if there is hemodynamic concern. The suggested dosage is 0.1 to 0.3 mg/kg intravenously.

Propofol. Although propofol has some ICP-reducing properties,[32,36] it also decreases blood pressure significantly.[41] Thus, its use for elevated ICP is generally limited to its sedative benefit in the neurologic intensive care unit (ICU). Idiosyncratic adverse metabolic acidosis[42] and hypertriglyceridemia[43] are significant concerns with its prolonged use, particularly in children, adolescents, and young adults.[44] In vitro data indicate that propofol has some tendency to interfere with mitochondrial respiration.[45]

Lidocaine. Like barbiturates, lidocaine decreases ICP by decreasing CBF and CMR, but it does not produce as much CNS depression.[37,38] It is not as potent or reliable as barbiturates in decreasing ICP, but it can be useful when there is hemodynamic instability or when barbiturates are not tolerated hemodynamically. It can be useful prior to airway manipulations.[38] It is not typically used in prolonged therapy of intracranial hypertension but is most useful when administered in 0.5- to 1.5-mg/kg doses intravenously or intratracheally for acute treatment of high ICP, particularly that associated with airway manipulation.

Mannitol. Mannitol, long a mainstay of the therapy for elevated ICP, probably works via a dual mechanism. Initially, possibly accounting for its rapid action, it decreases blood viscosity.[46,47] The effect of this is to prompt vasoconstriction in normally autoregulating brain areas to decrease CBV and, secondarily, ICP. Subsequently, it may induce a further decrease in ICP through fluid shifts from brain to blood in areas with an intact blood–brain barrier (BBB)[48-50] (see Mannitol, under Hyperosmolar Therapy, later). Hypertonic saline may exert similar effects.[51]

CSF Drainage

CSF volume is reduced by removal via a ventricular drain (Fig. 24-8). This can be effected by setting the drainage apparatus at a prescribed height above the midbrain, or by opening the drain whenever the ICP exceeds 20 to 25 mm Hg. Leaving a drain open risks excessive CSF drainage when the patient coughs or when the drain is manipulated in the course of routine nursing procedures, and it can contribute to collapse of the ventricles. Excessive and abrupt decrease in local pressure around the drain can produce intracranial gradients, leading to a herniation syndrome. Leaving the drain clamped and monitored, however, risks the development of untreated intracranial hypertension.

Hyperosmolar Therapy

Mannitol. Mannitol is the traditional mainstay of hyperosmolar therapy. After initial hypoviscosity-mediated autoregulatory vasoconstriction, it may induce a further decrease in ICP through brain dehydration in areas with an intact BBB.[48-50] However, this may be limited by the generation of intracellular "idiogenic osmoles,"[52,53] which equalize transmembrane osmolar gradients. This effect might be limited, theoretically, through concomitant administration of a loop diuretic.[54]

Unfortunately, mannitol can have delayed effects on increased ICP. There are four mechanisms. First, as a potent diuretic, mannitol can have a secondary effect if decreasing blood volume, thus decreasing cardiac output and blood pressure. This can result in normal reflex autoregulatory increases in CBV, which can increase ICP.[3] Second, the increased urine output, if not replaced with commensurate intravenous fluid therapy, can elevate the hematocrit, thus opposing the initial mannitol-induced decrease in viscosity.[55] Third, mannitol can cross the BBB in an unpredictable manner, with the

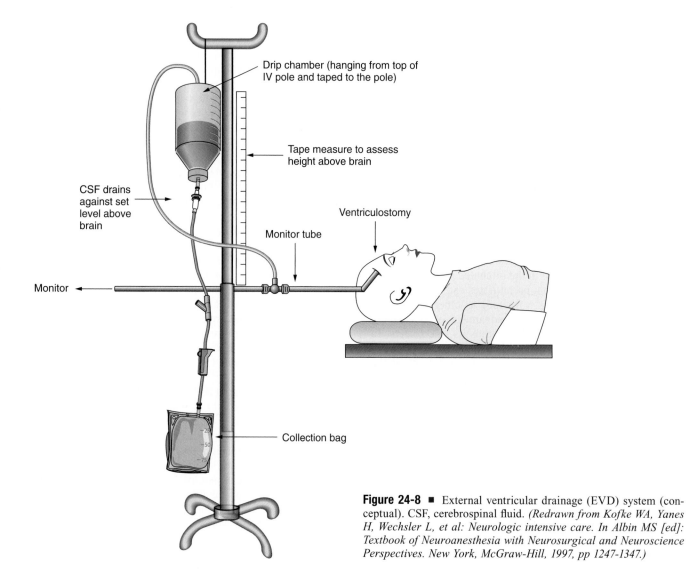

Drip chamber (hanging from top of IV pole and taped to the pole)

Tape measure to assess height above brain

CSF drains against set level above brain

Ventriculostomy

Monitor tube

Monitor

Collection bag

Figure 24-8 ■ External ventricular drainage (EVD) system (conceptual). CSF, cerebrospinal fluid. *(Redrawn from Kofke WA, Yanes H, Wechsler L, et al: Neurologic intensive care. In Albin MS [ed]: Textbook of Neuroanesthesia with Neurosurgical and Neuroscience Perspectives. New York, McGraw-Hill, 1997, pp 1247-1347.)*

possibility of a rebound increase in ICP, similar to that observed with urea.[55,56] This is partly because the reflection coefficient of the BBB is 0.9, indicating that mannitol can slowly diffuse into even a normal brain.[57] Finally, it is theoretically possible that increased intracellular osmolarity can be generated via idiogenic osmoles, which may predispose the patient to a rebound increase in brain volume with discontinuation of mannitol.[52,53] These complications are probably lessened if urine output is replaced with balanced crystalloid infusion and if, once blood osmolarity is increased, it is not allowed to decrease to the prior level, unless clinical improvement indicates that weaning of ICP-reducing therapy is appropriate. This should be considered in any patient demonstrating periodic abrupt increases in ICP.

Hypertonic Saline. Hypertonic saline (HTS) is a recently revisited alternative to mannitol. With a reflection coefficient of 1.0,[57] and with no potential to produce deleterious diuresis and undesired hypovolemia, HTS has properties that make it an attractive hyperosmolar agent. Moreover, clinical reports indicate that it is an effective ICP-reducing drug with a very useful niche in the group of patients who are refractory to mannitol. It may find a place as a first-line drug, replacing mannitol in that role.

HTS has undergone scrutiny in many laboratory and clinical studies, with virtually all indicating a beneficial effect in decreasing ICP. However, this is not a new observation, having been initially reported in 1919 by Weed and McKibben.[58] Studies generally have employed 3%, 7.5%, or 23.4% saline, with a colloid, typically dextran or hetastarch, or without.

In normal animals, early studies indicated that HTS produces brain dehydration while augmenting CBF.[51] This led to work evaluating the mechanisms and therapeutic potential of HTS in animal models of intracerebral hemorrhage (ICH), subarachnoid hemorrhage (SAH), and traumatic brain injury (TBI). Animals with TBI and shock were studied by Prough and coworkers,[59,60] who reported a lower ICP when HTS was used instead of lactated Ringer's solution. Battistella and Wisner[61] and Anderson and colleagues[62] made similar observations in sheep. Moreover, in normotensive sheep with focal cryogenic injury, HTS produced lower ICP with improved oxygen delivery.[63] Rats with SAH treated with HTS/dextran had lower ICP and better outcome than when treated with 0.9% saline.[64] In dogs with ICH treated with either mannitol or HTS, both drugs effectively decreased ICP, although the duration of action of HTS was longer.[65] HTS was associated with decreased intraparenchymal pressure throughout the brain, including the perihematoma region.[65]

In humans, the effect of HTS has been reported in ischemic stroke, ICH, SAH, TBI, and hepatic encephalopathy. All studies show that HTS effectively and reproducibly reduces ICP with concomitant improvement in CPP. Indeed, Suarez and coworkers[66] showed one important effect: 23.4% HTS effectively decreased ICP in eight patients when all other medical therapies did not work (Fig. 24-9). Similar observations in patients with refractory intracranial hypertension were reported by Horn and associates.[67]

Early case reports by Worthley and colleagues[68] on patients with refractory ICP elevations supported the thera-

peutic potential for this therapy and supported the many studies that followed. A retrospective study by Qureshi and coworkers[69] showed that HTS decreases ICP in head trauma and postoperative brain edema, but not nontraumatic ICH or ischemic stroke. Schatzmann and colleagues[70] performed a prospective nonrandomized evaluation of HTS in patients with severe head injury, also finding that it effectively reduced ICP. A subsequent prospective randomized study by Vialet and coworkers[71] in patients with TBI found better ICP control than with mannitol. Another prospective randomized study did not show better ICP control with HTS than with standard therapy, but in that study the sample size was relatively small, and the HTS patients were sicker on entry into the study.[72] Three studies report that HTS can be safely and effectively used in children to decrease ICP after TBI.[73-75] Suarez and colleagues,[66] studying severe SAH patients, reported that HTS therapy effectively decreased ICP while concomitantly increasing CBF (see Fig. 24-9). Schatzmann and coworkers[70] evaluated HTS-plus-hetastarch therapy in ischemic stroke patients with high ICP, compared with mannitol. Both therapies decreased ICP, but the HTS group had better control.

Patients with intracranial hypertension associated with hepatic encephalopathy have been demonstrated by Murphy and associates[76] to sustain ICP decrements after HTS. Given the presumed diffuse nature of this disease, this is perhaps surprising, as diffuse BBB dysfunction might have been expected to attenuate any positive effect.

Although many studies show the efficacy of HTS in improving ICP and other parameters, no one has yet evaluated the impact of its use on ultimate outcome other than in prehospital studies. In 1991, Vassar and colleagues[77] evaluated this hypothesis, showing a trend for better outcome in the HTS-treated patients. However, another, more recent and larger study by Cooper and coworkers[78] found no effect of HTS when compared with isotonic therapy given once in the prehospital setting. This study did not assess the impact of systematic use of HTS throughout the hospital course. We can thus conclude it will not produce a breakthrough outcome effect from a one-time use. More studies are needed to assess the impact on outcome when it is employed in a more systematic manner to control ICP throughout the post-insult hospital course. Given the widespread belief that controlling ICP is associated with better outcome, and the multiple studies reporting that HTS can rescue ICP in patients in whom all therapies, including mannitol and barbiturates, are futile, it may be very difficult to find investigators with equipoise who can ethically conduct such a study.

From a mechanistic perspective, several reports, including a review by Suarez,[79] indicate that HTS most likely decreases ICP by several interacting mechanisms:

- HTS decreases brain water, with the most salient effect in noninjured brain,[61,63,80-82] indicating that the main ICP-reducing effect is not on injured brain, and that some normal BBB is necessary for it to work effectively.[79] One study by Berger and colleagues[82] suggests that mannitol therapy produces less water in the lesion, but that HTS produces less brain water in the normal

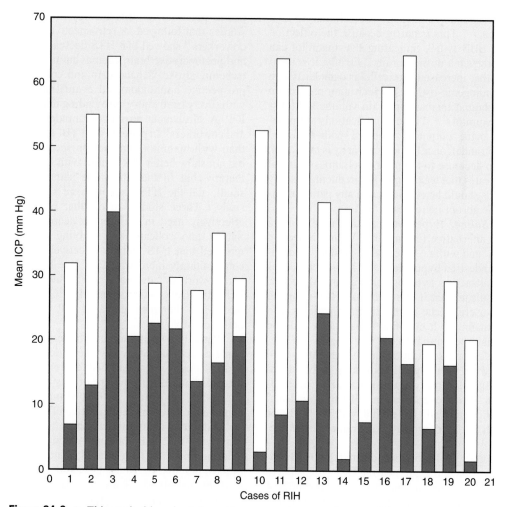

Figure 24-9 ■ This stacked-bar chart shows the mean pretreatment intracranial pressure (ICP) and the mean ICP 1 hr after treatment with 23.4% saline for every episode of refractory intracranial hypertension (RIH). Patient distribution is as follows: *1,* spontaneous basal ganglia hemorrhage; *2,* subarachnoid hemorrhage; *3,* subarachnoid hemorrhage; *4 to 6,* traumatic head injury; *7 to 8,* subarachnoid hemorrhage; *9,* subarachnoid hemorrhage; *10 to 12,* subarachnoid hemorrhage; *13 to 20,* brain tumor. *(Redrawn from Suarez JI, Qureshi AI, Bhardwaj A, et al: Crit Care Med 1998;26:1118-1122.)*

brain. This was confirmed in a case report by Saltarini and coworkers,[83] who provided magnetic resonance imaging confirmation of decreased cerebral water content after infusion of 18% saline in a patient with refractory ICH.

- HTS improves CBF[62,63,63a] (Fig. 24-10) and O$_2$ delivery.[63] One suggested mechanism of increased regional perfusion is dehydration and shrinkage of cerebral endothelial cells, in addition to viscosity and other effects.[79]

- In vitro, hypertonic solutions cause cells to shrink, but they rapidly return to their previous volume,[54] presumably because of an autoregulated increase in intracellular osmolarity to maintain normal cell volume (via idiogenic osmoles). This underscores the notion that hypertonic therapy can have a temporary effect, and that rebound intracranial hypertension can arise if systemic hyperosmolarity is allowed to normalize too quickly. Notably, this cell volume autoregulation can

be inhibited significantly in vitro with concomitant application of the loop diuretic bumetanide.[54] The clinical relevance of this observation remains to be evaluated.

- Reduced blood viscosity is an expected side effect of intravascular volume expansion and decreased hematocrit, produced with HTS administration.[51] Reduced viscosity with some intact autoregulation is thought to produce a decrease in ICP through cerebral vasoconstriction.[47,79]

- HTS may produce more rapid absorption of CSF through increased plasma tonicity.[79,84]

- There may be a diminished inflammatory response to brain injury with HTS.[79]

HTS clearly has the potential to exert a positive impact in the management of ICH. However, there are concerns about possible deleterious effects, and perhaps the most worrisome is renal failure, as mentioned in a report by Peterson

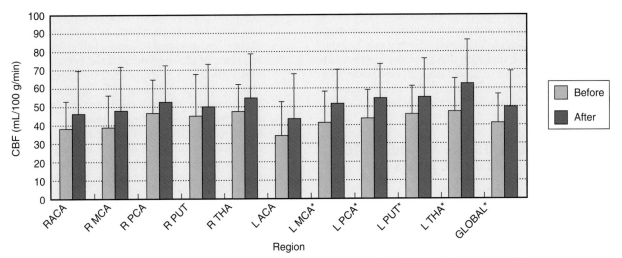

Figure 24-10 ■ Changes in regional and global cerebral blood flow (CBF) in six patients with poor-grade subarachnoid hemorrhage (SAH) given hypertonic saline (HTS). Abbreviations: R, right; L, left; ACA, anterior cerebral artery distribution; MCA, middle cerebral artery distribution; PCA, posterior cerebral artery distribution; PUT, putamen; THA, thalamus. *$P < 0.05$ (t test). *(Redrawn from Tseng M-Y, Al-Rawi PG, Pickard JD, et al: Effect of hypertonic saline on cerebral blood flow in poor-grade patients with subarachnoid hemorrhage. Stroke 2003;June:1390-1397.)*

and coworkers,[75] wherein 2 out of 10 children developed reversible renal failure; however, it was also related to multiorgan failure and sepsis. Nonetheless, the issue of renal failure was further underscored in editorials by Valadka and Robertson[85] and by Dominguez and coworkers,[86] but with disagreement about this as a significant risk expressed by Bratton and colleagues.[87] Other potential adverse effects were nicely reviewed by Suarez[79] and include intracranial complications such as the following:

- Rebound edema
- Disruption of the BBB ("osmotic opening")
- Excess neuronal death. Postulated after continuous infusion of 7.5% saline in a rat model resulted in worsened outcome after transient ischemia.[88] This has not been found to be clinically relevant.
- Alterations in the level of consciousness associated with hypernatremia[89]
- Central pontine myelinolysis. This is typically associated with too-rapid correction of (typically chronic) hyponatremia.[90] It has not been associated with the use of HTS in humans.

Systemic complications include the following:

- Congestive heart failure[79]
- Transient hypotension has been reported in animals after rapid intravenous hypertonic fluid infusions.[91,92]
- Decreased platelet aggregation and coagulation factor abnormalities[93]
- Hypokalemia and hyperchloremic metabolic acidosis with large quantities of HTS.[94]
- Phlebitis. Infusion should be done via a central venous catheter.[79]
- Renal failure.[75,85-87] As discussed earlier, the relationship to HTS is not clear; there are no reports of renal failure in animals or humans in the absence of more common etiologies of renal failure, such as sepsis and organ failure.

Resection of Brain Tissue

Resection of brain tissue is occasionally performed for malignant intracranial hypertension. Because of the proximity of the temporal lobe to the brainstem, one approach is to resect part of this lobe in an effort to avert a herniation syndrome.[95] An alternative approach, suggested specifically for malignant ICH caused by stroke, is to resect dead and swelling infarcted tissue, leaving noninfarcted tissue intact.[96] However, the difficulties of identifying such tissue intraoperatively create a risk of inadvertent resection of viable tissue.

Resection of Non-neural Masses or Hematomas

When clinical examination indicates a global decrement in level of consciousness, indicating elevated ICP, and imaging studies show the presence of a mass lesion, then urgent surgical removal of the mass is thought to be indicated.[95] Nonetheless, there is some controversy about this. With intracerebral hematomas, there is no evidence of improvement in long-term outcome using the aggressive approach of surgically resecting the hematoma.[97] However, resection can be lifesaving for cerebellar hematomas or epidural hematomas with abrupt neurologic deterioration.[97] The case for subdural hematoma (SDH) is less clear, although acute SDH in the context of a recent injury and neurologic deterioration seems to respond well to surgery.

Surgical Removal of Skull and Dura

Decompressive craniectomy to allow brain swelling after a large stroke or head injury is somewhat controversial. Reports have been published supporting its use for ischemic stroke,[98-101] subarachnoid hemorrhage,[102] massive intracerebral hemorrhage,[103] cerebral venous/sinus thrombosis,[104] and traumatic brain injury.[101,105] Notably, Jaeger and coworkers[106] reported that decompressive craniectomy, while decreasing ICP, also produced a significant increase in brain PO_2, which increased from 6 to 23 mm Hg in three SAH patients. However, all of the reports on its use are in nonrandomized case series, and it has never undergone prospective randomized investigation. Nonetheless, although functional recovery may be poor, it remains an attractive approach that seems to improve survival, and its small chance of acceptable outcome renders the procedure worthy of consideration.[101,105] This aggressive approach is in need of a prospective randomized trial.

■ CEREBROVASCULAR RESERVE AND THE ACUTELY INJURED BRAIN: PHYSIOLOGIC ISSUES

Satisfactory perioperative care of the acutely injured brain requires a physiologic and biochemical milieu that will promote a good recovery, and issues related to cerebrovascular reserve are central to these considerations. The brain must have the ability to successfully compensate for physiologic stresses such as hypoglycemia, hypoxemia, hypotension, and anemia. In all of these situations, vasodilation arises to provide a compensatory increase in CBF.

Animal experiments indicate that it is possible to produce a condition in which cerebrovascular reserve is compromised to the point at which there is an increased tendency to cerebral infarction.[107] For example, symptoms are not produced when one carotid artery is occluded or when moderate hypoxemia is produced, because cerebral vasodilatation occurs to compensate. (Indeed, some contend that arterial hypoxemia, when it occurs with normal cerebrovascular compensatory mechanisms, does not cause brain damage. Of course, one contributing factor to this notion is that hypoxic myocardial dysfunction produces organismic death, so that isolated neuronal injury cannot occur.) However, when hypoxemia and carotid occlusion happen together, a stroke occurs because compensatory mechanisms, already fully utilized, cannot accommodate the further decrease in O_2 supply.[107] Examples of variants of this situation abound clinically.[108-111] Examples of attenuated cerebrovascular reserve include cerebral edema, hypoxemia, anemia, carotid stenosis, peri-infarct penumbra, and so on. In each of these situations, although it is not easy to quantitate, it is clear that added compromise of O_2 supply to the brain risks neuronal injury.[111]

■ AIRWAY EVALUATION AND MANAGEMENT IN THE PATIENT WITH ACUTE CNS INJURY

In the CNS-injured patient, the first concern with respect to airway management is that, if there is intracranial pathophysiology, the hemodynamic or respiratory changes associated with airway manipulation can lead to elevated ICP, exacerbated brain edema, or worsened intracranial hemorrhage. If there is spinal cord injury, which initially may not be clinically apparent, cervical spine manipulation risks producing or worsening any acute plegic deficits. Most head-injured patients are assumed to have an unstable cervical spine until definitive clearance is obtained.

The airway evaluation is similar to most preanesthetic evaluations. The following specific items need to be sought in the history and physical examination:

- NPO (nil per os) status. This is helpful history, but it has little impact on plans, as most acutely injured patients are assumed to have a full stomach.
- Evidence of elevated intracranial pressure. This may affect the choice of drugs used to support intubation.
- History of the incident. The approach may vary depending on whether the cause of the injury was direct trauma or a medical problem.
- Other medical history, if available.
- Presence of neurologic deficits, especially paraplegia or quadriplegia. This may have an impact on the choice of drugs to support intubation and the method by which intubation is performed. It may suggest the possibility of autonomic dysfunction. Quadriplegic patients have a significant attenuation of the catecholamine response to intubation.[112]
- Evidence of airway injury.
- Evidence of aspiration or other impediments to gas exchange. An associated lung injury or aspiration related to altered mental status leads to faster desaturation during intubation and is likely to worsen the neurologic outcome.

Therapeutic Options

The main options in airway management have to do with whether and how deeply to produce CNS depression, and which tool will be used to effect intubation of the trachea. There are pros and cons to each approach, and considerable clinical judgment is needed to match the spectrum of benefits and risks to the underlying disease processes.

Awake versus Asleep

The anesthetic states that may be employed are on a continuum from awake and unsedated to fully anesthetized with neuromuscular blockade. In the context of possible intracranial hypertension or hemorrhage, the side effects of anesthetic drugs can be used to control systemic and intracranial hypertension. Although the full spectrum of effects of anesthetic drugs is beyond the scope of this chapter, some of them—thiopental, propofol, and etomidate—have direct ICP-reducing qualities that can be of use during intubation, which is known to produce intracranial hypertension.[113,114] Attenuation of systemic hypertension can be augmented with judicious use of an opioid such as fentanyl, in addition to a blood pressure–reducing drug such as thiopental or propofol. Neuromuscular blockade can be achieved with vecuronium or rocuronium, neither of which has any reported cerebrovascular effects.[115] Succinylcholine can also be used, although concerns remain about increasing ICP, probably related to the increased CBF induced by afferent spindle stimulation.[116] However, given after a large bolus of one of the aforementioned induction drugs, succinylcholine seems to be associated with no significant problems. Moreover, its use is theoretically safe with hyperacute-onset paraplegia or quadriplegia (i.e., before nicotinic receptor upregulation), but I refrain from using it with spinal cord injury patients because of concern about the speed of receptor upregulation or an inaccurate history leading to fatal hyperkalemia.[117]

In patients with cervical cord injuries, it is generally better to employ little or no anesthetic, except as needed for safe conscious sedation, and to then use fiberoptic bronchoscopy with good topical anesthesia. This does require the cooperation of the patient, and if that is not possible or if the intubation needs to be done emergently, direct laryngoscopy, possibly with in-line immobilization,[118] has not been associated with apparent neurologic complications, although its anatomic efficacy has been questioned. However, Lennarson and colleagues[119] reported that neither traction nor in-line immobilization in fresh cadavers prevented distraction or angulation of the C4-5 injured cervical spine with laryngoscopy by Macintosh blade. Thus, concern persists that this approach produces or exacerbates cervical spine injury, and it is reserved for emergencies or for the uncooperative patient in whom general anesthesia with rapid intubation by laryngoscopy is the only viable option.

There have been many reports of approaches to endotracheal intubation, with various endpoints. Some are simply case reports indicating that a given technique worked in a given patient with cervical vertebral instability. However, there is no published prospective randomized study that provides conclusive outcome data favoring any one approach. Nonetheless, some studies that used other reasonable surrogate endpoints can provide an element of evidentiary support for some approaches.

Fiberoptic Scope versus Laryngoscopy versus Other

Turkstra and coworkers,[120] in normal anesthetized patients, performed a fluoroscopic evaluation of neck extension produced by bag-valve-mask (BVM) ventilation, Macintosh blade laryngoscopy, light wand, and GlideScope. They found minimal movement during BVM ventilation, with the most extension noted by Macintosh blade laryngoscopy. Both light wand and GlideScope produced much less neck extension than Macintosh blade laryngoscopy, with the light wand taking an equivalent time and the GlideScope taking longer.

Rudolph and colleagues[121] compared Macintosh laryngoscopy with a rigid Bonfils fiberoptic scope and reported less cervical spine motion with the rigid fiberoptic scope; however, it was not zero. Hastings and coworkers[122] evaluated external extension without fluoroscopy and reported very little neck extension with the Bullard laryngoscope as compared with Miller and Macintosh blades.

Waltl and colleagues[123] compared cervical spine radiographic cervical movement between the intubating laryngeal mask airway (LMA) and direct laryngoscopy. They reported that the amount of excursion was acceptably low with the intubating LMA.

Brimacombe and coworkers[124] compared the effects of facemask application, esophageal/tracheal Combitube, laryngoscopy-guided intubation, flexible fiberoptic–guided intubation, intubating LMA, and maximal head/neck flexion and extension in cadavers with C3 instability. Displacement was negligible with the fiberscope, moderate with LMA and facemask/chin lift, worse with laryngoscopy, and worst with the Combitube. Data on extension of the neck as a percent of the maximum that was seen with purposeful neck extension are presented in Figure 24-11.

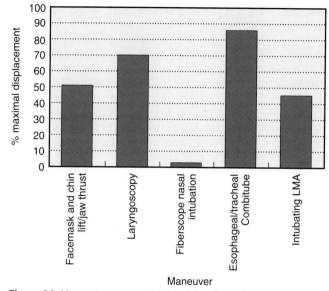

Figure 24-11 ■ Summary of effects of various airway maneuvers on fresh cadavers with experimentally induced cervical instability. LMA, laryngeal mask airway. *(From data of Brimacombe J, Keller C, Kunzel K, et al: Anesth Analg 2000;91:1274-1278.)*

In another fluoroscopic study of cervical spine–injured cadavers, Gerling and colleagues[125] compared laryngoscope blades combined with in-line immobilization and reported that the Miller blade produced less cervical vertebral displacement than the Macintosh blade, and that manual immobilization is superior to cervical collar during intubation.

These data, taken altogether and summarized, suggest that flexible fiberoptic techniques remain the gold standard for intubation of the trachea in the patient with an unstable neck. Intubating LMA, light wand, and Bullard scopes seem to be reasonable alternatives. In-line immobilization is not the optimal technique for immobilizing the airway, but it is better than nothing. If laryngoscopy is required, Miller blades appear to be superior to Macintosh blades. The esophageal-tracheal Combitube does not appear to be better than laryngoscopy.

In applying these data to an individual patient, considerable judgment may be needed. Often, the best evidence-based method may not fit the individual patient's situation. Nonetheless, fiberoptic visualization of the airway with intubation of the trachea is the gold standard and is associated with a near-zero risk of exacerbation of spinal cord injury. However, in the real world, the brain-injured patient is typically not cooperative, and the agitation that may ensue with fiberoptic attempts can produce unacceptable patient-induced neck movement. This results in the need for increasing amounts of sedation, in the context of a full stomach. This may not produce sufficient sedation, putting the patient in an unacceptable in-between state of pharmacologically depressed sensorium with persisting agitation and an unprotected airway. The situation may be emergent enough that the use of a fiberoptic technique, in a setting of developing hypoxemia, full stomach, and possible airway injury with associated secretions, elevates the planned nonexpeditious intubation to a level of unacceptable risk of hypoxemia or aspiration.

For these reasons, in such situations many clinicians advocate direct laryngoscopy with appropriate dosages of CNS depressants and neuromuscular blockade with immobilization or in-line traction. If a difficult airway problem arises in this situation, there should be no extreme laryngoscopy attempts that would clearly risk quadriplegia. Rather, the algorithm should move quickly to LMA to at least establish oxygenation, followed by securing the airway via LMA, followed by intubation or tracheostomy.

Oxygenation

PaO₂ Physiology. The relationship between CBF and PaO_2 is conceptualized in Figure 24-12. Hypoxemia, usually below a PaO_2 of approximately 50 to 60 mm Hg, is associated with vasodilation.[126] At the opposite extreme, Floyd and coworkers[127] demonstrated the vasoconstrictive effect of hyperoxemia and its accompanying hypocapnia in a group of healthy normal volunteers (Fig. 24-13). Nakajima and colleagues[128] evaluated this phenomenon in patients with cerebrovascular disease, finding that areas of the brain with impaired cerebrovascular reserve were not adversely affected by hyperoxia.

Outcome Data. The optimal PaO_2 to seek in a brain-injured patient is unclear. Some data support hyperoxic therapy, and other data suggest that such an approach is deleterious. In addition, the bedside decision about PaO_2 management is coupled to cerebrovascular reserve issues, as previously discussed. Thus, a low PaO_2 that would normally be tolerated through vasodilation may not be well tolerated if vasodilatory reserve is compromised with, for example, carotid occlusion, brain edema, or anemia.

Fiskum and colleagues,[129] among others, have reported in laboratory studies that hyperoxic therapy promotes generation of free radicals, and that such oxidative stress causes mitochondrial injury, which impairs neurologic recovery. This notion from in vitro studies is supported by in vivo studies in rodents and dogs, which demonstrated worse neu-

rologic outcome when hyperoxia was employed before or after an ischemic insult.[130-132]

On the other hand, with the advent of reports supporting the feasibility and reliability of brain tissue PO_2 monitoring,[133] these data are mounting and they demonstrate that normoxemic therapy, in the context of cerebral hypoxia, may promote ischemic injury. Indeed, many recent reports have described nonrandomized retrospective and prospective series of both traumatic and SAH patients in whom brain tissue PO_2 of less than 20 to 30 mm Hg was associated with a worsened neurologic outcome (Fig. 24-14).[134-138] However, these studies did not examine the effects of hyperoxia, which is the negative situation identified by Fiskum and associates[129]; rather, these studies point out the value of avoiding tissue hypoxia, perhaps at the cost of systemic hyperoxia but not intracranial hyperoxia. However, one side observation that arises from these studies is the impact of avoiding hyperoxia, as brain tissue oxygen monitoring allows the provision of the minimal fraction of inspired CO_2 ($FICO_2$) that permits the optimal (not too high, not too low) brain tissue oxygen level.

Given these potentially conflicting therapeutic priorities, the most sensible approach at this time may be as follows: If a brain tissue PO_2 monitor is available, adjust physiologic parameters to keep $P_{br}O_2$ greater than 20 mm Hg. This may entail the use of a fraction of inspired O_2 (FIO_2) greater than 60%, with a concomitant risk of pulmonary oxygen toxicity.[139] It seems that this risk can be incurred for 1 to 2 days. However, past this point, dependence on pulmonary-toxic oxygen concentrations should prompt caregivers to decrease FIO_2, even if this means using higher airway pressure or allowing $P_{br}O_2$ to decrease after a few days.

In the absence of a $P_{br}O_2$ monitor, the clinician must base therapy on assumptions about the brain's oxygenation. If it is felt that many brain areas are well perfused and at risk for hyperoxia, pulmonary management should aim for a PaO_2 just sufficient to produce an O_2 saturation (SaO_2) of greater than 95%. On the other hand, if there are areas of brain hypoperfusion or elevated ICP, then a reasonable empiric approach would be to utilize an FIO_2 of 0.60. This will maximize PaO_2 and $P_{br}O_2$ but without significant risk of acute pulmonary injury.

PEEP and Intracranial Hypertension. Positive end-expiratory pressure (PEEP) can increase ICP (Fig. 24-15).[140] Two mechanisms can be posited. The first is that it occurs through impedance of cerebral venous return to increase cerebral venous pressure and ICP. The second is that it occurs through decreased blood pressure and a reflex increase in cerebral blood volume, which leads to an increase in ICP. The data of Huseby and associates[141] suggest that direct cerebral venous effects occur only with very high PEEP.

Shapiro and Marshall[140] demonstrated increases in ICP in head-injured humans with intracranial hypertension with application of PEEP (see Fig. 24-15). Examination of their data suggests that the most profound decreases in CPP occurred in patients with PEEP-induced decrements in mean arterial pressure, consistent with the notion put forth by Rosner and Becker[3] that decreases in blood pressure increase CBV, leading to an increase in ICP. Aidinis and colleagues[142] confirmed these observations in a more controlled setting. In

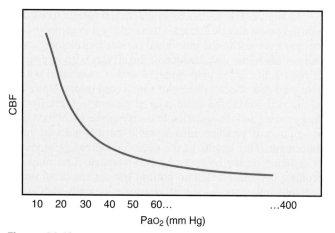

Figure 24-12 ■ Hyperoxia vasoconstricts the brain, whereas hypoxemia produces significant vasodilation. CBF, cerebral blood flow.

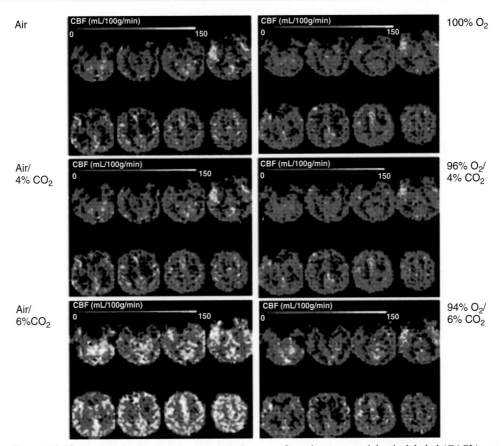

Figure 24-13 ■ Colorized magnetic resonance images of continuous arterial spin-labeled (CASL)-perfusion with scale depicting cerebral blood flow (CBF) changes in response to air, air plus 4% CO_2, air plus 6% CO_2, 100% O_2, 96% O_2 plus 4% CO_2, and 94% O_2 plus 6% CO_2. *(Reproduced with permission from Floyd T, Clark J, Gelfand R, et al: J App Physiol 2003;95:2453-2461.)*

Figure 24-14 ■ Restricted cubic spline functions of the relative risk of death as related to initial low values categorized into less than 5, less than 10, and less than 15 mm Hg. The ordinal characterization follows from the layering of the curves, less than 5 being worse than less than 10, which is worse than less than 15. Note that the curves stabilize at long durations of hypoxia. $P_{br}O_2$, oxygen tension of brain tissue. *(Redrawn from van den Brink W, van Santbrink H, Steyerberg E, et al: Neurosurgery 2000;46:876-878.)*

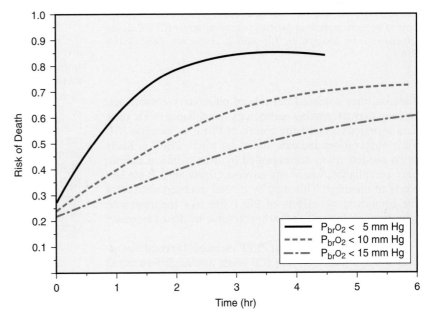

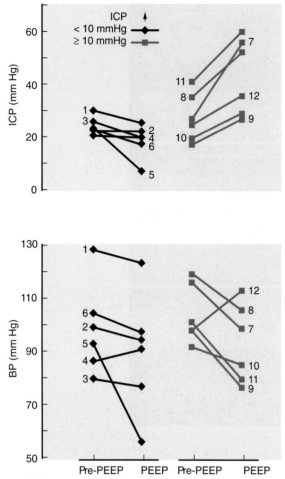

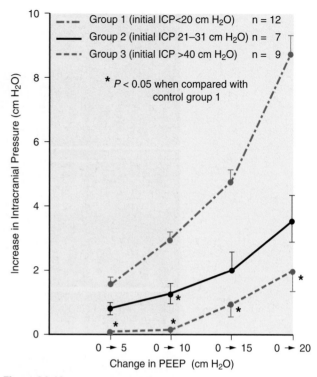

Figure 24-16 ■ Increases in intracranial pressure (ICP) with positive end-expiratory pressure (PEEP) in dogs. Values are mean ± standard error of the mean. Group 1 included 12 animals with initial ICP less than 20 cm H_2O; group 2 included 7 animals with initial ICP of 21 to 39 cm H_2O; group 3 included 9 animals with initial ICP greater than 40 cm H_2O. Blood pressure was maintained constant in all animals. Note that with blood pressure maintained constant, the most significant increases in PEEP occurred in the animals with the lowest starting PEEP level. *(Redrawn from Huseby J, Luce J, Cary J, et al: J Neurosurg 1981;55:704-707.)*

Figure 24-15 ■ Intracranial pressure (ICP) and arterial blood pressure (BP) before and with the application of positive end-expiratory pressure (PEEP) (4 to 8 cm H_2O) in severely head-injured patients. The patients are arbitrarily divided into two groups: those with an ICP increase of ≥10 mm Hg, and those with ICP gains of <10 mm Hg. Note that PEEP-induced blood pressure decreases appear to be more marked in patients sustaining larger ICP increases. *(Redrawn from Shapiro H, Marshall L: J Trauma 1978;18:254-256.)*

addition, they assessed the role of pulmonary compliance, finding that decreasing pulmonary compliance with oleic acid injections lessens the ability of PEEP to increase ICP. Such observations indicate situations where PEEP is likely to be needed, often accompanied by decrements in pulmonary compliance, where any adverse effects on ICP are less likely to manifest. This may be related to observations that the hemodynamic effects of PEEP are less apparent with noncompliant lungs,[143] so that hypotensive-mediated increases in CBV do not occur.

The intuitive notion that PEEP increases cerebral venous pressure and thus increases ICP is not as straightforward as it might seem. For PEEP to increase cerebral venous pressure to levels that will increase ICP, the cerebral venous pressure must equal at least the ICP. Thus, the higher the ICP, the higher PEEP must be to have such a direct hydraulic effect

on ICP. This concept was nicely proven by Huseby and coworkers[141] in studies in which PEEP was increased progressively with different starting levels of ICP (Fig. 24-16). It is important to note that they prevented PEEP-induced decrements in blood pressure, thus avoiding any reflex increases in cerebral blood volume. They suggested a hydraulic model for better conceptualization (Fig. 24-17). Thus, for example, if all of a 10 cm H_2O PEEP application were transmitted to the cerebral vasculature, which is unlikely given the decreased pulmonary compliance associated with the need for such PEEP, then ICP would be affected only if it is *less than* 10 cm H_2O (7.7 mm Hg), increasing to a level no higher than the applied PEEP. Such observations are consistent with the notion that there is a Starling resister regulating cerebral venous outflow.[144]

Ventilation

PaCO₂ Physiology. $PaCO_2$ is determined by the balance between CO_2 production and elimination. CO_2 production is determined by metabolic rate and respiratory quotient (CO_2 production divided by O_2 consumption) and is ordinarily 0.8. Factors that may increase CO_2 production are

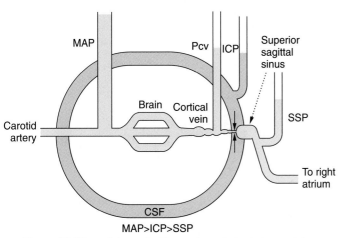

Figure 24-17 ■ Schematic illustration of the intracranial space during raised intracranial pressure (ICP). The *arrows* indicate the position of the hypothesized Starling resistor. Here, the mean arterial pressure (MAP) is greater than ICP, which is greater than sagittal sinus pressure (SSP). Cortical vein pressure (Pcv) cannot fall below ICP, and thus flow is dependent on MAP-ICP, and independent of small changes in SSP. CSF, cerebrospinal fluid. *(Redrawn from Huseby J, Luce J, Cary J, et al: J Neurosurg 1981;55: 704-707.)*

hyperthyroidism, fever, elevated catecholamines, exercise, sepsis, and some pharmacologic stimulants. The respiratory quotient is affected by energy metabolism, so that intake of calories in excess of needs results in lipogenesis, which is a CO_2-producing process that leads to more CO_2 produced than oxygen consumed.[145]

CO₂ elimination is determined by minute ventilation and dead space. The linear relationship between minute ventilation and $PaCO_2$ is such that a simple proportion can be used to predict the $PaCO_2$ that will result with a given change in minute ventilation. Dead space effects are more complex. There are two types of dead space: anatomic and physiologic. Anatomic dead space is that portion of the airways that does not participate in gas exchange because it has no proximity to pulmonary capillaries. Such structures include the mouth, trachea, bronchi, and other large airways. Notably, anatomic dead space is roughly halved via endotracheal intubation and halved again by conversion from translaryngeal intubation to tracheostomy. Physiologic dead space is that portion of non–gas-exchanging ventilation that occurs in alveoli that are suboptimally perfused. Thus, physiologic dead space is increased by anything that increases the amount of gas in alveoli without a commensurate increase in alveolar perfusion, or it is increased by anything that may decrease perfusion to alveoli without commensurate decrease in ventilation. Physiologic situations associated with elevated physiologic dead space include the use of PEEP in compliant lungs, pulmonary emboli, and shock. A more detailed overview of this physiology can be found in West.[145]

In the healthy brain, CBF varies linearly, with $PaCO_2$ between about 20 and 60 mm Hg.[146] The mechanism of effect is thought to be related to the effects of $PaCO_2$ on the pH of CSF.[147] Thus, patients who are chronically hypercapnic and who sustain pH adjustment of the CSF may not be hyperemic.

These patients, of course, may be expected to sustain even more profound decreases in CBF with decrements in $PaCO_2$ to equivalent levels.

Hyperventilation

The $PaCO_2$-mediated changes in CBF are generally without any neurologic import in health. However, in the context of head injury or other cause of ICP elevation, the effects can be profound, as the changes in CBF induce changes in intracranial blood volume. In the brain with little capacitance for such a change in intracranial contents, the change in $PaCO_2$ can have a significant impact on the intracranial pressure.

Thus, for many years hyperventilation was embraced as a mainstay of treatment of intracranial hypertension.[148] However, such therapy was observed to produce a significant cerebral oligemia with the lowered ICP,[149] often developed from a low CBF baseline. On the other hand, at times, elevated $PaCO_2$ in patients with brain injury was noted to produce both high ICP and high CBF, producing a therapeutic quandary. Moreover, adding to the dilemma were observations from the basic science literature of some neuroprotective side effects associated with hypercapnic cerebral acidosis.[150]

Optimal $PaCO_2$. Relatively recent studies debunked what was previously accepted as verity—that hyperventilation is an automatic element of treatment of head injury. Muizelaar and colleagues[27] did a prospective randomized study of the efficacy of hyperventilation in traumatic brain injury (see Fig. 24-16). Because their outcome data showed a persuasively negative impact of hyperventilation, it has been abandoned as a routine therapy in TBI. However, in some situations it is still accepted. Some authors suggest that brain oxygen monitoring by either jugular oximetry or tissue $P_{br}O_2$ can be used to guide the use of hyperventilation.[151] Direct CBF-measuring techniques could also be employed. Such information can allow the clinician to identify whether the patient has an element of hyperemia that contributes to the elevated ICP, a situation that logically seems appropriate for hyperventilation therapy, although this notion has not undergone rigorous scrutiny. Nonetheless, Coles and associates[149] elegantly demonstrated the potential for hypocapnia to produce ischemic areas throughout an injured brain (Figs. 24-18 and 24-19).

Temperature

Temperature has a profound effect on the brain. Fever is convincingly associated with worsened outcomes, with greater release of and toxicity of neurotoxic amino acids, mismatch between flow and metabolism, oxidative stress, and many other probably unknown processes.[152,153] In the normal brain, hypothermia produces a 7% reduction in cerebral metabolic rate for oxygen with every 1° C reduction in brain temperature,[154] thus decreasing consumption of energy metabolites and increasing the time until a hypoxic stress leads to high energy phosphate depletion, and thus increasing the time that the hypoxia can be tolerated.[155] This reduction in cerebral metabolic rate for oxygen cannot entirely explain the neuroprotective effect of mild hypothermia, which must be caused by synergism of many physicochemical mechanisms.

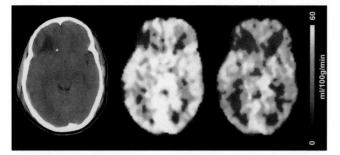

Figure 24-18 ■ Effect of hyperventilation on the burden of hypoperfusion. Radiographic computed tomography *(left)* and grayscale positron-emission tomographic imaging of cerebral blood flow obtained from a 31-year-old man 7 days after injury at relative normocapnia *(middle)*, PaCO$_2$ 35 mm Hg (4.7 kPa), and hypocapnia *(right)*, 26 mm Hg (3.5 kPa). Voxels with a cerebral blood flow of less than 10 mL/100 g/min are shaded in *black*. Note the right frontal contusion and small parietal subdural hematoma. Baseline intracranial pressure (ICP) was 21 mm Hg, and baseline cerebral perfusion pressure (CPP) was 74 mm Hg. Baseline jugular venous saturation (SjvO$_2$) values of 70% and arteriovenous oxygen difference (AVDO$_2$) of 3.7 mL/dL are consistent with hyperemia and support the use of hyperventilation for ICP control. Hyperventilation did result in a reduction in ICP to 17 mm Hg and an increase in CPP to 76 mm Hg, with maintenance of SjvO$_2$ and AVDO$_2$ within desirable ranges (58% and 5.5 mL/mL, respectively). However, despite these SjvO$_2$ and AVDO$_2$ figures, baseline hypoperfused brain volume (HypoBV) was 141 mL and increased to 428 mL with hyperventilation. These increases were observed in both perilesional and normal regions of brain tissue. *(Reproduced with permission from Coles J, Minhas P, Fryer T, et al: Crit Care Clin 2002;30:1950-1959.)*

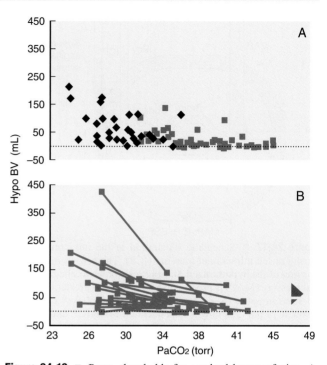

Figure 24-19 ■ PaCO$_2$ thresholds for cerebral hypoperfusion. **A,** Plot of hypoperfused brain volume (HypoBV) versus PaCO$_2$ in healthy volunteers *(blue squares)*, and after hyperventilation *(blue diamonds)*. **B,** Relationship of HypoBV to PaCO$_2$ in patients imaged at baseline *(blue squares)* and after hyperventilation *(blue diamonds)*. The 95% confidence interval for HypoBV in healthy volunteers is shown in *hatched gray area*. (Redrawn from Coles J, Minhas P, Fryer T, et al: Crit Care Med 2002;30:1950-1959.)

A comparison between the neuroprotective efficacy of hypothermia and that produced by an anesthetic producing an equivalent decrement in cerebral metabolic rate always shows greater protection by hypothermia. This is thought to be somehow related to the differential effects of hypothermia and anesthetics on the compartments of brain energy metabolism.[156] Anesthetics decrease metabolic processes related to the work of the neuron (e.g., neurotransmitter synthesis and metabolism), whereas hypothermia also affects the compartment responsible for constitutive activities of the cell (e.g., membrane integrity, ionic concentration homeostasis, and so on). In addition, other biochemical processes contribute to hypothermic protection. For example, with mild hypothermia, there is a substantial blunting of the release of neurotoxic dicarboxylic amino acids such as glutamate and aspartate.[157]

It is thus not surprising that there are countless case reports and basic science studies showing the neuroprotective potential of hypothermia across a broad range of neurologic insults. It is of interest that clinical studies do not uniformly show comparable efficacy.

Hypothermia has been studied and clinically employed for much of the 20th century and to the present. This arose from anecdotes describing miraculous recovery from drowning and other brain ischemia situations in cold environments. Deep hypothermic conditions have been employed for many

years for neuroprotection during cardiac surgery, and during therapeutically induced deep hypothermic cardiac arrest for a variety of procedures.[158,159] At less extreme levels, hypothermia has also been reported to be neuroprotective, although not uniformly so in recent studies. This discussion focuses on moderate hypothermia (30° to 34°C).

In traumatic brain injury, there have been many reports of neuroprotection with hypothermia (Table 24-1), but these were all single-institution studies. When hypothermia was examined in multi-institutional studies, protection could not be demonstrated.[160] However, in a study by Clifton and associates, neuroprotection was reported if the patient was hypothermic on arrival, and rapid rewarming may have contributed to some of the negative findings.[161,162] This supports the notion that speed of induction and suspension of hypothermia may not have been uniformly applied across the participating institutions in the multi-institutional studies. Clifton and coworkers[162] make a persuasive argument in this regard, asserting that significant degradation of the signal-to-noise ratio may have made detection of hypothermic neuroprotection very difficult. The factors contributing to this, which they documented, are the extensive practice variation that occurs across the United States in the approach to management of head trauma, many of which very likely have an

| **24-1** | **Prospective Randomized Clinical Trials of Hypothermia for Traumatic Brain Injury** |

Primary Author, Year	Setting	Patients (N)	Depth/Duration of Cooling	Follow-up	GOOD OUTCOME		P Value
					Hypothermia (%)	Normothermia (%)	
Shiozaki,[281] 1993	Single hospital	33	34°C/48 hr	6 mo	38	6	>.05
Clifton,[282] 1993	Single hospital	46	32°-33°C/48 hr	3 mo	52	36	>.29
Marion,[169] 1997	Single hospital	82	32°-33°C/24 hr	6 mo	56	33	=.05
Jiang,[283] 2000	Single hospital	87	33°-35°C/3-14 days	1 yr	46.5	27	<.05
Shiozaki,[284] 2001	11 hospitals	91	34°C/48 hr	3 mo	46	59	>.99
Clifton,[160] 2001	11 hospitals	392	33°C/48 hr	6 mo	43	43	=.99
Gal,[285] 2002	Single hospital	30	34°C/72 hr	6 mo	87	47	=.08
Zhi,[286] 2003	Single hospital	396	32°-35°C/1-7 days	6 mo	62	38	<.05
Qiu,[287] 2005	Single hospital	86	33°-35°C/3-5 days	2 yr	65	37	<.05

Data complied by Don Marion.

| **24-2** | **Summary of Two Studies Showing a Neuroprotective Effect of Moderate Hypothermia Applied to Patients Sustaining Out-of-Hospital Cardiac Arrest** |

Study	EUROPE*		AUSTRALIA[†]	
	Cold	Warm	Cold	Warm
Patients (N)	136	137	43	34
Good neurologic outcome (%)	55	39	49	26
Time of assessment	6 mo		Discharge	
Target temperature (°C)	32-34	Normal	33	—
How cooled	Custom cold air mattress; ice	Nothing	Cold packs	—
Time to target temperature	4 hr	—	2 hr	—
Duration of cold	24 hr	—	12 hr	—
Mode of rewarming	Passive	—	Active at 18 hr	—

*From Bernard S, Gray T, Buist M, et al: N Engl J Med 2002;346:557-563.
[†]From Minamisawa H, Nordstrom C, Smith M, Siesjo B: J Cereb Blood Flow Metab 1990;10:365-374.

impact on outcome, and differences in admission temperature. The latter factor may have important geographic and climatic origins. Moreover, with respect to the hypothermia itself, it requires an attentive multidisciplinary approach for it to be rapidly and safely induced. Hypothermia is associated with coagulopathy, immune suppression, and pneumonia, among other factors.

Many basic science studies support the use of hypothermia before and, importantly, after cardiac arrest. This led to the concurrent *New England Journal of Medicine* publication of two studies showing that moderate hypothermia had a neuroprotective effect when applied to patients who sustained out-of-hospital cardiac arrest.[163,164] These patients sustained a return of spontaneous circulation, but on initial examination were not responsive, and thus were randomized to the protocol. The protection was identified when the target hypothermic temperature was successfully achieved up to 6 hours after the return of spontaneous circulation. The Advanced Cardiac Life Support (ACLS) guidelines now include this as a recommended practice for coma after cardiac arrest. A summary of these two studies is presented in Table 24-2.

Focal ischemia can be categorized as temporary or permanent. Temporary ischemia occurs often during aneurysm clipping surgery, when a large cerebral artery may be temporally occluded to facilitate clipping of the aneurysm. Typi-

cally, this lasts only a few minutes, but occasionally it can last longer than 15 minutes, risking the development of ischemic injury. Ample animal data support the potential value of hypothermia in this context,[165-167] which was the reason most neuroanesthesiologists in the United States employed it prophylactically in patients undergoing cerebral aneurysm clipping until 2005. However, another multi-institutional study, the IHAST trial with over 1000 patients randomized to moderate hypothermia or normothermia, was unable to detect a difference in either stroke rate or cognitive deficits.[168] Thus, moderate hypothermia for this clinical context has been largely abandoned.

However, one critique of the IHAST study[168] suggests that by examining all aneurysm patients without any measurement of the degree of intraoperative ischemia, there may also exist a signal-to-noise problem, an issue similar to some of the problems seen in the TBI study by Clifton and coworkers. Only a small subset of the study group may have had a risk of stroke-inducing ischemia. In this case, the argument against this was the scrupulous oversight given to the physiologic support of all of the patients at the various sites, and the power analysis done on the pilot data from patients who were presumably reflective of the entire group. Notably, the pilot data came from a single-institution study, which showed a protective effect. Nonetheless, this negative study supports not using moderate hypothermia routinely in unselected cases.

It remains unresolved whether rapid induction of moderate hypothermia could be of value in the patient in whom significant focal ischemia is occurring. I believe that a neuroprotective effect in such a situation may have been missed in the IHAST study. Taking into account the many neuroprotective animal studies and the possible therapeutic gain versus expected outcome, as well as the risks of the intervention, this seems a reasonable approach in cases where temporary focal ischemia is thought to be very likely. Whether to estimate the probability of such an occurrence and implement hypothermia in advance, or to wait for it to arise and emergently induce hypothermia, remains an open question.

Fever is the opposite situation, and it has been convincingly associated with exacerbation of neurologic outcome in the injured brain in both animal and clinical studies. Many neurologic ICU patients have recurrent problems with significant fever in excess of 39°C in the absence of identifiable sepsis. Indeed, in a prospective quantification of 428 consecutive patients admitted to the neurovascular or neurotrauma ICU, 46.7% had at least one febrile episode.[169] This is most likely a sequela of the neurologic process, thought by one group of authors to at times reflect autonomic dysfunction induced by the neurologic injury.[170] SAH is an independent risk factor for development of fever without identifiable cause.[171] The notion that fever kills neurons is gaining widespread acceptance, and it is based on many clinical studies showing an improvement in neurologic outcome associated with prevention of fever.

The mortality rate in patients who had hyperthermia within the first 72 hours after stroke was 15.8%, and the rate was 1% in patients who were normothermic during that time.

Hyperthermia that occurred with the first 24 hours after stroke, without respect to infectious or noninfectious origin, was independently related to a larger infarct volume, worse neurologic deficits, and dependency 3 months after the injury.[172] Azzimondi and Bassein[173] reported that temperature of 37.9°C or greater proved to be an independent risk factor predicting a worse outcome; patients with high fever were far more likely to die with the first 10 days than those with lower temperatures. A prospective study by Reith and associates[174] of 390 consecutive cases of acute stroke classified patients into three groups based on temperature at admission: hypothermic (36.5°C or less), normothermic (36.6° to 37.5°C), and hyperthermic (greater than 37.5°C). They showed that body temperature at admission was highly correlated with initial stroke severity, size of the infarct, mortality rate, and poor outcome. For a 1°C difference in body temperature, the relative risk of poor outcome was more than doubled. This was supported by Ginsberg and Busto,[175] who reported that in stroke patients, fever that occurs soon after the development of stroke is most strongly associated with poor outcome. Body temperature was significantly higher in patients who died within 3 days after admission than in the rest of the study population. Moreover, in ICH patients surviving the first 72 hours after hospital admission, the duration of fever is associated with poor outcome and seems to be a prognostic

factor in these patients.[176] In SAH, fever is associated with vasospasm and poor outcome independently of hemorrhage severity or the presence of infection.[177]

Pharmacologic methods can be employed to control fever. Such modalities include acetaminophen[178] and ibuprofen,[179] although there is some evidence suggesting that ibuprofen is not efficacious in the context of ischemic stroke.[180] Acetaminophen's value can be limited by hepatotoxicity and the theoretical concern that it is an oxidizing agent that even at subhepatotoxic levels may decrease glutathione to lessen potentially helpful free radical scavenging processes.[181] Ibuprofen is linked to issues with gastric ulceration and bleeding.[182]

An alternative method is to use a hypothermia blanket or indwelling hypothermia catheters.[183] Both techniques are based on a servo-controlled system wherein the cooling bath temperature decreases when the patient's temperature starts to rise. In our neurologic ICU, we have generated temperature curves (Fig. 24-20), indicating that it is possible to virtually eliminate fever from the pathophysiology of severe brain injury. Examination of this Figure 24-20 reveals a new vital sign, $T_{bathmin}$, indicating the minimum bath temperature needed to prevent fever in a given patient. Ascertaining the $T_{bathmin}$ that indicates a need to investigate for infection remains to be elucidated.

Glycemic Control

Hyperglycemia has been associated with exacerbation of brain damage with both head trauma and cerebral ischemia.[184-187] However, it is not a straightforward issue. Clearly, neuronal damage after global cerebral ischemia is exacerbated with hyperglycemia.[185,188-191] Some studies have suggested that a blood glucose level greater than 120 mg% is deleterious in stroke patients.[184] However, subsequent studies have suggested a threshold of around 180 mg% with subhuman primates subjected to global ischemia.[191] Clearly, blood glucose levels of greater than 400 mg% cause significant worsening of neurologic outcome with global ischemia.[185,190] Moreover, the general critical care literature also supports prevention of hyperglycemia, based on overall mortality, with a suggested goal of 120 mg%.[192,193] This is such tight control that there is concern about diminishing returns because of hypoglycemic complications.[194]

With focal cerebral ischemia, the picture is a good deal less clear. Animal and human studies have shown that brain damage is worsened (not affected, or lessened) with hyperglycemia.[184,195-212] One report by Prado and colleagues[209] using rats suggested that the discriminating factor in whether brain damage is worsened with hyperglycemia is whether there is collateral flow. Areas of the brain with minimal collaterals were not affected, or were improved, with hyperglycemia. Brain areas with a continued trickle of flow sustained worsened brain damage. Presumably, the continued substrate supply in oligemic (not ischemic) areas allowed greater accumulation of organic acids in the cells, leading to worsening of brain damage.[186,200] Unfortunately, these observations are difficult to apply clinically to patients with focal ischemia.

Even if low levels of hyperglycemia were deleterious, it would not be straightforward to treat. Aggressive therapy of

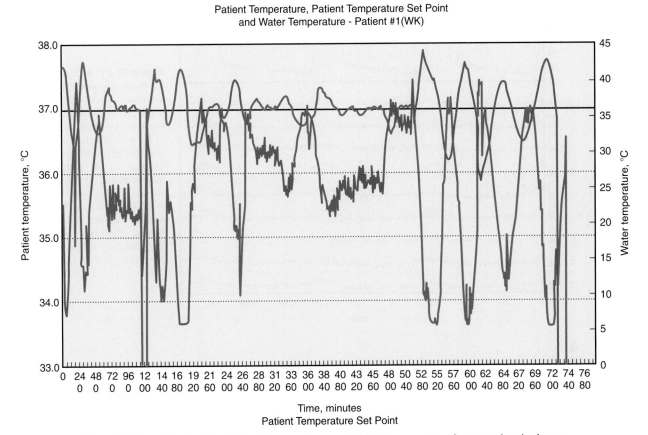

Patient Temperature, Patient Temperature Set Point
and Water Temperature - Patient #1(WK)

Time, minutes
Patient Temperature Set Point

Figure 24-20 ■ Cooling blanket bath temperatures and patient temperatures from a patient in the neurologic ICU of the University of Pennsylvania. A servo-controlled homeothermic blanket system can effectively eliminate fever. Bath temperature required to maintain normal temperature is a new vital sign. *Blue line,* patient temperature; *red line,* bath temperature.

hyperglycemia would impose a risk of hypoglycemia, with its deleterious effects.[194] Thus, given the data in the general critical care literature, it seems that a reasonable approach is to aim for a blood glucose level of approximately 120 to 150 mg% in all acutely ill hyperglycemic patients at risk for cerebral ischemia, but to be less stringent in blood glucose control, perhaps aiming for 150 to 180 mg% in less acutely ill patients who are expected to be in the ICU for less than 3 days. In any event, the blood glucose level should not be allowed to undergo wide variations in concentration, to avoid having it swing to less than 100 mg% or greater than 400 mg%.

Thus, an insulin infusion with frequent glucose assessment should be used in acutely ill patients at risk of cerebral anaerobic metabolism who develop hyperglycemia with a level greater than 150 mg%, with the infusion titrated to keep blood glucose at about 120 to 150 mg%. Once the hyperacute phase has resolved, the intensity of glucose monitoring can be lessened somewhat to match the decreased acuteness of the situation (e.g., decreased concern about hyperglycemic exacerbation of ischemic injury), and somewhat less stringent goals can be used as the patient is readied for discharge from the ICU.

Hyperglycemia has not been shown to have deleterious or protective effects in two animal models of status epilepticus.[213,214] The model used by Swan and colleagues[214] produced limbic system damage, whereas Kofke and coworkers[213] used a model producing substantia nigra damage. Nigral damage in this model is associated with hypermetabolic lactic acidosis,[215] which should have been exacerbated with hyperglycemia. The fact that nigral damage was not exacerbated with hyperglycemia suggests that metabolic acidosis may not be an important factor in the development of brain damage after seizure.

■ CARDIOVASCULAR EVALUATION AND MANAGEMENT IN THE PATIENT WITH ACUTE CNS INJURY

Blood Pressure Effects

In 1960, Lundberg[216] monitored ICP in hundreds of patients and identified characteristic pressure waves. Plateau waves are one type known to be associated with increased cerebral blood volume (Fig. 24-21).[2] Such waves occur when the ICP abruptly increases to nearly systemic levels for about 15 to 30 minutes, occasionally accompanied by neurologic deterioration. Rosner and Becker[3] provided data and a synthesis of the data that convincingly suggests that intracranial blood

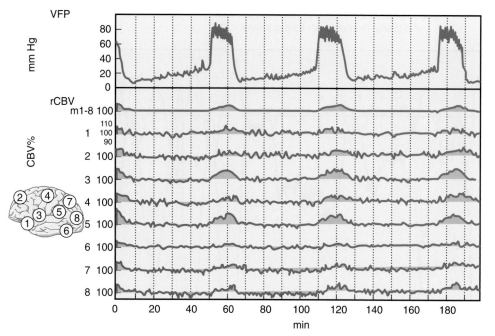

Figure 24-21 ■ Simultaneous recordings of regional cerebral blood volume (rCBV) and ventricular fluid pressure (VFP) during three consecutive plateau waves. The rCBF was measured in eight regions over the left hemisphere. The mean changes in the eight regions are shown in the uppermost curve of the rCBF diagram. Note that the rCBV and VFP curves show very similar courses during the three waves. *(Redrawn from Risberg J, Lundberg N, Ingvar D: J Neurosurg 1969;31:303-310.)*

volume dysautoregulation is responsible for plateau waves. They induced mild head trauma in cats and then intensively monitored the animals after the insult. With normal fluctuations in blood pressure in the normal range, they observed that mild blood pressure decrements to approximately 70 to 80 mm Hg preceded the development of plateau waves (Fig. 24-22). Cerebral blood volume in normally autoregulating brain tissue increases as a result of vasodilation with decreasing blood pressure and, moreover, the increase in CBV is nonlinear. The increase in CBV is exponential as blood pressure decreases to below 80 mm Hg (Fig. 24-23).[217] A small decrease in blood pressure, although in the normotensive range, produces exponential increases in CBV in a setting of abnormal intracranial compliance with the ICP at the elbow of the ICP–intracranial volume relationship (see Fig. 24-2). Thus, a small decrease in blood pressure introduces an exponential CBV change into an exponential ICP relationship, with the result that ICP increases abruptly and to a significant extent. Plateau waves spontaneously resolve with a hypertensive response or with hyperventilation or other vasoconstrictive therapy, which acts to oppose the increase in CBV. Clearly, to develop a plateau wave there must be a portion of the brain with normally reactive vasculature and, at the same time, other brain areas with a mass effect and elevated ICP, a situation of heterogeneous autoregulation (Fig. 24-24). Such data indicate that in patients with high ICP, it is probably important to maintain MAP in the 80 to 100 mm Hg range, in addition to preventing and treating plateau waves.

On the other hand, hypertension can also increase ICP. Normally, within the normal autoregulatory range and at normal ICP, changes in blood pressure have no effect on ICP. However, with brain injury and associated vasoparalysis, increases in blood pressure mechanically produce cerebral vasodilation and thus increase ICP (see Fig. 24-24).[218]

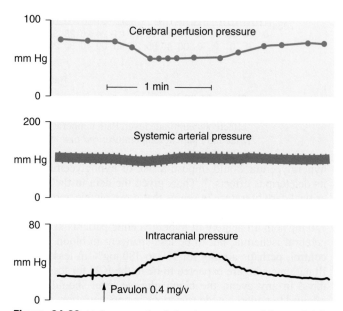

Figure 24-22 ■ In an animal head trauma model, a trivial-appearing and transient decrease in systemic arterial blood pressure in the setting of borderline cerebral perfusion pressure (CPP) precipitates sufficient cerebral vasodilation to markedly increase the intracranial pressure. Restoration of CPP is associated with abolition of the plateau wave. *Arrow* indicates pancuronium (Pavulon) administered. *(Redrawn from Rosner M, Becker D: J Neurosurg 1984;60:312-324.)*

Notably, the Lund group (in Sweden) suggests that hypertension-induced exacerbation of brain edema increases ICP. The increase in ICP then acts to occlude venous outflow, increasing venous pressure, which in turn further worsens the brain edema, constituting a positive feedback cycle initially started by arterial hypertension.[219]

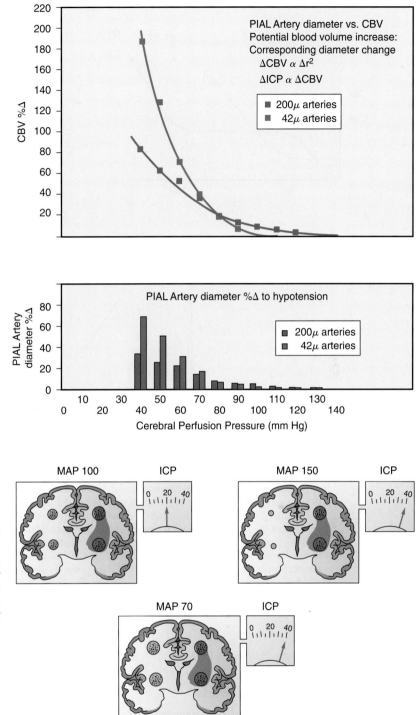

Figure 24-23 ■ Vasodilation occurs at a logarithmic rate as cerebral perfusion pressure (CPP) is reduced. Intracranial pressure (ICP) increases at a proportional rate within each pressure range, with the most rapid increase occurring below a CPP of 80 mm Hg. CBV, cerebral blood volume. *(Redrawn from Rosner MJ, Becker DP: The etiology of plateau waves: A theoretical model and experimental observations. In Ishii S, Nagai H, Brock M (eds): Intracranial Pressure. New York, Springer-Verlag, 1983, pp 301-306.)*

Figure 24-24 ■ In the setting of heterogeneous autoregulation in the brain, conditions may predispose to cerebral blood volume–mediated increases in intracranial pressure with either increases or decreases in blood pressure. *(Redrawn from Kofke WA, Yanes H, Wechsler L, et al: Neurologic intensive care. In Albin MS [ed]: Textbook of Neuroanesthesia with Neurosurgical and Neuroscience Perspectives. New York, McGraw-Hill, 1997, pp 1247-1347.)*

It thus appears that both increasing and decreasing blood pressure can increase ICP, suggesting the presence of a CPP optimum for ICP. In the absence of any patient-specific physiologic information, this is probably about 80 to 100 mm Hg, although this has not been definitively determined experimentally (Fig. 24-25, and see Fig. 24-24).

These considerations underlie a current controversy with respect to blood pressure management in the context of elevated ICP. One argument is that blood pressure should be maintained at a level high enough to ensure adequate CBF and to minimize the probability of plateau waves. The contrary argument is for ample fluids and low blood pressure to promote CBF primarily, rather than pressure. It is my opinion that the preferred approach is to induce the lowest blood pressure that allows sufficient CBF, as indicated by repeated (preferably bedside) measurements. However, lacking such

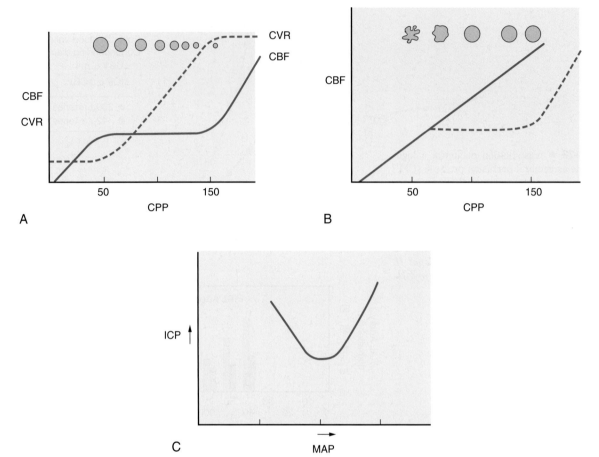

Figure 24-25 ■ Cerebral perfusion pressure (CPP) versus cerebral blood flow (CBF) and cerebrovascular resistance (CVR). **A,** Blood flow is normally maintained constant through changes in CVR, depicted as changes in vascular diameter (and therefore cerebral blood volume [CBV] in the figure). CBV varies inversely with CPP. **B,** With vasoparalysis caused by injury, CVR does not change with CPP variations, so CBF and CBV vary directly with CPP. **C,** In the situation of decreased intracranial compliance, both of the factors in **A** and **B** can interact to increase intracranial pressure (ICP). Normally autoregulating tissue as in **A** will predispose to CBV-mediated ICP elevation with decreasing blood pressure, whereas vasoparalyzed tissue **(B)** will predispose to CBV-mediated ICP elevations with increasing blood pressure, leading to the notion of an ICP optimum (probably about 80 to 100 mm Hg) with varying CPP. MAP, mean arterial pressure. *(Redrawn from Kofke WA, Yanes H, Wechsler L, et al: Neurologic intensive care. In Albin MS [ed]: Textbook of Neuroanesthesia with Neurosurgical and Neuroscience Perspectives. New York, McGraw-Hill, 1997, pp 1247-1347.)*

technology, it seems best to aim for a CPP in the 80 mm Hg range.

Blood Pressure Management

Blood pressure management is an important issue in most neurologic ICU patients. There is concern that systemic hypertension may exacerbate cerebral edema or intracranial hemorrhage, or have deleterious cardiopulmonary effects, such as pulmonary edema or myocardial ischemia. On the other hand, blood pressure decreases can lead to insufficient perfusion, even at a pressure in the normal range of autoregulation. Moreover, mild blood pressure decreases have been implicated in the genesis of plateau waves. Several important principles apply to management of blood pressure in neurologic ICU patients.

Hypertension

When blood pressure is high, the first question is whether the pressure is elevated as a result of normal homeostatic mechanisms to maintain adequate perfusion. For example, with conditions of inadequate brainstem perfusion, a compensatory hyperadrenergic state may occur, resulting in increased blood pressure, thus maintaining sufficient perfusion to maintain aerobic metabolism in the brainstem. If a decision is made to decrease blood pressure, then brainstem failure and death may ensue.

Animal data with cerebral ischemia models provide strong support for the notion that sympatholytic drugs should be used to decrease blood pressure if cerebral ischemia is a possibility. Compared with hemorrhage-induced hypotension, ischemic damage was decreased with the use of ganglionic blockade with hexamethonium,[220] central adrenergic blockade with alpha-2 agonists,[221] and angiotensin-converting enzyme inhibition.[222] Hemorrhaged controls were noted to sustain an increase in exogenous catecholamine concentrations. To test the hypothesis that these catecholamines contributed to brain damage, some of the animals treated with hexamethonium also received intravenous catecholamine infusions. Reversal of the hexamethonium brain protective effect was observed in these animals (Fig. 24-26).[220] Similarly, brain protection has been observed in laboratory studies with pre-ischemic[223] and pre-seizure[224] treatment with reserpine, a drug that depletes presynaptic catecholamine stores. Finally, in a report by Neil-Dwyer and associates,[225] subarachnoid hemorrhage patients received therapy with phentolamine/propranolol or no sympatholytic therapy (Fig. 24-27). Patients who received sympatholytic therapy had significantly better neurologic outcome than controls. In addition, beta-adrenergic blocking drugs have not been reported to produce cerebral vasodilatation or to increase ICP.[226-228]

Calcium channel antagonist drugs, which may also have brain protective effects, are available for antihypertensive therapy. Nimodipine and nicardipine, developed specifically for brain protection purposes, have been assessed in numerous studies, and several reports have shown them to confer protection against delayed ischemic brain damage.[229-235] Solely on the basis of these observations, they appear to be reasonable choices for antihypertensive drugs. They are vasodilators and can modestly increase ICP.[236,237] As vasodilators they also may be expected to produce compensatory catecholamine release,[238] and, on the basis of the previous discussion, this may obviate some of their protective qualities. Moreover, nimodipine has been observed to decrease brain tissue PO_2.[239] Whether this can alter outcome is not known.

Peripheral vasodilators such as nitroprusside, nitroglycerin, and hydralazine all have the potential to induce cerebral vasodilatation and thus cause hyperemic intracranial hypertension.[240-243] Moreover, they are associated with a

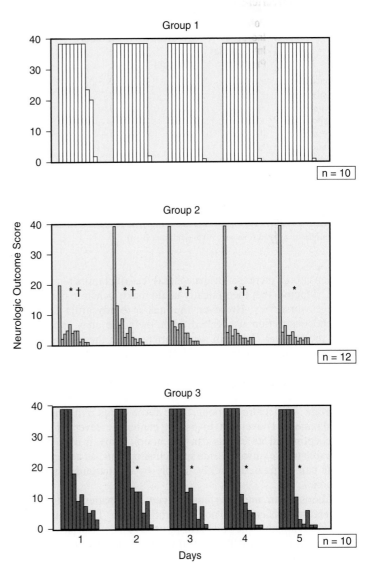

Figure 24-26 ■ Neurologic deficit scores after incomplete focal cerebral ischemia in rats over a 5-day examination period. Each *bar* represents the neurologic score for each rate (*$P < .05$ versus group 1; †$P < .05$ versus group 3). The rats are ranked according to total outcome score in descending order (0 = normal). Cerebral ischemia was induced with occlusion of one carotid artery with hemorrhagic hypotension. Group 1 rats received no vasoactive drugs; group 2 rats received pre-ischemic hexamethonium, and group 3 rats received hexamethonium plus intravenous epinephrine and norepinephrine. Protection was conferred by hexamethonium in a catecholamine-reversible manner. *(Redrawn from Werner C, Hoffman W, Thomas C, et al: Anesthesiology 1990;73: 923-929.)*

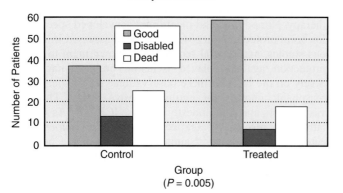

One-year outcome

Figure 24-27 ■ Patients with subarachnoid hemorrhage (SAH) were randomly treated with propranolol or placebo. Neurologic outcome was better in patients undergoing beta-blockade.

24-3	Considerations* in the Choice of an Antihypertensive Drug		
Drug	**Potential to Increase Intracranial Pressure**	**Brain-Protective Side Effects**	**Sympatholytic Effects**
Nitroprusside	+++	0	0
Nitroglycerin	++	0	0
Hydralazine	+++	0	0
Enalapril	+	++	+
Trimethaphan	0	+++	+++
Labetalol	0	+	+++
Propranolol	0	+	+++
Esmolol	0	+	+++
Nifedipine	++	+	0
Nicardipine	++	+++	0
Clonidine		+++	+++

*Considerations rated from none (0) to significant (+++).

compensatory increase in peripheral catecholamines and renin,[238] factors that theoretically could make ischemic brain damage worse.[220,223] However, the lack of bradycardia and bronchoconstriction associated with their use may make them the optimal choice in some patients with these conditions. If such a drug is chosen and the patient is at risk of neurologic deterioration from ischemia or high ICP, close clinical observation is indicated. Any deterioration would mandate discontinuation of the drug. Such concerns are important for deciding among these three drugs. Although hydralazine is convenient to use, it cannot be reversed at the receptor and its effects can last hours. Thus, it may be preferable to use nitroprusside in such situations, as adverse effects can be treated quickly, simply by discontinuing the infusion.

Choosing an antihypertensive agent for a patient at risk for cerebral ischemia is not straightforward. Therapeutic urgency, sympatholytic and brain-protective side effects, and potential to increase ICP are all important considerations in the choice of an antihypertensive drug (Table 24-3).

If it is deemed that blood pressure must be decreased very quickly (i.e., within minutes), nicardipine in 100- to 500-μg boluses is very effective and safely titratable. Once the blood pressure is reduced, a maintenance regimen of nicardipine or another drug can be started. Alternatively, sodium nitroprusside can be started, although its deleterious side effects (as discussed in preceding paragraphs) make it less preferred as an antihypertensive agent for a neurologic patient. However, it is perhaps the most potent and reliable antihypertensive drug available.

Plateau waves, first reported by Lundberg[216] and associated with neurologic deterioration, were demonstrated by Risberg and colleagues[2] to be associated with cerebral vasodilation. Rosner and Becker[3] reported that mild decreases in blood pressure to the 60 to 80 mm Hg range can be associated with plateau waves. Presumably, the decrease in blood pressure prompts vasodilatation in normally autoregulating tissue. The increase in cerebral blood volume, which is an exponential function, versus cerebral perfusion pressure,[3] superimposed on the exponential ICP versus intracranial volume relationship, is associated with an explosive hyperemic increase in ICP, a plateau wave (see Figs. 24-20 to 24-22). This, then, introduces a concern with the use of any antihypertensive agent—that, aside from having specific, direct cerebrovascular effects, normal autoregulation may also increase ICP as cerebral perfusion pressure decreases to about 80 mm Hg or below.

Clearly, any time hypotensive therapy is employed in a patient with altered intracranial compliance, edema, or ischemia, very close and continuous observations of the patient are mandatory. Deterioration should prompt consideration of one of the above processes occurring, with corrective therapy then introduced along with concomitant reconsideration of the need to lower blood pressure.

Hypotension Treatment and Induced Hypertension
When a patient is hypotensive, efforts should focus not only on treating the low blood pressure but also on ascertaining the cause of the hypotension. In patients with head trauma, consideration needs to be given to other injuries that may be causing hemorrhage or spinal shock. Loss of blood flow to the brainstem can also be associated with hypotension, which can be quite difficult to treat. In addition, usual non-neurologic causes of hypotension in an ICU (e.g., pneumothorax, sepsis, and cardiogenic causes) should also be considered.

When therapy to increase blood pressure (to treat vasospasm) is contemplated, the need for it must be seriously considered. Excessive increases in blood pressure can exacerbate cerebral edema.[244-248] This presumably occurs in brain areas with dysautoregulation and BBB disruption, so that increasing blood pressure, rather than producing vasoconstriction and no change in rCBF, causes vascular distention, increased rCBF, and transudation of fluid across the damaged BBB. In addition, increases in blood pressure risk producing or exacerbating intracranial hemorrhage.

Catecholamines used to increase blood pressure are either neurotransmitters or chemically similar to neurotransmitters. It is thus to be expected, if they cross the BBB, that neural effects will arise secondary to their use. Normally, exogenously administered catecholamines do not cross the BBB and have no effect on CBF or metabolism.[249] However, it has been demonstrated that when there is BBB disruption, catecholamine infusion leads to increased blood flow and metabolism.[250] In patients with subarachnoid hemorrhage, catecholamine infusions produce a variety of disparate and unpredictable effects on CBF,[251] and adrenergic blockade confers neurologic protection.[225] Finally, catecholamines have direct neurotoxic potential, as indicated by data showing neurotoxicity with application directly to the cortex in vivo.[252] Unfortunately, catecholamines are the only clinically accepted routine means of increasing blood pressure pharmacologically in neurologic ICU patients.

Increasing preload to the heart is one nonpharmacologic way to increase blood pressure. With crystalloid or colloid infusion, this is generally associated with hemodilution, and the effects on the patient's status should be considered. The hemodilution may improve flow to areas where microcirculation is compromised. However, it may be associated with increased CBV and hyperemic intracranial hypertension if hematocrit decreases excessively with compensatory vasodilatation.

Whether to use crystalloid or colloid for this purpose is controversial. The BBB is functionally an osmometer.[253-258] Thus, the added trivial increase in osmolarity with colloid is not a sufficient reason to use it, unless one expects the BBB to be permeable to electrolytes and less so to colloid. Using an iso-osmolar or a slightly hyperosmolar fluid to increase blood pressure has a smaller likelihood of producing brain edema, and this approach is supported by animal studies.

Some advocate the use of induced systemic hypertension with high ICP to prevent plateau waves. As blood pressure increases, incremental increases in vasoconstriction occur in normally reactive tissue to decrease CBV and thus ICP. However, the advantage of this therapy may be offset by increased edema in injured brain regions.[219]

SAH is particularly notable for catecholamine effects, but these effects also occur with other intracranial processes, including increased ICP, stroke, head trauma, or any situation of compromised midbrain or hindbrain O_2 delivery. Serum catecholamine levels increase dramatically after SAH, peaking at the same time as the peak incidence of post-SAH vasospasm, with symptom development corresponding to serum catecholamine levels.[259-262] This leads to the notion that hypothalamic injury with excess catecholamine release may be an important factor in the genesis of post-SAH spasm and stroke,[260-262] observations that may be relevant to other intracranial processes previously elaborated. Several lines of evidence further support this hypothesis:

- The cerebral vasculature is somewhat invested with adrenergic nerves. With SAH, the number of adrenergic receptors in the cerebral vessels decreases.[262,263] This suggests that denervation hypersensitivity may be occurring, so that the increase in humoral catecholamines with SAH produces spasm in hyper-reacting vessels.

- Catecholamine release after SAH is sufficient to produce electrocardiographic changes[259] with ventricular wall motion abnormalities[260] and myocardial injury.[261]
- Treatment of humans with SAH with beta- and alpha-adrenergic antagonists is associated with an improvement in neurologic outcome (see Fig. 24-27)[261] and in electrocardiographic abnormalities.[259]
- In animal models, selective destruction of hindbrain adrenergic nuclei with cephalad projections prevents the development of vasospasm.[262] Moreover, laboratory studies indicate an important role for vasopressin in vasospasm, as vasospasm cannot be produced in vasopressin-deficient rats.[263]
- Animal data with cerebral ischemia models provide strong support for the notion that catecholamines can exacerbate cerebral ischemia. Compared with hemorrhage-induced hypotension, ischemic damage was decreased with hypotension induced through the use of ganglionic blockade with hexamethonium,[220] central adrenergic blockade with alpha-2 agonists,[221] and angiotensin-converting enzyme inhibition.[222] Hemorrhaged controls were noted to sustain an increase in exogenous catecholamine concentrations. To test the hypothesis that these catecholamines contributed to brain damage, some of the animals treated with hexamethonium also received intravenous catecholamine infusions. Reversal of the hexamethonium brain-protective effect was observed in these animals (see Fig. 24-26).[220]
- Brain protection has been observed in laboratory studies with pre-ischemic[223] and pre-seizure[224] treatment using reserpine, a drug that depletes presynaptic catecholamine stores.
- Application of catecholamines directly to nonischemic cortical tissue has also been observed to have neurotoxic potential.[252] In addition, intravenous administration can exacerbate brain swelling after head trauma, although this is most likely a direct effect of blood pressure on a dysautoregulating brain (see Fig. 24-25), rather than a manifestation of biochemical neurotoxicity.[290]

Optimal Hemoglobin Level

Anemia is generally well tolerated neurologically except at extreme levels. This indicates the enormous cerebrovascular reserve that, in health, is in place to compensate for this and similar physiologic stresses. Observations by Borgstrom and coworkers[275] indicate that, in rodents, decreasing Hb levels produce an increase in CBF that is initially caused primarily by decreased viscosity, but as Hb continues to decrease to below 10 gm%, active vasodilation arises (Fig. 24-28). If the brain vasculature is already maximally vasodilated because of other stresses such as hypoxemia or low cerebral perfusion pressure, then the anemic stress may not be well tolerated and may produce hypoxic/ischemic brain damage.

Supporting observations of anemia-associated cerebral vasodilation have been observed in humans after cardiac surgery (Fig. 24-29).[276] Dexter and Hindman[277] modeled these competing issues mathematically, and their data agreed with laboratory[275] and empiric observations that an Hb con-

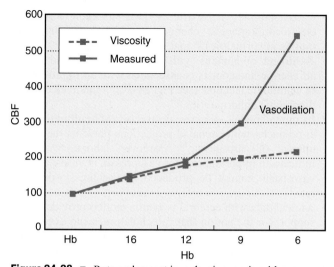

Figure 24-28 ■ Rats underwent isovolemic anemia with measurement of change in global cerebral blood flow (CBF). The theoretical CBF that would arise solely from change in viscosity is indicated by the viscosity curve. The measured CBF follows this line until hemoglobin (Hb) falls to less than 10, after which active vasodilation was observed. *(Adapted from Borgstrom L, Johannsson H, Siesjo B: Acta Physiol Scand 1975;93:505-514.)*

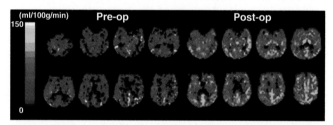

Figure 24-29 ■ Continuous arterial spin-labeled perfusion magnetic resonance images obtained before (PRE-OP) and after (POST-OP) cardiac surgery, showing cerebral blood flow (CBF) with color scale for an 81-year-old man. Global CBF increased from baseline of 36 to 62 mL/100 g/min on the 5th day after surgery. Multiple regression analysis over all subjects in the study revealed a significant and inverse relationship between CBF and hematocrit. *(Reproduced with permission from Floyd T, McGarvey M, Ochroch E, et al: Ann Thoracic Surg 2003;76:2037-2042.)*

centration of less than 10 gm% associated with vasodilation can be expected to be deleterious in conditions of altered cerebrovascular reserve. Kim and Kang's[278] observations of anemia-associated stroke after GI hemorrhage support Dexter and Hindman's calculations. Another supporting point is the observation in brain-injured patients of increased brain tissue P_{O_2} with transfusion to exceed an Hb of 10 gm%.[279] Indeed, one of the approaches to managing low $P_{br}O_2$ is to transfuse to an Hb of greater than 10 gm%, based on observations that such therapy can significantly improve brain oxygenation in the context of severe brain injury.

Notwithstanding reports that 7 gm% is optimal in a general critical care population,[280] these observations taken altogether suggest that transfusion to a goal of 10 gm% is reasonable in the context of impaired cerebrovascular reserve.

■ REFERENCES

1. Cushing H: Concerning a definite regulatory mechanism of the vasomotor centre which controls blood pressure during cerebral compression. Johns Hopkins Hosp Bull 1901;126:290-292.
2. Risberg J, Lundberg N, Ingvar D: Regional cerebral blood volume during acute rises in the intracranial pressure (plateau waves). J Neurosurg 1969;31:303-310.
3. Rosner M, Becker D: Origin and evolution of plateau waves: Experimental observations and a theoretical model. J Neurosurg 1984;50:312-324.
4. Greenberg J, Alavi A, Reivich M, et al: Local cerebral blood volume response to carbon dioxide in man. Circ Res 1978;43:324.
5. Sakai F, Nakaazawa K, Tazaki, et al: Regional cerebral blood volume and hematocrit measured in normal human volunteers by single photon emission computed tomography. J Cereb Blood Flow Metab 1985;5:207.
6. Strandgaard S, Olesen J, Skinhoj E, et al: Autoregulation of brain circulation in severe arterial hypertension. Br Med J 1973;3:507.
7. Miller J, Becker D, Ward J, et al: Significance of intracranial hypertension in severe head injury. J Neurosurg 1977;47:503.
8. Lundberg N, Troupp H, Lorin H: Continuous recording of ventricular fluid pressure in patients with severe acute traumatic brain injury: A preliminary report. J Neurosurg 1965;22:581.
9. Giulioni M, Ursino M, Alvis IC: Correlations among intracranial pulsatility, intracranial hemodynamics, and transcranial Doppler wave form: Literature review and hypothesis for future studies. Neurosurgery 1988;22:807.
10. Hassler W, Steinmetz H, Gawlowski J: Transcranial Doppler ultrasonography in raised intracranial pressure and in intracranial circulatory arrest. J Neurosurg 1988;68:745-751.
11. Greitz T, Gordon E, Kolmodin G, Widen L: Aortocranial and carotid angiography in determination of brain death. Neuroradiology 1973;5:13-19.
12. Langfitt T, Weinstein J, Kassell N: Cerebral vasomotor paralysis produced by intracranial hypertension. Neurology 1965;15:622.
13. Langfitt T, Weinstein J, Kassell N, Simeone FA: Transmission of increased intracranial pressure: I. Within the craniospinal axis. J Neurosurg 1964;21:989-997.
14. Jalan R, Olde Damink S, Deutz N, et al: Moderate hypothermia prevents cerebral hyperemia and increase in intracranial pressure in patients undergoing liver transplantation for acute liver failure. Transplantation 2003;75:2034-2039.
15. Kofke W, Dong M, Bloom M, et al: Transcranial Doppler ultrasonography with induction of anesthesia for neurosurgery. J Neurosurg Anesthesiol 1994;6:89.
16. Aggarwal S, Kramer D, Yonas H, et al: Cerebral hemodynamic and metabolic changes in fulminant hepatic failure: A retrospective study. Hepatology 1994;19:80.
17. Michenfelder J: The 27th Rovenstine Lecture: Neuroanesthesia and the achievement of professional respect. Anesthesiology 1989;70:695.
18. Wilkins R: Cerebral vasospasm. Crit Rev Neurobiol 1990;6:51.
19. Jaggi J, Obrist W, Gennarelli T, Langfitt T: Relationship of early cerebral blood flow and metabolism to outcome in acute head injury. J Neurosurg 1990;72:176-182.
20. Castillo J, Davalos A, Noya M: Timing for fever-related brain damage in acute ischemic stroke. Stoke 1998;29:2455-2460.
21. Raichle M, Posner J, Plum F: Cerebral blood flow during and after hyperventilation. Arch Neurol 1970;23:394-403.
22. Lassen N: Control of cerebral circulation in health and disease. Circ Res 1974;34:749.
23. Shapiro H: Intracranial hypertension: Therapeutic and anesthetic considerations. Anesthesiology 1975;43:445.
24. Shenkin H, Bouzarth W: Clinical methods of reducing intracranial pressure. N Engl J Med 1970;282:1465.
25. Raichle M, Plum F: Hyperventilation and cerebral blood flow. Stroke 1972;3:566-575.
26. Stringer W, Hasso A, Thompson J, et al: Hyperventilation-induced cerebral ischemia in patients with acute brain lesions: Demonstration by xenon-enhanced CT. Am J Neurorad 1993;14:475-484.

27. Muizelaar J, Marmarou A, Ward J, et al: Adverse effects of prolonged hyperventilation in patients with severe head injury: A randomized clinical trial. J Neurosurg 1991;75:731.

28. Chater S, Simpson K: Effect of passive hyperventilation on seizure threshold in patients undergoing electroconvulsive therapy. Br J Anaesth 1988;60:70-73.

29. Cruz J, Miner M, Allen S, et al: Continuous monitoring of cerebral oxygenation in acute brain injury: Injection of mannitol during hyperventilation. J Neurosurg 1990;73:725.

30. Pierce E, Lambertsen C, Deutsch S: Cerebral circulation and metabolism during thiopental anesthesia and hyperventilation in man. J Clin Invest 1962;41:1664-1671.

31. Marshall L, Shapiro H, Rauscher A, et al: Pentobarbital therapy for intracranial hypertension in metabolic coma: Reye's syndrome. Crit Care Med 1978;6:105.

32. Hartung H: [Intracranial pressure after propofol and thiopental administration in patients with severe head trauma.] Anaesthesist 1987;36:285-287.

33. Larsen R, Hilfiker O, Radke J, et al: [The effects of midazolam on the general circulation, the cerebral blood-flow and cerebral oxygen consumption in man.] Anaesthesist 1981;30:18-21.

34. Renou A, Vernhiet J, Macrez P, et al: Cerebral blood flow and metabolism during etomidate anaesthesia in man. Br J Anaesth 1978;50:1047-1051.

35. Prior J, Hinds C, Williams J, et al: The use of etomidate in the management of severe head injury. Int Care Med 1983;9:313-320.

36. Vandesteene A, Trempont V, Engelman E, et al: Effect of propofol on cerebral blood flow and metabolism in man. Anaesthesia 1988;45(Suppl):42-43.

37. Sakabe T, Maekawa T, Ishikawa T, et al: The effects of lidocaine on canine metabolism and circulation related to the electroencephalogram. Anesthesiology 1974;40:433-441.

38. Yano M, Nishiyama H, Yokota H, et al: Effect of lidocaine on ICP response to endotracheal suctioning. Anesthesiology 1986;64:651-653.

39. Michenfelder J: The interdependency of cerebral functional and metabolic effects following massive doses of thiopental in the dog. Anesthesiology 1974;41:231-236.

40. Preziosi P, Vacca M: Adrenocortical suppression and other endocrine effects of etomidate. Life Sci 1988;42:477.

41. Skues M, Prys-Roberts C: The pharmacology of propofol. J Clin Anesth 1989;1:387.

42. Burow B, Johnson M, Packer D: Metabolic acidosis associated with propofol in the absence of other causative factors. Anesthesiology 2004;101:239-241.

43. Devlin J, Lau A, Tanios M: Propofol-associated hypertriglyceridemia and pancreatitis in the intensive care unit: An analysis of frequency and risk factors. Pharmacotherapy 2005;25:1348-1352.

44. Parke T, Stevens J, Rice A, et al: Metabolic acidosis and fatal myocardial failure after propofol infusion in children: Five case reports. BMJ 1992;305:613-616.

45. Schenkman K, Yan S: Propofol impairment of mitochondrial respiration in isolated perfused guinea pig hearts determined by reflectance spectroscopy. Crit Care Clin 2000;28:172-177.

46. Muizelaar JP, Lutz HA 3rd, Becker DP: Effect of mannitol on ICP and CBF and correlation with pressure autoregulation in severely head-injured patients. J Neurosurg 1984;61:700-706.

47. Muizelaar J, Wei E, Kontos H, Becker D: Cerebral blood flow is regulated by changes in blood pressure and in blood viscosity alike. Stroke 1986;17:44-48.

48. Reichenthal E, Kaspi T, Cohen M, et al: The ambivalent effects of early and late administration of mannitol in cold-induced brain oedema. Acta Neurochir 1990;51(Suppl):110.

49. Rosenberg G, Barrett J, Estrada E, et al: Selective effect of mannitol-induced hyperosmolality on brain interstitial fluid and water content in white matter. Metab Brain Dis 1988;3:217.

50. Bell B, Smith M, Kean D, et al: Brain water measured by magnetic resonance imaging: Correlation with direct estimation and changes after mannitol and dexamethasone. Lancet 1987;1:66.

51. Todd M, Tommasino C, Moore S: Cerebral effects of isovolemic hemodilution with a hypertonic saline solution. J Neurosurg 1985;63:944-948.

52. Chan P, Fishman R: Elevation of rat brain amino acids, ammonia and idiogenic osmoles induced by hyperosmolality. Brain Res 1979;161:293.

53. Pollock A, Arieff A: Abnormalities of cell volume regulation and their functional consequences. Am J Physiol 1980;239:F195.

54. McManus M, Strange K: Acute volume regulation of brain cells in response to hypertonic challenge. Anesthesiology 1993;78:1132-1137.

55. Kofke W: Mannitol: Potential for rebound intracranial hypertension? J Neurosurg Anesth 1993;5:1-3.

56. Rudehill A, Gordon E, Ohman G, et al: Pharmacokinetics and effects of mannitol on hemodynamics, blood and cerebrospinal fluid electrolytes, and osmolality during intracranial surgery. J Neurosurg Anesth 1993;5:4-12.

57. Zornow M: Hypertonic saline as a safe and efficacious treatment of intracranial hypertension. J Neurosurg Anesth 1996;8:175-177.

58. Weed LH, McKibben PS: Pressure changes in the cerebrospinal fluid following intravenous injection of solutions of various concentrations. Am J Physiol 1919;48:512-530.

59. Prough D, Johnson J, Poole GJ, et al: Effects on intracranial pressure of resuscitation from hemorrhagic shock with hypertonic saline versus lactated Ringer's solution. Crit Care Med 1985;13:407-411.

60. Prough D, Whitley J, Taylor C, et al: Regional cerebral blood flow following resuscitation from hemorrhagic shock with hypertonic saline: Influence of a subdural mass. Anesthesiology 1991;75:319-327.

61. Battistella F, Wisner D: Combined hemorrhagic shock and head injury: Effects of hypertonic saline (7.5%) resuscitation. J Trauma 1991;31:182-188.

62. Anderson JT, Wisner DH, Sullivan PE, et al: Initial small-volume hypertonic resuscitation of shock and brain injury: Short- and long-term effects. J Trauma 1997;42:592-600.

63. Shackford S, Zhuang J, Schmoker J: Intravenous fluid tonicity: Effect on intracranial pressure, cerebral blood flow, and cerebral oxygen delivery in focal brain injury. J Neurosurgery 1992;76:91-98.

63a. Tseng M-Y, Al-Rawi PG, Pickard JD, et al: Effect of hypertonic saline on cerebral blood flow in poor-grade patients with subarachnoid hemorrhage. Stroke 2003;June:1390-1397.

64. Zausinger S, Thal S, Kreimeier U, et al: Hypertonic fluid resuscitation from subarachnoid hemorrhage in rats. Neurosurgery 2004;55:679-687.

65. Qureshi AI, Wilson DA, Traystman RJ: Treatment of elevated intracranial pressure in experimental intracerebral hemorrhage: Comparison between mannitol and hypertonic saline. Neurosurgery 1999;44:1055-1063.

66. Suarez JI, Qureshi AI, Bhardwaj A, et al: Treatment of refractory intracranial hypertension with 23.4% saline. Crit Care Med 1998;26:1118-1122.

67. Horn P, Munch E, Vajkoczy P, et al: Hypertonic saline solution for control of elevated intracranial pressure in patients with exhausted response to mannitol and barbiturates. Neurol Res 1999;21:758-764.

68. Worthley L, Cooper D, Jones N: Treatment of resistant intracranial hypertension with hypertonic saline: Report of two cases. J Neurosurg 1988;68:478-481.

69. Qureshi AI, Suarez JI, Bhardwaj A, et al: Use of hypertonic (3%) saline/acetate infusion in the treatment of cerebral edema: Effect on intracranial pressure and lateral displacement of the brain. Crit Care Med 1998;26:440-446.

70. Schatzmann C, Heissler H, Konig K, et al: Treatment of elevated intracranial pressure by infusions of 10% saline in severely head injured patients. Acta Neurochir 1998;71:31-33.

71. Vialet R, Albanèse J, Thomachot L, et al: Isovolume hypertonic solutes (sodium chloride or mannitol) in the treatment of refractory posttraumatic intracranial hypertension: 2 mL/kg 7.5% saline is more effective than 2 mL/kg 20% mannitol. Crit Care Med 2003;31:1683-1687.

72. Shackford SR, Bourguignon PR, Wald SL, et al: Hypertonic saline resuscitation of patients with head injury: A prospective, randomized clinical trial. J Trauma 1998;44:50-58.

73. Simma B, Burger R, Falk M, et al: A prospective, randomized, and controlled study of fluid management in children with severe head

injury: Lactated Ringer's solution versus hypertonic saline. Crit Care Med 1998;26:1265-1270.

74. Khanna S, Davis D, Peterson B, et al: Use of hypertonic saline in the treatment of severe refractory posttraumatic intracranial hypertension in pediatric traumatic brain injury. Crit Care Med 2000;28: 1144-1151.

75. Peterson B, Khanna S, Fisher B, Marshall L: Prolonged hypernatremia controls elevated intracranial pressure in head-injured pediatric patients. Crit Care Med 2000;28:1136-1143.

76. Murphy N, Auzinger G, Bernel W, Wendon J: The effect of hypertonic sodium chloride on intracranial pressure in patients with acute liver failure. Hepatology 2004;39:464-470.

77. Vassar M, Perry C, Gannaway W, Holcroft J: 7.5% sodium chloride/ dextran for resuscitation of trauma patients undergoing helicopter transport. Arch Surg 1991;126:1065-1072.

78. Cooper DJ, Myles PS, McDermott FT, et al: Prehospital hypertonic saline resuscitation of patients with hypotension and severe traumatic brain injury: A randomized controlled trial. JAMA 2004;291: 1350-1357.

79. Suarez JI: Hypertonic saline for cerebral edema and elevated intracranial pressure. Cleve Clin J Med 2004;71(Suppl 1):S9-13.

80. Zornow M, Scheller M, Shackford S: Effect of a hypertonic lactated Ringer's solution on intracranial pressure and cerebral water content in a model of traumatic brain injury. J Trauma 1989;29:484-488.

81. Gunnar W, Jonasson O, Merlotti G, et al: Head injury and hemorrhagic shock: Studies of the blood brain barrier and intracranial pressure after resuscitation with normal saline solution, 3% saline solution, and dextran-40. Surgery 1988;103:398-407.

82. Berger S, Schurer L, Hartl R, et al: Reduction of post-traumatic intracranial hypertension by hypertonic/hyperoncotic saline/dextran and hypertonic mannitol. Neurosurgery 1995;37:98-107.

83. Saltarini M, Massarutti D, Baldassarre M, et al: Determination of cerebral water content by magnetic resonance imaging after small volume infusion of 18% hypertonic saline solution in a patient with refractory intracranial hypertension. Eur J Emerg Med 2002;9: 262-265.

84. Paczynski R: Osmotherapy: Basic concepts and controversies. Crit Care Clin 1997;13:105-129.

85. Valadka A, Robertson C: Should we be using hypertonic saline to treat intracranial hypertension? Crit Care Med 2000;28:1245-1246.

86. Dominguez T, Priestley M, Huh J: Caution should be exercised when maintaining a serum sodium level >160 meq/L. Crit Care Med 2004;32:1438-1439.

87. Dominguez TE, Priestley M, Huh W: Caution should be exercised when maintaining a serum sodium level >160 meq/L. Crit Care Med 2004;32:1438-1439.

88. Bhardwaj A, Harukuni I, Murphy S: Hypertonic saline worsens infarct volume after transient focal ischemia in rats. Stroke 2000;31:1694-1701.

89. Swanson P: Neurological manifestations of hypernatremia. In Vinken P, Bruyn G (eds): Handbook of Clinical Neurology. Amsterdam, North-Holland, 1976, pp 443-461.

90. Sterns R, Riggs J, Schochet S: Osmotic demyelination syndrome following correction of hyponatremia. N Engl J Med 1986;314: 1535-1542.

91. Kien N, Kramer G, White D: Acute hypotension caused by rapid hypertonic saline infusion in anesthetized dogs. Anesth Analg 1991;73:597-602.

92. Cote C, Greenhow D, Marshall B: The hypotensive response to rapid intravenous administration of hypertonic solutions in man and in the rabbit. Anesthesiology 1979;50:30-35.

93. Reed R, Johnston T, Chen Y, Fischer R: Hypertonic saline alters plasma clotting times and platelet aggregation. J Trauma 1991;31: 8-14.

94. Kolsen-Petersen J, Nielsen J, Tonnesen E: Acid base and electrolyte changes after hypertonic saline (7.5%) infusion: A randomized controlled clinical trial. Scand J Clin Lab Invest 2005;65:13-22.

95. Gudeman S, Young H, Miller J, et al: Indications for operative treatment and operative technique in closed head injury. In Becker D, Gudeman S (eds): Textbook of Head Injury. Philadelphia, WB Saunders, 1989, pp 138-181.

96. Kalia K, Yonas H: An aggressive approach to massive middle cerebral artery infarction. Arch Neurol 1993;50:1293.

97. Manno E, Atkinson J, Fulgham J, Wijdicks E: Emerging medical and surgical management strategies in the evaluation and treatment of intracerebral hemorrhage. Mayo Clin Proc 2005;80:420-433.

98. Kondziolka D, Fazl M: Functional recovery after decompressive craniectomy for cerebral infarction. Neurosurgery 1988;23:143.

99. Adams H, Brott T, Crowell R, et al: Guidelines for the management of patients with acute ischemic stroke: A statement for healthcare professionals from a special writing group of the Stroke Council, American Heart Association. Stroke 1994;25:1901-1914.

100. Forsting M, Reith W, Schabitz W, et al: Decompressive craniectomy for cerebral infarction: An experimental study in rats. Stroke 1995;26:259-264.

101. Kilincer C, Asil T, Utku U, et al: Factors affecting the outcome of decompressive craniectomy for large hemispheric infarctions: A prospective cohort study. Acta Neurochir 2005;147:587-594.

102. Thal G, Szabo M, Lopez-Bresnahan M, Crosby G: Exacerbation or unmasking of focal neurologic deficits by sedative medication. J Neurosurg Anesthesiol 1993;5:291.

103. Murthy J, Chowdary G, Murthy T, et al: Decompressive craniectomy with clot evacuation in large hemispheric hypertensive intracerebral hemorrhage. Neurocrit Care 2005;2:258-262.

104. Keller E, Pangalu A, Fandino J, et al: Decompressive craniectomy in severe cerebral venous and dural sinus thrombosis. Acta Neurochir 2005;94:177-183.

105. Albanese J, Leone M, Alliez J, et al: Decompressive craniectomy for severe traumatic brain injury: Evaluation of the effects at one year [see comment]. Crit Care Clin 2003;31:2535-2538.

106. Jaeger M, Soehle M, Meixensberger J: Effects of decompressive craniectomy on brain tissue oxygen in patients with intracranial hypertension. J Neurol Neurosurg Psychiatry 2003;74:513-515.

107. Levine S: Anoxic-ischemic encephalopathy in rats. Am J Pathol 1960;36:1.

108. Schroeder T: Cerebrovascular reactivity to acetazolamide in carotid artery disease: Enhancement of side-to-side cerebral blood flow asymmetry indicates critically reduced perfusion pressure. Neurol Res 1986;8:231.

109. Hojer-Pedersen E: Effect of acetazolamide on cerebral blood flow in subacute and chronic cerebrovascular disease. Stroke 1987;18: 887.

110. Nemoto E, Yonas H, Kuwabara H, et al: Identification of hemodynamic compromise by cerebrovascular reserve and oxygen extraction fraction in occlusive vascular disease. J Cereb Blood Flow Metab 2004;24:1081-1089.

111. Yonas H, Pindzola R: Clinical application of cerebrovascular reserve assessment as a strategy for stroke prevention. Keio J Med 2000;49: A4-10.

112. Yoo K, Lee J, Kim H, Im W: Hemodynamic and catecholamine responses to laryngoscopy and tracheal intubation in patients with complete spinal cord injuries. Anesthesiology 2001;95:647-651.

113. Moss E, Powell D, Gibson R, et al: Effects of tracheal intubation on intracranial pressure following induction of anaesthesia with thiopentone or althesin in patients undergoing neurosurgery. Br J Anaesth 1978;50:353-360.

114. Hamill J, Bedford R, Weaver D, et al: Lidocaine before endotracheal intubation: Intravenous or laryngotracheal? Anesthesiology 1981;55: 578-581.

115. Kofke W, Shaheen N, McWhorter J, et al: Transcranial Doppler ultrasonography with induction of anesthesia and neuromuscular blockade in surgical patients. J Clin Anesth 2001;13:335-338.

116. Lanier W, Milde J, Michenfelder J: Cerebral stimulation following succinylcholine in dogs. Anesthesiology 1986;64:551-559.

117. Greenawalt JW 3rd: Succinylcholine-induced hyperkalemia 8 weeks after a brief paraplegic episode. Anesth Analg 1992;75:294-295.

118. Hastings R, Wood P: Head extension and laryngeal view during laryngoscopy with cervical spine stabilization maneuvers. Anesthesiology 1994;80:825-831.

119. Lennarson P, Smith D, Sawin P, et al: Cervical spinal motion during intubation: Efficacy of stabilization maneuvers in the setting of complete segmental instability. J Neurosurg 2001;94(Suppl 2):265-270.

120. Turkstra T, Craen R, Pelz D, Gelb A: Cervical spine motion: A fluoroscopic comparison during intubation with lighted stylet, GlideScope, and Macintosh laryngoscope. Anesth Analg 2005;101:1011.

121. Rudolph C, Schneider J, Wallenborn J, Schaffranietz L: Movement of the upper cervical spine during laryngoscopy: A comparison of the Bonfils intubation fibrescope and the Macintosh laryngoscope. Anaesthesia 2005;60:668-672.

122. Hastings R, Vigil A, Hanna R, et al: Cervical spine movement during laryngoscopy with the Bullard, Macintosh, and Miller laryngoscopes. Anesthesiology 1995;82:859-869.

123. Waltl B, Melischek M, Schuschnig C, et al: Tracheal intubation and cervical spine excursion: Direct laryngoscopy vs. intubating laryngeal mask. Anaesthesia 2001;56:221-226.

124. Brimacombe J, Keller C, Kunzel K, et al: Cervical spine motion during airway management: A cinefluoroscopic study of the posteriorly destabilized third cervical vertebrae in human cadavers. Anesth Analg 2000;91:1274-1278.

125. Gerling M, Davis D, Hamilton R, et al: Effects of cervical spine immobilization technique and laryngoscope blade selection on an unstable cervical spine in a cadaver model of intubation. Ann Emerg Med 2000;36:293-300.

126. Brown M, Wade J, Marshall J: Fundamental importance of arterial oxygen content in the regulation of cerebral blood flow in man. Brain 1985;108(Pt 1):81-93.

127. Floyd T, Clark J, Gelfand R, et al: Independent cerebral vasoconstrictive effects of hyperoxia and accompanying arterial hypocapnia at 1 ATA. J Appl Physiol 2003;95:2453-2461.

128. Nakajima S, Meyer J, Amano T, et al: Cerebral vasomotor responsiveness during 100% oxygen inhalation in cerebral ischemia. Arch Neurol 1983;40:271-276.

129. Fiskum G, Rosenthal R, Vereczki V, et al: Protection against ischemic brain injury by inhibition of mitochondrial oxidative stress. J Bioenerg Biomembr 2004;36:347-352.

130. Halsey JH Jr, Conger K, Garcia J, Sarvary E: The contribution of reoxygenation to ischemic brain damage. J Cereb Blood Flow Metab 1991;11:994-1000.

131. Mickel H, Kempski O, Feuerstein G, et al: Prominent white matter lesions develop in Mongolian gerbils treated with 100% normobaric oxygen after global brain ischemia. Acta Neuropathol (Berl) 1990;79:465-472.

132. Marsala J, Marsala M, Vanicky I, Galik J, Orendacova J: Post cardiac arrest hyperoxic resuscitation enhances neuronal vulnerability of the respiratory rhythm generator and some brainstem and spinal cord neuronal pools in the dog. Neurosci Lett 1992;146:121-124.

133. Dings J, Meixensberger J, Jager A, Roosen K: Clinical experience with 118 brain tissue oxygen partial pressure catheter probes. Neurosurgery 1998;43:1982-1995.

134. van den Brink W, van Santbrink H, Steyerberg E, et al: Brain oxygen tension in severe head injury. Neurosurgery 2000;46:876-878.

135. Valadka A, Gopinath S, Contant C, et al: Relationship of brain tissue PO_2 to outcome after severe head injury. Crit Care Clin 1998;26:1576-1581.

136. van Santbrink H, vd Brink W, Steyerberg E, et al: Brain tissue oxygen response in severe traumatic brain injury. Acta Neurochir (Wien) 2003;145:429-438.

137. Stiefel M, Spiotta A, Gracias V, et al: Reduced mortality rate in patients with severe traumatic brain injury treated with brain tissue oxygen monitoring. J Neurosurg 2005;103:805-811.

138. Meixensberger J, Vath A, Jaeger M, et al: Monitoring of brain tissue oxygenation following severe subarachnoid hemorrhage. Neurol Res 2003;25:445-450.

139. Klein J: Normobaric pulmonary oxygen toxicity. Anesth Analg 1990;70:195-207.

140. Shapiro H, Marshall L: Intracranial pressure responses to PEEP in head-injured patients. J Trauma 1978;18:254-256.

141. Huseby J, Luce J, Cary J, et al: Effects of positive end-expiratory pressure on intracranial pressure in dogs with intracranial hypertension. J Neurosurg 1981;55:704-707.

142. Aidinis S, Lafferty J, Shapiro H: Intracranial responses to PEEP. Anesthesiology 1976;45:275-286.

143. Harken A, Brennan M, Smith B, et al: The hemodynamic response to positive end-expiratory ventilation in hypovolemic patients. Surgery 1974;76:786-793.

144. Luce J, Huseby J, Kirk W, Butler J: A Starling resistor regulates cerebral venous outflow in dogs. J App Physiol 1982;53:1496-1503.

145. West J: Respiratory Physiology: The Essentials. Baltimore, Williams and Wilkins, 1974.

146. Harper A, Glass H: Effect of alterations in the arterial carbon dioxide tension on the blood flow through the cerebral cortex at normal and low arterial blood pressures. J Neurol Neurosurg Psychiatry 1965;28:449-452.

147. Koehler R, Traystman R: Bicarbonate ion modulation of cerebral blood flow during hypoxia and hypercapnia. Am J Physiol 1982;243:H33-40.

148. Heffner J, Sahn S: Controlled hyperventilation in patients with intracranial hypertension: Application and management. Arch Intern Med 1983;143:765-769.

149. Coles J, Minhas P, Fryer T, et al: Effect of hyperventilation on cerebral blood flow in traumatic head injury: Clinical relevance and monitoring correlates. Crit Care Clin 2002;30:1950-1959.

150. Simon R, Niro M, Gwinn R: Brain acidosis induced by hypercarbic ventilation attenuates focal ischemic injury. J Pharmacol Exp Ther 1993;267:1428-1431.

151. Gopinath S, Valadka A, Uzura M, Robertson C: Comparison of jugular venous oxygen saturation and brain tissue Po_2 as monitors of cerebral ischemia after head injury. Crit Care Clin 1999;27:2337-2345.

152. Thompson H, Tkacs N, Saatman K, et al: Hyperthermia following traumatic brain injury: A critical evaluation. Neurobiol Dis 2003;12:163-173.

153. Suehiro E, Fujisawa H, Ito H, et al: Brain temperature modifies glutamate neurotoxicity in vivo. J Neurotrauma 1999;16:285-297.

154. Rosomoff H, Holaday D: Cerebral blood flow and cerebral oxygen consumption during hypothermia. Am J Physiol 1954;179:85-88.

155. Michenfelder J, Theye R: The effects of anesthesia and hypothermia on canine cerebral ATP and lactate during anoxia produced by decapitation. Anesthesiology 1970;33:430-439.

156. Nemoto E, Klementavicius R, Melick J, Yonas H: Suppression of cerebral metabolic rate for oxygen ($CMRO_2$) by mild hypothermia compared with thiopental. J Neurosurg Anesth 1996;8:52-59.

157. Busto R, Globus M, Dietrich W, et al: Effect of mild hypothermia on ischemia-induced release of neurotransmitters and free fatty acids in rat brain. Stroke 1989;20:904-910.

158. Wypij D, Newburger J, Rappaport L, et al: The effect of duration of deep hypothermic circulatory arrest in infant heart surgery on late neurodevelopment: The Boston Circulatory Arrest Trial. J Thorac Cardiovasc Surg 2003;126:1397-1403.

159. Haverich A, Hagl C: Organ protection during hypothermic circulatory arrest. J Thorac Cardiovasc Surg 2003;125:460-462.

160. Clifton G, Miller E, Choi S, et al: Lack of effect of induction of hypothermia after acute brain injury. N Engl J Med 2001;344:556-563.

161. Marion D: Moderate hypothermia in severe head injuries: The present and the future. Curr Opin Crit Care 2002;8:111-114.

162. Clifton G, Choi S, Miller E, et al: Intercenter variance in clinical trials of head trauma: Experience of the National Acute Brain Injury Study—Hypothermia. J Neurosurg 2001;95:751-755.

163. Hypothermia after Cardiac Arrest Study Group: Mild therapeutic hypothermia to improve the neurologic outcome after cardiac arrest. N Engl J Med 2002;346:549-556.

164. Bernard S, Gray T, Buist M, et al: Treatment of comatose survivors of out-of-hospital cardiac arrest with induced hypothermia. N Engl J Med 2002;346:557-563.

165. Minamisawa H, Nordstrom C, Smith M, Siesjo B: The influence of mild body and brain hypothermia on ischemic brain damage. J Cereb Blood Flow Metab 1990;10:365-374.

166. Dietrich W, Busto R, Valdes I, Loor Y: Effects of normothermic versus mild hyperthermic forebrain ischemia in rats. Stroke 1990;21:1318-1325.

167. Minamisawa H, Smith M, Siesjo B: The effect of mild hyperthermia and hypothermia on brain damage following 5, 10, and 15 minutes of forebrain ischemia. Ann Neurol 1990;28:26-33.

168. Todd M, Hindman B, Clarke W, Torner J: Intraoperative Hypothermia for Aneurysm Surgery Trial (IHAST) Investigators. Mild intraoperative hypothermia during surgery for intracranial aneurysm. N Engl J Med 2005;352:135-145.

169. Marion D, Penrod L, Kelsey S, et al: Treatment of traumatic brain injury with moderate hypothermia. N Engl J Med 1997;336:540-546.

170. Rossitch EJ, Bullard D: The autonomic dysfunction syndrome: Aetiology and treatment. Br J Neurosurg 1988;2:471-478.

171. Commichau C, Scarmeas N, Mayer S: Risk factors for fever in the neurologic intensive care unit. Neurology 2003;60:837-841.

172. Castillo J, Davalos A, Noya M: Timing for fever-related brain damage in acute ischemic stroke. Stroke 1998;29:2455-2460.

173. Azzimondi G, Bassein L, Nonino F, et al: Fever in acute stroke worsens prognosis: A prospective study. Stroke 1995;26:2043-2050.

174. Reith J, Jorgensen H, Pedersen P, et al: Body temperature in acute stroke: relation to stroke severity, infarct size, mortality, and outcome. Lancet 1996;347:422-425.

175. Ginsberg M, Busto R: Combating hypothermia in acute stroke: A significant clinical concern. Stroke 1998;29:529-534.

176. Schwarz S, Häfner K, Aschoff A, Schwab S: Incidence and prognostic significance of fever following intracerebral hemorrhage. Neurology 2000;54:354-361.

177. Oliveira-Filho J, Ezzeddine MA, Segal AZ, et al: Fever in subarachnoid hemorrhage: Relationship to vasospasm and outcome. Neurology 2001;56:1299-1304.

178. Bachert C, Chuchalin A, Eisebitt R, et al: Aspirin compared with acetaminophen in the treatment of fever and other symptoms of upper respiratory tract infection in adults: A multicenter, randomized, double-blind, double-dummy, placebo-controlled, parallel-group, single-dose, 6-hour dose-ranging study. Clin Ther 2005;27:993-1003.

179. Grebe W, Ionescu E, Gold M, et al: A multicenter, randomized, double-blind, double-dummy, placebo- and active-controlled, parallel-group comparison of diclofenac-K and ibuprofen for the treatment of adults with influenza-like symptoms. Clin Ther 2003;25:444-458.

180. Dippel D, van Breda E, van der Worp H, et al, PISA Investigators: Effect of paracetamol (acetaminophen) and ibuprofen on body temperature in acute ischemic stroke: PISA, a phase II double-blind, randomized, placebo-controlled trial [ISRCTN98608690]. BMC Cardiovasc Disord 2003;3:2.

181. Johnston S, Pelletier L: Enhanced hepatotoxicity of acetaminophen in the alcoholic patient: Two case reports and a review of the literature. Medicine 1997;75:185-191.

182. Lewis S, Langman M, Laporte J, et al: Dose-response relationships between individual nonaspirin nonsteroidal anti-inflammatory drugs (NANSAIDs) and serious upper gastrointestinal bleeding a meta-analysis based on individual patient data. Br J Clin Pharmacol 2002;54:320-326.

183. Diringer M, Neurocritical Care Fever Reduction Trial Group: Treatment of fever in the neurologic intensive care unit with a catheter-based heat exchange system. Crit Care Clin 2004:559-564.

184. Pulsinelli W, Levy D, Sigsbee B, et al: Increased damage after ischemic stroke in patients with hyperglycemia with or without established diabetes mellitus. Am J Med 1983;74:540.

185. Siemkowicz E: Hyperglycemia in the reperfusion period hampers recovery from cerebral ischemia. Acta Neurolog Scand 1981;64:207.

186. Rehncrona S, Rosen I, Siesjo B: Brain lactic acidosis and ischemic cell damage: 1. Biochemistry and neurophysiology. J Cereb Blood Flow Metab 1981;1:297-311.

187. De Salles A, Muizelaar J, Young H: Hyperglycemia, cerebrospinal fluid lactic acidosis, and cerebral blood flow in severely head-injured patients. Neurosurgery 1987;21:45.

188. Li P, Shamloo M, Smith M, et al: The influence of plasma glucose concentrations on ischemic brain damage is a threshold function. Neurosci Lett 1994;177:63.

189. Warner D, Gionet T, Todd M, McAllister A: Insulin-induced normoglycemia improves ischemic outcome in hyperglycemic rats. Stroke 1992;23:1775.

190. Siemkowicz E, Gjedde A: Post-ischemic coma in rat: Effect of different pre-ischemic blood glucose levels on cerebral metabolic recovery after ischemia. Acta Physiol Scand 1980;110:225.

191. Lanier W, Stangland K, Scheithauer B, et al: The effects of dextrose infusion and head position on neurologic outcome after complete cerebral ischemia in primates: Examination of a model. Anesthesiology 1987;66:39.

192. Van den Berghe G, Wouters P, Weekers F, et al: Intensive insulin therapy in critically ill patients. N Engl J Med 2001;345:1359-1367.

193. Van den Berghe G, Wouters P, Bouillon R, et al: Outcome benefit of intensive insulin therapy in the critically ill: Insulin dose versus glycemic control. Crit Care Clin 2003;31:359-366.

194. Bhatia A, Cadman B, Mackenzie I: Hypoglycemia and cardiac arrest in a critically ill patient on strict glycemic control. Anesth Analg 2006;102:549-551.

195. Broderick J, Hagen T, Brott T, Tomsick T: Hyperglycemia and hemorrhagic transformation of cerebral infarcts. Stroke 1995;26:484.

196. Murros K, Fogelholm R, Kettunen S, Vuorela A: Serum cortisol and outcome of ischemic brain infarction. J Neurol Sci 1993;116:12-17.

197. Murros K, Fogelholm R, Kettunen S, et al: Blood glucose, glycosylated haemoglobin, and outcome of ischemic brain infarction. J Neurol Sci 1992;111:59-64.

198. Matchar D, Divine G, Heyman A, Feussner J: The influence of hyperglycemia on outcome of cerebral infarction. Ann Intern Med 1992;117:449.

199. de Courten-Myers G, Kleinholz M, Holm P, et al: Hemorrhagic infarct conversion in experimental stroke. Ann Emerg Med 1992;21:120.

200. Sieber F, Traystman R: Special issues: Glucose and the brain. Crit Care Med 1992;20:104.

201. Yip P, He Y, Hsu C, et al: Effect of plasma glucose on infarct size in focal cerebral ischemia-reperfusion. Neurology 1991;41:899.

202. Vazquez-Cruz J, Marti-Vilalta J, Ferrer I, et al: Progressing cerebral infarction in relation to plasma glucose in gerbils. Stroke 1990;21:1621-1624.

203. Kushner M, Nencini P, Reivich M, et al: Relation of hyperglycemia early in ischemic brain infarction to cerebral anatomy, metabolism, and clinical outcome. Ann Neurol 1990;28:129.

204. Kraft S, Larson CJ, Shuer L, et al: Effect of hyperglycemia on neuronal changes in a rabbit model of focal cerebral ischemia. Stroke 1990;21:447.

205. Zasslow M, Pearl R, Shuer L, et al: Hyperglycemia decreases acute neuronal ischemic changes after middle cerebral artery occlusion in cats. Stroke 1989;20:519.

206. de Courten-Myers G, Myers R, Schoolfield L: Hyperglycemia enlarges infarct size in cerebrovascular occlusion in cats. Stroke 1988;19:623.

207. Duverger D, MacKenzie E: The quantification of cerebral infarction following focal ischemia in the rat: Influence of strain, arterial pressure, blood glucose concentration, and age. J Cereb Blood Flow Metab 1988;8:449.

208. Nedergaard M: Mechanisms of brain damage in focal cerebral ischemia. Acta Neurol Scand 1988;77:81.

209. Prado R, Ginsberg M, Dietrich W, et al: Hyperglycemia increases infarct size in collaterally perfused but not end-arterial vascular territories. J Cereb Blood Flow Metab 1988;8:186.

210. Ginsberg M, Prado R, Dietrich W, et al: Hyperglycemia reduces the extent of cerebral infarction in rats. Stroke 1987;18:570.

211. Nedergaard M: Transient focal ischemia in hyperglycemic rats is associated with increased cerebral infarction. Brain Res 1987;408:79.

212. Nedergaard M, Astrup J: Infarct rim: Effect of hyperglycemia on direct current potential and [14C]2-deoxyglucose phosphorylation. J Cereb Blood Flow Metab 1986;6:607-615.

213. Kofke W, Ahdab-Barmada M, Rose M, et al: Substantia nigra damage after flurothyl-induced seizures in rats worsens after post seizure recovery: No exacerbation with hyperglycemia. Neurol Res 1993;15:333.

214. Swan J, Meldrum B, Simon R: Hyperglycemia does not augment neuronal damage in experimental status epilepticus. Neurology 1986;36:1351.

215. Ingvar M, Folbegrova J, Siesjo B: Metabolic alterations underlying the development of hypermetabolic necrosis in the substantia nigra in status epilepticus. J Cereb Blood Flow Metab 1987;7:103.

216. Lundberg N: Continuous recording and control of ventricular fluid pressure in neurosurgical practice. Acta Psychiatr Neurol Scand 1960;36(Suppl 149):1.

217. Rosner M, Becker D: The etiology of plateau waves: A theoretical model and experimental observations. In Ishii S, Nagai H, Brock M (eds): Intracranial Pressure. New York, Springer-Verlag, 1983, pp 301-306.

218. Matakas F, Von Waechter R, Knupling R, Potolicchio SJ: Increase in cerebral perfusion pressure by arterial hypertension in brain swelling: A mathematical model of the volume-pressure relationship. J Neurosurg 1975;42:282.

219. Grande P, Asgeirsson B, Nordstrom C: Volume-targeted therapy of increased intracranial pressure: The Lund concept unifies surgical and non-surgical treatments. Acta Anaesth Scand 2002;46:929-941.

220. Werner C, Hoffman W, Thomas C, et al: Ganglionic blockade improves neurologic outcome from incomplete ischemia in rats: Partial reversal by exogenous catecholamines. Anesthesiology 1990; 73:923-929.

221. Hoffman W, Kochs E, Werner C, et al: Dexmedetomidine improves neurologic outcome from incomplete ischemia in the rat: Reversal by the alpha 2-adrenergic antagonist atipamezole. Anesthesiology 1991; 75:328.

222. Werner C, Hoffman W, Kochs E, et al: Captopril improves neurologic outcome from incomplete cerebral ischemia in rats. Stroke 1991; 22:910.

223. Busto R, Harik S, Yoshida S, et al: Cerebral norepinephrine depletion enhances recovery after brain ischemia. Ann Neurol 1985; 18:329.

224. Kofke W, Garman R, Garman RH, Rose M: Opioid neurotoxicity: Role of neurotransmitter systems. Neurol Res 2000;22:733-737.

225. Neil-Dwyer G, Walter P, Cruickshank J: Beta-blockade benefits patients following a subarachnoid hemorrhage. Eur J Clin Pharmacol 1985;28:25.

226. Schroeder T, Schierbeck J, Howardy P, et al: Effect of labetalol on cerebral blood flow and middle cerebral arterial flow velocity in healthy volunteers. Neurol Res 1991;13:10.

227. Orlowski J, Shiesley D, Vidt D, et al: Labetalol to control blood pressure after cerebrovascular surgery. Crit Care Med 1988;16:765.

228. Van Aken H, Puchstein C, Schweppe M-L, et al: Effect of labetalol on intracranial pressure in dogs with and without intracranial hypertension. Acta Anaesth Scand 1982;26:615.

229. Kakarieka A, Schakel E, Fritze J: Clinical experiences with nimodipine in cerebral ischemia. J Neural Transm Suppl 1994;43:13-21.

230. Rosenbaum D, Zabramski J, Frey J, et al: Early treatment of ischemic stroke with a calcium antagonist. Stroke 1991;22:437-441.

231. A multicenter trial of the efficacy of nimodipine on outcome after severe head injury. The European Study Group on Nimodipine in Severe Head Injury. J Neurosurg 1994;80:797.

232. Pickard J, Murray G, Illingworth R, et al: Effect of oral nimodipine on cerebral infarction and outcome after subarachnoid haemorrhage: British aneurysm nimodipine trial. BMJ 1989;298:636.

233. Kucharczyk J, Chew W, Derugin N, et al: Nicardipine reduces ischemic brain injury: Magnetic resonance imaging/spectroscopy study in cats. Stroke 1989;20:268.

234. Alps B, Calder C, Hass W, Wilson A: Comparative protective effects of nicardipine, flunarizine, lidoflazine and nimodipine against ischaemic injury in the hippocampus of the Mongolian gerbil. Br J Pharmacol 1988;93:877.

235. Grotta J, Spydell J, Pettigrew C, et al: The effect of nicardipine on neuronal function following ischemia. Stroke 1986;17:213.

236. Bedford R, Dacey R, Winn H, Lynch CD: Adverse impact of a calcium entry-blocker (verapamil) on intracranial pressure in patients with brain tumors. J Neurosurg 1983;59:800.

237. Hayashi M, Kobayashi H, Kawano H, et al: Treatment of systemic hypertension and intracranial hypertension in cases of brain hemorrhage. Stroke 1988;19:314-321.

238. Stanek B, Zimpfer M, Fitzal S, Raberger G: Plasma catecholamines, plasma renin activity and haemodynamics during sodium nitroprusside-induced hypotension and additional beta-blockade with bunitrolol. Eur J Clin Pharmacol 1981;19:317-322.

239. Stiefel M, Heuer G, Abrahams J, et al: The effect of nimodipine on cerebral oxygenation in patients with poor-grade subarachnoid hemorrhage. J Neurosurg 2004;101:594-599.

240. Overgaard J, Skinhoj E: A paradoxical cerebral hemodynamic effect of hydralazine. Stroke 1975;6:402.

241. Griswold W, Roznik V, Mendoza S: Nitroprusside induced intracranial hypertension. JAMA 1981;246:2679.

242. Marsh M, Shapiro H, Smith R, et al: Changes in neurologic status and intracranial pressure associated with sodium nitroprusside administration. Anesthesiology 1979;51:336.

243. Dohi S, Matsumoto M, Takahashi K: The effects of nitroglycerin on cerebrospinal fluid pressure in awake and anesthetized humans. Anesthesiology 1981;54:511.

244. Meinig G, Reulen H, Hadjidimos A, et al: Induction of filtration edema by extreme reduction of cerebrovascular resistance associated with hypertension. Eur Neurol 1972;8:97-103.

245. Langfitt T, Marshall W, Kassell N, Schutta H: The pathophysiology of brain swelling produced by mechanical trauma and hypertension. Scand J Clin Lab Invest Suppl 1968;102:XIV:B.

246. Marshall W, Jackson J, Langfitt T: Brain swelling caused by trauma and arterial hypertension: Hemodynamic aspects. Arch Neurol 1969;21:545-553.

247. Schutta H, Kassell N, Langfitt T: Brain swelling produced by injury and aggravated by arterial hypertension: A light and electron microscopic study. Brain 1968;91:281.

248. Marshall W, Weinstein J, Langfitt T: The pathophysiology of brain swelling produced by mechanical trauma and hypertension. Surg Forum 1968;19:431.

249. Olesen J: The effect of intracarotid epinephrine, norepinephrine, and angiotensin on the regional cerebral blood flow in man. Neurology 1972;22:978-987.

250. MacKenzie E, McCulloch J, Harper A: Influence of endogenous norepinephrine on cerebral blood flow and metabolism. Am J Physiol 1976;231:489.

251. Darby J, Yonas H, Marks E, et al: Acute cerebral blood flow response to dopamine-induced hypertension after subarachnoid hemorrhage. J Neurosurg 1994;80:857.

252. Stein S, Cracco R: Cortical injury without ischemia produced by topical monoamines. Stroke 1982;13:74.

253. Hindman B, Funatsu N, Cheng D, et al: Differential effect of oncotic pressure on cerebral and extracerebral water content during cardiopulmonary bypass in rabbits. Anesthesiology 1990;73: 951.

254. Kaieda R, Todd M, Warner D: Prolonged reduction in colloid oncotic pressure does not increase brain edema following cryogenic injury in rabbits. Anesthesiology 1989;71:554.

255. Kaieda R, Todd M, Cook L, Warner D: Acute effects of changing plasma osmolality and colloid oncotic pressure on the formation of brain edema after cryogenic injury. Neurosurgery 1989; 24:671.

256. Zornow M, Scheller M, Todd M, Moore S: Acute cerebral effects of isotonic crystalloid and colloid solutions following cryogenic brain injury in the rabbit. Anesthesiology 1988;69:180.

257. Tommasino C, Moore S, Todd M: Cerebral effects of isovolemic hemodilution with crystalloid or colloid solutions. Crit Care Med 1988;16:862.

258. Zornow M, Todd M, Moore S: The acute cerebral effects of changes in plasma osmolality and oncotic pressure. Anesthesiology 1987;67: 936.

259. Cruickshank J, Neil-Dwyer G, Lane J: The effect of oral propranolol upon the ECG changes occurring in subarachnoid hemorrhage. Cardiovasc Res 1975;9:236.

260. Kono T, Morita H, Kuroiwa T, et al: Left ventricular wall motion abnormalities in patients with subarachnoid hemorrhage: Neurogenic stunned myocardium. J Am Coll Cardiol 1994;24:636.

261. Kolin A, Norris J: Myocardial damage from acute cerebral lesions. Stroke 1984;15:990.

262. Svengaard N, Brismar J, Delgado T, Rosengren E: Subarachnoid haemorrhage in the rat: Effect on the development of vasospasm of selective lesions of the catecholamine systems in the lower brain stem. Stroke 1985;16:602.

263. Svendgaard NA, Delgado TJ, Arbab MA: Catecholaminergic and peptidergic systems underlying cerebral vasospasm: CBF and CMRgl changes following an experimental subarachnoid hemorrhage in the rat. Proceedings of the Charlottesville Conference, April 29-May 1, 1987. In Wilkins RH (ed): Cerebral Vasospasm. New York, Raven Press, 1988, pp 175-186.

264. Oldendorf W, Kitano M: Radioisotope measurement of brain blood turnover time as a clinical index of brain circulation. J Nucl Med 1967;8:570.

265. Karpman H, Sheppard J: Effect of papaverine hydrochloride on cerebral blood flow as measured by forehead thermograms. Angiology 1975;26:592.

266. Griffith D, James I, Newbury P, Woollard M: The effect of beta-adrenergic receptor blocking drugs on cerebral blood flow. Br J Clin Pharmacol 1979;7:491.

267. Schmidt J: Changes in human cerebral blood flow estimated by the (A-V) O_2 difference method. Dan Med Bull 1992;39:335-342.

268. Dickman C, Carter LP, Baldwin H, et al: Continuous regional cerebral blood low monitoring in acute craniocerebral trauma. Neurosurgery 1991;28:467-472.

269. Pearson R, Griffity D, Woollard M, et al: Comparisons of effects on cerebral blood flow of rapid reduction in systemic arterial pressure by diazoxide and labetalol in hypertensive patients: Preliminary findings. Br J Clin Pharmacol 1979;8(Suppl 2):195S.

270. Olesen J, Hougard K, Hertz M: Isoproterenol and propranolol: Ability to cross the blood-brain barrier and effects on cerebral circulation in man. Stroke 1978;9:344.

271. Merrick M, Ferrington C, Cowen S: Parametric imaging of cerebral vascular reserves: 1. Theory, validation and normal values. Eur J Nucl Med 1991;18:171.

272. Gould R: Perfusion quantitation by ultrafast computed tomography. Invest Radiol 1992;27(Suppl 2):S18.

273. Hartmann A, Dettmers C, Schuler F, et al: Effect of stable xenon on regional cerebral blood flow and the electroencephalogram in normal volunteers. Stroke 1991;22:181.

274. Burcar P, Norenberg M, Yarnell P: Hyponatremia and central pontine myelinolysis. Neurology 1977;27:223.

275. Borgstrom L, Johannsson H, Siesjo B: The influence of acute normovolemic anemia on cerebral blood flow and oxygen consumption of anesthetized rats. Acta Physiol Scand 1975;93:505-514.

276. Floyd T, McGarvey M, Ochroch E, et al: Perioperative changes in cerebral blood flow after cardiac surgery: Influence of anemia and aging. Ann Thoracic Surg 2003;76:2037-2042.

277. Dexter F, Hindman BJ: Effect of haemoglobin concentration on brain oxygenation in focal stroke: A mathematical modelling study. Br J Anaesth 1997;79:346-351.

278. Kim J, Kang S: Bleeding and subsequent anemia: A precipitant for cerebral infarction. Eur Neurol 2000;43:201-208.

279. Smith M, Stiefel MF, Magge S, et al: Packed red blood cell transfusion increases local cerebral oxygenation. Crit Care Clin 2005;33:1104-1108.

280. McIntyre L, Hebert P, Wells G, et al, Canadian Critical Care Trials Group: Is a restrictive transfusion strategy safe for resuscitated and critically ill trauma patients? J Trauma 2004;57:563-568.

281. Shiozaki T, Sugimoto H, Taneda M, et al: Effect of mild hypothermia on uncontrollable intracranial hypertension after severe head injury. J Neurosurg 1993;79:363-368.

282. Clifton G, Allen S, Barrodale P, et al: A phase II study of moderate hypothermia in severe brain injury. J Neurotrauma 1993;10:263-271.

283. Jiang J, Yu M, Zhu C: Effect of long-term mild hypothermia therapy in patients with severe traumatic brain injury. J Neurosurg 2000;93:546-549.

284. Shiozaki T, Hayakata T, Taneda M, et al: A multicenter prospective randomized controlled trial of the efficacy of mild hypothermia for severely head injured patients with low intracranial pressure. Mild Hypothermia Study Group in Japan. J Neurosurg 2001;94:50-54.

285. Gal R, Cundrle I, Zimova I, Smrcka M: Mild hypothermia therapy for patients with severe brain injury. Clin Neurol Neurosurg 2002;104:318-321.

286. Zhi D, Zhang S, Lin X: Study on therapeutic mechanism and clinical effect of mild hypothermia in patients with severe head injury. Surg Neurol 2003;59:381-385.

287. Qiu W, Liu W, Shen H, et al: Therapeutic effect of mild hypothermia on severe traumatic head injury. Chin J Traumatol 2005;8:27-32.

288. Ropper A, Kennedy S: Postoperative neurosurgical care. In Ropper A (ed): Neurological and Neurosurgical Intensive Care, ed 3. New York, Raven Press, 1993, pp 185-191.

289. Suarez JI, Qureshi AI, Bhardwaj A, et al: Treatment of refractory intracranial hypertension with 23.4% saline. Crit Care Med 1998;26:1118-1122.

290. Kofke WA, Yanes H, Wechsler L, et al: Neurologic intensive care. In Albin MS (ed): Textbook of Neuroanesthesia with Neurosurgical and Neuroscience Perspectives. New York, McGraw-Hill, 1997, pp 1247-1347.

Gastrointestinal System

Chapter

25 Prevention and Treatment of Gastrointestinal Morbidity

Duane Funk and Tong J. Gan

Undergoing general anesthesia for an elective operation has become exceedingly safe and is now rarely associated with mortality. With the improvements in perioperative screening, risk reduction, and intraoperative management, we can now focus on and improve the quality of postoperative recovery. For example, gastrointestinal morbidity is frequent after elective surgery. In the past decade, there has been a vast increase in the understanding of the risk factors and therapeutic modalities associated with postoperative nausea and vomiting and with postoperative ileus. Further study has targeted interventions to specific patient populations to reduce the risk for these complications. This chapter will highlight several common causes of gastrointestinal morbidity and provide strategies to reduce the risk for adverse gastrointestinal outcomes. Using this information will allow the clinician to improve the quality of postoperative recovery, increase patient satisfaction, and decrease the length of hospital stay.

■ ASPIRATION OF GASTRIC CONTENTS

Incidence, Etiology, and Pathogenesis

The aspiration of gastric contents under anesthesia is fortunately a rare event but one that can be associated with serious morbidity and even mortality. Despite a greater understanding of the risk factors, prevention, and management, there has been no appreciable decrease in its incidence or associated mortality over the past several decades. The consequences of aspiration include bronchospasm, laryngospasm, aspiration pneumonitis, aspiration pneumonia, and the acute respiratory distress syndrome.

Historically, the syndrome of aspiration pneumonitis was first described by Mendelson in 1946 in a group of obstetric patients undergoing general anesthesia.[1] He was also the first to describe the role of the acidity of gastric contents in the pathogenesis of this syndrome. Installation of gastric contents into the lung was indistinguishable pathologically from the effect of the introduction of 0.1N hydrochloric acid.[1] Later, it was shown that neutralization of gastric acid prior to aspiration reduced the damage to the lungs.[2] In experimental studies, the degree of pulmonary injury increased significantly with a decrease in pH and an increase in volume.

The commonly cited values of a gastric volume of 0.3 to 0.4 mL/kg and a gastric pH of lower than 2.5 for the development of aspiration pneumonitis come from animal studies that involved the direct installation of acid into the lungs of Rhesus monkeys.[3,4] However, gastric contents are not purely liquid, and the presence of particulate matter can cause inflammation and lung injury, even with a pH higher than 2.5.[5,6] Also, the volume of gastric fluid present does not seem to correlate to the risk for aspiration or the amount aspirated, Many appropriately fasted patients have gastric volumes that exceed 0.4 mL/kg and demonstrate no evidence of aspiration.[7,8] Extrapolating gastric volume to the potential aspirated volume is therefore speculative at best, and it is further complicated by the difficulty of accurately measuring gastric volumes. The current fasting recommendation of most hospitals is nil per os (NPO) for at least 8 hours preoperatively for adults to reduce gastric volumes. The Cochrane Database review on perioperative fasting found some studies that show an increase in gastric emptying with the ingestion of clear fluids.[9]

The anatomic and physiologic mechanisms that prevent reflux include the upper esophageal sphincter (UES), the lower esophageal sphincter (LES), and the laryngeal reflexes. Alteration of any of these can increase the risk for aspiration. The LES forms a barrier between the stomach and the esophagus that prevents aspiration. When gastric pressure exceeds the LES barrier pressure, aspiration is possible.[10] A decrease in the LES pressure is the most significant physiologic derangement in patients who aspirate during anesthesia and in those who suffer from gastroesophageal reflux disease (GERD). Many of the drugs used in anesthesia can alter the LES pressure, thus affecting the risk for aspiration. In general, opiates, anesthetic induction agents, volatile anesthetics, and anticholinergics all cause a decrease in LES pressure, whereas cholinergics, prokinetics, and alpha agonists all increase LES pressure (Table 25-1).[10]

The UES is composed of the cricopharyngeal muscle. It extends around the pharynx, and in healthy conscious adults it prevents the entrance of gastric contents from the esophagus into the hypopharynx. The tone of the UES, like that of the LES, is altered by many of the anesthetic induction agents as well as by neuromuscular blockers and sleep. These factors may combine and further increase the risk for aspiration.[11] Of particular importance is the effect of residual neuromuscular blockade on the UES. In a study using fluoroscopy and manometry, it was shown that at a train-of-four (TOF) ratio of 0.8, resting UES and pharyngeal muscle tone was decreased significantly.[12] These investigators were also able to demonstrate alterations in swallowing and found discordant activity of the pharyngeal muscles and the UES. These alterations in UES and pharyngeal tone could be clinically significant and could lead to an increased risk for aspiration in the postoperative period.

Risk Factors

The best defined risk factor for aspiration is an emergent operation. There are several theories as to why this should be the case. First, patients scheduled for emergent surgeries are not appropriately fasted and thus have increased gastric volumes. The sympathetic response to pain also decreases gastric motility.[13] Second, any opiate administered to such patients in the preoperative period will slow gastric emptying.[14] Finally, traumatic brain or spinal cord injuries have been shown to cause gastroparesis.

Late-term pregnancy, with its alterations in gastric morphology, increases in intra-abdominal pressure, and increases in progesterone levels, predisposes patients to passive regurgitation. There is controversy, however, over whether there is a delay in gastric emptying in parturient women.[15] Obstetric labor is also known to delay gastric emptying. This most likely results from the effect of pain and the administration of central neuraxial opiates, both of which are known to slow gastric transit time.[16] In addition to having these physiologic and anatomic factors, parturient women may also have increased upper airway edema and tissue mass, which may necessitate multiple attempts to perform a laryngoscopy and a longer duration of that procedure, leaving the pregnant patient with an unprotected airway for a longer time than a nonpregnant patient.

Obese patients are also thought to be at higher risk for aspiration. Although no decrease in the rate of gastric emptying has been demonstrated, the airway difficulties of obese patients could place them at increased risk for aspiration for the same reasons as pregnant patients.[17]

Other systemic diseases such as scleroderma, diabetes mellitus type I, and Parkinson's disease are all known to cause either delays in gastric emptying or alterations in the LES, leading to an increased risk for aspiration (Box 25-1).

Risk Reduction

Knowledge of the risk factors for aspiration allows the clinician to alter the anesthetic plan to reduce the perioperative risk for this condition. The clinician can employ four broad strategies to facilitate this. First, decrease the chance of gastric contents entering the hypopharynx. Second, inhibit the passage of the contents from the pharynx and esophagus into the trachea and lungs. Third, alter the pH of the gastric fluid (by the use of histamine-2 [H_2] blockers, proton pump inhibitors, and particulate antacids). And finally, decrease the volume of gastric fluid.

The most common way to prevent the gastric contents from entering the hypopharynx, trachea, and lungs is by using cricoid pressure, first described by Sellick in 1961. The anatomic theory behind this maneuver is that pressure on the circular cricoid ring will occlude the esophagus against the fifth cervical vertebrae, thus inhibiting gastric contents from entering the tracheobronchial tree.[18] Although this technique is attractive in theory, its application has many pitfalls. There is evidence that the application of cricoid pressure can cause a decrease in LES tone, perhaps through a mechanoreceptor-mediated reflex mechanism.[19] The suggested force of 44 newtons (N) of pressure has been shown in endoscopic studies to cause cricoid deformation, airway closure, and

25-1	Perioperative Dugs That Lower the Tone of the Lower Esophageal Sphincter
Drug Class	**Example**
Anticholinergics	Glycopyrrolate, atropine
Catecholamines	Dopamine
Volatile anesthetics	Isoflurane, desflurane, sevoflurane
Opioids	Morphine, fentanyl, sufentanil
Induction agents	Propofol, thiopental

25-1	Diseases and Conditions Known to Increase the Risk of Aspiration

- Pain
- Pregnancy
- Trauma
- Diabetes
- Head injury or altered level of consciousness
- Spinal cord injury
- Scleroderma (or CREST syndrome [acronym for calcinosis, Raynaud's phenomenon, esophageal dysmotility, sclerodactyly, and telangiectasia])
- Parkinson's disease
- Obesity
- Amyotrophic lateral sclerosis
- Zenker's diverticulum
- Pyloric stenosis

increased difficulty in ventilation.[20] Further, most anesthesia assistants misapply the cricoid pressure (with variations in force between 10 and 90 N), and this can lead to difficulties in visualizing the glottic opening.[21] The maneuver itself is not without risk, and there have been reports of esophageal rupture when cricoid pressure has been applied to a patient who is vomiting.[22]

Alteration of the pH of gastric fluid is the most common pharmacologic method to reduce morbidity should aspiration occur. The three classes of drugs used to accomplish this goal are H_2-receptor blockers, proton pump inhibitors (PPIs), and nonparticulate antacids. None of these has been subjected to a rigorous clinical trial. With the actual event rate of aspiration being so small, surrogate measures such as gastric fluid volume have been used instead, but some question the use of gastric fluid volume as a clinically significant endpoint.

H_2-receptor antagonists are the most commonly used agents to increase gastric pH. They bind the histamine type 2 receptor on gastric parietal cells and inhibit gastric acid secretion. Pharmacologic features of these drugs that should be recognized, however, include the lack of correlation between acid suppression and peak plasma concentration, significant interindividual variation in the degree of acid suppression, and the development of tolerance.

PPIs are a newer class of medications that form a covalent bond with the H^+,K^+-ATPase of the parietal cell. To be effective in increasing gastric pH in the preoperative period, these medications must be given the night before and the morning of surgery.[23]

Many head-to-head studies of the H_2-receptor antagonists and PPIs have shown an increase in gastric pH and a decrease in gastric volume.[24] Whether these surrogate endpoints are clinically relevant has engendered much debate. Even if a reduction in morbidity or mortality could be demonstrated, the number needed to treat (see later) would be too large to recommend wide-scale adoption of this practice for all patients. In fact, the American Society of Anesthesiologists (ASA) task force has not endorsed the use of H_2 antagonists for patients who are not at risk for aspiration.[25]

Nonparticulate antacids (e.g., sodium citrate, sodium bicarbonate) have been shown to increase the pH of gastric fluid but to have no effect on gastric volume. These agents are attractive because they increase gastric pH rapidly, making their use with the emergency surgical patient more feasible than that of the PPIs or H_2 blockers.

Decreasing the volume of gastric fluid can be accomplished by either pharmacologic means or by the use of preoperative fasting. Pharmacologically, the prokinetic metoclopramide is the most common drug used, but the lack of published data relating the risk for pulmonary aspiration with the use of this drug led the ASA task force not to recommend it for those not at risk for aspiration.[25]

The theory behind fasting is that, should aspiration occur on induction of anesthesia, the volume would be minimal and there would be no particulate matter. The traditional guideline for NPO after midnight has been challenged recently on the basis of inconsistent efficacy and patient discomfort (including dehydration and hypoglycemia). The guideline has been liberalized to allow the intake of clear liquids for up to 2 hours before entering the operating room. This is based on evidence that patients who were allowed clear fluids up to 2 hours prior to their surgery had similar gastric fluid volumes and pH when compared with those who fasted longer.[26]

The ingestion of a light meal (such as toast with a clear liquid) on the morning of surgery and its relation to gastric volume and emptying has been investigated. Although gastric volume was not increased, particulate matter was still present in the stomach up to 4 hours after ingestion,[27] which is particularly worrisome because particulate material in the lung elicits a profound inflammatory response. Heavy meals (such as those containing fried foods) took up to 9 hours to exit the stomach.[28] The ASA taskforce on perioperative fasting has therefore recommended that a period of 6 hours elapse before the conduct of general anesthesia in patients who have had a light meal, and up to 8 hours for those who have consumed a meal that contains fatty foods.[28]

These guidelines, however, apply only to patients without gastrointestinal (GI) pathology. Patients with type I diabetes, with small bowel obstruction or ileus, or receiving tube feeds, or those in whom airway management might be difficult, warrant special consideration, and the ASA guidelines do not have any clear recommendations for this subset of individuals.

As mentioned previously, pregnant patients are another group for whom preoperative fasting has been extensively investigated. Parturients are a unique subset of patients, as they might need an operative intervention at some time during the course of their labor, but keeping them NPO for a procedure that might not occur is not practical. Most obstetric units allow patients clear fluids (including gelatin) while in labor, recognizing that this may place them at increased risk for aspiration should they require a regional or general anesthetic.

Management Strategy

The spectrum of clinical problems encountered when a patient aspirates ranges from asymptomatic aspiration, bronchospasm, laryngospasm, aspiration pneumonitis, aspiration pneumonia, and acute respiratory distress syndrome.

The initial management of the patient who has aspirated focuses on suctioning the oropharynx of any aspirated material and on urgent airway control (Fig. 25-1). Once the airway has been secured, a tracheal suction catheter should be passed down the endotracheal tube to try to remove any particulate matter from the lungs. At this point, a decision must be made as to whether surgery should proceed. Several factors influence this decision, such as the duration of the case, the emergent nature of the procedure, and the patient's respiratory stability. Early hypoxemia, bronchospasm, or high peak airway pressures are all signs that portend an aspiration event, and they are likely to worsen over the ensuing several hours. Clinicians should have a low threshold for canceling elective cases in this scenario. Emergent cases (when most aspiration events occur) pose more of a problem, and many times the anesthesiologist is left little choice but to proceed with the case, knowing the potential for a worsening pulmonary status.

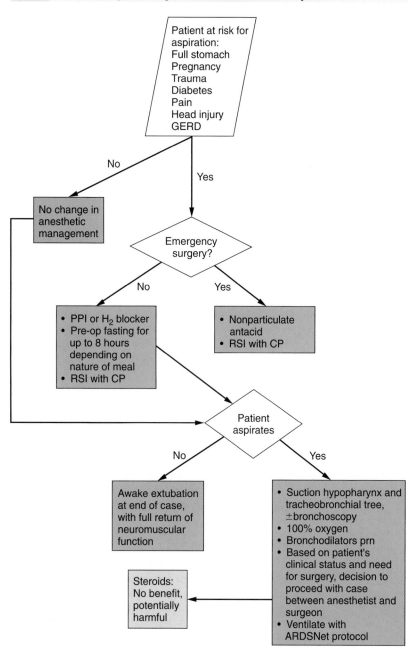

Figure 25-1 ■ Algorithm for the treatment of the patient at risk for aspiration. GERD, gastroesophageal reflux disease; PPI, proton pump inhibitor; prn, as needed; RSI with CP, rapid sequence induction with cricoid pressure.

Aspiration of gastric contents results in a severe chemical burn of the tracheobronchial tree with an ensuing inflammatory response. The lung injury is usually biphasic: initially (in the first 1 to 2 hours) the gastric fluid has direct acidic effects on the alveoli, and then, approximately 4 to 6 hours later, the condition is worsened by the migration of neutrophils and the inflammatory cytokines that are liberated. Several adhesion molecules, complement, tumor necrosis factor-α, and a myriad of other mediators are responsible for this delayed reaction, which can be demonstrated histologically as an acute inflammatory response.

Because the stomach is acidic, the gastric contents are usually sterile, and early pneumonia of the patient who has

aspirated is uncommon. Those patients who have a bowel obstruction and aspirate feculent material are clearly more likely to have bacterial contamination of their lungs. Interestingly, increasing the gastric pH with H_2 blockers may increase the rate of colonization of the stomach by pathogenic bacteria, increasing the risk for early pneumonia.[29]

Despite the lack of evidence of efficacy, prophylactic antibiotics are commonly prescribed for patients who have aspirated. This is not recommended, as the early institution of antimicrobial therapy serves only to select for resistant organisms. The exception is the patient in whom the aspiration has occurred in the setting of a small bowel obstruction, or those in whom gastric colonization is suspected. The development of a fever, radiographic infiltrate, and leukocytosis often prompts clinicians to initiate antibiotics. This is also discouraged, as the clinical patterns of aspiration pneumonitis and pneumonia have significant overlap. Antibiotics should be instituted only in those cases where the pneumonitis persists for 48 hours, or where there is documented evidence of infection. Documenting the infection has the further advantage of allowing the clinician to tailor the antibiotic regimen and of reducing the incidence of selecting for resistant organisms. Should antibiotics become necessary, broad-spectrum agents active against both gram-positive and gram-negative organisms are suggested. Empiric anaerobic coverage is not usually necessary. Levofloxacin, ceftazidime, ceftriaxone, and piperacillin-tazobactam are all good first-line agents to treat this condition.

For several decades, steroids have been a mainstay of treatment for aspiration pneumonitis despite a lack of evidence showing their benefit. Theoretically, corticosteroids should help to reduce the inflammation caused by the aspiration event. One prospective placebo-controlled study showed an earlier improvement in radiographically evident aspiration pneumonitis, but these patients had longer stays in the intensive care unit (ICU) and had no change in overall outcome.[30]

Very few patients develop an aspiration syndrome serious enough to result in acute respiratory distress syndrome (ARDS). Patients with ARDS are identified by having a ratio of the partial pressure of oxygen in arterial blood to the fraction of inspired oxygen (PaO_2/FIO_2) of less than 200 mm Hg, the presence of bilateral infiltrates on a chest radiograph, and a pulmonary artery occlusion pressure of less than 18 mm Hg or the absence of clinical evidence of left atrial hypertension. However, if the anesthesiologist suspects ARDS, the management is largely supportive, and early transfer to an ICU is recommended. While awaiting transfer, the ventilatory strategy used in the ARDSNet trial has been shown to decrease mortality in this condition.[31] This study showed that using a low tidal volume approach of 6 mL/kg ideal bodyweight, with the goal of limiting plateau pressures to less than 30 cm H_2O, mortality was decreased by 22% from the control group where 10 to 12 mL/kg tidal volumes were used. In this study, up to 24 cm H_2O of positive end-expiratory pressure (PEEP) was allowed if the FIO_2 was 1.0.

■ POSTOPERATIVE NAUSEA AND VOMITING

Background and Incidence

Postoperative nausea and vomiting (PONV) is a relatively common condition, occurring in 20% to 30% of patients.[32] In certain high-risk populations, the incidence can approach 70%. The etiology of PONV is multifactorial, with patient, surgical, and anesthetic factors playing a role (Box 25-2). PONV is among the 10 most undesirable outcomes for surgical patients, and Gan and colleagues found that patients were willing to pay up to $100 at their own expense to avoid it.[33] Universal antiemetic prophylaxis is not cost effective; however, identifying high-risk patients allows cost-effective antiemetic prophylaxis to be used in the most economical fashion.

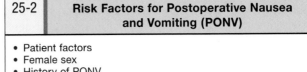

25-2	Risk Factors for Postoperative Nausea and Vomiting (PONV)

- Patient factors
- Female sex
- History of PONV
- History of motion sickness
- Nonsmoking history
- Anesthetic factors
- Opioids
- Volatile anesthetic agents
- High-dose neostigmine
- Nitrous oxide
- Surgical factors
- Emetogenic surgery (breast, ear-nose-and-throat, laparoscopic, intra-abdominal, gynecologic, strabismus)
- Long surgical procedures

25-3	Evidence-Rating Scales for the Management of Postoperative Nausea and Vomiting

Level of Evidence Based on Study Design

I Large randomized, controlled trial, $n \geq 100$ per group
II Systematic review
III Small randomized, controlled trial, $n < 100$ per group
IV Nonrandomized, controlled trial or case report
V Expert opinion

Strength of Conclusion or Recommendation

A Good evidence to support the conclusion or recommendation
B Fair evidence to support the conclusion or recommendation
C Insufficient evidence to recommend for or against

In general, the management of PONV includes (1) the identification of patients at risk, (2) the reduction of baseline risk factors, (3) the appropriate prophylaxis of PONV on the basis of risk stratification, and (4) the treatment of established PONV in patients who did not receive antiemetics or in whom prophylaxis with antiemetics failed. Most of the evidence-based data on prophylaxis and treatment comes from a recent PONV consensus statement.[34] This document was composed by an international panel of experts who reviewed the evidence for prophylaxis and treatment of PONV and, by rating the level of evidence (I to V), were able to suggest recommendations based on the strength of this evidence (Box 25-3).

Risk Factors

Several scoring systems have been developed to try to identify patients at high risk. The most commonly cited patient risk factors for PONV are female sex, need for opioids for postoperative pain, nonsmoking history, and a history of either PONV with prior anesthetics or of motion sickness. The presence of none, one, two, three, or four risk factors leads to an incidence of 10%, 21%, 39%, 61%, or 79%, respectively.[35]

Surgical factors may also play in a role in the development of PONV. An increase in surgery time is directly correlated with an increase in PONV. Furthermore, ear-nose-and-throat (ENT), strabismus, gynecologic, and laparoscopic surgery have all been associated with an increase in the risk for PONV.[36] The recent PONV consensus guidelines on the prevention and treatment of PONV classify the type of surgery as only level B evidence in the development of this condition.[37] It is possible that female sex may be a greater determinant than the type of surgery.

The type of anesthetic can also influence the likelihood of PONV. Nitrous oxide and opioids have been the most consistently implicated agents in the development of this condition. However, more recent data suggest that nitrous oxide increases the risk only minimally.[38] Regional anesthesia, because of its opioid-sparing effects, the frequent use of benzodiazepines (which may have antiemetic effects), and the avoidance of volatiles and nitrous oxide, has also been shown to decrease the incidence of PONV.

Management of PONV

Pharmacologic Prophylaxis and Treatment

The four major receptor classes that have been implicated in the generation of PONV are serotonergic (5-HT3), cholinergic, dopaminergic (D_2), and histaminergic (H_2). Box 25-4 summarizes the different methods used to treat PONV. Numerous studies have looked at the various antiemetics both alone and in combination for the treatment and prophylaxis of PONV, and numerous meta-analyses have examined both the number needed to treat (NNT) and the number needed to harm (NNH) to determine which antiemetic regimen is the most efficacious. With respect to the antiemetics, the NNT is the number of patients who would have to be treated with a particular drug to prevent an episode of nausea or vomiting that would have occurred had the drug not been administered. The NNH is the number of patients who would have to receive the drug and demonstrate an adverse event that would not have occurred had they not received the medication.

5-HT3 Receptor Antagonists

The 5-HT3 receptor antagonists ondansetron, granisetron, dolasetron, and tropisetron bind very specifically to their receptors in the chemoreceptor trigger zone and have a very favorable side-effect profile. They are virtually devoid of the sedative effects commonly seen with other antiemetics, making them ideal for the ambulatory surgery setting.[39]

Ondansetron was the first agent in this class to be marketed in the United States, and it is the most widely used agent in this class. It is a much better antivomiting agent than antinauseant, and it is most effective when given toward the end of surgery.[34,40] The recommended dosage of ondansetron is 4 to 8 mg, and the NNT is 5 to 6. Common side effects include headache (NNH = 36), dizziness, flushing, elevated liver enzymes, and constipation.

Granisetron has been used in both the treatment and prophylaxis of PONV. For prophylaxis, a dosage of 1.0 mg has been recommended, although more recent studies have found that lower dosages are efficacious, especially when

25-4	Options Available for the Management of Postoperative Nausea and Vomiting

Pharmacologic Techniques

A. Monotherapy
1. Older generation antiemetics
   a. Phenothiazines: aliphatic [promethazine, chlorpromazine], heterocyclic [perphenazine, prochlorperazine].
   b. Buterophenones: droperidol, haloperidol.
   c. Benzamides: metoclopramide, domperidone.
   d. Anticholinergics: scopolamine.
   e. Antihistamines: ethanolamines [dimenhydrinate, diphenhydramine], piperazines [cyclizine, hydroxyzine, meclizine].
2. Newer generation antiemetics:
   a. Serotonin (5-HT3) receptor antagonists: ondansetron, granisetron, dolasetron, tropisetron.
   b. NK-1 receptor antagonists (aprepitant)
3. Other antiemetics: dexamethasone, propofol, ephedrine
B. Combination of two or more of the above antiemetics
1. 5-HT3 receptor antagonists + droperidol
2. 5-HT3 receptor antagonists + dexamethasone
3. Other combinations

Nonpharmacologic Techniques

1. Acupuncture
2. Acupressure
3. Laser stimulation of the P6 point
4. Transcutaneous Acupoint Electrical Stimulation
5. Hypnosis

Additional Measures with Potential Antiemetic Effects

1. Supplemental oxygen
2. Benzodiazepines
3. Adequate hydration
4. Good pain relief
5. α-2-Adrenergic agonists

Multimodal Approach

combined with dexamethasone. For established PONV, a dosage of only 0.1 mg has been found to be efficacious.[41]

Dolasetron is structurally related to granisetron and tropisetron. Unlike ondansetron, the timing of the administration of this drug seems to have little effect on the prevention of PONV.[42]

Of the several head-to-head comparisons of the 5-HT3 antagonists, none has demonstrated any difference between the agents with regard to their efficacy in the prevention and treatment of PONV. For example, in patients undergoing ENT procedures, there was no difference in the incidence of PONV between ondansetron dosages of 4 mg or 8 mg, and between dolasetron dosages of 12.5 mg and 25 mg.[43]

Dopamine Receptor Antagonists

Droperidol. Droperidol has been used extensively in the past for the treatment of PONV. It is as effective as ondansetron in the prevention of PONV (with an NNT of 5). The advantage of droperidol over the other antiemetic agents is in its duration of action, which can extend up to 24 hours even though its half-life is only 3 hours.[44]

In 2001, the U.S. Food and Dug Administration (FDA) issued a "black box" warning for droperidol based on 10 case reports of QTc-interval prolongation and the development of torsades de pointes when dosages of less than 1.25 mg were used.[45] It is important to note that these case reports span over 30 years of use of droperidol, and that the estimated incidence of cardiac adverse events is somewhere in the range of 6.7/1 million. Furthermore, no case reports have appeared in peer-reviewed journals linking droperidol to torsades, QTc prolongation, or cardiac arrest in the dosages commonly used in the prevention and treatment of PONV. This is impressive considering all the other drugs used during the course of a general anesthetic that could prolong the QT interval. Were it not for the black box warning, the PONV consensus panel would have made droperidol their overwhelming first choice for the prophylaxis of PONV based on its efficacy and cost.

Metoclopramide. Metoclopramide has been used for years in the treatment of chemotherapy-induced nausea and vomiting in dosages of 10 to 20 mg in adults. Its use in the treatment of PONV is much more controversial. Despite widespread use, approximately 50% of the studies performed with metoclopramide have shown it to be no more effective than placebo. A meta-analysis of all the metoclopramide studies has identified an NNT of between 9 and 10. The PONV consensus panel could not recommend the use of metoclopramide as an antiemetic, but there was not consensus on this issue.

Anticholinergics and Antihistaminergics
The most commonly used cholinergic for the treatment of PONV is scopolamine. The transdermal preparation when applied either the night before or 4 hours before the conclusion of surgery has been shown to have an NNT of 3.8.[46] Some of the drawbacks of this drug, however, include dry mouth, visual disturbances, dizziness, and agitation (with NNHs of 5.6, 12.5, 50, and 100, respectively).[41] Other disadvantages of scopolamine include the long time for its peak effect (2 to 4 hours) and its associated medical contraindications.

Antihistamines are also commonly used for the treatment of PONV. Their use is limited by various side effects, such as sedation, urinary retention, blurred vision, and dry mouth. They have also been shown to delay recovery-room discharge. However, the NNT compares well with other antiemetics with a prophylactic NNT of 6 for a dosage of 1 to 2 mg/kg for dimenhydrinate, and an NNT of 5 for established PONV.[47]

Other Antiemetics
Dexamethasone. Dexamethasone has long been used as an effective antiemetic for chemotherapy patients. Its use has been studied in the surgical population, and it has been found that in dosages ranging from 2.5 to 10 mg, its NNT was 4.3 (level IIA evidence for use).[34] It appears that dexamethasone is most effective when given prior to the induction of general anesthesia. There are no reported side effects when dexamethasone is used in antiemetic dosages for short duration; however, some patients complain of a burning perineal pain when the drug is injected. It has been hypothesized that this reaction is caused by the phosphate ester of the corticosteroid, because perineal irritation has been described with hydrocortisone-21-phosphate sodium and prednisolone phosphate.[48]

Propofol. When compared with volatile anesthesia, propofol total intravenous anesthesia (TIVA) has been associated with a decreased risk of developing PONV (level IIIa evidence).[49] This risk reduction seems to be most prominent in the early postoperative period, and it is not present if propofol is used only as a bolus for the induction of anesthesia. Recently, it has been discovered that subhypnotic dosages of propofol can be used to treat established PONV. The dosages required to achieve this antiemetic effect are several magnitudes lower than those needed for sedation and anesthesia.[50]

Benzodiazepines. Benzodiazepines have been used for the treatment of PONV when other forms of treatment have failed. This evidence is based only on small randomized trials and, as such, was graded as level IIIB by the PONV consensus task force. Alpha-2-adrenergic agonists have also been found to reduce the incidence of PONV in adults and children (level IIIA). It is thought that their anesthetic and opioid-sparing effects might explain their usefulness in this condition.[51]

Neurokinin-1 Antagonists. Another emerging pharmacologic strategy is neurokinin-1 (NK-1) inhibitors. The NK-1 antagonist class of drugs acts on the final common pathway from the emetic center. These compounds are known to inhibit the effects of substance P in the brainstem regions associated with emesis. In humans, NK-1 receptor antagonists are effective for the prophylaxis and treatment of PONV. In one study of women undergoing gynecologic surgery, the NK-1 receptor antagonist CP-122,721 provided better prophylaxis against vomiting than ondansetron. The combination of both agents also significantly prolongs the time to administration of rescue antiemetics compared with either drug alone and is associated with a very low incidence of emesis (2%). Cost may, however, be an issue when considering routine use of these newer drugs for PONV. Aprepitant is the only drug of this class approved in the United States for chemotherapy-induced nausea and vomiting, and emerging data suggest it has excellent efficacy for preventing emesis.[52]

The choice of intraoperative fluid may also play a role in the genesis of PONV. Although differences between crystalloids and colloids are difficult to demonstrate in terms of mortality and morbidity, the quality of the recovery may be different. In a recent study, the intraoperative use of colloids was associated with a decrease in the rates of PONV and the use of rescue antiemetics.[53] It is possible that the use of colloids results in less bowel edema, and this might be the reason for the observed decrease in PONV.

Nonpharmacologic Therapies

The use of nonpharmacologic therapies, such as acupressure, acupoint stimulation, transcutaneous nerve stimulation, and acupuncture (at the P6 point), have been reviewed recently.[54] These therapies have shown a significant reduction in PONV when compared with placebo. When acupuncture techniques were compared with conventional antiemetics (not including the 5-HT3 antagonists), there was a comparable decrease in the incidence of PONV. A recent placebo-controlled study comparing the use of transcutaneous acupoint electrical stimulation and ondansetron showed comparable results between these two strategies and significantly superior results to placebo.[55] These nonpharmacologic approaches are interesting, but the lack of familiarity with the techniques by most practitioners and the need for additional equipment limit their use.

Strategy for the Prevention of PONV

PONV is frequently encountered in anesthesia, but it is not cost effective to provide prophylaxis with antiemetics for all patients. Instead, a risk stratification of patients should be undertaken that includes patient, anesthetic, and surgical risk factors. On the basis of the presence of these risk factors, different levels of prophylaxis can be suggested. The treatment of established nausea and vomiting depends on what type of antiemetic (if any) the patient has received.

Patients who have no risk factors (neither surgical nor patient related) for the development of PONV should not receive prophylaxis, as this has been shown to be not cost effective, unless vomiting might compromise the patient in some way (e.g., because of raised intracranial pressure or a wired jaw). Those patients with risk factors for PONV should receive prophylaxis according to the algorithm in Figure 25-2. Those patients at the highest risk for PONV (i.e., those who have had PONV repeatedly in the past) should receive double prophylaxis, and consideration should be given to performing the surgery under a regional anesthetic technique. Should this not be practical, a general risk-reduction strategy should be considered, including reducing opioid dosage by using multimodal analgesia, ensuring adequate hydration, avoiding high-dose neuromuscular reversal agents, and the use of propofol for induction and maintenance of anesthesia (level IIIA evidence).

Treatment of Established PONV

Evidence supporting a definitive treatment for those patients with established PONV (with or without prophylaxis) is less clear. The patient in whom prophylaxis has failed presents a difficult problem. Factors such as the use of postoperative opioids, blood entering the throat, or a mechanical bowel obstruction should be ruled out before the institution of pharmacologic therapy. In those patients in whom prophylaxis has failed, the use of an agent from another class is recommended (level IIA to IVB, depending on the prophylaxis). In the trials for rescue therapy, the 5-HT3 receptor antagonists are the most commonly studied medications. As seen when their role is prophylaxis, their antiemetic effect is stronger than their antinauseant effect. There is no reported dose–response effect, so smaller dosages of these agents have been used. The recommended dosages are ondansetron, 1 mg; dolasetron, 12.5 mg; granisetron, 0.1 mg; and tropisetron, 0.5 mg.[56]

The data on the efficacy or the optimal dosage of the other agents for the treatment of established PONV are limited. This is because to obtain the required number of

patients who actually experienced PONV, the number that would need to be recruited would have to be quite large.

■ POSTOPERATIVE ILEUS

Postoperative ileus (POI) is an impairment of GI motility after abdominal or other forms of surgery. It is characterized by the lack of bowel sounds, accumulation of gas and fluids in the bowel, abdominal distention, and intolerance to enteral feeding.[57] This condition generally lasts for 3 to 5 days and is usually self-limiting. POI should be differentiated from mechanical small bowel obstruction, as the etiology and management are very different.

Reducing length of hospital stay is paramount in the current climate of health-care cost minimization. POI serves only to lengthen the average stay after a laparotomy from 3 to 10 days. This is associated with increased costs and the potential for other morbidity such as delayed mobility, delayed absorption of food and medications, and the increased risk for infectious and pulmonary complications.

Etiology

Normal bowel motility depends on many factors, including the enteric and central nervous systems and hormones. Motility of the small intestine and the stomach also depends on whether the patient is in the fasted or fed state. The perturbation of gastric motility in the postoperative period is likewise the result of many interrelated and overlapping factors. In the normal state, the balance between the excitatory parasympathetic and inhibitory sympathetic nervous systems is such that antegrade motility is preserved. Increased activity of the sympathetic nervous system (which is common in postoperative states because of pain and the stress response) causes activation of the α-2-adrenoreceptors on cholinergic neurons, which leads to a dominant parasympathetic effect on the intestines, thereby reducing motility.[58]

Nitric oxide (NO) also plays a role in the development of POI, and it is the most important nonadrenergic noncholinergic neurotransmitter. NO plays an inhibitory role with respect to bowel motility. Administration of an NO synthase inhibitor reverses the lack of bowel motility caused by surgical manipulation in rats.[59]

The release of endogenous opioids secondary to surgical trauma of the abdomen may have a role in the development of POI. In animal studies, the infusion of an endogenous opiate peptide has been shown to slow bowel motility. What role these endogenous opioids play in humans is questionable, as the administration of synthetic opioids probably dominates.

The stress response to the surgery may also play a role in the development of POI. Hypothalamic liberation of corticotrophin-releasing factor (CRF) is the most important factor in this response. Exogenous administration of CRF is known to slow gastric emptying, and the infusion of a CRF antagonist partially prevents POI in rats.[60]

Intuitively, the inflammatory cascade that is initiated with surgery should also play a role in the development of POI. The resultant edema and liberation of cytokines could

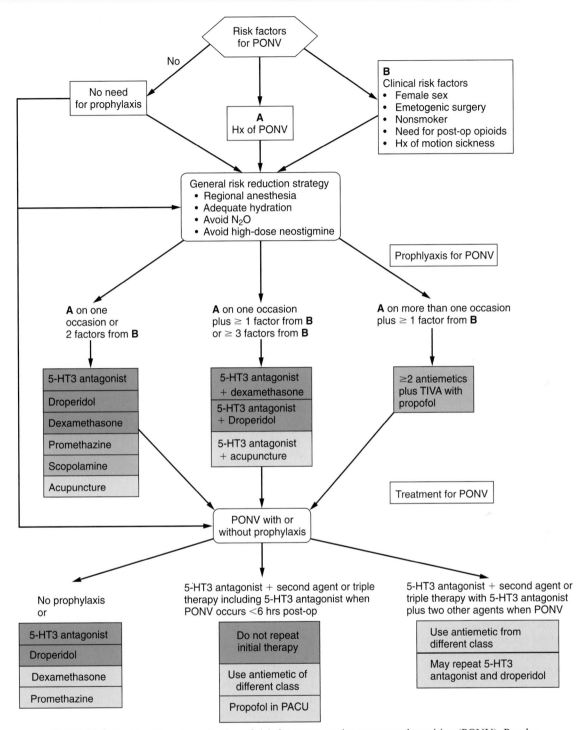

Figure 25-2 ■ Algorithm for reduction of risk for postoperative nausea and vomiting (PONV). Prophylaxis depends on both patient and surgical risk factors. A treatment strategy for established PONV based on the presence or absence of prophylaxis is presented at the bottom of the figure. PACU, postanesthesia care unit; TIVA, total intravenous anesthesia.

also explain the pathogenesis, but its role in humans has not been studied adequately.

In the end, the development of POI is most probably caused by multiple overlapping factors. This is demonstrated by the lack of any antagonist to the previously mentioned factors to completely reverse or prevent POI.

Role of Postoperative Opioids

Opioids are the most common and efficacious treatment for postoperative pain. Their use, however, is associated with a decrease in intestinal transit time. In 1972, opioid receptors that affect bowel motility were discovered in the GI tract. The central opioid receptors also play a role in bowel motility. The site in the GI tract where opioids have their most profound effect is the colon. Opioids increase the basal muscle tone in the colon to the level of spasm, thereby reducing the propulsive forces. This slows the passage of feces through the lumen, which causes drying and hardening of the contents, further slowing passage.[61]

Role of General Anesthesia

Administration of anesthesia to patients alters bowel motility. Induction agents, nitrous oxide, and inhalation agents all have been implicated. Of these, nitrous oxide is the best described. Diffusion of this gas into the bowel lumen distends the bowel and has been shown to cause a delay in the return of gastric function. Its use also results in longer hospital stays when compared with an air–oxygen mixture.[62]

Treatment of Postoperative Ileus

Nonpharmacologic Methods

Nasogastric Drainage

Decompression of the stomach by a nasogastric (NG) tube has been the mainstay of therapy for POI since the late 1800s. Although this therapy does reduce patient discomfort, there is no evidence that it hastens the return of normal motility. Among patients who were given a colonic resection, no difference in duration of ileus or hospital stay was observed between those who received an NG tube and those who did not.[63]

Early Enteral Nutrition

It is common for patients to be maintained in an NPO status after a major laparotomy. Traditionally, patients are not fed until after bowel sounds return. Unfortunately, this practice might be flawed, as the lack of bowel sounds is less pathologic than it is a response to fasting. The presence of food in the GI tract stimulates the release of hormones that initiate intestinal propulsive activity. Early enteral nutrition has therefore been proposed as a safe and effective way of preventing or reducing the duration of POI, and the maintenance of NPO status may be detrimental to the patient. Fasting causes a catabolic state at a time when patients need to be anabolic. Furthermore, translocation of bacteria and endotoxin across the paracellular space from the gut lumen into the circulation may be responsible for the development of postoperative infections and multiple organ dysfunction syndrome.[64] There is some evidence that early enteral feeding reduces this translocation. Some studies also show a decrease

in the duration of POI when early enteral nutrition is implemented. Recent trials, however, have shown no change in the duration of ileus or hospital stay.[65] Still, it is important to note that in all of these trials, early nutrition was not associated with any adverse effects, challenging the dogma that patients should be fasted until the return of bowel sounds.

Postoperative Fluid Administration

The amount and type of fluid administered in the perioperative period also plays a role in the development and duration of POI. When a goal-directed fluid protocol titrated to esophageal Doppler cardiac output was used in patients undergoing major surgery, those who received fluid optimization demonstrated a decrease in the rates of PONV, an earlier return of bowel function, and a shorter hospital stay.[66] Indices of tissue perfusion such as gastric pH and base excess are correlated with the development of postoperative complications, so titrating therapy might be expected to reduce GI morbidity. On the other hand, some studies have demonstrated that excess fluid in the perioperative period is associated with the development of POI. Theoretically, this may be the result of the development of bowel wall edema and subsequent dysfunction. In a study by Moretti and coworkers, it was shown that the administration of intraoperative colloid was associated with a decrease in the amount of GI complications.[53] The clinician is thus faced with a dilemma of how much fluid to give. It would seem prudent, therefore, to optimize fluid administration by titrating to specific endpoints such as gastric pH, base excess, or (if it is available) esophageal Doppler cardiac output (see later).

Mobilization

There is no known benefit to immobilization after surgery but there are many potential hazards. In theory, early postoperative ambulation should help induce gastric motility, and this is commonly practiced. Unfortunately, this has not been demonstrated in clinical studies.[67] Despite a lack of benefit to the GI system, the reduction in the incidence of deep vein thrombosis and postoperative pulmonary complications (such as atelectasis and pneumonia) argue for its continued use as part of facilitated recovery from surgery.

Pharmacologic Therapies for the Treatment of POI

The effects of various drugs on POI are listed in Table 25-2.

Agents Acting on the Autonomic Nervous System

As mentioned previously, normal GI motility depends on a delicate balance between the sympathetic and parasympathetic nervous systems. The enhanced activity of the sympathetic nervous system in the postoperative state is very likely a factor contributing to POI. This has led several investigators to suggest that the alteration of this balance with agents that act on the adrenergic or cholinergic nervous systems might have a role in the prevention or treatment of POI.

Some older evidence indicates that the cholinergic agonists of the muscarinic receptor, such as bethanechol, carbachol, and methacholine, would stimulate gastric motility via intestinal receptors. More recent and larger studies have focused on the role of cholinesterase inhibitors such as

25-2 | **Drug Effects on Postoperative Ileus**

Drug	Mechanism of Action	Effect on Postoperative Ileus
Atenolol, esmolol, propranolol	β-Receptor antagonist	Decreased or none
Dihydroergotamine	α-Receptor antagonist	Decreased or none
Neostigmine	Acetylcholinesterase inhibitor	Decreased or none
Erythromycin	Motilin agonist	None
Cisapride	Acetylcholine and serotonin receptor agonist	Decreased or none
Metoclopramide	Cholinergic stimulant, peripheral dopamine antagonist	None
Cholecystokinin	Prokinetic peptide	None
Vasopressin	Defecation stimulant	None

From Mythen MG: Anesth Analg 2005;100:196-204.

neostigmine in the treatment of ileus. Several studies have shown neostigmine to be effective in the reduction of the duration of ileus.[68] However, neostigmine has some significant untoward side effects, such as the development of profound bradycardia and bronchorrhea, that mandate its being given in a monitored setting, which is not always possible or cost effective. Higher dosages of neostigmine (>2.5 mg) are also associated with an increase in PONV.

Adrenergic blockade is another attractive pharmacologic target for the treatment of POI. However, as with agents that act on the cholinergic system, sympathetic blockade of postoperative patients is associated with sufficient deleterious cardiovascular effects to make its administration impractical in the clinical setting.

Prokinetic Agents
Metoclopramide has been in use for over 40 years for the treatment of PONV and is used as a prokinetic (see Dopamine Receptor Antagonists, earlier). It has both central and peripheral sites of action. The peripheral sites of action cause an increase in gastric contractions, increased gastric emptying, and increased transit time in the GI tract. It has been extensively studied with several different clinical endpoints and has not been shown to reduce the severity, duration, or incidence of POI. Side effects such as dystonic reactions and prolongation of the QTc further limit its use in clinical medicine.

Laxatives
Historically, laxatives are also widely used in the treatment of POI. However, blinded randomized trials have not been conducted, so their potential benefit is unproven.

Opioid Antagonists
The presence of both endogenous and exogenous opioids is known to play a role in postoperative bowel dysfunction. The administration of opioid antagonists is therefore an attractive intervention to decrease morbidity. The ideal therapeutic agent would be one that antagonizes only the peripheral opiate receptors in the GI tract but is not able to cross the GI lumen to affect central receptors causing increased postoperative pain. Several compounds accomplish this, including alvimopan and methylnaltrexone.

Alvimopan is a new μ-receptor antagonist that has been studied in a randomized controlled trial of patients undergoing colonic resection or abdominal hysterectomy. It was found that patients given 6 mg alvimopan 2 hours before major abdominal surgery had a decrease in the median time to first flatus and bowel movement of about 18 hours. Patients in the treatment group were also ready for hospital discharge 1 day earlier than those given placebo.[69]

Methylnaltrexone is a quaternary derivative of the μ-receptor antagonist naltrexone that is poorly lipid soluble and does not cross into the central nervous system. It has recently been investigated in humans, demonstrating an improvement in colonic motility in patients receiving elective colon surgery and given postoperative morphine.[70]

Nonsteroidal Anti-inflammatory Agents
The prostaglandin is another pathway that plays a role in POI and is subject to pharmacologic modification. The initial step in prostaglandin synthesis is catalyzed by the enzyme cyclooxygenase (COX). There are two isoforms of COX, designated COX-1 and COX-2. COX-1 is constitutively expressed and is necessary for platelet aggregation, maintenance of renal function in hypovolemic states, and gastrointestinal protection. COX-2 is inducible and responsible for the inflammation, pain, and fever seen after tissue trauma.

Prostaglandins E_2 and I_2 lower the threshold for stimulation of afferent nerves by noxious chemical stimuli such as histamine and bradykinin. Some prostaglandins also decrease smooth muscle activity in the GI tract and thus decrease transit time. Inhibition of prostaglandins is thus another way of potentially reversing POI. Ketorolac (a nonselective COX inhibitor) administered preoperatively was shown to reverse the delay in gastric transit seen in patients with POI.[71] The authors hypothesized that the inhibition of all prostaglandin synthesis resulted in the dominant inhibitory effects being reversed.

One of the potential drawbacks of using nonselective COX inhibitors on postoperative patients is the potential for the increased risk for GI ulceration and bleeding, the potential for increased blood loss secondary to the effects on platelet aggregation, and the detrimental effects of renal function. These drawbacks led to the development of selective inhibitors of COX-2 such as celecoxib, rofecoxib, and valdecoxib. There have been no published studies on their effect on POI.

Recently, many studies have linked COX-2 inhibitors to an increase in adverse cardiac events such as myocardial infraction, stroke, congestive heart failure, and cardiac death.[72] It is thought that because of the selective inhibition of prostacyclin synthesis with no effect on thromboxane A_2

synthesis, a prothrombotic state is created when these drugs are administered. It is important to note that these studies were on patients who were taking COX-2 inhibitors long term for the prevention of colorectal adenomas. What role these agents might play in the incidence of perioperative myocardial infarction with short-term use has not been studied, but is probably not of significant clinical magnitude.[73]

It is likely that any beneficial effect of nonsteroidal anti-inflammatory drugs (NSAIDs) on bowel motility and the incidence of POI is more a result of their opioid-sparing effect than of prostaglandin balance. Their contribution to a multimodal approach to postoperative pain is significant. With the previously noted adverse cardiac effects of the COX-2 inhibitors and the effects of nonselective NSAIDs on platelets, renal function, and GI ulceration, the use of these drugs will have to be better defined with more studies on their risk-to-benefit ratio.

Epidural Analgesia

Epidural analgesia is perhaps the ideal method of reducing the incidence of postoperative bowel dysfunction. It reduces the amount of parenteral opioid used, and implementing a blockade of the thoracolumbar sympathetic nervous system while leaving the craniosacral parasympathetic nervous system intact creates a favorable balance, promoting GI motility. There is also evidence to show that epidurals increase GI blood flow, and that local anesthetics themselves have anti-inflammatory properties.[74]

The benefit of epidural analgesia on GI motility appears to be significant only when the catheter is placed above the level of the 12th thoracic vertebrae. There appears to be less effect when a lumbar epidural is placed for abdominal surgery.[75]

Goal-Directed Therapy and Gastrointestinal Outcome

The administration of fluids to surgical patients is quite variable between centers and across the decades. The initial thought in the 1950s and 1960s was that because of the obligatory water and sodium conservation that occurred after surgical trauma, fluid restriction was required, as first proposed by Moore.[76] This view was later challenged by Shires and colleagues, who introduced the concept of third-space losses.[75] Their recommendation was that this third-space fluid be replaced aggressively with crystalloid administration. This theory was supported by studies during the Korean War in which it was shown that aggressive fluid resuscitation led to improved outcomes in trauma patients. Modern clinical practice has been more influenced by Shires, as patients are often resuscitated with fluid in excess of their deficit. With the current preoperative fasting guidelines and with the introduction of bowel regimens, patients often have a fluid deficit at the beginning of an anesthesia.

The type of surgery itself often influences how much fluid patients receive. It is not uncommon for patients undergoing abdominal aortic reconstructive surgery to receive 4 to 6 L of fluid (in addition to the replacement of blood loss). The same aggressive fluid regimen, however, has been shown to be detrimental in flap surgery, where the increase in venous pressure secondary to postoperative edema decreases flap survival.

With regard to the GI system, "dry" and "wet" strategies can both lead to postoperative complications and morbidity. A fluid replacement regimen that is conservative has the potential for a decrease in cardiac output and in perfusion to the splanchnic bed. This can lead to intestinal acidosis, POI, and the translocation of bacteria and endotoxin into the vascular system, potentially causing sepsis or multiple system organ failure (MSOF).

On the other hand, the use of an aggressive, or wet, approach to fluid replacement is known to increase bowel edema, decrease the tolerance for enteral feeding, and increase the incidence of POI. The liberal administration of fluid is also known to increase the venous pressure in the intestines (secondary to the edema) and therefore to cause a decrease in splanchnic oxygenation by reducing the perfusion pressure. This can also lead to the transmigration of bacteria and endotoxin into the circulation.

Furthermore, some data suggest that the administration of vasopressors and inotropes to the surgical patient with the goal of maximizing oxygen delivery can improve outcome.[77]

The clinician is thus faced with choosing the fluid replacement strategy that will best improve outcome and lessen GI morbidity. Recently, the concept of goal-directed therapy—that is, titrating fluid and vasoactive medications to specified clinical and hemodynamic endpoints—has increased in popularity. Goal-directed therapy was first proposed by Shoemaker and Bland, who found that the hemodynamic patterns of patients who did not survive major surgery were different from those of survivors.[78] They found that those patients who died after major surgery had lower cardiac indices, oxygen consumption, and oxygen delivery. They speculated that nonsurvivors had an oxygen debt, and that this was the cause of their death. This led to the practice of identifying supranormal physiologic goals to be achieved in these high-risk patients to avoid the oxygen debt and potentially reduce mortality. Although the idea is controversial, variations of this therapy have been shown to be effective in reducing the postoperative mortality of selected high-risk patients.[77] This practice has largely been supplanted by trying to maintain normality of cardiac index, oxygen delivery (DO_2), and volume of oxygen consumption (VO_2), and by looking at other indices of tissue perfusion such as gastric mucosal pH and central mixed venous oxygen saturation ($S_{cv}O_2$).

Role of Fluid Composition

The debate as to whether crystalloid or colloid is the better replacement fluid began shortly after the introduction of colloids. Colloid proponents point to the increased edema and large volumes of fluid that are required in surgical patients as evidence of the inferiority of crystalloids. Crystalloid proponents suggest that hemostatic effects and the potential of anaphylactic reactions to colloids limit their use. Most of the studies comparing crystalloids and colloids have been conducted on critically ill patients in the ICU or on patients undergoing resuscitation from trauma and have not looked specifically at GI outcome. Perhaps the right question is not being asked in the crystalloid-versus-colloid debate. Measuring the quality of outcomes from resuscitation using secondary endpoints such as incidence of PONV, POI, postoperative edema, and length of stay might be more practical.[79]

In a study with patients who underwent major noncardiac surgery, patients were randomized to receive 6% hetastarch in either a balanced salt solution, normal saline, or lactated Ringer's solution.[56] Hemodynamic targets such as blood pressure, heart rate, and urine output were maintained within a predefined range. Patients in the colloid group had less PONV and need for rescue antiemetics. They also reported less severe pain, periorbital edema, and double vision.[56] This study did not consider length of stay or incidence of POI.

■ SUMMARY

Modern anesthetic practice has made mortality after elective surgery in healthy patients an exceedingly rare event. The goal of today's anesthesiologist is to improve the quality of recovery by avoiding aspiration and reducing the incidence of PONV and POI. When applied in a systematic fashion, several interventions, such as PONV prophylaxis and goal-directed fluid therapy, have been shown to decrease patient morbidity and length of stay. These outcomes are becoming increasingly important in today's cost-saving culture. Still, further research is needed to further define strategies that can decrease the GI morbidity associated with anesthetic practice.

■ REFERENCES

1. Mendelson CL: The aspiration of stomach contents into the lungs during obstetric anesthesia. Am J Obstet Gynecol 1946;52:191-205.
2. Teabeaut JR: Aspiration of gastric contents: An experimental study. Am J Pathol 1952;28:51-67.
3. Exarhos ND, Logan WD Jr, Abbott OA, Hatcher CR Jr: The importance of pH and volume in tracheobronchial aspiration. Dis Chest 1965;47:167-169.
4. James CF, Modell JH, Gibbs CP, et al: Pulmonary aspiration, effects of volume and pH in the rat. Anesth Analg 1984;63:665-668.
5. Schwartz DJ, Wynne JW, Gibbs CP, et al: The pulmonary consequences of aspiration of gastric contents at pH values greater than 2.5. Am Rev Respir Dis 1980;121:119-126.
6. Knight PR, Rutter T, Tait AR, et al: Pathogenesis of gastric particulate lung injury: A comparison and interaction with acidic pneumonitis. Anesth Analg 1993;77:754-760.
7. Ingebo KR, Rayhorn NJ, Roxanne M, et al: Sedation in children: Adequacy of two-hour fasting. J Pediatr 1997;131:155-158.
8. Schwartz DA, Connelly NR, Theroux CA, et al: Gastric contents in children presenting for upper endoscopy. Anesth Analg 1998;87:757-760.
9. Brady M, Kinn S, Stuart P: Preoperative fasting for adults to prevent perioperative complications. Cochrane Database Syst Rev 2003:CD004423.
10. Ng A, Smith G: Gastroesophageal reflux and Aspiration of Gastric contents in Anesthetic practice. Anesth Analg 2001;93:494-515.
11. Kahrilas PJ, Dodds WJ, Dent J, et al: Effect of sleep, spontaneous gastroesophageal reflux, and a meal on upper oesophageal sphincter pressure in normal human volunteers. Gastroenterology 1987;92:466-471.
12. Eriksson LI, Sundman E, Olsson R, et al: Functional assessment of the pharynx at rest and during swallowing in partially paralysed humans. Anesthesiology 1997;87:1035-1043.
13. Carlin CB, Scanlon PG, Wagner DA, et al: Gastric emptying in trauma patients. Dig Surg 1999;16:192-196.
14. Crighton IM, Margin PH, Hobbs GJ, et al: A comparison of the effects of intravenous tramadol, codeine and morphine on gastric emptying in human volunteers. Anesth Analg 1999;89:80-89.
15. Chiloiro M, Darconza G, Piccioli E, et al: Gastric emptying and orocecal time in pregnancy. J Gastroenterol 2001;36:538-543.
16. Porter JS, Bonello E, Reynolds F: The influence of epidural administration of fentanyl infusion on gastric emptying in labor. Anesthesia 1997;52:1151-1156.
17. Harter RL, Kelly WB, Kramer MG, et al: A comparison of the volume and pH of gastric contents of obese and lean surgical patients. Anesth Analg 1998;86:147-152.
18. Sellick BA: Cricoid pressure to control regurgitation of stomach contents during induction of anaesthesia. Lancet 1961;2:404-406.
19. Tournadre JP, Chassard D, Berrada KR, Bouletreau P: Cricoid cartilage pressure decreases lower esophageal sphincter tone. Anesthesiology 1997;86:7-9.
20. MacG Palmer JH, Ball DR: The effect of cricoid pressure on the cricoid cartilage and vocal cords: An endoscopic study in anaesthetised patients. Anaesthesia 2000;55:263-268.
21. Meek T, Gittins N, Duggan JE: Cricoid pressure: Knowledge and performance amongst anaesthetic assistants. Anaesthesia 1999;54:51-85.
22. Ralph SJ, Wareham CA: Rupture of the esophagus during cricoid pressure. Anesthesia 1991;46:40-41.
23. Nishina K, Mikawa K, Maekawa N, et al: A comparison of lansoprazole, omeprazole and ranitidine for reducing preoperative gastric secretion in adult patients undergoing elective surgery. Anesth Analg 1996;82:832-836.
24. Kulkarni PN, Batra YK, Wig J: Effects of different combinations of H2 receptor antagonist with gastrokinetic drugs on gastric fluid pH and volume in children: A comparative study. Int J Pharmacol Ther 1997;35:561-564.
25. American Society of Anesthesiologists Task Force on Preoperative Fasting: Practice guidelines for preoperative fasting and the use of pharmacologic agents to reduce the risk of pulmonary aspiration: Application to healthy patients undergoing elective procedures. Anesthesiology 1999;90:896-905.
26. Splinter WM, Schaefer JD: Unlimited clear fluid ingestion two hours before surgery in children does not affect volume or pH or stomach contents. Anaesth Intensive Care 1990;18:522-526.
27. Soreide E, Hausken T, Soreide JA, Steen PA: Gastric emptying of a light hospital breakfast: A study using real time ultrasonography. Acta Anaesthesiol Scand 1996;40:549-553.
28. Moore JG, Christian PE, Coleman RE: Gastric emptying of varying meal weight and composition in man: Evaluation of dual liquid and solid phase isotopic method. Dig Dis Sci 1981;26:16-22.
29. Bonten MJ, Gaillard CA, van der Geest S, et al: The role of intragastric acidity and stress ulcus prophylaxis on colonization and infection in mechanically ventilated ICU patients: A stratified, randomized, double-blind study of sucralfate versus antacids. Am J Respir Crit Care Med 1995;152:1825-1834.
30. Sukumaran M, Granada MJ, Berger HW, et al: Evaluation of corticosteroid treatment in aspiration of gastric contents: A controlled clinical trial. Mt Sinai J Med 1980;47:335-340.
31. The Acute Respiratory Distress Syndrome Network: Ventilation with lower tidal volumes as compared with traditional tidal volumes for acute lung injury and the acute respiratory distress syndrome. N Engl J Med 2000;342:1301-1308.
32. Cohen MM, Duncan PG, DeBoer DP, Tweed WA: The postoperative interview: Assessing risk factors for nausea and vomiting. Anesth Analg 1994;78:7-16.
33. Gan T, Sloan F, Dear Gde L, El-Moalem HE, Lubarsky DA: How much are patients willing to pay to avoid postoperative nausea and vomiting? Anesth Analg 2001;92:393-400.
34. Tramer MR, Reynolds DJ, Moore RA, McQuay HJ: Efficacy, dose-response, and safety of ondansetron in prevention of postoperative nausea and vomiting: A quantitative systematic review of randomized placebo controlled trials. Anesthesiology 1997;87:1277-1289.
35. Apfel CC, Laara E, Koivuranta M, et al: A simplified risk score for predicting postoperative nausea and vomiting: Conclusions from cross-validations between two centers. Anesthesiology 1999;91:693-700.

36. Sinclair DR, Chung F, Mezei G: Can postoperative nausea and vomiting be predicted? Anesthesiology 1999;91:109-118.

37. Gan TJ, Meyer T, Apfel CC, et al: Consensus guidelines for managing postoperative nausea and vomiting. Anesth Analg 2003;97:62-71.

38. Apfel CC, Korttila K, Abdalla M, et al: A factorial trial of six interventions for the prevention of postoperative nausea and vomiting. N Engl J Med 2004;350:2441-2451.

39. Habib AS, Gan TJ: Evidence-based management of postoperative nausea and vomiting: A review. Can J Anaesth 2004;51:326-341.

40. Tang J, Wang B, White PF, et al: The effect of timing of ondansetron administration on its efficacy, cost-effectiveness, and cost-benefit as a prophylactic antiemetic in the ambulatory setting. Anesth Analg 1998;86:274-282.

41. Taylor AM, Rosen M, Diemunsch PA, et al: A double-blind, parallel-group, placebo-controlled, doe-ranging, multicenter study of intravenous granisetron in the treatment of postoperative nausea and vomiting in patients undergoing surgery with general anesthesia. J Clin Anesth 1997;9:658-663.

42. Chen X, Tang J, White PF, et al: The effect of timing of dolasetron administration on its efficacy as a prophylactic antiemetic in the ambulatory setting. Anesth Analg 2001;93:906-911.

43. Zarate E, Watcha MF, White PF, et al: A Comparison of the costs and efficacy of ondansetron versus dolasetron for antiemetic prophylaxis. Anesth Analg 2000;90:1352-1358.

44. Fischler M, Bonnet F, Trang H, et al: The pharmacokinetics of droperidol in anesthetized patients. Anesthesiology 1986;64:486-489.

45. FDA strengthens warnings for droperidol. Available at http://www.fda.gov/bbs/topics/ANSWERS/2001/ANS01123.html.

46. Kranke P, Morin AM, Roewer N, et al: The efficacy and safety of transdermal scopolamine for the prevention of postoperative nausea and vomiting: A quantitative systematic review. Anesth Analg 2002;95:133-143.

47. Kranke P, Morin AM, Roewer N, Eberhart LH: Dimenhydrinate for prophylaxis of postoperative nausea and vomiting: A meta-analysis of randomized controlled trials. Acta Anaesthesiol Scand 2002;46:238-244.

48. Perron G, Dolbec P, Germain J, Bechard P: Perineal pruritus after iv dexamethasone administration. Can J Anesth 2003;50:749-750.

49. Price ML, Walmsley A, Swaine C, Ponte J: Comparison of a total intravenous anaesthetic technique using a propofol infusion, with an inhalational technique using enflurane for day case surgery. Anaesthesia 1988;43:84-87.

50. Gan TJ, Glass PSA, Howell ST, et al. Determination of plasma concentrations of propofol associated with 50% reduction in postoperative nausea. Anesthesiology 1997;87:779-784.

51. Oddby-Muhrbeck E, Eksborg S, Bergendahl HT, et al: Effects of clonidine on postoperative nausea and vomiting in breast cancer surgery. Anesthesiology 2002;96:1109-1114.

52. Gan TJ, Apfel C, Kovac A, et al: The NK1 receptor antagonist aprepitant for prevention of postoperative nausea and vomiting. Anesthesiology 2005;A769.

53. Moretti EW, Robertson KM, El-Moalem H, Gan TJ: Intraoperative colloid administration reduces postoperative nausea and vomiting and improves postoperative outcomes compared with crystalloid administration. Anesth Analg 2003;96:611-617.

54. Lee A, Done ML: The use of nonpharmacologic techniques to prevent postoperative nausea and vomiting: A meta-analysis. Anesth Analg 1999;88:1362-1369.

55. Gan TJ, Jiao KR, Zenn M, Georgiade G: A randomized controlled comparison of electro-acupoint stimulation or ondansetron versus placebo for the prevention of postoperative nausea and vomiting. Anesth Analg 2004;99:1070-1075.

56. Moretti EW, Robertson KM, El-Moalem H, Gan TJ: Intraoperative colloid administration reduces postoperative nausea and vomiting and improves postoperative outcomes compared with crystalloid administration. Anesth Analg 2003;96:611–617.

57. Holte K, Kehlet H: Postoperative ileus: A preventable event. Br J Surg 2000: 87:1480-1493.

58. Livingston EH, Passaro EP: Postoperative Ileus. Digest Dis Soc 1990;35:121-132.

59. DeWinter BY, Boeckxstaens GE, DeMan JG, et al: Effect of adrenergic and nitrergic blockade on experimental ileus in rats. Br J Pharmacol 1997;120:464-468.

60. Tache Y, Monnikes H, Bonaz B, Rivier J: Role of CRF in stress related alterations of gastric and colonic motor function. Ann NY Acad Sci 1993;697:233-243.

61. Borody TJ, Quigley EM, Phillips EF, et al: Effects of morphine and atropine on motility and transit in the human ileum. Gastroenterology 1985;89:562-570.

62. Scheinin B, Lindgren L, Scheinin TM: Perioperative nitrous oxide delays bowel function after colonic surgery. Br J Anaesth 1990;64:154-158.

63. Colvin DB, Lee W, Eisenstat TE, et al: The role of nasointestinal intubation in elective colonic surgery. Dis Colon Rentum 1986;29:295-299.

64. Swank GM, Deitch EA: Role of the gut in multiple organ failure: Bacterial translocation and permeability changes. World J Surg 1996;20:411-417.

65. Heslin MJ, Latkany L, Leung D, et al: A prospective randomized trial of early enteral feeding after resection of upper gastrointestinal malignancy. Ann Surg 1997;226:567-577.

66. Gan TJ, Soppitt A, Maroof M, et al: Goal-directed intraoperative fluid administration reduces length of hospital stay after major surgery. Anesthesiology 2002;97:820-826.

67. Waldhausen JH, Schirmer BD: The effect on ambulation on recovery from postoperative ileus. Ann Surg 1990;212:671-677.

68. Kreis ME, Kasparek M, Zittel TT, et al: Neostigmine increases postoperative colonic motility in patients undergoing colorectal surgery. Surgery 2001;130:449-456.

69. Taguchi A, Sharma N, Saleem RM, et al: Selective postoperative inhibition of gastrointestinal opioid receptors. N Engl J Med 2001;345:935-940.

70. Viscusi E, Rathmell J, Fichera A, et al: A double-blind, randomized, placebo-controlled trial of methylnaltrexone (MNTX) for postoperative bowel dysfunction in segmental colectomy patients. Anesthesiology 2005;A893.

71. Kelly MC, Hocking MP, Marchand SD, et al: Ketorolac prevents postoperative small intestine ileus in rats. Am J Surg 19993;165:107-111.

72. Solomon SD, McMurray JJ, Pfeffer MA, et al: Cardiovascular risk associated with celecoxib in a clinical trial for colorectal adenoma prevention. N Engl J Med 2005;352:1071-1080.

73. Mamdani M, Rochon P, Juurlink DN, et al: Effect of selective cyclooxygenase 2 inhibitors and naproxen on short-term risk of acute myocardial infarction in the elderly. Arch Intern Med 2003;163:481-486.

74. Steinbrook RA: Epidural anesthesia and gastrointestinal motility. Anesth Analg 1998;86:837-844.

75. Shires T, Williams J, Brown F: Acute change in extracellular fluids associated with major surgical procedures. Ann Surg 1961;154:803-810.

76. Moore FD: Metabolic Care of the Surgical Patient. Philadelphia, WB Saunders, 1959.

77. Kern JW, Shoemaker WC: Meta-analysis of hemodynamic optimization in high-risk patients. Crit Care Med 2002;30:1686-1692.

78. Bland RD, Shoemaker WC, Abraham E, Cobo JC: Hemodynamic and oxygen transport patterns in surviving and nonsurviving postoperative patients. Crit Care Med 1985;13:85-90.

79. Moretti EW, Robertson KM, Gan TJ: The colloid crystalloid debate: Are we asking the right question? TATM 2003;5:378-391.

80. Mythen MG: Postoperative gastrointestinal tract dysfunction. Anesth Analg 2005;100:196-204.

Hematology and Coagulation

Chapter

26 Prevention and Management of Deep Vein Thrombosis and Pulmonary Embolism

Jagajan Karmacharya and Edward Y. Woo

The prevalence of deep vein thrombosis in the United States is about 500,000 patients per year. More than 50,000 deaths are the result of pulmonary embolism. Current data indicate that almost 300,000 venous thrombosis–related deaths occur in the United States each year. Approximately 10% of hospital deaths are caused by pulmonary embolism (Fig. 26-1). Approximately 1% of Medicare inpatients were discharged with a diagnosis of deep vein thrombosis or pulmonary embolism.

The economic cost of venous thrombosis is enormous and runs into billions of dollars. Adequate prophylactic measures could reduce this burden to the health-care system. A recent database of over 5000 patients indicated that less then 50% of the patients received deep vein thrombosis (DVT) prophylaxis within 1 month of the DVT diagnosis. Without any prophylaxis, about 50% to 60% of patients develop postoperative venous thrombosis, which could result in fatal pulmonary embolism (PE) or other chronic problems associated with post-thrombotic events, such as chronic venous insufficiency. Pulmonary embolism is often lethal, and 11% of symptomatic patients die within the first hour of onset of symptoms. Adequate anticoagulation and appropriate recognition can save more than 90% of the patients who survive this initial period. The majority of pulmonary emboli resolves over 30 days, but about 4% of patients develop chronic pulmonary hypertension within 2 years of diagnosis of the initial pulmonary event. This disabling condition carries a poor prognosis and is prevalent in patients with recurrent pulmonary embolic events. Chronic venous insufficiency develops in 30% to 50% of patients with diagnosed DVT. Furthermore, chronic leg swelling, discomfort, dermatitis, development of venous stasis ulcers, reduction in quality of life, and adverse socioeconomic effects are complications associated with the post-thrombotic state. Failure to prevent venous thromboembolism (VTE) results not only in a high incidence of such morbid conditions but also in long hospital stays, frequent readmissions, failure of anticoagulation, and recurrent thrombosis. Clearly, early recognition, appropriate prophylaxis, and institution of appropriate anticoagulation are important.

■ PATHOLOGY AND PATHOPHYSIOLOGY

In 1856, Rudolph Virchow suggested the mechanism of venous thrombosis. He recognized that pulmonary thrombi originate in the periphery. The three main reasons for venous thrombosis are hypercoagulability, presence of injured endothelium, and stasis. This constellation of predisposing factors is also known as Virchow's triad. The initial response to endothelial injury or stasis is aggregation of platelets, subsequent activation of procoagulants, and suppression of the fibrinolytic system. Hypercoagulability and stasis-inducing thrombosis usually start in the calf veins, specifically the soleal vein. Vessel manipulation and direct trauma to the vessels lead to direct endothelial injury and are thought to be at the center of thrombotic events. This process is evident in patients with vein compression from femoral or popliteal aneurysms, and after pelvic surgery and other orthopedic procedures. Early studies of postoperative patients demonstrated that DVT usually starts in the calf veins and does not propagate. However, in approximately 15% of patients, DVT occurs 3 weeks after surgery, particularly after hip replacement. The highest incidence of fatal PE is in patients with hip fracture. Approximately 13% of these patients sustain fatal PE. Autopsies of 1200 surgical patients in the United Kingdom who died during their hospital stay (within 1 month) after a surgical procedure indicated that PE was the cause of death in 29% of cases. Modern care in the intensive care unit (ICU), aging population of hospitalized patients, prevalence of advanced malignancy, many trauma patients with long

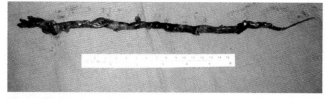

Figure 26-1 ■ Large pulmonary embolus removed from the right pulmonary artery.

26-1	**Risk Factors for Deep Vein Thrombosis and Pulmonary Embolism**

- Age greater than 40
- Congestive heart failure
- Familial and acquired hypercoagulable states
- Malignancy
- Major surgery
- Myocardial infarction
- Major fracture
- Obesity
- Prolonged immobility
- Paralysis
- Presence of indwelling femoral catheters
- Stroke
- Inflammatory bowel disease
- Estrogen use

stays in the ICU, and complex and extensive surgical procedures are some of the factors that might contribute to an even higher prevalence of VTE. However, failure of the calf muscle pump begins in the intraoperative period under anesthesia.

The known risk factors for DVT and PE include age greater then 40 years, prolonged immobility or paralysis, prior VTE, malignancy, major surgery, obesity, presence of varicose veins, congestive heart failure, myocardial infarction, stroke, major fractures, inflammatory bowel disease, nephritic syndrome, the use of estrogen, the presence of indwelling femoral catheters, and familial and acquired hypercoagulable states (Box 26-1). Familial hypercoagulable conditions include deficiencies of protein C, protein S, and various fibrinolytic factors such as antithrombin III. Other heritable conditions include mutations of clotting factors such as factor V Leiden. These patients are 10 times more likely to develop venous thrombosis than the general population. Factor V Leiden deficiency exists in both heterozygous and homozygous forms. The homozygous variant of factor V Leiden deficiency is associated with a very high incidence of venous thrombosis (80 times the incidence in the general population). Other genetic predisposing factors, such as prothrombin 20210A, non-O blood group, methylene tetrahydrofolate reductase 677T, or hyperhomocysteinemia, render certain patients more vulnerable to venous thrombosis. These conditions often become apparent during or after surgical intervention. Patients with antiphospholipid antibodies are 10 times more likely to develop venous thrombosis than patients without these antibodies. Other hematologic conditions that

are associated with VTE are thrombotic thrombocytopenia, hemolytic uremic syndrome, polycythemia vera, heparin-induced thrombocytopenia (HIT), and various myeloproliferative disorders.

Physiologic conditions such as pregnancy lead to a hypercoagulable state and, thus, are associated with DVT and its sequelae. The prevalence of venous thrombosis is greater during the puerperium. This relationship is related to hypercoagulability, hypofibrinolysis, platelet activation, venous smooth muscle relaxation, and venous compression. However, when sex differences are evaluated, men are more prone to develop recurrent DVT. Recurrent VTE after adequate treatment varies from 3% to 30%, depending on inherent risk factors and etiology. If the risk factor is reversible, the incidence of recurrence is 3% at 1 year after the venous thromboembolic event and 10% after 5 years. However, recurrent thromboembolism is higher if the etiology is unknown (10% at 1 year and 30% at 5 years). Patients who have had multiple traumas have a higher incidence of DVT. Sepsis and the presence of malignancy (3% to 20%) predispose patients to DVT. Obese patients also have a higher incidence of venous disease and subsequent VTE. The incidence of PE is higher after surgical interventions in these patients.

■ PREVENTION OF DEEP VEIN THROMBOSIS AND PULMONARY EMBOLISM

Prevention denotes avoiding or circumventing the situation by intervention in the form of diagnostic tests, by pharmacology, or by mechanical methodology. However, current diagnostic techniques are not widely adopted for screening because of their inherent limitations. Screening tools include fibrinogen-uptake testing, impedence plethysmography, contrast venography, and Doppler ultrasonography. Fibrinogen leg scanning is no longer used because of the risk of viral transmission and because of its lack of sensitivity and specificity for detecting DVT. Similarly, impedence plethysmography is no longer used because of its inability to detect asymptomatic DVT in high-risk patients. Contrast venography was the gold standard and was used widely in the initial trials that laid the foundation for today's approach to venous thromboprophylaxis, but this test is no longer routinely recommended because of its cost, the dye load, its limited availability, and patient discomfort. Further limitations include interobserver variability, the clinical relevance of the small thrombi it detects, and its high rate of incomplete and nondiagnostic results.

In recent large trials, Doppler ultrasound has gained popularity because of its high accuracy in detecting symptomatic DVT. Ultrasound is noninvasive and repeatable and includes Doppler flow analysis and B-mode scanning. The images are not highly specific or sensitive for detecting asymptomatic cases (20% to 70%). Nevertheless, it is very sensitive for detecting symptomatic cases. The sensitivity of color-flow duplex below the knee in acute symptomatic DVT is 93%. The ultrasonic findings that suggest an acute DVT are enlarged affected veins, lack of intraluminal echoes, and lack of significant collaterals. The most important finding consistent with DVT is lack of compressibility. In chronic

DVT, the veins are much smaller with intraluminal echoes, and they have developed significant collaterals (Fig. 26-2).

A scoring system can also be used to estimate the likelihood of estimating the presence of lower extremity DVT. The following factors are scored: presence of active cancer, paralysis, paresis, recent immobilization with a plaster cast, recent bedridden status, major surgery, localized tenderness along the distribution of the deep venous system, swelling of the entire leg, calf swelling at least 3 cm larger than the asymptomatic side, pitting edema confined to the symptomatic leg, and previously documented DVT. If the score is less than 2, the likelihood of DVT is low. Laboratory assessment of circulating D-dimer concentration for the assessment of PE is 96% to 98% accurate but with a specificity of only 39% to 52%. *This simple blood test can rule out with high sensitivity and specificity the presence of DVT.* The presence of PE can be detected with ventilation–perfusion (V/Q) scans in only a

third of patients with the disease. It is specific in only 10% of patients and sensitive in about 98%. A strong clinical suspicion with a high-probability finding in a V/Q scan increases the sensitivity. There is a growing body of evidence indicating the superiority of multidetector computed tomographic (CT) scanners to detect acute segmental and subsegmental PE (Fig. 26-3).

Current methods for the prevention of DVT and PE include the routine use of duplex imaging to screen all patients with multiple traumas, and the use of a combination of mechanical and pharmacologic techniques. Early ambulation and the use of pneumatic compression devices, unfractionated heparin, low-molecular-weight heparin, and Coumadin are well-tried methods for preventing venous thromboembolic events. Since the introduction of the Greenfield filter (Boston Scientific, Boston, Mass), prophylactic caval filters have gained increasing popularity for reducing

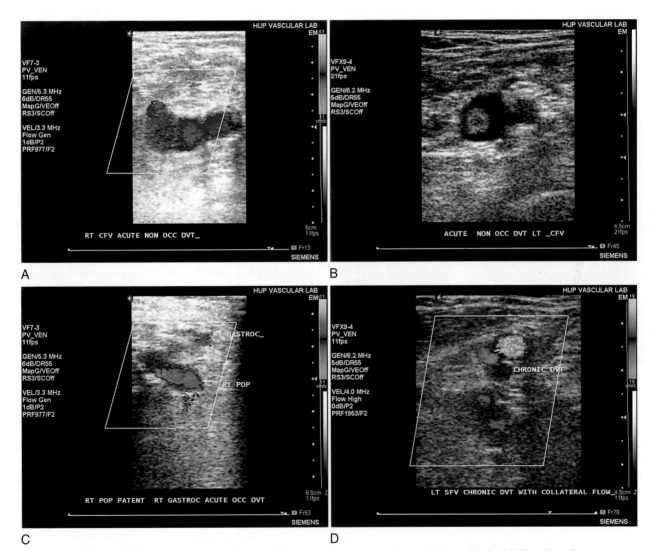

Figure 26-2 ■ **A, B,** Doppler ultrasound demonstrating an acute, deep vein thrombosis (DVT)-enlarged superficial femoral artery, lack of intraluminal echoes, and lack of significant collaterals. **C,** The most important finding consistent with acute DVT is lack of compressibility. **D,** In chronic DVT, the veins are much smaller; they have intraluminal echoes and significant collaterals.

fatal PE. Newer medications such as fondaparinux (a synthetic pentasaccharide) have increased our pharmacologic armamentarium to prevent venous embolic events. Oral heparin and a new oral low-molecular-weight heparin may be available in the near future.

The American College of Chest Physicians (ACCP) consensus guidelines on antithrombotic therapy categorize patients into low, moderate, high, and highest risk for DVT and recommend the appropriate type of prophylaxis. The patients with the lowest risk are those with no risk factors who are less than 40 years old and undergoing uncomplicated minor surgery. Patients at moderate risk include those between the ages of 40 and 60 years, and those less than 40 years old who are undergoing major surgery or minor surgery with additional risk factors. The patients in the high-risk category are those older than 60 years (with no additional risk factors) or 40 to 60 years of age undergoing major surgery (with additional risk factors). Patients at highest risk for DVT are older than 40 years and undergoing major surgery, with a prior history of VTE, malignancy, or a hypercoagulable state. Other highest-risk patients include those undergoing major lower extremity orthopedic procedures, and those with hip fractures, stroke, or multiple trauma or spinal cord injuries. General surgery patients have a 25% risk

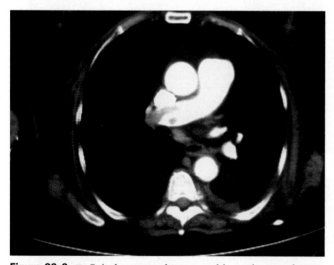

Figure 26-3 ■ Spiral computed tomographic angiogram demonstrating an acute pulmonary embolus in the right pulmonary artery.

of DVT without any prophylaxis, whereas the risk for DVT is as high as 60% in orthopedic surgery patients. Approximately a third of these thrombi are from the proximal deep veins, as mentioned earlier.

Mechanical methods of prevention of venous thrombosis include pneumatic compression devices (PCD) and stockings (TED). Mechanical venous thromboprophylaxis approaches work by increasing lower extremity blood flow and thus preventing venous stasis. It is also thought that natural fibrinolytic factors are enhanced by pneumatic compression. Although a reduction in DVT is seen with these devices, their ability to prevent PE is unknown. These devices are clearly indicated for all patients except low-risk patients, who should be treated by early ambulation only. Moderate-risk patients should be treated with any of the following: PCD, elastic stockings, low-dose heparin (5000 units twice a day), or low-molecular-weight heparin (LMWH, 3400 U daily). Unfractionated low-dose heparin binds antithrombin III and accelerates its effect on factors IIa, Xa, and IXa. It also functions by binding to von Willebrand factor. The dosage of 5000 U of low-dose unfractionated heparin should be given subcutaneously at least 2 hours before surgery and every 8 to 12 hours after the procedure until the patient is ambulating adequately. However, there is some risk of bleeding, especially with the preoperative dosing. Low-dose heparin has been shown to reduce the risk of DVT from 25% to 8% and to reduce fatal PE by 50% in several studies of general, gynecologic, and urologic surgical patients. Depolymerization and fractionation of standard heparin yields LMWH, which has been shown to reduce PE at about the same rate as standard heparin, with fewer bleeding complications. In addition, LMWH has better bioavailability, as heparin-binding proteins do not neutralize it. Low-dose heparin (5000 U three times a day), LMWH (3400 U daily), or PCD can be used for high-risk patients. However, a combination of PCD and either low-dose heparin (5000 U three times a day) or LMWH (3400 U daily) is recommended for highest-risk patients (Table 26-1). The use of aspirin alone is not recommended in surgery to prevent venous thrombosis. Warfarin is effective in the prevention of venous thromboembolism, but it is associated with a high risk of bleeding because of its long half-life. Many surgeons are very reluctant to use warfarin for this reason.

The risk of DVT is very high in neurosurgical patients as well as those with traumatic injuries to the spinal cord and pelvis. The combination of low-dose heparin (5000 U three

26-1	Venous Thromboembolic Prophylaxis: Current Recommendations	
Risk	**Surgical Status**	**Method of Prophylaxis**
Low	Minor surgery in patients <40 yr with no additional risk factors	Ambulation
Moderate	Minor surgery in patients with additional risk factors; non–major surgery in patients 40 to 60 yr with no additional risk factors; major surgery in patients <40 with no additional risk factors	LDH or LMWH or PCD or TED
High	Non–major surgery in patients >60 yr or with additional risk factors; major surgery in patients >40 yr with additional risk factors	LDH or LMWH or PCD
Highest	Major surgery in patients >40 yr plus prior venous thromboembolism, cancer, or hypercoagulable states; hip or knee replacement, hip fracture surgery; major trauma, spinal cord injury	LDH and PCD LMWH and PCD

LDH, low-dose heparin; LMWH low-molecular-weight heparin; PCD, pneumatic compression devices; TED, compression stockings.

times a day) or LMWH (3400 U daily) with PCD is recommended. If there are contraindications to the use of heparin, such as intracranial bleeding, paraspinal hematoma, ongoing bleeding, or coagulopathy, early placement of an inferior vena cava (IVC) filter is recommended.

■ MANAGEMENT OF VENOUS THROMBOSIS AND PULMONARY EMBOLISM

The diagnosis of DVT can be confirmed by phlebography, impedance plethysmography, radiolabeled fibrinogen scanning, magnetic resonance venography, duplex ultrasound imaging, or a handheld venous Doppler. Being aware of risk factors and being on the lookout for the signs and symptoms of DVT may prevent many fatal pulmonary emboli.

Once acute DVT is diagnosed, adequate anticoagulation is the standard of care (Fig. 26-4). The rate of recurrent thrombosis is 29% to 47%. If adequate anticoagulation is instituted, recurrent thrombosis falls to between 4.7% and 7.1%. The incidence of fatal PE after the diagnosis of DVT is 0.3% to 0.4% when patients are adequately anticoagulated with systemic heparin. The standard dose is an 80 U/kg intravenous bolus followed by continuous infusion of 18 U/kg/hr. Heparin activity against factor IIa is determined by measuring the activated partial thromboplastin (aPTT) time. A therapeutic level is achieved when the aPTT is 1.5 times to 2.5 times greater than normal. This level of anticoagulation should be maintained for 5 days or longer, followed by the gradual introduction of therapy with warfarin. Warfarin is a coumarin derivative and functions by inhibiting protein C, protein S, and the vitamin K–dependent coagulation factors II, VII, IX, and X. The use of warfarin alone without heparin is associated with a hypercoagulable state for the first 24 to 48 hours because of the depletion of factor VII and protein C. This effect is especially dangerous in patients with protein C deficiency, and cases of severe skin necrosis have been reported. Heparin should be discontinued once therapeutic levels of warfarin are achieved as reflected by measuring an International Normalized Ratio (INR) of 2 to 3. Warfarin should be continued for 6 months to a year after the first episode of DVT in the lower extremity. Recurrent events mandate evaluation for the presence of a hypercoagulable state and potentially lifelong anticoagulation. The risk of standard heparinization is bleeding (about 10% in reported series). Bleeding can lead to minor, major, or even fatal complications. Other important complications are heparin-associated thrombocytopenia, osteoporosis, and alopecia. There is also a need for intravenous administration and the need for frequent monitoring, as the biological half-life of heparin, which ranges from 30 minutes to 4 hours, is not linear, does not follow first-order kinetics, and is not dose dependent.

LMWH also has been shown in many trials to be an effective form of primary therapy for the management of DVT. LMWH has a better pharmacokinetic profile than standard unfractionated heparin. The half-life is not dose

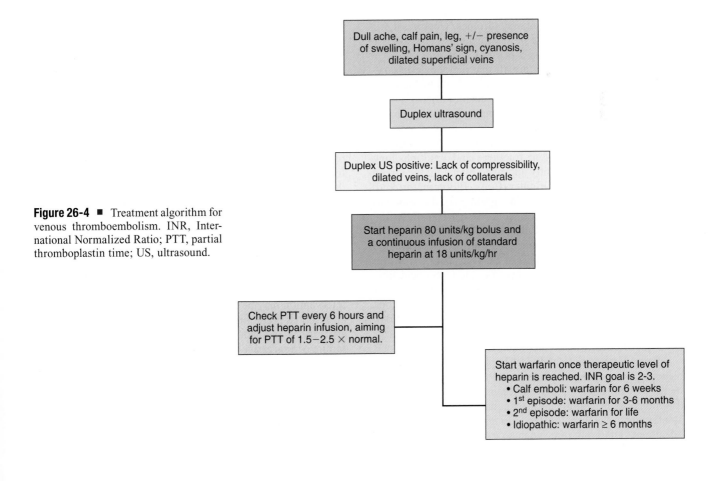

Figure 26-4 ■ Treatment algorithm for venous thromboembolism. INR, International Normalized Ratio; PTT, partial thromboplastin time; US, ultrasound.

dependent, and LMWH has less antiplatelet activity than conventional heparin. LMWH has more constant anti–factor Xa activity, less effect on protein C levels, less complement activation, and less inhibition of platelet aggregation. It can be administered subcutaneously and does not require frequent laboratory monitoring. LMWH, when compared with unfractionated heparin for the treatment of DVT, is associated with fewer hemorrhagic complications, and it is also effective for the treatment of VTE. Treatment with LMWH results in similar improvements for both symptomatic and asymptomatic cases of PE. The cost of outpatient treatment with LMWH in randomized trials is lower than the cost of unfractionated heparin for inpatients. LMWH is approved in the United States for acute DVT. The formulation that is approved is enoxaparin (Lovenox). The dosage is 1 mg/kg subcutaneously every 12 hours. Twice-daily administration of LMWH was compared with daily dosing in a study of over 1500 patients and there was no significant difference in recurrence, thrombus size, hemorrhagic events, or mortality. However, twice-daily dosing is recommended in obese patients and those with malignancy. Frequent monitoring may be necessary in patients with renal failure and in the morbidly obese.

Ambulation is very important after the treatment of VTE. Fear about early ambulation exists in many centers. The rate and severity of post-thrombotic syndrome after proximal DVT can be reduced by 50% by the use of compression stockings. Numerous studies have demonstrated that early ambulation with good compression does not increase the risk of PE, but it significantly decreases the incidence and severity of the post-thrombotic syndromes. Compression is required only up to the knee in most patients. The key is to reduce edema. Compression stockings that provide 30 to 40 mm Hg of ankle gradient are all that may be necessary.

Indications for placement of vena caval filters are failure of anticoagulation and contraindications for anticoagulation, including hemorrhage, thrombocytopenia, large free-floating thrombi, plans to undergo hip or knee replacement or gastric bypass surgery for morbid obesity, pregnancy, high-risk trauma with complex pelvic fractures and, multiple long-bone fractures. The currently approved filters are the Greenfield filter, the Gunther tulip filter (Cook, Bloomington, Ind), the Simon-Nitinol filter (Bard Covington, Ga), the Vena tech filter (B. Braun/VenaTech, Evanston, Ill), the Trap-Ease filter (Cordis, Europa N.V., L. J. Roden, The Netherlands), and the bird's nest filter (Cook, Bloomington, Ind). All these devices are effective for the prevention of PE (Fig. 26-5). However, the device with longest track record is the Greenfield filter. Temporary and retrievable filters are also available, and the currently approved ones are the Gunther Tulip filter (Cook, Bloomington, Ind), the Bard Recovery Nitinol filter (Bard Covington, Ga), and the Cordis Opteases (Cordis, Europa N.V., L. J. Roden, The Netherlands).

Immediate complications after placement of a filter are bleeding, device misplacement, and PE at the time of deployment. PE can occur if the device is deployed through the thrombus. This complication can be avoided by accurate assessment of the thrombus and cavography. Long-term complications, although rare, include caval thrombosis, filter

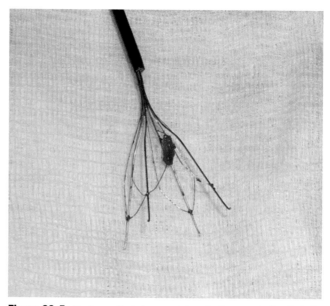

Figure 26-5 ■ A small clot was retrieved after prophylactic inferior vena cava (IVC) filter placement.

migration, device failure, strut fracture, and vessel penetration. The overall caval thrombosis rate after placement of a Greenfield filter is about 2% to 4%. This complication is treated with anticoagulation. Catheter-directed thrombolysis also may be indicated. Stents may be used to recanalize the IVC by pushing the filter against the wall.

Routine use of systemic thrombolytic therapy has no advantage over standard anticoagulation therapy for DVT. Indeed, the incidence of bleeding complications is higher. However, early thrombolysis in certain situations may be effective and is associated with fewer bleeding complications, and it may reduce the risk of post-thrombotic syndromes. Early catheter-directed thrombolysis (within 1 week) of massive iliofemoral DVT is very promising, with venous patency of 85% after 2 years. Catheter-directed thrombolysis for PE has been shown to reduce right heart strain and to decrease pulmonary hypertension and perfusion deficits in some patients. Tissue plasminogen activator and urokinase have also been used with similar results. However, the time required for the embolic obstruction to lyse may worsen the hemodynamically unstable patient with a massive PE. In these situations, careful fluid management; mechanical ventilation; use of inotropic agents such as dobutamine, isoprotenol, or, in some cases, inhaled nitric oxide; and operative intervention may be necessary. Bedside echocardiography is an essential prerequisite before taking the patient to the operating room. Indications for pulmonary embolectomy include failure of aggressive management, persistent hypoxemia, and persistent hypotension. Pulmonary embolectomy is associated with a high mortality (30%). This figure is even higher (70%) if cardiac arrest has occurred. An arrest before reaching the hospital and age greater than 80 years are significant factors in predicting mortality after pulmonary embolectomy.

■ SUGGESTED READINGS

1. Ageno W, Turpie AG: Low molecular weight heparin in the treatment of pulmonary embolism. Semin Vasc Surg 2000;13:189-193.
2. Aklog L, Williams, CS, Byrne JG, et al: Acute pulmonary embolectomy: A contemporary approach. Circulation 2002;105:1416-1419.
3. Bauer KA, Rosendaal FR, Heit JA: Hypercoagulability: Too many tests, too much conflicting data. Hematology 2002;1:353-368.
4. Bjarnason H, Kruse JR, Asinger DA, et al: Iliofemoral deep vein thrombosis: Safety and efficacy outcome during 5 years of catheter-directed thrombolytic therapy. J Vasc Interv Radiol 1997;8:405-418.
5. Geerts WH, Pineo GF, Heit JA, et al: Prevention of venous thromboembolism. The Seventh ACCP Conference on Antithrombotic and Thrombolytic Therapy. Chest 2004;126:338S-400.
6. Goldhaber SZ: Thrombolytic therapy in venous thromboembolism. Clin Chest Med 1995;16:307-320.
7. Greenfield LJ, Proctor MC: Recurrent thromboembolism in patients with vena caval filters. J Vasc Surg 2001;33:510-514.
8. Henke PK, Schmaier A, Wakefield TW: Thrombosis due to hypercoagulable states. In Rutherford RB (ed): Rutherfords Textbook of Vascular Surgery, ed 6. Philadelphia, Elsevier, 2004.
9. Hyers TM, Agnelli G, Hall RI, et al: Antithrombotic therapy for venous thromboembolic disease. Chest 2001;119:176S-193S.
10. Joshi A, Carr J, Chrisman H, et al: Filter-related, thrombolic occlusion of the inferior vena cava treated with a Gianturro stent. J Vasc Interv Radiol 2003;14:381-385.
11. Keraron C, Julian JA, Newman TE, et al: Noninvasive diagnosis of deep venous thrombosis. Ann Intern Med 1998;128:663-677.
12. Levine MN, Raskob G, Landerfelod S, et al: Hemorrhagic complications of anticoagulant treatment. Chest 1998;114:511S-523.
13. Lindblad B, Eriksson A, Bergqvist D: Autopsy verified pulmonary embolism in surgical department: analysis of the period 1951 to 1968. Br J Surg 1991;78:849-852.
14. Rectenwald JE, Wakefield TW: Prophylaxis for deep venous thrombosis. In Zelenock GB, Huber TS, Messina LM (eds): Mastery of Vascular and Endovascular Surgery. Lippincott Williams & Wilkins, Philadelphia, 2006, pp 527-537.
15. Ridker PM, Goldhaber SZ, Danielson E, et al: Long-term, low-intensity warfarin therapy for the prevention of recurrent venous thromboembolism. N Engl J Med 2003l;348:1425-1434.
16. Wakefield TW, Henke PK: Complications of venous disease and therapy. In Mulholland MW, Doherty GA (eds): Lippincott Williams & Wilkins, 2006, pp 337-356.

27 Perioperative Management of Bleeding and Transfusion

Steven E. Hill and Richard C. D'Alonzo

Transfusion therapy is necessary and can be lifesaving in some surgical patients. However, despite being the standard of care for blood loss and anemia, it has never undergone the rigorous, randomized testing required of a new therapeutic agent, including assessment of adverse events and risk assessment. Since the outbreak of acquired immunodeficiency syndrome (AIDS) in the 1980s, it has become apparent that the full extent of the risk of allogeneic transfusion therapy is unknown. More recently, the British National CJD Surveillance Unit identified 48 individuals who received a blood component from 15 donors who later developed variant Creutzfeldt-Jakob disease (vCJD).[3] One of these individuals developed symptoms 6.5 years after a transfusion of packed red blood cells (PRBCs) from an asymptomatic donor and died of vCJD in December 2003. Considering these risks, it becomes apparent that alternatives to transfusion must be developed in combination with blood conservation measures. The goal of these measures should be to limit transfusion to clinical scenarios in which allogeneic blood product administration is clearly necessary to maintain adequate oxygen delivery and reduce mortality.

■ HISTORY OF TRANSFUSION

Transfusion therapy was not a viable option for patient care prior to the 20th century. Before the discovery of the major blood group antigens on the surface of red blood cells, recipients of allogeneic blood transfusions were at high risk for rapid hemolytic transfusion reactions and rapid death. In 1901, Karl Landsteiner described the basic human blood groups, which were later named A, B, and O, and was awarded the Nobel Prize for physiology and medicine in 1930.[4,5] During World War I, the British military developed the first human blood depot in which phlebotomized blood was stored with anticoagulant at refrigerated temperatures. However, transfusion therapy was not practical until after World War I, largely because of the logistical problems associated with delivering adequately stored, anticoagulated, and compatible blood to patients on the battlefield.

Specialized blood donor services first evolved in the 1920s, and in 1937, Bernard Fantus coined the phrase *blood bank* when he established the first United States unit at Cook County Hospital in Chicago. In 1940, with the development of cold ethanol fractionation by Ethan Cohn, albumin, gamma globulin, and fibrinogen became available for clinical use. By the start of World War II, delivery of blood and blood products to military hospitals was a reality. After World War II, use of transfusion therapy became widespread as the Red Cross introduced the first nationwide civilian blood program, which now supplies nearly 50% of the blood and blood products in the United States. Additionally, the American Association of Blood Banks (AABB) was formed to promote common goals among blood-banking practitioners and the blood-donating public by providing quality control and maximizing distribution.[6]

The unintended consequence of widespread enthusiasm for saving lives with the dramatic option of transfusion was that it quickly became the standard of care for a myriad of situations. In fact, transfusion therapy became indicated for a wide variety of disease states that involved acute or chronic anemia, without being tested with any scientific rigor. The treatment of acute exsanguination with replacement of a portion of the lost blood volume by compatible allogeneic blood undoubtedly saves lives in traumatic injury and high-blood-loss surgery. On the other hand, the indiscriminate administration of transfusion therapy, which is a biologically active and complex therapy, in situations that have never been studied in a randomized and controlled fashion very likely results in harm to patients through known and unknown risks that are only now undergoing investigation. Not until patient groups, most notably the Jehovah's Witnesses Church, refused transfusion therapy was the ability to tolerate, and recover from, severe anemia widely appreciated. These patients, along with the realization of the lay public that AIDS could be contracted from blood transfusion, caused the medical profession to take a critical look at longstanding practices and realize that the true risk of transfusion as a standard-of-care treatment was not completely known.

Blood banking has enjoyed great success in minimizing the risk of transmitting diseases and agents such as human immunodeficiency virus (HIV), hepatitis B, and hepatitis C. However, identification of the infectious agent responsible for the AIDS epidemic that began in the 1980s took several years. Retrospective testing of donors in 1984 and 1985 revealed an incidence of 16 cases of donor HIV infection per 10,000 donations prior to the development of the anti-HIV-1 enzyme-linked immunosorbent assay (ELISA), with a subsequent disease transmission rate of 90%.[7,8] The most dangerous infectious agent in the blood supply is the next one. This point emphasizes the need to develop discriminating transfusion practice and eliminate unnecessary blood product administration to patients who would tolerate anemia or respond to an agent other than allogeneic blood. According to Goodnough and Despotis, even after development of widely accepted transfusion guidelines by the American College of American Pathologists in 1994[9] and the American Society of Anesthesiologists (ASA) in 1996,[10] unnecessary transfusion still occurred in up to 50% of cases of cardiac surgery.[11] The development of evidence-based protocols for targeted transfusion therapy with the support of point-of-care testing and reproducible clinical assessment promises to benefit future patients and clinicians. Administration of a therapy with risk, but with unknown benefit, in many cases is clearly a situation to avoid. The goal of modern transfusion therapy is to reliably identify the patient who would benefit from a transfusion in spite of the risk. Through a multidisciplinary effort combining basic science and clinical research, that goal should be attainable.

PREOPERATIVE ASSESSMENT OF BLEEDING RISK

Common Disease States Associated with Excessive Bleeding

Hepatic Insufficiency

Patients with hepatic failure have an increased risk for perioperative hemorrhage due to factor deficiency and portal venous obstruction. In the event of portal venous obstruction, development of esophageal varices and potential venous engorgement around the operative field can produce enhanced blood loss. Deficiencies of liver-dependent factors, including factors II, VII, IX, and X, result in a coagulopathy most frequently characterized by prolongation of the prothrombin time (PT). Vitamin K may be indicated in the preoperative period if malnutrition is a component of the coagulopathy in a patient with liver failure. On the other hand, factor deficiency due to inadequate hepatic synthesis is likely to be unresponsive to vitamin K, and direct repletion of clotting factors with fresh-frozen plasma (FFP) or pooled factor concentrates may be necessary to prevent life-threatening hemorrhage. In this case, the goal of therapy is to achieve a prothrombin time of 1.2 times normal.

Accelerated fibrinolysis probably also plays a role in the coagulopathy seen in patients with liver failure. This acceleration is evidenced by D-dimer levels that are normal or slightly elevated in severe liver disease. One mechanism for the increased fibrinolysis in patients with chronic liver failure is the reduced clearance of tissue plasminogen activator (t-PA).[12] Another potential mechanism is related to decreased synthesis of hepatic regulating plasma proteins. For example, alpha-2-antiplasmin is a hepatically synthesized enzyme[13] that may be deficient in liver failure and, when deficient, may result in increased plasmin activity.[14] Alpha-2-antiplasmin inhibits plasmin-mediated fibrinolysis by rapidly inactivating circulating plasmin and by crosslinking to fibrin, making clots that are resistant to plasmin degradation. Although plasminogen (the precursor to plasmin) and alpha-2-antiplasmin are both synthesized in the liver, alpha-2-antiplasmin is present in lower concentrations than plasminogen and may

be depleted even when plasminogen is not. Another liver-synthesized molecule, fibrinogen, may also become depleted in liver failure and may merit measurement.[15,16] However, pure fibrinogen deficiency is uncommon.

Factor VIII is not made in the liver and is present in normal to high levels in liver disease. Because cryoprecipitate contains predominately factor VIII, von Willebrand factor (vWF), and fibrinogen, but not factor VII, administration of this product is not indicated in hepatic failure, and fresh-frozen plasma is the blood product component of choice. Large doses of FFP (6 to 8 units) are frequently required to adequately reverse the coagulopathy associated with liver failure. Platelet count is often low in liver failure, as a result of either splenic sequestration or increased consumption. Measures of platelet count and function may be useful to guide platelet transfusion therapy in this setting. Although no randomized controlled trials are yet available to test the efficacy of activated factor VII in the setting of acute hemorrhage and liver failure, some reports suggest that this agent may prove beneficial.[17,18]

Renal Failure

The most common blood clotting abnormality in uremic renal failure is platelet dysfunction. The defect is a function of uremia and is not intrinsic to the platelets. Therefore, transfusion of allogeneic platelets is not indicated except for patients with documented low platelet counts. Primary treatment for uremic platelet dysfunction is treatment of the underlying renal failure, with dialysis if necessary. Desmopressin (DDAVP; 1-deamino-8-D-arginine vasopressin) may help platelet function by stimulating endothelial cell release of vWF.[167] A one-time dose of 0.3 μg/kg delivered intravenously may be indicated to help offset life-threatening hemorrhage while efforts are made to correct the underlying uremia.[21] However, lack of prospective, randomized evidence for safety and efficacy limits recommendation for this mode of treatment.

Clotting Factor Deficiency

Deficiency of individual clotting factors can be the result of inherited defects such as those found in hemophilia A (factor VIII) and hemophilia B (factor IX). Deficiency can also result from acquired deficiencies, such as the abnormal platelet consumption occasionally observed in patients after cardiopulmonary bypass. A history of excessive bleeding with prior surgical or dental procedures or development of hemarthrosis should raise awareness of a possible bleeding diathesis. Often, screening tests such as partial thromboplastin time (PTT) can identify factor deficiencies in the intrinsic arm of the coagulation cascade (factors VIII and IX) and alert practitioners to perioperative risk for bleeding. In the case of cardiopulmonary bypass, measured levels of factor activity decrease because of contact activation of the clotting cascade, with a resulting consumption of multiple factors. After cardiopulmonary bypass, elevation of prothrombin time is common and is not predictive of postoperative bleeding unless severely elevated (>1.5 times normal).

Treatment of specific clotting factor deficiencies requires identification and replacement of the missing factors. Both factor VIII and IX are available as recombinant products that are effective but expensive. In general, more than 40% of normal clotting factor activity is required to prevent bleeding, and higher levels may be necessary to stop active bleeding.[22] Recently, recombinant activated factor VII has been approved for use in life-threatening hemorrhage in patients with hemophilia who have developed inhibitors against factor VIII or factor IX.[17] Use of this product bypasses the factor VIII pathway by stimulating the final common pathway directly, thereby initiating clot formation. The recommended dosage is 90 μg/kg administered every 2 hours until bleeding ceases. Although effective in this clinical setting, case reports suggest that activated factor VII may also help treat non-hemophilic bleeding that is refractory to transfusion of FFP. In theory, the use of activated factor VII should help in refractory hemorrhage, but the effectiveness of its use and its potential risk for hypercoagulability have not been studied in randomized, controlled clinical trials. Furthermore, the cost of this therapy can be extreme.[19] Currently, it costs $0.83 per unit, with 90 units required per kilogram (more than $5000 for a 70-kg patient).

Patients with vitamin K deficiency or those who have experienced a warfarin overdose usually respond to vitamin K administration within 12 to 24 hours. Intramuscular, subcutaneous, or intravenous administration of 10 mg of vitamin K often corrects the prothrombin time to an International Normalized Ratio (INR) of less than 1.3. Smaller doses of 1 to 2 mg allow partial correction in the absence of active bleeding for patients who need reinstitution of warfarin. Acute treatment of life-threatening hemorrhage from vitamin K deficiency or warfarin overdose may be treated with FFP, but 6 to 8 units are frequently required to slow active bleeding. Factor IX complex, also called prothrombin complex concentrate, is also available. This solution contains vitamin K clotting factors, including factors II, VII, and X, and proteins C and S, in addition to factor IX. Prothrombin complex concentrate is first isolated from pooled plasma and then filtered and heat treated to reduce the risk of infectious transmission to negligible levels. Unlike activated factor VII, prothrombin complex solutions are not yet available as a recombinant product.

When treating the coagulopathy initiated by cardiopulmonary bypass, it is necessary to differentiate between a clotting factor deficiency and a platelet defect caused by decreased platelet count or function. Traditional screening tests such as PT and PTT that are commonly used to screen for bleeding diatheses in the preoperative setting are less useful in the postoperative cardiac surgical patient. The PT and PTT tests require too much time to process, and there is a lack of correlation between test abnormalities and clinical bleeding. A more rapid, point-of-care coagulation test is required that targets therapy to a specific deficiency.[11] For example, the use of a protocol involving thromboelastography to guide postoperative therapy for bleeding after cardiopulmonary bypass effectively limits unnecessary transfusion and decreases costs without an adverse effect on clinical outcome.[2] Incorporation of a stepwise, evidence-based transfusion protocol with rapid feedback for clinicians promises to improve patient outcome while decreasing cost.

Platelet Deficiency

Deficiency of platelet number or function has multiple potential etiologies, many of which require interventions other than transfusion. Primary bone marrow failure or drug-induced bone marrow suppression can cause a deficiency in platelet production. Conversely, immune-mediated mechanisms, mechanical destruction, or drugs can cause a deficiency due to increased platelet consumption. Idiopathic thrombocytopenic purpura (ITP) is caused by presence of a platelet antibody of unknown etiology. This condition does not respond well to transfusion and is treated with steroids and/or large doses of intravenous immune globulin when there is life-threatening bleeding. Patients with chronic ITP may be treated with immune suppression or splenectomy. Thrombotic thrombocytopenic purpura (TTP) is a syndrome characterized by a pentad of fever, thrombocytopenia, microangiopathic hemolytic anemia, central nervous system dysfunction, and renal failure. TTP is most likely the result of an inborn or acquired deficiency of a plasma protease that normally cleaves vWF multimers.[20] Presumably, when vWF multimers are not cleaved they promote spontaneous aggregation of platelets in the circulation, producing thrombi rich in platelets and vWF, with a resultant consumptive deficiency. Patients with TTP usually maintain a normal fibrinogen level and a normal disseminated intravascular coagulation (DIC) screen. In fact, TTP is characterized by thrombi that are rich in platelets and vWF but low in fibrin and fibrinogen content.[23] This condition must be treated aggressively with plasmapheresis or plasma exchange: patients have an 80% chance of survival if treated early and aggressively. Awareness and identification of this condition in the perioperative period is essential, given the increased usage of drugs known to be offending agents. Important drugs that can cause acquired TTP include ticlopidine, quinine, clopidogrel, and calcineurin inhibitors such as cyclosporine A.

In addition to the disruptive processing of vWF seen with TTP, deficient production and function of vWF, as seen with von Willebrand disease (vWD), also lead to excessive bleeding perioperatively. Although not an intrinsic platelet disorder, vWD leads to a reduction in the adhesion and aggregation of platelets. This condition is frequently diagnosed in patients with a history of abnormal bleeding associated with surgical and dental procedures, who often present with an elevated PTT. Appropriate therapy of this condition requires identification of the disease type through an activity assay in conjunction with input from a hematology specialist. Patients with type 1 vWD are most effectively treated by the administration of DDAVP in a dose of 0.3 μg/kg.[24] This therapy is most useful in patients who have vWF that is stored and can be released. Other types of vWD respond to administration of cryoprecipitate (not FFP) that is rich in vWF. The large volume of FFP required to correct the bleeding problems in patients with vWD severely limits its use. Cryoprecipitate is rich in the "labile" clotting factors VIII, XIII, and vWF. It is also a concentrated source of fibrinogen for patients with fibrinogen deficiency who are unable to tolerate large volumes of fresh-frozen plasma. Cryoprecipitate is prepared by flash-freezing plasma and thawing it at 1° to 6° C. The cold insoluble portion of the thawed plasma is expressed off the top, collected into separate collection bags, and refrozen to become the cryoprecipitate product.

Heparin-induced thrombocytopenia (HIT) is a spectrum of diseases resulting from the formation of antiplatelet antibodies in response to prolonged heparin therapy. Mild thrombocytopenia develops in 10% of patients on heparin in the first 2 to 5 days and is usually self-limited. Life-threatening HIT occurs with prolonged therapy or with reexposure in 1% to 2% of hospitalized patients on heparin. It is characterized by bleeding associated with a low platelet count or "white clot" thrombosis caused by abnormal platelet aggregation. Bovine heparin is reported to be associated with a higher rate of HIT than porcine heparin. Because of the frequency with which heparin is used in the hospitalized patient population, vigilance for the formation of this potentially lethal adverse drug reaction must be maintained. Diagnosis is made by the detection of antiplatelet antibodies or the abnormal aggregation of platelets in response to heparin exposure.[25] Because these tests are relatively insensitive and frequently not immediately available, initiation of therapy may need to proceed on the basis of clinical suspicion while awaiting definitive diagnosis. If HIT is suspected, heparin therapy must be discontinued and other agents used for anticoagulation.[26] Direct thrombin inhibitors, including argatroban and lepirudin, are acceptable alternatives to heparin therapy but lack the safety benefit of reversibility with protamine. Bivalirudin, also a direct thrombin inhibitor, has been successfully used for patients with HIT on cardiopulmonary bypass. However, because no reversal agent exists for bivalirudin, postoperative bleeding after cardiac surgery is frequently excessive until the bivalirudin is cleared. For patients with a vague history of heparin-induced thrombocytopenia without life-threatening bleeding or thrombotic complications, the use of heparin for anticoagulation during cardiopulmonary bypass may still be the safest therapy. If antiplatelet antibody titers are not detectable with screening, bolus-dose heparin therapy prior to bypass with prompt reversal at the end of bypass may be indicated. The advice of a consulting hematologist is recommended to assist with the risk-to-benefit analysis of short-term heparin exposure in a patient with a history of HIT. Low-molecular-weight heparin can also stimulate antiplatelet antibodies and should not be used for patients with suspicion of HIT. If long-term anticoagulation is required for a patient with HIT, administration of therapeutic warfarin therapy is recommended. However, warfarin should be started and adjusted to therapeutic levels while other forms of anticoagulation are in place and already at therapeutic levels. Warfarin has the potential to inhibit production of the antithrombotic, vitamin K–dependent factors protein C and protein S prior to therapeutic depression of factors II, VII, IX, and X.

Drug-Induced Clotting Deficiency

Increased interest in alternatives to traditional medical therapy with dietary supplements has created the potential for unanticipated perioperative hemostatic defects. Some herbal remedies such as garlic, ginseng, and ginkgo biloba possess anticoagulant activity that could prove problematic in the perioperative period.[27-29] Herbal remedies are often not considered to be drugs by the patient and may not be volunteered when a list of current medications is requested. A careful history of all medications and dietary supplements consumed is necessary to identify these agents. Recent practice guidelines announced by the American Society of Anesthesiologists recommend that patients should be advised that certain supplements could potentially influence the need for transfusion perioperatively.[1] Specific agents listed in these guidelines include agents that decrease platelet aggregation such as bilberry, bromelain, don quoi, feverfew, fish oil, flaxseed oil, garlic, ginger, ginkgo biloba, grape seed extract, and saw palmetto. Additional herbs and vitamins that inhibit clotting include chamomile, dandelion root, dong quoi, horse chestnut, vitamin K, and vitamin E. Our institution recommends that these agents should be discontinued at least 2 days prior to surgery to help eliminate their adverse effects on clotting.

The advent of therapeutic agents to prevent pathologic blood clot formation in the setting of coronary artery and peripheral vascular disease has significantly improved outcome in the settings of cardiac and cerebrovascular ischemia. The beneficial effect of drugs such as aspirin and clopidogrel for coronary artery disease and aspirin/dipyridamole for stroke prevention has been validated in randomized, controlled trials.[26,30,31] Although these medications should be discontinued for as brief a time as possible in the perioperative period, they do increase perioperative bleeding, and the benefit of therapy must be weighed against the risk for incomplete hemostasis for each patient and procedure.

Aspirin

Aspirin (salicylic acid) is an irreversible inhibitor of platelet cyclooxygenase-1 (COX-1). Inhibition of COX-1 prevents the transformation of arachidonic acid to the platelet-aggregating substance thromboxane A_2[31] (Fig. 27-1). The effect persists for the life of the platelet, resulting in an effective duration of action of 7 to 10 days. Aspirin therapy clearly benefits the treatment of acute myocardial ischemia and prevention of recurrent myocardial infarction.[26,32] Alone, and in combination with dipyridamole (Aggrenox), aspirin reduces the incidence of stroke for patients with transient ischemic attacks.[33] Although aspirin does increase bleeding after coronary artery bypass surgery,[34,35] the effect is mild, and the beneficial antiplatelet effect of aspirin for maintenance of graft patency in the perioperative period[36-39] generally outweighs the risk for clinically significant hemorrhage caused by this agent.[40] Effective intraoperative hemostasis can overcome the clotting defect caused by aspirin. When the theoretical risk for epidural hematoma formation was studied in patients undergoing epidural catheter placement, continued aspirin therapy was not found to be associated with significant adverse outcome.[41] Therefore, aspirin therapy should generally be continued throughout the perioperative period. If the patient is at risk for life-threatening perioperative hemorrhage, such as in cardiac surgery, reduction of the aspirin dosage to 81 mg/day should be considered 7 to 10 days prior to surgery. Once hemostasis is ensured postoperatively, the dosage should again be increased to 325 mg daily.

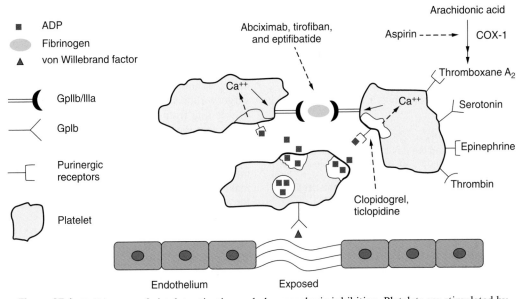

Figure 27-1 ■ Diagram of platelet activation and pharmacologic inhibition. Platelets are stimulated by agents such as epinephrine, serotonin, thrombin, exposed collagen, and thromboxane A_2 to release calcium and adenosine diphosphate (ADP), which stimulate glycoprotein (Gp) IIb/IIIa activity. GpIIb/IIIa receptors bind to fibrinogen and are essential to formation of a platelet plug at the site of a breach in vessel wall integrity. GpIIb/IIIa receptor activity can be inhibited by the use of noncompetitive and competitive receptor antagonists (abciximab, tirofiban, and eptifibatide). Platelet ADP-receptor inhibitors (clopidogrel, ticlopidine) also reduce activation of GpIIb/IIIa receptors. Aspirin, an irreversible inhibitor of platelet cyclooxygenase-1 (COX-1), prevents the transformation of arachidonic acid to the platelet-aggregating substance, thromboxane A_2. (Adapted from Bayer Pharmaceutical Corporation database.)

Glycoprotein IIb/IIIa Inhibitors

Glycoprotein (GP) IIb/IIIa is a platelet surface receptor essential to formation of a platelet plug at the site of a breach in vessel wall integrity (see Fig. 27-1). This integrin family receptor is the "final common pathway" of platelet aggregation. Expression and activation of this receptor on the cell surface of circulating platelets enables platelet binding of fibrinogen and other proteins found in a developing clot.[42] Lack of expression or inhibition of glycoprotein IIb/IIIa prevents platelet-to-platelet binding. Without proper platelet binding, weak or nonfunctional clots form at areas of vessel trauma and lead to bleeding. Therapeutic applications of these agents vary depending on persistence of effect and the clinical scenario.

Noncompetitive Glycoprotein IIb/IIIa Inhibition. Abciximab is a noncompetitive inhibitor of glycoprotein IIb/IIIa that forms a high-avidity bond to the receptor for the life of the platelet. Abciximab-bound platelets become ineffective, and regeneration of new platelets is required before the prolonged bleeding time returns to baseline. Abciximab has a plasma elimination half-life of approximately 30 minutes, but the half-life is highly variable from patient to patient. Abciximab is also highly protein bound and has a strong affinity to the GP IIb/IIIa receptor. Because of its high affinity to the receptor, it has a prolonged antiplatelet effect, leading to a gradual recovery of platelet function over 24 to 48 hours after discontinuation of the medication. The stoichiometry for abciximab is approximately one and a half molecules of drug to every molecule of GP IIb/IIIa integrin. Its use is generally restricted to the cardiac catheterization laboratory in conjunction with angioplasty procedures with or without stent placement.[43,44] If a patient requires emergent surgery after receiving therapeutic doses of abciximab (0.15 to 0.3 mg/kg), bleeding should be anticipated and can be life-threatening. If possible, major surgery should be delayed at least 24 hours to allow clearance of unbound drug from the plasma and recovery of platelet function (Box 27-1). It has been demonstrated that, because the drug is a noncompetitive inhibitor and does not persist in excess in the plasma space, infusion of allogeneic platelets can reverse the pharmacologic effect of abciximab and halt hemorrhage caused by this agent.[45,46] Although abciximab is tightly bound to the IIb/IIIa integrin, secondary redistribution may occur and can result in delayed "re-inhibition" of platelet aggregation several hours after platelet transfusion. This re-inhibition may necessitate additional platelet transfusion if recurrent hemorrhage occurs. With the advent of shorter-acting competitive inhibitors of GP IIb/IIIa, use of abciximab is less common.

Competitive Glycoprotein IIb/IIIa Inhibition. Eptifibatide and tirofiban are concentration dependent, competitive inhibitors of GP IIb/IIIa that produce profound inhibition of platelet aggregation. These agents have a rapid onset and a relatively short duration of action (6 to 8 hours) after discontinuation compared with abciximab. Because of these properties, they are now widely used to augment heparin and aspirin therapy in the setting of acute coronary syndrome. Furthermore, they are used to prevent acute occlusion after angioplasty with or without stent placement, especially when

---

27-1 | **Guidelines for the Pharmacologic Management of Patients Awaiting Coronary Artery Bypass Graft Surgery**

Recommendations should consider patient-specific issues (e.g., indications, allergies, sensitivities, presence of thrombocytopenia, overall health status, contraindications) in the administration of these agents.

Oral Antiplatelet Agents

- Aspirin: 81 mg daily, including the day of surgery. The dosage should be reduced to 81 mg daily as early as possible before surgery.
- Ticlopidine: None before diagnostic cardiac catheterization; discontinue at least 5 days before the day of surgery.
- Clopidogrel: None before diagnostic cardiac catheterization; discontinue for at least 5 days before the day of surgery.
- Aspirin with dipyridamole: Continue therapy, including the day of surgery.

Platelet Glycoprotein IIb/IIIa Receptor (Integrin) Blockers

- Abciximab: Discontinue ReoPro more than 24 hours before induction.
- Eptifibatide: Discontinue at 4 hours before induction.
- Tirofiban: Discontinue at 4 hours before induction.

Antithrombins

- Heparin: When indicated, continue heparin by IV infusion up through induction.
- Enoxaparin: Discontinue more than 12 hours before induction; administer unfractionated heparin for pump run.
- Bivalirudin: Continue through induction; request coagulation consult to assist with perioperative management.
- Argatroban, hirudin, heparinoid: Request coagulation consult to assist with perioperative management.

Miscellaneous Agents

- Herbal supplements: Discontinue 2 days before the day of surgery.
- Vitamins (vitamin E): Discontinue 2 days before the day of surgery.
- Glucophage: Discontinue 2 days before the day of surgery.

---

emergent surgical intervention may be required. Use of these drugs has been demonstrated to be efficacious for prevention of reocclusion after interventional treatment of a thrombosed coronary artery.[47,48] At therapeutic concentrations, more than 100 molecules of the drug are present for every molecule of GP IIb/IIIa integrin; hence, platelet transfusion does *not* reverse the pharmacologic effect of these agents. Allogeneic platelet transfusion results only in the inhibition of both transfused and native platelets. Although eptifibatide and tirofiban are primarily cleared via renal mechanisms and can dialyze across membranes, there is no practical way to reverse their effect other than by discontinuation. Because the elimination half-life of both of these agents is approximately 2 to 2.5 hours, their clinical effect should subside within 4 to 8 hours, with platelet function returning to normal. Dialysis may be indicated in patients with bleeding and renal failure because of the inability of their kidneys to eliminate these antiplatelet medications.

Although reversible only with elimination, eptifibatide and tirofiban may prove beneficial in cardiac surgical patients, and they certainly provide a desirable alternative to abciximab in this patient group. Because the platelet inhibition effect persists for only up to 8 hours, discontinuation of these drugs 4 hours before induction of anesthesia for cardiac surgery allows platelets to recover function around the time of weaning from cardiopulmonary bypass. In fact, evidence exists that the presence of eptifibatide in the plasma during cardiopulmonary bypass actually protects the platelet from activation in the bypass circuit and reduces the thrombasthenia associated with cardiac surgery.[49,50] This protective action makes these the preferred agents, along with heparin therapy, for acute coronary syndrome if emergent cardiac surgery is possible.

Platelet ADP-Receptor Inhibitors

Thienopyridines are oral agents capable of irreversible platelet inhibition. Clopidogrel and ticlopidine are the drugs in this class originally approved for oral prophylaxis against arterial thrombosis. Because of concerns related to severe neutropenia with ticlopidine, clopidogrel has emerged as the agent used in combination with aspirin to prevent recurrent coronary artery thrombosis.[51] The use of clopidogrel is becoming increasingly common in an aging population susceptible to coronary artery disease, cerebral vascular disease, and peripheral vascular disease.[52] The beneficial effect of clopidogrel on reducing mortality and morbidity has been proven in randomized, controlled clinical trials to treat patients in many situations such as coronary stenting,[53-57] therapy for myocardial infarction with ST-segment elevation,[58] and non-ST-elevation acute coronary syndrome.[59] Guidelines by the American College of Cardiology (ACC) and the American Heart Association (AHA) recommend 75 mg/day of therapy for 1 month after bare stent implantation, for 3 to 6 months after drug-eluting stent implantation, and for up to 12 months for patients who are not at high risk for bleeding.[60,61] Although of proven benefit, these agents pose a significant risk for perioperative hemorrhage in the surgical patient.[62,63] The thienopyridines are more potent than aspirin in inhibiting platelet function. They work by irreversibly modifying and deactivating the low-affinity platelet type 2 adenosine diphosphate (ADP) receptor, thereby inhibiting activation of the GP IIb/IIIa complex[30] (see Fig. 27-1). The onset of biological activity is within a few hours of treatment, but maximal inhibition requires approximately 5 days of therapy. At steady state (75 mg/day of clopidogrel by mouth), the thienopyridines produce 40% to 60% inhibition of platelet aggregation and extend the bleeding time approximately twofold. The antiplatelet activity of the thienopyridines lasts for 7 to 10 days, which corresponds to the average life span of the circulating platelet. However, significant functional recovery of platelets occurs 5 days after discontinuation of usual therapeutic dosages because of the formation of new uninhibited platelets. Concomitant aspirin and thienopyridine therapy results in synergistic platelet inhibition. On the basis of high-avidity binding and relatively quick plasma clearance (half-life elimination of 8 hours for clopidogrel, 0.25 hours for parent aspirin, 2 to 6 hours for salicylates), platelet transfusion with uninhibited allogeneic platelets should reverse the pharmacologic effects of the thienopyridines as well as concomitant aspirin therapy for patients with life-threatening clinical bleeding. Recent data suggest that full-dose aprotinin results in reduced blood loss associated with coronary artery bypass graft (CABG) surgery for cardiopulmonary bypass patients taking clopidogrel therapy within 5 days before surgery.[64]

Anticoagulant Medications

Medications designed to prevent undesired thrombosis have had extensive clinical use for a variety of medical conditions, including treatment and prevention of deep venous thrombosis, treatment of acute myocardial ischemia, and prophylactic anticoagulation for prevention of thrombosis on mechanical prosthetic heart valves. Although anticoagulant medications can treat and prevent potentially fatal conditions such as pulmonary embolus, these medications have a narrow therapeutic window with a significant risk for iatrogenic bleeding. Unlike the thrombolytic medications that dissolve existing clots, anticoagulant medications prevent formation of further thrombosis and allow the patient's intrinsic thrombolytic mechanisms to remove existing clots.

Heparin

Heparin sodium is a naturally occurring anticoagulant medication derived from pork intestine or bovine lung. It produces its anticoagulant effects by stimulating native antithrombin III activity, which then leads to inhibition of thrombin and decreased activation of factors V, VIII, and XIII.[65] Unfractionated heparin is widely used in many inpatient settings as an intravenous infusion for full anticoagulation such as treating acute myocardial ischemia. Furthermore, subcutaneous unfractionated heparin injections are used for prophylaxis against deep venous thrombosis in the perioperative period.[66] Heparin has the advantage of a short half-life (mean, 1.5 hours) and is inexpensive. It is readily titratable and can be monitored with routine laboratory testing of the PTT with a usual therapeutic activated PTT (aPTT) of 1.5 to 2.5 times the patient's baseline. Adjusted-dose subcutaneous heparin can be used to obtain therapeutic anticoagulation in the outpatient setting, such as during pregnancy. However, with widespread and frequent use of heparin therapy, the incidence, or at least the frequency of diagnosis, of heparin-induced thrombocytopenia is increasing. As a result, alternatives to traditional heparin therapy are under development and in clinical use. Because of the short half-life of heparin, infusions can be run safely for up to 4 hours prior to surgery. Holding the subcutaneous heparin dose on the morning of surgery allows resolution of the heparin effect for the operation. Depending on the type of procedure, heparin therapy should be reinstituted once the risk for significant bleeding has subsided.

Low-Molecular-Weight Heparin

Enoxaparin is a low-molecular-weight heparin that has a longer half-life than unfractionated heparin, is at least as effective for treatment and prevention of venous thromboembolism,[67] and can be safely administered as an outpatient drug.[68,69] It is commonly used for deep venous thrombosis

prophylaxis in major orthopedic surgery.[70] Enoxaparin is also useful as a means of maintaining therapeutic anticoagulation in the perioperative period yet allowing a brief window for hemostasis during surgery, for patients requiring therapeutic warfarin. Enoxaparin, like unfractionated heparin, binds to antithrombin and converts it to a rapid inactivator of coagulation factors, particularly factor Xa. Unlike unfractionated heparin, enoxaparin has decreased inhibitory effects on thrombin, and its effects cannot be readily measured with standard assay techniques such as the activated clotting time or the aPTT.[71] The elimination half-life of subcutaneous enoxaparin is approximately 4.5 to 7 hours, with some degree of antithrombotic effect expected for approximately 12 hours after a subcutaneous dose. Enoxaparin is only partially reversed with protamine.[72] A hemostatic defect exists after protamine reversal until factor Xa activity normalizes. On the basis of biological plausibility, factor replacement (with FFP) therapy will help to reverse the pharmacologic effects of enoxaparin. For surgical procedures with a high risk for bleeding, enoxaparin therapy should be discontinued for a minimum of 12 hours before induction of anesthesia. Enoxaparin is not a substitute for unfractionated heparin in patients with heparin-induced thrombocytopenia or for anticoagulation in those on cardiopulmonary bypass.[73]

Direct Thrombin Inhibitors

Bivalirudin, lepirudin, and argatroban are synthetic, nonimmunogenic direct thrombin inhibitors with dose-dependent action. Lepirudin and argatroban are indicated in patients with heparin-induced thrombocytopenia, and bivalirudin is an effective substitute for heparin therapy in patients undergoing percutaneous coronary intervention (PCI).[74-76] The pharmacologic effect of bivalirudin can be measured with standard activated clotting time (ACT) devices, although therapeutic reference ranges are not well established. The half-life of intravenous bivalirudin is quite short (30 minutes). Therefore, the drug should be reversed simply by terminating the infusion. Bivalirudin is cleared predominantly by the kidneys, and caution should be used in patients with renal failure. Discontinuation of bivalirudin before induction of anesthesia should allow sufficient time for recovery of adequate operative hemostasis in patients with normal renal function.

Argatroban, unlike bivalirudin, is hepatically metabolized and presents more reliable pharmacokinetics in renal failure patients.[77] On the other hand, it should be used with caution in patients with hepatic impairment. Therapeutic levels of argatroban are monitored using the aPTT.[78] The prothrombin time is unreliable in patients receiving argatroban and should not be used to guide therapy with this agent. Although PT does elevate further with the addition of therapeutic doses of warfarin than with argatroban alone, confirmation of sufficient suppression of factor Xa activity is a more reliable marker of adequacy of warfarin therapy before discontinuation of argatroban infusion. Discontinuation of argatroban infusion 4 to 6 hours before induction of anesthesia for a surgical procedure should allow sufficient recovery of coagulation for intraoperative hemostasis in the absence of hepatic impairment. Normalization of the aPTT can be used to confirm the reversal of the argatroban effect.

Lepirudin, a recombinant hirudin derived from yeast cells, is a 65-amino-acid polypeptide almost identical to the naturally occurring antithrombin compound produced by leeches. Therapeutic effect is monitored with aPTT. In healthy adults, lepirudin has a terminal half-life of 1.3 hours, but elimination half-lives can be prolonged up to 2 days in patients with renal failure. Antihirudin antibodies develop in about 40% to 70% of patients with heparin-induced thrombocytopenia who are treated with lepirudin for more than 5 days.[79] Interestingly, these antibodies may enhance the action of hirudin, possibly by delaying elimination.[80] Serious anaphylactic reactions have been reported on initial and repeat exposure with this agent.[81] On the basis of the terminal half-life in patients with normal renal function, therapeutic lepirudin infusion should be discontinued 8 hours before scheduled surgical procedures with potential for blood loss. This allows the aPTT to correct to normal before the operative period.

Although successful use of direct antithrombins for anticoagulation during cardiopulmonary bypass has been reported in patients with heparin-induced thrombocytopenia, consultation with a hematologist familiar with the management of this condition should be obtained before using direct antithrombins in cardiac surgery. Unlike heparin, these agents do not reverse with protamine, and severe bleeding can be expected in the perioperative period while awaiting resolution of the clinical effect of these drugs through elimination. To determine the best therapy for a patient on cardiopulmonary bypass and with a history of HIT, the risk for clinically significant heparin-induced thrombocytopenia on reexposure to heparin must be weighed against the risk for hemorrhage or insufficient anticoagulation. This risk-to-benefit analysis can be aided by testing for antiplatelet antibody titers and platelet aggregation on heparin exposure in the laboratory, by estimating the severity of the past clinical presentation, and by assessing the accuracy of the diagnosis. If no antibodies are measurable and the past diagnosis of HIT is questionable, a one-time, repeat exposure to heparin for anticoagulation during cardiopulmonary bypass may be the safest course of action.

Warfarin Sodium

Warfarin sodium is an inhibitor of the synthesis of vitamin K–dependent clotting factors, including factors II, VII, IX, and X, as well as protein C and protein S.[82] Vitamin K is an essential cofactor in the gamma-carboxylation of these proteins. Warfarin produces declines in vitamin K–dependent factor activities that are proportional to their plasma half-lives. For example, there is a sequential depression of factor VII (half-life, about 4 to 6 hours), IX (half-life, about 24 hours), X (half-life, about 48 hours), and then II (half-life, about 60 hours), with dose-dependent prolongation of prothrombin time. Because the half-lives of the anticoagulant proteins C and S are about 8 and 30 hours, respectively, care must be taken when converting patients from intravenous anticoagulation to warfarin. The initial anticoagulation

should not be stopped until the PT (or decrement in Xa activity) is therapeutic.

Beginning oral warfarin therapy alone could potentially result in transient hypercoagulability because of deficiencies of proteins C and S that result prior to a drop in total clotting factor activity. Warfarin therapy is indicated in the following situations: prophylaxis and treatment of deep venous thrombosis and pulmonary embolus, prophylaxis and treatment of thromboembolic complications of atrial fibrillation, cardiac valve replacement with a mechanical prosthesis, and prophylaxis against recurrent myocardial infarction or the thromboembolic complications associated with myocardial infarction. Because of these many indications, warfarin therapy is common in the patient population and is frequently encountered during preparation for surgical procedures. If the indication for warfarin is strong, such as in patients with mechanical cardiac valves or known intracardiac thrombus, initiation of an anticoagulant bridge with therapeutic subcutaneous heparin or enoxaparin is required on discontinuation of warfarin therapy. The benefit of this method is that these bridging agents can be held for the immediate perioperative period, allowing a brief period of normal hemostasis with resumption of therapeutic anticoagulation once the risk for surgical hemorrhage has subsided.

For patients on warfarin requiring urgent surgical intervention with a high risk for bleeding, administration of 10 mg of intravenous vitamin K will reverse the warfarin effect within approximately 24 hours for patients with normal hepatic synthetic function.[83] However, reestablishing therapeutic warfarin anticoagulation may require more than a week, necessitating interim intravenous or therapeutic subcutaneous anticoagulation. If the risk for bleeding with the procedure is not great, reversal of warfarin with 1 to 2 mg of vitamin K often results in a decline of the PT with less protracted warfarin therapy necessary for regaining therapeutic anticoagulation.[84] For patients requiring emergent surgery with significant risk for blood loss, administration of fresh-frozen plasma transiently replenishes depleted stores of vitamin K–dependent clotting factors. However, 6 to 8 units of FFP are frequently required to adequately reverse warfarin in the immediate preoperative period, and the effect lasts only until plasma factor VII activity drops below about 40% of normal, usually in 6 to 8 hours.

If a patient (e.g., one with atrial fibrillation) has an INR of 2.0 to 3.0 and a low risk for thrombosis after discontinuation of warfarin therapy, therapy should be stopped at least 4 days before the surgical procedure and reinstituted once the risk for surgical bleeding has abated.[85] Normalization of preoperative INR levels greater than 3.0 may require withholding the warfarin for more than 4 days. Special consideration of the risks and benefits of neuraxial anesthesia is essential for the patient on warfarin therapy. After discontinuation of warfarin, factor VII activity recovers quickly and results in a decrease in the measured PT/INR. Although the PT/INR is lower, the patient may still be at risk for bleeding, as factor II and X activities recover more slowly than factor VII.[41] To prevent the rare but catastrophic complication of a spinal hematoma, central neuraxial blockade should be avoided until the PT/INR has normalized.[41] Any indwelling catheters should be removed while the PT/INR is 1.5 or less.

Dextran

Dextran is a large-molecule polysaccharide used for prophylaxis of deep venous thrombosis and to enhance blood flow to transplanted tissues by decreasing blood viscosity and inhibiting platelet aggregation.[86] Although the exact mechanism of the antiplatelet effect of dextran solutions is unknown, it is likely to be related to interference with platelet adhesion to traumatized vessels and other platelets. Discontinuation of dextran 40 infusion 12 hours before surgery and dextran 70 infusion 24 hours before surgery should eliminate excessive bleeding caused by these agents. However, for procedures with a low risk for bleeding or in which mild anticoagulation may be indicated to offset a high risk for deep venous thrombosis (e.g., total hip or knee arthroplasty), continuation of dextran infusion throughout the perioperative period may be indicated.

Activated Protein C

Drotrecogin alfa is a recombinant form of human activated protein C used to help treat the massive systemic inflammatory response associated with severe sepsis.[87] Because activated protein C inhibits factors Va and VIIIa and also displays indirect profibrinolytic activity, the major side effect of treatment with drotrecogin alfa is bleeding. Drotrecogin alfa variably prolongs the aPTT but has minimal effect on prothrombin time. Effective treatment with this agent requires an infusion over 96 hours, during which time critically ill, septic patients may require surgical intervention. For surgical or other invasive procedures with a risk for bleeding, the drotrecogin alfa infusion should be stopped 2 hours before the procedure. If the procedure proves to be minimally invasive and uncomplicated, the infusion may be restarted immediately. For surgery with significant risk for continued bleeding, reinstitution of the infusion should be considered only after 12 hours of achieving adequate hemostasis. There is no effective antidote for the bleeding associated with drotrecogin alfa other than discontinuation of the infusion.

Hydroxyethyl Starch

Hydroxyethyl starch solutions are plasma expanders used to restore and maintain intravascular volume, increase right heart filling, and improve tissue perfusion.[88] Controversy exists in the medical literature as to the potential for adverse effects of these agents on coagulation in the perioperative period. With large-volume infusions, dilutional effects on platelets and clotting factor activity from starch solutions are possible. Decreased vWF and factor VIII activity has been observed with the use of slowly degradable hydroxyethyl starch solutions,[88-91] which may impair adhesion of platelets to subendothelial collagen and diminish activation of factor X in the coagulation cascade. Platelet surface coating by hydroxyethyl starch molecules may also impair the binding of GP IIb/IIIa receptors to their ligands, which include soluble fibrinogen and vWF, thus reducing platelet aggregation.[88,92,93] Desmopressin has been demonstrated to increase factor VIII levels after hydroxyethyl starch therapy and has been suggested as a therapy for mild coagulopathies resulting from hydroxyethyl starch administration.[90] Although the clinical sequelae of these reported effects are debatable, thromboelastography and platelet function analysis suggest that slowly degradable hydroxyethyl starch solutions do impair platelet function.[88,89,94,95] Depending on the clinical scenario, this may be an undesirable effect, and limitation of the volume of these solutions for patients with significant clinical bleeding is indicated.

■ TRANSFUSION IN CARDIAC SURGERY

Prior database studies have suggested that hematocrit values less than 23% are associated with elevated mortality in cardiac surgical patients.[96] Fang and colleagues reported that mortality doubled in low-risk patients whose lowest hematocrit fell below 14% on cardiopulmonary bypass or in high-risk patients whose lowest hematocrit fell below 17%.[97] Hardy and coworkers reported an inverse relationship between hemoglobin levels in postoperative cardiac surgical patients and major morbidity.[98] In a recently reported database study of 5000 cardiac surgical procedures with cardiopulmonary bypass, perioperative vital organ dysfunction, as well as short-term and intermediate-term mortality, significantly increased when the lowest perioperative hematocrit was less than 22%.[99] Although they identify an association between low hemoglobin levels and adverse outcome in cardiac surgery, these studies are retrospective database investigations and are unable to assess the cause of the association. Specifically, no adjustment was made for low preoperative hemoglobin levels. Low preoperative hemoglobin very likely represents a marker for chronic disease, and it is an independent source of elevated perioperative morbidity and mortality.[100,101] Also, these studies did not assess the potential adverse impact that the transfusions may have had on morbidity and mortality.

A well-publicized study appearing in the New England Journal of Medicine[102] reported a decreased 30-day mortality for patients diagnosed with an acute myocardial infarction if they were transfused for an admission hematocrit below 30%. This study was also a retrospective, database study, and its results have little bearing on postoperative cardiac surgical patients with adequate revascularization. Furthermore, variance between the transfused and nontransfused patient populations alone may have been responsible for the reported results. Patients with an admission hematocrit of less than 30% were twice as likely to have a do-not-resuscitate order written, and they underwent acute intervention for revascularization at only half the rate of the patients with a hematocrit greater than 30%. Once again, low hematocrit may be a marker for the underlying chronic disease that elevates mortality. A more recent database study of 24,112 patients with acute coronary syndrome found a strong association between increased mortality and transfusion in patients undergoing treatment for myocardial ischemia.[103] These results suggest an adverse impact of transfusion on outcome in these patients.

Review of the literature also reveals data supporting the use of a restrictive transfusion policy for cardiac surgical patients. When adjusting for preoperative risk factors, including preoperative hematocrit, no association existed between lowest hematocrit on cardiopulmonary bypass and mortality.[101] Data collected from 2202 patients in the McSpi database suggested an association between higher hematocrit on admission to the intensive care unit (ICU) and perioperative myocardial infarction after CABG. In high-risk patients, higher hematocrit on ICU admission was associated with increased mortality.[104] This study suggests that the transfusion itself, rather than the low hematocrit that led to transfusion, may be the factor contributing to elevated mortality.[105] In a randomized, prospective clinical trial of transfusion strategy for ICU patients admitted for treatment of conditions other than coronary artery ischemia, restrictive RBC transfusion only for hemoglobin less than 7 g/dL was associated with a lower 30-day mortality than liberal RBC transfusion for a hemoglobin of less than 10 g/dL in the cohort of patients with Apache II scores of 20 or less.[106] These data collected in a randomized, prospective fashion strongly suggest an adverse effect of liberal transfusion in patients without active coronary ischemia. In a prospective, randomized trial of 428 consecutive primary CABG patients at the Texas Heart Institute, lowering the transfusion trigger from 9 g/dL to 8 g/dL resulted in a significant decrease in transfusion rate and associated cost without objective or subjective difference in clinical outcome.[107] Although not yet conclusive, prospective and randomized studies of transfusion tend to favor a restrictive strategy.

Recent outcome studies have suggested a detrimental effect of transfusion on both short- and long-term mortality. In a European study of anemia in the ICU, 3534 patients were followed in a prospective, observational manner. A propensity-to-transfuse score was developed, including age, sex, admission urgency, admission diagnosis, Sequential Organ Failure Assessment (SOFA) score, Apache II score, day-1 hemoglobin level, recent history of anemia, recent acute blood loss, shock on ICU admission, and hospital length of stay. When matched for propensity score, transfused patients had an overall 28-day mortality rate of 22.7% compared with a mortality rate of 17.1% for nontransfused patients ($P = .02$).[108] For patients undergoing cardiac surgery, transfusion may significantly and adversely affect long-term survival. In a retrospective database study of 1915 patients surviving at least 30 days after primary CABG surgery, 5-year mortality was twice as high for patients who received a transfusion during hospitalization than for nontransfused patients. To adjust for preexisting disease, a propensity score for transfusion was developed that included age, sex, body mass, hospital length of stay, cardiopulmonary bypass time, and the Society of Thoracic Surgeons' risk stratification score. Five hundred forty-six patients transfused during hospitalization were matched by propensity score with 546 nontransfused patients, and mortality was again compared. After correction for comorbidity, 5-year mortality remained 70% higher in the transfused group ($P < .001$).[109] Although these data are from a retrospective database, they strongly suggest that transfusion should be administered only when absolutely necessary.

Limited data exist to determine the best hemoglobin trigger for RBC transfusion. Data collected in Jehovah's Witnesses patients suggest that mortality resulting from anemia increases once hemoglobin levels fall below 5.0 g/dL,[110] and that mortality exceeds 95% if hemoglobin falls to less than 3.0 g/dL.[111] In a later retrospective cohort study of 300 patients with postoperative hemoglobin levels of 8 g/dL or lower who declined RBC transfusion, the odds of death increased 2.5 times for each gram decrease in hemoglobin level.[112] In conscious, resting, healthy humans, global tissue oxygenation was not compromised at a hemoglobin level of 5.0 g/dL.[113] However, cognitive function in this same study population became impaired at a hemoglobin concentration of less than 5.7 g/dL.[114] The cognitive dysfunction was reversible with supplemental oxygen, suggesting this level as a minimum acceptable hemoglobin concentration for healthy individuals. The minimum acceptable level for cardiac surgical patients has yet to be conclusively determined but is probably somewhat higher than that for healthy individuals. In a dog model of normothermic cardiopulmonary bypass, oxygen delivery and whole-body oxygen uptake were significantly reduced when hematocrit fell to less than 18%, suggesting a level above 18% as optimal.[115]

If transfusion increases mortality and morbidity and the minimum acceptable hemoglobin concentration for the cardiac surgical patient is unknown, what is the best practice? The ASA transfusion guidelines,[10] updated in July, 2006,[1] remain the standard of care—the most comprehensive set of recommendations for best practice. They include the following points:

- RBC transfusion should be for inadequate tissue oxygenation and not on a rigid trigger.
- RBC transfusion is rarely indicated when hemoglobin concentration is greater than 10 g/dL.
  - Autologous blood should not be routinely administered to patients who pre-donated if the hemoglobin concentration is greater than 10 g/dL.
- RBC transfusion is almost always indicated when the hemoglobin concentration is less than 6 g/dL.
- Surgical patients with microvascular bleeding usually require platelet transfusion if the count is less than 50,000 and rarely if it is greater than 100,000.
  - Platelet transfusion may be needed in the setting of microvascular bleeding with normal platelet counts if there is known or suspected platelet dysfunction, as seen with cardiopulmonary bypass and antiplatelet agents.
  - Prophylactic platelet transfusion is ineffective if the etiology is increased platelet destruction.
- FFP is indicated for microvascular bleeding when the PT is greater than 1.5, the INR is greater than 2.0, or the aPTT is greater than 2.0 times normal.
- FFP is indicated for urgent reversal of warfarin or for correction of known factor deficiency for which specific concentrate is unavailable.
- FFP is indicated for correction of microvascular bleeding when more than one blood volume has been transfused and the PT, INR, or aPTT value cannot be obtained quickly.

- FFP is indicated for treating heparin resistance in a patient receiving heparin.
- FFP is contraindicated for augmentation of plasma volume or albumin concentration.
- Cryoprecipitate is rarely indicated when fibrinogen levels are greater than 150 mg/dL.
- Cryoprecipitate is indicated for bleeding patients with fibrinogen levels less than 80 to 100 mg/dL, for massively transfused patients when fibrinogen cannot be measured quickly, or for patients with congenital fibrinogen deficiencies.
- Cryoprecipitate is indicated for bleeding patients with von Willebrand disease when specific concentrates are not available.
- Desmopressin or topical hemostatics should be considered with excessive bleeding.
- Recombinant factor VII should be considered in patients with excessive bleeding when traditional methods to stop bleeding have failed.

If adopted for cardiac surgical patients when using point-of-care testing to rapidly identify specific deficiencies in heparin reversal, platelet function, or clotting factor activity,[11] these guidelines should result in restriction of unnecessary transfusion and have a favorable impact on morbidity and mortality.

Based on review of literature to date, avoidance of severe anemia without allogeneic transfusion is the strategy most likely to result in improved outcome. In a recent report from a successful blood management program at Englewood Hospital in New Jersey, 89% of patients undergoing coronary artery bypass, valve surgery, and combined coronary and valve surgery avoided transfusion of any type of blood product. The reported techniques used in this program included preoperative optimization of hemoglobin, intraoperative acute normovolemic hemodilution, autotransfusion of mediastinal blood, tolerance of anemia (hematocrit of 20% on coronary artery bypass and 24% immediately after), meticulous surgical technique, endovascular vein harvesting, on-site coagulation monitoring, and targeted pharmacotherapy.[116] Consumer data released by the state of New Jersey for the time period reported by Moskowitz and colleagues showed risk-adjusted mortality for coronary artery bypass surgery patients at Englewood to be the lowest in the state while transfusing only 11% of their patients.[117] These results demonstrate that, although difficult to perform, a randomized prospective trial of outcome is needed to compare a comprehensive blood management program with a more liberal transfusion practice.

Transfusion in Noncardiac Surgery

Targeted and judicious transfusion practice for noncardiac surgical patients, as for cardiac surgery patients, optimizes benefits and limits the known and unknown risks of allogeneic blood administration. If given a choice, most patients prefer management that includes specific therapies designed to reduce or avoid allogeneic blood. Development of a comprehensive, evidence-based, multidisciplinary plan for procedure-specific blood management has been shown to reduce

transfusion with associated reductions in deep wound infection rate.[118]

■ BLOOD MANAGEMENT TECHNIQUES

Optimization of Preoperative Hemoglobin

Probably the single most important technique of effective blood management in the perioperative period is to ensure identification and adequate treatment of preoperative anemia (total hemoglobin concentration, ≤13.0 g/dL). As discussed earlier, low preoperative hemoglobin is associated with poor outcome. It is also a marker for perioperative transfusion, which is an independent predictor of poor outcome.[96-99] By optimizing preoperative hemoglobin for surgery with significant anticipated blood loss, the probability of avoiding low hemoglobin in the perioperative period is improved.[119-122]

Iron-Deficiency Anemia

The identification and correction of iron deficiency is relatively inexpensive and effective, especially when compared with the cost of RBC transfusion. However, to be effective, the iron-deficiency anemia needs to be recognized early enough to allow adequate time for iron therapy to stimulate bone marrow production of new erythrocytes with increased hemoglobin concentrations. The presence of hypochromic (decreased mean corpuscular hemoglobin concentration), microcytic (decreased mean corpuscular volume) anemia on a routine blood count is an effective screen for iron deficiency. The diagnosis is confirmed by measurement of serum iron level, total iron-binding capacity (TIBC), and serum ferritin. If serum iron and ferritin are low and TIBC is elevated, iron deficiency is one source of the patient's anemia. Low serum ferritin levels are specific for iron deficiency, but the test is not sensitive, as ferritin is an acute-phase reactant and may be present in higher levels in patients with inflammatory, malignant, or liver disease.[123] In the presence of a nondiagnostic ferritin level, the Fe/TIBC ratio can also be used. If the ratio is less than 0.1, iron deficiency is strongly suggested, even in the presence of a normal to high serum ferritin.

Iron deficiency is most commonly treated with oral ferrous sulfate at a dosage of 325 mg three times daily (195 mg of elemental iron per day) prior to surgery or until follow-up iron studies normalize. If the patient has severe iron deficiency or is unable to tolerate oral iron, intravenous administration of 5 mL iron sucrose (20 mg/mL of elemental iron) or 10 mL of sodium ferric gluconate (12.5 mg/mL of elemental iron) one to three times weekly for a maximum of 10 doses is effective to reverse iron deficiency.

Macrocytic Anemia

Macrocytic anemia presents another potentially reversible cause of preoperative hemoglobin deficiency. Patients with cyanocobalamin (vitamin B_{12}) or folic acid deficiency present with low total hemoglobin concentrations but enlarged red blood cells (increased mean corpuscular volume). The diagnosis can be confirmed by measurement of serum vitamin levels. Vitamin replacement therapy with oral folic acid or B_{12} is indicated for deficiency. Patients with low B_{12} levels caused by decreased gut absorption (intrinsic factor deficiency or gastric resection) require B_{12} injections for treatment.

Autologous Pre-Donation

When blood loss in a scheduled elective surgery is expected to be significant, the technique of autologous pre-donation allows a patient to donate units of his or her own whole blood to be stored for use in the perioperative period if needed. Assuming absence of clerical error, reinfusion of autologous whole blood or PRBCs avoids the immune response complications of allogeneic blood, including hypersensitivity reactions, immune suppression, and systemic inflammation. However, because the blood is collected by phlebotomy and stored for the patient, the risks of clerical error and bacterial contamination persist, leaving the two greatest risk factors for acute transfusion-related mortality unchanged. Because of preparation factors (in the case of PRBCs) or to length of storage (in the case of autologous whole blood), platelet function and clotting factor activity are eliminated in the autologous unit.[6] Although autologous pre-donation has the theoretical benefit of stimulating bone marrow production and allowing recovery of RBC mass prior to the operation, the number of units pre-donated is limited by the individual's rate of erythropoiesis and the shelf-life of the product. The technique often results in phlebotomy-induced anemia on the day of surgery, which can offset the intended benefit.

Although extensively used in the past, especially for orthopedic and urologic procedures in otherwise healthy individuals, there is little evidence from prospective randomized, controlled clinical trials that proves efficacy over preoperative optimization of hemoglobin alone or intraoperative hemodilution. Currently, usage of autologous pre-donation is decreasing, largely for two reasons: first, the technique is inconvenient for the patient; and second, patients with an RBC mass large enough to allow pre-donation of 2 or more units of RBCs without becoming anemic are likely to tolerate most procedures without transfusion. Autologous pre-donation is also expensive and wasteful. Because the autologous pre-donation units are not screened in the same fashion as regular donor units, the red blood cells cannot be released for general use and must be discarded if not infused into the autologous donor. In certain procedures, 40% to 60% of units are discarded.[124,125] In terms of cost, both the patient and the hospital must bear substantial administrative fees. For example, patients are currently charged about $180 for each unit. The hospital is also charged by the collecting agency for each unit, but the cost of the autologous unit (about $300 per unit) is reimbursed only if the unit is reinfused. Therefore, the cost of the unit is absorbed by the institution if the patient does not clinically need the autologous unit and it is discarded. Because of the many disadvantages associated with autologous pre-donation, other blood management techniques are gaining in popularity.

Anemia of Chronic Disease

For patients with anemia of chronic disease, preoperative therapy with epoetin alfa, a recombinant form of human erythropoietin, can effectively stimulate bone marrow erythropoiesis. In randomized, controlled trials of patients scheduled for major orthopedic surgery, therapy with epoetin alfa resulted in a significant increase in preoperative hemoglobin levels and decreased the requirement for allogeneic transfusion.[119-121] Reticulocytosis develops in 5 to 9 days in response to therapy with epoetin alfa. This reticulocytosis is accompanied by an increase in hemoglobin concentration of an average of 1 g/dL per week with continued therapy. As with treatment of iron deficiency anemia, effective therapy requires early identification and treatment prior to scheduled surgery. If reticulocytosis is inadequate in response to recommended doses of epoetin alfa, iron supplementation may be necessary to optimize the response.

To limit the expense of treatment with epoetin alfa, Medicare-approved indications have been established based on results of randomized, controlled trials that prove efficacy. Medicare guidelines support epoetin alfa therapy in the preoperative period to treat noncardiac, nonvascular surgical procedures with an anticipated blood loss of 2 units or more of whole blood in patients who are not candidates for autologous pre-donation. Preoperative hemoglobin levels measured within 1 week of starting epoetin alfa therapy must be greater than 10.0 g/dL and less than or equal to 13.0 g/dL. Furthermore, the anemia must result from chronic disease and not from an easily correctable cause such as iron deficiency. Accepted treatment regimens are (1) 600 units/kg weekly for 3 weeks, with a fourth dose on the day of surgery, or (2) 300 units/kg daily for 10 days, with a dose on the day of surgery and for the first 4 postoperative days.

Although studies suggest that erythropoietin therapy is effective in increasing hematocrit levels in preparation for cardiac surgery,[126-131] results from one study involving epoetin alfa administration to CABG surgery patients in the perioperative period showed an increased mortality in the treatment group.[126] In this study, four deaths resulted from thrombotic vascular events that occurred during therapy. Although a causative role of epoetin alfa was not definitively determined, these results suggest that caution is indicated in this patient population. Therefore, unless the risk for life-threatening hemorrhage is markedly elevated, epoetin alfa is not recommended for use in major cardiac or vascular procedures. An example of a case in which epoetin alfa may be indicated in cardiac or vascular procedures is the patient who refuses transfusion (e.g., a member of Jehovah's Witnesses) but who would poorly tolerate a required procedure without correction of anemia.[132] Although not approved by the U.S. Food and Drug Administration (FDA) in this setting, the benefit may outweigh the risk in select cases as long as the increase in hemoglobin is monitored closely.[116] If hemoglobin levels increase faster than 1 g/dL per week, or the level exceeds 14 g/dL, epoetin alfa therapy should be discontinued.

■ INTRAOPERATIVE MANAGEMENT

By far, the single most important component of effective blood management is surgical hemostasis. Meticulous attention to detail by the surgeon is essential to prevent postoperative morbidity related not only to blood loss but also to hematoma formation around the surgical site. New devices that may provide enhanced hemostasis when compared with traditional electrocautery are being developed and tested.[133]

Intraoperative Normovolemic Hemodilution

Conservation of RBC mass via intraoperative autologous donation is a technique that has been studied in orthopedic, cardiac, and urologic surgery patients with varying results.[134] The concept of normovolemic hemodilution involves harvest of a predetermined volume of autologous whole blood into anticoagulant-containing blood donation bags identical to those used in blood banks. The harvested blood may be removed via a central venous catheter, an arterial catheter, or a large-bore peripheral intravenous catheter, but flow must be reliable and at an adequate flow rate to prevent clot formation prior to reaching the anticoagulant in the donor bag. The autologous blood is then kept at room temperature with gentle mixing for up to 8 hours prior to reinfusion.[135] Harvested volume is replaced with colloid or crystalloid via a separate peripheral intravenous line to maintain normovolemia. Box 27-2 contains one method of calculating the autologous harvest volume to reach a target hemoglobin level based on the patient's estimated blood volume and starting hemoglobin level.[101] After hemodilution, subsequent blood lost in the surgical field has a reduced RBC mass, and fluid replacement at the end of the case consists of fresh whole blood instead of intravenous fluid.

Intraoperative normovolemic hemodilution essentially reverses fluid administration for a major surgical procedure. The majority of intravenous colloid and crystalloid adminis-

tration occurs prior to significant blood loss instead of intravenous fluid administration as replacement for blood lost in the surgical field. The net effect is a loss of dilute blood and replacement with harvested blood containing a higher hemoglobin concentration. To conserve a significant volume of whole blood, the patient's starting hemoglobin and blood volume needs to be great enough to allow harvest of a large volume of whole blood, and the surgical loss of diluted blood needs to be extensive enough to make the procedure worthwhile.[134,136] For example, normovolemic harvest of 2000 mL of whole blood from a patient with a starting hemoglobin of 15 g/dL and an estimated blood volume of 6000 mL followed by a 2000 mL intraoperative blood loss results in a nadir intraoperative hemoglobin of 6.7 g/dL. Overall, 1.5 units of whole blood with the same hemoglobin content as the average hemoglobin content of the harvested blood are preserved. Although this extent of blood conservation may improve the chances that allogeneic transfusion can be avoided, the procedure involves significant alteration of intravascular oxygen-carrying capacity, which could be a problem for patients with limited physiologic reserve.

Results of hemodilution efficacy trials have been mixed. In a meta-analysis of normovolemic hemodilution, including 24 prospective, randomized, controlled trials with 1218 patients undergoing major surgery such as cardiac and orthopedic procedures, the overall likelihood of exposure to allogeneic blood was reduced (odds ratio, 0.31 [0.15-0.62]).[134] However, institution of a perioperative transfusion protocol eliminated the beneficial effect of hemodilution, which could suggest that the reduction of exposure was the result of biased study design. In a prospective, randomized trial of 79 patients undergoing radical prostatectomy, intraoperative hemodilution resulted in similar allogeneic exposure rates and lower costs when compared with autologous pre-donation, or with preoperative epoetin alfa plus intraoperative hemodilution.[137] Similar allogeneic exposure rates were also found in a prospective, randomized trial of 46 patients undergoing total hip arthroplasty when intraoperative hemodilution of up to 3 units of whole blood was compared with autologous pre-donation of 3 units.[138] A more recent randomized, controlled trial of 78 patients undergoing major hepatic resection revealed that allogeneic exposure at 72 hours after resection was significantly reduced for hemodiluted patients with a target post-harvest hematocrit of 24% and a minimum hematocrit of 20%.[139]

Compared with autologous pre-donation, intraoperative hemodilution has practical advantages. For example, the technique requires minimal preparation and equipment. It is far more convenient than pre-donation of multiple units and can be performed at significantly lower cost. The returned whole blood also contains functional platelets and clotting factors not present in stored autologous units. However, although moderate degrees of hemodilution may prove effective in selected patient populations, the results of extreme hemodilution studies with nadir intraoperative hematocrits less than 20% have shown increased rates of perioperative morbidity that may be caused in part by complications of acute hemodilution.[140] Thus, it is prudent to avoid extreme levels of hemodilution in patients. Currently (as of 2006), a

---

27-2	**Sample Calculation of Whole-Blood Volume Conserved with Normovolemic Hemodilution**

Assume an 86-kg man with an estimated blood volume of 6000 mL and preoperative hemoglobin of 15 g/dL. With a harvest volume of 2000 mL and an intraoperative blood loss of 2000 mL, what would be the hemoglobin mass and whole blood volume preserved by normovolemic hemodilution?

Harvest volume of 2000 mL replaced by equivalent intravascular volume of crystalloid or colloid would result in a 33% drop in hemoglobin concentration, from 15 to 10 g/dL, with a mean hemoglobin concentration of 12.5 g/dL in the harvested blood.

- Subsequent intraoperative blood loss of 2000 mL replaced by an equivalent intravascular volume of crystalloid or colloid would result in a 33% drop in hemoglobin concentration, from 10 g/dL to 6.7 g/dL, with a mean hemoglobin concentration of 8.3 g/dL in the blood lost from the surgical field.
- Hemoglobin mass returned to patient = 20 dL harvest volume × 12.5 g/dL, mean hemoglobin concentration in harvested blood = 250 g hemoglobin reinfused.
- Hemoglobin mass lost from surgical field = 20 dL blood loss × 8.33 g/dL, mean hemoglobin concentration in surgical blood loss = 167 g hemoglobin lost.
- Preserved hemoglobin mass = 250 g − 167 g = 83 g hemoglobin preserved.
- Hemoglobin mass per unit of harvested blood = 12.5 g/dL × 4.5 dL per unit whole blood = 56 g hemoglobin per unit.
- Units whole blood preserved by hemodilution = 83 g preserved ÷ 56 g per unit = 1.5 units.

randomized, prospective, controlled clinical trial with sufficient power to definitively determine safety and efficacy of acute intraoperative hemodilution has yet to be done. If the therapy is used as part of a blood management program, care must be taken to avoid procedural complications, as definitive benefit has not been proved.

Cell Salvage

Intraoperative cell salvage is a widely used blood conservation technique in which shed blood from the surgical field is aspirated into a sterile collection canister containing anticoagulant (heparin or citrate). The shed blood is then processed by washing with normal saline and spinning in a centrifuge to separate RBCs from other blood components and cellular debris. The recovered RBCs are resuspended in normal saline and pumped into a sterile storage bag for reinfusion, usually through a lipid-reduction filter. Benefits of this technique include the recovery of shed RBCs that would otherwise be discarded, and preparation of fresh, concentrated, autologous RBCs for reinfusion. In cardiac surgical patients, use of cell salvage devices in lieu of aspiration of shed blood from the sternotomy site has been reported to decrease the embolic load of lipid-containing particles to the brain compared with arterial filters alone.[141] Disadvantages of cell salvage include expense, with a current disposable cost of about $350 for each cell salvage use and loss of platelets and plasma proteins (including clotting factors) during processing. Excessive use of cell salvage can contribute to a dilutional coagulopathy, particularly in patients (e.g., those undergoing cardiopulmonary bypass procedures) prone to this complication.

Data supporting cell salvage are convincing for several procedures involving significant blood loss. In a 1999 meta-analysis of 29 studies involving cardiac or orthopedic surgical patients that used avoidance of allogeneic RBC transfusion as the outcome measure, cell salvage decreased the risk of exposure for orthopedic patients (relative risk, 0.39 [0.30-0.51]) but not for cardiac surgical patients.[142] The discrepancy between the two types of surgeries is most likely the result of cardiopulmonary bypass–induced platelet and clotting factor deficiency combined with the dilutional coagulopathy that results from reinfusion of large volumes of salvaged RBCs depleted of platelets and plasma proteins in cardiac surgical patients.

In our institution, we limit immediate reinfusion of salvaged RBCs to 2 units for cardiopulmonary bypass patients to help avoid an acute dilutional effect. Reinfusion of additional salvaged RBCs can be considered over the first 4 hours after processing. Risks of cell salvage include bacterial contamination, inadvertent air embolus (caused by failure to remove air from the reinfusion bag), dilutional coagulopathy, and the theoretical risk for tumor cell dissemination or amniotic fluid embolus. According to Waters and coworkers, administration of tumor cells or the products of conception with properly processed salvaged RBCs infused through a Pall RS leukoreduction filter (Pall Medical, East Hills, NY) is minimal.[143-146] This position is supported by follow-up studies of patients who received radical prostatectomies in which intraoperative cell salvage was used. These studies showed that the rate of prostate cancer recurrence was no different from the recurrence rate of patients undergoing the same procedure without intraoperative cell salvage.[147,148] The cost of cell salvage is easily offset if the volume of RBCs processed and returned to the patient is sufficient to decrease the requirement for allogeneic red blood cell administration by at least 1 unit. The cost of disposable cell salvage equipment can be reduced when the blood loss is unpredictable by using only the anticoagulant-containing reservoir (about $70) for collection of shed blood from the field and opening the remainder of the processing disposables only if the volume of shed blood is sufficient to result in at least 1 full unit of salvaged RBCs (about $300). If used judiciously, cell salvage is a vital component of any effective blood management program.

Antifibrinolytic Therapy

Fibrinolysis, caused either by excessive native plasmin or urokinase activity or by the activity of pharmacologic fibrinolytic therapy, can result in bleeding complications in the perioperative period. With the introduction of tissue plasminogen activator as therapy for acute coronary thrombosis, intracranial hemorrhage secondary to excessive fibrinolysis was quickly identified as the most dreaded complication of this therapy. During prostate resection, fibrinolytic activity caused by urokinase release can result in excessive bleeding. Enhanced activity of fibrinolytic pathways combined with a reduction in clotting factor activity and fibrinogen levels around the time of cardiopulmonary bypass produces excessive bleeding after cardiac surgery.[12,149]

Lysine analogs, including epsilon-aminocaproic acid and tranexamic acid, block binding of plasminogen, tissue plasminogen activator, and plasmin to lysine sites on fibrin. Both agents have been studied for use in reducing postoperative bleeding associated with cardiac surgery and have been found to be effective for controlling perioperative fibrinolysis in low-risk primary coronary artery surgery patients.[150,151] In a 1999 meta-analysis of antifibrinolytic therapy in cardiac surgery, epsilon-aminocaproic acid and tranexamic acid both decreased reexploration rate and increased avoidance of transfusion without an increase in the rate of perioperative myocardial infarction.[152]

When studied in pediatric patients undergoing elective spinal instrumentation with fusion for scoliosis, both tranexamic acid and epsilon-aminocaproic acid significantly reduced blood loss in the perioperative compared with saline control but failed to reduce transfusion requirements.[153,154] Although these trials were randomized, double-blinded, and controlled, the number of subjects was too small ($n = 44$ for the tranexamic acid trial[153]; $n = 36$ for the epsilon-aminocaproic acid trial[154]) to establish a clear difference between groups with relation to transfusion avoidance. Larger trials are probably necessary to establish efficacy of these agents in high-blood-loss spine surgery.

Aprotinin

Aprotinin is a nonselective, serine-protease inhibitor approved by the FDA for use as prophylaxis against excessive bleeding after primary and repeat CABG surgery with cardiopulmonary bypass. The use of this agent as part of an effective blood management program is supported by multicenter, randomized, double-blinded, placebo-controlled trials. When compared with placebo, the use of aprotinin as prophylaxis against perioperative bleeding in repeat CABG surgery significantly reduced total allogeneic blood product requirements and percentage of patients receiving allogeneic red blood cells.[155,156] When dose effectiveness was compared in this same patient population, full-dose aprotinin (2 million kallikrein-inhibiting units as a bolus, followed by 500,000 units per hour infusion during surgery, with 2 million units in the bypass pump prime) was more effective in reducing thoracic drainage and total allogeneic units transfused than was half-dose aprotinin.[156] Use of full-dose aprotinin for primary CABG surgery also resulted in significantly lower thoracic drainage volume and allogeneic units transfused.[155] However, although the transfusion rate was lower postoperatively, the primary coronary artery bypass group had an overall lower transfusion requirement than the repeat surgery group. Because of this lower transfusion requirement, less clinical difference was noted between the control and aprotinin-treated patients, and less cost effectiveness was noted when compared with the repeat coronary artery surgery. In a meta-analysis of antifibrinolytic therapies for coronary artery surgery, aprotinin not only reduced reexploration rate and increased transfusion avoidance, but it also reduced overall mortality by 45% when compared with placebo.[152]

A recent observational study of 4374 coronary artery bypass surgery patients showed an association between aprotinin use and increased mortality as well as increased cardiovascular, cerebrovascular, and renal complications when compared with control patients. The same associations were not observed for patients treated with aminocaproic acid or tranexamic acid when compared with the control group.[157] These findings conflict with previous results from randomized, double-blinded, placebo-controlled trials that showed efficacy in reduction of transfusion requirements with an acceptable risk profile. In this observational database study, significant differences in baseline health characteristics were seen between patients receiving placebo and those receiving aprotinin for 64% of the variables examined. Although an attempt was made to adjust for dissimilar patient populations using propensity scoring, completely correcting for selection bias in any retrospective study is impossible. Of the patients in this analysis, only 46% (596 of 1295) in the aprotinin group received one of the FDA-approved doses previously studied in randomized, controlled trials. Although database studies are capable of identifying associations that may merit further study, conclusions relating association to causation are invalid. However, the database study does provide evidence that, as with any complex pharmacologic agent, caution and further study are needed to fully evaluate the risk for aprotinin. This is especially true for renal risks of aprotinin, which had not been well established by previous studies.

Because aprotinin is a nonspecific serine protease inhibitor, its pharmacologic effect extends beyond inhibition of plasmin. Subsequent studies of aprotinin's effect on inhibiting activation of the PAR-1 (protease-activated receptor-1) molecule on the platelet surface suggest a protective effect on platelet function during cardiopulmonary bypass that may contribute to postoperative hemostasis in this patient group.[158-160] As discussed earlier, recent data suggest that full-dose aprotinin reduces blood loss for patients on clopidogrel therapy prior to CABG surgery with cardiopulmonary bypass.[64] Aprotinin also inhibits kallikrein, bradykinin, activated complement factor 5, and elastase. Its ability to inhibit these inflammatory molecules suggests that it may help attenuate the systemic inflammatory response to bypass.[161] Aprotinin may also reduce the incidence of postoperative stroke. In Levy's 1995 trial that studied the use of aprotinin in repeat coronary artery surgery, a statistically significant reduction in stroke events was noted in the treated group ($P = .01$).[156] A significant decrease in stroke was again noted in a 1996 database study of all coronary artery surgery patients treated with aprotinin in randomized, prospective, controlled trials, when compared with placebo for full-dose, but not reduced-dose, aprotinin ($P = .027$).[162] This effect, combined with the reduction in transfusion observed with aprotinin use, was studied in a lifetime cost analysis of aprotinin use in coronary artery bypass surgery. Full-dose aprotinin was cost neutral for primary coronary surgery and resulted in an average lifetime cost reduction of $6044 when used for repeat coronary artery bypass procedures.[162]

Although not FDA approved for use in high-blood-loss surgical procedures other than CABG surgery, aprotinin has been studied in randomized, controlled trials of orthopedic surgical procedures. In a randomized, double-blinded, placebo-controlled trial of 44 pediatric patients undergoing elective spinal fusion for scoliosis, patients receiving aprotinin demonstrated statistically significant reduction in blood loss and mean number of RBC units transfused.[163] In a randomized, double-blinded, placebo-controlled trial of 53 patients undergoing bilateral or revision hip arthroplasty, patients received either 3.8×10^6 kallikrein inactivation units (KIU) aprotinin or saline placebo.[164] Aprotinin-treated patients in this trial showed a significant reduction of blood loss and RBC units transfused. In another study, the transfusion rate in 301 patients undergoing primary unilateral total hip replacement was lower in all aprotinin-treated patients compared with controls.[165] However, the results were not statistically significant because multiple dosing regimens of aprotinin were used, which led to sample sizes that were inadequate to find differences between any one dosing regimen and placebo. Theoretical concern over potential for aprotinin-induced thrombosis in the orthopedic patient population has prompted close scrutiny for deep venous thrombosis development in the trials of major orthopedic surgery. When all studies of aprotinin use in major orthopedic surgery from 1995 to 2002 were combined ($N = 466$), the deep venous thrombosis rate for placebo patients was 9%, and the rate for patients receiving aprotinin was 6.5%, suggesting that aprotinin does not enhance likelihood of this complication in orthopedic surgery. The results of further, randomized, controlled trials of aprotinin use in hip and spine surgery will help define the role of this agent in noncardiac surgical blood conservation. Enrollment in a trial of high-dose aprotinin use in primary total hip arthroplasty has recently been completed with results pending analysis.

Desmopressin

Desmopressin acetate is a synthetic analog of naturally occurring 8-arginine vasopressin and is FDA approved for treatment of diabetes insipidus, type 1 vWD, and mild hemophilia A (factor VIII activity, <5%). Desmopressin's effect on hemostasis is mediated by its indirect stimulation of endothelial cell release of the factor VIII–vWF complex, leading to enhanced platelet adhesion.[166] For patients with end-stage renal disease, this therapy has been used to offset uremia-induced platelet dysfunction with some success.[168] However, results of desmopressin use to enhance hemostasis in cardiac surgery have not been favorable.[169,170] When compared with other pharmacologic agents for reduction of blood loss in a meta-analysis of cardiac surgical patients, desmopressin was associated with an increased rate of perioperative myocardial infarction but no change in mortality when compared with placebo.[152] Although the risk of its generalized use in cardiac surgery may outweigh the benefit, its use as part of a blood management protocol using point-of-care coagulation monitoring to identify and treat isolated platelet dysfunction in the setting of clinical bleeding may prove beneficial.[171]

Activated Factor VII

Activated factor VII is a recombinant version of the naturally occurring enzyme that is the crucial factor in the extrinsic pathway of the clotting cascade. This product is FDA approved for treatment of bleeding secondary to hemophilia A and B. It is capable of bypassing the deficiency in the intrinsic pathway in these disease states by directly stimulating the common pathway leading to fibrin deposition.[17] Because of the strength of its effect, this agent has been used in other disease states with refractory, life-threatening hemorrhage and has been reported to be effective in individual cases.[172-174] However, other than in hemophilia patients, activated factor VII has not been studied in prospective trials, and the potential for a life-threatening prothrombotic effect is a concern. Although this agent has a theoretical advantage of binding to exposed collagen and activating clot formation only in regions of vessel trauma without triggering systemic coagulation, it must be tested in a randomized, blinded, placebo-controlled trial of refractory hemorrhage to know whether the benefit outweighs the risk. Also, it must be determined whether the effect is worth the cost of approximately $5000 per dose, with multiple doses often necessary to stop active hemorrhage.

■ GUIDELINES FOR EFFECTIVE BLOOD MANAGEMENT

Although unnecessary transfusion is wasteful and harmful, effective transfusion therapy designed to support oxygen-carrying capacity and replace essential components of normal coagulation in the setting of acute hemorrhage is supported by decades of battlefield, civilian trauma, and high-blood-loss surgical experience. Because transfusion therapy is an accepted standard of care, large prospective, randomized, blinded trials of transfusion versus no transfusion would be difficult to perform and would be criticized as unethical. Therefore, guidance for effective blood management is imperfect and relies on consensus expert opinion gleaned from available evidence. An additional problem arises in that, even though consensus opinion is published and widely accepted,[9,10] the presence of rational guidelines has not translated into consistent practice or reduction in unnecessary transfusion.[11,104] Protocol-driven therapy is necessary to standardize effective therapy and must be supported by point-of-care testing with timely feedback to the clinicians to guide treatment decisions at the bedside. Only in this manner can the effect of blood management techniques be adequately studied and outcome improved.[175] The remainder of this chapter discusses our institutional blood management strategy for limiting unnecessary transfusion in cardiac surgery to demonstrate the use of this concept. The protocols discussed incorporate the ASA guidelines for transfusion therapy with point-of-care testing to guide therapy at the bedside. Although many point-of-care coagulation tests are either not available or are under development, thromboelastogram (TEG) (Fig. 27-2) and activated clotting time are available and were selected as the tests used to guide therapy.

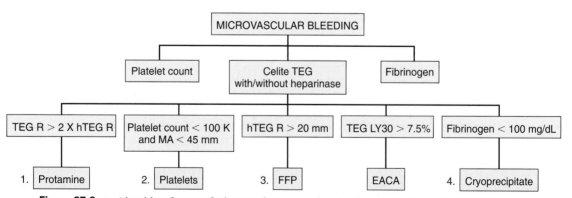

Figure 27-2 ■ Algorithm for transfusion requirements using the thromboelastography (TEG) test as a guide. EACA, ε-aminocaproic acid; FFP, fresh-frozen plasma; hTEG, heparinase-activated TEG; LY30, lysis index at 30 minutes; MA, maximum amplitude; R, reaction time. (*Redrawn from Shore-Lesserson L, Manspeizer HE, DePerio M, et al: Anesth Analg 1999;88:312-319.*)

These tests were selected for ease of use and because of published evidence supporting their use in this setting.[2,176]

Packed Red Blood Cell Transfusion

Most transfusions containing RBCs consist of packed red blood cells separated from plasma at the time of donation. Passage through a leukoreduction filter is commonly done to decrease the incidence of febrile transfusion reactions, and recent outcome data support this practice.[177] However, a prospective, randomized clinical trial of leukoreduction failed to show significant benefit.[178] PRBCs may be stored at 4° C for up to 42 days.[6] Special red blood cell preparations include frozen RBCs and irradiated RBCs. Freezing may be used to store cells with rare blood types for up to 10 years and is also used by the military as a means of stockpiling cells. Irradiation serves to inactivate any lymphocytes in the red cell preparation to prevent graft-versus-host disease in severely immunosuppressed patients such as those undergoing bone marrow transplantation or receiving chemotherapy that causes extreme bone marrow suppression. Although fresh whole blood administration may have benefits as a replacement for acute hemorrhage, this product is difficult to collect and screen for use in emergent situations. Stored whole blood has few advantages over RBCs, as platelets become inactivated when refrigerated, and clotting factor activity diminishes rapidly with storage unless frozen. Therefore, packed red cell transfusion is the recommended therapy for restoring diminished oxygen-carrying capacity in most circumstances.

The goals of therapy with RBCs are twofold: (1) to increase the oxygen-carrying capacity of blood to meet tissue demand, and (2) to replace the oxygen-carrying elements of the intravascular volume lost during acute hemorrhage. Several pieces of evidence demonstrate that stored RBCs are not as efficient as native cells for oxygen delivery. Stored RBCs become deficient in 2,3-diphosphoglycerate, resulting in hemoglobin with increased oxygen affinity (i.e., a left shift in its oxyhemoglobin dissociation curve).[179] However, this effect is transient, as the 2,3-diphosphoglycerate content of stored RBCs recovers over 24 hours after transfusion. In addition to the effects of 2,3-diphosphoglycerate depletion, evidence from animal studies shows that blood cells stored for prolonged periods of time are less efficient than native cells in meeting tissue oxygen demand.[180,181] Stored cells are less compliant, have increased osmotic fragility, and demonstrate impaired flow through microcirculation.[182] Therefore, if the patient tolerates anemia well, transfusion of stored, allogeneic red blood cells is unlikely to improve outcome and exposes the patient to unnecessary risk.

According to a single multicenter, randomized, controlled clinical trial comparing transfusion triggers in critically ill patients, associated comorbidities affect an individual's ability to tolerate anemia.[183] In this trial, patients were randomized into two groups with different hemoglobin transfusion triggers (7 g/dL or 10 g/dL) on admission to the ICU. Overall, there was no difference in 30-day mortality between the groups. However, a subgroup analysis that separated the patients into two groups depending on health status prior to the acute illness (Apache II score ≤20 versus >20)

revealed that healthier patients benefited from a restrictive RBC transfusion strategy. When this healthier group was treated with a restrictive transfusion strategy (transfused for hemoglobin ≤7 g/dL), their 30-day outcome was significantly improved compared with those treated with a liberal transfusion strategy (Fig. 27-3). Outcome was unchanged when the two transfusion strategies were compared in patients with Apache II scores greater than 20 on admission to the ICU. These results suggest that when a patient group is less able to tolerate anemia, they are not harmed by maintaining hemoglobin at a higher level with transfusion.

To divide cardiac surgical patients into low-risk and high-risk groups, a modification of the ICU severity-of-illness score, developed by Higgins and colleagues,[184] was applied to our patients on arrival in our cardiac surgery recovery unit (Table 27-1). The severity-of-illness score reported by Higgins

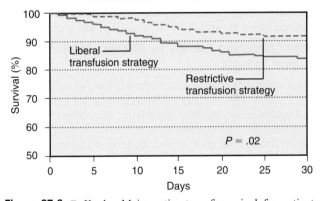

Figure 27-3 ■ Kaplan-Meier estimates of survival for patients with an APACHE II score less than 20. The survival curve includes the 30 days after admission to the intensive care unit for patients treated with a restrictive or liberal transfusion strategy. *(Redrawn from Hebert PC, Wells G, Blajchman MA, et al: N Engl J Med 1999;340:409-417. Erratum in N Engl J Med 1999;340:1056.)*

27-1	**Calculating* the Severity of Illness Score at Admission to Intensive Care**	
Condition		**Points**
Intra-aortic balloon pump in place		7
Preoperative albumin <3.5 g/dL, or hematocrit < 35%		5
Preoperative creatinine >1.9 mg/dL		4
Admission arterial HCO_3^- <21 mmol/L		4
Admission central venous pressure >17 mm Hg		4
Age >70 years		3
History of peripheral vascular disease or vascular surgery		3
Cardiopulmonary bypass time >160 minutes		3
Admission heart rate >100 beats/min		3
Admission cardiac index <2.1 L/min/m²		3
Admission alveolar-arterial gradient >250 mm Hg		2
More than one prior heart operation		2
Body surface area <1.72 m²		1
One prior heart operation		1

*Cumulative point total represents the Severity of Illness score.
Adapted from Higgins TL, Estafanous FG, Loop FD, et al: Ann Thorac Surg 1997;64:1050-1058.

and coworkers incorporated low serum albumin level as a risk factor for poor outcome.[185] This low preoperative albumin correlated with low preoperative hematocrit in the data set.[184] Because preoperative hematocrit was uniformly available in all patients scheduled for cardiac surgery but serum albumin was not otherwise measured, a preoperative hematocrit of less than 35% was substituted for serum albumin less than 3.5 g/dL in our model. According to Higgins and colleagues, 30-day mortality increased markedly if the postoperative severity-of-illness score was 10 or greater. Therefore, we combined this score with physiologic parameters indicative of adequate tissue oxygen delivery to divide patients into high- and low-risk groups (Box 27-3). A hemoglobin level of less than 8.0 g/dL was used as a trigger for RBC transfusion in the low-risk patient group, and a hemoglobin level of less than 9.3 g/dL was used as a trigger in the high-risk group after cardiac surgery. If postoperative hemorrhage was present with a chest tube output greater than 400 mL/hr, the hemoglobin trigger for transfusion was less than 10.0 g/dL. Once determination of treatment group was made, patients were managed according to the algorithm in Figure 27-4.

Blood Component Therapy for Bleeding Cardiac Surgical Patients

Blood component therapy is commonly used to replace functional platelets or clotting factor activity after hemorrhage, cardiopulmonary bypass, pathologic consumption states, drug-induced bone marrow suppression, or hepatic suppression. Randomized, prospective, controlled clinical trials of component therapy are lacking in the literature, and the risk of transfusion of multiple allogeneic blood components is significant, especially for platelets. Therefore, component therapy must be used judiciously and targeted to specific, identified defects in coagulation for patients with clinically significant bleeding. For postoperative cardiac surgical patients, clinically significant bleeding can be defined in any of the following ways:

- Greater than 300 mL of chest tube output in any 1 hour

- Greater than 400 mL of chest tube output in any 2 hours
- Greater than 100 mL/hr for 2 hours of chest tube output after the first 2 hours

Currently (as of 2006), published consensus guidelines (ASA and College of American Pathologists) are the best available evidence to guide non–red blood cell component therapy and should be combined with point-of-care testing to target therapy. Our institution's cardiac surgical algorithm for component therapy is contained in Figure 27-5.

Heparin Reversal

Inadequate protamine administration or the mobilization of heparin from poorly perfused capillary beds during hypothermic cardiopulmonary bypass represents an easily reversible cause of postoperative bleeding after cardiac surgery. The activated clotting time or heparin concentration titration can be used to ascertain the correct dose of protamine. Protamine sulfate may be administered in doses of 25 to 50 mg by slow intravenous infusion in the ICU if the activated clotting time is prolonged.

Additional protamine should *not* be given if a history of protamine reaction is present or total protamine dose exceeds 1 mg protamine per 100 units of heparin administered.

Platelet Transfusion

The decision to transfuse platelets should be made only after evidence of significant nonsurgical bleeding is identified and laboratory evidence supports functional platelet deficiency as the source of the bleeding. Transfusion of platelets is not benign and carries several identifiable risks. Platelets are stored at room temperature, unlike other blood components that are refrigerated or frozen, and platelet transfusion carries the highest risk of bacterial contamination and possible fatal bacterial sepsis.[186] Furthermore, this bacterial contamination is difficult to detect. With a short shelf-life of 5 days, positive culture results obtained from a contaminated unit may not return until after the unit is infused. Febrile nonhemolytic transfusion reactions resulting from platelet transfusion are also possible. These febrile reactions are believed to result from accumulation of bioreactive substances during storage.[187] For example, because platelet activation occurs during storage,[188] some cytokine levels in a 5-day-old unit of platelets can exceed 1000 times that of normal plasma.[187] Other clinical evidence demonstrates that platelet transfusion is associated with poor outcome in cardiac surgery and may contribute to multiorgan dysfunction in the postoperative period as a result of stimulation of a systemic inflammatory response syndrome.[189]

However, despite the risks of platelet transfusion, patients undergoing cardiac surgery with cardiopulmonary bypass often require transfusion because of a reduction in platelet count and platelet function. Although a platelet count of greater than 50,000/mm[3] is usually acceptable for most surgeries, postcardiopulmonary bypass bleeding caused by thrombasthenia may not cease without transfusion of functional allogeneic platelets, even at normal platelet counts. The decision to transfuse platelets is aided by the finding of a

---

27-3	**Risk Stratification of Postoperative Cardiac Surgical Patients**

Low-Risk Criteria for Postoperative Morbidity or Mortality

- Intensive care unit admission severity of illness score (Higgins II score) <10
- Chest tube output ≤200 mL in first hour after intensive care unit arrival
- Cardiac index ≥2 L/min/m[2]
- Venous oxygen saturation (SvO$_2$) ≥60%
- Mean arterial pressure ≥60 mm Hg
- Dopamine infusion ≤5 μg/kg/min
- Epinephrine infusion ≤0.02 μg/kg/min

High-Risk Criteria for Postoperative Morbidity or Mortality

- Incomplete surgical revascularization
- Low-risk criteria not met

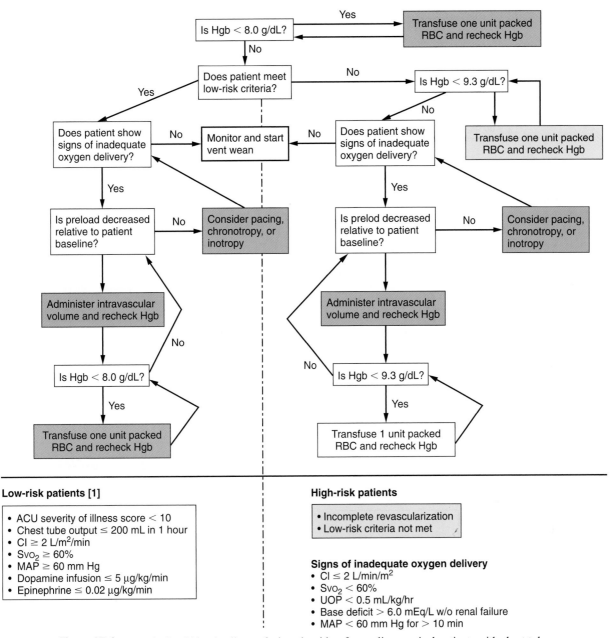

Figure 27-4 ■ Packed red blood cell transfusion algorithm for cardiac surgical patients with chest tube output of less than 400 mL/hr and no ongoing ischemia. ACU, acute care unit; CI, cardiac index; Hgb, hemoglobin; MAP, mean arterial pressure; RBC, red blood cell; Svo₂, venous oxygen saturation; UOP, urine output.

decreased maximum amplitude on thromboelastography with an underlying normal fibrinogen level. These findings suggest decreased platelet function and signify the need for platelet transfusion in the bleeding cardiac surgery patient. If bleeding persists without measurable clotting factor deficiency and the patient has a history of long-acting, nonaspirin platelet inhibitor therapy, such as clopidogrel, ticlopidine, or abciximab, then platelet transfusion is also indicated. A post-transfusion platelet count should be obtained to ensure effective therapy. Pretreatment for platelet reaction is seldom necessary, as long as the platelets are infused over 20 to 30

minutes and not given as a bolus. Platelet transfusion is ineffective for platelet dysfunction because of competitive GP IIb/IIIa inhibitors such as eptifibatide or tirofiban; transfused platelets are inactivated as long as these agents are present. Native platelet function returns to normal once the competitive GP IIb/IIIa inhibitors are eliminated, which occurs 4 to 6 hours after discontinuation.

Fresh-Frozen Plasma

Fresh-frozen plasma contains significant quantities of factors II, V, VII, IX, X, and XI, as well as antithrombin III. The

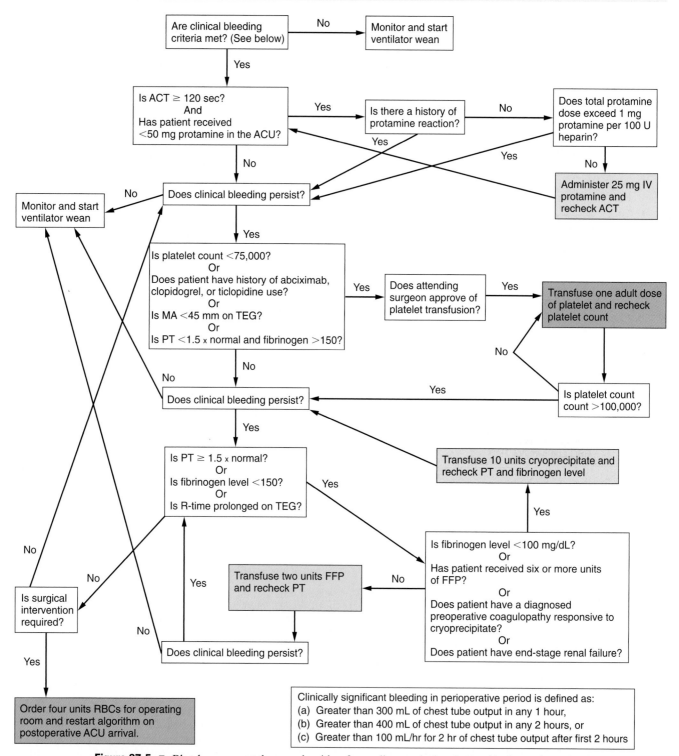

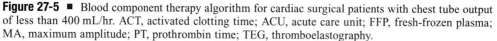

Figure 27-5 ■ Blood component therapy algorithm for cardiac surgical patients with chest tube output of less than 400 mL/hr. ACT, activated clotting time; ACU, acute care unit; FFP, fresh-frozen plasma; MA, maximum amplitude; PT, prothrombin time; TEG, thromboelastography.

half-life of clotting factors in FFP is shorter than that of native factors. Fresh-frozen plasma contains significant amounts of fibrinogen (up to 700 mg per unit) and renders cryoprecipitate unnecessary in most cardiac surgical patients. It is effective at reversing the coagulopathy induced by warfarin sodium or liver failure in the setting of acute hemorrhage but must be given in large quantities (6 to 8 units) to raise factor activity levels effectively. FFP is indicated for treatment of coagulopathy resulting from massive transfusion or cardiopulmonary bypass as long as factor deficiency is documented and clinical bleeding persists. It is also the treatment of choice for thrombotic thrombocytopenic purpura in combination with plasmapheresis. FFP should be administered as a bolus and not as a continuous infusion to acutely raise factor activity to an effective level.

Fresh-frozen plasma is not an appropriate intravascular volume expander, and it carries the same risk for viral transmission as other allogeneic blood components. Because plasma contains donor antibodies, it is a potential source of graft-versus-host disease and has been identified as a source of transfusion-related acute lung injury (TRALI).[190] TRALI, defined as new acute lung injury occurring during a transfusion or within 6 hours afterward, is now a leading cause of transfusion-associated mortality.[191] Laboratory evidence that supports the transfusion of FFP in bleeding cardiac surgical patients includes a prothrombin time greater than 1.4 times normal, a fibrinogen level between 100 and 150 mg/dL, and a prolonged R-time on a thromboelastogram. If the R-time is prolonged, heparinase must be added to the TEG to remove residual heparin before the test can support the decision to transfuse FFP. The presence of aprotinin also prolongs R-time on TEG. Thus, a normal angle of deflection on the TEG in a patient with a prolonged R-time on aprotinin suggests that FFP is not necessary. In this case, prolonged prothrombin time should be documented before administering plasma.

Cryoprecipitate

Cryoprecipitate is prepared by slowly thawing a bag of fresh-frozen plasma to 60° F, at which point a precipitate develops that is expressed from the remainder of the plasma and is refrozen. The precipitate is composed of factor VIII, von Willebrand factor, fibrinogen (about one-third the fibrinogen content of a unit of whole blood), and fibronectin. Cryoprecipitate is indicated for specific types of vWD, for hemophilia A (if monoclonal factor VIII is not available), and for patients with afibrinogenemia or dysfibrinogenemia. It is the product of choice for replacement of fibrinogen in consumption states such as disseminated intravascular coagulation. Cryoprecipitate is rarely necessary in cardiac surgery. However, for bleeding cardiac surgical patients with severely decreased levels of fibrinogen (<100 mg/dL), the small volume (10 to 15 mL per bag containing 200 to 300 g fibrinogen) allows a large amount of fibrinogen to be administered without producing volume overload. Bleeding cardiac surgical patients may benefit from cryoprecipitate if their bleeding is unresponsive to 6 or more units of FFP, and if they exhibit an abnormal prothrombin time or a TEG that shows a markedly prolonged R-time and a narrow angle of deflection. Any preoperative history of bleeding suggestive of vWD should be evaluated by a hematologist to correctly treat this condition with cryoprecipitate or desmopressin acetate if necessary.

Surgical Reexploration

An unligated vessel does not respond to pharmacologic or transfusion therapy, and it exposes the patient to increased risk for postoperative infection and to the stress of a second surgical procedure. Therefore, every effort should be made to distinguish surgical bleeding from coagulopathy prior to leaving the operating theater. According to a database study by Spiess and coworkers,[176] if a patient has clinically significant bleeding after cardiac surgery and has a normal thromboelastogram, then a surgically correctable source is predicted with greater than 90% accuracy. Additionally, if a patient bleeds more that 400 mL in the first hour or meets the criteria listed previously for clinical bleeding, yet has a prothrombin time less than 1.5 times normal, a platelet count greater than 150, and normal maximum amplitude on thromboelastography, surgical reexploration is probably necessary.

Effect of Multidisciplinary, Protocol-Driven Care

Although patient variation and practitioner bias make compliance with any complex algorithm in a large institution imperfect, attention to the clinical problem and standardization of practice can improve care and clinical outcomes. Figure 27-6 shows the change in transfusion practice at our institution over the first 2 years after enactment of the clinical guidelines outlined here. Exposure to allogeneic blood products dropped 60% in valvular surgery and 40% in coronary artery surgery. Independent assessment of surgical mortality

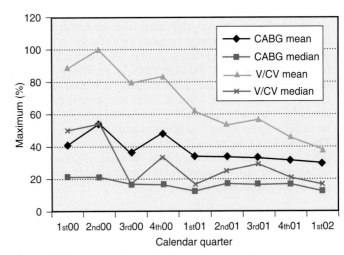

Figure 27-6 ■ Trend in Duke Heart Center patient exposure to allogeneic blood products from January 2000 through March 2002. Linear plots represent the mean and median exposures per patient for all units of allogeneic blood products administered for isolated coronary artery bypass grafting (CABG) as well as for valve repair or replacement procedures or combined coronary and valve procedures (V/CV), graphed as a percentage (%) of maximum mean exposure to allogeneic blood products. Plots do not differentiate between primary and repeat sternotomy procedures or between cardiopulmonary bypass or off-pump procedures. If CABG was performed in conjunction with valve procedures, data were included with isolated valve surgery.

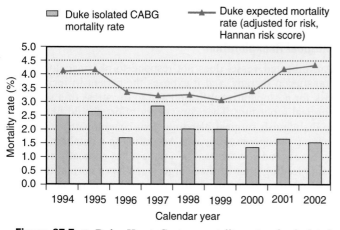

Figure 27-7 ■ Duke Heart Center mortality rates for isolated coronary artery bypass grafting (CABG) surgery by calendar year. The *linear plot* represents the expected mortality rate for primary coronary artery bypass surgical patients when adjusted for risk using the Hannan preoperative risk stratification score.[192] *Box plots* represent actual mortality rate.

over the same time period (fiscal years 2000 through 2002) revealed that mortality remained unchanged. Surprisingly, mortality remained unchanged despite the fact that expected mortality rose because of a patient population with increased comorbidity (Fig. 27-7). Therefore, initiation of evidence-based, protocol-driven care favorably affected transfusion practice without an adverse effect on mortality.

Transfusion Algorithms in Noncardiac Surgery

Although the transfusion algorithm discussed thus far was designed for use in cardiac surgical patients, the principles demonstrated apply to other high-blood-loss surgical procedures. Modification of the algorithm by removing heparin reversal and substituting other clinical indicators of postoperative blood loss in place of chest tube output make the algorithm generally applicable. The details of the algorithm must be adapted to each institution and patient population. The specifics of the protocol are less important than development of a rational, evidence-based standard of practice that addresses the risk-to-benefit ratio of each unit of allogeneic blood component transfused.

■ CONCLUSION

Very low hemoglobin is harmful. Unnecessary transfusion is harmful. The best clinical practice is to prevent low hemoglobin in the first place. To avoid the complications of allogeneic blood products while maintaining adequate oxygen delivery to overcome the stress of major surgery, attention must be paid to (1) timing of surgery in relation to antithrombotic agent administration (especially clopidogrel, ticlopidine, and abciximab), (2) minimizing effects of acute, severe hemodilution on initiation of cardiopulmonary bypass, (3) use of aprotinin for cardiac surgical patients at high risk for excessive bleeding or antifibrinolytic therapy (aminocaproic acid, tranexamic acid) in low-risk patients, (4) meticulous

attention to hemostasis in the operating theater, (5) use of point-of-care testing to guide directed transfusion therapy, and (6) clinical monitoring of patient-specific adequacy of oxygen delivery. Continued research into blood conservation and alternatives to transfusion therapy is necessary for improved care of the cardiac surgical patient.

■ ACKNOWLEDGMENTS

The authors of this chapter thank Mary Lee Campbell, BS, and Pamela J. Pennigar, BSN, MSN, FNP, for their contributions to this manuscript.

■ REFERENCES

1. Practice Guidelines for Perioperative Blood Transfusion and Adjuvant Therapies: An updated report by the American Society of Anesthesiologists Task Force on Perioperative Blood Transfusion and Adjuvant Therapies. Anesthesiology 2006;105:198-208.
2. Shore-Lesserson L, Manspeizer HE, DePerio M, et al: Thromboelastography-guided transfusion algorithm reduces transfusions in complex cardiac surgery. Anesth Analg 1999;88:312-319.
3. Llewelyn CA, Hewitt PE, Knight RS, et al: Possible transmission of variant Creutzfeldt-Jakob disease by blood transfusion. Lancet 2004;363:417-421.
4. Landsteiner K: Ueber agglutinationserscheinungen normalen menschlichen blutes. Wien Klin Wochenschr 1901;14:1132-1134.
5. Owen R: Karl Landsteiner and the first human marker locus. Genetics 2000;155:995-998.
6. Brecher ME (ed): Technical Manual, ed 15. Bethesda, American Association of Blood Banks, 2005.
7. Kleinman SH, Niland JC, Azen SP, et al: Prevalence of antibodies to human immunodeficiency virus type 1 among blood donors prior to screening. The Transfusion Safety Study/NHLBI Donor Repository. Transfusion 1989;29:572-580.
8. Donegan E, Stuart M, Niland JC, et al: Infection with human immunodeficiency virus type 1 (HIV-1) among recipients of antibody-positive blood donations [see comment]. Ann Intern Med 1990;113:733-739.
9. Practice parameter for the use of fresh-frozen plasma, cryoprecipitate, and platelets. Fresh-Frozen Plasma, Cryoprecipitate, and Platelets Administration Practice Guidelines Development Task Force of the College of American Pathologists [see comment]. JAMA 1994;271:777-781.
10. Stehling LC, Doherty DC, Faus RJ: Practice guidelines for blood component therapy: A report by the American Society of Anesthesiologists Task Force on Blood Component Therapy [see comments]. Anesthesiology 1996;84:732-747.
11. Goodnough LT, Despotis GJ: Future directions in utilization review: The role of transfusion algorithms. Transfus Sci 1998;19:97-105.
12. Hunt BJ, Segal H: Hyperfibrinolysis. J Clin Path 1996;49:958. Erratum in J Clin Pathol 1997;50:357.
13. Favier R, Aoki N, de Moerloose P: Congenital alpha-plasmin inhibitor deficiencies: A review. Br J Haematol 2001;114:4-10.
14. Meijer C, Wiezer MJ, Hack CE, et al: Coagulopathy following major liver resection: The effect of rBPI21 and the role of decreased synthesis of regulating proteins by the liver. Shock 2001;15:261-271.
15. Francis JL, Armstrong DL: Acquired dysfibrinogenaemia in liver disease. J Clin Pathol 1982;35:667-672.
16. Kamath S, Lip GY: Fibrinogen: Biochemistry, epidemiology and determinants [see comment]. QJM 2003;96:711-729.
17. Goodnough LT, Lublin DM, Zhang L, et al: Transfusion medicine service policies for recombinant factor VIIa administration. Transfusion 2004;44:1325-1331.
18. Shami VM, Caldwell SH, Hespenheide EE, et al: Recombinant activated factor VII for coagulopathy in fulminant hepatic failure compared with conventional therapy. Liver Transpl 2003;9:138-143.

19. Wysocki B: Wonder drug stops bleeding, but cost is high. Wall Street Journal 2004;Mar 17:Section B1.
20. Tsai HM: Advances in the pathogenesis, diagnosis, and treatment of thrombotic thrombocytopenic purpura. J Am Soc Nephrol 2003;14: 1072-1081.
21. Shapiro MD, Kelleher SP: Intranasal deamino-8-D-arginine vasopressin shortens the bleeding time in uremia. Am J Nephrol 1984;4:260-261.
22. Xi M, Beguin S, Hemker HC: The relative importance of the factors II, VII, IX and X for the prothrombinase activity in plasma of orally anticoagulated patients. Thromb Haemost 1989;62:788-791.
23. Allford SL, Machin SJ: Current understanding of the pathophysiology of thrombotic thrombocytopenic purpura. J Clin Pathol 2000;53: 497-501.
24. Mannucci PM: How I treat patients with von Willebrand disease. Blood 2001;97:1915-1919.
25. Warkentin TE: Heparin-induced thrombocytopenia: Diagnosis and management. Circulation 2004;110:e454-458.
26. Antithrombotic Trialists Collaboration: Collaborative meta-analysis of randomised trials of antiplatelet therapy for prevention of death, myocardial infarction, and stroke in high risk patients. BMJ 2002;324: 71-86. Erratum in BMJ 2002;324:141.
27. Evans V: Herbs and the brain: Friend or foe? The effects of ginkgo and garlic on warfarin use. J Neurosci Nurs 2000;32:229-232.
28. Vaes LP, Chyka PA: Interactions of warfarin with garlic, ginger, ginkgo, or ginseng: Nature of the evidence. Ann Pharmacother 2000;34:1478-1482.
29. Ang-Lee MK, Moss J, Yuan CS: Herbal medicines and perioperative care. JAMA 2001;286:208-216.
30. Sharis PJ, Cannon CP, Loscalzo J: The antiplatelet effects of ticlopidine and clopidogrel. Ann Intern Med 1998;129:394-405.
31. Schror K: Antiplatelet drugs: A comparative review. Drugs 1995;50: 7-28.
32. Hennekens CH, Dyken ML, Fuster V: Aspirin as a therapeutic agent in cardiovascular disease: A statement for healthcare professionals from the American Heart Association. Circulation 1997;96: 2751-2753.
33. Diener HC, Cunha L, Forbes C, et al: European Stroke Prevention Study: 2. Dipyridamole and acetylsalicylic acid in the secondary prevention of stroke. J Neurol Sci 1996;143:1-13.
34. Sethi GK, Copeland JG, Goldman S, et al: Implications of preoperative administration of aspirin in patients undergoing coronary artery bypass grafting. Department of Veterans Affairs Cooperative Study on Antiplatelet Therapy. J Am Coll Cardiol 1990; 15:15-20.
35. Goldman S, Copeland J, Moritz T, et al: Starting aspirin therapy after operation: Effects on early graft patency. Department of Veterans Affairs Cooperative Study Group [see comment]. Circulation 1991;84: 520-526.
36. Sanz G, Pajaron A, Alegria E, et al: Prevention of early aortocoronary bypass occlusion by low-dose aspirin and dipyridamole. Grupo Espanol para el Seguimiento del Injerto Coronario (GESIC). Circulation 1990;82:765-773.
37. Gavaghan TP, Gebski V, Baron DW: Immediate postoperative aspirin improves vein graft patency early and late after coronary artery bypass graft surgery: A placebo-controlled, randomized study. Circulation 1991;83:1526-1533.
38. Stein PD, Schunemann HJ, Dalen JE, Gutterman D: Antithrombotic therapy in patients with saphenous vein and internal mammary artery bypass grafts: The Seventh ACCP Conference on Antithrombotic and Thrombolytic Therapy. Chest 2004;126(3 Suppl):S600-608.
39. Mangano DT: Multicenter Study of Perioperative Ischemia Research: Aspirin and mortality from coronary bypass surgery. N Engl J Med 2002;347:1309-1317.
40. Sun JC, Crowther MA, Warkentin TE, et al: Should aspirin be discontinued before coronary artery bypass surgery. Circulation 2005; 112:e85-90.
41. Horlocker TT, Wedel DJ, Benzon H, et al: Regional anesthesia in the anticoagulated patient: Defining the risks (Second ASRA Consensus Conference on Neuraxial Anesthesia and Anticoagulation). Reg Anesth Pain Med 2003;28:172-197.
42. Plow EF, Ginsberg MH: Cellular adhesion: GPIIb-IIIa as a prototypic adhesion receptor. Prog Hemost Thromb 1989;9:117-156.
43. Use of a monoclonal antibody directed against the platelet glycoprotein IIb/IIIa receptor in high-risk coronary angioplasty. The EPIC Investigation. N Engl J Med 1994;330:956-961.
44. Simoons ML, GUSTO IV-ACS Investigators: Effect of glycoprotein IIb/IIIa receptor blocker abciximab on outcome in patients with acute coronary syndromes without early coronary revascularisation: The GUSTO IV-ACS randomised trial. Lancet 2001;357: 1915-1924.
45. Lemmer JH Jr, Metzdorff MT, Krause AH Jr, et al: Emergency coronary artery bypass graft surgery in abciximab-treated patients. Ann Thorac Surg 2000;69:90-95.
46. Kereiakes DJ, Essell JH, Abbottsmith CW, et al: Abciximab-associated profound thrombocytopenia: Therapy with immunoglobulin and platelet transfusion. Am J Cardiol 1996;78:1161-1163.
47. Effects of platelet glycoprotein IIb/IIIa blockade with tirofiban on adverse cardiac events in patients with unstable angina or acute myocardial infarction undergoing coronary angioplasty. Randomized Efficacy Study of Tirofiban for Outcomes and REstenosis. Circulation 1997;96:1445-1453.
48. Randomised placebo-controlled trial of effect of eptifibatide on complications of percutaneous coronary intervention: IMPACT-II. Integrilin to Minimise Platelet Aggregation and Coronary Thrombosis-II. Lancet 1997;349:1422-1428.
49. Uthoff K, Zehr KJ, Geerling R, et al: Inhibition of platelet adhesion during cardiopulmonary bypass reduces postoperative bleeding. Circulation 1994;90(5 Pt 2):II269-274.
50. Suzuki Y, Hillyer P, Miyamoto S, et al: Integrilin prevents prolonged bleeding times after cardiopulmonary bypass. Ann Thorac Surg 1998;66:373-381.
51. Hass WK, Easton JD, Adams HP Jr, et al: A randomized trial comparing ticlopidine hydrochloride with aspirin for the prevention of stroke in high-risk patients. Ticlopidine Aspirin Stroke Study Group. N Engl J Med 1989;321:501-507.
52. A randomised, blinded, trial of clopidogrel versus aspirin in patients at risk of ischaemic events (CAPRIE). CAPRIE Steering Committee. Lancet 1996;348:1329-1339.
53. Bertrand ME, Rupprecht HJ, Urban P, et al: Double-blind study of the safety of clopidogrel with and without a loading dose in combination with aspirin compared with ticlopidine in combination with aspirin after coronary stenting: The clopidogrel aspirin stent international cooperative study (CLASSICS). Circulation 2000;102: 624-629.
54. Moussa I, Oetgen M, Roubin G, et al: Effectiveness of clopidogrel and aspirin versus ticlopidine and aspirin in preventing stent thrombosis after coronary stent implantation. Circulation 1999;99:2364-2366.
55. Dangas G, Mehran R, Abizaid AS, et al: Combination therapy with aspirin plus clopidogrel versus aspirin plus ticlopidine for prevention of subacute thrombosis after successful native coronary stenting. Am J Cardiol 2001;87:470-472.
56. Berger PB, Bell MR, Rihal CS, et al: Clopidogrel versus ticlopidine after intracoronary stent placement. J Am Coll Cardiol 1999;34: 1891-1894.
57. Mishkel GJ, Aguirre FV, Ligon RW, et al: Clopidogrel as adjunctive antiplatelet therapy during coronary stenting. J Am Coll Cardiol 1999;34:1884-1890.
58. Sabatine MS, Cannon CP, Gibson CM, et al: Addition of clopidogrel to aspirin and fibrinolytic therapy for myocardial infarction with ST-segment elevation. N Engl J Med 2005;352:1179-1189.
59. Yusuf S, Zhao F, Mehta SR, et al: Effects of clopidogrel in addition to aspirin in patients with acute coronary syndromes without ST-segment elevation [see comment]. N Engl J Med 2001;345:494-502. Erratum in N Engl J Med 2001;345:1716.
60. Braunwald E, Antman EM, Beasley JW, et al: ACC/AHA 2002 guideline update for the management of patients with unstable angina and non-ST-segment elevation myocardial infarction—summary article: A report of the American College of Cardiology/American Heart Association task force on practice guidelines (Committee on the Management of Patients with Unstable Angina). J Am Coll Cardiol 2002;40:1366-1374.

61. Antman EM, Anbe DT, Armstrong PW, et al: ACC/AHA guidelines for the management of patients with ST-elevation myocardial infarction—executive summary: A report of the American College of Cardiology/American Heart Association Task Force on Practice Guidelines (Writing Committee to Revise the 1999 Guidelines for the Management of Patients with Acute Myocardial Infarction). Circulation 2004;110:588-636.

62. Cannon CP, Mehta SR, Aranki SF: Balancing the benefit and risk of oral antiplatelet agents in coronary artery bypass surgery. Ann Thorac Surg 2005;80:768-779.

63. Ray JG, Deniz S, Olivieri A, et al: Increased blood product use among coronary artery bypass patients prescribed preoperative aspirin and clopidogrel. BMC Cardiovasc Disord 2003;3:3.

64. van der Linden J, Lindvall G, Sartipy U: Aprotinin decreases postoperative bleeding and number of transfusions in patients on clopidogrel undergoing coronary artery bypass graft surgery. Circulation 2005;112:I276-280.

65. Hirsh J, Anand SS, Halperin JL, et al: Guide to anticoagulant therapy: Heparin—A statement for healthcare professionals from the American Heart Association. Circulation 2001;103:2994-3018.

66. Hirsh J, Raschke R: Heparin and low-molecular-weight heparin: The Seventh ACCP Conference on Antithrombotic and Thrombolytic Therapy. Chest 2004;126(3 Suppl):S188-203.

67. Dolovich LR, Ginsberg JS, Douketis JD, et al: A meta-analysis comparing low-molecular-weight heparins with unfractionated heparin in the treatment of venous thromboembolism: Examining some unanswered questions regarding location of treatment, product type, and dosing frequency. Arch Intern Med 2000;160:181-188.

68. Levine M, Gent M, Hirsh J, et al: A comparison of low-molecular-weight heparin administered primarily at home with unfractionated heparin administered in the hospital for proximal deep-vein thrombosis [see comment]. N Engl J Med 1996;334:677-681.

69. Koopman MM, Prandoni P, Piovella F, et al: Treatment of venous thrombosis with intravenous unfractionated heparin administered in the hospital as compared with subcutaneous low-molecular-weight heparin administered at home. The Tasman Study Group. N Engl J Med 1996;334:682-687. Erratum in N Engl J Med 1997;337:1251.

70. Nurmohamed MT, Rosendaal FR, Buller HR, et al: Low-molecular-weight heparin versus standard heparin in general and orthopaedic surgery: A meta-analysis. Lancet 1992;340:152-156.

71. Schafer AI: Low-molecular-weight heparin: An opportunity for home treatment of venous thrombosis. N Engl J Med 1996;334:724-725.

72. Massonnet-Castel S, Pelissier E, Bara L, et al: Partial reversal of low molecular weight heparin (PK 10169) anti-Xa activity by protamine sulfate: In vitro and in vivo study during cardiac surgery with extracorporeal circulation. Haemostasis 1986;16:139-146.

73. Warkentin TE, Greinacher A: Heparin-induced thrombocytopenia: Recognition, treatment, and prevention: The Seventh ACCP Conference on Antithrombotic and Thrombolytic Therapy. Chest 2004;126(3 Suppl):S311-337. Erratum in Chest 2005;127:416.

74. Mahaffey KW: Anticoagulation for acute coronary syndromes and percutaneous coronary intervention in patients with heparin-induced thrombocytopenia. Curr Cardiol Rep 2001;3:362-370.

75. Lincoff AM, Bittl JA, Harrington RA, et al: Bivalirudin and provisional glycoprotein IIb/IIIa blockade compared with heparin and planned glycoprotein IIb/IIIa blockade during percutaneous coronary intervention: REPLACE-2 randomized trial. JAMA 2003;289:853-863. Erratum in JAMA 2003;289:1638.

76. Di Nisio M, Middeldorp S, Buller HR: Direct thrombin inhibitors. N Engl J Med 2005;353:1028-1040.

77. Swan SK, Hursting MJ: The pharmacokinetics and pharmacodynamics of argatroban: Effects of age, gender, and hepatic or renal dysfunction. Pharmacotherapy 2000;20:318-29.

78. Sheth SB, DiCicco RA, Hursting MJ, et al: Interpreting the International Normalized Ratio (INR) in individuals receiving argatroban and warfarin. Thromb Haemost 2001;85:435-440. Erratum in Thromb Haemost 2001;86:727.

79. Eichler P, Friesen HJ, Lubenow N, et al: Antihirudin antibodies in patients with heparin-induced thrombocytopenia treated with lepirudin: Incidence, effects on aPTT, and clinical relevance. Blood 2000;96:2373-2378.

80. Fischer KG, Liebe V, Hudek R, et al: Anti-hirudin antibodies alter pharmacokinetics and pharmacodynamics of recombinant hirudin. Thromb Haemost 2003;89:973-982.

81. Greinacher A, Lubenow N, Eichler P: Anaphylactic and anaphylactoid reactions associated with lepirudin in patients with heparin-induced thrombocytopenia [see comment]. Circulation 2003;108:2062-2065.

82. Freedman MD: Oral anticoagulants: Pharmacodynamics, clinical indications and adverse effects. J Clin Pharmacol 1992;32:196-209.

83. Ansell J, Hirsh J, Dalen J, et al: Managing oral anticoagulant therapy. Chest 2001;119(1 Suppl):S22-38.

84. Hanley JP: Warfarin reversal. J Clin Pathol 2004;57:1132-1139.

85. White RH, McKittrick T, Hutchinson R, Twitchell J: Temporary discontinuation of warfarin therapy: Changes in the international normalized ratio. Ann Intern Med 1995;122:40-42.

86. Kakkar VV: Deep vein thrombosis: Detection and prevention. Circulation 1975;51:8-19.

87. Bernard GR, Vincent JL, Laterre PF, et al: Efficacy and safety of recombinant human activated protein C for severe sepsis [see comment]. N Engl J Med 2001;344:699-709.

88. Kozek-Langenecker SA: Effects of hydroxyethyl starch solutions on hemostasis. Anesthesiology 2005;103:654-660.

89. Jamnicki M, Bombeli T, Seifert B, et al: Low- and medium-molecular-weight hydroxyethyl starches: Comparison of their effect on blood coagulation. Anesthesiology 2000;93:1231-1237.

90. Conroy JM, Fishman RL, Reeves ST, et al: The effects of desmopressin and 6% hydroxyethyl starch on factor VIII:C. Anesth Analg 1996;83:804-807.

91. Claes Y, Van Hemelrijck J, Van Gerven M, et al: Influence of hydroxyethyl starch on coagulation in patients during the perioperative period. Anesth Analg 1992;75:24-30.

92. Stogermuller B, Stark J, Willschke H, et al: The effect of hydroxyethyl starch 200 kD on platelet function. Anesth Analg 2000;91:823-827.

93. Franz A, Braunlich P, Gamsjager T, et al: The effects of hydroxyethyl starches of varying molecular weights on platelet function. Anesth Analg 2001;92:1402-1407.

94. Boldt J, Haisch G, Suttner S, et al: Effects of a new modified, balanced hydroxyethyl starch preparation (Hextend) on measures of coagulation. Br J Anaesth 2002;89:722-728.

95. Niemi TT, Kuitunen AH: Artificial colloids impair haemostasis: An in vitro study using thromboelastometry coagulation analysis. Acta Anaesthesiol Scand 2005;49:373-378.

96. DeFoe GR, Ross CS, Olmstead EM, et al: Lowest hematocrit on bypass and adverse outcomes associated with coronary artery bypass grafting. Ann Thorac Surg 2001;73:769-776.

97. Fang WC, Helm RE, Krieger KH, et al: Impact of minimum hematocrit during cardiopulmonary bypass on mortality in patients undergoing coronary artery surgery. Circulation 1997;96(9 Suppl):II194-199.

98. Hardy JF, Martineau R, Couturier A, et al: Influence of haemoglobin concentration after extracorporeal circulation on mortality and morbidity in patients undergoing cardiac surgery. Br J Anaesth 1998;81(1 Suppl):38-45.

99. Habib RH, Zacharias A, Schwann TA, et al: Adverse effects of low hematocrit during cardiopulmonary bypass in the adult: Should current practice be changed? J Thorac Cardiovasc Surg 2003;125:1438-1450.

100. van Wermeskerken GK, Lardenoye JW, Hill SE, et al: Intraoperative physiologic variables and outcome in cardiac surgery: Part II. Neurologic outcome. Ann Thorac Surg 2000;69:1077-1083.

101. Hill SE, van Wermeskerken GK, et al: Intraoperative physiologic variables and outcome in cardiac surgery: Part I. In-hospital mortality. Ann Thorac Surg 2000;69:1070-1075; discussion 1075-1076.

102. Wu WC, Rathore SS, Wang Y, et al: Blood transfusion in elderly patients with acute myocardial infarction. N Engl J Med 2001;345:1230-1236.

103. Rao SV, Jollis JG, Harrington RA, et al: Relationship of blood transfusion and clinical outcomes in patients with acute coronary syndromes. JAMA 2004;292:1555-1562.

104. Stover EP, Siegel LC, Parks R, et al: Variability in transfusion practice for coronary artery bypass surgery persists despite national consensus

guidelines: A 24-institution study. Institutions of the Multicenter Study of Perioperative Ischemia Research Group. Anesthesiology 1998;88:327-333.

105. Spiess BD: Blood transfusion: The silent epidemic. Ann Thorac Surg 2001;72:S1832-1837.

106. Freilich D, Branda R, Hacker M, et al: Decreased lactic acidosis and anemia after transfusion of o-raffinose cross-linked and polymerized hemoglobin in severe murine malaria. Am J Trop Med Hyg 1999;60:322-328.

107. Bracey AW, Radovancevic R, Riggs SA, et al: Lowering the hemoglobin threshold for transfusion in coronary artery bypass procedures: Effect on patient outcome. Transfusion 1999;39:1070-1077.

108. Vincent JL, Baron JF, Reinhart K, et al: Anemia and blood transfusion in critically ill patients. JAMA 2002;288:1499-1507.

109. Engoren MC, Habib RH, Zacharias A, et al: Effect of blood transfusion on long-term survival after cardiac operation [see comment]. Ann Thorac Surg 2002;74:1180-1186.

110. Viele MK, Weiskopf RB: What can we learn about the need for transfusion from patients who refuse blood? The experience with Jehovah's Witnesses. Transfusion 1994;34:396-401.

111. Spence RK, Costabile JP, Young GS, et al: Is hemoglobin level alone a reliable predictor of outcome in the severely anemic surgical patient? Am Surg 1992;58:92-95.

112. Carson JL, Noveck H, Berlin JA, Gould SA: Mortality and morbidity in patients with very low postoperative Hb levels who decline blood transfusion. Transfusion 2002;42:812-818.

113. Weiskopf RB, Viele MK, Feiner J, et al: Human cardiovascular and metabolic response to acute, severe isovolemic anemia. JAMA 1998;279:217-221.

114. Weiskopf RB, Kramer JH, Viele M, et al: Acute severe isovolemic anemia impairs cognitive function and memory in humans. Anesthesiology 2000;92:1646-152.

115. Liam BL, Plochl W, Cook DJ, et al: Hemodilution and whole body oxygen balance during normothermic cardiopulmonary bypass in dogs. J Thorac Cardiovasc Surg 1998;115:1203-1208.

116. Moskowitz DM, Klein JJ, Shander A, et al: Predictors of transfusion requirements for cardiac surgical procedures at a blood conservation center. Ann Thorac Surg 2004;77:626-634.

117. New Jersey Department of Health and Senior Services, Lacy CR (Commissioner): Cardiac Surgery in New Jersey 2001: A Consumer Report. 2004:1-21. Available at www.state.nj.us/health/hcsa/documents/cardconsumer01.pdf.

118. Slappendel R, Dirksen R, Weber EW, van der Schaaf DB: An algorithm to reduce allogenic red blood cell transfusions for major orthopedic surgery. Acta Orthop Scand 2003;74:569-575.

119. Goldberg MA, McCutchen JW, Jove M, et al: A safety and efficacy comparison study of two dosing regimens of epoetin alfa in patients undergoing major orthopedic surgery. Am J Orthop 1996;25:544-552.

120. de Andrade JR, Jove M, Landon G, et al: Baseline hemoglobin as a predictor of risk of transfusion and response to epoetin alfa in orthopedic surgery patients. Am J Orthop 1996;25:533-542.

121. Faris PM, Ritter MA, Abels RI: The effects of recombinant human erythropoietin on perioperative transfusion requirements in patients having a major orthopaedic operation. The American Erythropoietin Study Group. J Bone Joint Surg Am 1996;78:62-72.

122. Pierson JL, Hannon TJ, Earles DR: A blood-conservation algorithm to reduce blood transfusions after total hip and knee arthroplasty. J Bone Joint Surg Am 2004;86-A:1512-1518.

123. Provan D: Mechanisms and management of iron deficiency anaemia. Br J Haematol 1999;105(1 Suppl):19-26.

124. Goodnough LM, Grishaber JE, Birkmeyer JD, et al: Efficacy and cost-effectiveness of autologous blood predeposit in patients undergoing radical prostatectomy procedures. Urology 1994;44:226-231.

125. Monk TG, Goodnough LT, Brecher ME, et al: Acute normovolemic hemodilution can replace preoperative autologous blood donation as a standard of care for autologous blood procurement in radical prostatectomy. Anesth Analg 1997;85:953-958.

126. D'Ambra MN, Gray RJ, Hillman R, et al: Effect of recombinant human erythropoietin on transfusion risk in coronary bypass patients. Ann Thorac Surg 1997;64:1686-1693.

127. Goodnough LT, Despotis GJ, Parvin CA: Erythropoietin therapy in patients undergoing cardiac operations. Ann Thorac Surg, 1997;64:1579-1580.

128. Kyo S, Omoto R, Hirashima K, et al: Effect of human recombinant erythropoietin on reduction of homologous blood transfusion in open-heart surgery: A Japanese multicenter study. Circulation 1992;86(5 Suppl):II413-418.

129. Omoto R, Kyo S, Furuse A, et al: [Effects of subcutaneous administration of erythropoietin on autologous blood predonation in open heart surgery: Japanese multicenter double-blinded dose-study]. Rinsho Kyobu Geka 1994;14:510-521.

130. Sowade O, Warnke H, Scigalla P, et al: Avoidance of allogeneic blood transfusions by treatment with epoetin beta (recombinant human erythropoietin) in patients undergoing open-heart surgery. Blood 1997;89:411-418.

131. Sowade O, Ziemer S, Sowade B, et al: The effect of preoperative recombinant human erythropoietin therapy on platelets and hemostasis in patients undergoing cardiac surgery. J Lab Clin Med 1997;129:376-383.

132. Gaudiani VA, Mason HD: Preoperative erythropoietin in Jehovah's Witnesses who require cardiac procedures. Ann Thorac Surg 1991;51:823-824.

133. Spence RK: Current concepts and issues in blood management. Orthopedics 2004;27(6 Suppl):S643-651.

134. Bryson GL, Laupacis A, Wells GA: Does acute normovolemic hemodilution reduce perioperative allogeneic transfusion? A meta-analysis. The International Study of Perioperative Transfusion. Anesth Analg 1998;86:9-15.

135. American Association of Blood Banks, Perioperative Standards Program Unit: Standards for perioperative autologous blood collection and administration, ed 1. Bethesda, AABB, 2001.

136. Helm RE, Klemperer JD, Rosengart TK, et al: Intraoperative autologous blood donation preserves red cell mass but does not decrease postoperative bleeding. Ann Thorac Surg 1996;62:1431-1441.

137. Monk TG, Goodnough LT, Brecher ME, et al: A prospective randomized comparison of three blood conservation strategies for radical prostatectom. Anesthesiology 1999;91:24-33.

138. Goodnough LT, Despotis GJ, Merkel K, Monk TG: A randomized trial comparing acute normovolemic hemodilution and preoperative autologous blood donation in total hip arthroplasty. Transfusion 2000;40:1054-1057.

139. Matot I, Scheinin O, Jurim O, Eid A: Effectiveness of acute normovolemic hemodilution to minimize allogeneic blood transfusion in major liver resections. Anesthesiology 2002;97:794-800.

140. Hill SE, Grocott HP, Leone BJ, et al: Cerebral physiology of cardiac surgical patients treated with the perfluorocarbon emulsion, AF0144. Ann Thorac Surg 2005;80:1401-1407.

141. Kincaid EH, Jones TJ, Stump DA, et al: Processing scavenged blood with a cell saver reduces cerebral lipid microembolization. Ann Thorac Surg 2000;70:1296-1300.

142. Huet C, Salmi LR, Fergusson D, et al: A meta-analysis of the effectiveness of cell salvage to minimize perioperative allogeneic blood transfusion in cardiac and orthopedic surgery. International Study of Perioperative Transfusion (ISPOT) Investigators. Anesth Analg 1999;89:861-869.

143. Kongsgaard UE, Wang MY, Kvalheim G: Leucocyte depletion filter removes cancer cells in human blood. Acta Anaesthesiol Scand 1996;40:118-120.

144. Waters JH, Lee JS, Karafa MT: A mathematical model of cell salvage compared and combined with normovolemic hemodilution. Transfusion 2004;44:1412-1416.

145. Edelman MJ, Potter P, Mahaffey KG, et al: The potential for reintroduction of tumor cells during intraoperative blood salvage: Reduction of risk with use of the RC-400 leukocyte depletion filter. Urology 1996;47:179-181.

146. Perseghin P, Vigano M, Rocco G, et al: Effectiveness of leukocyte filters in reducing tumor cell contamination after intraoperative blood salvage in lung cancer patients. Vox Sang 1997;72:221-224.

147. Davis M, Sofer M, Gomez-Marin O, et al: The use of cell salvage during radical retropubic prostatectomy: Does it influence cancer recurrence? BJU Int 2003;91:474-476.

148. Gray CL, Amling CL, Polston GR, et al: Intraoperative cell salvage in radical retropubic prostatectomy. Urology 2001;58:740-745.

149. Teufelsbauer H, Proidl S, Havel M, Vukovich T: Early activation of hemostasis during cardiopulmonary bypass: Evidence for thrombin mediated hyperfibrinolysis. Thromb Haemost 1992;68:250-252.

150. Despotis GJ, Avidan MS, Hogue CW Jr. Mechanisms and attenuation of hemostatic activation during extracorporeal circulation. Ann Thorac Surg 2001;72:S1821-1831.

151. Nuttall GA, Oliver WC, Ereth MH, et al: Comparison of blood-conservation strategies in cardiac surgery patients at high risk for bleeding. Anesthesiology 2000;92:674-682.

152. Levi M, Cromheecke ME, de Jonge E, et al: Pharmacological strategies to decrease excessive blood loss in cardiac surgery: A meta-analysis of clinically relevant endpoints. Lancet 1999;354:1940-1947.

153. Sethna NF, Zurakowski D, Brustowicz RM, et al: Tranexamic acid reduces intraoperative blood loss in pediatric patients undergoing scoliosis surgery. Anesthesiology 2005;102:727-732.

154. Florentino-Pineda I, Thompson GH, Poe-Kochert C, et al: The effect of Amicar on perioperative blood loss in idiopathic scoliosis: The results of a prospective, randomized double-blind study. Spine 2004;29:233-238.

155. Lemmer JH Jr, Stanford W, Bonney SL, et al: Aprotinin for coronary bypass operations: Efficacy, safety, and influence on early saphenous vein graft patency: A multicenter, randomized, double-blind, placebo-controlled study. J Thorac Cardiovasc Surg 1994;107:543-551; discussion 551-553.

156. Levy JH, Pifarre R, Schaff HV, et al: A multicenter, double-blind, placebo-controlled trial of aprotinin for reducing blood loss and the requirement for donor-blood transfusion in patients undergoing repeat coronary artery bypass grafting. Circulation 1995;92:2236-2244.

157. Mangano DT, Tudor IC, Dietzel C: The risk associated with aprotinin in cardiac surgery. N Engl J Med 2006;354:353-365.

158. Poullis M, Manning R, Laffan M, et al: The antithrombotic effect of aprotinin: Actions mediated via the protease-activated receptor 1. J Thorac Cardiovasc Surg 2000;120:370-378.

159. Landis RC, Asimakopoulos G, Poullis M, et al: The antithrombotic and antiinflammatory mechanisms of action of aprotinin. Ann Thorac Surg 2001;72:2169-2175.

160. Day JR, Punjabi PP, Randi AM, et al: Clinical inhibition of the seven-transmembrane thrombin receptor (PAR1) by intravenous aprotinin during cardiothoracic surgery. Circulation 2004;110:2597-2600.

161. Mojcik CF, Levy JH: Aprotinin and the systemic inflammatory response after cardiopulmonary bypass. Ann Thorac Surg 2001;71:745-754.

162. Smith PK, Muhlbaier LH: Aprotinin: Safe and effective only with the full-dose regimen. Ann Thorac Surg 1996;62:1575-1577.

163. Cole JW, Murray DJ, Snider RJ, et al: Aprotinin reduces blood loss during spinal surgery in children. Spine 2003;28:2482-2485.

164. Murkin JM, Shannon NA, Bourne RB, et al: Aprotinin decreases blood loss in patients undergoing revision or bilateral total hip arthroplasty. Anesth Analg 1995;80:343-348.

165. Murkin JM, Haig GM, Beer KJ, et al: Aprotinin decreases exposure to allogeneic blood during primary unilateral total hip replacement. J Bone Joint Surg Am 2000;82:675-684.

166. Zeigler ZR, Megaludis A, Fraley DS: Desmopressin (d-DAVP) effects on platelet rheology and von Willebrand factor activities in uremia. Am J Hematol 1992;39:90-95.

167. Kaufmann JE, Vischer UM: Cellular mechanisms of the hemostatic effects of desmopressin (DDAVP). J Thromb Haemost 2003;1:682-689.

168. Mannucci PM, Remuzzi G, Pusineri F, et al: Deamino-8-D-arginine vasopressin shortens the bleeding time in uremia. N Engl J Med 1983;308:8-12.

169. Pleym H, Stenseth R, Wahba A, et al: Prophylactic treatment with desmopressin does not reduce postoperative bleeding after coronary surgery in patients treated with aspirin before surgery. Anesth Analg 2004;98:578-584.

170. Ozkisacik E, Islamoglu F, Posacioglu H, et al: Desmopressin usage in elective cardiac surgery. J Cardiovasc Surg 2001;42:741-747.

171. Despotis GJ, Levine V, Saleem R, et al: Use of point-of-care test in identification of patients who can benefit from desmopressin during cardiac surgery: A randomised controlled trial. Lancet 1999;354:106-110.

172. Holcomb JB: Use of recombinant activated factor VII to treat the acquired coagulopathy of trauma. J Trauma 2005;58:1298-1303.

173. Almeida AM, Khair K, Hann I, Liesner R: The use of recombinant factor VIIa in children with inherited platelet function disorders [see comment]. Br J Haematol 2003;121:477-481.

174. Roberts HR, Monroe DM, White GC: The use of recombinant factor VIIa in the treatment of bleeding disorders. Blood 2004;104:3858-3864.

175. Van der Linden P, De Hert S, Daper A, et al: A standardized multidisciplinary approach reduces the use of allogeneic blood products in patients undergoing cardiac surgery. Can J Anaesth 2001;48:894-901.

176. Spiess BD, Gillies BS, Chandler W, Verrier E: Changes in transfusion therapy and reexploration rate after institution of a blood management program in cardiac surgical patients. J Cardiothorac Vasc Anesth 1995;9:168-1673.

177. Hebert PC, Fergusson D, Blajchman MA, et al: Clinical outcomes following institution of the Canadian universal leukoreduction program for red blood cell transfusions. JAMA 2003;289:1941-1949.

178. Dzik WH, Anderson JK, O'Neill EM, et al: A prospective, randomized clinical trial of universal WBC reduction. Transfusion 2002;42:1114-1122.

179. Valeri CR, Hirsch NM: Restoration in vivo of erythrocyte adenosine triphosphate, 2,3-diphosphoglycerate, potassium ion, and sodium ion concentrations following the transfusion of acid-citrate-dextrose-stored human red blood cells. J Lab Clin Med 1969;73:722-733.

180. Fitzgerald RD, Martin CM, Dietz GE, et al: Transfusing red blood cells stored in citrate phosphate dextrose adenine-1 for 28 days fails to improve tissue oxygenation in rats. Crit Care Med 1997;25:726-732.

181. van Bommel J, de Korte D, Lind A, et al: The effect of the transfusion of stored RBCs on intestinal microvascular oxygenation in the rat. Transfusion 2001;41:1515-1523.

182. Ho J, Sibbald WJ, Chin-Yee IH: Effects of storage on efficacy of red cell transfusion: When is it not safe? Crit Care Med 2003;31(12 Suppl):S687-697.

183. Hebert PC, Wells G, Blajchman MA, et al: A multicenter, randomized, controlled clinical trial of transfusion requirements in critical care. Transfusion Requirements in Critical Care Investigators, Canadian Critical Care Trials Group. N Engl J Med 1999;340:409-417. Erratum in N Engl J Med 1999;340:1056.

184. Higgins TL, Estafanous FG, Loop FD, et al: ICU admission score for predicting morbidity and mortality risk after coronary artery bypass grafting. Ann Thorac Surg 1997;64:1050-1058.

185. Higgins TL, Estafanous FG, Loop FD, et al: Stratification of morbidity and mortality outcome by preoperative risk factors in coronary artery bypass patients. A clinical severity score. JAMA 1992;267:2344-2348. Erratum in JAMA 1992;268:1860.

186. Centers for Disease Control and Prevention: Fatal bacterial infections associated with platelet transfusions—United States, 2004. MMWR Morb Mortal Wkly Rep 2005;54:168-170.

187. Ferrer F, Rivera J, Corral J, et al: Evaluation of pooled platelet concentrates using prestorage versus poststorage WBC reduction: Impact of filtration timing. Transfusion 2000;40:781-788.

188. Muylle L: The role of cytokines in blood transfusion reactions. Blood Rev 1995;9:77-83.

189. Spiess BD, Royston D, Levy JH, et al: Platelet transfusions during coronary artery bypass graft surgery are associated with serious adverse outcomes. Transfusion 2004;44:1143-1148.

190. Silliman CC, Boshkov LK, Mehdizadehkashi Z, et al: Transfusion-related acute lung injury: Epidemiology and a prospective analysis of etiologic factors. Blood 2003;101:454-462.

191. Toy P, Popovsky MA, Abraham E, et al: Transfusion-related acute lung injury: Definition and review. Crit Care Med 2005;33:721-726.

192. Hannan EL, Kilburn H Jr, Racz M, et al: Improving the outcomes of coronary artery bypass surgery in New York State. JAMA 1994;271:761-766.

Infections

Chapter

28 | Prevention of Perioperative and Surgical Site Infection

Carlene A. Muto and Marian Pokrywka

Each year, health-care facilities report increases in the number of surgical procedures that occur. Data from the National Center for Health Statistics reported a 4% increase in surgical procedures from 1995 to 1996, and, according to the most recent data reported, 46.5 million surgical procedures were performed in 1996.[1,2] Surgical site infections (SSIs) are the second most common cause of hospital-acquired infections, accounting for approximately 17% of them.[3] Two decades ago, the Centers for Disease Control and Prevention (CDC) estimated that approximately 500,000 SSIs occur annually in the United States.[4] The CDC National Nosocomial Infections Surveillance System (NNIS) report for 1986-1996 described an SSI rate of 2.6% for all operations at the reporting hospitals.[3] If the rate of SSIs has remained stable, then we can expect that greater than 1 million SSIs now occur annually.

SSIs are associated with increased costs and worse outcomes for hospital inpatients. SSIs prolong hospital stay by an average of 7.4 days and add $400 to $2600 to hospital costs.[5-11] SSIs following cardiac surgery have been associated with significantly higher costs, ranging from $8200 to $42,000.[12-15] Table 28-1 shows estimates of the annual financial impact for a variety of types of SSIs.

All surgical wounds are contaminated by bacteria, but only a minority actually demonstrate clinical infection. In most patients, infection does not develop because innate host defenses are quite efficient in eliminating contaminants at the surgical site. Whether an SSI develops after surgery depends on a complex interaction between (1) patient-related factors such as age, obesity, host immunity, nutritional status, and the presence or absence of diabetes; (2) procedure-related factors such as placement of a foreign body, duration of operation, skin antisepsis, and the magnitude of tissue trauma; (3) microbial factors that mediate tissue adherence

and invasion or that enable the bacterium to survive the host immune response and to concurrently colonize or infect the host; and (4) perioperative antimicrobial prophylaxis.

■ INFECTION CLASSIFICATION

Classification of wounds can be based on the degree of bacterial load or contamination that they contain. Since the landmark 1964 National Academy of Sciences' National Research Council study on the use of ultraviolet lights in the operating room (OR), wounds have been classified by the level of risk for contamination. The four categories are clean, clean/contaminated, contaminated, and dirty/infected.[16] This classification of the degree of contamination in the surgical site during surgery has become the traditional system for predicting infection risk in surgical wounds.

Surgical site infections are classified into two groups: (1) incisional and (2) organ and organ/space. The incisional SSIs are further divided into those involving only skin and subcutaneous tissue (superficial incisional SSI) and those involving deeper soft tissues of the incision (deep incisional SSI). Organ/space SSIs involve any part of the anatomy (e.g., organ or space) other than incised body wall layers that was opened or manipulated during an operation.[17,18] The criteria used for defining an SSI are listed in Box 28-1. The identification of SSI involves interpretation of clinical and laboratory data. The CDC has derived standardized surveillance definitions, and these criteria must be applied consistently when classifying an SSI.

■ MICROBIOLOGY

The risk for infection increases once the site has been contaminated with greater than 10^5 organisms per gram of

28-1	Estimated Annual Financial Impact of Surgical Site Infection (SSI) by Specific Procedure			
	CABG	**Colorectal**	**THR**	**TKR**
Procedures *(N)*	383,000	250,000	293,000	324,000
SSI *(n)*	14,975	15,075	4,109	3,726
Deaths *(n)*	11,107	11,500	3,809	648
Cost per SSI	$5,576	$8,425	$47,700	$16,908
Total cost (in millions)	$83.5	$127	$196	$63

CABG, coronary artery bypass grafting; THR, total hip replacement; TKR, total knee replacement.

From Centers for Disease Control and Prevention National Nosocomial Infections Surveillance System data.

tissue.[19] The bacterial burden necessary to inflict infection is significantly reduced when foreign material is in place (i.e., only 100 staphylococci per gram of tissue when introduced on silk sutures).[20-22] Risk is also proportional to the toxins produced by the specific pathogen, as these agents can facilitate host invasion, can damage tissues, and can interfere with host defenses.

The pathogens responsible for SSIs have not significantly changed over time. Table 28-2 lists the distribution of pathogens isolated from SSIs. *Staphylococcus aureus,* coagulase-negative staphylococci, and *Enterococcus* species represent nearly 50% of the pathogens associated with SSIs. Recently, there has been an increase in the proportion of SSIs that are caused by antimicrobial-resistant pathogens, such as methicillin-resistant *S. aureus* (MRSA) and *Candida albicans.*[23-25]

Sources of Pathogens

The primary source of SSI pathogens is the endogenous flora of the patient's skin, mucous membranes, or hollow viscera.[26]

28-2	Distribution of Pathogens Isolated* from Surgical Site Infections, National Nosocomial Infections Surveillance System, 1986-1996	
	% OF ISOLATES	
Pathogen	**1986-1989** **N = 16,727**	**1990-1996** **N = 11,724**
Staphylococcus aureus	17	20
Coagulase-negative staphylococci	12	14
Enterococcus species	13	12
Escherichia coli	10	8
Pseudomonas aeruginosa	8	8
Enterobacter species	8	7
Proteus mirabilis	4	3
Klebsiella pneumoniae	3	3
Other *Streptococcus* species	3	3
Candida albicans	2	3
Group D streptococci (nonenterococci)	—	2
Other gram-positive aerobes	—	2
Bacteroides fragilis	—	2

*Pathogens representing less than 2% of isolates are excluded.

28-1	Criteria for Defining a Surgical Site Infection (SSI)

Superficial Incisional SSI

- Occurs within 30 days after the operation
- Involves only the skin or subcutaneous tissue
- At least one of the following:
  - Purulent drainage, with or without laboratory confirmation, from the superficial incision
  - Organisms isolated from an aseptically obtained culture of fluid or tissue from the superficial incision
  - At least one of the following signs or symptoms of infection: pain or tenderness, localized swelling, redness, or heat, *and* the superficial incision is deliberately opened by surgeon, *unless* incision is culture negative
  - Diagnosis of superficial incisional SSI by the surgeon or attending physician

Deep Incisional SSI

- Occurs within 30 days after the operation if no implant is left in place, or within 1 year if implant is in place and the infection appears to be related to the operation
- Involves deep soft tissues (e.g., fascial and muscle layers) of the incision
- At least one of the following:
  - Purulent drainage from the deep incision but not from the organ/space component of the surgical site
  - A deep incision spontaneously dehisces or is deliberately opened by a surgeon when the patient has at least one of the following signs or symptoms: fever (>38°C), localized pain or tenderness, unless site is culture negative
  - An abscess or other evidence of infection involving the deep incision is found on direct examination, during reoperation, or by histopathologic or radiologic examination
  - Diagnosis of a deep incisional SSI by a surgeon or attending physician

Organ/Space SSI

- Infection occurs within 30 days after the operation if no implant is left in place or within 1 year if implant is in place and the infection appears to be related to the operation
- Involves any part of the anatomy (e.g., organs or spaces) other than the incision, which was opened or manipulated during an operation and involves anatomic structures not opened or manipulated during the operation
- At least one of the following:
  - Purulent drainage from a drain that is placed through a stab wound into the organ/space
  - Organisms isolated from an aseptically obtained culture of fluid or tissue in the organ/space
  - An abscess or other evidence of infection involving the organ/space that is found on direct examination, during reoperation, or by histopathologic or radiologic examination
  - Diagnosis of an organ/space SSI by a surgeon or attending physician

From National Nosocomial Infections Surveillance (NNIS) System Report, data summary from January 1992 to June 2002, issued August 2002. Atlanta, Centers for Disease Control, and available at www.cdc.gov/ncidod/dhqp/pdf/guidelines/SSI.pdf.

When the mucous membrane or skin is incised, the exposed tissues are at risk for contamination with endogenous flora.[27] These organisms are usually aerobic gram-positive cocci (e.g., staphylococci). When an organ system is entered, endogenous flora specific to it may be the source of the pathogen (e.g., enteric flora such as *Escherichia coli* or other gram-negative rods when bowel surgery is performed).

Surgical pathogens can also be derived from exogenous sources. Examples include surgical personnel (especially members of the surgical team), the OR environment (including air), and materials on the sterile field (such as instruments, equipment, containers) during an operation. Exogenous flora are primarily aerobes, especially gram-positive organisms (e.g., staphylococci and streptococci).[28-32] Although *S. aureus* is usually from an endogenous source, evidence suggests exogenous pathways as well.[33] Fungal SSIs are infrequent but can be endogenously or exogenously derived.[34] Infections in patients undergoing clean surgical procedures are usually derived from airborne exogenous microorganisms.[35]

Nevertheless, there are over two dozen reports of *Candida* infections in prosthetic joints,[36] and a growing number of studies report *Candida* infections after cardiac surgery.[37-43] Although these infections are infrequent, they are associated with serious problems. Mortality is greater than 50%.[41-46] One outbreak was traced to a member of the surgical team.[42]

■ RISK AND PREVENTION: PATIENT CHARACTERISTICS

A *risk factor* is a characteristic statistically associated with, although not necessarily causally related to, an increased risk for a particular outcome. Risk of developing an SSI is directly proportional to the size of the bacterial inoculum and the virulence of the organism(s) and inversely proportional to the resistance of the host. A number of host factors must be considered. Factors that increase a patient's risk of developing an SSI include extremes of age,[6,47-53] steroid use,[54-56] cigarette smoking,[47,57-61] obesity (>20% ideal bodyweight),[55,57,62-66] a low preoperative serum albumin level or malnutrition,[48,57,63,67-69] the presence of remote infection at the time of surgery,[70-79] perioperative transfusion,[80-83] preoperative nares colonization,[84-86] hypoxemia,[87] and diabetes.[54,55,57,62,88-90] Most potential host factors have not been well studied, or the studies done have not been able to consistently and independently link the potential risk factor to an increased SSI risk. However, a few host factors deserve special attention.

Diabetes

Diabetes mellitus is a well-known risk factor for adverse medical events. Historically, the independent contribution of diabetes to SSI risk was not clear because of many confounders. More recently, poor glucose control has been associated with increased SSI risk.[91-95] Increased risk for infection is thought to result from a combination of the long-term effects of hyperglycemia (e.g., macrovascular and microvascular disease) and the poor wound healing associated with neutrophil dysfunction.[96-102] Hyperglycemia may also impair the function of complement and antibodies, thus impairing phagocytosis and further reducing barriers to infection.[103,104] Although many of the long-term effects of diabetes cannot be reversed, some evidence suggests that improving glucose control can improve immunologic function and reduce the

incidence of SSIs.[96-98,102] Recent prospective randomized studies showed that tight glucose control during the perioperative period in diabetic patients undergoing cardiac surgery is associated with reduced infection risk.[89,105] Aggressive glucose control in the perioperative period was achieved using a continuous intravenous insulin infusion, and serum glucose was maintained at a level of less than 200 mg/dL. Furnary and colleagues found that the effect of the aggressive glucose control remained statistically significant in a logistic regression model adjusting for multiple potential confounding variables, and they found that no patient experienced a hypoglycemic event.[105]

Perioperative Normothermia

Hypothermia causes numerous adverse outcomes, including morbid myocardial events, coagulopathy with increased blood loss and transfusion requirement, postsurgical wound infections, and prolonged hospitalization.[106] The primary connection between thermoregulation and postsurgical resistance to infection is that hypothermia triggers thermoregulatory vasoconstriction, which, in turn, decreases tissue oxygenation. Hyperthermia reduces the production of superoxide radicals and other oxygen intermediates at a given level of tissue oxygenation,[107] thereby mediating neutrophil oxidative killing of microorganisms. According to one recent trial, better intraoperative and postoperative temperature control of patients may reduce the risk for SSI.[108] This study, designed to determine whether normothermia during colorectal resection decreases the incidence of surgical wound infections or length of hospital stay, was a randomized, double-blind, controlled trial with follow-up for 2 weeks after discharge. Elective surgical patients ($N = 200$) undergoing colon resection were randomized to routine intraoperative thermal care (core body temperature $\geq 34.5°$ C) or additional warming (core body temperature maintained at greater than $36.5°$ C). Other variables of care were standardized between groups. Patients maintained at the higher core temperature had an SSI rate of 6%, whereas those in the lower core temperature group had an SSI rate of 19% ($P < .009$). The study concluded that normothermia during colorectal resection was associated with decreased surgical wound infections and shorter length of hospital stay.

Supplemental Perioperative Oxygen

A prospective, randomized trial of elective colon surgery provided evidence that administering supplemental oxygen has a favorable influence in the prevention of infection.[87] Patients were randomized to receive 30% or 80% inspired oxygen during the procedure and for 2 hours postoperatively in the recovery area. All patients received standardized care, including mechanical bowel preparation and systemic antibiotics. Patients in the 30% inspired oxygen group had an SSI rate of 11% compared with an SSI rate of 5% ($P < .05$) in the 80% inspired oxygen group. It is presumed that increased oxygen availability is a positive host factor, perhaps via enhanced production of oxidant products that facilitate phagocytic eradication of microbes. The authors concluded that the perioperative administration of supplemental oxygen is a practical method of reducing the incidence of surgical wound infections.[87]

Several potential issues have been cited regarding this study. Alonso-Echanove and colleagues at the CDC noted that the surveillance period for SSIs was abbreviated to 15 postoperative days and suggested that supplemental oxygen may have delayed, rather than prevented, infections.[109] Lee raised the issue that specific timing and dosages of prophylactically administered antibiotics were not reported, and if there were differences, other variables could have explained the reported outcomes.[110] A more recent randomized controlled trial by Pryor and colleagues[111] attempted to study the effects of hyperoxia in the general surgical population, whereas the earlier study included only patients having colorectal resection. This study was terminated prematurely, as an interim analysis of the first 160 patients (of a planned 300) unexpectedly showed a significantly higher rate of SSI in the group receiving a fractional concentration of carbon dioxide in inspired gas (FIO_2) of 0.80 (25.0%) than in the group receiving an FIO_2 of 0.35 (11.3%). They concluded that the routine use of high perioperative FIO_2 in a general surgical population does not reduce the overall incidence of SSI and may have predominantly deleterious effects. Until additional well-designed studies can elucidate the risks and benefits of hyperoxia, routine implementation of this strategy should not occur. Instead, oxygen should continue to be administered with the goals of maintaining adequate hemoglobin oxygen saturation and ensuring adequate oxygen transport.

Preoperative Nares Colonization with S. aureus

Nasal carriage of *S. aureus* has been known as a risk factor for the development of surgical wound infection for nearly half a century. In 1959, Williams and associates reported an increased risk for wound infection in patients carrying *S. aureus* in their nose preoperatively.[112] Weinstein[113] found that patients with preoperative colonization of nasal pathogens who were undergoing major surgery were 2.3 times more likely to acquire an infection than those patients with negative nasal cultures. Over the past dozen years, several studies have conclusively demonstrated that nasal carriage of *S. aureus* is a risk factor for wound infection among cardiothoracic surgery patients.[86,114,115] Additionally, genotypically identical strains of *S. aureus* have been recovered from the nose and from the surgical wound infection of patients.[86,116,117] Treatment with topical mupirocin has been suggested as a strategy to eradicate nasal *S. aureus* and to decrease SSIs. Numerous studies have reported lower *S. aureus* SSI rates among patients who received preoperative treatment with mupirocin,[118-120] but methodologic concerns have been raised. The double-blinded, randomized, controlled MARS (Mupirocin and the Risk of *Staphylococcus aureus*) study failed to find a significant decrease in the incidence of *S. aureus* surgical site infections.[121] Paterson and colleagues demonstrated a lack of efficacy of mupirocin in prevention of *S. aureus* infections in the liver transplant population they studied.[122]

Routine treatment of all patients and personnel with nasal carriage of MRSA has been done in some parts of Europe and Australia and has been proposed in the United States. However, several institutions have found that mupirocin resistance increased after its use. Miller and coworkers, for example, reported an increase in mupirocin resistance from 2.7% to 65%.[123] Investigators in Brazil also found the University Hospital in Rio de Janeiro had a mupirocin resistance rate of 63% after the hospital began to use mupirocin daily in colonized or infected patients.[124] The efficacy of the routine use of mupirocin to reduce SSIs requires further study.

■ PREOPERATIVE ISSUES

Preoperative Antiseptic Showering

A preoperative antiseptic shower or bath reduces skin colonization and decreases the risk for contamination at the surgical site. More than 2 decades ago, Cruse and Foord reported that the SSI rate (2.3%) was nearly double among patients who did not shower compared with those who showered with chlorhexidine (1.3%).[6] Hayek and colleagues[125] and Paulson[126] also found that chlorhexidine-containing products lowered SSI rates. Garibaldi reported a ninefold reduction of cutaneous bacterial colony counts in patients who received chlorhexidine preoperative antiseptic showers, whereas povidone-iodine or triclocarban-medicated soap reduced colony counts by 1.3- and 1.9-fold, respectively.[127] However, in this study, no difference in SSI rates was observed. Similar results were reported by Rotter and colleagues[128] and others.[127-134] Rotter and coworkers reported no significant difference in SSI rates after conducting a large prospective, double-blinded trial randomizing patients to perioperative baths with or without chlorhexidine. Maximal benefit is achieved after several applications of chlorhexidine gluconate–containing products, so repeated antiseptic showers are recommended.[135]

Preoperative Hair Removal

Although the origin of the practice of removing hair from the operative site has not been clearly documented, this surgical practice dates back to at least the 1850s at Bellevue Hospital in New York City,[136] and it has been an established practice since the beginning of the 20th century.[137] Numerous studies have demonstrated, however, that razor shaving is associated with a decrease in skin integrity because of the nicks and cuts that occur on the skin surface. These gross and microscopic razor injuries liberate resident dermal bacteria into the operative field and make the skin environment more favorable to bacterial proliferation.[138]

The Guideline for Prevention of Surgical Site Infection, published in 1999 by the CDC,[139] advises that if hair is to be removed, it should be done so immediately before surgery and preferably with electric hair clippers. Despite this recommendation and the consistent outcomes of 30 years of repetitive studies demonstrating that preoperative shaving is a risk factor for the development of SSIs, razor shaving, on either wet or dry skin, remains the most common method of preoperative hair removal. Seropian and Reynolds[140] conducted the first prospective randomized studies that challenged this practice. Their study evaluated the rate of SSI after either razor hair removal or a depilatory or no hair removal in 406 patients. These investigators found that the SSI rate was nearly 10 times higher when hair was removed by razors (5.6%) than when no hair was removed or a depilatory was used (0.6%). In 1967, Cruse and Foord[48] conducted a large prospective study of all surgical wounds at the Foothills Hospital in Calgary, Alberta, Canada. Hair removal technique was evaluated on 23,649 patients. Shaved patients had an SSI rate of 2.3%, whereas clipped patients had an SSI rate of 1.7%. The SSI rate was lowest (0.9%) for the patients who had no hair removal. A landmark 10-year prospective study found the SSI rate was higher when hair was removed by electric clippers (1.4%) and highest when hair was removed by razors (2.5%) compared with no hair removal (0.9%).[141] Other studies have confirmed these findings.[50,93,142-145]

The timing of the hair removal is also important. Hair removal immediately prior to the operation is associated with decreased SSI rates when compared with hair removal within 24 hours preoperatively. Preoperative shaving of the surgical site the night before the surgery was found to be associated with a significantly higher SSI risk than either the use of depilatory agents or no hair removal.[6,50,146-148] Clipping hair immediately before an operation has been associated with an even lower risk for SSI than shaving or clipping the night before an operation (1.8% versus 4.0%).[142,144,145,149] Other studies have shown increased SSI risk with any means of hair removal and advocate that that no hair be removed.[50,93,143]

Preoperative Antisepsis for Surgical Team Members

Hand and Forearm Scrubbing

An antiseptic is defined as a germicidal that is used on skin or living tissue for the purpose of inhibiting or destroying microorganisms. Surgical hand scrubs have been known to play a vital part in preventing surgical site infections for many years, beginning with the pioneering work of Ignaz Philipp Simmelweiss[150] and Joseph Lister in the 1860s. Six commercially available antimicrobial ingredients in the United States are approved antiseptic agents for surgical hand/forearm antisepsis. They include alcohols, chlorhexidine gluconate, iodine/iodophors, parachlorometaxylenol (PCMX), hexachlorophene, and triclosan. Chlorhexidine gluconate, the iodophors (e.g., povidone-iodine), and alcohol-containing products are the most commonly used agents.[151-153] The U.S. Food and Drug Administration (FDA) requires that products for surgical hand scrubs provide a one-log reduction on day 1, a two-log reduction on day 2, a three-log reduction on day 5, and show persistent activity for at least 6 hours on each of the 3 test days.[154] Although the data on the efficacy of microbial killing by these antiseptics demonstrate decreased bacterial colony counts on hands, the impact of the choice of scrub agent on SSI risk has not been evaluated.[152,155-159]

Alcohol is the primary agent for surgical hand antisepsis in several European countries.[150,160,161] It has been found to be more effective than washing hands with plain soap in all studies, and the majority of alcohols were more effective than povidone-iodine or chlorhexidine in reducing microbial counts.[152,162-172] Historically, alcohol-containing products were used less frequently in the United States, probably because

of concerns about flammability and drying of skin. A fire associated with an alcohol-based hand rub was recently reported in the United States.[173] However, alcohol-based preparations for surgical hand antisepsis are gaining popularity because they are waterless, they involve less scrub time, they have a broad spectrum of activity, and, perhaps most importantly, no brushes are needed.[174] Povidone-iodine and chlorhexidine gluconate are the current agents of choice for most U.S. surgical team members.[175] These agents are more active than triclosan or plain soap. One of the most important attributes of chlorhexidine is its persistence. Because of its strong affinity for skin, it remains active for at least 6 hours, which makes it the best agent for an activity of long duration, and it is not inactivated by blood or serum proteins. The greatest sustained activity was achieved when alcoholic chlorhexidine (60% isopropanol and 0.5% chlorhexidine gluconate in 70% isopropanol) was tested.[176,177] Studies reporting PCMX efficacy have yielded contradictory results.[152,169,174]

Factors other than the choice of antiseptic agent influence the effectiveness of the surgical scrub. Scrubbing technique, the duration of the scrub, the condition of the hands, and the techniques used for drying and gloving are examples of such factors. Surgical hand-antisepsis protocols have required personnel to scrub with a brush or sponge. Scrubbing with these products is associated with equally reduced bacterial counts,[178-180] but this practice is damaging to the skin and results in increased shedding of bacteria from the hands.[181,182] Data now suggest that neither a brush nor a sponge is necessary to reduce bacterial counts on the hands of surgical personnel to acceptable levels, especially when alcohol-based products are used.[172,183-187]

Duration of Scrub Time

Traditionally, a scrub time of 10 minutes was typical. Recent data suggest that a shortened scrub time of 2 or 3 minutes is as effective as the longer scrub time in reducing hand bacterial colony counts,[184,188-194] but the optimal duration of scrubbing is still not clear.

Artificial nails should not be worn by a surgical team member, as this may increase microbial hand colonization despite performing an adequate hand scrub[195,196] and increase risk for infection.[197] Nails should be kept short so as to not compromise the integrity of the surgical gloves.[175,195,198]

Management of Infected or Colonized Surgical Personnel

A limited number of SSI outbreaks have been linked to surgical personnel who have active infections or are colonized with certain microorganisms.[95,199-215] Health-care facilities should implement policies to prevent transmission of microorganisms from personnel to patients. Infected or colonized health-care workers should be prohibited from work until they are deemed no longer infectious, without being penalized with loss of wages, benefits, or job status.[216]

Patient Skin Preparation in the Operating Room

The primary aim of patient skin antisepsis is to kill or incapacitate microorganisms and reduce the risk for postoperative infection.[217] The FDA requires skin preparations to be safe and fast-acting, to have a broad spectrum of activity, and to significantly reduce microbial skin counts.[218] The operative site should be prepared by thoroughly washing the incision site to remove gross contamination before performing antiseptic skin preparation.[219] Five commercially available antimicrobial ingredients in the United States are approved antiseptic agents for surgical site disinfection. They include alcohols, chlorhexidine gluconate, iodine/iodophors, PCMX, and triclosan. Chlorhexidine gluconate, the iodophors (e.g., povidone-iodine), and alcohol-containing products are the most commonly used agents. There have been no well-controlled studies to determine the superiority of any agent.

As mentioned, alcohol is readily available and inexpensive, and it is the most effective and rapid-acting skin antiseptic.[220] Although it has excellent germicidal activity against bacteria, fungi, and viruses, spores can be resistant.[175,220] Chlorhexidine gluconate and iodophors have broad spectra of antimicrobial activity.[175,221,222] Compared with iodophors, chlorhexidine gluconate has been shown to have a greater microflora reductive effect, to have greater residual activity after a single application,[223-225] and to not be inactivated by blood or serum proteins.[220,221,226,227]

An evolution of antiseptics has influenced perioperative practices. Historically, antiseptic agents progressed from the era of alcohol and carbolic acid to hexachlorophene and PCMX, then to povidone iodine, followed by chlorhexidine gluconate agents. Each agent is characterized by advantages and disadvantages, requiring knowledge of its proper use. Now, newer formulations of these antiseptics as well as advanced technologies offer an enhanced, prolonged, persistent efficacy with low toxicity to the patient when used properly. Historically, the patient's skin was prepared by applying the antiseptic in concentric circles, beginning in the area of the proposed incision.[175,219] Eighty percent of resident and transient skin flora reside in the first five epidermal layers of the skin barrier, so the antiseptic should be applied with mechanical friction. Friction can be best achieved with a side-to-side application, which allows the solution to penetrate the cracks and fissures of the epidermal layer of the skin. This technique may be recommended by the manufacturer.[228]

The application may need to be modified, depending on the condition of the skin (e.g., burns) or the location of the incision site (e.g., face). Suggested modifications of the preoperative skin preparation procedure include (1) removing or wiping off the antiseptic agent after application, (2) using an antiseptic-impregnated adhesive drape, (3) merely painting the skin with an antiseptic in lieu of the full skin preparation procedure described, or (4) using a "clean" instead of a sterile surgical skin preparation kit.[229-232] None of these modifications has been shown to offer an advantage.

Antimicrobial Prophylaxis

Antimicrobial prophylaxis (AMP) refers to a short course of an antibiotic. The first dose should be administered prior to the surgery.[233-235] The goal is to reduce the number of organisms that could contaminate the operative site to a level that will not overwhelm host defenses. Several decades ago, it

was determined that such contaminants, including *S. aureus*, can be recovered from the operative site prior to closure.[236,237] Burke demonstrated that prevention of SSI required that antibiotics be at an effective concentration in the tissue at the time of contamination.[238] Systemic antibiotics given after the contaminating event had no appreciable effect on the natural history of infection.

For AMP to be fully effective, an appropriate antimicrobial agent is selected on the basis of the type of surgery. Recommendations for surgical AMP are listed in Table 28-3,[239] and these follow current national guidelines.[240-242] Optimal surgical AMP depends on adequate concentrations being present in the serum, tissue, and wound during the entire time that the incision is open and at risk for contamination. The antimicrobial should be active against all potential contaminants. The agent should be safe and inexpensive and should have the least effect on the normal flora of the body.

Timing of AMP Infusion

The initial dose of the AMP agent should be infused so that its bactericidal concentration is established in serum and tissues by the time the skin is incised, and so that it remains at a therapeutic concentration until the incision is closed.[241-245] Classen and associates found that SSI rates ranged from 0.6% to 3.8% depending on the timing on the infusion. The highest rates were seen when antibiotics were infused more than 2 hours before and again 3 hours after the incision. Rates were lowest (at 0.6%) among patients who were infused within 2 hours of the incision.[246]

Over the past few years, appropriate AMP infusion timing has undergone significant discussion, and several surgical guidelines have been published.[233,240,247-251] The Medicare National Surgical Infection Prevention Project (SIPP) committee thoroughly reviewed these surgical AMP guidelines and found variation in AMP timing recommendations.[252] They concluded that the infusion of the first antimicrobial dose should begin within 60 minutes before incision (120 minutes if a fluoroquinolone or vancomycin is indicated). There was no consensus that the infusion must be completed before incision.

Duration of Surgical AMP

The majority of the published evidence demonstrates that AMP after wound closure is unnecessary. A variety of clinical studies have found no difference in SSI rates when single-dose and multiple-dose regimens have been compared.[233,240,245,247,248,250,253-255] Extended use may be associated with adverse events, such as *Clostridium difficile* colitis and the emergence of resistant bacterial strains.[256-258] The recommendation that AMP should be discontinued within 24 hours after the operation is supported by the published literature and is endorsed by the Centers for Medicare and Medicaid Services and the CDC-implemented SIPP.[259]

A recent study showed that preoperative *S. aureus* nasal carriage is the most important risk factor for development of sternal wound infection with *S. aureus* after sternotomy.[260] It was hypothesized that perioperative elimination of nasal carriage might reduce SSI rates. Intranasal mupirocin has been

28-3 Recommendations for Surgical Antimicrobial Prophylaxis (AMP)

Surgical Procedure	Recommended Agent	Likely Pathogens	Strength of Evidence for Prophylaxis[a]
Cardiac			
Valve surgery Coronary artery bypass Other open heart surgery	Cefazolin[b] or vancomycin[b]	*Staphylococcus aureus,* *Staphylococcus epidermidis,* *Corynebacterium,* enteric gram-negative bacilli	A
Heart transplant	Cefazolin[b] or vancomycin[b]	*S. aureus, S. epidermidis,* *Corynebacterium,* enteric gram-negative bacilli	A
Thoracic			
Pulmonary or mediastinal surgery	Cefazolin[b] or vancomycin[b]	*S. aureus, S. epidermidis,* streptococci, enteric gram-negative bacilli	A
Esophagectomy	Ampicillin/sulbactam,[b] or vancomycin[b]	*S. aureus, S. epidermidis,* streptococci, enteric gram-negative bacilli	A
Lung transplantation (nonseptic)	Ampicillin/sulbactam,[b] vancomycin + aztreonam	*S. aureus, S. epidermidis,* streptococci, enteric gram-negative bacilli, *Pseudomonas aeruginosa* (transplant recipients)	A
Lung transplantation (septic)	Individualize antimicrobials to infective flora and/or pre-transplant culture and sensitivity results	*S. aureus, S. epidermidis,* streptococci, enteric gram-negative bacilli, *P. aeruginosa* (transplant recipients)	B
Neurosurgery			
Neurosurgical procedures	Cefazolin[b,c] or vancomycin	*S. aureus, S. epidermidis*	A
Orthopedic			
Hip fracture repair Total joint replacement	Cefazolin[b] or vancomycin	*S. aureus, S. epidermidis*	A
Internal fixation of fractures	Cefazolin[b] or vancomycin	*S. aureus, S. epidermidis*	C
Peripheral Vascular			
Arterial surgery involving the abdominal aorta, a prosthesis, or a groin incision	Cefazolin[b] or vancomycin	*S. aureus, S. epidermidis,* enteric gram-negative bacilli	A
Lower-extremity amputation for ischemia	Cefazolin[b,d] or vancomycin	*S. aureus, S. epidermidis,* enteric gram-negative bacilli, *Clostridia* species	A
Ophthalmic			
Ophthalmic procedures	Polytrim, gentamicin, or fluoroquinolone drops or cefazolin conjunctivally	*S. aureus, S. epidermidis,* enteric gram-negative bacilli, *Pseudomonas* species	C
Head and Neck			
Head and neck procedures	Cefazolin[d]	*S. aureus,* anaerobes, enteric gram-negative bacilli	A
Abdominal			
Gastroduodenal For high-risk patients when lumen is entered: bleeding gastric or duodenal ulcer, obstructive duodenal ulcer, gastric cancer, percutaneous gastrostomy, morbid obesity[e]	Cefotetan or metronidazole + gentamicin	Group B streptococcus, enterococci, enteric gram-negative bacilli, staphylococci, anaerobes	A, C

Continued

28-3   Recommendations for Surgical Antimicrobial Prophylaxis (AMP)—cont'd

Surgical Procedure	Recommended Agent	Likely Pathogens	Strength of Evidence for Prophylaxis[a]
Appendectomy	Cefotetan or metronidazole + gentamicin	Enterococci, enteric gram-negative bacilli, staphylococci, anaerobes	A
Biliary tract For high-risk patients: age >70 yr, obstructive jaundice, nonfunctioning gall bladder, acute cholecystitis, biliary obstruction, or common bile duct stones	Cefotetan or metronidazole + gentamicin	Enterococci, enteric gram-negative bacilli, *Clostridia* species	A
ERCP For high-risk patients: those with artificial heart valves, known valvular heart disease or prostheses, history of bacterial endocarditis, or biliary obstruction	Piperacillin/tazobactam or clindamycin + gentamicin	Enterococci, enteric gram-negative bacilli, *Clostridia* species	B
Colorectal	Oral neomycin base + erythromycin base or IV cefotetan, cefoxitin, or cefazolin + metronidazole	Enterococci, enteric gram-negative bacilli, anaerobes	A
Genitourinary For high-risk patients: preoperative or prolonged postoperative catheterization, positive or unavailable urine culture, transrectal prostatic biopsy	Oral: trimethoprim/sulfamethoxazole or quinolone IV: cefazolin[c]	Enterococci, enteric gram-negative bacilli (especially *Escherichia coli*)	A
Abdominal Transplant			
Liver or multivisceral	Ampicillin/sulbactam[c,d] or vancomycin + aztreonam	Gram-negative aerobic bacilli, staphylococci, enterococci	B
Kidney	Cefazolin[b,c] or vancomycin + aztreonam	Staphylococci, enteric gram-negative aerobic bacilli (especially *E. coli* and *Klebsiella* species)	A
Kidney-pancreas	Cefotetan[b,c] or vancomycin + aztreonam	Staphylococci, enteric gram-negative aerobic bacilli (especially *E. coli* and *Klebsiella* species)	B
Gynecologic and Obstetric			
Cesarean delivery	Cefazolin[b] or vancomycin	Enteric gram-negatives, anaerobes, enterococci, streptococci, staphylococci	A
Hysterectomy	Cefazolin[b] or vancomycin	Enteric gram-negatives, anaerobes, enterococci, streptococci, staphylococci	A
Abortion, 1st trimester, high risk[f]	Penicillin or doxycycline	Enteric gram-negatives, anaerobes, enterococci, streptococci, staphylococci	A
Penetrating Abdominal Trauma			
Laparotomy	Cefotetan	Enteric gram-negative bacilli, anaerobes, enterococci	B

28-3 | **Recommendations for Surgical Antimicrobial Prophylaxis (AMP)—cont'd**

Surgical Procedure	Recommended Agent	Likely Pathogens	Strength of Evidence for Prophylaxis[a]
Ruptured viscus	Cefotetan + gentamicin or clindamycin + gentamicin	Enteric gram-negative bacilli, anaerobes, enterococci	B
Traumatic wound	IV: cefazolin[b] Oral: amoxicillin/clavulanate (Augmentin)	Staphylococci, streptococci, Clostridia species	B
Orthopedic trauma: closed fractures	Cefazolin[b,c] or vancomycin or clindamycin	Staphylococci, streptococci, Clostridia species	A
Orthopedic trauma: open fractures	Grade I: see closed fracture	Staphylococci, streptococci, Clostridia species	B
	Grade II: add gentamicin	Staphylococci, streptococci, Clostridia species	B
	Grade III: same as grade II Where soil contamination or very large amounts of soft tissue damage, add penicillin	Staphylococci, streptococci, Clostridia species	B

a. Strength of evidence supports using or not using prophylaxis as A (levels I-III), B (levels IV-VI), or C (level VII). Level 1 evidence is from large, well-conducted, randomized, controlled trials. Level II evidence is from small, well-conducted, randomized, controlled trials. Level III evidence is from well-conducted cohort studies. Level IV evidence is from well-conducted case-control studies. Level V, VI, and VII evidence is from poorly constructed uncontrolled studies, conflicted evidence that tends to support the opinion, and expert opinion, respectively.

b. Vancomycin may be used for patients with documented penicillin or cephalosporin allergy. Routine use of vancomycin for surgical prophylaxis should be discouraged because it promotes the emergence of resistant enterococci. When used, vancomycin must be infused over 60 minutes.

c. If surgery is >3 hr, an additional dose is necessary every 4 to 6 hr during the length of the surgery.

d. If colonization or infection with gram-negative organisms is expected, consider adding an aminoglycoside to the clindamycin regimen: gentamicin 80 mg IV (1.7 mg/kg) at induction of anesthesia. Addition of metronidazole 500 mg IV to cefazolin regimen increases coverage against anaerobic organisms.

e. For gastric bypass surgery, duration may be up to 24 hr.

f. Previous pelvic inflammatory disease, previous gonorrhea, or multiple sex partners.

ERCP, endoscopic retrograde cholangiopancreatography; IV, intravenous.

Adapted from Skledar S, Gross P, Hamilton L: University of Pittsburgh recommendations for surgical antimicrobial prophylaxis. In Potoski B (ed): Guide to Antimicrobial Chemotherapy. Pittsburgh, Pa, University of Pittsburgh Medical Center, Presbyterian, 2005, pp 40-45.

studied in a variety of operations to evaluate its impact on SSIs. Kluytmans and associates[261] did an unblended interventional study with historical controls. Those in the intervention group were given topical mupirocin for 5 days, with the first dose given the day before surgery. They found that the overall SSI rate was 4.5% lower (68/928 [7.3%] versus 24/868 [2.8%], $P < .0001$) than in the historical controls. They concluded that routine use of mupirocin was effective in reducing SSIs.

More recently, a prospective randomized, double-blinded, placebo-controlled trial looked at the efficacy of preventing S. aureus nosocomial infections associated with cardiothoracic, general, and neurosurgical surgeries.[262] All patients were screened, and 891 of 4030 (22%) were colonized with S. aureus. Placebo was given to 436 of the 891, and 429 received mupirocin. At the time of analysis, 409 of 436 (93.8%) in the control group were still positive for S. aureus, but only 87 of 429 (4.6%) of the treated group were positive ($P < .0001$). In the treatment group, 57 of 411 (13.9%) had SSI, and in the placebo group, 72 of 425 (16.9%) had SSI (P = not significant). Of the 129 infections, 51 were caused by S. aureus; 17 of 398 (4.3%) were in the treatment group, and 34 of 418 (8.1%) were in the placebo group ($P = .03$).

A group from the Netherlands did an unblinded historical controlled interventional trial in which 1044 patients undergoing orthopedic surgery received mupirocin and 1260 patients did not.[120] The SSI rate was 14 of 1044 (1.3%) in the intervention group and 34 of 1260 (2.7%) in the control group ($P = .02$). The rates of infection caused by S. aureus were 7 of 1044 (0.7%) in the intervention group and 14 of 1260 (1.1%) in the control group ($P = .3$). This study did not reach statistical significance. Although the use of intranasal mupirocin has been effective at reducing nasal carriage of S. aureus, the majority of studies do not demonstrate a reduction in SSI rates.[121,263,264]

Are Cephalosporins Adequate as AMP in the Era of Methicillin-Resistant S. aureus?

The routine use of vancomycin for AMP is not recommended for any kind of surgery. However, CDC guidelines[250] suggest that vancomycin can be considered in certain clinical situations, such as when a cluster of MRSA infections has been detected. The threshold to support the decision to use vancomycin has not been scientifically defined. Additionally, there is no evidence that routine use of vancomycin for AMP will result in fewer SSIs than when other agents are used, even in institutions with perceived high rates of MRSA infection. Finkelstein and colleagues, in an institution with a perceived high rate of MRSA infection, randomized 885 cardiac surgery patients to AMP with cefazolin or vancomycin.[265] SSI rates were not statistically different (9.0% of patients who received cefazolin and 9.5% of patients who received vancomycin, respectively; *P* = .8). However, cefazolin-treated patients who later developed an SSI were more likely to be infected with MRSA, and vancomycin-treated patients were more likely to be infected with methicillin-susceptible *S. aureus*. Manian and associates[266] did not find that the use of a non–vancomycin-containing AMP regimen was associated with risk for MRSA SSI. Vancomycin might be considered an appropriate AMP agent in patients known to be colonized by MRSA. According to the recent Society for Healthcare Epidemiology of America guideline, colonization status of patients at high risk for carriage of MRSA should be routinely determined at the time of admission.[267]

OPERATING ROOM ENVIRONMENT

The operating room (OR), a controlled environment designed for the performance of surgical procedures, is the most highly regulated of all the patient service areas in the hospital. Its operation and maintenance are governed by the state department of health, the Joint Commission on Accreditation of Healthcare Organizations (JCAHO), recommendations from the CDC, the American Institute of Architects, and clinical practice guidelines developed by professional organizations such as the American College of Surgeons, the American Society of Anesthesiologists, and the Association of Operating Room Nurses. Together, these associations and organizations have outlined strict controls for the design and mechanical function of the OR.

Ventilation

Microorganisms in the air of the OR can be a potential source of surgical wound contamination. Airflow is therefore directed and balanced to maintain positive pressure in the OR rooms with respect to corridors and adjacent areas.[268] Conventional OR ventilation systems are required to provide a minimum of 15 air exchanges of filtered air per hour, 20% of which must be fresh air. Hospital ventilation systems use filters in series to filter fresh air, and the internal ventilation system employs a filter at each room with greater than 90% efficiency. Air is introduced at the level of the ceiling and exhausted near the floor.[269]

Laminar airflow with high-efficiency particulate air (HEPA) filters has been shown to be useful primarily in orthopedic and implant surgery, where infection rates have been significantly reduced.[270] Laminar airflow is designed to move particle-free air (ultra-clean) over the sterile field at a uniform velocity of 0.3 to 0.5 μm/sec. The ultra-clean recirculated air passes through HEPA filters and can be directed vertically or horizontally in the room.[271] A large multicenter study compared infection rates among total hip and knee replacement procedures that were performed in conventionally ventilated rooms, with infection rates after procedures done in rooms with ultra-clean air that was provided by special ventilation systems or by body-exhaust suits in conventionally ventilated rooms. The results showed that the SSI rates and the amount of airborne contamination measured by air sampling were significantly less in the ultra-clean air rooms.[272]

To determine the effect of the ventilation system on infection rates after total hip and total knee arthroplasties performed in operating rooms with and without a horizontal unidirectional filtered air-flow system and antibiotic prophylaxis, Salvati and coworkers studied a cohort of 3175 patients.[273] From this cohort, 57 matched pairs for a case-control study were established. A reduced infection rate after total hip replacement (from 1.4% to 0.9%) and an increased infection rate after total knee replacement (from 1.4% to 3.9%) were found when patients operated on in the filtered laminar air-flow operating room were compared with those whose operations were done in two conventional rooms. This pattern was statistically significant and was believed to result from the positions of the operating team and of the wound with respect to the air flow.[273]

Ultraviolet lighting, despite its known bactericidal effects, has no demonstrable effect on decreasing surgical site infections.[274,275] Factors such as control of traffic in and out of OR rooms and protective clothing that may be required make this technology limited in application.

Traffic Control

Traffic within the operating suite must be controlled to ensure that only authorized personnel are entering restricted zones, to maintain the separation of clean from dirty areas, and to segregate clean equipment areas from contaminated workrooms.[276] Surgical attire (scrub suit, hair covering, OR shoes or shoe covers) is required for trafficking in semi-restricted zones such as hallways, offices, or supply rooms that are adjacent to an OR, and a face mask is required when entering a room while a procedure is in progress. Attempts are made to limit the number of personnel in an OR during a procedure. Traffic is controlled to decrease the bacterial load of the room by negating both air turbulence and bacterial shedding by personnel in the room.[277]

Cleaning and Disinfection of Environmental Surfaces

Although environmental surfaces are not routinely implicated in surgical site infections, it is important to maintain a hygienic work environment within the confines of the OR. Routine cleaning of environmental surfaces should be performed between cases and at the end of the workday by hospital housekeeping staff trained in the proper techniques of OR cleaning. The decontamination process begins at the highest level in the room (light tracks, ceiling fixtures) and progresses downward to the level of shelves, tables, kickstands, and the floor. Hospital disinfectants approved by the Environmental Protection Agency (EPA) should be employed for routine cleaning.[198] The Occupational Safety and Health Administration (OSHA) requires the environmental cleaning of all surfaces that have come in contact with blood or body fluids.[278]

The Association of Operating Room Nurses (AORN) has developed recommended practices for environmental cleaning in the surgical practice setting, taking into consideration the varied types of settings in which invasive procedures may be performed (e.g., traditional ORs, ambulatory surgery units, cardiac catheterization suites).[279] The following six practices are recommended by the AORN:

1. Patients should be provided with a safe, clean environment. Operating rooms should be cleaned before and after each surgical procedure.
2. During surgical procedures, contamination should be confined and contained within the immediate vicinity of the surgical field to the degree possible.
3. After each surgical procedure, a safe, clean environment should be reestablished. Disposable items should be disposed of according to local, state, and federal regulations.
4. Surgical procedure rooms and scrub/utility areas should be terminally cleaned daily. Cleaning should include all equipment and areas of the OR, including fixed and ceiling-mounted equipment; all furniture including wheels, casters, and stools; hallways and floors; cabinets; ventilation faceplates; substerile areas; and scrub/utility areas and scrub sinks.
5. All areas and equipment in the surgical practice setting should be cleaned according to an established schedule. These include ducts and filters, heating grills, closets, warmers, refrigerators, ice machines, offices, lounges, restrooms, and locker rooms.
6. Policies and procedures for environmental cleaning should be written, reviewed annually, and readily available in the surgical practice setting.

No data support a need for special or separate cleaning procedures, or for closing an OR, after a case has been labeled dirty or contaminated.[280]

Microbiologic Sampling

According to the CDC Guideline for the Prevention of Surgical Site Infections,[250] there are no standardized parameters for the evaluation and comparison of microbial counts from air sampling or environmental cultures in ORs. Therefore, routine culturing of the OR environment should not be done. Microbiologic sampling of the environment should take place only if an epidemiologic investigation is being conducted that implicates some area as a potential source of an outbreak or a cluster of infections.

Sterilization of Surgical Instruments

Instruments used during surgical procedures that are not disposable must undergo physical cleaning (i.e., washer sterilizer or manual cleaning/soak in an enzymatic detergent) followed by sterilization using steam under pressure, dry heat, ethylene oxide, or some other approved chemical sterilization or high-level disinfection method.[195] The most critical issue with regard to instrument reprocessing is the required monitoring of the functional parameters (time, temperature, and pressure) of the sterilization process. Microbiologic and chemical testing of sterilization methods must be performed on a scheduled basis.[198] Microbiologic testing used to require 48 to 72 hours for results, but new rapid testing

methods can provide verification of sterilization status within 4 hours

Newer methods of sterilization for surgical equipment include hydrogen peroxide plasma sterilization. Hydrogen peroxide plasma has been found to be efficient in disinfecting material contaminated with bacteria.[281] This process produces an unstable reactive cloud of ions, electrons, and neutral particles, forming free radicals within the plasma and interacting with vital cell components, such as cell membranes, enzymes, and nucleic acids. Nonlumened and, recently, lumened instruments can undergo plasma sterilization.[282]

Flash Sterilization

Flash sterilization is the processing of patient care items by steam sterilization when the item is intended for immediate use in a patient procedure. This situation arises when a critical instrument has been inadvertently dropped or another necessary piece of equipment is emergently needed. Flash sterilization is not appropriate for implantable items and it is not to be considered for the convenience or time saving of the operating room schedule. The problems with flash sterilization include a lack of biological monitoring, an absence of protective packaging, an increased possibility of contamination, and shortened or minimal sterilization cycles. In steam sterilization, the parameters of time, temperature, and pressure are critical for adequately reprocessing a surgical instrument.[250] The use of rapid biological and chemical indicators has been evaluated by Rutala and associates and found to be acceptable.[283] It is advisable, however, that flash sterilization be restricted to specific times and events.

Surgical Attire

Appropriate surgical attire helps contain bacterial shedding and promotes environmental control within the OR. *Surgical attire* typically refers to reusable scrub suits consisting of pants and shirt, and sterile gowns. The term can also be extended to the disposable masks, gloves, surgical caps and hoods, and shoe covers that are utilized in the OR. The reusable attire must be made of reusable woven fabric or single-use, nonwoven fabric that is low-linting. Low-linting fabrics minimize bacterial shedding and provide comfort and safety for OR personnel. As personnel move, friction between their bodies and clothing frees bacteria that can become airborne. The use of surgical attire provides protection to personnel from splashes of blood and body fluids in cases of gross contamination. Surgical attire should be changed daily or whenever it becomes visibly soiled, contaminated, or wet. OSHA regulations dictate that if a garment is penetrated by blood or body fluids, it is to be removed immediately or as soon as possible. OSHA also requires that masks in combination with protective eyewear such as goggles, glasses with eye shields, or face shields be worn in anticipation of bloodborne pathogen exposures.[278] Recommended practices for appropriate surgical attire and care of scrubs are outlined by the AORN in their Practice Guidelines updated in 2005[284] and in their 1999 Standards.[195]

The AORN guidelines emphasize the following practices:

1. All individuals who enter the semi-restricted and restricted areas of the surgical suite should wear freshly laundered surgical attire intended for use only within the surgical suite.
2. Personnel should cover head and facial hair, including sideburns and necklines, when in the semi-restricted and restricted areas of the surgical suite.
3. All individuals entering restricted areas of the OR suite should wear a mask when open sterile items and equipment are present.
4. All personnel entering the semi-restricted and restricted areas of the surgical suite should confine or remove all jewelry and watches.
5. Fingernails should be kept short, clean, natural, and healthy.
6. Protective barriers must be made available to reduce the risk of exposure to potentially infectious materials.
7. Policies and procedures for surgical attire should be developed, reviewed periodically, and readily available in the practice setting. These policies and procedures should include, but not be limited to, definition of areas where surgical attire must be worn, appropriate attire within those defined areas, and the choice for the use of cover apparel outside the surgical suite.

Sterile Gowns and Drapes

In an attempt to isolate the sterile field from contamination, the use of sterile gowns and drapes is indicated.[285] These items provide a physical barrier between the sterile field and the surrounding sources of microbial contamination such as skin and hair. Regardless of the many materials used for gowns and drapes, the items should be impermeable to liquids and viruses.[286] To meet the standards of the American Society for Testing Materials, the fabrics must be reinforced with films, coatings, or membranes to prevent breakthrough of fluids. As such materials create increased body heat and may be uncomfortable, surgeons and staff must decide what materials should be selected for their practice.[287]

Asepsis and Surgical Technique

Asepsis is defined as the freedom from infection and the prevention of contact with any microorganism that could cause infection. Aseptic technique refers to the practices that are employed by the surgical team to prevent infection during medical procedures. The basic principles of aseptic technique prevent contamination of the open wound, isolate the operative site from the surrounding unsterile physical environment, and create and maintain a sterile field in which the surgery can be performed. Many factors come into play to affect asepsis in the OR including the surgical scrub, appropriate gowning and ungowning, gloving technique, site preparation to reduce the normal flora of the patient, hair removal if necessary, and surgical draping.[288]

The most critical aspect of surgery is the technical and aseptic skills of the primary surgeon. It is the technique of the surgeon that has the most dramatic effect on the risk for surgical site infection.[198,221] That technique encompasses preventing hypothermia, maintaining hemostasis, handling tissues correctly, preserving blood supply, avoiding entries into a hollow viscus, removing devitalized tissue, placing drains appropriately, suturing appropriately, eradicating dead space, and managing the postoperative wound.[250]

Inflammation of the surgical site because of the presence of a foreign body, whether it be a prosthesis, a drain, or suture material, can increase the probability of infection. The type of suture used can affect outcome. Monofilament sutures are associated with lower infection rates.[63,198,221,289]

AORN recommends seven practices for asepsis in the OR[195]:

1. Scrubbed persons should wear sterile gowns and gloves.
2. Sterile drapes should be used to establish a sterile field.
3. Items used within a sterile field should be sterile.
4. All items introduced onto a sterile field should be opened, dispensed, and transferred by methods that maintain sterility.
5. A sterile field should be constantly monitored and maintained.
6. All personnel moving within or around a sterile field should do so in a manner that maintains the integrity of the sterile field.
7. Policies and procedures for basic aseptic technique should be written, reviewed annually, and readily available in the practice setting.

■ SURVEILLANCE

The JCAHO has identified nosocomial infection rates as an indicator of the quality of care in hospitals. Accredited hospitals perform surgical site surveillance by systematic review of surgical patient charts, microbiology culture results, pharmacy data, radiology reports, communications from surgeons and nurses, and other sources of reliable information, such as pathology reports, autopsy reports, clinic visit reports, emergency room reports, and quality improvement databases operated by individual surgical services. To calculate meaningful SSI rates, data should be collected on all patients undergoing a surgical procedure of interest. Surveillance is best performed by an individual trained in hospital epidemiology and infection control—for example, the infection control practitioner—who is guided by the practices of the Association for Professionals in Infection Control and Epidemiology (APIC). Monitoring of inpatient and outpatient surgeries should be performed along with postdischarge surveillance. Currently there is no consensus on the best method of postdischarge surveillance; hospitals may choose methods that best fit their unique mix of procedures, personnel resources, and data needs.[250] Reporting the results of the SSI surveillance directly to the surgeon has been shown to affect behavior and thus reduce infection rates. SSI surveillance is an important component of strategies to reduce postsurgical infection.[290,291]

Historically, hospitals have reported SSI rates using the single risk category of bacterial contamination in the OR (class I, clean; class II, clean and contaminated; and class III/IV, contaminated and dirty). The surgical wound index includes both intrinsic and extrinsic measurements of surgical patient risk. A member of the surgical team makes the determination of wound class. This index has been used by the National Nosocomial Infections Surveillance (NNIS) system, which collects and disseminates SSI rates compiled voluntarily from several hundred U.S. hospitals. The CDC uses the data that are reported by participating hospitals to estimate the magnitude of nosocomial infection problems in the United States and to monitor trends in infections and risk factors.[292-294]

RISK STRATIFICATION

SSI data on risk factors in the population of patients being monitored by CDC criteria provide SSI risk stratification for the calculation of risk-specific infection rates. The following data points are collected by the NNIS system: operation date, NNIS operative procedure category, surgeon identifier, patient identifier, age and sex, duration of operation, wound class, use of general anesthesia, American Society of Anesthesiologists (ASA) Physical Status Classification, emergency status, trauma, multiple procedures, endoscopic approach, and discharge date. An infection risk index is then established using the wound class, the ASA Physical Status Classification, and the length of the surgery. The index values range from 0 to 3 points, depending on the three independent and equally weighted variables. Adjustments for variables known to confound infection rate estimates are essential to provide any valid benchmarks and comparisons of SSI rates between surgeons or hospitals. Risk stratification is useful but does depend on the reliability of surveillance personnel to correctly and consistently record the data.[295,296] Recently, the NNIS has been converted to the National Safety Health Network (NSHN), which continues to collect and monitor nosocomial SSI data for the monitoring of SSI trends, with a new emphasis on patient safety and medication error reporting in hospitals.

PRION DISEASE AND THE OPERATING ROOM

Prion diseases such as Creutzfeldt-Jakob disease (CJD), variant Creutzfeldt-Jakob disease (vCJD), and bovine spongiform encephalopathy (BSE) (or mad cow disease) represent a unique infection control problem because prions exhibit an unusual resistance to conventional chemical and physical decontamination methods. Because the CJD prion is not readily inactivated by conventional disinfection and sterilization procedures, and because of the invariably fatal outcome of CJD, the procedures for disinfection and sterilization have been both conservative and controversial for many years.

Iatrogenic cases of prion disease have occurred as a result of direct inoculation of prion particles into the brain or spinal cord of patients undergoing procedures in the hospital setting.[297] Contaminated surgical equipment or electrodes in the brain have also transmitted infectious prions from one patient to another.[298] Recommendations to prevent transmission of infection from medical devices contaminated by the CJD prion have been based primarily on prion inactivation studies. Recommendations for enhanced cleaning and sterilization (274°C for 18 minutes) of instruments used on

patients suspected of having or confirmed to have CJD, have been provided by the World Health Organization (WHO)[299] and are cited in the APIC disinfectant guideline.[300]

In 2001, the JCAHO reported two incidents at accredited hospitals where a total of 14 patients may have been exposed to CJD through instruments used during brain surgeries on patients of unsuspected cases of CJD.[301] The following lessons were learned from these events:

1. A patient with CJD or a prion disease does not always present with symptoms of CJD.
2. The time interval between biopsy and pathology report should be monitored and reviewed to ensure the shortest time from biopsy to results.
3. Instruments used in brain biopsy procedures should not be reused when the patient's diagnosis is uncertain at the time of the procedure.

More recently, another facility reported potential exposure to more than 3600 patients after a patient with unsuspected CJD had undergone a craniotomy. The diagnosis was not made until autopsy nearly a year later.[302] Potential CJD exposures after an unsuspected case can have an enormous emotional and financial impact. As a result, this institution has mandated the enhanced cleaning and sterilization of all OR instruments to ensure that future unintentional CJD exposures do not occur.

BSE is a progressive neurologic disorder of cattle first identified about 3 decades ago in Europe. By 2005, more than 184,000 cattle cases had been confirmed. VCJD is thought to result from eating BSE-contaminated food. There have been two cases of BSE in U.S. cows, one of which was known to have come from Canada.[303] Three other cases of BSE-infected cows were identified in or linked to Canada.[304]

In April 2002, the Florida Department of Health and the CDC announced the occurrence of a likely case of vCJD in a Florida resident believed to have contracted variant CJD years ago in England.[305] Over the past 10 years, 147 human cases of vCJD were reported in the United Kingdom (UK), seven in France, and one each in Canada, Ireland, Italy, and the United States.[306]

As prion diseases continue to increase in the United States and Europe, the potential for human-to-human iatrogenic spread of vCJD will probably increase. Infected individuals, like the rest of the population, will undergo medical and surgical procedures, and in these cases, the result may be contamination of equipment.[247] If it develops that there are large numbers of unidentified prion-infected persons, extending disinfectant protocols in the medical setting may be a strategy that deserves further investigation.

REFERENCES

1. U.S. Department of Health and Human Services, Centers for Disease Control and Prevention, National Center for Health Statistics: Vital and Health Statistics: Ambulatory and in-patient procedures in the United States, 1995. Series 13: Data from the National Health Care Survey, No. 135, DHHS publ. no. (PHS). Hyattsville, Md, 1998: 98-1796.
2. U.S. Department of Health and Human Services, Centers for Disease Control and Prevention, National Center for Health Statistics: Vital

and Health Statistics: Ambulatory and in-patient procedures in the United States, 1996. Series 13: Data from the National Health Care Survey, No. 139, DHHS publ. no. (PHS). Hyattsville, Md, 1996:98-1798.

3. National Nosocomial Infections Surveillance (NNIS) System: National Nosocomial Infections Surveillance (NNIS) Report, data summary from October 1986-1996, issued May 1996. Am J Infect Control 1996;24:380-388.

4. Haley R, Culver D, White J, et al: The efficacy of infection surveillance and control programs in preventing nosocomial infections in U.S. hospitals. Am J Epidemiol 1985;121:182-205.

5. Cruse P: Wound infection surveillance. Rev Infect Dis 1981;4: 734-737.

6. Cruse P, Foord R: The epidemiology of wound infection: A 10-year prospective study of 62,939 wounds. Surg Clin North Am 1980;60: 27-40.

7. Martone W, Jarvis W, Culver D, Haley R: Incidence and nature of endemic and epidemic nosocomial infections. In Bennett JV, et al (eds): Hospital Infections. Boston, Little, Brown, 1992, pp 577-596.

8. Boyce J, Potter-Bynoe G, Dziobek L: Hospital reimbursement patterns among patients with surgical wound infections following open heart surgery. Infect Control Hosp Epidemiol 1990;11:89-93.

9. Poulsen K, Bremmelgaard A, Sorensen A, et al: Estimated costs of postoperative wound infections: A case control study of marginal hospital and social security costs. Epidemiol Infect 1994;113:283-295.

10. Vegas A, Jodra V, Garcia M: Nosocomial infection in surgery wards: A controlled study of increased duration of hospital stays and direct cost of hospitalization. Eur J Epidemiol 1993;9:504-510.

11. Brachman P, Dan B, Haley R, et al: Nosocomial surgical infections: Incidence and cost. Surg Clin North Am 1980;60:15-25.

12. Nelson DB, Kien CL, Mohr B, et al: Dressing changes by specialized personnel reduce infection rates in patients receiving central venous parenteral nutrition. JPEN J Parenter Enteral Nutr 1986;10:220-222.

13. Taylor G, Mikell F, Moses H, et al: Determinants of hospital charges for coronary artery bypass surgery: The economic consequences of postoperative complications. Am J Cardiol 1990;65:309-313.

14. Hall R, Ash A, Ghali W, Moskowitz M: Hospital cost of complications associated with coronary artery bypass graft surgery. Am J Cardiol 1997;79:1680-1682.

15. Holtz T, Wenzel R: Postdischarge surveillance for nosocomial wound infection: A brief review and commentary. Am J Infect Control 1992;20:206-213.

16. Howard JM, Beskid G, Grotziuger PJ: Ultraviolet radiation in the operating room: A historical review. Ann Surg 1964;160:1-192.

17. Horan T, Gaynes R: Surveillance of nosocomial infections. In Mayhall C (ed): Hospital Epidemiology and Infection Control. Philadelphia, Lippincott Williams & Wilkins, 2004, pp 1659-1702.

18. Horan T, Gaynes R, Martone W, et al: CDC definitions of nosocomial surgical site infections, 1992: A modification of CDC definitions of surgical wound infections. Infect Control Hosp Epidemiol 1992;13:606-608.

19. Krizek T, Robson M: Evolution of quantitative bacteriology in wound management. Am J Surg 1975;130:579-584.

20. Elek S, Conen P: The virulence of *Staphylococcus pyogenes* for man: A study of problems with wound infection. Br J Exp Pathol 1957;38:573-586.

21. Noble W: The production of subcutaneous staphylococcal skin lesions in mice. Br J Exp Pathol 1965;46:254-262.

22. James R, MacLeod C: Induction of staphylococcal infections in mice with small inocula introduced on sutures. Br J Exp Pathol 1961;42:266-277.

23. Schaberg D: Resistant gram-positive organisms. Ann Emerg Med 1994;24:462-464.

24. Schaberg D, Culver D, Gaynes R: Major trends in the microbial etiology of nosocomial infection. Am J Med 1991;91:72S-75.

25. Jarvis W: Epidemiology of nosocomial fungal infections, with emphasis on *Candida* species. Clin Infect Dis 1995;20:1526-1530.

26. Altemeier W, Culbertson W, Hummel R: Surgical considerations of endogenous infections: Sources, types, and methods of control. Surg Clin North Am 1968;48:227-240.

27. Wiley A, Ha'eri G: Routes of infection: A study of using "tracer particles" in the orthopedic operating room. Clin Orthop 1979;139: 150-155.

28. Calia F, Wolinsky E, Mortimer EJ, et al: Importance of the carrier state as a source of *Staphylococcus aureus* in wound sepsis. J Hyg (Lond) 1969;67:49-57.

29. Dineen P, Drusin L: Epidemics of postoperative wound infections associated with hair carriers. Lancet 1973;2:1157-1159.

30. Mastro T, Farley T, Elliott J, et al: An outbreak of surgical-wound infections due to group A *Streptococcus* carried on the scalp. N Engl J Med 1990;323:968-972.

31. Ford C, Peterson D, Mitchell C: An appraisal of the role of surgical face masks. Am J Surg 1967;113:787-790.

32. Letts R, Doermer E: Conversation in the operating theater as a cause of airborne bacterial contamination. J Bone Joint Surg [Am] 1983;65:357-362.

33. Jakob H, Borneff-Lipp M, Bach A, et al: The endogenous pathway is a major route for deep sternal wound infection. Eur J Cardiothoracic Surg 2000;17:154-160.

34. Giamarellou H, Antoniadou A: Epidemiology, diagnosis, and therapy of fungal infections in surgery. Infect Control Hosp Epidemiol 1996;17:558-564.

35. Nichols R: Techniques known to prevent postoperative wound infection. Infect Control 1982;3:34-37.

36. Bruce ASW, Kerry RM, Norman P, Stockley I: Fluconazole-impregnated beads in the management of fungal infection of prosthetic joints. J Bone Joint Surg Br 2001;83:183-184.

37. Siegman-Igra Y, Shafir R, Weiss J, et al: Serious infectious complications of mid-sternotomy: A review of bacteriology and antimicrobial therapy. Scand J Infect Dis 1990;22:633-643.

38. Grossi E, Culliford A, Krieger K, et al: A survey of 77 major infectious complications of median sternotomy: A review of 7,949 consecutive operative procedures. Ann Thorac Surg 1985;40:214-223.

39. Munoz P, Menasalvas A, Bernaldo de Quiros J, et al: Post-surgical mediastinitis: A case-control study. Clin Infect Dis 1997;25: 1060-1064.

40. Thomas F, Martin C, Fisher R, Alford RH: *Candida albicans* infection of sternum and costal cartilages: Combined operative treatment and drug therapy with 5-fluorocytosine. Ann Thorac Surg 1977;23: 163-166.

41. Isenberg H, Tucci V, Sintron F, et al: Single source outbreak of *Candida tropicalis* complicating coronary bypass surgery. J Clin Microbiol 1989;27:2426-2428.

42. Pertowski C, Baron R, Lasker B, et al: Nosocomial outbreak of *Candida albicans* sternal infections following cardiac surgery traced to a scrub nurse. J Infect Dis 1995;172:817-822.

43. Petrikkos G, Skiada A, Sabatakou H, et al: Successful treatment of two cases of post-surgical sternal osteomyelitis due to *Candida krusei* and *Candida albicans*, respectively, with high doses of triazoles (fluconazole, itraconazole). Mycoses 2001;44:422-425.

44. Clancey C, Nguyen M, Morris A: Candidal mediastinitis: An emerging clinical entity. Clin Infect Dis 1997;25:608-613.

45. Glower D, Douglas J, Gaynor J, et al: *Candida* mediastinitis after a cardiac operation. Ann Thorac Surg 1990;49:157-163.

46. Thomas F, Martin C, Fisher R, Alford R: *Candida albicans* infection of sternum and costal cartilages: Combined operative treatment and drug therapy with 5-fluorocytosine. Ann Thorac Surg 1977;23: 163-166.

47. Beitsch P, Balch C: Operative morbidity and risk factor assessment in melanoma patients undergoing inguinal lymph node dissection. Am J Surg 1992;164:462-6; discussion 465-466.

48. Cruse P, Foord R: A five-year prospective study of 23,649 surgical wounds. Arch Surg 1973;107:206-210.

49. Claesson B, Holmlund D: Predictors of intraoperative bacterial contamination and postoperative infection in elective colorectal surgery. J Hosp Infect 1988;11:127-135.

50. Mishriki S, Law D, Jeffery P: Factors affecting the incidence of postoperative wound infection. J Hosp Infect 1990;16:223-230.

51. Culver D, Horan T, Gaynes R, et al: Surgical wound infection rates by wound class, operative procedure, and patient risk index. National Nosocomial Infections Surveillance System. Am J Med 1991;91: 152S-157.

52. Doig C, Wilkinson A: Wound infection in a children's hospital. Br J Surg 1976;63:647-650.

53. Sharma L, Sharma P: Postoperative wound infection in a pediatric surgical service. J Pediatr Surg 1986;21:889-891.

54. Gil-Egea M, Pi-Sunyer M, Verdaguer A, et al: Surgical wound infections: Prospective study of 4,486 clean wounds. Infect Control 1987; 8:277-280.

55. Slaughter M, Olson M, Lee JJ, Ward H: A fifteen-year wound surveillance study after coronary artery bypass. Ann Thorac Surg 1993;56: 1063-1068.

56. Post S, Betzler M, vonDitfurth B, et al: Risks of intestinal anastomoses in Crohn's disease. Ann Surg 1991;213:37-42.

57. Nagachinta T, Stephens M, Reitz B, Polk B: Risk factors for surgical wound infection following cardiac surgery. J Infect Dis 1987;156: 967-973.

58. Bryan A, Lamarra M, Angelini G, et al: Median sternotomy wound dehiscence: A retrospective case control study of risk factors and outcome. J R Coll Surg Edinb 1992;37:305-308.

59. Jones J, Triplett R: The relationship of cigarette smoking to impaired intraoral wound healing: A review of evidence and implications for patient care. J Oral Maxillofac Surg 1992;50:237-239; discussion 239-240.

60. Vinton A, Traverso L, Jolly P: Wound complications after modified radical mastectomy compared with tylectomy with axillary lymph node dissection. Am J Surg 1991;161:584-588.

61. Holley D, Toursarkissian B, Vansconez H, et al: The ramifications of immediate reconstruction in the management of breast cancer. Am Surg 1995;61:60-65.

62. Lilienfeld D, Vlahov D, Tenney J, McLaughlin J: Obesity and diabetes as risk factors for postoperative wound infections after cardiac surgery. Am J Infect Control 1988;16:3-6.

63. Berard F, Gandon J: Postoperative wound infections: The influence of ultraviolet irradiation of the operating room and of various other factors. Ann Surg 1964;160(Suppl 1):1-192.

64. Nystrom P, Jonstam A, Hojer H, Ling L: Incisional infection after colorectal surgery in obese patients. Acta Chir Scand 1987;153:225-227.

65. He G, Ryan W, Acuff T, et al: Risk factors for operative mortality and sternal wound infection in bilateral internal mammary artery grafting. J Thorac Cardiovasc Surg 1994;107:196-202.

66. Barber G, Miransky J, Brown A, et al: Direct observations of surgical wound infections at a comprehensive cancer center. Arch Surg 1995;130:1042-1047.

67. Casey J, Flinn W, Yao J, et al: Correlation of immune and nutritional status with wound complications in patients undergoing vascular operations. Surgery 1983;93:822-827.

68. Greene K, Wilde A, Stulberg B: Preoperative nutritional status of total joint patients. Relationship to postoperative wound complications. J Arthroplasty 1991;6:321-325.

69. Weber T: A prospective analysis of factors influencing outcome after fundoplication. J Pediatr Surg 1995;30:1061-1063; discussion 1063-1064.

70. Slaughter L, Morris J, Starr A: Prosthetic valvular endocarditis: A 12-year review. Circulation 1973;47:1319-1326.

71. Carlsson A, Lidgren L, Lindberg L: Prophylactic antibiotics against early and late deep infections after total hip replacements. Acta Orthop Scand 1977;48:405-410.

72. Hunter J, Padilla M, Cooper-Vastola S: Late *Clostridium perfringens* breast implant infection after dental treatment. Ann Plast Surg 1996;36:309-312.

73. Stuesse D, Robinson J, Durzinsky D: A late sternal wound infection caused by hematogenous spread of bacteria. Chest 1995;108:1742-1743.

74. Howe C: Experimental wound sepsis from transient *Escherichia coli* bacteremia. Surgery 1969;66:570-574.

75. Velasco E, Thuler L, Martins C, et al: Risk factors for infectious complications after abdominal surgery for malignant disease. Am J Infect Control 1996;24:1-6.

76. Bruun J: Post-operative wound infection: Predisposing factors and the effect of a reduction in the dissemination of staphylococci. Acta Med Scand Suppl 1970;514(Suppl):3-89.

77. Simchen E, Rozin R, Wax Y: The Israeli Study of Surgical Infection of drains and the risk of wound infection in operations for hernia. Surg Gynecol Obstet 1990;170:331-337.

78. Edwards L: The epidemiology of 2056 remote site infections and 1966 surgical wound infections occurring in 1865 patients: A four year study of 40,923 operations at Rush-Presbyterian-St. Luke's Hospital, Chicago. Ann Surg 1976;184:758-766.

79. Valentine R, Weigelt J, Dryer D, Rodgers C: Effect of remote infections on clean wound infection rates. Am J Infect Control 1986;14: 64-67.

80. Vamvakas E, Carven J: Transfusion of white-cell-containing allogeneic blood components and postoperative wound infection: Effect of confounding factors. Transfus Med 1998;8:29-36.

81. Vamvakas E, Carven J, Hibberd P: Blood transfusion and infection after colorectal cancer surgery. Transfusion 1996;36:1000-1008.

82. Jensen L, Kissmeyer-Nielsen P, Wolff B, Qvist N: Randomised comparison of leucocyte-depleted versus buffy-coat-poor blood transfusion and complications after colorectal surgery. Lancet 1996;348: 841-845.

83. Heiss M, Mempel W, Jauch K, et al: Beneficial effect of autologous blood transfusion on infectious complications after colorectal cancer surgery. Lancet 1993;342:1328-1333.

84. Perl T, Golub J: New approaches to reduce *Staphylococcus aureus* nosocomial infection rates: Treating *S. aureus* nasal carriage. Ann Pharmacotherapy 1998;32:S7-16.

85. Perl T, Cullen J, Pfaller M, et al: A randomized, double-blind, placebo-controlled clinical trial of intranasal mupirocin ointment (IM) for prevention of *S. aureus* surgical site infections (SSI). Abstracts of the IDSA 36th Annual Meeting 1998;91:88.

86. Kluytmans JA, Mouton JW, Ijzerman EPF, et al: Nasal carriage of *Staphylococcus aureus* as a major risk factor for wound infections after cardiac surgery. J Infect Dis 1995;171:216-219.

87. Greif R, Akca O, Horn E, et al: Supplemental perioperative oxygen to reduce the incidence of surgical-wound infection. Outcomes Research Group. N Engl J Med 2000;342:161-167.

88. Furnary A: Continuous intravenous insulin infusion reduces the incidence of deep sternal wound infection in diabetic patients after cardiac surgical procedures [discussion]. Ann Thorac Surg 1999;67:360-362.

89. Lazar H, Chipkin S, Fitzgerald C, et al: Tight glycemic control in diabetic coronary artery bypass graft patients improves perioperative outcomes and decreases recurrent ischemic events. Circulation 2004;109:1497-1502.

90. Cohen O, Dankner R, Chetrit A, et al: Multidisciplinary intervention for control of diabetes in patients undergoing coronary artery bypass graft (CABG). Cardiovasc Surg 2003;11:195-200.

91. Medina-Cuadros M, Sillero-Arenas M, Martinez-Gallego G, Delgado-Rodriguez M: Surgical wound infections diagnosed after discharge from hospital: Epidemiologic differences with in-hospital infections. Am J Infect Control 1996;24:421-428.

92. Kanat A: Risk factors for neurosurgical site infections after craniotomy: A prospective multicenter study of 2944 patients. Neurosurgery 1998;43:189-190.

93. Moro M, Carrieri M, Tozzi A, et al: Risk factors for surgical wound infections in clean surgery: A multicenter study. Italian PRINOS Study Group. Ann Ital Chir 1996;67:13-19.

94. Barry B, Lucet J, Kosmann M, Gehanno P: Risk factors for surgical wound infections in patients undergoing head and neck oncologic surgery. Acta Otorhinolaryngol Belg 1999;53:241-244.

95. Richet H, Chidiac C, Prat A, et al: Analysis of risk factors for surgical wound infections following vascular surgery. Am J Med 1991;91: 170S-172.

96. Marhoffer W, Stein M, Schleinkofer L, Federlin K: Monitoring of polymorphonuclear leukocyte functions in diabetes mellitus: A comparative study of conventional radiometric function tests and low-light imaging systems. J Biolumin Chemilumin 1994;9:165-170.

97. Terranova A: The effects of diabetes mellitus on wound healing. Plast Surg Nurs 1991;11:20-25.

98. Allen D, Maguire J, Mahdavian M, et al: Wound hypoxia and acidosis limit neutrophil bacterial killing mechanisms. Arch Surg 1997;132: 991-996.

99. Nolan C, Beaty H, Bagdade J: Further characterization of the impaired bactericidal function of granulocytes in patients with poorly controlled diabetes. Diabetes 1978;27:889-894.

100. Bagdade J, Walters E: Impaired granulocyte adherence in mildly diabetic patients: Effects of tolazamide treatment. Diabetes 1980;29:309-311.

101. Mowat A, Baum J: Chemotaxis of polymorphonuclear leukocytes from patients with diabetes mellitus. N Engl J Med 1971;284:621-627.

102. MacRury S, Gemmell C, Paterson K, MacCuish A: Changes in phagocytic function with glycaemic control in diabetic patients. J Clin Pathol 1989;42:1143-1147.

103. Hennessey P, Black C, Andrassy R: Nonenzymatic glycosylation of immunoglobulin G impairs complement fixation. JPEN J Parenter Enteral Nutr 1991;15:60-64.

104. Black C, Hennessey P, Andrassy R: Short-term hyperglycemia depresses immunity through nonenzymatic glycosylation of circulating immunoglobulin. J Trauma 1990;30:830-832.

105. Furnary A, Zerr K, Grunkemeier G, Starr A: Continuous intravenous insulin infusion reduces the incidence of deep sternal wound infection in diabetic patients after cardiac surgical procedures. Ann Thorac Surg 1999;67:352-360.

106. Sessler D, Akca O: Nonpharmacological prevention of surgical wound infections. Clin Infect Dis 2002;35:1397-1404.

107. Wenisch C, Narzt E, Sessler D, et al: Mild intraoperative hypothermia reduces production of reactive oxygen intermediates by polymorphonuclear leukocytes. Anesth Analg 1996;82:810-816.

108. Kurz A, Sessler D, Lenhardt R: Perioperative normothermia to reduce the incidence of surgical-wound infection and shorten hospitalization. Study of Wound Infection and Temperature Group. N Engl J Med 1996;334:1209-1215.

109. Alonso-Echanove J, Richards C Jr, Horan TC: Response to: Supplemental perioperative oxygen to reduce surgical-wound infections. N Engl J Med 2000;342:1613-1614.

110. Lee J: Response to: Supplemental perioperative oxygen to reduce surgical-wound infections. N Engl J Med 2000;342:1613-1614.

111. Pryor K, Fahey TI, Lien C, Goldstein P: Surgical site infection and the routine use of perioperative hyperoxia in a general surgical population: A randomized controlled trial. JAMA 2004;291:79-87.

112. Williams REO, Jevons MP, Shooter RA: Nasal staphylococci and sepsis in hospital patients. Br Med J 1959;2:658-663.

113. Weinstein HJ: The relation between the nasal-staphylococcal-carrier state and the incidence of postoperative complications. N Engl J Med 1959;260:1303-1310.

114. Parisian Mediastinitis Study Group: Risk factors for deep sternal wound infection after sternotomy: A prospective, multicenter study. J Thorac Cardiovasc Surg 1996;111:1200-1207.

115. Kalmeijer M: Nasal carriage of *Staphylococcus aureus* is a major risk factor for surgical-site infections in orthopedic surgery. Infect Control Hosp Epidemiol 2000;21:319-323.

116. Ruef C, Fanconi S, Nadal D: Sternal wound infection after heart operations in pediatric patients associated with nasal carriage of *Staphylococcus aureus*. J Thorac Cardiovasc Surg 1996;112:681-686.

117. Corbella X, Dominguez MA, Pujol M, et al: Staphylococcus aureus nasal carriage as a marker for subsquent staphylococcal infections in intensive care unit patients. Eur J Clin Microbiol Infect Dis 1997;16:351-357.

118. Kluytmans J, Mouton JW, VandenBergh MF, et al: Reduction of surgical-site infections in cardiothoracic surgery by elimination of nasal carriage of *Staphylococcus aureus*. Infect Control Hosp Epidemiol 1996;17:780-785.

119. Cimochowski G, Harostock MD, Brown R, et al: Intranasal mupirocin reduces sternal wound infection after open heart surgery in diabetics and nondiabetics. Ann Thorac Surg 2001;71:1572-1579.

120. Gernaat-van der Sluis A, Hoogenboom-Verdegaal AM, Edixhoven PJ, Spies-van Rooijen NH: Prophylactic mupirocin could reduce orthopedic wound infections: 1,044 patients treated with mupirocin compared with 1,260 historical controls. Acta Orthop Scand 1998;69:412-414.

121. Perl T, Cullen JJ, Wenzel RP, et al., and the Mupirocin and the Risk of *Staphylococcus aureus* Study Team: Intranasal mupirocin to prevent postoperative *Staphylococcus aureus* infections. N Engl J Med 2002;346:1871-1877.

122. Paterson DL, Rihs JD, Squier C, et al: Lack of efficacy of mupirocin in the prevention of infections with *Staphylococcus aureus* in liver transplant recipients and candidates. Transplantation 2003;75:194-198.

123. Miller M, Dascal A, Portnoy J, Mendelson J: Development of mupirocin resistance among methicillin-resistant *Staphylococcus aureus* after widespread use of nasal mupirocin ointment. Infect Control Hosp Epidemiol 1996;17:811-813.

124. Netto dos Santos KR, de Souza Fonseca L, Gontijo Filho PP: Emergence of high-level mupirocin resistance in methicillin-resistant *Staphylococcus aureus* isolated from Brazilian university hospitals. Infect Control Hosp Epidemiol 1996;17:813-816.

125. Hayek L, Emerson J, Gardner A: A placebo-controlled trial of the effect of two preoperative baths or showers with chlorhexidine detergent on postoperative wound infection rates. J Hosp Infect 1987;10:165-172.

126. Paulson D: Efficacy evaluation of a 4% chlorhexidine gluconate as a full-body shower wash. Am J Infect Control 1993;21:205-209.

127. Garibaldi R: Prevention of intraoperative wound contamination with chlorhexidine shower and scrub. J Hosp Infect 1988;11(Suppl B):5-9.

128. Rotter M, Larsen S, Cooke E, et al: A comparison of the effects of preoperative whole-body bathing with detergent alone and with detergent containing chlorhexidine gluconate on the frequency of wound infections after clean surgery. The European Working Party on Control of Hospital Infections. J Hosp Infect 1988;11:310-320.

129. Leigh D, Stronge J, Marriner J, Sedgwick J: Total body bathing with "Hibiscrub" (chlorhexidine) in surgical patients: A controlled trial. J Hosp Infect 1983;4:229-235.

130. Ayliffe G, Noy M, Babb J, et al: A comparison of pre-operative bathing with chlorhexidine-detergent and non-medicated soap in the prevention of wound infection. J Hosp Infect 1983;4:237-244.

131. Lynch W, Davey P, Malek M, et al: Cost-effectiveness analysis of the use of chlorhexidine detergent in preoperative whole body disinfection in wound infection prophylaxis. J Hosp Infect 1992;21:179-191.

132. Brady L, Thomson M, Palmer M, Harkness J: Successful control of endemic MRSA in a cardiothoracic surgical unit. Med J Aust 1990;152:240-245.

133. Tuffnell D, Croton R, Hemingway D, et al: Methicillin-resistant *Staphylococcus aureus*: The role of antisepsis in the control of an outbreak. J Hosp Infect 1987;10:255-259.

134. Bartzokas CA, Paton JH, Gibson MF, et al: Control and eradication of methicillin-resistant *Staphylococcus aureus* on a surgical unit. N Engl J Med 1984;10:255-259.

135. Kaiser A, Kernodle D, Barg N, Petracek M: Influence of preoperative showers on staphylococcal skin colonization: A comparative trial of antiseptic skin cleansers. Ann Thorac Surg 1988;45:35-38.

136. Wangensteen O, Wangensteen S: The rise of surgery: Emergence from empiric craft to scientific discipline. Minneapolis, University of Minnesota Press, 1978.

137. Esmarch F, Kowalzig E: Surgical Technic: A Textbook on Operative Surgery. New York, Macmillan, 1901.

138. Tkach J, Shannon A, Beastrom R: Pseudofolliculitis due to preoperative shaving. AORN J 1979;30:881-884.

139. Mangram AJ, Horan TC, Pearson ML, et al: The Hospital Infection Control Practices Advisory Committee. Guideline for Prevention of Surgical Site Infection, 1999. Infect Control Hosp Epidemiol 1999;20:247-278.

140. Seropian R, Reynolds B: Wound infections after preoperative depilatory versus razor preparation. Am J Surg 1971;121:251-254.

141. Powis S, Waterworth T, Arkell D: Preoperative skin preparation: Clinical evaluation of depilatory cream. Br Med J 1976;2:1166-1168.

142. Alexander J, Fischer J, Boyajian M, Palmquist J: The influence of hair removal methods on wound infections. Arch Surg 1983;118:347-352.

143. Winston K: Hair and neurosurgery. Neurosurgery 1992;31:320-329.

144. Sellick J, Stelmach M, Mylotte J: Surveillance of surgical wound infection following open heart surgery. Infect Control Hosp Epidemiol 1991;12:591-596.

145. Ko W, Lazenby D, Zelano J, et al: Effects of shaving methods and intraoperative irrigation on suppurative mediastinitis after bypass operations. Ann Thorac Surg 1992;53:301-305.

146. Hamilton H, Hamilton K, Lone F: Preoperative hair removal. Can J Surg 1977;20:269-271, 274-275.

147. Olson M, MacCallum J, McQuarrie D: Preoperative hair removal with clippers does not increase infection rate in clean surgical wounds. Surg Gynecol Obstet 1986;162:181-182.

148. Mehta G, Prakash B, Karmoker S: Computer assisted analysis of wound infection in neurosurgery. J Hosp Infect 1988;11:244-252.

149. Masterson T, Rodeheaver G, Morgan R, Edlich R: Bacteriologic evaluation of electric clippers for surgical hair removal. Am J Surg 1984;148:301-302.

150. Rotter M: Hygienic hand disinfection. Infect Control 1984;5:18-22.

151. Gravens D, Butcher HJ, Ballinger W, Dewar N: Septisol antiseptic foam for hands of operating room personnel: An effective antibacterial agent. Surgery 1973;73:360-367.

152. Babb J, Davies J, Ayliffe G: A test procedure for evaluating surgical hand disinfection. J Hosp Infect 1991;18(Suppl B):41-49.

153. Larson E, Butz A, Gullette D, Laughon B: Alcohol for surgical scrubbing? Infect Control Hosp Epidemiol 1990;11:139-143.

154. Food and Drug Administration: Topical antimicrobial drug products for over-the-counter human use: Tentative final monograph for healthcare antiseptic drug products—Proposed rule (21 CFR Parts 333 and 369). Fed Reg 1994;59:31441-31452.

155. Rubio P: Septisol antiseptic foam: A sensible alternative to the conventional surgical scrub. Int Surg 1987;72:243-246.

156. Holloway P, Platt J, Reybrouck G, et al: A multi-centre evaluation of two chlorhexidine-containing formulations for surgical hand disinfection. J Hosp Infect 1990;16:151-159.

157. Kobayashi H: Evaluation of surgical scrubbing. J Hosp Infect 1991;18(Suppl B):29-34.

158. Nicoletti G, Boghossian V, Borland R: Hygienic hand disinfection: A comparative study with chlorhexidine detergents and soap. J Hosp Infect 1990;15:323-337.

159. Rotter M, Koller W: Surgical hand disinfection: Effect of sequential use of two chlorhexidine preparations. J Hosp Infect 1990;16:161-166.

160. Lowbury E, Lilly H, Ayliffe GA: Preoperative disinfection of surgeons' hands: Use of alcoholic solutions and effects of gloves on skin flora. Br Med J 1974;4:369-372.

161. Lilly H, Lowbury E, Wilkins M, Zaggy A: Delayed antimicrobial effects of skin disinfection by alcohol. J Hyg (Lond) 1979;82:497-500.

162. Larson E, Morton H: Alcohols. In Block SS (ed): Disinfection, Sterilization and Preservation, ed 4. Philadelphia, Lea and Febiger, 1991, pp 642-654.

163. Price P: Ethyl alcohol as a germicide. Arch Surg 1939;38:528-542.

164. Harrington C, Walker H: The germicidal action of alcohol. Boston Med Surg J 1903;148:548-552.

165. Jarvis J, Wynne C, Enwright L, Williams J: Handwashing and antiseptic-containing soaps in hospital. J Clin Pathol 1979;32:732-737.

166. Pereira L, Lee G, Wade K: An evaluation of five protocols for surgical handwashing in relation to skin condition and microbial counts. J Hosp Infect 1997;36:49-65.

167. Aly R, Maibach H: Comparative study on the antimicrobial effect of 0.5% chlorhexidine gluconate and 70% isopropyl alcohol on the normal flora of hands. Appl Environ Microbiol 1979;37:610-613.

168. Rosenberg A, Alatary S, Peterson A: Safety and efficacy of the antiseptic chlorhexidine gluconate. Surg Gynecol Obstet 1976;143:789-792.

169. Ayliffe G, Babb J, Bridges K, et al: Comparison of two methods for assessing the removal of total organisms and pathogens from the skin. J Hyg (Lond) 1975;75:259-274.

170. Blech M, Hartemann P, Paquin J: Activity of non antiseptic soaps and ethanol for hand disinfection. Zentralbl Bakteriol Hyg [B] 1985;181:496-512.

171. Berman R, Knight R: Evaluation of hand antisepsis. Arch Environ Health 1969;18:781-783.

172. Hobson D, Woller W, Anderson L, Guthery E: Development and evaluation of a new alcohol-based surgical hand scrub formulation with persistent antimicrobial characteristics and brushless application. Am J Infect Control 1998;26:507-512.

173. Bryant KA, Pearce J, Stover B: Flash fire associated with the use of alcohol-based antiseptic agent [letter]. Am J Infect Control 2002;30:256-257.

174. Boyce J, Pittet D: Guideline for hand hygiene in health-care settings. Recommendations of the Healthcare Infection Control Practices Advisory Committee and the HICPAC/SHEA/APIC/IDSA Hand Hygiene Task Force. Society for Healthcare Epidemiology of America/Association for Professionals in Infection Control/Infectious Diseases Society of America. MMWR Morb Mortal Wkly Rep 2002;51:1-45.

175. Hardin W, Nichols R: Handwashing and patient skin preparation. In Malangoni MA (ed): Critical Issues in Operating Room Management. Philadelphia, Lippincott-Raven, 1997, pp 133-149.

176. Nichols R, Smith J, Garcia R, et al: Current practices of preoperative bowel preparation among North American colorectal surgeons. Clin Infect Dis 1997;24:609-619.

177. Wade J, Casewell M: The evaluation of residual antimicrobial activity on hands and its clinical relevance. J Hosp Infect 1991;18(Suppl B):23-28.

178. Dineen P: The use of a polyurethane sponge in surgical scrubbing. Surg Gynecol Obstet 1966;123:595-598.

179. Bornside G, Crowder VJ, Cohn IJ: A bacteriological evaluation of surgical scrubbing with disposable iodophor-soap impregnated polyurethane scrub sponges. Surgery 1968;64:743-751.

180. McBride M, Duncan W, Knox JM: An evaluation of surgical scrub brushes. Surg Gynecol Obstet 1973;137:934-936.

181. Meers P, Yeo G: Shedding of bacteria and skin squames after handwashing. J Hyg (Lond) 1978;81:99-105.

182. Kikuchi-Numagami K, Saishu T, Fukaya M, et al: Irritancy of scrubbing up for surgery with or without a brush. Acta Derm Venereol 1999;79:230-232.

183. Eitzen H, Ritter M, French M, Gioe T: A microbiological in-use comparison of surgical hand-washing agents. J Bone Joint Am 1979;61A:403-406.

184. Galle P, Homesley H, Rhyne A: Reassessment of the surgical scrub. Surg Gynecol Obstet 1978;147:215-218.

185. Larson E, Aiello A, Heilman J, et al: Comparison of different regimens for surgical hand preparation. AORN J 2001;73:412-420.

186. Dewar N, Gravens D: Effectiveness of Septisol antiseptic surgical scrub agent. Appl Microbiol 1973;26:544-549.

187. Mulberry G, Snyder A, Heilman J, et al: Evaluation of waterless, scrubless chlorhexidine gluconate/ethanol surgical scrub for antimicrobial efficacy. Am J Infect Control 2001;29:377-382.

188. Dineen P: An evaluation of the duration of the surgical scrub. Surg Gynecol Obstet 1969;129:1181-1184.

189. O'Farrell D, Kenny G, O'Sullivan M, et al: Evaluation of the optimal hand-scrub duration prior to total hip arthroplasty. J Hosp Infect 1994;26:93-98.

190. Lowbury E, Lilly H: Disinfection of the hands of surgeons and nurses. Br Med J 1960;1:1445-1450.

191. Hingst V, Juditzki I, Heeg P, Sonntag H: Evaluation of the efficacy of surgical hand disinfection following a reduced application time of 3 instead of 5 min. J Hosp Infect 1992;20:79-86.

192. Pereira L, Lee G, Wade K: The effect of surgical handwashing routines on the microbial counts of operating room nurses. Am J Infect Control 1990;18:354-364.

193. O'Shaughnessy M, O'Malley V, Corbett G, Given H: Optimum duration of surgical scrub-time. Br J Surg 1991;78:685-686.

194. Wheelock S, Lookinland S: Effect of surgical hand scrub time on subsequent bacterial growth. AORN J 1997;65:1087-1092, 1094-1098.

195. Association of Operating Room Nurses: Standards, Recommended Practices, Guidelines. Denver, Association of Operating Room Nurses, 1999.

196. Pottinger J, Burns S, Manske C: Bacterial carriage by artificial versus natural nails. Am J Infect Control 1989;17:340-344.

197. Passaro D, Waring L, Armstrong R, et al: Postoperative *Serratia marcescens* wound infections traced to an out-of-hospital source. J Infect Dis 1997;175:992-995.

198. Committee on Control of Surgical Infections of the Committee on Pre- and Postoperative Care: American College of Surgeons. Manual on Control of Infections in Surgical patients. Philadelphia, JB Lippincott, 1984.

199. Richet H, Craven P, Brown J, et al: A cluster of *Rhodococcus (Gordona) bronchialis* sternal-wound infections after coronary-artery bypass surgery. N Engl J Med 1991;324:104-109.

200. Wenger P, Brown J, McNeil M, Jarvis W: *Nocardia farcinica* sternotomy site infections in patients following open heart surgery. J Infect Dis 1998;178:1539-1543.

201. Centers for Disease Control: Epidemic keratoconjunctivitis in an ophthalmology clinic—California. MMWR Morb Mortal Wkly Rep 1990;39:598-601.

202. Ford E, Nelson K, Warren D: Epidemiology of epidemic keratoconjunctivitis. Epidemiol Rev 1987;9:244-261.

203. Jernigan J, Lowry B, Hayden F, et al: Adenovirus type 8 epidemic keratoconjunctivitis in an eye clinic: Risk factors and control. J Infect Dis 1993;167:1307-1313.

204. Boyce J, Opal S, Potter-Bynoe G, Mederios A: Spread of methicillin-resistant *Staphylococcus aureus* in a hospital and after exposure to a health-care worker with chronic sinusitis. Clin Infect Dis 1993;17:496-504.

205. Belani A, Sherertz R, Sullivan M, et al: Outbreak of staphylococcal infection in two hospital nurseries traced to a single nasal carrier. Infect Control 1986;7:487-490.

206. Kreiswirth B, Kravitz G, Schlievert P, Novick R: Nosocomial transmission of a strain of *Staphylococcus aureus* causing toxic shock syndrome. Ann Intern Med 1986;105:704-707.

207. Weber D, Rutala W, Denny FJ: Management of healthcare workers with pharyngitis or suspected streptococcal infections. Infect Control Hosp Epidemiol 1996;17:753-761.

208. Viglionese A, Nottebart V, Bodman H, Platt R: Recurrent group A streptococcal carriage in a health care worker associated with widely separated nosocomial outbreaks. Am J Med 1991;91:329S-333.

209. Paul S, Genese C, Spitalny K: Postoperative group A beta-hemolytic streptococcus outbreak with the pathogen traced to a member of a healthcare worker's household. Infect Control Hosp Epidemiol 1990;11:643-646.

210. Berkelman R, Martin D, Graham D, et al: Streptococcal wound infection caused by a vaginal carrier. JAMA 1982;247:2680-2682.

211. Ridgway E, Allen K: Clustering of group A streptococcal infections on a burns unit: Important lessons in outbreak management. J Hosp Infect 1993;25:173-182.

212. Schaffner W, Lefkowitz LJ, Goodman J, Koenig M: Hospital outbreak of infections with group A streptococci traced to an asymptomatic anal carrier. N Engl J Med 1969;280:1224-1225.

213. Richman D, Breton S, Goldman D: Scarlet fever and group A streptococcal surgical wound infection traced to an anal carrier. J Pediatr 1977;90:387-390.

214. Stromberg A, Schwan A, Cars O: Throat carrier rates of beta-hemolytic streptococci among healthy adults and children. Scand J Infect Dis 1988;20:411-417.

215. Stamm W, Feeley J, Facklam R: Wound infection due to group A streptococcus traced to a vaginal carrier. J Infect Dis 1978;138:287-292.

216. Bolyard E, Tablan O, Williams W, et al: Guideline for infection control in healthcare personnel, 1998. Hospital Infection Control Practices Advisory Committee. Am J Infect Control 1998;26:289-354.

217. Bruch M: Methods of testing antiseptics: Antimicrobials used topically in humans and procedures for hand scrubs. In Block SS (ed): Disinfection, Sterilization, and Preservation. Philadelphia, Lea & Febiger, 1991, pp 1028-1046.

218. Ascenzi JM (ed): Handbook of Disinfectants and Antiseptics. New York, Marcel Dekker, 1996.

219. Association of Operating Room Nurses: Recommended practices for skin preparation of patients. AORN J 1996;64:813-816.

220. Larson E: Guideline for use of topical antimicrobial agents. Am J Infect Control 1988;16:253-266.

221. Mayhall C: Surgical infections including burns. In RP Wenzel (ed): Prevention and Control of Nosocomial Infections. Baltimore, Williams & Wilkins, 1993, pp 614-664.

222. Hardin W, Nichols R: Aseptic technique in the operating room. In Fry D (ed): Surgical Infections. Boston, Little, Brown, 1995, pp 109-118.

223. Lowbury E, Lilly H: Use of 4 percent chlorhexidine detergent solution (Hibiscrub) and other methods of skin disinfection. Br Med J 1973;1:510-515.

224. Aly R, Maibach H: Comparative antibacterial efficacy of a 2-minute surgical scrub with chlorhexidine gluconate, povidone-iodine, and chloroxylenol sponge-brushes. Am J Infect Control 1988;16:173-177.

225. Peterson A, Rosenberg A, Alatary S: Comparative evaluation of surgical scrub preparations. Surg Gynecol Obstet 1978;146:63-65.

226. Brown T, Ehrlich C, Stehman F, et al: A clinical evaluation of chlorhexidine gluconate spray as compared with iodophor scrub for preoperative skin preparation. Surg Gynecol Obstet 1984;158:363-366.

227. Lowbury E, Lilly H: The effect of blood on disinfection of surgeons' hands. Br J Surg 1974;61:19-21.

228. Mediflex Chlorap: Website at www.medi-flex.com/chloraprep_com/Swabstick_Sell_Sheet.pdf.

229. Kutarski P, Grundy H: To dry or not to dry? An assessment of the possible degradation in efficiency of preoperative skin preparation caused by wiping skin dry. Ann R Coll Surg Engl 1993;75:181-185.

230. Gauthier D, O'Fallon P, Coppage D: Clean vs sterile surgical skin preparation kits: Cost, safety, effectiveness. AORN J 1993;58:486-495.

231. Hagen K, Treston-Aurand J: A comparison of two skin preps used in cardiac surgical procedures. AORN J 1995;62:393-402.

232. Shirahatti R, Joshi RM, Vishwanath Y, et al: Effect of pre-operative skin preparation on post-operative wound infection. J Postgrad Med 1993;39:134-136.

233. Page C, Bohnen J, Fletcher J, et al: Antimicrobial prophylaxis for surgical wounds: Guidelines for clinical care. Arch Surg 1993;128:79-88.

234. Platt R: Guidelines for perioperative antibiotic prophylaxis. In Abrutyn E, Goldmann D, Scheckler W (eds): Saunders Infection Control Reference Service. Philadelphia, WB Saunders, 1997, pp 229-234.

235. Sanderson P: Antimicrobial prophylaxis in surgery: Microbiological factors. J Antimicrob Chemother 1993;31(Suppl B):1-9.

236. Culbertson W, Altemeir W, Gonzalez L, et al: Studies on the epidemiology of postoperative wounds. Ann Surg 1961;154:599-610.

237. Burke J: Identification of the sources of staphylococci contaminating the surgical wound during operation. Ann Surg 1963;158:898-904.

238. Burke J: The effective period of preventive antibiotic action in experimental incisions and dermal lesions. Surgery 1961;50:161.

239. Skledar S, Gross P, Hamilton L: University of Pittsburgh recommendations for surgical antimicrobial prophylaxis. In Potoski B (ed): Guide to Antimicrobial Chemotherapy. Pittsburgh, Pa, University of Pittsburgh Medical Center, Presbyterian, 2005, pp 40-45.

240. American Society of Health-System Pharmacists: ASHP therapeutic guidelines on antimicrobial prophylaxis in surgery. Am J Health-Syst Pharm 1999;56:1839-1888.

241. Nichols R: Antibiotic prophylaxis in surgery. J Chemother 1989;1:170-178.

242. Trilla A, Mensa J: Perioperative antibiotic prophylaxis. In Wenzel R (ed): Prevention and Control of Nosocomial Infections. Baltimore, Williams & Wilkins, 1993, pp 665-682.

243. Nichols R: Surgical antibiotic prophylaxis. Med Clin North Am 1995;79:509-522.

244. Scher K: Studies on the duration of antibiotic administration for surgical prophylaxis. Am Surg 1997;63:59-62.

245. McDonald M, Grabsch E, Marshall C, Forbes A: Single- versus multiple-dose antimicrobial prophylaxis for major surgery: A systematic review. Aust N Z J Surg 1998;68:388-396.

246. Classen D, Evans R, Pestotnik S, et al: The timing of prophylactic administration of antibiotics and the risk of surgical-wound infection. N Engl J Med 1992;326:281-286.

247. Antimicrobial prophylaxis in surgery. Med Lett Drugs Ther 2001;43:92-97.

248. Dellinger E, Gross P, Barrett T, et al: Quality standard for antimicrobial prophylaxis in surgical procedures. Infectious Diseases Society of America. Clin Infect Dis 1994;18:422-427.

249. Gilbert D, Moellering R, Sande M: The Sanford guide to antimicrobial therapy. Hyde Park, Vt, Antimicrobial Therapy, 2003.

250. Mangram A, Horan T, Pearson M, et al: Guideline for prevention of surgical site infection, 1999. Hospital Infection Control Practices Advisory Committee. Infect Control Hosp Epidemiol 1999;20:250-278.

251. American College of Obstetricians and Gynecologists: Antibiotic prophylaxis for gynecologic procedures. ACOG Committee on Practice Bulletins. ACOG Practice Bulletin 23. 2001.

252. Bratzler D, Houck P, for the Surgical Infection Prevention Guidelines Writers Workgroup: Antimicrobial prophylaxis for surgery: An advisory statement from the National Surgical Infection Prevention Project. Clin Infect Dis 2004;38:1706-1715.

253. Auerbach A: Prevention of surgical site infections. In Shojania K, Duncan B, McDonald K, et al (eds): Making Health Care Safer: A Critical Analysis of Patient Safety Practices. Evidence Report/ Technology Assessment no. 43. AHRQ publication no. 01-E058. Rockville, Md, Agency for Healthcare Research and Quality, 20 July 2001, pp 221-244.

254. Meijer W, Schmitz P, Jeekel J: Meta-analysis of randomized, controlled clinical trials of antibiotic prophylaxis in biliary tract surgery. Br J Surg 1990;77:283-290.

255. Kreter B, Woods M: Antibiotic prophylaxis for cardiothoracic operations: Meta-analysis of thirty years of clinical trials. J Thorac Cardiovasc Surg 1992;104:590-599.

256. Harbarth S, Samore M, Lichtenberg D, Carmeli Y: Prolonged antibiotic prophylaxis after cardiovascular surgery and its effect on surgical site infections and antimicrobial resistance. Circulation 2000;101: 2916-2921.

257. Eggimann P, Pittet D: Infection control in the ICU. Chest 2001;120: 2059-2093.

258. Hecker M, Aron D, Patel N, et al: Unnecessary use of antimicrobials in hospitalized patients: Current patterns of misuse with an emphasis on the antianaerobic spectrum of activity. Arch Intern Med 2003;163:972-978.

259. Centers for Medicare & Medicaid Services: Surgical Infection Prevention Project description. Available at www.medqic.org/sip, 2004.

260. Wenzel R, Perl T: The significance of nasal carriage of *Staphylococcus aureus* and the incidence of postoperative wound infection. J Hospital Infection 1995;31:13-24.

261. Kluytmans J, van Belkum A, Verbrugh H: Nasal carriage of *Staphylococcus aureus*: Epidemiology, underlying mechanisms, and associated risk. Clin Microbiol Rev 1997;10:505-520.

262. Perl TM, Cullen JJ, Wenzel RP, et al: Intranasal mupirocin to prevent postoperative *Staphylococcus aureus* infections. N Engl J Med 2002; 13:1871-1877.

263. Laupland K, Conly J: Treatment of *Staphylococcus aureus* colonization and prophylaxis for infection with topical intranasal mupirocin: An evidence-based review. Clin Infect Dis 2003;37:933-938.

264. Suzuki Y, Kamigaki T, Fujino Y, et al: Randomized clinical trial of preoperative intranasal mupirocin to reduce surgical-site infection after digestive surgery. Br J Surg 2003;90:1072-1075.

265. Finkelstein R, Rabino G, Mashiah T, et al: Vancomycin versus cefazolin prophylaxis for cardiac surgery in the setting of a high prevalence of methicillin-resistant staphylococcal infections. J Thorac Cardiovasc Surg 2002;123:326-332.

266. Manian F, Meyer P, Setzer J, Senkel D: Surgical site infections associated with methicillin-resistant *Staphylococcus aureus*: Do postoperative factors play a role? Clin Infect Dis 2003;36:863-868.

267. Muto C, Jernigan J, Ostrowsky B, et al: SHEA guideline for preventing nosocomial transmission of multidrug-resistant strains of *Staphylococcus aureus* and *Enterococcus*. Infect Control Hosp Epidemiol 2003;24:362-386.

268. American Institute of Architects: Guidelines for Design and Construction of Hospitals and Health Care Facilities. Washington, DC, American Institute of Architects Press, 2001.

269. Nichols R: The operating room. In Bennet J, Brachman P (eds): Hospital Infections. Boston, Little Brown, 1992, pp 461-473.

270. Dharan S, Pittet D: Environmental controls in operating theatres. J Hosp Infect 2002;51:79-84.

271. Friberg B: Ultraclean laminar airflow in ORs. AORN J 1998;67: 841-851.

272. Lidwell O, Lowbury E, Whyte W, et al: Airborne contamination of wounds in joint replacement operations: The relationship to sepsis rates. J Hosp Infect 1983;4:111-131.

273. Salvati E, Robinson R, Zeno SM, et al: Infection rates after 3175 total hip and total knee replacements performed with and without a horizontal unidirectional filtered air-flow system. J Bone Joint Surg Am 1982;64:525-535.

274. Brown IW Jr, Moor GF, Hummel BW, et al: Toward further reducing wound infections in cardiac operations. Ann Thorac Surg 1996;62: 1783-1789.

275. Taylor G, Chandler J: Ultraviolet light in the orthopedic operating theatre. Br J Theat Nurs 1997;6:10-14.

276. AORN Recommended Practices Committee: Recommended practices for traffic patterns in the perioperative practice setting. In Standards, Recommended Practices and Guidelines, 2000.

277. Pryor F, Messmer P: The effect of traffic patterns in the OR on surgical site infections. AORN J 1998;68:649-660.

278. Department of Labor OSHA: Occupational exposure to bloodborne pathogens: Final rule (29 CRF Part 1910.1030). Fed Reg 1991;56: 64004-64182.

279. The Association of Perioperative Nurses: Recommended practices for environmental cleaning in the surgical practice setting. AORN J 2002;76:1071-1076.

280. Laufman H: The operating room. In Bennett J, Brachman P (eds): Hospital Infections. Boston, Little, Brown, 1986, pp 315-323.

281. Crow S, Smith J: Gas plasma sterilization-application of space-age technology. Infect Control Hosp Epidemiol 1995;16:483-487.

282. Okpara-Hofmann J, Knoll M, Dürr M, et al: Comparison of low-temperature hydrogen peroxide gas plasma sterilization for endoscopes using various Sterrad models. J Hosp Infect 2005;59: 280-285.

283. Rutala W, Jones S, Weber D: Comparison of a rapid readout biological indicator for steam sterilization with four conventional biological indicators and five chemical indicators. Infect Control Hosp Epidemiol 1996;17:423-428.

284. Association of Perioperative Nurses: Recommended practice for surgical attire. AORN J 2005;81:413-416, 418-420.

285. Garibaldi R, Maglio S, Lere T, et al: Comparison of non-woven and woven gown and drape fabric to prevent intraoperative wound contamination and postoperative infection. Am J Surg 1986;152: 505-509.

286. American Society for Testing Material: Standard test method for resistance of materials used in protective clothing to penetrations by synthetic blood. American Society for Testing Materials, 1998: F1670-1698.

287. Granzow J, Smith J, Nichols R, et al: Evaluation of the protective value of hospital gowns against blood strike-through and methicillin-resistant *Staphylococcus aureus* penetration. Am J Infect Control 1998;26:85-93.

288. Association of Professionals in Infection Control and Epidemiology (APIC): APIC Text of Infection Control and Epidemiology. Washington, DC, APIC, 2005.

289. Garner J: The CDC Hospital Infection Control Practices Advisory Committee. Am J Infect Control 1993;21:160-162.

290. Kluytmans J: Surgical infections including burns. In Wenzel R, Pine J (eds): Prevention and Control of Nosocomial Infections. Baltimore, Md, Williams & Wilkins, 1997, pp 841-856.

291. Haley R, Culver D, Morgan W: Identifying patients at high risk of surgical wound infection: A simple multivariate index of patient susceptibility and wound contamination. Am J Epidemiol 1985;121: 206-215.

292. Emori T, Culver D, Horan T: National Nosocomial Infections Surveillance System (NNIS): Description of surveillance methods. Am J Infect Control 1991;19:19-35.

293. Horan T, Emori T: Definitions of key terms used in the NNIS System. Am J Infect Control 1997;25:112-116.

294. Horan T, Gaynes R, Martone W, et al: CDC definitions of nosocomial surgical site infections, 1992. Am J Infect Control 1992;20:271-274.

295. Cardo D, Falk P, Mayhall C: Validation of surgical wound surveillance. Infect Control Hosp Epidemiol 1993;14:211-215.

296. Horan T, Gaynes R, Culver D: National Nosocomial Infection Surveillance System (NNIS), CDC: Development of predictive risk factors for nosocomial surgical site infections (SSI). Infect Control Hosp Epidemiol 1994;15(suppl):P46(M72).

297. Blattler T: Implications of prion diseases for neurosurgery. Neurosurg Rev 2002;25:195-203.

298. Will RG, Matthews WB: Evidence for case-to-case transmission of Creutzfeldt-Jakob disease, J Neurol Neurosci Psychiatry 1982;45: 235-238.

299. Ayliffe GA: Recommendation for the control of methicillin-resistant *Staphylococcus aureus* (MRSA). In Control DoEaOCDSa (ed): Geneva, Switzerland, World Health Organization, 1996.

300. Rutala W: APIC guideline for selection and use of disinfectants. Am J Infect Control 1996;24:313-342.

301. Joint Commission on Accreditation of Healthcare Organizations: Sentinel event alert: Exposure to Creutzfeldt-Jakob disease. 2001;20.

302. Pokrywka M, Andro R, Bingham P, Muto C: Creutzfeldt Jacob Disease (CJD): Impact of an unsuspected case. 13th Annual Meeting of the Society for Healthcare Epidemiology of America, Washington, DC, 2003.

303. Centers for Disease Control: Bovine spongiform encephalopathy in a dairy cow: Washington State, 2003. MMWR Morb Mortal Wkly Rep 2004;52:1280-1285.

304. Canadian Food Inspection Agency: Bovine spongiform encephalopathy (BSE) in North America. Available at: www.inspections.gc.ca.

305. Centers for Disease Control: Probable Variant Creutzfeldt-Jakob disease in a U.S. resident: Florida, 2002. MMWR Morb Mortal Wkly Rep 2002;51:927.

306. Calfee DP, Giannetta E, Durbin LJ, Farr BM: MRSA and VRE prevalence among patients being transferred from primary and secondary care facilities. 2000.

Obstetric

29 Perioperative Protection of the Pregnant Woman

Theodore G. Cheek

Contemporary expectations are that the degree of maternal safety in pregnancy is high, yet within living memory, nearly 1 in 100 women in the United States died as a result of events associated with pregnancy and childbirth. In parts of Africa, maternal mortality remains at nearly 1 in 50 births. Without continued effort on the part of the medical community, the causes of mortality and morbidity may increase and the gains in maternal safety may not endure. This chapter reviews causes of perioperative maternal risk and suggests a number of ways to protect the mother from these risks. *Perioperative* refers primarily to surgery but here also includes delivery.

At the beginning of the 20th century, for every 1000 live births, six to nine women in the United States died of pregnancy-related complications, and approximately 100 infants died before the age of 1 year.[1,2] From 1900 through 1997, the maternal mortality rate declined almost 99%, to less than 0.1 reported deaths per 1000 live births (7.7 deaths per 100,000 live births in 1997) (Fig. 29-1).[3,4] Environmental interventions, improvements in nutrition, advances in clinical medicine, improvements in access to health care, improvements in surveillance and monitoring of disease, increases in education levels, and improvements in standards of living contributed to this remarkable decline.[1] Despite these improvements in maternal mortality rates, significant preventable causes of maternal death still persist.

Information on anesthesia and maternal safety has been historically hard to obtain. This chapter relies on data gathered from the United Kingdom since the 1950s and, more recently, in the 1990s from the U.S. Centers for Disease Control (CDC). An effort has been made to summarize available literature, task force opinions, and practice advisories regarding best perioperative care of the pregnant patient at high risk. Where possible, prospective randomized trials and evidence-based data such as Cochrane and other meta-

analyses are used, along with controlled studies and published standards. For certain types of maternal risk, such as thromboembolism, thrombophilia, hypertension, and some cardiac diseases, more outcome data are available than for others. Hypoxia, resulting from inability to control the airway, gastric content aspiration, and maternal hemorrhage, is widely reported on, but limited prospective randomized outcome data are available because this type of study is rarely feasible. This chapter offers recommendations toward what authorities consider best practice.

■ WHY MOTHERS DIE

Since 1952, the most thorough and reliable data on maternal mortality have come from the Confidential Enquiry into Maternal Death, now called Confidential Enquiry into Maternal and Child Health (CEMACH).[5,6] Another useful source is the ongoing Maternal Mortality Survey conducted at the CDC under the direction of Dr. Cindy Berg.[7]

The most recent period reviewed by CEMACH incorporated the years 2000 through 2002 and was published in 2005. Out of nearly 2 million deliveries, there were 391 obstetric deaths, with 106 caused by pregnancy within 42 days of delivery (direct) (Fig. 29-2) and 155 caused by pre-existing conditions (indirect) (Fig. 29-3). A further 130 deaths were coincidental or occurred more than 42 days after delivery. Major risk factors for maternal death included poor antenatal care, obesity, domestic violence, and substance abuse. Socioeconomic pressures such as poverty, unemployment, and minority status measurably increased maternal mortality risk.

Among direct causes of maternal death, thromboembolism continues as a leading cause, and its incidence is not decreasing (see Fig. 29-2). The data suggest that late or

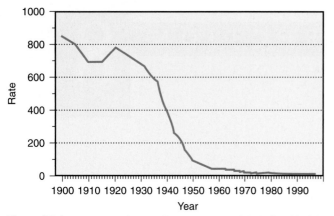

Figure 29-1 ■ Maternal mortality rate (per 100,000 live births) by year, United States, 1900-1997. In 1900, approximately 100 infants died for every 1000 births. This has decreased to 7.2 per 1000 in 1997. *(Redrawn from Centers for Disease Control and Prevention: Healthier mothers and babies. MMWR Morb Mortal Wkly Rep 1999;48:850.)*

inadequate treatment by uninformed practitioners is a root cause. Severe hemorrhage has increased as a cause of mortality. Seven deaths were reported in 1997-99, and 17 were reported in 2000-2002. The majority were postpartum hemorrhages that occurred in small hospitals that were not prepared to treat severe bleeding. The association of placenta previa and low anterior placenta over a previous scar with massive blood loss was ignored or not known. Young age of the patient and her ability to tolerate blood loss and hypovolemia may have led to delayed diagnosis and treatment. Clinicians must be experienced enough to recognize the risks, to prepare blood and have the means to deliver it rapidly, and to assess patient response. Demise resulting from hypertensive disease (preeclampsia or eclampsia) was unchanged, but

this is still a leading cause of death. The evidence pointed to inadequate or late treatment of high blood pressure.

Data on maternal mortality from the CDC, although slightly older, agree closely with statistics coming from the United Kingdom (Fig. 29-4).

Anesthetic Causes of Death

From the early 1980s until the 1999 triennium, anesthetic deaths decreased from 12 per year to less than 4 per year (Fig. 29-5). In the most recent period (2000 to 2002), the risk of death regressed to 1/20,000 anesthetic procedures, similar to the 1982-84 period. There was an increase of six deaths from anesthetic causes, and most of these were the result of poor airway management. Three deaths resulted from esophageal intubation, two from hypoventilation leading to hypoxia, and one from an inability to resuscitate a woman with severe anaphylaxis. Of the six cases, all but one were isolated cases performed by inexperienced anesthetists. Obesity, aspiration, and lack of capnography were associated with one or more of the cases.

Reduction of Maternal Mortality from Thromboembolism

Pregnancy and its hormonal changes are known to promote coagulation and are reviewed elsewhere.[8-10] Clotting factors increase with gestational age, and together with rapid myometrial contraction at delivery, help prevent excessive blood loss. Platelet production, consumption, and activation increase. Thromboelastography demonstrates accelerated clot formation,[11] which further increases risk of thromboembolism in pregnancy.

Risk factors associated with maternal thromboembolism include older age, immobility, prolonged travel,[12] surgery, family history, patient history, oral contraceptive use, and obesity.[13] The question arises as to whether there is a role for thromboembolic prophylaxis in postpartum women,

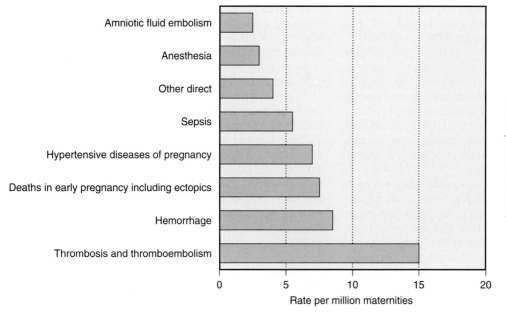

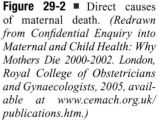

Figure 29-2 ■ Direct causes of maternal death. *(Redrawn from Confidential Enquiry into Maternal and Child Health: Why Mothers Die 2000-2002. London, Royal College of Obstetricians and Gynaecologists, 2005, available at www.cemach.org.uk/publications.htm.)*

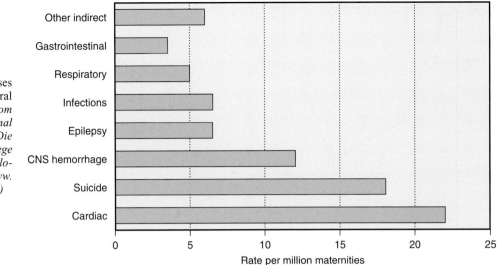

Figure 29-3 ■ Indirect causes of maternal death. CNS, central nervous system. *(Redrawn from Confidential Enquiry into Maternal and Child Health: Why Mothers Die 2000-2002. London, Royal College of Obstetricians and Gynaecologists, 2005, available at www. cemach.org.uk/publications.htm.)*

especially after cesarean section. It is common for patients to receive thromboprophylaxis after appendectomy and gallbladder surgery. Why not a similar policy after cesarean section? The risk of asymptomatic deep vein thrombosis (as found by ultrasound examination) is about 0.5%. The incidence of some clot being found in pelvic veins after cesarean delivery is more frequent (up to 65% of cesarean sections examined by magnetic resonance imaging). Maternal death due to thromboembolism decreased from 1950 to 1980, but the rate has remained fairly steady since that time (Figs. 29-6 and 29-7).

Recent recommendations have included using heparin prophylaxis after a cesarean section for women with other risk factors (smoking, obesity, age greater than 40 years, previous or family history of thromboembolic disease). There may also be a role for aspirin therapy, stockings, and inter-

mittent compression stockings. At present, routine prophylaxis for all postpartum women is not recommended (Table 29-1 and Box 29-1). No large-scale trials have looked at therapeutic outcome for thromboembolism.

Thrombophilia

Thrombophilia is emerging as an important cause of maternal thromboembolic risk. It is found in up to 17% of white North Americans. Thrombophilias can be divided into three general categories: familial, acquired, and mixed. Familial causes include protein C, protein S, and antithrombin III deficiencies, as well as factor V Leiden and prothrombin gene polymorphism. Conditions that increase the risk of thrombophilia include antiphospholipid antibodies and lupus anticoagulant. Mixed thrombophilia risk includes methylene tetrahydrofolate reductase polymorphism and hyperhomocysteinemia. The incidence in the general population and estimated risk for deep venous thrombosis (DVT) and pulmonary embolism (PE) in pregnancy can be reviewed in Table 29-2. Genetic thrombophilia is associated with other complications of pregnancy such as pregnancy-induced hypertension (PIH), intrauterine growth restriction (IUGR), abruption, and stillbirth.[14-16] In one study,[15] 52% of women with severe PIH and associated problems also had thrombophilia. There are no well-designed trials that address the effects of aspirin therapy or heparin prophylaxis on the outcome of this disease.[17] An ongoing study in Canada (TIMTS) is attempting to answer some of these questions regarding treatment.

Hypertension in Pregnancy

Chronic hypertension complicates 1% to 5% of pregnancies. It is defined as a blood pressure greater than 140/90 mm Hg that either predates pregnancy or develops before 20 weeks of gestation. PIH develops after 20 weeks of gestation and complicates 5% to 10% of pregnancies. Gestational hypertension, which is PIH in isolation, may reflect a familial predisposition to chronic hypertension, or it may be an early manifestation of preeclampsia. Preeclampsia is PIH in

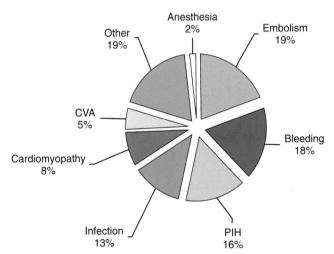

Figure 29-4 ■ Causes of maternal death in the United States. CVA, cerebrovascular accident; PIH, pregnancy-induced hypertension. *(Redrawn from Berg CJ, Chang J, Callaghan WM, Whitehead SJ: Obstet Gynecol 2003;101:289-296.)*

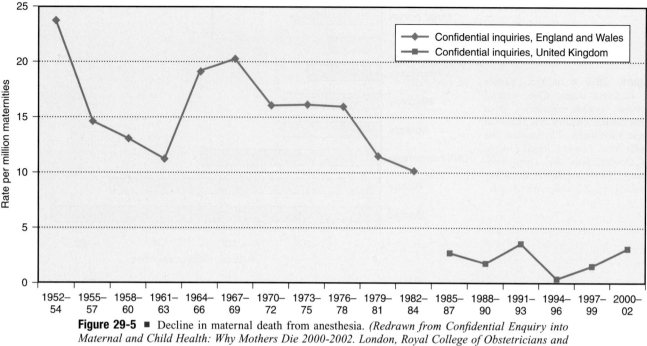

Figure 29-5 ■ Decline in maternal death from anesthesia. *(Redrawn from Confidential Enquiry into Maternal and Child Health: Why Mothers Die 2000-2002. London, Royal College of Obstetricians and Gynaecologists, 2005, available at www.cemach.org.uk/publications.htm.)*

association with proteinuria or edema, or both, and virtually any organ system may be affected.

PIH, in contrast to chronic hypertension, arises *after* the 20th week of gestation and is primarily seen as preeclampsia, which may progress to eclampsia (and seizures) or hemolysis, elevated liver enzymes, and low platelets (HELLP). Pre-

eclampsia is the most common disease that is unique to human gestation, occurring in 6% to 8% of pregnancies. Classically, PIH was described by Young as EPH gestosis, in which EPH stood for the observed edema, proteinuria, and hypertension. Present-day authorities use the term *preeclampsia* when PIH includes renal involvement and

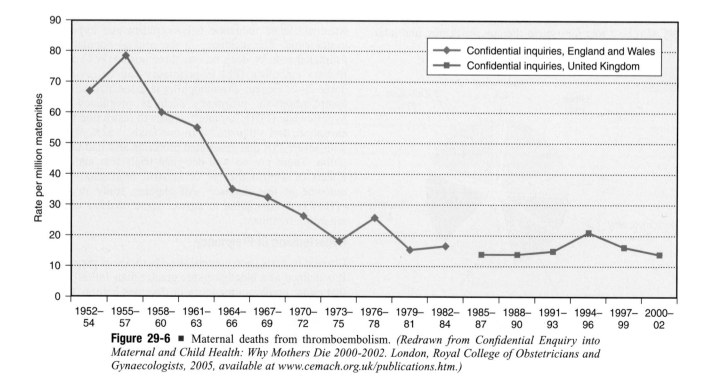

Figure 29-6 ■ Maternal deaths from thromboembolism. *(Redrawn from Confidential Enquiry into Maternal and Child Health: Why Mothers Die 2000-2002. London, Royal College of Obstetricians and Gynaecologists, 2005, available at www.cemach.org.uk/publications.htm.)*

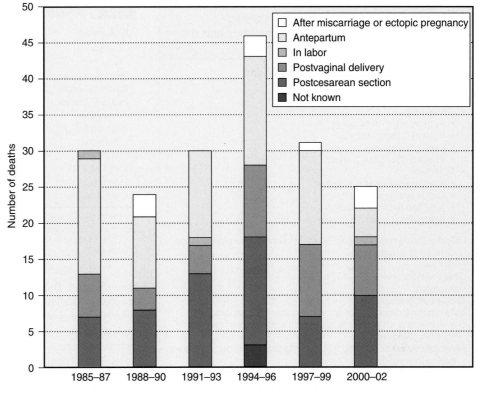

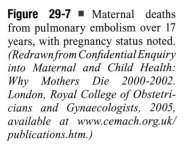

Figure 29-7 ■ Maternal deaths from pulmonary embolism over 17 years, with pregnancy status noted. *(Redrawn from Confidential Enquiry into Maternal and Child Health: Why Mothers Die 2000-2002. London, Royal College of Obstetricians and Gynaecologists, 2005, available at www.cemach.org.uk/publications.htm.)*

29-1   Thromboprophylaxis Guidelines

Evidence Levels IIa, IIb, and III*

Women with previous venous thromboembolism (VTE) should be screened for inherited and acquired thrombophilia, ideally before pregnancy.

Women with previous VTE and thrombophilia should be offered thromboprophylaxis with low-molecular-weight heparin (LMWH) antenatally and for at least 6 postpartum weeks.

Antenatal thromboprophylaxis should begin as early in pregnancy as practical.

Postpartum prophylaxis should begin as soon as possible after delivery (but after regional anesthesia, see precautions).

LMWHs are the agents of choice for antenatal thromboprophylaxis. They are as effective as and safer than unfractionated heparin in pregnancy.

Warfarin should usually be avoided during pregnancy. It is safe after delivery and during breastfeeding.

Evidence Level IV*

All women should undergo an assessment of risk factors for VTE in early pregnancy or before pregnancy. This assessment should be repeated if the woman is admitted to the hospital or develops other intercurrent problems.

Women with previous VTE should be offered postpartum thromboprophylaxis with LMWH. It may be reasonable not to use antenatal thromboprophylaxis with heparin in women with a single previous VTE associated with a temporary risk factor that has now resolved.

Women with asymptomatic inherited or acquired thrombophilia may qualify for antenatal or postnatal thromboprophylaxis, depending on the specific thrombophilia and the presence of other risk factors.

Good-Practice Points†

Regardless of the risk of VTE, immobilization of women during pregnancy, labor, and the puerperium should be minimized and dehydration should be avoided.

Women with three or more persisting risk factors should be considered for thromboprophylaxis with LMWH antenatally and for 3 to 5 postpartum days.

Women should be reassessed before or during labor for risk factors for VTE. Age greater than 35 years and body mass index greater than 30 (or bodyweight greater than 90 kg) are important independent risk factors for postpartum VTE, even after vaginal delivery.

The combination of either of these risk factors with any other risk factor for VTE (such as preeclampsia or immobility) or the presence of two other persisting risk factors should lead the clinician to consider the use of LMWH for 3 to 5 postpartum days.

Once the woman is in labor or thinks she is in labor, she should be advised not to inject any further heparin. She should be reassessed on admission to the hospital and further doses should be prescribed by medical staff.

---

*Evidence levels IIa, IIb, and III require the availability of well-controlled clinical studies but no randomized clinical trials on the topic of recommendations. Evidence level IV requires evidence obtained from expert committee reports or opinions and/or clinical experiences of respected authorities. This level indicates an absence of directly applicable clinical studies of good quality.

†Good practice points are recommended best practice based on the clinical experience of the guideline development group.

Reproduced from RCOG green-top guideline no. 37: Thromboprophylaxis during pregnancy, labour and after vaginal delivery, January 2004, with the permission of the Royal College of Obstetricians and Gynaecologists.

29-1	Risk Factors for Venous Thromboembolism in Pregnancy and the Puerperium*

Preexisting Venous Thromboembolism

Thrombophilia

- Congenital
  - Antithrombin deficiency
  - Protein C deficiency
  - Factor V Leiden
  - Prothrombin gene variant
- Acquired
  - Antiphospholipid syndrome
  - Lupus anticoagulant
  - Anticardiolipin antibodies
  - Age greater than 35 years

Obesity (body mass index >30 kg/m^2 either before pregnancy or in early pregnancy)
Parity >4
Gross varicose veins
Paraplegia
Sickle cell disease
Inflammatory disorders (e.g., inflammatory bowel disease)
Some medical disorders (e.g., nephritic syndrome, certain cardiac diseases)
Myeloproliferative disorders (e.g., essential thrombocythemia, polycythemia vera)

New-Onset or Transient Venous Thromboembolism[†]

Surgical procedure in pregnancy or puerperium (e.g., evacuation of retained products of conception, postpartum sterilization)
Hyperemesis
Dehydration
Severe infection (e.g., pyelonephritis)
Immobility (>4 days of bedrest)
Preeclampsia
Excessive blood loss
Long-distance travel
Prolonged labor
Midcavity instrumental delivery[‡]
Immobility after delivery[‡]

*Although these are all accepted as thromboembolic risk factors, there are few data to support the degree of increased risk associated with many of them.

[†]These risk factors are potentially reversible and may develop at later stages in gestation than the initial risk assessment, or they may resolve. An ongoing individual risk assessment is important.

[‡]Risk factors specific to postpartum venous thromboembolism only.

Reproduced from RCOG green-top guideline no. 37: Thromboprophylaxis during pregnancy, labour and after vaginal delivery, January 2004, with the permission of the Royal College of Obstetricians and Gynaecologists.

29-2	Thrombophilia Prevalence and Risk		

Risk Factor	% in General Population	% Risk for First DVT/PE in Pregnancy (Background of 0.03%)
Decreased protein S	6.6	?
Decreased protein C	3.3	0.1
Factor V Leiden mutation	7.7	0.25
Prothrombin gene mutation G2021A	1.3	0.5
FVL and PTG	0.1	4.6
Decreased antithrombin	1.5	0.4

DVT, deep-vein thromboembolism; FVL, Factor V Leiden; PE, pulmonary embolism; PTG, prothrombin gene mutation.

From Kupferminc MJ, Eldor A, Steinman N, et al: N Engl J Med 1999;340:9-13.

then released. Blood vessel narrowing and decreased elasticity are associated with increased vascular resistance. Women who become preeclamptic, unlike those with a normal pregnancy, do not lose sensitivity to angiotensin and catecholamines. Uterine Doppler studies show evidence of high vascular resistance and flow abnormalities (Fig. 29-8).

An immune reaction involving trophoblast material and basement membrane, prostacyclin imbalance, and vascular nitric oxide dysfunction have all been suggested as important parts of the puzzle. A genetic analysis of its aspects is underway.[20,21] General risk factors for the development of PIH can be found in Table 29-3. A new urine test for urinary placental growth factor may allow early prediction of the development of preeclampsia.[22]

Maternal mortality due to hypertensive disease has decreased since 1952 (Fig. 29-9). In 2000 to 2002 in the United Kingdom, there were 14 maternal deaths attributable to hypertension. The specific causes included nine from intracranial hemorrhage, two from coagulopathy, two from multiorgan failure (including hepatic), and one from adult respiratory distress syndrome. Five were before 30 weeks gestation and nine after 34 weeks. Eight of these hypertensive deaths were accompanied by HELLP syndrome.

Recommendations that grew out of examining these maternal deaths included (1) better educating patients and practitioners to recognize the warning signs of hypertensive disease, (2) applying a standard systolic blood pressure threshold at which treatment should begin (i.e., 140/90), (3) streamlining and standardizing care whenever possible, and (4) increasing the use of magnesium. (Magnesium use in preeclampsia is not as widespread in the United Kingdom as it is in the United States.)

Management of Maternal Hypertension and Preeclampsia

There is disagreement over the benefits of hospitalization, bedrest, and antihypertensive medications. However, a growing number of randomized trials and meta-analyses are shedding light on these issues.[23,24] Hospitalization is no longer necessary, except in the presence of severe preeclampsia. Bedrest, though often advocated, has not been subjected to

proteinuria. Hyperreflexia and liver function disturbance are also included in the diagnosis. Sixteen percent of maternal deaths in the United States are associated with PIH (see Fig. 29-4). Detailed discussions of obstetric[18] and anesthesia[19] management are available.

The etiology is unknown, but the defining feature of preeclampsia is vasospasm affecting organs throughout the body. Cellular damage can be seen in endothelium, platelets, and trophoblasts. Vasoactive amines and prostaglandins are

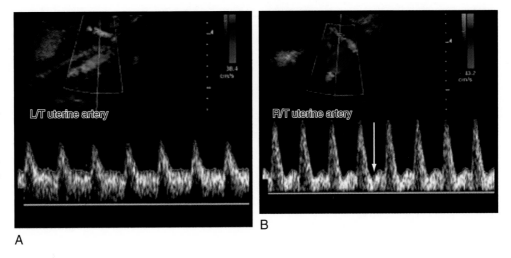

Figure 29-8 ■ Doppler uterine artery assessment showing normal flow velocity waveform with low resistance (**A**), and abnormal flow velocity waveform with an early diastolic notch (*arrow*) and a high resistance index (**B**). *(From James PR, Nelson-Piercy C: Heart 2004;90:1499-1504.)*

randomized trials that compare it with restricted activity. A number of randomized trials compare antihypertensive drugs with placebo or no treatment. In summary, these studies showed slower and less development of severe disease but no protection to the fetus.[23] With the exception of those involving magnesium, the trials were not of sufficient size to estimate the incidence of abruptio placenta, maternal outcome, or perinatal death.

Obstetric maternal monitoring should be done in all women with gestational hypertension and preeclampsia. The object in mild gestational hypertension is to watch for progression to severe hypertension or preeclampsia.[17,25] In women with severe preeclampsia, the goal is to detect and avoid organ dysfunction.[26]

Women with mild disease are followed closely as outpatients. Diet is controlled and activity is limited, fetal movement is monitored, and patients are schooled to look for signs of worsening disease. They are usually seen twice a week for evaluation.

Severe preeclampsia indicates immediate hospitalization. Most obstetricians start magnesium immediately. Obstetric management and speed of delivery are determined by the severity of the disease and the maturity of the fetus. Detailed descriptions of accepted management are available from Sibai[26] and American College of Obstetricians and Gynecologists (ACOG).[17,27]

Magnesium Sulfate

The use of magnesium sulfate is considered a best practice in this country for the control of seizures in preeclampsia and eclampsia.[26,28] The recent Magpie Trial (Magnesium Sulfate for the Prevention of Eclampsia), a large, worldwide, placebo-controlled study, looked at this drug's effectiveness (Fig. 29-10).[29] The nearly 10,000 women in 33 countries who were recruited had exhibited at least two blood pressure readings of greater than 140/90 and had at least 1+ proteinuria. Of these, 4999 received an intravenous (IV) loading dose of 4 g and then maintenance dosages of 1 g/hr intravenously or 5 g intramuscularly every 5 hours, and 4993 women received a placebo.

There were fewer eclamptic convulsions among women given magnesium sulfate than among those receiving placebo (40 [0.8%] versus 96 [1.9%]); that is, 11 fewer women convulsed per 1000 preeclamptic patients (confidence interval [CI], 7 to 16; $P < .0001$). Maternal mortality was lower among women given magnesium sulfate than among those given placebo (11 [0.2%] versus 20 [0.4%]; relative risk (RR) reduction, 45%; 95% CI, 0.26 to 1.14; $P = .11$) (see Fig. 29-10). Of interest, one third of the patients in this trial received nifedipine while receiving magnesium, and the rates of hypotension among these women were not higher than the rates seen in the placebo group. Further trials are needed to determine the minimum effective dose of magnesium sulfate and the optimal time to give it.

Blood Pressure Control

Treatment of high blood pressure is indicated if systolic pressure exceeds 180 mm Hg or if diastolic pressure exceeds 110 mm Hg despite magnesium therapy and bedrest. It is not clear how much of a decrease in maternal blood pressure is safe for the fetus. Some authorities recommend decreasing the systolic pressure to below 150 mm Hg, the diastolic pressure to below 100 mm Hg, and the mean blood pressure to below 125 mm Hg.[26]

29-3	Risk Factors for the Development of Pregnancy-Induced Hypertension	
Risk Factor		**Risk Ratio**
Nulliparity		3 : 1
Age >40 yr		3 : 1
African-American race		1.5 : 1
Family history of pregnancy-induced hypertension		5 : 1
Chronic hypertension		10 : 1
Chronic renal disease		20 : 1
Antiphospholipid syndrome		10 : 1
Diabetes mellitus		2 : 1
Twin gestation		4 : 1
Angiotensin gene T235		
Homozygous		20 : 1
Heterozygous		4 : 1

From American College of Obstetricians and Gynecologists: Hypertension in pregnancy. Technical Bulletin No. 219, 1996.

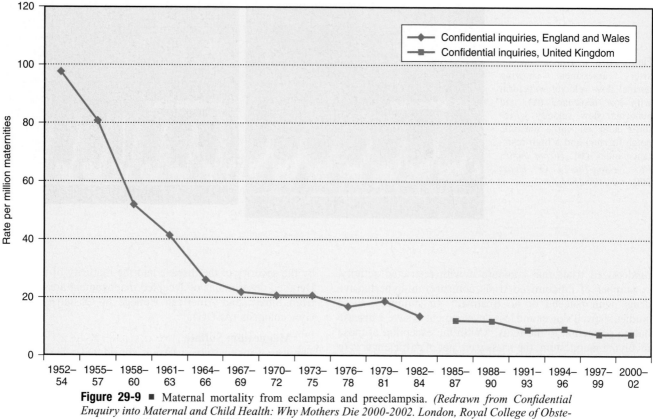

Figure 29-9 ■ Maternal mortality from eclampsia and preeclampsia. *(Redrawn from Confidential Enquiry into Maternal and Child Health: Why Mothers Die 2000-2002. London, Royal College of Obstetricians and Gynaecologists, 2005, available at www.cemach.org.uk/publications.htm.)*

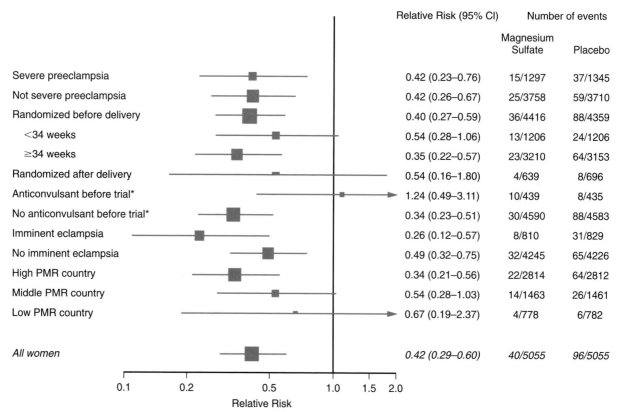

Figure 29-10 ■ The effects of magnesium sulfate treatment on preeclampsia/eclampsia. CI, confidence interval; PMR, perinatal mortality rate. *Not known whether previous anticonvulsant was given to 2 of 25 babies allocated magnesium sulfate and to 7 of 36 babies allocated placebo. *(Redrawn from the Magpie Trial Collaborative Group: Lancet 2002;359:1877-1890.)*

Hydralazine versus Labetalol and Nifedipine

Hydralazine given intravenously has been recommended for over 30 years to control severe hypertension in pregnancy. However, in 11 trials involving 570 participants, hydralazine was compared with other antihypertensives for control of severe hypertension in pregnancy.[30] The authors found that parenteral hydralazine is not the drug of first choice for acute severe hypertension later in pregnancy, as it is associated with more maternal and perinatal adverse effects than other drugs, particularly IV labetalol or oral or sublingual nifedipine. The trials compared IV hydralazine (5- to 10-mg bolus, followed by an infusion at 3 to 10 mg/hr [maximum, 15 to 80 mg/hr] or 20 to 40 mg intramuscularly) with other antihypertensives such as IV labetalol (four trials; 10- to 20-mg bolus over 2 minutes and every 10 minutes as needed) or oral sublingual nifedipine (four trials; 5 to 10 mg orally every 30 minutes, as needed). Figure 29-11 demonstrates that labetalol and nifedipine compared with hydralazine caused less hypotension, fewer cesarean sections, less placental abruption, and fewer low Apgar scores. Hydralazine was 3.2 times more likely to be associated with maternal hypotension than labetalol and nifedipine. Neonatal bradycardia was more common in the labetalol group, but only one neonate required treatment. A clinical advantage of nifedipine is that it is given by mouth; nursing staff may give it on an as-needed basis (every 30 minutes).[31] Caution is advised because an interaction between nifedipine and magnesium sulfate has been reported to produce profound maternal muscle weakness, as well as maternal hypotension and fetal distress.[32]

Other Antihypertensives

Clonidine and prazosin have been used with good results for preeclampsia, but no large clinical trials are available.[33]

Nitroglycerin and nitroprusside infusions are recommended for acute hypertensive crisis and to attenuate or treat hypertension associated with the induction and emergence of general anesthesia. Both are rapid acting and somewhat unpredictable, usually requiring an intra-arterial catheter to avoid overshoot. Although effective, nitroprusside is associated with cyanide toxicity in large doses. Nitroglycerin is a venodilator and is less reliable in controlling severe hypertension. Detailed descriptions of clinical use of these drugs are available.[19]

Central Monitoring

Because the vast majority of women with PIH have adequate left ventricular function and normal pulmonary artery pressures, clinicians must weigh the risk of pulmonary artery catheterization against the usefulness of any additional information beyond that of standard monitoring and hemodynamic data. There are no large randomized trials showing improved maternal outcome with or without pulmonary artery monitoring in severe preeclampsia. Until such evidence is available, conservative indications for pulmonary artery catheterization (modified from Clark and Cotton[34]) include refractory hypertension or oliguria, cardiac lesions, or signs of congestive heart failure. The American Society of Anesthesiologists (ASA) taskforce on obstetric anesthesia states, "It is not necessary to routinely use central invasive hemodynamic monitoring for severe preeclamptic parturients."[35]

Anesthetic Considerations

Old obstetric concerns that epidural and spinal analgesia in preeclampsia could lead to sudden maternal hypotension with maternal and fetal deterioration[36] have not been borne

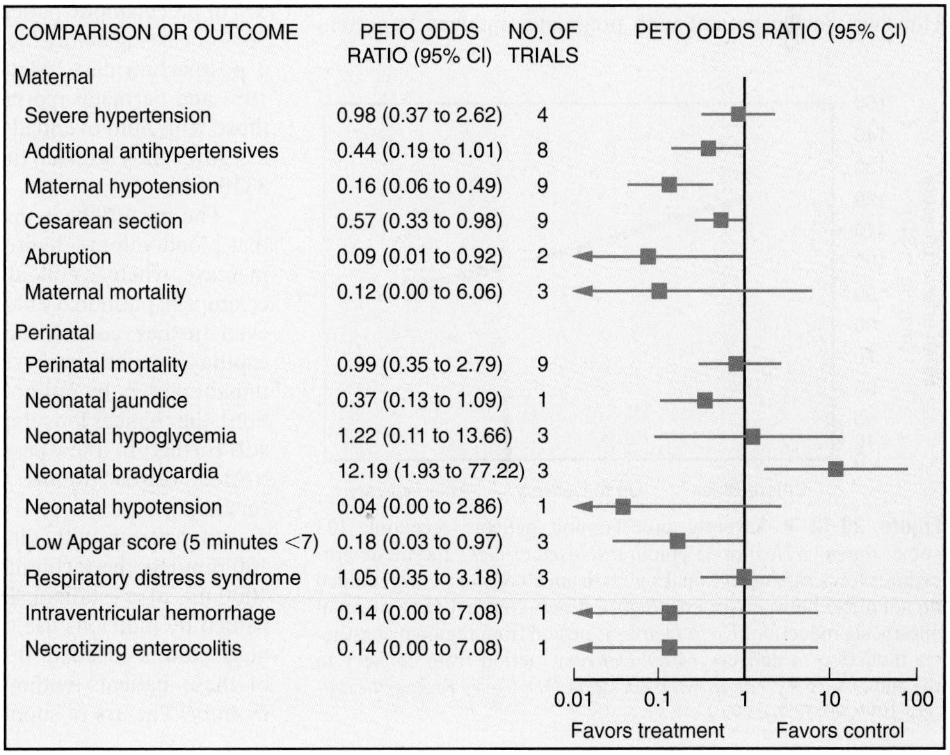

Figure 29-11 ■ Summary odds ratios (95% confidence intervals [CI]) for parenteral antihypertensive medications and for hydralazine for severe hypertension presenting later in pregnancy from 11 trials. *(Redrawn from Magee LA, Ornstein MP, von Dadelszen P: BMJ 1999;318:1332-1336.)*

COMPARISON OR OUTCOME	PETO ODDS RATIO (95% CI)	NO. OF TRIALS	PETO ODDS RATIO (95% CI)
Maternal			
Severe hypertension	0.98 (0.37 to 2.62)	4	
Additional antihypertensives	0.44 (0.19 to 1.01)	8	
Maternal hypotension	0.16 (0.06 to 0.49)	9	
Cesarean section	0.57 (0.33 to 0.98)	9	
Abruption	0.09 (0.01 to 0.92)	2	
Maternal mortality	0.12 (0.00 to 6.06)	3	
Perinatal			
Perinatal mortality	0.99 (0.35 to 2.79)	9	
Neonatal jaundice	0.37 (0.13 to 1.09)	1	
Neonatal hypoglycemia	1.22 (0.11 to 13.66)	3	
Neonatal bradycardia	12.19 (1.93 to 77.22)	3	
Neonatal hypotension	0.04 (0.00 to 2.86)	1	
Low Apgar score (5 minutes <7)	0.18 (0.03 to 0.97)	3	
Respiratory distress syndrome	1.05 (0.35 to 3.18)	3	
Intraventricular hemorrhage	0.14 (0.00 to 7.08)	1	
Necrotizing enterocolitis	0.14 (0.00 to 7.08)	1	

0.01   0.1   1   10   100

Favors treatment   Favors control

out. Although no large randomized trial or meta-analysis addresses the effect of an anesthetic on maternal outcome in preeclampsia, a number of small trials, some prospective and randomized, are available for review. Thirteen trials involving 544 women with preeclampsia who received either regional or general anesthesia have been published.[37-49] Three trials involved laboring preeclamptic patients ($N = 24$). Ten trials involved preeclamptic patients who received a cesarean section ($N = 520$), and five of these compared regional anesthesia with general anesthesia ($N = 291$). One trial compared spinal with epidural block in patients with severe preeclampsia ($N = 138$) (Fig. 29-12). Two trials looked solely at spinal anesthesia ($N = 72$) and general anesthesia techniques ($N = 39$). Overall, the incidence of maternal hypotension in these series was not considered to have an adverse clinical effect on either maternal or fetal outcome. In those trials where general anesthesia was used, four trials[38,39,41,43] found peri-induction hypertension difficult to control, whereas two[44,48] found the incidence and severity of hypertension to be clinically acceptable. One series found the incidence of hypotension to be less in preeclamptic patients receiving spinal anesthesia than among normal women.[49] These trials are summarized in Table 29-4.

Risk of Coagulopathy and Low Platelet Count

The longstanding practice of withholding regional block if a woman's platelet count is below 100,000 is unwarranted and not supported by the available science. The ASA guidelines[35] state, "A platelet count may indicate the severity of a patient's pregnancy-induced hypertension. However, the literature is insufficient to assess the predictive value of a platelet count for anesthesia-related complications in either uncomplicated parturients or those with pregnancy-induced hypertension. The Consultants and Task Force both agree that a routine platelet count in the healthy parturient is not necessary. However, in the patient with pregnancy-induced hyperten-

sion, the Consultants and Task Force both agree that the use of a platelet count may reduce the risk of anesthesia-related complications."

Recommendations

A specific platelet count predictive of regional anesthetic complications has not been determined. According to the ASA Guidelines, "The anesthesiologist's decision to order or require a platelet count should be individualized and based upon a patient's history, physical examination, and clinical signs of a coagulopathy."[35]

Fluid Management

Intravenous fluid prior to regional block is part of standard anesthetic care. In the patient with preeclampsia, this should be done with certain precautions. Decreased colloid oncotic pressure, increased hydrostatic pressure, and damaged capillary endothelium predispose to development of pulmonary edema. Before an epidural is started for labor, most patients tolerate a 500-mL normal saline fluid load. This decreases the incidence of hypotension if the patient is not already dehydrated. Likewise, for cesarean section, a fluid preload of 1000 to 1500 mL is well tolerated by most preeclamptic patients. However, some patients with severe preeclampsia may be subject to early signs of pulmonary volume overload.

Prevention of Pulmonary Edema

The incidence of pulmonary edema in pregnancy is 80 to 500 per 100,000 pregnancies. It is responsible for about 25% of pregnancy-related transfers to the intensive care unit. Sciscione and colleagues[50] divide the causes of pregnancy-related pulmonary edema into tocolytic (36%), fluid overload (31%), PIH (26%), infection (4%), and other (3%). Approximately 3% of preeclamptic patients develop pulmonary edema, with 30% occurring before the birth and 70% occurring in the first 3 postpartum days. Maternal mortality may be as high as 10% and perinatal mortality as high as 50%. In this study, those with fluid overload identified as the likely etiology had a significantly greater mean positive fluid balance (6022 ± 3340 mL).

The parturient is predisposed to pulmonary edema, in that blood volume, hydrostatic pressure, and cardiac output increase, whereas colloid oncotic pressure decreases. In preeclampsia, pulmonary blood pressure and blood flow increase even further, colloid oncotic pressure decreases more, and capillary endothelium sustains damage. If lymph flow is impaired (e.g., by pulmonary tissue swelling and inflammation), the chances for symptomatic pulmonary edema increase still further. In a few cases, when preeclampsia has not been treated, cardiac failure exacerbates these conditions even further.

In patients with diastolic blood pressure greater than 100 mm Hg, the recommendation is to limit prehydration to 1000 mL of crystalloid. The block is then performed, accompanied by judicious use of vasopressors and further intravenous fluid, as needed. It is usually possible to care for most of these patients without a central venous or pulmonary monitor. The use of supplemental intravenous 25% albumin,

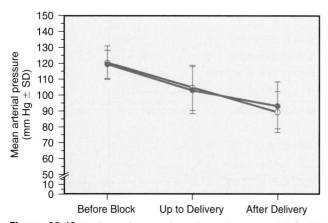

Figure 29-12 ■ Severely preeclamptic patients receiving 103 spinal *(open circles)* or 35 epidural *(closed circles)* anesthetic procedures for cesarean section. Lowest mean blood pressures recorded do not differ between groups. *Before Block,* 20 min before regional anesthesia induction; *Up to Delivery,* period from regional anesthesia induction to delivery; *After Delivery,* period from delivery to the end of surgery. *(Redrawn from Hood DD, Curry R: Anesthesiology 1999;90:1276-1292.)*

29-4   **Trials of Effect of Anesthetic Choice on Maternal Outcome in Pre-eclampsia**

Author (ref.)	Technique	N	Finding
Labor Analgesia			
Greenwood and Lilford (39)	Epidural 1st stage labor Pregnancy-induced hypertension (PIH)	66	No change in the maximum systolic or diastolic blood pressure after epidural analgesia
Jouppila et al. (40)	Labor: essential hypertension Severe preeclampsia	6 11	Xenon: intervillous blood flow (IVBF) After epidural, IVBF improved in all preeclamptic patients, and half of essential hypertension patients
Jouppila et al. (42)	Labor: severe preeclampsia	7	Xenon: IVBF After epidural, IVBF improved in 6/7 preeclampsia patients
Cesarean Anesthesia			
Hodgkinson et al. (37)	Epidural vs general anesthesia (GA)	12 8	No significant hypotension w/epidural Significant hypertension w/GA
Moore et al. (38)	Epidural vs GA	100	No significant hypotension w/epidural Significant hypertension w/GA despite vigorous therapy
Ramanathan et al. (41)	Epidural vs GA	11 10	Neuroendocrine stress response after GA
Wallace et al. (44)	General Epidural or spinal	26 27 27	GA not associated w/severe hypertension Regional not associated with significant hypotension
Hood and Curry (47)	Spinal Epidural	103 35	Severe preeclamptic patients Magnitude of hypotension similar between groups Ephedrine doses similar IV fluid greater in patients w/subarachnoid block (SAB)
Dyer et al. (48)	Spinal vs general	35 35	Preeclamptic patients w/nonreassuring fetal heart rate Maternal hemodynamics similar between groups Fetal pH lower and base deficit higher in SAB neonates but not clinically significant
Karinen et al. (45)	Spinal	12	Preeclamptic patients, 2/12 had decrease in blood pressure <80% baseline Changes in umbilical artery velocity not significant during hypotensive episodes
Aya et al. (49)	Spinal normals vs severe preeclampsia	30 30	Less hypotension in preeclamptic patients than normal patients. However, PIH patients received IV hydration prior to block
Ramanathan et al. (43)	GA preeclampsia control vs labetalol therapy	10 15	Labetalol 1 mg/kg controlled hypertensive response to laryngoscopy
Ramanathan et al. (46)	General preeclampsia vs normals	8 6	Significant increase in middle cerebral artery velocity after intubation in PIH

recommended in the past, is not widely used now. Decreasing vital capacity and a decrease in oxygen saturation by pulse oximetry may be indicative of developing pulmonary edema.

■ CARDIAC DISEASE IN PREGNANCY

The differential diagnosis for sudden hemodynamic deterioration in a pregnant woman includes thrombopulmonary embolism, hemorrhage, sepsis, preeclampsia, and cardiac disease. Maternal cardiac disease causes approximately 16% of all maternal deaths.[51] The most common single cause of maternal mortality is cardiac disease. Cardiomyopathy, myocardial infarction, and aortic dissection are the most commonly reported conditions, with chronic and acquired diseases such as pulmonary hypertension, and valvular and congenital diseases being less common.[52]

The most recent CEMACH data show that between 2000 and 2002, there were 44 maternal deaths, with 35 from acquired causes and nine from congenital causes (Fig. 29-13). Specific causes can be further broken down into cardiomyopathy (23%), aortic dissection (19%), myocardial infarction (18%), pulmonary hypertension (15%), and other (25%).

Cardiomyopathy

Peripartum cardiomyopathy occurs in 1:1500 to 1:4000 deliveries. There is no clear medical cause, and onset can be 1 month prior to delivery and up to 5 months after parturition.[53] Multiparity, older age, African heritage, and birth of twins appear to result in a higher incidence of cardiomyopathy.[54] Authorities still do not agree on an etiology, although viral and immune responses have been implicated.[55]

Of the eight women in the most recent report,[5] all presented with cardiomyopathy after the birth, three of them

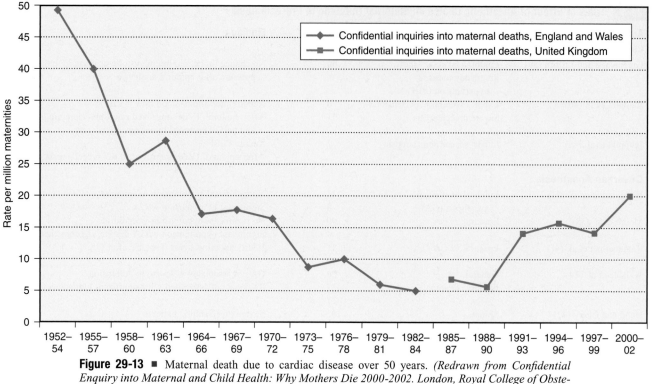

Figure 29-13 ▪ Maternal death due to cardiac disease over 50 years. *(Redrawn from Confidential Enquiry into Maternal and Child Health: Why Mothers Die 2000-2002. London, Royal College of Obstetricians and Gynaecologists, 2005, available at www.cemach.org.uk/publications.htm.)*

within 48 hours. All had risk factors, which included obesity, advanced age, multiparity, and hypertension.

The onset of peripartum cardiomyopathy is usually within the last month of pregnancy and up to 5 months after delivery. There is usually no history of heart disease. Perhaps most unsettling to the clinician, the onset of signs and symptoms is nonspecific and easily confused with normal changes of pregnancy, such as breathlessness, or with a viral chest infection.

The diagnosis of peripartum cardiomyopathy can be difficult. Easy fatigue, dyspnea, and ankle edema can be normal or abnormal. Clinicians should not ignore a patient who has dyspnea at rest or orthopnea, paroxysmal nocturnal dyspnea, chest pain, nocturnal cough, pulmonary rales, jugular venous distention, or regurgitant murmur. The electrocardiogram is often nondiagnostic, although findings may be consistent with cardiomegaly and include arrhythmias and ST changes. Most agree that an echocardiogram is the strongest diagnostic tool (Box 29-2).[56]

Patients with peripartum cardiomyopathy are best followed by a cardiologist familiar with the changes of pregnancy. Therapy includes diuretics, salt restriction, and volume overload avoidance. Vasodilation is aided with hydralazine, nitrates, or amlodipine. Angiotensin-converting enzyme (ACE) inhibitors are avoided because of reported teratogenic effects, fetal renal failure, and death.[57] Amiodarone and verapamil are rarely used because of their potentially deleterious fetal effects.[58] Most calcium channel blockers are associated with negative inotropy,[59] but carvedilol may improve overall

survival rate in parturient women with dilated cardiomyopathy, and perhaps patients with peripartum cardiomyopathy.[60] Recent successful use of polyclonal human antibody to improve left ventricular function has been reported in peripartum cardiomyopathy.[61] Patients with low ejection fractions (<35%) may be given thromboprophylaxis with unfractionated or low-molecular-weight heparin.

Delivery of the fetus, if viable, improves cardiac function in women with cardiomyopathy. Induction of labor can be done safely in most cases if cardiac stabilization can be achieved. Early consultation with an anesthesiologist is expected. Less blood loss, lower infection rate, decreased surgical stress and occurrence of respiratory complications,

29-2	**Clinical Definition of Peripartum Cardiomyopathy**

1. Heart failure within the last month of pregnancy or 5 months postpartum
2. Absence of prior heart disease
3. No determinable cause
4. Strict echocardiographic indication of left ventricular dysfunction:
   - Ejection fraction <45% and/or fractional shortening <30%
   - End-diastolic dimension >2.7 cm per square meter of body surface area

From Hibbard JU, Lindheimer M, Lang RM: Obstet Gynecol 1999;94:311-316.

and improved hemodynamic stability are advantages of vaginal delivery. The addition of a regional block decreases the variation in blood pressure, decreases the preload and afterload on the heart, and provides ideal conditions should instrumental delivery be required. Cesarean delivery may be necessary if the mother is in extremis or fetal indications are present.

For cesarean section, either regional block or general anesthesia is an acceptable approach, depending on the patient's coagulation status and ability to cooperate. In patients with symptomatic cardiomyopathy, direct arterial and central venous monitoring are advised. Some very ill patients who are gasping for breath may require induction in the sitting position, converting to supine once consciousness is lost. Etomidate for induction is advised if myocardial function is impaired. If there is time before induction, a digitalis load should also be considered. Clearly, some of these patients will require respiratory and inotropic support postoperatively, and intensive medical care will be necessary. No large-scale studies on anesthesia outcomes exist, but descriptions of anesthesia with satisfactory outcome are available.[62] In patients with severe myocardial impairment, a left ventricular assist device (LVAD) may be necessary, and consideration should be given to transplantation if ventricular function does not improve.[62] Those who improve usually do so within 6 months after pregnancy.[63] Mortality from peripartum cardiomyopathy ranges from 18% to 56%,[55] and persistent cardiomegaly is associated with an 85% mortality.[53]

Myocardial Infarction

Myocardial infarction is rare in this population; it occurs about 1 : 10,000 deliveries.[64] Risk factors are familiar and include increased age, diabetes, smoking, hypertension, cardiomyopathy, and obesity. However, 78% have no apparent risk factors.[65] Myocardial infarction is more common during the third trimester of pregnancy, and mortality is high if it occurs within 2 weeks of delivery. Symptoms are classic, including anginal-type chest pain, diagnostic electrocardiographic changes, and increased plasma enzymes, such as cardiac-specific troponin I (to >0.15 ng/mL). Labor may mask these symptoms, and muscle creatinine kinase is normally elevated. Chest pain can also be caused by hemorrhage/shock, sickle cell crisis, severe preeclampsia, pulmonary embolism, and aortic dissection.

Immediate treatment may include oxygen therapy, sublingual nitroglycerin, aspirin ingestion, heparinization, and coronary angiography with possible stenting.[66] Tissue plasminogen activator (TPA) and assessment for emergency coronary artery bypass graft (CABG) have also been suggested.[66,67] TPA and anticoagulants predispose to increased bleeding in the immediate postpartum period and are not advised during that period. These drugs also increase the risk of bleeding associated with regional block.

If possible, the use of ergot alkaloids (Methergine) is avoided in these patients. Reports of puerperal myocardial infarction following ergot administration are frequent.[68-70] If ischemia occurs, it is usually rapid, and treatment with sublingual or intravenous nitroglycerin (400 μg/min) is recommended.[70]

Aortic Dissection

Although rare, aortic dissection is associated with severe hypertension and inherited disorders such as Marfan's syndrome. If symptoms are present, intrascapular or chest pain are most common. Increasing severity is associated with signs of cerebral, cardiac, renal, or limb ischemia and heart failure caused by aortic regurgitation or hemopericardium.

Vaginal delivery with regional block and postpartum repair is advocated if the fetus is viable and the lesion is a descending (Stanford type B) dissection. If the lesion is larger and the fetus is less than 28 weeks, attempted repair with the fetus in situ has been done. If the fetus is viable, and because of the life-threatening nature of nonoperative treatment (80% mortality[71,72]), surgical repair and concomitant cesarean delivery should be anticipated.

Anesthetic goals include a reduction in pressure-flow gradient across the dissection. Epidural analgesia is suggested to reduce the wall tension, mean arterial blood pressure (MABP), and vessel shear stresses (cardiac output) seen in labor.[73] Acute blood pressure control can be accomplished with labetalol (1 to 10 μg/kg/min). For cesarean section, general anesthesia may be necessary if anticoagulation increases the risk of regional block.[74] The risk of hypertension during induction of general anesthesia is well known. Arterial and central venous lines are recommended to provide beat-to-beat control of blood pressure and volume control as needed.

Chronic Cardiac Disease

Women with a history of cardiac disease in previous pregnancies or congenital heart disease with prior cardiac surgery can be identified, assessed, and counseled before becoming pregnant. In some cases, such as when severe pulmonary hypertension or Eisenmenger physiology is involved, pregnancy termination is advised.[75] Ready assessment and communication between cardiologist, obstetrician, and anesthesiologist should be the norm. New York Heart Association (NYHA) functional class may not predict how the patient will adapt to pregnancy, and regular echocardiographic assessment of the mother and fetal assessment are desirable.

Congenital Heart Disease

Because of improvements in diagnosis and treatment in recent years, women with repaired congenital heart disease (CHD) are reaching childbearing age in increasing numbers, and there is widespread encouragement in the literature for them to consider pregnancy.[52,76] Pregnancy in women with CHD not complicated by Eisenmenger syndrome is associated with a low mortality.[76-78] However, potential risk factors for maternal morbidity include poor maternal functional class, poorly controlled arrhythmias, heart failure, cyanosis, significant left heart obstruction, and a history of cerebral ischemia. Cyanosis is a risk factor for fetal and neonatal complications. On the basis of these risk factors, patients can be stratified into low-, intermediate-, or high-risk categories.[78] An absence of these risk factors generally places patients into a low-risk category. The highest risk is associated with Eisenmenger syndrome, with which postnatal maternal mortality can exceed 50%. Because the current data are mainly based on retrospective case series from tertiary care institutions, caution should be exercised in risk stratification of pregnant women with uncommon conditions such as Mustard/Senning or of those who have had a Fontan procedure.[79-81] Patients with these lesions or procedures should be placed in the intermediate-risk category until additional data become available. Medical or surgical termination of pregnancy in intermediate- or high-risk patients requires careful monitoring and should be done in a regional adult congenital heart disease center.[82]

■ PULMONARY HYPERTENSION

Primary pulmonary hypertension, which is rare, affects young women by reducing nitric oxide and prostacyclin synthesis in pulmonary vessels, and it increases endothelin and thromboxane production. Histologically, medial thickening and intimal fibrosis are seen. There is no clear etiology, and pulmonary artery pressures are greater than 25 mm Hg. The chief problem is the cardiopulmonary system's inability to adapt to the hydremia and hyperdynamic state of pregnancy. The greatest risk is in the peripartum period, and the majority of maternal deaths occur in the first week after delivery, usually from right ventricular failure that manifests as increasing shortness of breath, cough, easy fatigue, occasional hemoptysis, cyanosis, and fainting. Echocardiography and right heart catheterization are useful in differentiating the symptoms from pulmonary embolism. Treatment includes high-flow oxygen and pulmonary vasodilators such as nifedipine, prostacyclin, and nitric oxide. Anticoagulation may be necessary.

If pregnancy is carried toward viability and the maternal condition does not improve, delivery is achieved as soon as possible (32 to 34 weeks). During this time, the obstetrician and the anesthesiologist endeavor to avoid conditions that increase pulmonary vascular resistance (pain, hypothermia, hypoxia, hypercarbia, acidosis, high intrathoracic pressure, excessive use of catecholaminergic drugs). It is also important to maintain right ventricular preload, left ventricular afterload, and right ventricular contractility. Anesthetic management is challenging. There are no large-scale series, but a review of case reports supports the use of regional block, either by epidural local anesthetic or a combination of epidural or spinal opioids.[83,84] The mother must be monitored closely, with a rapid-cycling automated blood pressure device or arterial line during regional block. Decreased peripheral vascular resistance may be treated with volume replacement and appropriate doses of phenylephrine or ephedrine. Phenylephrine has been shown to increase pulmonary vascular resistance. Oxytocin for induction of labor and postpartum involution is recommended, with the caveat that it can cause peripheral vasodilation and may slightly elevate pulmonary vascular tone. Prostaglandin $F_{2\alpha}$ and carboprost (Hemabate) are potent pulmonary vasoconstrictors and not advised in this condition.

Outcome studies have shown an increase in maternal mortality with cesarean section.[85] Both general anesthesia and regional block have risks and advantages.[86,87] Regional block allows the benefits of an awake patient and largely avoids the pitfalls of catecholamine surges of general anesthesia, but it runs the risk of catastrophic afterload reduction. General anesthesia maintains peripheral vascular tone and preload while providing a conduit for inhaled nitric oxide, but it risks severe pulmonary hypertension and marked myocardial depression.

The need for pulmonary artery monitoring is also debated. Some authors argue that an increase of morbidity is associated with Swan-Ganz catheters. Others argue that measurement of pulmonary artery pressures and cardiac output is useful when vasodilators can be directly infused. However, the data are insufficient, so the need for central monitoring is made on a case-by-case basis.

■ REDUCTION OF PERIOPERATIVE ANESTHESIA RISK

Decreasing Maternal Hypotension During Regional Block

During the 1940s, spinal shock (after spinal anesthesia) was the most common anesthetic cause of maternal mortality in the United States.[88] The discovery, physiologic description, and avoidance of the supine hypotensive syndrome, the development of pre-block IV infusions (prehydration), and the judicious use of vasopressors such as ephedrine have widely attenuated, if not extinguished, hypotension as a maternal risk during regional, especially spinal, anesthesia. In recent years, both the use of prehydration to avoid hypotension and the use of ephedrine (as opposed to phenylephrine) to treat it have been subject to closer scrutiny and to meta-analysis with regard to outcome and best practices. The utility of left uterine displacement has not been subject to recent statistical reevaluation, perhaps because of the robust early physiologic studies by Kerr and colleagues[89] and Bieniarz and coworkers.[90]

Ephedrine versus Phenylephrine

Since the 1960s, ephedrine has been recommended as the vasopressor of choice during pregnancy, based in part on studies by Shnider and associates,[91] primarily because it maintained maternal blood pressure with the least decrease in uterine blood flow. Gutsche recommended prophylactic ephedrine to avoid spinal hypotension during induction for cesarean section.[92] A recent quantitative systematic review by Lee and coworkers[93] supports these early findings that prophylactic ephedrine prevents or decreases the intensity and incidence of spinal hypotension during cesarean section but does not significantly change neonatal parameters (Fig. 29-14).[92,94-103]

Phenylephrine until recently was considered only a last-resort drug to treat maternal spinal hypotension because of feared effects on decreasing uteroplacental perfusion. Ramanathan[103a] found that small (50-μg) IV increments of phenylephrine were not associated with a deterioration in neonatal blood gases compared with those whose mothers received ephedrine for hypotension control. This led to debate among clinicians, many studies, and some prospective randomized trials.

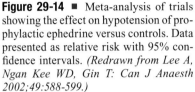

Figure 29-14 ■ Meta-analysis of trials showing the effect on hypotension of prophylactic ephedrine versus controls. Data presented as relative risk with 95% confidence intervals. *(Redrawn from Lee A, Ngan Kee WD, Gin T: Can J Anaesth 2002;49:588-599.)*

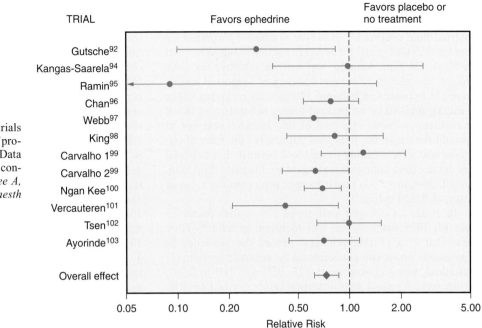

Recent quantitative systematic reviews of randomized controlled trials between ephedrine and phenylephrine for maternal treatment of spinal hypotension have produced some surprising and noteworthy findings.[104] It was *not* surprising that ephedrine and phenylephrine were equally effective in prevention and treatment of maternal hypotension (RR, 1.00; 95% CI, 0.96 to 1.06). Maternal bradycardia was also more likely to occur with phenylephrine than with ephedrine. What *was* surprising was that women given phenylephrine had neonates with higher umbilical arterial pH values than those given ephedrine (weighted mean difference, 0.03; 95% CI, 0.02 to 0.04) (Fig. 29-15). However, closer inspection of the data revealed that there was no true difference between groups in the incidence of clinical acidosis. Nevertheless, the conclusion of this meta-analysis contradicts the traditional belief that ephedrine is the best clinical choice for treating maternal hypotension caused by spinal anesthesia for cesarean section. Postulated mechanisms for this finding included the suggestions that the placental vascular bed is not as sensitive to alpha agonists and that ephedrine may increase fetal metabolism and CO_2 production. Many clinicians, including this author, are now using phenylephrine routinely, along with ephedrine, to control maternal hypotension in this setting.

An intriguing explanation for the lack of fetal acidosis seen after phenylephrine is given to treat spinal hypotension is that during pregnancy, sympathetic vasoconstrictor response tends to be attenuated in the mother, especially in the areas of the uterus and periplacental vasculature. This might explain why a relatively pure alpha agonist given in modest doses might increase maternal blood pressure while preserving placental perfusion. Unfortunately, this does not explain why ephedrine is associated with a slightly lower fetal cord gas pH compared with phenylephrine, unless it is

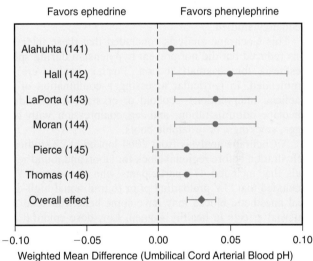

Figure 29-15 ■ Meta-analysis of trials. The effect of phenylephrine compared with ephedrine on umbilical cord arterial blood pH. Data are mean difference with 95% confidence intervals. *(Redrawn from Lee A, Ngan Kee WD, Gin T: Anesth Analg 2002;94: 920-926.)*

found ultimately to not be as effective a preserver of placental perfusion.

Pre-Block Fluid Loading to Decrease Hypotension

In 1950, Assali and Prystowsky published remarkable data from humans demonstrating profound hypotension in pregnant women who were given total or near total sympathectomies while kept supine without fluid loading or vasopressor therapy.[105] Wollman and Marx showed that 1 to 2 L of crystalloid before spinal block for cesarean section decreased the incidence of hypotension and did not result in maternal fluid overload.[106] However, studies of hydration for labor block[107] and spinal for cesarean section[108] suggested that pre-block IV fluid loading was not as effective as once thought. Specifically, Rout and colleagues[108] reported no difference in hypotension between 140 patients receiving either 20 mL/kg preload or no preload before subarachnoid block for cesarean section. The goal of this research was not to discredit the use of the fluid load but to allay the fears of clinicians who were avoiding spinal block because they believed they did not have enough time to give an adequate fluid load. Nevertheless, there was much disagreement over the value of prespinal fluid-loading.

In 2002, a Cochrane analysis of 229 studies found 25 trials (of 1477 women) that met inclusion criteria.[109] They found that 4 of 15 interventions reduced the incidence of hypotension under spinal anesthesia for cesarean section: (1) crystalloid versus control (RR, 0.78; 95% CI, 0.63 to 0.98), (2) preemptive colloid administration versus crystalloid (RR, 0.54; 95% CI, 0.37 to 0.78), (3) ephedrine versus control (RR, 0.69; 95% CI, 0.57 to 0.84), and (4) lower limb compression versus control (RR, 0.70; 95% CI, 0.59 to 0.83). Ephedrine was associated with dose-related maternal hypertension and tachycardia, as well as fetal acidosis of uncertain clinical significance. The effect of left uterine displacement was not adequately studied.

This Cochrane analysis concluded that these interventions reduced but did not prevent hypotension during spinal anesthesia for cesarean section. Further trials were recommended, in particular assessing a combination of the beneficial interventions—colloid or crystalloid preloading, ephedrine administration, and leg compression with bandages, stockings, or inflatable boots.

A Cochrane analysis from 2004 looked at 22 studies of prehydration before regional block for labor, and found seven trials that included 473 participants who met criteria.[110] It concluded that "IV preloading prior to traditional high-dose local anesthetic blocks may have some beneficial fetal and maternal effects in healthy women. Low-dose epidural and CSE [combined spinal epidural] analgesia techniques may reduce the need for preloading."

In a survey of 588 anesthesiologists, it was found that a large majority (87%) use some form of fluid load prior to spinal anesthesia for cesarean section.[111] It is also the author's practice to use a fluid load before spinal block for cesarean section. However, the lack of time for a preload does not contraindicate the use of this anesthetic technique.

■ THE OBESE PARTURIENT: RISKS AND MANAGEMENT

Obesity is widespread to the point of being called an epidemic by a recent ACOG committee opinion.[112] The World Health Organization (WHO) and the National Institutes of Health (NIH) define normal weight as a body mass index (BMI) of 25 to 29.9. Obesity is a BMI of 30 or more, with class II obesity as BMI of 35 to 39.9, and class III (extreme obesity) as greater than 40.[113,114] Calculation of BMI can be

found online at www.nhlbisupport.com/bmi. The most recent national health data report says that nearly one third of American women exceed the definition of obesity.[115] A recent comprehensive review of obesity and pregnancy reveals that obesity in pregnancy notably increases the risk of diabetes, hypertensive disorders, thromboembolic complications, cephalopelvic disproportion, increased cesarean section rate, and an increase in anesthetic morbidity and mortality.[116] A recent prospective multicenter study of more than 16,000 subjects found class I (BMI 30 to 34.9) and class II (BMI 35 to 39.9) obesity was associated with an increased risk of gestational hypertension (odds ratios [OR], 2.5 and 3.2, respectively), preeclampsia (OR, 1.6 and 3.3) and gestational diabetes (OR, 2.6 and 4.0), compared with a BMI of less than 30.[117] From the same study, the cesarean section rate for women with a BMI of 29.9 or less was 20.7%, for a BMI of 30 to 34.9 it was 33.8%, and for a BMI of 35 to 39.9 it was 47.4%. These findings are further supported by several prospective studies.[118-121] Operative and postoperative problems associated with obesity during pregnancy include excessive blood loss, operative time greater than 2 hours, wound infection, and endometritis.[122-124]

Anesthetic risk is clearly shown to increase in many categories for the obese parturient. Technical difficulty with regional block and the induction of general anesthesia resulting in failed airway management, aspiration, and postoperative hypoventilation are well documented.[124-126] In some U.S. studies, anesthesia mortality has been associated with maternal obesity in 80% of cases reported.[127] Of the 106 maternal deaths directly caused by pregnancy from 2000 to 2002, fully 35% were listed as obese. A consistent association with obesity and maternal airway mishaps leading to death has also been reported triennially from CEMACH in the United Kingdom.[5,6] It has been recommended that all women with a body mass of more than 35 kg/m^2 should receive an anesthetic assessment on admission, including an airway examination and discussion with the patient and surgeon regarding the best anesthetic approach. Especially important are IV access, the consideration of an early working epidural, and a discussion of how to approach emergency surgery.[128]

The increase in bariatric surgery has raised questions about its effect on future pregnancies. Both types of surgery (vertical banded gastroplasty and gastric banding) are associated with iron, vitamin B_{12}, folate, and calcium deficiencies. These patients are advised to wait 12 to 18 months after surgery before conception to avoid the rapid weight-loss period. These patients should be evaluated for nutritional deficiencies and supplementation before becoming pregnant. There are no large prospective trials comparing outcome in obesity and choice of anesthetic for labor or surgery.

■ AIRWAY MANAGEMENT

The closed claims review of obstetric complications found claims for anesthetic causes of maternal death accounting for 30% of cases in the 1970s, 15% in the 1980s, and 12% in the 1990s. They attributed this to the marked decrease in use of general anesthesia for cesarean section. This review did not specify the number of deaths caused by airway loss. However, it can be deduced that among the greatest risks avoided in this change was loss of airway during induction. A decrease in the use of 0.75% bupivacaine for women in labor in the United States also occurred during this time. Aspiration pneumonitis decreased from 9% of claims in 1970 to 1% of claims in the 1990s. Although direct evidence is not available, it is suggested that a decrease in the use of general anesthesia and an increase in the use of gastric emptying drugs, pH neutralizing efforts, and appropriate induction techniques may well have contributed to this decrease.[129,130]

Data from the CDC gathered since 1979 and extending to 1996 also show a marked decrease in the maternal death rate in both general and regional anesthesia but particularly associated with regional block (Table 29-5).[131] It is also clear that the risk of maternal mortality with general anesthesia is nearly seven times higher than with regional block. This may be a function of the technique, but it is also because general anesthesia is often chosen in emergencies when there is less time for patient preparation. It is also resorted to when regional block fails (obesity) or despite relative contraindications to a block (HELLP, coagulopathy in PIH). It is also possible that anesthesia residents get less training in general anesthesia for obstetrics than in former times. Samsoon and Young showed that the incidence of failed intubation was 1:2230.[132] The most recent follow-up survey of labor practices agrees with a number of previous studies over the past 20 years showing that failed intubation in obstetric patients remains at 1 in 238, or about a seven times higher failure rate.[133]

These sobering data have led to the reliance on national guidelines developed by the ASA for airway management dating from 1993,[134] and on more recent updates more specific to the pregnant patient.[130,135] In addition, many authorities recommend drills or practice of lost airway events which would include advance planning.

Advance Planning

Advance planning includes the following steps:

1. Put together a "difficult airway" box for labor and delivery. Recommend a prophylactic regional anesthetic when anticipating a difficult airway; administer aspiration prophylaxis as soon as operative delivery is anticipated; have extra, experienced hands available at induction of general anesthesia.

2. If you cannot ventilate after induction, awaken the patient, if possible. Have a laryngeal mask airway (LMA) or Combitube and jet ventilator available.

3. If you can ventilate and need to proceed, use a drying agent (such as glycopyrrolate), elevate the head of the bed, administer metoclopramide to increase gastroesophageal sphincter tone, consider spontaneous versus controlled ventilation, and decide whether to use inhaled or IV anesthesia after delivery (note uterine tone).[136]

Of the seven anesthetic deaths in the United Kingdom from 2000 to 2002, three were caused by unrecognized esophageal intubation. This has led to intensified efforts to establish protocols to rule out esophageal intubation, such as the following[128]:

- Maintain oxygenation as a priority.
- Always suspect the tube may not be in the trachea.
- Visualize the tube directly between the cords.
- Feel the lung recoil in the ventilation bag.
- Look at the chest and abdominal movement.
- Listen in the axillary line and epigastrium.
- Use capnography.
- Monitor oxygen saturation.
- Allow succinylcholine to wear off and observe spontaneous respiration.

Further precautions to take in the approach to the difficult airway include the following[130]:

- Use bougies or tube changers for the difficult airway with direct or indirect visualization.
- Even if an awake intubation is planned, the surgeon should be ready to do a tracheostomy.
- Reduce the use of jet ventilators in inexperienced hands.
- Avoid repeated (more than three) and frenzied attempts to intubate.
- LMA and Combitubes cannot be considered failsafe.

As yet, no large-scale trials have been conducted to test maternal outcomes with the interventions suggested here. Nevertheless, the decrease in maternal mortality due to airway disasters after the switch from a majority of general anesthetics for cesarean section to a majority of regional anesthetics strongly suggests that efforts to decrease maternal risk have led to a better outcome.

29-5	Maternal Morbidity and Mortality, 1979-1996								
	NUMBER OF DEATHS			CASE FATALITY RATE*			RISK RATIO		
	1979-1984	1985-1990	1991-1996	1979-1984	1985-1990	1991-1996	1979-1984	1985-1990	1991-1996
General anesthesia	33	32	1	20	32.3	16.8	2.3	16.7	6.7
Regional anesthesia	19	9	14	8.6	1.9	2.5	1	1	1

*Per million general or regional anesthesias.
From Hawkins JL: Can J Anaesth 2002;49:R1-R5 (Refresher Course Lecture).

■ HEMORRHAGE: RISK AND PROTECTION

Hemorrhage is still the leading cause of maternal mortality. Its early signs may be obscured by normal physiologic changes or by infection. The substantial uterine blood flow at term allows serious hemorrhage to progress to shock more rapidly. Recent successful therapy of maternal hemorrhage by interventional radiologists may not be widely available in primary centers.[137] Risk factors for intrapartum and postpartum hemorrhage include uterine atony (prolonged labor, or oxytocin augmentation, polyhydramnios, infection, grand multiparity, multiple gestation, fetal macrosomia, and, rarely, inhaled potent anesthetics), retained placenta, lacerations, fibroids, placenta previa, abruption, placenta accreta, and coagulopathy. In recent years, placenta accreta (an abnormally firm attachment of the placenta to the uterine wall, which leads to a 50% incidence of need for transfusion and a high incidence of emergency hysterectomy) has increased in incidence to as high as 1 in 540 pregnancies. This increase is associated with an increasing number of cesarean sections. The most important risk factor for placenta accreta is placenta previa, and there is a correlation with the number of previous cesarean sections (Table 29-6).[138] Other risk factors include maternal age over 35, placenta overlying previous uterine scar, previous multiple pregnancy, uterine scar, and previous dilatation and curettage (D and C).

Current reviews suggest that in addition to the usual precautions (timely obstetric notification of the operating room team, large-bore IV access, early blood bank involvement, and available ecbolic agents), improved outcome in women at risk for intraoperative and postpartum hemorrhage can be promoted with the use of erythropoietin-induced erythrocyte production, autologous donation, and preoperative isovolemic hemodilution and intraoperative cell saver use.[139] Intraoperative cell salvage may clear soluble protein but not cellular contents, even with ultrafiltration. Postpartum hemorrhage has been successfully treated with Sengstaken Blakemore tube tamponade and B-Lynch suturing.

Human recombinant factor VIIa, which promotes clotting by the extrinsic tissue factor pathway, has also been discussed of late. The dosage is 60 μg/kg, and the clinical effect occurs in 10 to 15 minutes and lasts about 2 hours. Side effects include hypertension, hypotension, bradycardia, and renal dysfunction. Currently, no large-scale trials are underway to test this drug in the general population or in pregnancy.[140]

29-6	Placenta Previa with Prior Uterine Incisions: Effect on Incidence of Placenta Accreta	
Number of Prior Uterine Incisions	**Percent with Placenta Accreta**	
0	5	
1	24	
2	47	
3	40	
4	67	

From Clark SL, Koonings PP, Phelan JP: Obstet Gynecol 1985;66:89-92.

■ REFERENCES

1. Meckel RA: Save the Babies: American Public Health Reform and the Prevention of Infant Mortality, 1850-1929. Baltimore, Johns Hopkins University Press, 1990.
2. Loudon I: Death in Childbirth: An International Study of Maternal Care and Maternal Mortality, 1800-1950. New York, Oxford University Press, 1992.
3. Hoyert DL, Kochanek KD, Murphy SL: Deaths: Final data for 1997. Natl Vital Stat Rep 1999;47:1-104.
4. Centers for Disease Control and Prevention: Achievements in public health, 1900-1999: Healthier mothers and babies. MMWR Morb Mortal Wkly Rep 1999;48:849-858, available at www.cdc.gov/mmwr/preview/mmwrhtml/mm4838a2.htm.
5. Confidential Enquiry into Maternal and Child Health: Why Mothers Die 2000-2002. London, Royal College of Obstetricians and Gynaecologists, 2005, available at www.cemach.org.uk/publications.htm.
6. Clyburn PA: Early thoughts on "Why Mothers Die 2000-2002." Anaesthesia 2004;59:1157-1159.
7. Berg CJ, Chang J, Callaghan WM, Whitehead SJ: Pregnancy-related mortality in the United States, 1991-1997. Obstet Gynecol 2003;101:289-296.
8. Stirling Y, Woolf L, North WRS, et al: Haemostasis in normal pregnancy. Thromb Haemost 1984;52:176-182.
9. Conklin K, Backus A: Physiologic changes of pregnancy. In Chestnut D (ed): Obstetric Anesthesia. St Louis, Mosby, 1999, pp 24-26.
10. Cheek T, Gutsche BB: Maternal physiologic alterations during pregnancy. In Hughes S, Levinson G, Rosen M (eds): Anesthesia for Obstetrics. Philadelphia, Lippincott, Williams & Wilkins, 2002, pp 11-19.
11. Sharma SK, Philip J, Wiley J: Thromboelastographic changes in healthy parturients and postpartum women. Anesth Analg 1997;85:94-98.
12. Scientific Advisory Committee of the Royal College of Obstetricians and Gynaecologists: Advice on preventing deep vein thrombosis for pregnant women travelling by air. Opinion Paper 1, October 2001; available at www.rcog.org.uk.
13. Clinical Green Top Guidelines: Thromboprophylaxis during pregnancy, labour and after normal vaginal delivery. Guideline no. 37, 2004. London, Royal College of Obstetricians and Gynaecologists, available at www.rcog.org.uk/index.asp?PageID = 535.
14. Rey E, Kahn SR, David M, Shrier I: Thrombophilic disorders and fetal loss: A meta-analysis. Lancet 2003;361:901-908.
15. Kupferminc MJ, Eldor A, Steinman N, et al: Increased frequency of genetic thrombophilia in women with complications of pregnancy. [Erratum appears in N Engl J Med 1999;341:384]. N Engl J Med 1999;340:9-13.
16. Lin J, August P: Genetic thrombophilias and preeclampsia: A meta-analysis. Obstet Gynecol 2005;105:182-192.
17. Walker MC, Ferguson SE, Allen VM: Heparin for pregnant women with acquired or inherited thrombophilias. Cochrane Database Syst Rev 2003:CD003580.
18. ACOG Committee on Practice Bulletins—Obstetrics: Diagnosis and management of preeclampsia and eclampsia. Obstet Gynecol 2001;98:159-167.
19. Gaiser RR, Gutsche BB, Cheek TG: Anesthetic considerations for the hypertensive disorders of pregnancy. In Hughes S, Levinson G (eds): Anesthesia for Obstetrics. Philadelphia, Lippincott, Williams & Wilkins, 2001, pp 297-322.
20. Levesque S, Moutquin JM, Lindsay C, et al: Implication of an AGT haplotype in a multigene association study with pregnancy hypertension. Hypertension 2004;43:71-78.
21. Broughton-Pipkin F: What is the place of genetics in the pathogenesis of pre-eclampsia? Biol Neonate 1999;76:325-330.
22. Levine RJ, Thadhani R, Qian C, et al: Urinary placental growth factor and risk of preeclampsia. JAMA 2005;293:77-85.
23. Magee LA, Ornstein MP, von Dadelszen P: Management of hypertension in pregnancy. BMJ 1999;318:1332-1336.
24. Barton JR, Witlin AG, Sibai BM: Management of mild preeclampsia. Clin Obstet Gynecol 1999;42:465-469.

25. National High Blood Pressure Education Program: Working group report on high blood pressure in pregnancy. Am J Obstet Gynecol 2000;183:S1-22.

26. Sibai B: Diagnosis and management of gestational hypertension and preeclampsia. Obstet Gynecol 2003;102:185-192.

27. Friedman SA, Lubarsky S, Schiff E: Expectant management of severe preeclampsia remote from term. Clin Obstet Gynecol 1999;42:470-478.

28. Duley L, Gülmezoglu AM, Henderson-Smart D: Anticonvulsants for women with pre-eclampsia. Cochrane Database Syst Rev 2000:CD000025.

29. The Magpie Trial Collaborative Group: Do women with pre-eclampsia, and their babies, benefit from magnesium sulphate? The Magpie Trial: A randomised placebo-controlled trial. Lancet 2002;359:1877-1890.

30. Magee LA, Cham C, Waterman EJ, et al: Hydralazine for treatment of severe hypertension in pregnancy: Meta-analysis. BMJ 2003;327;955-965.

31. Ales K: Magnesium plus nifedipine. Am J Obstet Gynecol 1990;162:288.

32. Brown MA, McCowan LME, North RA, Walters BN: Withdrawal of nifedipine capsules: Jeopardising the treatment of acute severe hypertension in pregnancy? Med J Aust 1997;166:640-643.

33. Horvath JS, Phippard A, Korda A, et al: Clonidine hydrochloride: A safe and effective antihypertensive in pregnancy. Obstet Gynecol 1985;66:634-638.

34. Clark SB, Cotton DB: Clinical indications for pulmonary artery catheterization in the patient with severe preeclampsia. Am J Obstet Gynecol 1988;158:453-458.

35. Practice Guidelines for Obstetric Anesthesia: An updated report by the American Society of Anesthesiologists Task Force on Obstetric Anesthesia. Anesthesiology 2007;166:843-863.

36. Hon EH, Reid BL, Hehre FW: The electronic evaluation of fetal heart rate: II. Changes with maternal hypotension. Am J Obstet Gynecol 1960;79:209-215.

37. Hodgkinson R, Husain FJ, Hayashi RH: Systemic and pulmonary blood pressure during caesarean section in parturients with gestational hypertension. Can Anaesth Soc J 1980;27:389-394.

38. Moore TR, Key TC, Reisner LS, et al: Evaluation of the use of continuous lumbar epidural anesthesia for hypertensive pregnant women in labor. Am J Obstet Gynecol 1985;152:404-412.

39. Greenwood PA, Lilford RJ: Effect of epidural analgesia on maximum and minimum blood pressures during first stage of labour in primigravidae with mild/moderate gestational hypertension. Br J Obstet Gynaecol 1986;93:260-263.

40. Jouppila R, Jouppila P, Hollmen A, et al: Epidural analgesia and placental blood flow during labour in pregnancies complicated by hypertension. Br J Ostet Gynaecol 1979;86:969-972.

41. Ramanathan J, Coleman P, Sibai B: Anesthetic modification of hemodynamic and neuroendocrine stress responses to cesarean delivery in women with severe preeclampsia [see comment]. Anesth Analg 1991;73:772-779.

42. Jouppila P, Jouppila R, Hollmen A, Koivula A: Lumbar epidural analgesia to improve intervillous blood flow during labor in severe preeclampsia. Obstet Gynecol 1982;59:158-161.

43. Ramanathan J, Sibai BM, Mabie WC, et al: The use of labetalol for attenuation of the hypertensive response to endotracheal intubation in preeclampsia. Am J Obstet Gynecol 1988;159:650-654.

44. Wallace DH, Leveno KJ, Cunningham FG, et al: Randomized comparison of general and regional anesthesia for cesarean delivery in pregnancies complicated by severe preeclampsia. Obstet Gynecol 1995;86:193-199.

45. Karinen J, Räsänen J, Alahuhta S, et al: Maternal and uteroplacental haemodynamic state in pre-eclamptic patients during spinal anaesthesia for caesarean section. Br J Anaesth 1996;76:616-620.

46. Ramanathan J, Angel JJ, Bush AJ, et al: Changes in maternal middle cerebral artery blood flow velocity associated with general anesthesia in severe preeclampsia. Anesth Analg 1999;88:357-361.

47. Hood DD, Curry R: Spinal versus epidural anesthesia for cesarean section in severely preeclamptic patients: A retrospective survey. Anesthesiology 1999;90 1276-1292.

48. Dyer RA, Els I, Farbas J, et al: Prospective, randomized trial comparing general with spinal anesthesia for cesarean delivery in preeclamptic patients with a nonreassuring fetal heart trace. Anesthesiology 2003;99:561-569.

49. Aya A, Mangin R, Vialles N, et al: Patients with severe preeclampsia experience less hypotension during spinal anesthesia for elective cesarean delivery than healthy parturients: A prospective cohort comparison. Anesth Analg 2003;97:867-872.

50. Sciscione AC, Ivester T, Largoza M, et al: Acute pulmonary edema in pregnancy. Obstet Gynecol 2003;101:511-515.

51. de Swiet M: Cardiac disease. In Lewis G, Drife J (eds): Why Mothers Die 1997-1999: The Confidential Enquiries into Maternal Deaths in the United Kingdom. London, Royal College of Obstetricians and Gynaecologists, 2001, pp 153-164.

52. Ray P, Murphy GJ, Shutt LE: Recognition and management of maternal cardiac disease in pregnancy. Br J Anaesth 2004;93:428-439.

53. Demakis JG, Rahimtoola SH, Sutton GC, et al: Natural course of peripartum cardiomyopathy. Circulation 1971;44:1053-1061.

54. Veille JC: Peripartum cardiomyopathies: A review. Am J Obstet Gynecol 1984;148:805-818.

55. Brown CS, Bertolet BD: Peripartum cardiomyopathy: A comprehensive review. Am J Obstet Gynecol 1998;178:409-414.

56. Hibbard JU, Lindheimer M, Lang RM: A modified definition for peripartum cardiomyopathy and prognosis based on echocardiography. Obstet Gynecol 1999;94:311-316.

57. Mastrobattista JM: Angiotensin converting enzyme inhibitors in pregnancy. Semin Perinatol 1997;21:124-134.

58. Page RL: Treatment of arrhythmias during pregnancy. Am Heart J 1995;130:871-876.

59. Packer M, O'Connor CM, Ghali JK, et al, for the PRAISE Study Group: Effect of amlodipine on morbidity and mortality in severe chronic heart failure. N Engl J Med 1996;335:1107-1114.

60. Packer M, Bristow MR, Cohn JN, et al: The effect of carvedilol on morbidity and mortality in patients with chronic heart failure. N Engl J Med 1996;334:1349-1355.

61. Bozkurt B, Villaneuva FS, Holubkov R, et al: Intravenous immune globulin in the therapy of peripartum cardiomyopathy. J Am Coll Cardiol 1999;34:177-180.

62. Colombo J, Lawal AH, Bhandari A, et al: Case 1-2002: A patient with severe peripartum cardiomyopathy and persistent ventricular fibrillation supported by a biventricular assist device. J Cardiothorac Vasc Anesth 2002;16:107-113.

63. Felker GM, Jaeger CJ, Klodas E, et al: Myocarditis and long-term survival in peripartum cardiomyopathy. Am Heart J 2000;140:785-791.

64. Hankins GDV, Wendel GD, Leveno KJ, Stoneham J: Myocardial infarction during pregnancy: A review. Obstet Gynecol 1985;65:139-146.

65. McKechnie RS, Patel D, Eitzman DT, et al: Spontaneous coronary artery dissection in a pregnant woman. Obstet Gynecol 2001;98:899-902.

66. Hoppe UC, Beukelmann DJ, Bohm M, Erdmann E: A young mother with severe chest pain. Heart 1998;79:205.

67. Lewis R, Mabie WC, Burlew B, Sibai BM: Biventricular assist device as a bridge to cardiac transplantation in the treatment of peripartum cardiomyopathy. South Med J 1997;90:955-958.

68. Sutaria N, O'Toole L, Northridge D: Postpartum acute MI following routine ergometrine administration treated successfully by primary PTCA. Heart 2000;83:97-98.

69. Mousa HA, McKinley CA, Thong K: Acute postpartum myocardial infarction after ergometrine administration in a woman with hypercholesterolaemia. Br J Obstet Gynaecol 2000;107:939-940.

70. Tsui BC, Stewart B, Fitzmaurice A, Williams R: Cardiac arrest and myocardial infarction induced by postpartum intravenous ergonovine administration. Anesthesiology 2001;94:363-364.

71. Weiss BM, von Segesser LK, Alon E, et al: Outcome of cardiovascular surgery and pregnancy: A systematic review of the period 1984-1996. Am J Obstet Gynecol 1998;179:1643-1653.

72. Zeebregts CJ, Schepens MA, Hameeteman TM, et al: Acute aortic dissection complicating pregnancy. Ann Thorac Surg 1997;64:1345-1348.

73. Child A: Management of pregnancy in Marfan syndrome, Ehlers-Danlos syndrome and the other heritable connective tissue diseases. In Oakley C (ed): Heart Disease in Pregnancy. London, BMJ, 1997, pp 153-163.

74. Kaufman I, Bondy R, Benjamin A: Peripartum cardiomyopathy and thromboembolism: Anesthetic management and clinical course of an obese diabetic patient. Can J Anaesth 2003;50:161-165.

75. Weiss BM, Hess OM: Pulmonary vascular disease and pregnancy: Current controversies, management strategies and perspectives. Eur Heart J 2000;21:104-115.

76. Whittemore R, Hobbins J, Engle M: Pregnancy and its outcomes in women with or without surgical treatment in congenital heart disease. Am J Cardiol 1982;50:641-651.

77. Shime J, Mocarski EJ, Hastings D, et al: Congenital heart disease in pregnancy: Short- and long-term implications. Am J Obstet Gynecol 1987;156:313-322.

78. Siu SC, Sermer M, Harrison DA: Risk and predictors for pregnancy-related complications in women with heart disease. Circulation 1997;96:2789-2794.

79. Genoni M, Jenni R, Hoerstrup SP, et al: Pregnancy after atrial repair for transposition of the great arteries. Heart 1999;81:276-277.

80. Canobbio MM, Mair DD, van der Velde M, Koos BJ: Pregnancy outcomes after the Fontan repair. J Am Coll Cardiol 1996;28:763-767.

81. Siu S, Chitayat D, Webb G: Pregnancy in women with congenital heart defects: What are the risks? Heart 1999;81:225-226.

82. Proceedings of the 32nd Bethesda Conference on Care of Adults with Congenital Heart Disease: Task Force Reports. J Am Coll Cardiol 2001;37:1161-1198.

83. Robinson DE, Leicht CH: Epidural analgesia with low dose bupivacaine and fentanyl for labor and delivery in a parturient with severe pulmonary hypertension. Anesthesiology 1988;68:285-288.

84. Smedstad KG, Cramb R, Morison DH: Pulmonary hypertension and pregnancy: A series of eight cases. Can J Anaesth 1994;41:502-512.

85. Weiss BM, Zemp L, Seifert B, Hess OM: Outcome of pulmonary vascular disease in pregnancy: A systematic overview from 1978-1996. J Am Coll Cardiol 1998;31:1650-1657.

86. Cole PJ, Cross MH, Dresner M: Incremental spinal anaesthesia for elective cesarean section in a patient with Eisenmenger's syndrome. Br J Anaesth 2001;86:723-726.

87. Lam GK, Stafford RE, Thorp J, et al: Inhaled nitric oxide for primary pulmonary hypertension in pregnancy. Obstet Gynecol 2001;98:895-898.

88. Bonica JJ: Principles and Practice of Obstetric Analgesia and Anesthesia. Baltimore, Williams & Wilkins, 1969.

89. Kerr MG, Scott DB, Samuel E: Studies of the inferior vena cava in late pregnancy. Br Med J 1964;1:532-533.

90. Bieniarz I, Crottogini JJ, Curachet E: Aortocaval compression by the uterus in late human pregnancy. Am J Obstet Gynecol 1968;100:203-217.

91. Ralston DH, Shnider SM, deLorimier AA: Effects of equipotent ephedrine, metaraminol, mephentermine and methoxamine on uterine blood flow in the pregnant ewe. Anesthesiology 1974;40:354-370.

92. Gutsche BB: Prophylactic ephedrine preceding spinal analgesia for cesarean section. Anesthesiology 1976;45:462-465.

93. Lee A, Ngan Kee WD, Gin T: Prophylactic ephedrine prevents hypotension during spinal anesthesia for cesarean delivery but does not improve neonatal outcome: A quantitative systematic review. Can J Anaesth 2002;49:588-599.

94. Kangas-Saarela T, Hollmén AI, Tolonen U, et al: Does ephedrine influence newborn neurobehavioural responses and spectral EEG when used to prevent maternal hypotension during caesarean section? Acta Anaesthesiol Scand 1990;34:8-16.

95. Ramin SM, Ramin KD, Cox K, et al: Comparison of prophylactic angiotensin II versus ephedrine infusion for prevention of maternal hypotension during spinal anesthesia. Am J Obstet Gynecol 1994;171:734-739.

96. Chan WS, Irwin MG, Tong WN, Lam YH: Prevention of hypotension during spinal anaesthesia for caesarean section: ephedrine infusion versus fluid preload. Anaesthesia 1997;52:896-913.

97. Webb AA, Shipton EA: Re-evaluation of IM ephedrine as prophylaxis against hypotension associated with spinal anaesthesia for caesarean section. Can J Anaesth 1998;45:367-369.

98. King SW, Rosen MA: Prophylactic ephedrine and hypotension associated with spinal anesthesia for cesarean delivery. Int J Obstet Anesth 1998;7:18-22.

99. Carvalho JC, Cardoso MM, Cappelli EL, et al: Prophylactic ephedrine during cesarean delivery spinal anesthesia: Dose-response study of bolus and continuous infusion administration [Portuguese]. Rev Bras Anestesiol 1999;49:309-314.

100. Ngan Kee WD, Khaw KS, Lee BB, et al: A dose-response study of prophylactic intravenous ephedrine for the prevention of hypotension during spinal anesthesia for cesarean delivery. Anesth Analg 2000;90:1390-1395.

101. Vercauteren MP, Coppejans HC, Hoffmann VH, et al: Prevention of hypotension by a single 5-mg dose of ephedrine during small-dose spinal anesthesia in prehydrated cesarean delivery patients. Anesth Analg 2000;90:324-327.

102. Tsen LC, Boosalis P, Segal S, et al: Hemodynamic effects of simultaneous administration of intravenous ephedrine and spinal anesthesia for cesarean delivery. J Clin Anesth 2000;12:378-382.

103. Ayorinde BT, Buczkowski P, Brown J, et al: Evaluation of pre-emptive intramuscular phenylephrine and ephedrine for reduction of spinal anaesthesia-induced hypotension during caesarean section. Br J Anaesth 2001;86:372-376.

103a. Ramanathan S, Grant GJ: Vasopressor therapy for hypotension due to epidural anesthesia for cesarean section. Acta Anaesth Scand 1988;32:559-565.

104. Lee A, Ngan Kee WD, Gin T: A quantitative, systematic review of randomized controlled trials of ephedrine versus phenylephrine for the management of hypotension during spinal anesthesia for cesarean delivery. Anesth Analg 2002;94:920-926.

105. Assali NS, Prystowsky H: Studies on autonomic blockade: I. Comparison between the effects of tetraethylammonium chloride (TEAC) and high selective spinal anesthesia on the blood pressure of normal and toxemic pregnancy. J Clin Invest 1950;29:1354-1366.

106. Wollman SB, Marx GF: Acute hydration for prevention of hypotension from spinal anesthesia in parturients. Anesthesiology 1968;29:374-380.

107. Cheek TG, Samuels P, Miller F, et al: Normal saline i.v. fluid load decreases uterine activity in active labour. Br J Anaesth 1996;77:632-635.

108. Rout CC, Rocke DA, Levin J, et al: A reevaluation of the role of crystalloid preload in avoiding hypotension associated with spinal anesthesia for elective cesarean section. Anesthesiology 1993;79:262-269.

109. Emmett RS, Cyna AM, Andrew M, Simmons SW: Techniques for preventing hypotension during spinal anaesthesia for caesarean section. Cochrane Database Syst Rev 2002:CD002251.

110. Hofmeyr GJ, Cyna AM, Middleton P: Prophylactic intravenous preloading for regional analgesia in labour. Cochrane Database Syst Rev 2004:CD000175.

111. Burns SM, Cowan CM, Wilkes RG: Prevention and management of hypotension during spinal anaesthesia for elective caesarean section: A survey of practice. Anaesthesia 2001;56:794-798.

112. American College of Obstetricians and Gynecologists Committee Opinion no. 315: Obesity in pregnancy. Obstet Gynecol 2005;106:671-675.

113. World Health Organization: Obesity: Preventing and managing the global epidemic. Geneva, World Health Organization, 2000, technical report series 894.

114. National Heart, Lung, and Blood Institute (NHLBI) and National Institute for Diabetes and Digestive and Kidney Diseases (NIDDK): Clinical guidelines on the identification, evaluation and treatment of overweight and obesity in adults: The evidence report. Obes Res 1998;6(suppl 2):51S-210.

115. Hedley AA, Ogden CL, Johnson CL, et al: Prevalence of overweight and obesity among US children, adolescents, and adults, 1999-2002. JAMA 2004;291:2847-2850.

116. Andreasen KR, Andersen ML, Schantz AL: Obesity and pregnancy. Acta Obstet Gynecol Scand 2004;83:1022-1029.

117. Weiss JL, Malone FD, Emig D, et al: Obesity, obstetric complications and cesarean delivery rate: A population-based screening study. FASTER Research Consortium. Am J Obstet Gynecol 2004;190:1091-1097.

118. Baeten JM, Bukusi EA, Lambe M: Pregnancy complications and outcomes among overweight and obese nulliparous women. Am J Public Health 2001;91:436-440.

119. Cedergren MI: Maternal morbid obesity and the risk of adverse pregnancy outcome. Obstet Gynecol 2004;103:219-224.

120. Sebire NJ, Jolly M, Harris JP, et al: Maternal obesity and pregnancy outcome: A study of 287,213 pregnancies in London. Int J Obes Relat Metab Disord 2001;25:1175-1182.

121. Young TK, Woodmansee B: Factors that are associated with cesarean delivery in a large private practice: The importance of prepregnancy body mass index and weight gain. Am J Obstet Gynecol 2002;187:312-318; discussion, 318-320.

122. Kabiru W, Raynor BD: Obstetric outcomes associated with increase in BMI category during pregnancy. Am J Obstet Gynecol 2004:191:928-932.

123. Myles TD, Gooch J, Santolaya J: Obesity as an independent risk factor for infectious morbidity in patients who undergo cesarean delivery. Obstet Gynecol 2002;100:959-964.

124. Perlow JH, Morgan MA: Massive maternal obesity and perioperative cesarean morbidity. Am J Obstet Gynecol 1994;170:560-565.

125. Hood DD, Dewan DM: Anesthetic and obstetric outcome in morbidly obese parturients. Anesthesiology 1993;79:1210-1218.

126. Maasilta P, Bachour A, Teramo K, et al: Sleep-related disordered breathing during pregnancy in obese women. Chest 2001;120:1448-1454.

127. Endler GC, Mariona FG, Sokol RJ, Stevenson LB: Anesthesia-related maternal mortality in Michigan, 1972 to 1984. Am J Obstet Gynecol 1988;159:187-193.

128. McClure J, Cooper G: Fifty years of confidential enquiries into maternal deaths in the United Kingdom: Should anesthesia celebrate or not? Int J Obstet Anaesth 2005;14:87-89.

129. Davies JM: Closed Claims Project focuses on 3 decades of obstetric complications. APSF (Anesthesia Patient Safety Foundation) Newsletter, 2004;49:49.

130. Peterson GN, Domino KB, Caplan RA, et al: Management of the difficult airway. Anesthesiology 2005;103:33-39.

131. Larson CP, Steadman RH: Management of the full stomach: A re-evaluation. Curr Rev Clin Anesth 2005;25:253-264.

132. Samsoon GLT, Young JRB: Difficult tracheal intubation: A retrospective study. Anaesthesia 1987;42:487-490.

133. Rahman K, Jenkins JG: Failed tracheal intubation in obstetrics: No more frequent but still managed badly. Anaesthesia 2005;60:168.

134. Practice Guidelines for Management of the Difficult Airway: A report by the American Society of Anesthesiologists Task Force on Management of the Difficult Airway. Anesthesiology 1993;78:597-602.

135. Kuczkowski KM, Reisner LS, Benumof JL: Airway problems and new solutions for the obstetric patient. J Clin Anesthesia 2003;15:552-563.

136. Hawkins JL: Maternal morbidity and mortality: Anesthetic causes. Can J Anaesth 2002;49:R1-R5 (Refresher Course Lecture).

137. Hansch E, Chitkara U, McAlpine J, et al: Pelvic arterial embolization for control of obstetric hemorrhage: A five-year experience. Am J Obstet Gynecol 1999;180:1454-1460.

138. Clark SL, Koonings PP, Phelan JP: Placenta previa/accreta and prior cesarean section. Obstet Gynecol 1985;66:89-92.

139. Esler MD, Douglas MJ: Planning for hemorrhage: Steps an anesthesiologist can take to limit and treat hemorrhage in the obstetric patient. Anesthesiol Clin No rth Am 2003;21:127-144.

140. Tsen L: Gerard W. Ostheimer "What's new in obstetric anesthesia?" lecture. Anesthesiology 2005;102:672-679.

141. Alahuhta S, Rasanen J, Jouppila P, et al: Ephedrine and phenylephrine for avoiding maternal hypotension due to spinal anaesthesia for caesarean section. Int J Obstet Anesth 1992;1:129-134.

142. Hall PA, Bennett A, Wilkes MP, Lewis M: Spinal anaesthesia for caesarean section: Comparison of infusions of phenylephrine and ephedrine. Br J Anaesth 1994;73:471-474.

143. LaPorta RF, Arthur GR, Datta S: Phenylephrine in treating maternal hypotension due to spinal anaesthesia for caesarean delivery: Effects on neonatal catecholamine concentrations, acid base status and Apgar scores. Acta Anaesthesiol Scand 1995;39:901-905.

144. Moran DH, Perillo M, LaPorta RF, et al: Phenylephrine in the prevention of hypotension following spinal anesthesia for cesarean delivery. J Clin Anesth 1991;3:301-305.

145. Pierce ET, Carr DB, Datta S: Effects of ephedrine and phenylephrine on maternal and fetal atrial natriuretic peptide levels during elective cesarean section. Acta Anaesthesiol Scand 1994;38:48-51.

146. Thomas DG, Robson SC, Redfern N, et al: Randomized trial of bolus phenylephrine or ephedrine for maintenance of arterial pressure during spinal anaesthesia for caesarean section. Br J Anaesth 1996;76:61-65.

30 Preservation of Fetal Viability in Noncardiac Surgery

Robert R. Gaiser and Mary K. McHugh

Caring for the pregnant patient is one of the most challenging and most rewarding aspects of anesthesia, as it involves two patients, the mother and the fetus, and both must be considered when making decisions. The mother is the primary patient, with the fetus secondary. Generally, optimal care of the mother provides good care of the fetus. Pregnancy alters maternal physiology. These changes must be considered when evaluating the pregnant patient, as must the effects of anesthetic agents on the fetus.

■ DOES ANESTHESIA HAVE A TERATOGENIC EFFECT?

One percent to 2% of pregnant women require anesthesia for surgery unrelated to the pregnancy. The greatest concern for the parturient is the effect of anesthetic agents on the fetus and whether there is an increase in the risk for congenital anomalies. All anesthetic agents have been implicated as teratogens in animal studies. However, the animal model does not replicate the clinical situation, as the majority of these studies involve exposures at amounts greater than would be used clinically. For a teratogenic effect to occur, the mother must be exposed to a given level of drug for a specific period at a specific point in the gestation. Thus, to assess the teratogenicity of general anesthesia, population studies must be used.

Snider and Webster were the first to study the effects of anesthesia and surgery during pregnancy.[1] These authors evaluated the medical records of 9073 women who delivered infants between July 1959 and August 1964. Of these women, 147 parturients (1.6%) had surgery during pregnancy. There was no increased incidence of congenital anomalies in the surgical group, but the authors noted that the majority of parturients received anesthesia during the second or third trimester (after the period of organogenesis, which occurs during the first trimester). For those parturients who had surgery during the first trimester, multiple techniques and agents were used, making it difficult to draw conclusions.

Brodsky and colleagues had a different approach, mailing a questionnaire to dentists and dental assistants to identify pregnant women who underwent surgery during pregnancy, and also to identify parturients who had occupational exposure to nitrous oxide or volatile agents.[2] They identified 287 women who had surgery during pregnancy. Of these women, 187 had surgery during the first trimester. A larger number, 3624 parturients, had occupational exposure only. There was no major difference in the incidence of congenital anomalies

in infants born to women who had surgery during pregnancy compared with a control group who did not have surgery. Also, there was no increase in congenital anomalies in infants born to women with occupational exposure. Duncan and coworkers reviewed the health insurance data from the province of Manitoba from 1971 to 1978.[3] These authors matched 2565 women who underwent surgery during pregnancy to those of similar height and weight who did not. There was no difference in the rate of congenital anomalies between the two groups.

Mazze and Kallen examined cases from three Swedish health care registries for the years 1973 to 1981.[4] These authors identified 5405 women who underwent surgery during pregnancy. Among these women, 65% received general anesthesia. Of these parturients, 2248 had surgery during the first trimester. This study is important because it was the largest to examine surgery during the period of organogenesis (the period of the greatest risk for teratogenicity). The authors found no increased incidence of congenital anomalies.

Another group sought to determine whether anesthetic agents result in an increase in congenital anomalies by examining anomalies and then seeing if there is a link to anesthesia.[5] Of the 20,830 pregnant women who had offspring with a congenital anomaly, 31 patients had had surgery and anesthesia. This fraction did not differ from the 35,727 women who had babies without defects, 73 of whom had surgery during pregnancy. There was no higher incidence of surgery and anesthesia for any congenital anomaly group.[5]

Despite these data, the status of nitrous oxide as a reproductive toxin continues to be debated. Nitrous oxide is a teratogen in animals. It inhibits methionine synthetase, an enzyme necessary for folate metabolism.[6] Despite the previous studies, other authors have postulated a link. Kallen and Mazze reexamined their database and noted six infants who had neural tube defects.[7] This number is much higher than the expected number, 2.2 (an incidence of 1 per 1000 births). The authors postulated nitrous oxide as a possible cause, although the numbers and exposure do not support this proposition. Another study examined infants born with central nervous system defects in Atlanta between 1968 and 1980 who were matched to controls by race, birth hospital, and period of birth.[8] Of the 694 mothers of infants with central nervous system defects, 12 reported first-trimester anesthetic exposure (34 of 2984 control mothers reported such exposure), yielding an odds ratio of 1.7 (confidence interval [CI],

0.8 to 33; not statistically significant). However, when examining infants with hydrocephalus and eye defects, the odds ratio increased to 39.6 (CI, 7.5 to 208.2). Although the odds ratio is high, it is important to examine the actual incidence. There were eight infants with this defect, three of whom had first-trimester exposure to anesthetic agents. Although this suggests a link, it is based on extremely small numbers.

In another study, which caused much concern, rats were exposed to typical amounts of common anesthetics for a normal period.[9] The anesthetics were midazolam, nitrous oxide, and isoflurane in dosages sufficient to maintain a surgical plane of anesthesia for 6 hours. The authors noted widespread apoptotic neurodegeneration in the developing brain. The greatest risk occurs during the synaptogenic period, also known as the brain growth-spurt period, which begins in the third trimester. Thus, the authors hint that anesthesia during the third trimester may have effects on the fetal brain.

The literature supporting the idea that there is a risk for congenital anomalies from anesthesia use is scant. No population study has found a link. Only two studies suggest a possible cause, both with extremely low numbers of affected children. It seems unlikely that a link exists. When discussing the risk of anesthesia with pregnant women scheduled for surgery, the anesthesia provider should remind the patient that there is a 3% baseline incidence of fetal anomalies among all pregnant women.

■ TREATING HYPOTENSION

The purpose of the placenta is to deliver oxygen and nutrients to the developing fetus. Uteroplacental perfusion is provided by the uterine and ovarian arteries, as they join and penetrate the myometrium to form the arcuate arteries. In the nonpregnant state, uterine blood flow accounts for less than 5% of the cardiac output. During pregnancy, uterine blood flow increases progressively, reaching approximately 500 to 800 mL/min (10% of the cardiac output) at term.[10] Uterine blood flow is directly proportional to the mean maternal arterial pressure and inversely proportional to uterine vascular resistance. Thus, it is important to maintain arterial blood pressure and to prevent increases in uterine vascular resistance. By maintaining arterial pressure, oxygen delivery to the fetus is ensured.

Wollman and Marx were the first to demonstrate the importance of avoiding hypotension when caring for the parturient.[11] Their original intent was to examine the effect of crystalloid prehydration on the incidence of hypotension after spinal anesthesia. In this study, no vasopressors were administered. In the five patients who received no prehydration prior to spinal anesthesia, all developed hypotension with a mean arterial pressure of 64 mm Hg. Apgar scores were lower in this group, infants took longer to initiate respiration, and the umbilical cord pH was lower (a reflection of decreased uterine blood flow). The authors confirmed that maternal hypotension is bad for the fetus.

Given that maternal hypotension is bad for the fetus, the rapid return of maternal blood pressure to baseline is desirable. When treating hypotension, the anesthesiologist may use a direct agonist (such as phenylephrine, which binds

directly to the alpha receptor) or an indirect acting sympathomimetic (such as ephedrine, which acts by causing the release of norepinephrine). The indirect acting drugs have both alpha and beta effects. When treating maternal blood pressure with these drugs, their effect on uterine blood flow must be considered as well as their effect on maternal blood pressure. The uterine artery vasoconstriction caused by the drug should not be sufficient to negate the effects of increased blood pressure.

The first study comparing different drugs for the treatment of blood pressure examined 14 pregnant ewes undergoing 80 treatments.[12] All the sheep received general and spinal anesthesia, and uterine blood flow was measured in all animals. The authors studied metaraminol (an alpha agonist), ephedrine (an indirect acting drug), and mephentermine (an indirect acting drug). In this model, a decrease in blood pressure resulted in a direct, proportional decrease in uterine blood flow. All three drugs increased blood pressure and uterine blood flow. However, mephentermine and ephedrine increased it much more than metaraminol. The authors concluded that spinal anesthesia decreases maternal blood pressure and uterine blood flow. Indirect acting agents restore uterine blood flow to a greater extent. If vasopressors are required, drugs whose mode of action lies in cardiac stimulation rather than peripheral vasoconstriction should be used. Hence, the idea that ephedrine is preferred over phenylephrine for the treatment of hypotension in the parturient was started.

A criticism of the study was that the ewes were intubated and ventilated during the spinal anesthesia, which is different from the spontaneous ventilation that accompanies regional anesthesia for cesarean section. In an attempt to correct this deficiency, 16 nonanesthetized pregnant ewes were studied to examine the effect on uterine blood flow when the blood pressure was increased to 50% greater than baseline.[13] In this study, uterine blood flow was unchanged with ephedrine, reduced 20% with mephentermine, reduced 45% with metaraminol, and reduced 62% with methoxamine. This study reaffirmed the use of ephedrine for the treatment of hypotension in parturients.

Ephedrine remained the standard of treatment for hypotension until 1988, when ephedrine was compared with phenylephrine to treat hypotension resulting from epidural anesthesia. In this study, parturients undergoing cesarean section during epidural anesthesia were randomized to receive either ephedrine (5 mg) or phenylephrine (100 μg) to treat hypotension.[14] An impedance cardiograph was used to measure stroke volume, ejection fraction, and end-diastolic volume. Both vasopressors restored maternal blood pressure. There was also no difference in neonatal Apgar scores and umbilical cord pH. Finally, despite ephedrine having a beta effect, there was no difference in stroke volume and ejection fraction between the two medications. It seems that phenylephrine was not as detrimental as had been thought (Fig. 30-1), and that the cardiac effects of ephedrine were not as important.

The previous study examined cesarean section during epidural anesthesia. A similar study was applied to spinal anesthesia.[15] In this study, there was no difference in effect

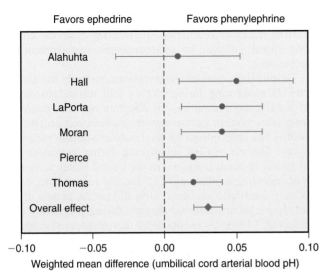

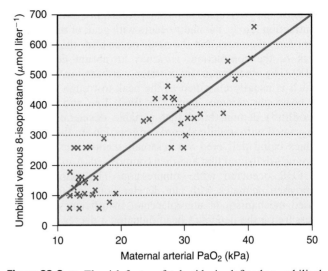

Figure 30-1 ■ Meta-analysis does not support the avoidance of phenylephrine for the treatment of hypotension accompanying regional anesthesia. In fact, there is a favorable (although small) effect on the umbilical arterial blood pH. *(Redrawn from Khaw KS, Wang CC, Ngan Kee WD, et al: Br J Anaesth 2002;88:18-23.)*

Figure 30-2 ■ The risk for true fetal acidosis, defined as umbilical arterial pH value of <7.20, was similar between the phenylephrine and ephedrine groups (relative risk, 0.78; 95% CI, 0.16-3.92). *(Redrawn from Lee A, Ngan K, Warwick DG, Gin T: Anesth Analg 2002;94:923-926.)*

on maternal blood pressure or neonatal Apgar scores. However, there was a difference in umbilical arterial pH, which was higher in the phenylephrine group (7.32 versus 7.28). This group of investigators was the first to show a difference in umbilical arterial pH. Subsequent studies comparing the two medications confirmed this finding.[16] In another study, Doppler echocardiography showed no difference in cardiac output between phenylephrine and ephedrine when used to treat hypotension occurring during spinal anesthesia.[17]

Subsequent studies have confirmed this statistically significant, but probably clinically insignificant, difference in umbilical cord arterial pH. The hypotension alone cannot be responsible for the additional acidosis. It has been postulated that rather than being caused by differences in uterine blood flow, the additional acidosis may be because ephedrine increases fetal catecholamine levels, as it readily crosses the placenta. This increase in catecholamine levels leads to an increase in oxygen consumption and an increase in lactate concentration.

A quantitative, systematic review of studies comparing phenylephrine and ephedrine was conducted.[18] Seven randomized controlled trials were identified, with a total of 292 patients. There was no difference between phenylephrine and ephedrine in ability to correct maternal hypotension, but a higher incidence of maternal bradycardia occurred if phenylephrine was used. In regard to the neonate, there was no difference in the incidence of true fetal acidosis (Fig. 30-2), but neonates whose mothers received phenylephrine had higher umbilical arterial pH values.

Clearly, the choice of vasopressor for treating hypotension in the parturient has undergone much study and change. All of the studies have investigated cesarean section. When discussing surgery during pregnancy, it must be assumed that

the same principles apply. The initial thought that ephedrine was the better agent was based on an animal model. Subsequent study on parturients did not support this finding. In fact, a statistically significant, but clinically insignificant, difference in umbilical arterial pH was found for phenylephrine. Either drug is acceptable for the treatment of hypotension. If multiple doses are required, phenylephrine is the preferred drug, as ephedrine readily crosses the placenta and increases lactate production. If the maternal heart rate is low, ephedrine is the better choice, as phenylephrine does slow the maternal heart rate further. It is important to treat the hypotension that occurs. The choice of drug, phenylephrine or ephedrine, is not as important.

■ MONITORING FETAL HEART RATE DURING NONOBSTETRIC SURGERY

The purpose of fetal heart rate (FHR) monitoring is to ensure that the fetus is well oxygenated. In the fetus, it is the brain that modulates the heart. It is thought that hypoxemia is reflected in the fetal heart rate. The FHR can be monitored externally or internally. The external monitor uses a Doppler device. When it is placed on the maternal abdomen and located over the fetal heart, a computerized program interprets and counts Doppler signals. The internal monitor involves the application of an electrode to the fetal scalp to record the heart rate, which requires that the amniotic membranes be ruptured. Continuous FHR was begun in the 1970s. By 1988, over half of all laboring women received it, and by 1998 this figure was 84%.[19] Current trends support a nearly universal use of FHR monitoring during labor.

In 1997, the National Institute of Child Health and Human Development proposed definitions for the interpretation of the FHR.[20] This group classified deceleration (a decrease in FHR) on the basis of its occurrence during uterine contraction (*early,* the nadir occurs with peak of the contraction; *late,* the onset and the nadir occur after the onset and peak of the contraction; *variable,* an abrupt decrease in FHR). The other important criterion was baseline variability, which is usually classified as the peak-to-trough amplitude in beats per minute (bpm). In 1963, Lee and Hon (see Goodlin[21]) demonstrated that variable decelerations were associated with umbilical cord compression. In this study of babies being delivered via cesarean section, the umbilical cord was delivered first and then compressed. A marked drop in FHR occurred with compression. The association of depressed neonates with late decelerations led to the proposed mechanism of uteroplacental insufficiency, whereas pressure on the neonate's head inducing a decrease in heart rate led to the association of head compression and early deceleration.

The purpose of FHR monitoring is to ensure the well-being of the fetus. A normal tracing (i.e., a baseline of 110 to 160 bpm, regular rate, presence of accelerations, presence of variability, and absence of periodic decelerations) is generally associated with a healthy, well-oxygenated fetus.[22] However, sometimes the tracing is not perfect. Fetal heart patterns that accurately predict asphyxia have not been specified. A nonreassuring tracing as an indication of fetal hypoxia has a false-positive rate greater than 99%.[23]

The use of continuous FHR monitoring was compared with intermittent auscultation during labor in 504 patients.[24] Intermittent auscultation was performed every 15 minutes during or immediately after a uterine contraction. In this study, there was no significant difference between the two groups in neonatal deaths, Apgar scores, maternal and neonatal morbidity, and cord blood gases. The only difference was the higher cesarean section rate in the continuously monitored group.[24] However, certain fetal patterns are associated with fetal acidosis and thus with decreased uterine perfusion and fetal hypoxemia. The perinatal outcomes of 301 term infants were correlated with the FHR tracings and umbilical cord gas analyses.[25] Late decelerations and variable decelerations during the first stage of labor were significant predictors of fetal acidosis.[25] The presence of late decelerations during the second stage correlated with fetal acidosis.[26] Finally, another FHR parameter associated with acidemia is decreased baseline variability. In 186 term gestations studied with continuous FHR monitoring, the presence of decreased variability in the 1 hour prior to delivery was significantly correlated with low pH.[27] Despite these strong associations with fetal acidemia, the role of FHR monitoring in reducing morbidity and mortality remains to be proven.

Because its efficacy in decreasing birth injury and reducing neonatal morbidity has not been proven, the use of fetal monitoring during maternal surgery is a much-debated topic. After 18 to 20 weeks of gestation, the fetal heart rate can be monitored. The argument for intraoperative fetal monitoring is that it can improve fetal outcome. Changes in the fetal heart rate may signal compromise of the uteroplacental circulation, allowing the anesthesia provider to take steps to improve uteroplacental perfusion and fetal oxygenation. These maneuvers may include increasing left uterine dis-

placement, increasing inspired concentration of oxygen, adjusting maternal ventilation, augmenting maternal circulating blood volume, or pharmacologic management of hypotension.

Despite these possible interventions, no study has examined FHR monitoring during surgery. Still, it stands to reason that if FHR monitoring has no effect on neonatal outcome during labor (except increasing the cesarean section rate), it probably has little impact on fetal outcome during maternal surgery. The use of FHR monitoring during surgery is not universally applied. Hospitals in the United States were surveyed regarding monitoring.[28] Of the 184 respondents, 60% routinely used fetal monitors; 40% did not. A review of all case reports of nonobstetric surgery during pregnancy was conducted.[29] The authors concluded that intraoperative monitoring by obstetric personnel was unnecessary, and they recommended that the FHR and uterine activity be checked before and after surgery. The American College of Obstetricians and Gynecologists (ACOG) recognized that there are no data regarding monitoring during surgery: "It is important for physicians to obtain obstetric consultation before performing nonobstetric surgery because obstetricians are uniquely qualified to discuss aspects of maternal physiology and anatomy that may affect intraoperative maternal and fetal well-being. The decision to use fetal monitoring should be individualized and, if used, may be based on gestational age, type of surgery, and facilities available. Ultimately, each case warrants a team approach for optimal safety of the woman and her baby."[30] Even ACOG agrees that the use of FHR monitoring during surgery is not mandatory (Fig. 30-3).

On the other hand, a recent case report questions this viewpoint.[31] A 27-year-old woman was undergoing cholecystectomy during general anesthesia, which was maintained with 100% oxygen, sevoflurane, and remifentanil. The patient was neither hypotensive nor hypercarbic. Prior to surgical incision, the fetal heart rate decreased rapidly to 70 bpm and did not return to baseline. The decrease did not respond to

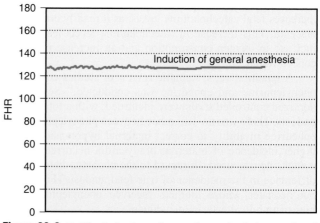

Figure 30-3 ■ The induction of general anesthesia is associated with a loss of beat-to-beat variability of the fetal heart rate (FHR). This is important to remember so that needless cesarean section is not performed.

increasing left uterine displacement. An emergency cesarean delivery was performed. The umbilical cord arterial gas values were PaO$_2$, 7 mm Hg; PaCO$_2$, 64 mm Hg; and pH 7.17. The Apgar scores were 1 and 5 at 1 and 5 minutes, respectively. This case report argues against the ACOG opinion, and the authors urge that all women having nonobstetric surgery have intraoperative fetal heart rate monitoring.

■ ASPIRATION DURING NONOBSTETRIC SURGERY

Because parturients are considered to have full stomachs, general anesthesia is induced by the rapid-sequence technique. Also, parturients frequently receive histamine (H$_2$)-blockers and oral nonparticulate antacids to prevent the development of pneumonitis if they should aspirate. Although these practices have become standard, the evidence on which these recommendations are based should be examined.

In 1946, Mendelson reported 66 cases of aspiration of stomach contents during obstetric anesthesia.[32] Of these patients, 5 aspirated solid material; 21 were subsequently diagnosed as having aspirated, and 40 aspirated liquid material. Mendelson further reported that these 40 parturients all had a stormy course for 36 to 48 hours, but all survived. The term *Mendelson's syndrome* was used to describe the pneumonitis accompanying aspiration. Researchers have focused on quantifying the volume and pH of a solution required to cause fatality in an animal model. This research led to the development of strategies to reduce gastric volume and increase gastric pH.[33]

Parturients are believed to be at risk for aspiration because of the physiologic changes of pregnancy. The enlarged gravid uterus displaces the stomach cephalad. This displacement alters the angle of the gastroesophageal junction, decreasing the competence of the gastroesophageal sphincter. The uterus also displaces the pylorus upward and posteriorly, resulting in delayed gastric emptying. Elevated concentrations of progesterone decrease gastrointestinal motility and food absorption. These changes facilitate the occurrence of gastric reflux and heartburn in as many as 70% of pregnant women.[34] Furthermore, the placenta secretes gastrin, a hormone that increases the acidity of the stomach contents.[35] The question is whether these changes place pregnant women at risk for regurgitation and aspiration of gastric contents during induction or maintenance of general anesthesia or during any loss of consciousness.

Recent studies have questioned whether the physiologic changes of pregnancy include delayed gastric emptying and increased gastrin concentration. The gastric emptying times of 11 women were measured during the first trimester, during the third trimester, and postpartum.[36] Although there was no difference between first trimester and postpartum, gastrointestinal transit time was significantly longer in the third trimester. Thus, despite hormonal changes, it seems that gastric emptying is affected only in the third trimester and during labor. This was further confirmed when the gastric contents were aspirated via a nasogastric tube prior to cesarean section.[37] The stomach contents of 100 term parturients were compared with the contents from 100 nonpregnant women scheduled for gynecologic surgery. The gastric volume in the pregnant group was greater than in the nonpregnant group, although serum gastrin levels did not differ between the groups. These studies confirm that parturients in the third trimester have risk factors.

Only one article suggests parturients have a greater incidence of aspiration. The Closed Claims Project Database includes all settled malpractice claims involving anesthesiologists.[38] Of the obstetric claims, 5% involved aspiration, as opposed to only 1% of the nonobstetric claims. However, there are shortcomings to this database. Only complications resulting in a malpractice claim are included, and because the database does not include a complication if it did not result in a lawsuit, the percentage does not represent an actual incidence. One conclusion from these data is that the incidence of aspiration in the parturient is increased. Another conclusion might be that obstetric patients are more likely to sue, or that general surgical patients are less likely to sue.

Another study suggesting a greater risk for the development of aspiration comes from The Netherlands.[39] A 4-year audit of gynecologic and obstetric patients who developed aspiration pneumonitis was performed. Aspiration pneumonitis was diagnosed on the basis of symptoms after a witnessed episode of gastric contents entering the trachea, or after an intraoperative episode making pulmonary aspiration likely. Eleven cases were identified, four in parturients and seven in women undergoing gynecologic procedures, yielding an incidence of developing aspiration pneumonitis of 0.11% in the obstetric population and 0.04% in the gynecologic population. Although it did not report the actual incidence of aspiration, this study suggests that parturients have a greater risk of developing aspiration pneumonitis if they do aspirate.

The most applicable study examined obstetric procedures performed in the peripartum period, excluding cesarean section. This study identified 1870 patients undergoing general anesthesia who were not intubated.[40] In this series, there was only a single case of mild aspiration. This incidence, 0.053%, is comparable with that in the general surgical population. This result challenges the concept that pregnant women undergoing general anesthesia (excluding cesarean section) require an endotracheal tube. It belies the belief that all pregnant patients undergoing nonobstetric surgery require rapid-sequence induction (RSI) and intubation.

Gastric emptying is not delayed until the third trimester. At term, a greater gastric volume occurs but not early in the pregnancy. Serum levels of gastrin are not elevated. Parturients during the first and second trimester should be treated like nonpregnant individuals. If the patient has symptomatic reflux, RSI and intubation should be done. If she is asymptomatic, RSI and intubation are not required. During the third trimester, it is prudent to perform RSI and intubation, although the literature does not support this contention.

■ USE OF 100% OXYGEN DURING NONOBSTETRIC SURGERY

Many anesthesia providers avoid nitrous oxide for parturients undergoing nonobstetric surgery because of concerns about teratogenicity. If nitrous oxide is avoided, the practitioner must decide whether to use 100% oxygen. Theoretically, the use of a lower inspired concentration of oxygen may be desirable.

The fetus is well adapted for a low blood oxygen concentration. Fetal hemoglobin accounts for 65% to 85% of the fetus's hemoglobin. Fetal hemoglobin has an increased affinity for oxygen (a shift to the left in the oxygen saturation curve), binding to it more avidly than adult hemoglobin. Furthermore, the fetus has a much higher hematocrit, typically 45%, allowing an increased oxygen-carrying capacity.

The purpose of using a high inspired oxygen concentration is to increase oxygen transfer to the fetus. Intraoperative fetal oxygen saturation was compared in 24 women undergoing cesarean section using sevoflurane with either 100% oxygen, or 50% oxygen and 50% nitrous oxide. Intraoperative fetal oxygen saturation was 57% in the 100% group, and 43% in the 50% group. Also, umbilical vein and artery PaO_2 were higher.[41] In a randomized study comparing maternal inspired oxygen concentrations of 30%, 50%, or 100%, there was no difference in arterial concentrations of oxygen between the 30% and the 50% groups. An inspired oxygen concentration of 100% resulted in the greatest umbilical arterial and venous oxygen concentrations.[42]

Clearly, an inspired concentration of 100% oxygen results in the greatest level of fetal oxygen. This level is not sufficient to cause retinopathy of prematurity. Despite this lack of effect on the fetal eye, are other toxic reactions to oxygen possible? Oxygen was discovered in 1772. It has two unpaired electrons and can exist as a free radical—a molecule capable of independent existence with one or more unpaired electrons. In 1969, it was shown that approximately 2% of the oxygen molecules in mammalian mitochondria form superoxide free radicals, or the dismutation product, hydrogen peroxide.[43] Oxygen free radicals have been implicated in the pathogenesis of inflammatory, toxic, and metabolic insults, ischemia-reperfusion injury, carcinogenesis, and atherosclerosis.

Is there a link between high inspired oxygen concentration and the formation of oxygen free radicals? Forty-four healthy parturients undergoing cesarean section during spinal anesthesia were randomized to breathe either 21% or 60% oxygen.[44] Direct detection of free radicals is difficult because of their brief life span. So, in this study, lipid hydroperoxides, the products of free radicals, were measured. There was a higher umbilical arterial and venous oxygen concentration in the 60% group. However, there were also greater concentrations of lipid peroxides in the fetus. Lipid peroxide concentrations were much greater in the umbilical vein than in the umbilical artery, suggesting that the main site of free radical activity was the placenta.[44] Clearly, administering a high concentration of inspired oxygen induces free radical generation in the fetus (Fig. 30-4). The clinical relevance of this increase is uncertain. Future research may reveal an adverse effect.

Increasing the maternal inspired oxygen concentration increases fetal oxygenation. This increase is not needed, as the fetus, with a high hematocrit and high percentage of fetal hemoglobin, is well adapted for the lower maternal oxygen

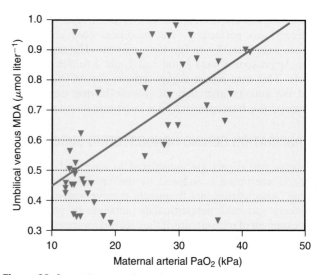

Figure 30-4 ▪ The use of supplemental oxygen during regional anesthesia during cesarean section is associated with the formation of oxygen free radicals in the fetus, even if hypotension and hypoxia are avoided. Although it is not possible to measure oxygen free radicals, there is a correlation between free radical products (lipid peroxides) and maternal PaO_2. (*Redrawn from Khaw KS, Wang CC, Ngan Kee WD, et al: Br J Anaesth 2002;88:18-23.*)

concentrations. A high maternal inspired oxygen concentration also increases fetal oxygen free radicals. Free radicals have been implicated in certain diseases but have not been shown to harm the fetus. It seems prudent to maintain mothers undergoing nonobstetric surgery at an inspired oxygen concentration necessary to maintain an oxygen saturation of 95% to 99%.

■ MANAGEMENT OF MATERNAL VENTILATION

An increase in minute ventilation represents one of the more profound physiologic adaptations to pregnancy. During the first trimester, altered chest wall dynamics and enhanced diaphragmatic excursion produce a significant increase in tidal volume. As pregnancy progresses, progesterone levels rise, stimulating central respiratory centers and further augmenting tidal volume. Ultimately, minute ventilation increases by 45% above prepregnant levels. As a consequence, the parturient experiences a mild, chronic respiratory alkalosis, and typical arterial carbon dioxide tension ranges from 28 to 32 mm Hg.[45]

Unlike the mild respiratory alkalosis characteristic of the parturient, the arterial carbon dioxide tension of the fetus typically approaches or surpasses 40 mm Hg. The difference in carbon dioxide tension between mother and fetus creates a transplacental concentration gradient, favoring elimination of carbon dioxide from the fetal unit to the maternal circulation. Mild degrees of hypercarbia are well tolerated by both mother and fetus; elimination of carbon dioxide from the fetus suffers when there is a significant increase in maternal carbon dioxide tension. Respiratory acidosis in the fetus initiates a downward spiral of fetal cardiac depression and hypotension.[46]

Maintenance of normocarbia in the parturient undergoing general anesthesia typically demands little more than subtle manipulation of minute ventilation. Laparoscopic surgery in the parturient presents greater challenges. For several decades, the general surgical community avoided laparoscopic procedures during pregnancy; untoward effects arising from the creation of pneumoperitoneum with carbon dioxide underscored this reluctance.[47]

In the 1990s, the first successful, nonobstetric-related laparoscopic procedure was performed during pregnancy.[48] Although many early cases argued its safety, others suggested caution. In 1996, Amos and colleagues reported a significant increase in fetal loss among women undergoing laparoscopic procedures as compared with a matched cohort undergoing laparotomy.[49] They suggested that the increased carbon dioxide levels predisposed both the mother and the fetus to unrecognized respiratory acidosis and increased fetal loss.

Several animal studies supported this, demonstrating that fetal respiratory acidosis ensues from the creation of carbon dioxide pneumoperitoneum.[50,51] Using the pregnant ewe model, Curet induced significant hypercarbia by the insufflation of carbon dioxide into the peritoneum.[51] Both the mother and the fetus experienced respiratory acidosis. However, the fetal increase in carbon dioxide tension dramatically exceeded the maternal increase, and it was associated with a significant increase in fetal heart rate and blood pressure. It was suggested that the fetal hypercarbia derived from two sources: (1) the disruption of the transplacental carbon dioxide gradient between mother and fetus, and (2) direct abdominal absorption. In spite of the physiologic perturbations associated with pneumoperitoneum, there was no increase in miscarriage in the pregnant sheep model.[52]

The management of maternal and fetal hypercarbia varies. Barnard hypothesized that the fetal respiratory acidosis is avoidable if the maternal–fetal concentration gradient for carbon dioxide elimination is preserved.[52] To maintain an appropriate transplacental concentration gradient during abdominal insufflation, pregnant ewes were hyperventilated to maintain normocarbia. In this situation, an increase in fetal carbon dioxide was not observed.

Using a similar approach, Cruz demonstrated an absence of fetal hypercarbia during abdominal insufflation if maternal carbon dioxide tension is maintained within normal limits.[53] Unlike in the previous study, both arterial and end-tidal carbon dioxide were monitored. There was a significant gradient from arterial to end-tidal carbon dioxide during abdominal insufflation, with end-tidal carbon dioxide grossly underestimating arterial concentration. Based on these results, end-tidal carbon dioxide monitoring was considered inadequate, and arterial concentrations should be obtained by blood gas analysis.

A significant discrepancy between end-tidal and arterial carbon dioxide tension was observed in other studies.[54,55] Given the deleterious effects of maternal hypercarbia, some authors have recommended placement of arterial catheters. Bhavani-Shankar studied the relationship between end-tidal and arterial carbon dioxide in parturients undergoing laparoscopy.[56] Unlike the animal models, parturients have a lower pre-insufflation gradient that remains low during abdominal insufflation. A lower alveolar dead space in the parturient compared with the pregnant ewe most likely accounts for this discrepancy. Thus, end-tidal carbon dioxide monitoring is adequate for the parturient.[56]

Since the 1990s, laparoscopy has become a standard of care for various procedures in the parturient, without adverse outcome. Normocarbia should be maintained during these procedures. Unlike for the animal model, monitoring carbon dioxide levels using end-tidal levels is adequate for the management of the parturient. Invasive monitoring is not required.

■ RISK FOR PRETERM LABOR OR MISCARRIAGE IN NONOBSTETRIC SURGERY

Although anesthesia providers accept that common anesthetics do not present a risk for teratogenic effects, the same cannot be stated for the risk for preterm labor and miscarriage. There is a strong belief that surgery with anesthesia carries a high risk for preterm labor and miscarriage. The incidence of each of these complications depends on the surgical procedure, with intra-abdominal and gynecologic procedures judged to have the highest risks. However, support for this contention is based on older data. With developments in surgical technique and newer anesthetic agents, this belief may need to be changed.

In the first study to examine pregnancy outcome, published in 1980, a questionnaire was mailed to 30,272 female dental assistants regarding surgery during pregnancy, and also regarding occupational exposure to anesthetic agents.[2] Occupational exposure resulted in an increase in spontaneous abortion in the first trimester (8.6/100 pregnancies versus 5.1/100 pregnancies) and in the second trimester (2.6/100 pregnancies versus 1.4/100 pregnancies). Surgery during pregnancy did not result in a further increase in the first trimester (8.0/100 pregnancies), but it did increase it further during the second trimester (6.9/100 pregnancies). There was an increase in spontaneous abortion in those women who had anesthesia and surgery during the first trimester. The rate for spontaneous abortion decreased during the second trimester, although surgery was associated with a proportionally greater risk for fetal loss compared with the first trimester. These rates were based on 187 women who had surgery during the first trimester and 100 women who had surgery during the second trimester. The confounding variable in this study was that all participants worked. Stress and increased time spent on one's feet increases the risk for both of these complications.

This increased risk was further verified when health insurance data from the province of Manitoba (1971 to 1978) was reviewed.[3] This database identified 2565 women undergoing nonobstetric surgery and then matched them to those not undergoing surgery. There were 181 abortions in the surgical group (7.1%) and 166 in the nonsurgical group (6.5%). Surgery and anesthesia during pregnancy did not increase the risk for abortion. However, there was a significant increase in abortion in those women who received a general anesthetic (relative risk, 1.58; CI, 1.19 to 2.09). When further analyzed, the cause was linked to the site of surgery rather than to the anesthesia. Gynecologic surgery had the greatest risk, and all of these procedures were performed during general anesthesia.

Since these two studies were published, advancements have been made in anesthetic agents and surgical techniques. Anesthetic agents have shorter half-lives and less residual effect. Surgical techniques are now less invasive. It is unclear whether the previous incidences of miscarriage and preterm labor are still applicable. A retrospective review of all cases of nonobstetric abdominal surgery from 1991 to 1998 at the Women's Hospital at the University of Southern California identified 106 cases of nonobstetric abdominal surgery (88 laparotomy and 18 laparoscopy).[57] The incidence of preterm delivery was 18%, which was not different from the institution's general incidence of 16%. Furthermore, there was no difference in pregnancy loss, suggesting no difference in preterm delivery or miscarriage in the surgical group compared with the nonsurgical group.

A review of 54 articles concerning nonobstetric surgery was conducted for a total of 12,452 patients.[58] The reported miscarriage incidence was 5.8% and the incidence of preterm labor was 8.2%. These percentages do not differ from the reported percentages in the general population. Still, it is difficult to evaluate because of the lack of a control group. The most frequent surgical procedure during pregnancy is appendectomy. There was a high percentage, 4.6%, of surgical-induced labor. The incidence of premature labor and delivery was higher for appendectomy than for other medical conditions. It appears that the effects of acute appendicitis and surgery on the patient are more severe than, and different from, other acute conditions requiring surgery during pregnancy.

With regard to long-term follow-up of the infant, the data are extremely sparse. Only one study examined infants whose mothers had surgery during pregnancy.[59] These infants were evaluated 1 to 8 years after laparoscopic surgery during the 16th to 28th week of gestation. There was no evidence of developmental or physical abnormalities in the infants. This area requires further study.

In former times, surgery during pregnancy increased the risk for miscarriage and preterm labor. With the development of newer, less invasive surgical techniques and of improved anesthetic agents, the risks of both of these complications are no different from the risks in those who have not had surgery. It is important to counsel parturients that there is a risk for miscarriage and preterm labor, but that it is not increased because of the surgery. This statement does not apply for appendectomy, where the risks are higher.

■ CONCLUSIONS

The evaluation of the parturient involves two patients, the mother and the fetus. Optimal care of the mother provides the best care for the fetus. The parturient undergoes various physiologic changes that vary depending on the stage of the gestation. These changes must be considered when devising an anesthetic plan, and when the parturient has an underlying disease. It appears that surgery during pregnancy does not increase the risk for preterm labor (except for appendectomy) or of teratogenicity (Table 30-1). The prompt treatment of hypotension is important; the choice of agent for the treatment is less important. The use of 100% oxygen has not been shown to harm the fetus, despite the production of oxygen free radicals. The use of fetal monitoring is at the discretion of the obstetrician.

30-1   Levels of Evidence for Optimal Care of Mother and Fetus for Surgery during Pregnancy

	Benefit >> Risk: Procedure/Treatment SHOULD BE PERFORMED/ ADMINISTERED	Benefit > Risk: Procedure/Treatment IS REASONABLE	Benefit ≥ Risk: Procedure/Treatment MAY BE CONSIDERED	Risk ≥ Benefit: Procedure/Treatment IS NOT HELPFUL AND MAY BE HARMFUL
Level of evidence: LOW	Maintenance of normocarbia	Rapid sequence induction (RSI) during first trimester RSI during second trimester	Use of 100% oxygen during surgery Nitrous oxide has been associated with neural tube defects	—
Level of evidence: MEDIUM	Anesthetic agents and surgery: not associated with teratogenicity	—	Laryngeal mask airway during first trimester Laryngeal mask airway during second trimester Fetal monitoring during surgical procedures Use of <100% inspired oxygen concentration	Laryngeal mask airway during third trimester Anesthetic agents with surgery (excluding appendectomy): not associated with preterm labor or miscarriage Maternal hypercarbia
Level of evidence: HIGH	Treatment of hypotension RSI during third trimester	Use of phenylephrine to treat hypotension Use of ephedrine to treat hypotension	—	Surgery with anesthesia for appendectomy: associated with preterm labor and miscarriage

■ REFERENCES

1. Shnider SM, Webster GM: Maternal and fetal hazards of surgery during pregnancy. Am J Obstet Gynecol 1965;92:891-900.
2. Brodsky JB, Cohen EN, Brown BW, et al: Surgery during pregnancy and fetal outcome. Am J Obstet Gynecol 1980;138:1165-1167.
3. Duncan PG, Pope WDB, Cohen MM, Greer N: Fetal risk of anesthesia and surgery during pregnancy. Anesthesiology 1986;64:790-794.
4. Mazze RI, Kallen B: Reproductive outcome after anesthesia and operation during pregnancy: A registry study of 5405 cases. Am J Obstet Gynecol 1989;161:1178-1185.
5. Czeizel AE, Pataki T, Rockenbauer M: Reproductive outcome after exposure to surgery under general anesthesia during pregnancy. Arch Gynecol Obstet 1998;261:193-199.
6. Koblin DD, Waskel L, Watson JE, et al: Nitrous oxide inactivates methionine synthetase in human liver. Anesth Analg 1982;61:75-78.
7. Kallen B, Mazze RI: Neural tube defects and first trimester operations. Teratology 1990;41:717.
8. Sylvester GC, Khoury MJ, Lu X, Erickson JD: First-trimester anesthesia exposure and the risk of central nervous system defects: A population based case-control study. Am J Public Health 1994;84:1757-1760.
9. Jevtovic-Todorovic V, Hartman RE, Izumi Y, et al: Early exposure to common anesthetic agents causes widespread neurodegeneration in the developing rat brain and persistent learning deficits. J Neurosci 2003;23:876-882.
10. Thaler I, Manor D, Itskovitz J, et al: Changes in uterine blood flow during human pregnancy. Am J Obstet Gynecol 1990;162:121-125.
11. Wollman SB, Marx GF: Acute hydration for prevention of hypotension of spinal anesthesia in parturients. Anesthesiology 1968;29:374-380.
12. James FM III, Greiss FC, Kemp RA: An evaluation of vasopressor therapy for maternal hypotension during spinal anesthesia. Anesthesiology 1970;33:25-34.
13. Ralston DH, Shnider SM, DeLorimier AA: Effects of equipotent ephedrine, metaraminol, mephentermine, and methoxamine on uterine blood flow in the pregnant ewe. Anesthesiology 1974;40:354-370.
14. Ramanathan S, Grant GJ: Vasopressor therapy for hypotension due to epidural anesthesia for cesarean section. Acta Anaestheiol Scand 1988;32:559-565.
15. Moran DH, Perillo M, LaPorta RF, et al: Phenylephrine in the prevention of hypotension following spinal anesthesia for cesarean delivery. J Clin Anesth 1991;3:301-305.
16. Thomas DG, Robson SC, Redfern N, et al: Randomized trial of bolus phenylephrine or ephedrine for maintenance of arterial pressure during spinal anaesthesia for caesarean delivery. Br J Anaesth 1996;76:61-65.
17. Saravanan S, Kocarev M, Wilson RC, et al: Equivalent dose of ephedrine and phenylephrine in the prevention of post-spinal hypotension in caesarean section. Br J Anaesth 2006;96:95-99.
18. Lee A, Ngan Kee WD, Gin T: A quantitative, systematic review of randomized controlled trails of ephedrine versus phenylephrine for the management of hypotension during spinal anesthesia for cesarean delivery. Anesth Analg 2002;94:920-926.
19. Albers LL: Monitoring the fetus in labor: Evidence to support the methods. J Midwifery Women's Health 2001;46:366-373.
20. Electronic Fetal Heart Rate Monitoring: Research Guidelines for Interpretation. National Institute of Child Health and Human Development Research Planning Workshop. Am J Obstet Gynecol 1997;177:1385-1390.
21. Goodlin RC: History of fetal monitoring. Am J Obstet Gynecol 1979;133:323-352.
22. Ellison PH, Foster M, Sheridan-Pereira M, MacDonald D: Electronic fetal heart monitoring: Auscultation and neonatal outcome. Am J Obstet Gynecol 1991;164:1281-1289.
23. American College of Obstetricians and Gynecologists: Intrapartum fetal heart rate monitoring, ACOG Practice Bulletin No. 62. Obstet Gynecol 2005;105:1161-1167.
24. Kelso IM, Parsons RJ, Lawrence GF, et al: An assessment of continuous fetal heart rate monitoring: A randomized trial. Am J Obstet Gynecol 1978;131:526-532.
25. Hadar A, Sheiner E, Hallak M, et al: Abnormal fetal heart rate tracing patterns during the first stage of labor: Effect on perinatal outcome. Am J Obstet Gynecol 2001;185:863-868.
26. Sheiner E, Hadar A, Hallak M, et al: Clinical significance of fetal heart rate tracings during the second stage of labor. Obstet Gynecol 2001;97:747-752.
27. Williams KP, Galerneau F: Fetal heart rate parameters predictive of neonatal outcome in the presence of a prolonged deceleration. Obstet Gynecol 2002;100:951-954.
28. Kendrick JM, Woodard CB, Cross SB: Surveyed use of fetal and uterine monitoring during maternal surgery. AORN 1995;62:386-392.
29. Horrigan TJ, Villarred R, Weinstein L: Are obstetrical personnel required for intraoperative fetal monitoring during nonobstetric surgery? J Perinatol 1999;19:124-126.
30. American College of Obstetricians and Gynecologists: Nonobstetric surgery in pregnancy, ACOG Committee Opinion 284. Obstet Gynecol 2003;102:431.
31. Ong BY, Baron K, Stearns EL, et al: Severe fetal bradycardia in a pregnant patient despite normal oxygenation and blood pressure. Can J Anesth 2003;50:922-925.
32. Mendelson CL: The aspiration of stomach contents into the lungs during obstetric anesthesia. Am J Obstet Gynecol 1946;52:191-204.
33. James C, Modell J, Gibbs C, et al: Pulmonary aspiration: Effects of volume and pH in the rat. Anesth Analg 1984;63:665-668.
34. O'Sullivan GM, Sutton AJ, Thompson SA, et al: Noninvasive measurement of gastric emptying in obstetric patients. Anesth Analg 1987;66:505-511.
35. Attia RR, Ebeid AM, Fischer JE, Goudsouzian NG: Maternal, fetal, and placental gastrin concentrations. Anaesthesia 1982;37:18-21.
36. Chiloiro M, Darconza G, Piccioli E, et al: Gastric emptying and oroccal transit time in pregnancy. J Gastroenterol 2001;36:538-543.
37. Hong JY, Park JW, Oh JI: Comparison of preoperative gastric contents and serum gastrin concentrations in pregnant and nonpregnant women. J Clin Anesth 2005;17:451-455.
38. Chadwick HS: Obstetric anesthesia closed claims update II. ASA Newsletter 1999;63:6.
39. Soreide E, Bjornestad E, Steen PA: An audit of perioperative aspiration pneumonitis in gynaecological and obstetric patients. Acta Anaesthesiol Scand 1996;40:14-19.
40. Ezri T, Szmuk P, Stein A, et al: Peripartum general anesthesia without tracheal intubation: Incidence of aspiration pneumonia. Anaesthesia 2000;55:421-426.
41. Parpaglioni R, Capogna G, Celleno D, Fusco P: Intraoperative fetal oxygen saturation during caesarean section: General anaesthesia using sevoflurane with either 100% oxygen or 50% nitrous oxide. Eur J Anaesth 2002;19:115-118.
42. Kee WDN, Khaw KS, Ma KC, et al: Randomized, double-blind comparison of different inspired oxygen fractions during general anaesthesia for caesarean section. Br J Anaesth 2002;89:556-561.
43. Saugstad OD: Is oxygen more toxic than currently believed? Pediatrics 2001;108:1203-1205.
44. Khaw KS, Wang CC, Kee WDN, et al: Effects of high inspired oxygen fraction during elective caesarean section under spinal anaesthesia on maternal and fetal oxygenation and lipid peroxidation. Br J Anaesth 2002;88:18-23.
45. Rosen M: Management of anesthesia for the pregnant surgical patient. Anesthesiology 1999;9:1159-1166.
46. Chestnutt AN: Physiology of normal pregnancy. Crit Care Clin 2004;20:609-615.
47. Holthausen UH, Mettler L, Troidl H: Pregnancy: A Contraindication? World J Surg 1999;23:856-862.
48. Reynolds JD, Booth JV, de la Fuente S, et al: A review of laparoscopy for non-obstetric-related surgery during pregnancy. Curr Surg 2003;60:164-173.
49. Amos JD, Schorr SJ, Norman PF, et al: Laparoscopic surgery during pregnancy: A word of caution. Am J Surg 1996;171:435-437.
50. Southerland LC, Duke T, Gollagher JM, et al: Cardiopulmonary effects of abdominal insufflation in pregnancy: Fetal and maternal parameters in the sheep model. Can J Anaesth 1994;41:A59.
51. Curet MJ, Vogt DA, Schob O, et al: Effects of CO_2 pneumoperitoneum in pregnant ewes. J Surg Res 1996;63:339-344.
52. Barnard JM, Chaffin D, Droste S, et al: Fetal response to carbon dioxide pneumoperitoneum in the pregnant ewe. Obstet Gynecol 1995;85:669-674.

53. Cruz A, Southerland L, Duke T, et al: Intraabdominal carbon dioxide insufflation in the pregnant ewe: Uterine blood flow, intraamniotic pressure and cardiopulmonary effects. Anesthesiology 1996;85:1395-1402.

54. Hunter G, Swanstrom L, Thournburg K: Carbon dioxide pneumoperitoneum induces fetal acidosis in a pregnant ewe model. Surg Endosc 1995;9:272-279.

55. Uemura K, McClaine R, de la Fuente S, et al: Maternal insufflation during the second trimester equivalent produces hypercapnia, acidosis and prolonged hypoxia in fetal sheep. Anesthesiology 2004;101:1332-1338.

56. Bhavani-Shankar K, Steinbrook RA, Brooks DC, Datta S: Arterial to end-tidal carbon dioxide pressure difference during laparoscopic surgery in pregnancy. Anesthesiology 2000;93:370-376.

57. Gerstenfeld TS, Chang DT, Pliego AR, Wing DA: Nonobstetrical abdominal surgery during pregnancy in women's hospital. J Matern Fetal Med 2000;9:170-172.

58. Cohen-Kerem R, Railton C, Oren D, et al: Pregnancy outcome following non-obstetric surgical intervention. Am J Surg 2005;190:467-473.

59. Rizzo AG: Laparoscopic surgery in pregnancy: Long-term follow up. J Laparoendosc Adv Surg Tech A 2003;13:11-15.

PART IV

Early Postoperative Care

Specific Operations

Chapter

31 Cardiac Surgery

G. Burkhard Mackensen

Each year, more than 500,000 cardiac surgery procedures are performed in the United States, and, until recently, this number continued to grow annually.[1] Cardiac surgical patients are routinely admitted to the intensive care unit (ICU) for monitoring of recovery from anesthesia and surgery, rewarming after cardiopulmonary bypass (CPB), optimization of hemodynamics, monitoring for possible complications, and weaning from ventilatory support. The ICU has emerged as the dominant area where the complex transition from the operating room to sophisticated care occurs. With high volumes of cardiac surgery procedures, the postoperative care of these patients accounts for a significant percentage of ICU admissions at many institutions. Cardiothoracic surgery intensive care units (CT-ICUs) have evolved as a separate entity from the general surgical ICU as management for cardiac surgery patients has become streamlined and algorithm driven. Critical care is best managed when the service is designed for a homogeneous population with a circumscribed set of medical and surgical issues.

Traditionally, cardiac surgery patients remained in the ICU for a few days before discharge to the ward or step-down unit. Over the past decade, ICU management has changed in response to changing patient populations, new surgical and anesthetic techniques, and the penetration of managed care. Patients presenting for cardiac surgery are significantly older as the number of patients undergoing angioplasty and stenting procedures increases. Aggressive medical therapy and nonsurgical revascularization techniques also result in patients' presenting for surgery at more advanced stages of disease and with substantially more comorbidities. Furthermore, given the current market of health maintenance organizations (HMOs) and other cost-containment strategies, there is an ongoing trend toward accelerated care (e.g., fast-tracking), clinical care pathways, immediate weaning of ventilatory support, and earlier discharge from intensive care.

With the development of minimally invasive cardiac surgery, warm bypass, and off-pump bypass techniques, cardiac surgeons have altered the requirements for conventional postoperative recovery. Movement away from the opioid-based anesthetic techniques of the past to newer forms of balanced anesthesia with shorter-acting induction agents (propofol and etomidate), volatile agents (isoflurane and sevoflurane), and opioids (remifentanil) allow accelerated patient recovery from anesthesia. Consequently, intensivists need to develop strategies to manage this ever-changing patient population in an efficient and cost-effective manner while maintaining quality and minimizing morbidity and mortality. Effective postoperative management depends highly on each patient's preoperative status, intraoperative events, and condition on ICU arrival. Although the majority of institutions utilize the surgical ICU or specialized CT-ICU for postoperative care, avoidance of ICU admission altogether may be the future: some institutions utilize step-down units or short-stay intensive care for the weaning process and high dependency care.[2-4]

■ TRANSPORT AND INITIAL ASSESSMENT

The transport of the freshly operated cardiac surgery patient from the operating room to the ICU is not without risks and should be as smooth as possible.[5] Problems encountered during transport include acute changes in physiology (with hypovolemia being the most prevalent), sudden awakening, or serious bleeding. Once surgery is complete and the patient is stabilized in the operating room, the patient is transported to the ICU while still emerging from anesthesia. To improve comfort and safety, the patient is routinely monitored (electrocardiography [ECG], invasive blood pressure monitoring, and pulse oximetry) and maintained on sedation with short-acting agents such as propofol or dexmedetomidine supplemented with morphine when needed. This allows the patient to wake up gradually in the ICU while necessary monitoring devices are being attached and the intensivist evaluates the patient. There is little evidence to support extubation in the operating room compared with early extubation in the ICU after 2 to 3 hours of stabilization.[6]

Admission

During the transition of care from the anesthesiologist to the ICU team, the intensivist must become familiar with the patient's past and current medical history. Both the anesthesiologist and the cardiac surgeon should participate in the initial report to the intensivist. Preoperative and intraoperative events vary in magnitude and duration but typically result in a myocardium of reduced contractility and compliance, which affects the postoperative management and eventual outcome.[7-9] Essential data include indication for surgery, the surgical procedure, preoperative cardiac function, cardiac catheterization findings, number of arterial and venous grafts, location of donor sites for the arterial grafts, valves repaired or replaced, bypass and cross-clamp times, difficulties weaning from the bypass pump, and post-bypass cardiac assessment with pulmonary arterial catheter measurements or transesophageal echocardiography (TEE). It is also important to know the adequacy of homeostasis, the patient's individual response to volume and vasoactive agents, the number and position of drains, whether cardiac pacing was required, and whether the procedure was a "redo." Redo procedures (repeat sternotomy or thoracotomy) are technically more challenging and tend to result in greater blood loss and higher complication rates. Finally, the amount and type of fluids and any blood products administered, the expected postoperative course, and any specific postoperative guidelines (e.g., blood pressure targets, time plan for weaning) should be communicated to the ICU team.

A standard admission includes routine admission orders (ideally using a computerized physician order entry system); the initiation of controlled ventilatory support; the transition of all transport monitoring to routine bedside monitoring; the inspection of all surgical sites; the position of the endotracheal tube, surgical drains, and invasive catheters; the conduct of a 12-lead ECG; a chest radiograph, and routine laboratory data. The patient's core and peripheral temperatures, the amount of drainage from the chest tubes, the oxygen saturation (SpO_2) and end-tidal partial pressure of carbon dioxide ($PETCO_2$), the fluid input and urinary output, and the hemodynamic status need to be assessed. The extent of hemodynamic monitoring depends on the patient's perioperative condition and anticipated complications during and after cardiac surgery. As a minimum, patients should have an arterial line, a central venous pressure (CVP) line, and a urinary catheter. The recent trend has been away from pulmonary artery (PA) catheterization, partly as a result of work by Connors and colleagues and partly because of the increased utilization of intraoperative TEE and other less invasive cardiac output monitors.[10-12] The data derived from these monitors are sufficient to address the majority of clinical situations.

Routine laboratory analysis on admission includes arterial blood gases to assess acid–base status and alveolar–arterial oxygen gradient, and blood chemistry. Potassium and magnesium plasma levels need to be kept above 4.0 and 2.0 mmol/L, respectively, to minimize the incidence of cardiac dysrhythmias.[13-16] Potassium repletion may not be successful without restoration of magnesium stores.[13,17,18] A complete blood count is required to guide transfusion therapy, and a coagulation profile is measured to assess potential clotting factor deficiency. An activated clotting time may also be used as a point-of-care test for adequate reversal of heparin given during surgery. The incorporation of thromboelastography (TEG) as a point-of-care monitor into a transfusion algorithm allows more specific diagnosis of bleeding problems and reduction of indiscriminant transfusion practices.[19] A routine chest radiograph is obtained to evaluate lung volume and to exclude pneumothorax or parenchymal infiltrates, as well as to confirm correct position of support equipment such as the endotracheal tube, invasive catheters, and chest tubes.[20]

■ RESPIRATORY MANAGEMENT

Mechanical Ventilation

In patients undergoing coronary artery bypass grafting (CABG), the traditional period of postoperative mechanical ventilation used to be less than 3 days but usually between 1 and 2 days.[21] Despite the introduction of clinical care pathways and novel organizational features of ICUs over the past decade, with resulting improved clinical outcomes, shortened mechanical ventilation, and decreased costs,[22-25] it is rare for patients to be extubated in the operating room. Immediate changes in respiratory function as a consequence of cardiac surgery and CPB include significant decreases in vital capacity, total lung capacity, and functional residual capacity, increased pulmonary edema correlating with the length of CPB, and atelectasis. Therefore, most patients require some ventilatory support for the first 4 to 8 postoperative hours. However, short-acting anesthetic agents such as propofol and dexmedetomidine facilitate a gradual low-stress emergence from anesthesia without the need for prolonged ventilation.[26] Early versus late endotracheal extubation after cardiac surgery has been shown to reduce the length of stay in the ICU and the hospital length of stay, to lower associated costs, to improve left ventricular function, and to decrease cardiopulmonary morbidity.[23,24,27]

With traditional protocols, the initial ventilator settings are aimed to provide complete support of the work of breathing for the patient. Traditionally, intermittent mandatory ventilation (IMV) with relatively high tidal volumes (8 to 10 cm^3/kg), low respiratory rates (8 to 10 breaths/min), and low positive end-expiratory pressure (PEEP) of 5 cm H_2O is initiated. The fraction of inspired oxygen (FIO_2) is normally set at 60% and is reduced as quickly as appropriate. The partial pressure of arterial carbon dioxide ($PaCO_2$) should be maintained at 40 to 44 mm Hg to maintain the CO_2-mediated stimulus to breathe. Patients arriving at the ICU with spontaneous breathing efforts can immediately be transitioned into some type of pressure support ventilation (PSV) mode with support levels of 10 to 15 cm H_2O. Early extubation soon

31-1	Criteria for Extubation after Cardiac Surgery
Central nervous system	Patient awake and following commands; pain controlled Neuromuscular blocking agents fully reversed or dissipated Cough and gag reflexes present; able to protect airway
Respiratory system	Adequate oxygenation and ventilation on minimal ventilatory support such as CPAP or T-piece (pH = 7.35; PaO_2 >80 mm Hg; $PaCO_2$ <50 mm Hg; FiO_2 <0.5; RR >10/min and <30/min; f/V_T ratio <100) Minimal secretions; chest radiograph within expectations
Hemodynamics	Hemodynamically stable with MAP >70 mm Hg, cardiac index >2.2/min/m^2, not on an IABP
Cardiac system	HR <110/min, stable cardiac rhythm
Renal system	Urine output >0.5 mL/kg/min
Hematologic system	No significant bleeding, with chest tube drainage <50 mL/hr
Temperature	Core temperature >36°C

CPAP, continuous positive airway pressure; FiO_2, fraction of inspired oxygen; f/V_T, respiratory rate/tidal volume; HR, heart rate; IABP, intraaortic balloon pump; MAP, mean arterial pressure; $PaCO_2$, partial pressure of arterial carbon dioxide; PaO_2, partial pressure of arterial oxygen; RR, respiratory rate.

31-2	Factors Predicting Successful Weaning from Mechanical Ventilation

Mechanical

Respiratory rate <25/min
Vital capacity >12-15 mL/kg
Maximal negative inspiratory pressure <–25 cm H_2O
Minute ventilation (V_m) <10 L/min
Maximal voluntary ventilation >2 × resting V_m
Respiratory rate (f) ÷ tidal volume (V_T) ratio <105

Gas Exchange

pH = 7.35
PaO_2 >60 mm Hg (FiO_2 <0.4)
PaO_2/FiO_2 ratio >200
Alveolar-arterial PO_2 <350 mm Hg

after admission to the ICU or extubation in the operating room is one essential component of fast-track protocols.

Routinely, weaning from ventilatory support can start once the patient spontaneously breathes over the rate set on the ventilator. Weaning should not be aggressive until the patient meets certain established criteria (Box 31-1).[28-30] These criteria relate to the patient's neurologic, hemodynamic, cardiac, respiratory, and renal status and define an awake, normothermic, and hemodynamically stable patient who most likely will not need to return to the operating room for cardiac tamponade or bleeding. One method of weaning is to gradually reduce the rate set on the ventilator by 2 breaths/min every 30 minutes until reaching a rate of zero with continuous positive airway pressure (CPAP) and 10 cm H_2O of pressure support. The patient who can maintain a reasonable gas exchange and is not tachypneic after 30 minutes on CPAP is ready to have the endotracheal tube removed. At some institutions, the patient's pulmonary mechanics (Box 31-2) are evaluated for further confirmation. An alternative weaning strategy is to attempt CPAP trials every 30 minutes until a certain set criterion is satisfied (see Box 31-2). Both methods are safe and neither has any clear advantage over the other. However, most patients undergoing cardiac surgery with normal pulmonary function preoperatively do not require a gradual wean from the ventilator. If the patient has remained stable during recovery from anesthesia and has no significant pulmonary disease, a rapid decrease in ventilator support to minimal levels can be safely instituted under close observation, and the patient can be

evaluated for extubation. The method of removal from ventilatory assistance varies between institutions depending on the characteristics of the individual ICU.

Long-term Ventilation and Weaning

The occurrence of respiratory complications and the duration of endotracheal intubation have been shown to correlate with mortality in patients who have undergone cardiac operations.[31,32] Because mechanical ventilation can have life-threatening complications, it should be discontinued at the earliest possible time. It is important to realize that prolonged intubation time may lead to respiratory tract mucociliary dysfunction, diminished clearing of secretions, additional sedation, and increased atelectasis and ventilator-associated pneumonia.[27,33] The process of discontinuing mechanical ventilation, termed weaning, is one of the most challenging problems in intensive care, and it accounts for a considerable proportion of the workload of ICU staff.[34]

Most cardiac surgical patients are expeditiously weaned from mechanical ventilation, but up to 6% of all patients undergoing CABG surgery require mechanical ventilation for more than 1 day, and approximately 2% remain on the ventilator for more than 2 weeks.[21] Identification of preoperative risk factors limiting the ability to wean from mechanical ventilation has been difficult, but common factors include age, marked neurologic deficits, acute renal failure with volume overload, limited perioperative cardiac function, unstable hemodynamics, and sepsis.[35,36] Other intraoperative and postoperative predictors of failure to wean include prolonged CPB, preexisting pulmonary disease (e.g., chronic obstructive pulmonary disease [COPD]), diaphragmatic paralysis, malnutrition, and high oxygen requirements.[27,37-39]

The difference in oxygen consumption between spontaneous and total mechanical ventilation can be substantial.[40] Routine preoperative pulmonary function tests have failed to serve as predictors for prolonged mechanical ventilation.[41] Risk stratification with established scoring systems has led to mixed results when predicting the length of endotracheal intubation after cardiac surgery.[42,43] Methods used to wean from mechanical ventilation include synchronized intermittent mandatory ventilation (SIMV), pressure support ventilation (PSV), and T-piece trials with spontaneous breathing. Until the early 1990s, all weaning methods were considered equally effective, and the intensivist's judgment was regarded as the critical determinant.[44] This has changed with the results of randomized controlled trials that revealed that the period of weaning is up to three times longer with IMV compared with trials of spontaneous breathing.[45,46] Spontaneous breathing trials may be as short as 30 minutes and appear to be as effective when performed once a day as several times a day.[46,47]

Protocol-driven weaning from mechanical ventilation or automated weaning protocols may facilitate the challenging task of weaning.[22,25,29] Scheduled assessment of respiratory mechanics may also predict successful weaning. Among patients who cannot be weaned, disconnection from the ventilator is followed almost immediately by an increase in respiratory rate and a fall in tidal volume—that is, rapid, shallow breathing.[48] The respiratory rate/tidal volume (f/V_T) ratio has been used with some success as a predictor of failure to wean. An f/V_T ratio greater than 105 resulted in 95% of patients failing to wean, whereas an f/V_T ratio less than 105 resulted in a weaning success of 80%.[38] In a randomized trial, a two-stage approach to weaning—systematic measurement of predictors, including f/V_T, followed by a single daily trial of spontaneous breathing—was compared with conventional management.[49] Although the patients assigned to the two-stage approach were generally sicker than those assigned to conventional weaning, they were weaned twice as rapidly. This approach was not only cost effective but also lowered the incidence of complications when compared with conventional management.

In addition to the increase in respiratory effort, an unsuccessful attempt at spontaneous breathing causes considerable cardiovascular stress.[35] Patients can have substantial increases in right and left ventricular afterload, with increases of 39% and 27% in pulmonary and systemic arterial pressures, respectively,[50] most likely because the negative swings in intrathoracic pressure are more extreme. One of the most common reasons for failure to wean is pulmonary edema, which worsens gas exchange and increases work of breathing. The correct diagnosis is made with a careful clinical examination, assessment of net fluid balance, and review of a chest radiograph. The etiology of the pulmonary edema will guide therapy. Careful attention to fluid balance and aggressive diuresis or use of ultrafiltration as indicated for patients with good cardiac function are essential components of therapy. Patients with poor cardiac function and pulmonary edema need afterload reduction and/or inodilator therapy in combination with diuresis in preparation for successful extubation.

Long-term management of failure to wean is facilitated by performing a tracheostomy, which allows better secretion control and utilization of intermittent ventilation but carries the risk of higher rates of mediastinitis.[51,52] A comparison of open versus bedside percutaneous dilatational tracheostomy in cardiothoracic surgical patients revealed no significant clinical differences but the potential for significant cost savings with the latter.[53]

■ STABILIZATION PHASE

Perfusion Pressure

Adequacy of perfusion and cardiac output (CO) can routinely be assessed with the clinical evaluation of heart rate (HR), heart rhythm, blood pressure (BP), skin perfusion, capillary refill, and urine output.[54] A patient with good skin perfusion and values within a normal range for mean arterial blood pressure (MAP), heart rate (HR), and urine probably has a normal CO and sufficient perfusion. However, these parameters remain insensitive indicators of dysoxia and are considered to be poor surrogates of markers for oxygen delivery at the tissue level, because tissue oxygenation is determined by the net balance between cellular oxygen supply and oxygen demand. Indirect measures of tissue perfusion and oxygenation include the calculation of oxygen delivery or the measurement of mixed venous oxygen saturation (SvO_2). SvO_2 can be readily measured from blood gas analysis derived at the bedside either intermittently or continuously with a fiberoptic PA catheter. The importance of monitoring arterial lactate levels in critically ill patients has been advocated, and concentrations of greater than 2 mmol/L are generally considered a biochemical marker of inadequate oxygenation.[55,56] Other methods to assess organ perfusion include gastrointestinal tonometry, near-infrared spectroscopy, and direct monitoring of tissue oxygenation with miniaturized implantable Clark electrodes.[57-59]

Blood Pressure

One of the most dynamic physiologic variables during the first hour of postoperative ICU care is the MAP, which changes rapidly as a result of dynamic alterations in both preload and ventricular compliance.[60] Significant vasodilation from a loss of vasomotor tone is also a frequent early contributor to a decreased MAP. Other less common causes for acute changes in MAP include a reduced heart rate, an acute deterioration of myocardial contractility, and a loss of atrioventricular synchrony. Although hypotension has no concrete definition, the general agreement is that the goal of therapy is a MAP of 70 to 80 mm Hg, and that a systolic BP of less than 90 mm Hg or a MAP of less than 60 mm Hg denotes hypotension. In older adult patients and those with preexisting cerebrovascular or renal disease, a higher MAP may be required. On the other hand, if the cardiac surgeon has determined the risk of bleeding to be greater than usual, the goals for MAP may be lowered. However, the patient's baseline BP must be considered, as that determines the range of autoregulation for end organs such as the brain or kidney. After CABG surgery, MAP needs to be high enough to ensure that newly placed bypass grafts remain patent. Also, diastolic BP is a major determinant of myocardial blood flow, so attention must be paid to diastolic BP if myocardial ischemia is evident.

Hypovolemia is the most common cause of hypotension in the postoperative patient. Peripheral rewarming causes vasodilation, requiring expansion of circulating blood volume for treatment. Ongoing bleeding requires intravascular volume replacement. Diagnosis of hypovolemia relies on both clinical observation (chest tube output) and invasive pressure measurements. Isolated measurements of CVP and pulmonary capillary occlusion pressure (PCOP) are less helpful than trends in these measurements or their response to a fluid bolus. Scientific investigation lacks sufficient evidence of the best resuscitation fluid to use in cardiac surgery patients. Blood products, albumin, or similar colloid and normal saline or hypertonic solutions are all being used, depending on the hemoglobin level and coagulation status. Hetastarch, up to 2 L, has been used successfully without excessive bleeding, although associated hemodilution and the possibility of coagulopathy need to be considered. Routinely, a rapidly administered fluid challenge of 250 to 500 mL tests the initial response to hypotension. This volume resuscitation should continue until the MAP responds. An intraoperative TEE provides valuable information about which CVPs, PA occlusion pressures, or PA diastolic pressures correspond with adequate left ventricular (LV) filling. These pressures are low in the presence of hypovolemia and high in the presence of LV dysfunction. Preoperative cardiac catheterization data, particularly LV end-diastolic pressure, is a useful predictor of postoperative LV systolic or diastolic dysfunction. Often, fluid resuscitation alone is fully successful in maintaining an effective MAP and perfusion.

Alternative diagnostic and therapeutic options need to be considered if preload resuscitation is not successful and MAP becomes significantly compromised or usual fluid resuscitation maximums (approximately 1 to 2 L) are exceeded. Vasodilation with associated, often severe, hypotension is a frequent complication occurring in up to 8% of patients after CPB and cardiac surgery.[61] Although the underlying mechanisms of this vasodilatory shock remain elusive, low ejection fraction and angiotensin-converting enzyme inhibitor use have been identified as predisposing factors, and anesthetic drugs, peripheral rewarming, anemia, and variable degrees of a systemic inflammatory response to the extracorporeal circuit may contribute.[61-63] Vasodilation, per se, is not undesirable and it is important to treat hypotension by addressing inadequate CO (preload, contractility, and HR) prior to increasing the systemic vascular resistance (SVR), except as a temporizing measure to maintain coronary perfusion while other therapy is initiated.[64] While volume resuscitation proceeds, vasopressor therapy is initiated with agents such as norepinephrine, phenylephrine, vasopressin, and (rarely) methylene blue.[61,65,66] When high-dose norepinephrine (>0.1 mg/kg/min) is required, arginine vasopressin has proven useful in increasing BP and reducing norepinephrine requirements, especially in patients undergoing placement of a left ventricular assist device (LVAD).[67] When vasoconstrictors are used for a prolonged period, it is essential to avoid hypovolemia, as severe peripheral hypoperfusion with gangrene may result.

Calcium increases BP without decreasing CO and has a negligible effect on HR. However, routine use of calcium to treat hypotension and low CO after cardiac surgery is controversial. Bolus administration of calcium may impair internal mammary artery (IMA) flow and potentially triggers vasospasm.[68] Furthermore, it is undesirable for ionized calcium levels to be abnormally high, so repeated administration should be guided by blood levels. Low blood levels

may result from rapid blood product transfusion and can reduce vascular responsiveness to catecholamines. A normal ionized calcium level is the goal.

Positive-pressure ventilation may produce relative hypovolemia, especially in patients with COPD, by eliminating the normal venous pressure gradient for filling of the right atrium. The presence of intrinsic positive end-expiratory pressure is diagnostic of this condition. Adjustment of ventilator settings to increase expiratory time will help alleviate this problem. The development of a tension pneumothorax as the result of chest tube obstruction or occult intraoperative lung injury on a side not drained by a chest tube (usually the right) can also acutely compromise right heart filling. Assurance that breath sounds are present and symmetric on arrival in the surgical ICU, as well as scrutiny of the initial postoperative chest radiograph, will identify this potential complication and guide the therapy (e.g., chest tube placement).

Some patients present with postoperative hypertension, instead of hypotension, in the ICU.[69] Systemic BP needs to be controlled, with a combination of nitroglycerin and nitroprusside infusion, to a mean BP range of 70 to 80 mm Hg because an excessive MAP may augment bleeding and create excessive afterload, whereas myocardial contractility and compliance are compromised and myocardial oxygen demand increases. Postoperative hypertension may be caused by increases in SVR, hypoxia, hypercarbia, pain, inadequate sedation, or hypothermia-induced shivering. Before therapy with vasodilating agents is initiated, these causes need to be ruled out or treated. Nitroprusside and nitroglycerin are routinely used, and alternative medications include nicardipine, labetalol, hydralazine, and esmolol. The vasodilation provided by propofol may also be helpful to modify blood pressure. Nitroprusside is widely used because it acts rapidly and can be easily titrated to effect and in response to sudden changes in preload and afterload. However, its use has been associated with the need for compensatory volume replacement, reflex tachycardia, toxicity, and metabolic acidosis. The hallmark of intravenous nicardipine is arterial specificity, which allows precise titration of blood pressure irrespective of intravascular volume.[70,71] This property is significant in perioperative hypertension, because arterial vasoconstriction with varying degrees of intravascular hypovolemia is a central characteristic. Nicardipine results in decreased mean arterial pressure (average drop, −18 mm Hg) and systemic vascular resistance, and an increase in cardiac output, but it does not affect filling pressures.[72,73]

Cardiac Output

The routine use of continuous or intermittent measurements of calculated hemodynamic indices is not necessary for low-risk patients undergoing routine CABG.[74] However, today's widespread use of PA catheters or other CO monitors allows most ICU teams to assess CO with a target cardiac index (CI, equal to CO per body surface area) of greater than 2.0 L/min/m^2. Manipulation of the CO is aimed at maximizing the pumping capacity of the cardiovascular system. A decreasing CI should be addressed before signs of overt hypoperfusion and tissue hypoxia develop, even if the baseline CI was similarly low. Clinical measures of right and left ventricular performance, such as preload or volume status, afterload (SVR), HR, and myocardial contractility, are essential to guide therapy toward a stable hemodynamic status.[54] Blood, crystalloid, or colloid may be infused to increase preload. CI can also be improved by optimizing afterload with a vasodilator such as nitroprusside. With an optimized preload and afterload, CI can sometimes be increased by atrial or atrioventricular (AV)-sequential pacing using epicardial pacing wires at a higher rate over the intrinsic HR. If preload and afterload are optimized, stroke volume (SV) would normally remain the same and a higher HR would increase the CI. If the target CI of greater than 2.0 $L/min/m^2$ is not achieved with optimization of preload, afterload, and HR, inotropic agents are usually required to improve cardiac contractility. There do not appear to be significant differences among the commonly used inotropes, but cardiac surgeons and intensivists often have personal preferences based on familiarity with the agent and clinical experience. One critical distinction to make in a hypotensive patient is between the relative intravascular hypovolemia from vasodilation during warming and the hypovolemia secondary to bleeding. Myocardial contractility may further diminish during the immediate postoperative period,[9,60] mandating continued inotropic support or augmentation of support with mechanical assistance (e.g., intra-aortic balloon pump [IABP]).

An array of inotropic agents exists, including epinephrine, milrinone, dobutamine, and dopamine. Intimate knowledge of each drug's inotropic, vasodilatory or vasoconstrictive, and chronotropic profile is warranted to achieve the desired effect. Combinations of inotropic and vasoconstrictive agents are selected when significantly reduced contractility is associated with severe hypotension. This is typical for phosphodiesterase inhibitors such as milrinone that often provide the wanted inotropic effect but not without significant vasodilation. Therefore, norepinephrine or vasopressin may be required in combination with milrinone to address the typical postoperative vasodilation and that related to the milrinone. Combining milrinone and epinephrine allows utilizing their different inotropic actions together with the vasoconstrictive effect of epinephrine for the treatment of hypotension. If the need for milrinone is anticipated in the operating room, it is ideally started during CPB to avoid a loading dose with its inherent hypotension. Dopamine is often selected as a first-choice agent to either increase CO or to allow weaning of epinephrine, but it might result in excessive tachycardia and increase the risk for atrial fibrillation. Dobutamine is generally associated with a positive chronotropic response and may be a good choice to increase CO if pulmonary artery pressures are elevated and baseline heart rate is low.[75]

Modes of Mechanical Support

Mechanical cardiac support is either initiated preemptively in the operating room or provided in the ICU when low CO persists despite adequate preload and afterload and maximized inotropic support. Insertion of an IABP is indicated for treatment of cardiogenic shock or low CO states, treatment of intractable angina, failure to wean from CPB, and, if indicated, as a prophylactic measure in patients at high risk

for cardiac failure. With optimized IABP and a normal sinus rhythm, cardiac output may rise by up to 20% while the diastolic pressure increases by 30%. Left and/or right ventricular assist devices (LVAD, RVAD) are placed when poor cardiac function demands either intermittent or long-term replacement therapy. Pulsatile (e.g., Abiomed or Heartmate I) and nonpulsatile (Heartmate II or Biomedicus centrifugal pump) assist devices are available. If an LVAD or RVAD is placed emergently, the goal of therapy is to achieve a stable CI of greater than 2.2 L/min. Weaning is ideally conducted in the operating room, and TEE allows assessing cardiac function while the pump's contribution is decreased. If adequate CO can be sustained and atrial pressures remain within acceptable limits while the assist device provides only minimal support, successful removal may be feasible. Frequently, continuation of IABP and increased inotropic support are essential to allow removal.

■ POSTOPERATIVE COMPLICATIONS

Bleeding

Patients undergoing cardiac surgery with CPB frequently have a variety of derangements of hemostasis (with striking interpatient variability poorly explained by clinical, procedural, biological, and genetic markers) that frequently result in transfusion of allogeneic blood products.[76] More than 12 million units of allogeneic red blood cells (RBCs) are administered in the United States annually, with more than 2 million units administered to patients undergoing cardiovascular surgery.[77] Institutions vary significantly in perioperative blood conservation and transfusion practices for cardiac surgery patients. Depending on the institution, between 27% and 92% of CABG patients are transfused, and the number of units of packed cells received ranges from 0 to 4.[77,78] Patients undergoing repeat sternotomy for cardiac surgery are approximately three times more likely to receive a perioperative transfusion than those undergoing primary cardiac surgery.[79] Transfusion-related complications have decreased significantly in the last 10 to 15 years but still remain a concern.

The transfusion of allogeneic RBCs has recently been described as a risk factor for decreased long-term survival after CABG surgery.[80] Another recent study showed that the storage duration of perioperatively transfused RBCs is associated with an increased risk of both short-term in-hospital and long-term out-of-hospital mortality, independent of the number of transfusions administered and other confounding factors.[81] Other risks include hepatitis C infection (approximately 1 in 50,000), transmission of the human immunodeficiency virus (less than 1 in 500,000), major ABO group incompatibility (less than 1 in 33,000), and minor transfusion reactions (approximately 1 in 5).[82,83]

According to the American Society of Anesthesiologists (ASA), the cost of transfusion therapy approaches 5 to 7 billion dollars per year in the United States, with up to 25% of RBC transfusions judged to be unnecessary. The ASA strongly advocates judicious use of blood products and has published a set of practice guidelines.[82] Although practice guidelines are imperfect and must not replace clinical judgment, the ASA guidelines provide a scientifically based model to assist decision making. However, in the cardiac surgical patient population, the ASA guidelines fail to account for platelet dysfunction known to occur after CPB. When major bleeding occurs in this patient group, platelet transfusion is indicated even when platelet count is greater than 100,000.[84]

Unfortunately, practice guidelines such as those from the ASA and the College of American Pathologists do not seem to change old transfusion habits, and inappropriate use of blood products has not been curtailed, especially in the cardiac surgical population.[85] One possible reason for lack of success is that the time delay until coagulation results return from the laboratory makes directed transfusion therapy difficult in a bleeding patient. In response to this problem, several rapid assay devices are being developed. When combined with goal-directed transfusion algorithms, such point-of-care tests may improve care and limit unnecessary transfusions (Fig. 31-1).[19,86] These algorithms usually incorporate some measure of platelet function, coagulation factor activity, and fibrinolysis as the stimulus for therapy. Although not perfect, thromboelastography appears to be a key component of such algorithms. Because its negative predictive value is greater than 90%, a normal TEG implies with greater than 90% certainty that a bleeding patient needs to return to the operating room and a surgical bleeder will be found. Incorporation of TEG produced a significantly reduced rate of reoperation for bleeding in a single-center study.[86]

Other strategies for limiting blood product requirements show some benefit in clinical trials. Antifibrinolytic therapy decreases the incidence of excessive postoperative bleeding caused by coagulopathy.[87-89] Effective antifibrinolytic agents include ε-aminocaproic acid, tranexamic acid, and aprotinin. Aprotinin is the only agent with class A level 1 evidence for reduction in rates of transfusion and return to operating room to control bleeding after heart surgery. However, data presented recently from a large observational database analysis suggested that aprotinin should be withdrawn from human use, as serious safety issues have been ignored or missed.[90] Primary safety issues raised over the years include an increased risk for thrombosis and renal dysfunction. The latter appears to be confirmed with a recent propensity-score case-control comparison of aprotinin and tranexamic acid in high-transfusion-risk cardiac surgery study by Karkouti and colleagues.[91] As the controversy about aprotinin versus other fibrinolytic agents continues, further insights can be expected from a large randomized prospective multicenter trial currently under way in Canada.[92]

Intraoperative autologous hemodilution has also demonstrated a blood-sparing effect in some studies,[93] but postoperative use of cell salvage has not proven to be effective in limiting the use of blood products in cardiac surgery.[94] Reinfusion of shed mediastinal blood may be associated with a greater frequency of wound infection.[95]

In current postoperative practice, hemostasis is assessed by measuring the amount of blood draining out of the chest tubes. Prothrombin time and activated partial thromboplastin time are normally slightly elevated after cardiac surgery. An activated clotting time may also be used as a point-of-care test for adequate reversal of heparin given during surgery. As outlined earlier, the incorporation of TEG as a point-of-care monitor into specific transfusion algorithm allows a more specific diagnosis of bleeding problems and a reduction of indiscriminant transfusion practices.[19] Fresh frozen plasma (FFP) is not required when there is no significant drainage from the chest tubes; if drainage from the chest tube exceeds 400 mL in the first 2 hours and 100 to 150 mL/hr after the first 2 hours, FFP is probably required to stop the bleeding. Infusion of 10 mL/kg of FFP normally restores the coagulation factors to an adequate level. It is also important to consider platelet transfusion in a bleeding patient after CPB even if the platelet count is greater than 100,000/μL, as platelet function might be impaired. In cases of most severe bleeding,

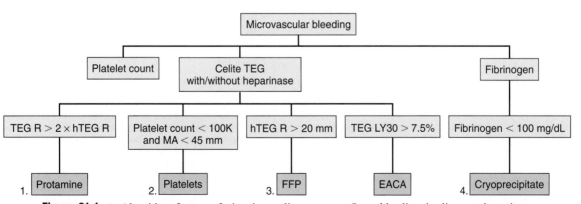

Figure 31-1 ■ Algorithm for transfusion in cardiac surgery. Once bleeding is diagnosed, patients receive blood transfusions based on the results of the tests in the algorithm. Because bleeding is often platelet related and the platelet count and thromboelastography (TEG) results are returned promptly, therapy is given in the numbered order of priority. EACA, ε-aminocaproic acid; FFP, fresh-frozen plasma; hTEG, heparinase-activated TEG; LY30, lysis index at 30 min; MA, maximum amplitude; R, reaction time. *(Adapted with permission from Shore-Lesserson L, Manspeizer HE, DePerio M, et al: Anesth Analg 1999;88:312-319.)*

cryoprecipitate and activated factor VII are added after platelet and FFP transfusion have failed. The value of activated factor VII in this setting needs to be further assessed in larger clinical trials.[96,97] The chest tubes need to be evaluated on a regular basis to avoid clogging by blood clots. When there is a sudden decrease in drainage from the chest tubes, the intensivist should exclude the possibility of concealed bleeding in the mediastinum and pericardial sac, which can lead to cardiac tamponade. If the response to the FFP and platelet infusion is not satisfactory, exploratory re-sternotomy should be seriously considered.[98,99]

Cardiac Dysrhythmia

Transient alterations in heart rate or conduction may contribute to postoperative hypotension or low cardiac output. When BP or CO is marginal, augmenting the heart rate should be considered, even if it is already in the normal range. Abnormal patterns within the first 24 hours include transient bradydysrhythmias, sinus tachycardia (>110 beats/min), and, in cases of valvular surgery, junctional tachycardia with atrioventricular interference or even heart block. Significant ventricular dysrhythmias are rare but if present may present a challenge to treatment.

Bradydysrhythmias are common after cardiac surgery, and atrial and ventricular epicardial pacing wires are typically placed to facilitate temporary pacing in the immediate postoperative period. Optimal pacing modalities have been investigated.[100] Dual-chamber pacing maximizes CO over a wide range of AV delay (100 to 225 msec). Conditions impairing diastolic filling (ventricular hypertrophy, cardiomyopathy, fibrosis) may benefit by extending the AV delay.

The rate of pacemaker dependency varies between studies and is approximately 1% after CABG, 2% after primary valve replacement, 7% after repeat valve replacement, and 10% after orthotopic heart transplant (OHT).[101-103] Identified risk factors include perivalvular calcification, older age, preoperative left bundle branch block, and increased CPB time. The etiology of bradydysrhythmia includes ischemia, edema, and irreversible surgical destruction of the conducting system. Recovery from the reversible causes can be considerably delayed. Permanent pacemakers are typically implanted for symptomatic sinus node dysfunction or AV block lasting beyond the fifth postoperative day. In the long term, up to 40% of patients with sinus node dysfunction and up to 100% of patients with complete AV block past day 5 remain pacemaker dependent.

For heart transplant patients, chronotropic medication may avoid the need for a permanent pacemaker.[104] Sinus node dysfunction is five times more likely than AV block to result in permanent pacemaker implantation in this group. Both types of dysfunction can be significantly reduced with bicaval rather than biatrial anastomoses.[103]

Atrial dysrhythmias (primarily atrial fibrillation [AF]) are by far the most common complication after cardiac surgery, with an incidence consistently reported to range between 27% and 40% and with little change over the past 2 decades.[105] AF most commonly occurs 2 to 3 days after surgery and can increase hospital stay, risk of stroke, risk of neurocognitive deficits, and mortality.[106-110] Those who have

undergone valvular surgery are at greatest risk. Patients with preexisting AF may return from the operating room in sinus rhythm and soon revert back to AF. If an atrial epicardial lead is in place, an atrial cardiogram cannot be conducted when the rhythm or conduction cannot otherwise be diagnosed.[111] Use of adenosine is another option for diagnosis and possible therapy when the atrial arrhythmia is not AF.[112] The exact pathogenesis of postoperative AF is unclear. Structural changes in the atria, reduced threshold for dysrhythmia generation, and a hyperadrenergic state after CPB and surgery are all suggested as mechanisms. Associated risk factors for the development of AF include advanced age, history of atrial fibrillation or chronic obstructive pulmonary disease, prolonged CPB and aortic cross-clamp times, left atrial enlargement, cardiomegaly, valve surgery, and postoperative withdrawal of a beta-blocker or an angiotensin-converting enzyme (ACE) inhibitor.[105,106,110]

Pharmacologic prophylaxis against AF is controversial. Prophylactic therapy includes supplemental magnesium and beta-blockade in the perioperative period to reduce the incidence of AF.[113,114] The American College of Cardiology and American Heart Association task force consensus recommendations for prevention and management of postoperative AF are summarized in Box 31-3.[115,116] In the largest trial of amiodarone in patients undergoing CABG surgery or valve replacement or repair surgery reported to date, prophylactic amiodarone was shown to effectively reduce the incidence of postoperative AF.[117] Management of postoperative

---

31-3	**Recommendations for Prevention and Management of Postoperative Atrial Fibrillation**

Class I

- Treat patients undergoing cardiac surgery with an oral beta-blocker to prevent postoperative atrial fibrillation (AF), unless contraindicated. (Level of evidence: A)
- In patients who develop postoperative AF, achieve rate control by administration of atrioventricular (AV) nodal blocking agents. (Level of evidence: B)

Class IIa

- Administer sotalol or amiodarone prophylactically to patients at increased risk of developing postoperative AF. (Level of evidence: B)
- Restore sinus rhythm in patients who develop postoperative AF by pharmacologic cardioversion with ibutilide or direct-current cardioversion, as recommended for nonsurgical patients. (Level of evidence: B)
- In patients with recurrent or refractory postoperative AF, attempt maintenance of sinus rhythm by administration of antiarrhythmic medications, as recommended for patients with coronary artery disease who develop AF. (Level of evidence: B)
- Administer antithrombotic medication in patients who develop postoperative AF, as recommended for nonsurgical patients. (Level of evidence: B)

Reproduced with permission from Fuster V, Ryden LE, Cannom DS, et al: Circulation 2006;114:e257-354.

supraventricular tachycardia (SVT) depends on the patient's clinical condition. If appropriate, a 12-lead ECG and an atrial rhythm strip via the atrial pacing electrodes aid diagnosis of the exact rhythm. Postoperative therapy of AF includes the correction of electrolyte abnormalities, empirical administration of magnesium and potassium, and amiodarone or beta-blockade. If pharmacologic restoration of sinus rhythm fails or if hemodynamic instability merits immediate synchronized direct current (DC) cardioversion, electrical cardioversion is attempted with an initial energy of 200 J for AF and 50 to 100 J for atrial flutter. Restitution of sinus rhythm rather than just rate control is the ultimate goal. After 48 hours of sustained AF, anticoagulation needs to be considered despite the recent cardiac surgery.

Premature ventricular complexes or ventricular arrhythmias are also common after surgery and often associated with electrolyte imbalances or may be introduced during pulmonary artery catheter placement. Other causes include hemodynamic instability, hypoxia, hypovolemia, ischemia, myocardial infarction, acute graft closure, proarrhythmic effects of inotropic drugs, and effects of antiarrhythmic drugs.[118] Sustained ventricular dysrhythmias after cardiac surgery are uncommon, with an incidence of about 1%.[119] Initial treatment of hemodynamically significant ventricular dysrhythmias is immediate defibrillation and administration of amiodarone or lidocaine. Prognosis of postoperative frequent premature ventricular complexes and nonsustained ventricular tachycardia in patients with normal ventricular function is no different from controls. However, patients with nonsustained ventricular dysrhythmias and an LV ejection fraction of less than 40% demonstrate a 75% mortality rate at 15-month follow-up.[118] Patients with sustained ventricular dysrhythmias have a poor short- and long-term prognosis, with a hospital mortality rate of 50%.[120] An additional 20% of the survivors have cardiac death within 24 months.[121] These poor outcomes merit aggressive therapy, particularly in the higher-risk patient with LV dysfunction. All electrolyte abnormalities should be corrected quickly. Ventricular fibrillation and pulseless ventricular tachycardia require immediate defibrillation in accordance with advanced cardiac life support (ACLS) guidelines. Synchronized DC cardioversion with 200 to 360 J is used for symptomatic sustained ventricular tachycardia with a pulse. Stable sustained monomorphic ventricular tachycardia may be treated initially with intravenous antidysrhythmic medication. Procainamide may be infused at a rate of 30 to 50 mg/min up to a maximum dose of 17 mg/kg or a widening of the QRS complex by 50%. The loading dose is followed by an intravenous continuous infusion of 1 to 4 mg/min. Dosage reductions are appropriate for older adult patients and patients with congestive heart failure or hepatic dysfunction. Lidocaine or amiodarone are good alternatives, especially in patients with LV dysfunction.

For patients with ventricular epicardial wires in place, conversion of stable ventricular tachycardia using overdrive ventricular pacing may be attempted by burst pacing the ventricle at rates greater than the native rate. Acceleration of the ventricular tachycardia may sometimes end in ventricular fibrillation, and it is important to have a defibrillator immediately available.

Long-term management of patients with dysrhythmia depends on the severity of the condition. With sustained ventricular dysrhythmias, electrophysiologic testing is performed to evaluate whether antidysrhythmic medication or implantation of an implantable cardioverter-defibrillator (ICD) or a defibrillator may be beneficial to the patient. A recent study demonstrated that ICD is superior to drug therapy for patients with hemodynamically significant ventricular dysrhythmias.[122]

Cardiac Tamponade

The clinical features of tamponade (unlike those of the more classical "primary" tamponade) after cardiac surgery are not specific, and this can delay diagnosis. In practice, the threshold for investigation must be low, and echocardiography (both transesophageal and transthoracic) has been invaluable in the detection and localization of pericardial collections.[123,124] Clinical and hemodynamic findings include hypotension, low CO, low urine output, and elevated CVP. This may be accompanied by a sudden decrease in drainage from the chest tubes. Concealed bleeding in the mediastinum and pericardial sac after excessive postoperative bleeding is the most likely etiology for cardiac tamponade after cardiac surgery. Immediate transport of the patient back to the operating room, reopening of the chest, and evacuation of the clot usually provides dramatic hemodynamic improvement. Cardiac tamponade typically occurs within the first 12 hours after cardiac surgery, although delayed-onset tamponade may present a week or more later, especially when patients are anticoagulated.[125]

Perioperative Myocardial Infarction

The risk of a perioperative myocardial infarction (MI) exists from immediately preoperatively through hospital discharge and thereafter. Postoperative myocardial ischemia as a result of incomplete revascularization or acute occlusion of either the native coronaries or the bypass grafts can result in a low output state. This condition is diagnosed by new segmental wall motion abnormalities on perioperative TEE or regional ECG changes. However, high peak enzyme level of postoperative creatine kinase MB, especially when 20 times the upper limit of normal (or more), is a stronger predictor of adverse outcomes than postoperative Q-wave myocardial infarction and also predicts increased mortality in this population.[126,127] Troponin I levels generally exceed those seen in myocardial infarction in noncardiac surgery settings.[128,129] Often, a combination of serial ECGs and enzyme profiles helps with the diagnosis, but specific diagnostic criteria do not exist. Inotropic agents tend to be less effective and are arrhythmogenic in ischemic areas. Nitroglycerine, milrinone, or an IABP may sufficiently improve myocardial perfusion, but reexploration (with or without diagnostic angiography) remains the definitive approach for an occluded bypass graft.

Oliguria

Acute renal impairment and renal failure are still significant medical problems, occurring in 7.2% of all hospital patients and 30% of those admitted to an ICU.[130,131] The incidence of acute renal failure (ARF) requiring dialysis after cardiac surgery is approximately 1% to 4%. Significant postoperative worsening of renal function is observed in approximately 7% of patients, and approximately 15% of these patients require dialysis. The importance of postoperative renal dysfunction lies in its consistent association with increased rates of in-hospital mortality, perioperative cost, and length of stay in the ICU, even after adjustment for other contributing factors.[132-135] Patients with renal dysfunction are also more likely to be discharged to an extended-care facility, with its associated financial and emotional costs.[136]

Many issues related to postoperative renal protection are similar to those discussed for the intraoperative period (e.g., intravenous fluid and inotrope selection). Pharmacologic interventions currently evaluated for renal protection are continued for an extended period as part of postoperative care. Of note, the protective benefits of insulin have been most convincingly demonstrated in the postoperative period.[137]

In the absence of effective treatment strategies to reverse renal injury, the major emphasis is on prevention (see Chapter 17). Identification of risk factors plays an important role in renal protection during cardiac surgery. One of the most powerful postoperative predictors of renal dysfunction is depressed cardiac function after CPB. Postoperative evidence of myocardial dysfunction, including low CO state and need for inotropic support, is associated with a twofold to fourfold increased risk of renal injury. Prolonged positive-pressure ventilation, preexisting cytomegalovirus infection, and postoperative sepsis present additional risks for renal dysfunction and acute renal failure.

Monitoring kidney function remains as a challenge, and no single test evaluates all renal activity. Despite its non-linear relationship with glomerular filtration rate (GFR), the test for serum creatinine is most commonly used to assess perioperative renal function. Plasma creatinine reflects a state of equilibrium between creatinine production and excretion and is influenced by sex, weight, and especially age. Creatine clearance and fractional excretion of sodium are probably better reflections of true renal function.

While the search for clinically proven renal protective drugs continues, current perioperative management of the cardiac surgical patient should include measures to ensure minimal renal stress, such as maintenance of adequate perfusion and intravascular volume and the prevention of hypoxemia. Although no firm evidence supports the use of any drug to protect the kidney, several "renal protective" regimens remain popular. These include activation of peripheral dopaminergic receptors (DA_1) with "renal dose" dopamine, which is based largely on the DA_1-mediated natriuretic, diuretic, and renal vasodilating properties of this drug at dosages of 0.5 to 3.0 µg/kg/min. Although dopamine has experimentally been shown to result in significant improvements in renal function after renal injury, human clinical studies have not demonstrated a similar benefit. Dopamine increases global renal blood flow without augmenting medullary blood flow and therefore does not prevent medullary hypoxia. Significant complications associated with intravenous dopamine, even at low dosages, need to be considered

if the drug is used solely for renal protection.[138,139] However, despite an overwhelming number of negative clinical trials, the use of dopamine for renoprotection remains controversial.

The potential usefulness of other clinically available DA_1-receptor agonists, such as fenoldopam and dopexamine, as renal protective agents has yet to be determined. Fenoldopam does seem to have some promise.[140] Studies examining its role in the setting of cardiac surgery are ongoing, but current data are insufficient to draw conclusions about its clinical potential as renal preservation therapy. Similarly, existing evidence is inconsistent and insufficient to recommend dopexamine for renoprotection for either high-risk surgical or critically ill patients.[141]

The rationale underlying renoprotection from diuretics relates to the induced diuresis and natriuresis and the decreased likelihood of tubular obstruction by casts after a renal insult. This may retain tubular patency and avoid oliguria or anuria and the need for dialysis. Osmotic diuretics, such as mannitol, also reduce tubular swelling to achieve this goal, but a secondary proposed protective property unique to loop diuretic agents, such as furosemide, is a reduction in medullary tubular oxygen consumption and a proposed anti-oxidant effect. Animal models of myoglobin uric and is-chemic renal failure demonstrate a protective effect from mannitol. However, with the exception of usefulness in the setting of early myoglobinuric ARF and renal transplantation, the clinical renoprotective effects of mannitol have not been confirmed.[136] There is similarly no convincing clinical evidence to advocate the use of furosemide for renoprotection. Importantly, despite the clinician's satisfaction at seeing the urine bag fill, the increased urine volume from diuretics does not ensure improved renal function.[142] In contrast, both furosemide and mannitol have been incriminated in aggravating renal injury in some settings. A deleterious property common to the use of all diuretics is that they can induce dehydration if intravascular volume status is not carefully monitored. Although there is some evidence that oliguric renal failure can be converted to nonoliguric renal failure by the use of diuretics, there is no proof that the reduced mortality seen with nonoliguric renal failure applies to patients receiving diuretics after cardiac surgery.

Absolute indications for initiating renal replacement therapy include fluid overload, refractory hyperkalemia or acidosis, and severe uremic symptoms.

Neurologic Complications

Neurologic injury after cardiac surgery ranges from incapacitating or life-ending stroke and coma to encephalopathy, delirium, and neurocognitive decline, which have been described by many investigators.[143-146] Although stroke after cardiac surgery is an important concern for both short- and long-term disability, more subtle neurologic deficits such as encephalopathy and neurocognitive dysfunction are also associated with an increase in medical costs and a decrease in short- and long-term cognitive function and quality of life.[143,147] Successful strategies for perioperative cerebral protection begin with accurate individual patient risk assessment. Although studies differ somewhat as to all the risk factors, certain patient characteristics consistently demonstrate an increased risk for cardiac surgery–associated neurologic injury. The factors representing key predictive variables in a recently validated model include advanced age, history of symptomatic neurologic disease, prior CABG surgery, vascular disease, unstable angina, diabetes, and pulmonary disease.[148]

Appropriately, most current strategies aimed toward risk reduction involve intraoperative and preventive measures. However, tailoring anesthetic technique to allow earlier postoperative awakening may play a significant role in assessment and treatment of patients with postoperative neurologic dysfunction.[149] Patients remaining comatose after surgery require early attention and the initiation of diagnostic steps. Metabolic abnormalities, drug side effect or overdose, and a primary central nervous system injury need to be ruled out. Management includes withholding of all sedatives, narcotics, and muscle relaxants, and assessment of peripheral neuromuscular function. An early computerized tomographic (CT) or magnetic resonance imaging (MRI) scan to rule out structural lesions or cerebral hemorrhage is warranted if the patient is hemodynamically stable. Electrophysiologic assessment includes electroencephalography (EEG) and evoked potential monitoring. Early assessment may also allow intervention through pharmacologic or other methods. Floyd and colleagues summarized a rational approach to postoperative neurologic assessment and management of the cardiothoracic patient (Fig. 31-2).[150] Postoperative delirium occurs in 32% to 73% of all patients undergoing cardiac surgery, and the incidence varies with patient risk factors, type of surgery, and method of assessment.[151,152] Initial management includes reassurance and orientation of the patient, and pain control and treatment of anxiety with opioids and benzodiazepines. For the patient who remains agitated and confused, haloperidol might be useful.

Postoperative Fever and Infections

Infection rates in patients undergoing cardiac surgery tend to be higher than those in patients undergoing general surgery. A number of factors are involved, including prolonged operative time, presence of indwelling catheters, deleterious effects of CPB on the immune system, poor tissue perfusion, hyperglycemia, and implantation of foreign material. The magnitude of the problem is significant, with one series reporting 71% of perioperative site cultures in patients undergoing open heart procedures as positive.[153,154] The overall incidence of postoperative infections has been reported to be between 2% and 20%, resulting in significantly prolonged hospitalization and substantial cost increases.[155-157]

Severe infectious complications include sepsis and deep sternal wound infections (DSWIs). DSWI is one of the most devastating infectious complications of cardiac surgery. Clinical features include redness and tenderness over the sternum, wound drainage or discharge (70% to 90% of cases), inability to wean, sternal instability, fever, and leukocytosis. Antibiotic therapy should be guided by culture results, but debridement and flap closure achieves healing in most cases. Indications for reoperation depend on the depth

and severity of the infection. Risk factors for DSWI include diabetes, low cardiac output, use of bilateral internal mammary artery grafts and reoperation for control of bleeding. A recent study suggested that uncontrolled hyperglycemia in diabetic patients after cardiac surgery, and not diabetes per se, is the true risk factor for DSWI.[158] Furthermore, this study demonstrated that tighter control of blood glucose levels throughout the perioperative period (levels maintained below 200 mg/dL) independently decreased the risk of DSWI by 66%.

Septic complications are difficult to predict or diagnose early in the immediate perioperative period after cardiac surgery. The proinflammatory state, triggered by CPB, induces a number of changes that may mimic a septic picture. Fever and temperatures exceeding 38.5°C are common during the first 24 hours after cardiac surgery, occurring in nearly 40% of patients. This often represents a spectrum of physiologic insults such as the activation of inflammatory cascades from CPB, basal atelectasis, and overly aggressive rewarming. There is some suggestion that scores such as the Acute Physiologic and Chronic Health Evaluation II (APACHE II) score or the EuroSCORE, or markers such as procalcitonin may help predict a significant infection.[159-161] Until the predictive value of these is confirmed, it is reasonable to treat increased temperatures symptomatically with an antipyretic drug during the first 24 hours after surgery. This appears to be even more important because postoperative hyperthermia has been associated with significant complications such as cognitive dysfunction.[162] If the patient is febrile beyond 24 hours, culture of urine, blood, and sputum as well as a white cell count are standard. Early antibiotic treatment is warranted if the patient has prosthetic material (valve or graft) or a preexisting infection (such as bacterial endocarditis). Nosocomial line infections are to be avoided by following strict protocols for intravenous and arterial lines. Nosocomial infections, which are common after cardiac surgery, are associated with prolonged lengths of hospitalization, the development of multiorgan dysfunction, and increased hospital mortality.[163]

■ GASTROINTESTINAL COMPLICATIONS

Gastrointestinal (GI) complications occur in about 2.5% of patients undergoing cardiac surgery, are associated with a high mortality (up to 33%), and account for nearly 15% of all postoperative deaths.[164] In a recent large study of 11,058 patients undergoing cardiac surgery, six independent predictors for GI complications were identified.[165] These include prolonged mechanical ventilation, postoperative renal failure, sepsis, valve surgery, preoperative chronic renal failure, and sternal wound infection. Other factors such as CPB time, ischemic time, and use of IABP are only marginally important. Monitoring for GI complications with a high level of vigilance, and instant diagnosis and treatment of GI complications are important means to decrease associated morbidity and mortality. Prophylactic measures such as optimization of postoperative hemodynamics, adaptation of early extubation protocols (e.g., fast tracking), and early mobilization might all contribute to prevent serious GI complications. Prevention

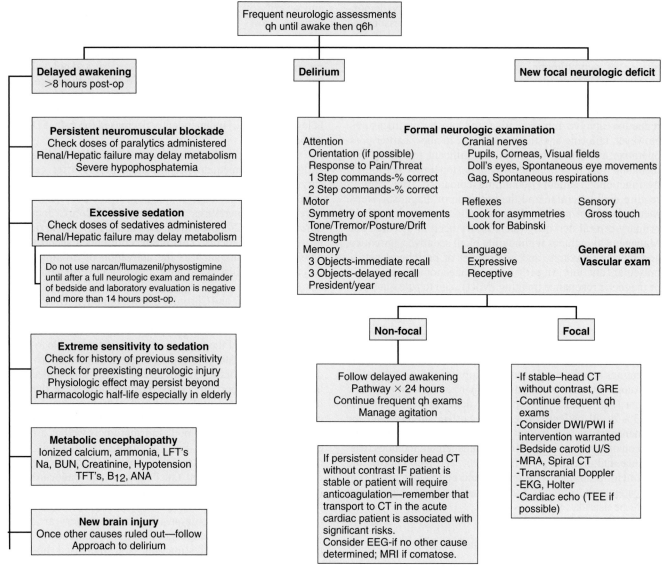

Figure 31-2 ■ Postoperative neurologic assessment and management of the cardiac surgical patient. ANA, antinuclear antibody; BUN, blood urea nitrogen; CT, computed tomography; DWI/PWI, diffusion-weighted imaging/perfusion-weighted imaging; EEG, electroencephalogram; ECG, electrocardiogram; GRE, gradient-recalled echo; LFT, liver function test; MRA, magnetic resonance angiography; post-op, postoperative; qh, every hr; q6h, every 6 hr; TEE, transesophageal echocardiogram; TFT, thyroid function test; Uls, ultrasound. *(Redrawn with permission from Floyd TF, Cheung AT, Stecker MM, et al: Semin Thorac Cardiovasc Surg 2000;12:337-348.)*

of perioperative infections and renal dysfunction, as well as tight control and monitoring of perioperative anticoagulation, should also be considered.

■ FAST TRACKING

In the past, cardiac surgery patients were traditionally maintained on sedation and mechanical ventilation until the morning after surgery. It was believed that the cardiovascular and other organ systems needed recovery time from the profound physiologic disturbances induced by CPB. More recently, clinical care pathways have been successfully

introduced for cardiac and thoracic procedures.[23,24,166] The idea of early extubation and minimization of ICU time, often termed fast tracking, has been suggested for many years.[167] The overall need for improved cost effectiveness in all areas of health care has supported the trend for early weaning from ventilator support and a shortened ICU and hospital length of stay after cardiac surgery.[168] Furthermore, organizational features of ICUs have been shown to have a major impact on clinical outcomes[169] and on the duration of mechanical ventilation.[22]

This new trend is made possible with innovative surgical and anesthetic techniques as well as improved postoperative sedative and analgesic agents. Shorter CPB times, improved myocardial protection, and modifications of anesthetic technique allow extubation 2 to 3 hours postoperatively, assuming hemodynamic stability.[170,171] Changes in surgical and anesthetic techniques include use of warmer core temperatures, reduction in invasive monitoring, and lower dosage of intraoperative opioids and benzodiazepines. Use of short-acting opioids and sedatives, such as remifentanil, propofol, and dexmedetomidine, and nonsedating analgesics, as well as use of intrathecal opioids or thoracic epidural catheters for postoperative pain, has hastened recovery from anesthesia and surgery.[172-174] User-friendly changes in ICU infrastructure, such as preconfigured management protocols and computerized physician order entries (CPOE), have enabled rapid transit of patients through the ICU.

The medical literature remains mixed on the virtue of fast-track protocols, including early extubation. No benefit exists for prolonged ventilation after CABG in low-risk patients, and such practice may be deleterious.[23,175] On the other hand, no benefit has been demonstrated from extubation in the operating room after CABG.[6] Recent series have supported a brief period of ventilation in the cardiac ICU postoperatively.[176] The success rate of early extubation and associated morbidity varies from 60%[177] to 85%.[23,178] Reintubation in conventionally weaned patients results in increased mortality and morbidity, including longer ICU length of stay, longer ventilator dependency, a higher incidence of nosocomial pneumonia, and a prolonged period of rehabilitation.[178,179] However, fast-track patients requiring reintubation do not seem to experience the same morbidity,[23,171] probably because of differences in the indications for reintubation in the two groups. Different criteria exist for selecting suitable fast-track patients. Patients determined to be suitable for fast-tracking have a low probability of needing circulatory or respiratory support postoperatively and an absence of significant comorbidity, corresponding with a low preoperative risk stratification score (e.g., the EuroSCORE).[3,180] Other important considerations include the patient's clinical condition after weaning from CPB[181] and on arrival in the ICU.[182] Factors associated with failure of early extubation include advanced age, requirement for inotropic or IABP therapy, persistent hypothermia, bleeding, and rapid atrial dysrhythmias.

Off-pump coronary artery bypass (OPCAB) procedures are CABG surgeries performed with partial to full heparinization of the beating heart and without the support of CPB. Routine immediate extubation and fast-tracking of patients undergoing OPCAB appears to be feasible and is probably safe. Maintenance of normothermia, use of appropriate anesthetic technique, and strict adherence to clinical care pathways appear to be essential in that patient population, and early extubation might even help to reduce certain complications of surgery.[183,184] Some authors found that port-access and minimally invasive valvular surgery, like OPCAB surgery, result in shorter lengths of ICU and hospital stays, faster return to normal activity (4 weeks versus 9 weeks) when compared with conventional median sternotomy, fewer blood transfusions, and lower rates of AF in the port-access group.[185-187]

Cost reduction is a major driving force behind accelerated recovery.[168,188] Short-stay intensive care after CABG surgery (maximum of 8 hours of ICU treatment) compared with conventional ICU care was documented as a safe and cost-effective approach in a recent prospective trial in Europe.[4] Cheng and coworkers reported a significant decrease of average ICU and hospital costs per patient by 53% and 25%, respectively, by introducing a fast-track recovery protocol, without change in morbidity.[24] Other benefits included a 15% increase in case volume and a decrease in cancellation. Besides potential cost reductions, early extubation offers increased patient satisfaction, earlier interaction between patient and relatives, earlier mobilization, earlier return to normal diet, improved pulmonary function with less postoperative pneumonia,[189] and improved perioperative mental status.[23] More recent data from Cheng and colleagues confirm the notion that fast-track cardiac anesthesia and surgery is a safe practice that decreases resource use after patient discharge over a 1-year follow-up period.[190]

ICU costs rank second to operating room costs, so early extubation protocols and fast-track recovery to allow earlier ICU and hospital discharge are economically appealing. Improvements in surgical and anesthetic techniques coupled with improved preoperative risk stratification and protocol-driven ICU care have allowed many medical centers to successfully implement fast-tracking protocols, and this trend is unlikely to be reversed.

SUMMARY

Postoperative management of today's complex cardiac surgery patients requires a well-prepared and vigilant ICU team with attention to detail, a multimodal monitoring infrastructure, and implementation of institutional clinical care pathways. These patients undergo major physiologic stress with limited perioperative reserve, making effective ICU care essential to their recovery. Detailed knowledge of the patient's preoperative history and baseline condition, instant and accurate assessment of the physiologic impact of perioperative events, immediate interpretation of trends in invasive monitoring data, and reasoned clinical judgment and initiation of therapy are required for optimization of patient care. Advances in ongoing research and discovery, along with improved risk stratification and continuous improvement of clinical care pathways, will allow perioperative physicians to provide optimized care at a tolerable cost with improved outcomes.

REFERENCES

1. DeFrances CJ, Podgornik MN:2004 National Hospital Discharge Survey. Adv Data 2006;(371):1-19.
2. Westaby S, Pillai R, Parry A, et al: Does modern cardiac surgery require conventional intensive care? Eur J Cardiothorac Surg 1993;7: 313-318; discussion 318.
3. Flynn M, Reddy S, Shepherd W, et al: Fast-tracking revisited: Routine cardiac surgical patients need minimal intensive care. Eur J Cardiothorac Surg 2004;25:116-122.

4. van Mastrigt GA, Heijmans J, Severens JL, et al: Short-stay intensive care after coronary artery bypass surgery: Randomized clinical trial on safety and cost-effectiveness. Crit Care Med 2006;34: 65-75.

5. Smith I, Fleming S, Cernaianu A: Mishaps during transport from the intensive care unit. Crit Care Med 1990;18:278-281.

6. Montes FR, Sanchez SI, Giraldo JC, et al: The lack of benefit of tracheal extubation in the operating room after coronary artery bypass surgery. Anesth Analg 2000;91:776-780.

7. Gray R, Maddahi J, Berman D, et al: Scintigraphic and hemodynamic demonstration of transient left ventricular dysfunction immediately after uncomplicated coronary artery bypass grafting. J Thorac Cardiovasc Surg 1979;77:504-510.

8. Czer L, Hamer A, Murphy F, et al: Transient hemodynamic dysfunction after myocardial revascularization: Temperature dependence. J Thorac Cardiovasc Surg 1983;86:226-234.

9. Stein KL, Breisblatt W, Wolfe C, et al: Depression and recovery of right ventricular function after cardiopulmonary bypass. Crit Care Med 1990;18:1197-1200.

10. Connors AF Jr, Speroff T, Dawson NV, et al: The effectiveness of right heart catheterization in the initial care of critically ill patients. SUPPORT Investigators. JAMA 1996;276:889-897.

11. Costachescu T, Denault A, Guimond JG, et al: The hemodynamically unstable patient in the intensive care unit: Hemodynamic vs. transesophageal echocardiographic monitoring. Crit Care Med 2002;30: 1214-1223.

12. Pearse RM, Ikram K, Barry J: Equipment review: An appraisal of the LiDCO plus method of measuring cardiac output. Crit Care 2004;8:190-195.

13. Gulker H, Haverkamp W, Hindricks G: [Ion regulation disorders and cardiac arrhythmia. The relevance of sodium, potassium, calcium, and magnesium.] Arzneimittelforschung 1989;39:130-134.

14. Jensen BM, Alstrup P, Klitgard NA: Postoperative arrhythmias and myocardial electrolytes in patients undergoing coronary artery bypass grafting. Scand J Thorac Cardiovasc Surg 1996;30:133-140.

15. Miller S, Crystal E, Garfinkle M, et al: Effects of magnesium on atrial fibrillation after cardiac surgery: A meta-analysis. Heart 2005;91: 618-623.

16. Cohen J, Kogan A, Sahar G, et al: Hypophosphatemia following open heart surgery: Incidence and consequences. Eur J Cardiothorac Surg 2004;26:306-310.

17. Ryan MP: Interrelationships of magnesium and potassium homeostasis. Miner Electrolyte Metab 1993;19:290-295.

18. Chadda KD: Clinical hypomagnesemia, coronary spasm and cardiac arrhythmia. Magnesium 1986;5:47-52.

19. Shore-Lesserson L, Manspeizer HE, DePerio M, et al: Thromboelastography-guided transfusion algorithm reduces transfusions in complex cardiac surgery. Anesth Analg 1999;88:312-319.

20. O'Brien W, Karski JM, Cheng D, et al: Routine chest roentgenography on admission to intensive care unit after heart operations: Is it of any value? J Thorac Cardiovasc Surg 1997;113:130-133.

21. Branca P, McGaw P, Light R: Factors associated with prolonged mechanical ventilation following coronary artery bypass surgery. Chest 2001;119:537-546.

22. Kollef MH, Shapiro SD, Silver P, et al: A randomized, controlled trial of protocol-directed versus physician-directed weaning from mechanical ventilation. Crit Care Med 1997;25:567-574.

23. Cheng DC, Karski J, Peniston C, et al: Morbidity outcome in early versus conventional tracheal extubation after coronary artery bypass grafting: A prospective randomized controlled trial. J Thorac Cardiovasc Surg 1996;112:755-764.

24. Cheng DC, Karski J, Peniston C, et al: Early tracheal extubation after coronary artery bypass graft surgery reduces costs and improves resource use: A prospective, randomized, controlled trial. Anesthesiology 1996;85:1300-1310.

25. Hendrix H, Kaiser ME, Yusen RD, Merk J: A randomized trial of automated versus conventional protocol-driven weaning from mechanical ventilation following coronary artery bypass surgery. Eur J Cardiothorac Surg 2006;29:957-963.

26. Higgins TL: Pro: Early endotracheal extubation is preferable to late extubation in patients following coronary artery surgery. J Cardiothorac Vasc Anesth 1992;6:488-493.

27. Higgins TL: Safety issues regarding early extubation after coronary artery bypass surgery. J Cardiothorac Vasc Anesth 1995;9:24-29.

28. Millbern SM, Downs JB, Jumper LC, Modell JH: Evaluation of criteria for discontinuing mechanical ventilatory support. Arch Surg 1978;113:1441-1443.

29. Frutos-Vivar F, Esteban A: When to wean from a ventilator: An evidence-based strategy. Cleve Clin J Med 2003;70:389, 392-393, 397.

30. Meade M, Guyatt G, Cook D, et al: Predicting success in weaning from mechanical ventilation. Chest 2001;120:400S-424.

31. Hammermeister KE, Burchfiel C, Johnson R, Grover FL: Identification of patients at greatest risk for developing major complications at cardiac surgery. Circulation 1990;82:IV380-389.

32. Kollef MH, Wragge T, Pasque C: Determinants of mortality and multiorgan dysfunction in cardiac surgery patients requiring prolonged mechanical ventilation. Chest 1995;107:1395-1401.

33. Tejerina E, Frutos-Vivar F, Restrepo MI, et al: Incidence, risk factors, and outcome of ventilator-associated pneumonia. J Crit Care 2006;21: 56-65.

34. Esteban A, Anzueto A, Alia I, et al: How is mechanical ventilation employed in the intensive care unit? An international utilization review. Am J Respir Crit Care Med 2000;161:1450-1458.

35. Lemaire F, Teboul JL, Cinotti L, et al: Acute left ventricular dysfunction during unsuccessful weaning from mechanical ventilation. Anesthesiology 1988;69:171-179.

36. Bando K, Sun K, Binford RS, Sharp TG: Determinants of longer duration of endotracheal intubation after adult cardiac operations. Ann Thorac Surg 1997;63:1026-1033.

37. Wilcox P, Baile EM, Hards J, et al: Phrenic nerve function and its relationship to atelectasis after coronary artery bypass surgery. Chest 1988;93:693-698.

38. Yang KL, Tobin MJ: A prospective study of indexes predicting the outcome of trials of weaning from mechanical ventilation. N Engl J Med 1991;324:1445-1450.

39. Wahba RW: Pressure support ventilation. J Cardiothorac Anesth 1990;4:624-630.

40. Nathan SD, Ishaaya AM, Koerner SK, Belman MJ: Prediction of minimal pressure support during weaning from mechanical ventilation. Chest 1993;103:1215-1219.

41. Habib RH, Zacharias A, Engoren M: Determinants of prolonged mechanical ventilation after coronary artery bypass grafting. Ann Thorac Surg 1996;62:1164-1171.

42. Kern H, Redlich U, Hotz H, et al: Risk factors for prolonged ventilation after cardiac surgery using APACHE II, SAPS II, and TISS: Comparison of three different models. Intensive Care Med 2001;27: 407-415.

43. Serrano N, Garcia C, Villegas J, et al: Prolonged intubation rates after coronary artery bypass surgery and ICU risk stratification score. Chest 2005;128:595-601.

44. Sivak ED: Management of ventilator dependency following heart surgery. Semin Thorac Cardiovasc Surg 1991;3:53-62.

45. Brochard L, Rauss A, Benito S, et al: Comparison of three methods of gradual withdrawal from ventilatory support during weaning from mechanical ventilation. Am J Respir Crit Care Med 1994;150: 896-903.

46. Esteban A, Frutos F, Tobin MJ, et al: A comparison of four methods of weaning patients from mechanical ventilation. Spanish Lung Failure Collaborative Group. N Engl J Med 1995;332:345-350.

47. Esteban A, Alia I, Tobin MJ, et al: Effect of spontaneous breathing trial duration on outcome of attempts to discontinue mechanical ventilation. Spanish Lung Failure Collaborative Group. Am J Respir Crit Care Med 1999;159:512-518.

48. Tobin MJ, Perez W, Guenther SM, et al: The pattern of breathing during successful and unsuccessful trials of weaning from mechanical ventilation. Am Rev Respir Dis 1986;134:1111-1118.

49. Ely EW, Baker AM, Dunagan DP, et al: Effect on the duration of mechanical ventilation of identifying patients capable of breathing spontaneously. N Engl J Med 1996;335:1864-1869.

50. Tobin MJ: Advances in mechanical ventilation. N Engl J Med 2001;344:1986-1996.

51. Curtis JJ, Clark NC, McKenney CA, et al: Tracheostomy: A risk factor for mediastinitis after cardiac operation. Ann Thorac Surg 2001;72: 731-734.

52. Frutos-Vivar F, Esteban A, Apezteguia C, et al: Outcome of mechanically ventilated patients who require a tracheostomy. Crit Care Med 2005;33:290-298.

53. Bacchetta MD, Girardi LN, Southard EJ, et al: Comparison of open versus bedside percutaneous dilatational tracheostomy in the cardiothoracic surgical patient: Outcomes and financial analysis. Ann Thorac Surg 2005;79:1879-1885.

54. Augoustides J, Weiss SJ, Pochettino A: Hemodynamic monitoring of the postoperative adult cardiac surgical patient. Semin Thorac Cardiovasc Surg 2000;12:309-315.

55. Mizock BA, Falk JL: Lactic acidosis in critical illness. Crit Care Med 1992;20:80-93.

56. Bakker J, Coffernils M, Leon M, et al: Blood lactate levels are superior to oxygen-derived variables in predicting outcome in human septic shock. Chest 1991;99:956-962.

57. Kolkman JJ, Otte JA, Groeneveld AB: Gastrointestinal luminal PCO2 tonometry: An update on physiology, methodology and clinical applications. Br J Anaesth 2000;84:74-86.

58. Wahr JA, Tremper KK, Samra S, Delpy DT: Near-infrared spectroscopy: Theory and applications. J Cardiothorac Vasc Anesth 1996;10:406-418.

59. Boekstegers P, Weidenhofer S, Kapsner T, Werdan K: Skeletal muscle partial pressure of oxygen in patients with sepsis. Crit Care Med 1994;22:640-650.

60. Breisblatt WM, Stein KL, Wolfe CJ, et al: Acute myocardial dysfunction and recovery: A common occurrence after coronary bypass surgery. J Am Coll Cardiol 1990;15:1261-1269.

61. Argenziano M, Chen JM, Choudhri AF, et al: Management of vasodilatory shock after cardiac surgery: Identification of predisposing factors and use of a novel pressor agent. J Thorac Cardiovasc Surg 1998;116:973-980.

62. Mekontso-Dessap A, Houel R, Soustelle C, et al: Risk factors for post-cardiopulmonary bypass vasoplegia in patients with preserved left ventricular function. Ann Thorac Surg 2001;71:1428-1432.

63. Boyle EM Jr, Pohlman TH, Johnson MC, Verrier ED: Endothelial cell injury in cardiovascular surgery: The systemic inflammatory response. Ann Thorac Surg 1997;63:277-284.

64. Christakis GT, Fremes SE, Koch JP, et al: Determinants of low systemic vascular resistance during cardiopulmonary bypass. Ann Thorac Surg 1994;58:1040-1049.

65. Morimatsu H, Uchino S, Chung J, et al: Norepinephrine for hypotensive vasodilatation after cardiac surgery: Impact on renal function. Intensive Care Med 2003;29:1106-1112.

66. Leyh RG, Kofidis T, Struber M, et al: Methylene blue: The drug of choice for catecholamine-refractory vasoplegia after cardiopulmonary bypass? J Thorac Cardiovasc Surg 2003;125:1426-1431.

67. Morales DL, Gregg D, Helman DN, et al: Arginine vasopressin in the treatment of 50 patients with postcardiotomy vasodilatory shock. Ann Thorac Surg 2000;69:102-106.

68. Janelle GM, Urdaneta F, Martin TD, Lobato EB: Effects of calcium chloride on grafted internal mammary artery flow after cardiopulmonary bypass. J Cardiothorac Vasc Anesth 2000;14:4-8.

69. Estafanous FG, Urzua J, Yared JP, et al: Pattern of hemodynamic alterations during coronary artery operations. J Thorac Cardiovasc Surg 1984;87:175-182.

70. Visser CA, Koolen JJ, van Wezel H, Dunning AJ: Hemodynamics of nicardipine in coronary artery disease. Am J Cardiol 1987;59:9J-12.

71. Levy JH: Management of systemic and pulmonary hypertension. Tex Heart Inst J 2005;32:467-471.

72. Singh BN, Josephson MA: Clinical pharmacology, pharmacokinetics, and hemodynamic effects of nicardipine. Am Heart J 1990;119:427-434.

73. Kwak YL, Oh YJ, Bang SO, et al: Comparison of the effects of nicardipine and sodium nitroprusside for control of increased blood pressure after coronary artery bypass graft surgery. J Int Med Res 2004;32:342-350.

74. Stewart RD, Psyhojos T, Lahey SJ, et al: Central venous catheter use in low-risk coronary artery bypass grafting. Ann Thorac Surg 1998;66:1306-1311.

75. Feneck RO, Sherry KM, Withington PS, Oduro-Dominah A: Comparison of the hemodynamic effects of milrinone with dobutamine in

76. Welsby IJ, Podgoreanu MV, Phillips-Bute B, et al: Genetic factors contribute to bleeding after cardiac surgery. J Thromb Haemost 2005;3:1206-1212.

77. Stover EP, Siegel LC, Parks R, et al: Variability in transfusion practice for coronary artery bypass surgery persists despite national consensus guidelines: A 24-institution study. Institutions of the Multicenter Study of Perioperative Ischemia Research Group. Anesthesiology 1998;88:327-333.

78. Stover EP, Siegel LC, Body SC, et al: Institutional variability in red blood cell conservation practices for coronary artery bypass graft surgery. Institutions of the MultiCenter Study of Perioperative Ischemia Research Group. J Cardiothorac Vasc Anesth 2000;14:171-176.

79. Litmathe J, Boeken U, Feindt P, Gams E: Predictors of homologous blood transfusion for patients undergoing open heart surgery. Thorac Cardiovasc Surg 2003;51:17-21.

80. Kuduvalli M, Oo AY, Newall N, et al: Effect of peri-operative red blood cell transfusion on 30-day and 1-year mortality following coronary artery bypass surgery. Eur J Cardiothorac Surg 2005;27:592-598.

81. Basran S, Frumento RJ, Cohen A, et al: The association between duration of storage of transfused red blood cells and morbidity and mortality after reoperative cardiac surgery. Anesth Analg 2006;103:15-20.

82. American Society of Anesthesiologists: Practice guidelines for blood component therapy: A report by the American Society of Anesthesiologists Task Force on Blood Component Therapy. Anesthesiology 1996;84:732-747.

83. Goodnough LT, Brecher ME, Kanter MH, AuBuchon JP: Transfusion medicine: First of two parts—Blood transfusion. N Engl J Med 1999;340:438-447.

84. Fresh-Frozen Plasma, Cryoprecipitate, and Platelets Administration Practice Guidelines Development Task Force of the College of American Pathologists: Practice parameter for the use of fresh-frozen plasma, cryoprecipitate, and platelets. JAMA 1994;271:777-781.

85. Goodnough LT, Despotis GJ: Future directions in utilization review: The role of transfusion algorithms. Transfus Sci 1998;19:97-105.

86. Spiess BD, Gillies BS, Chandler W, Verrier E: Changes in transfusion therapy and reexploration rate after institution of a blood management program in cardiac surgical patients. J Cardiothorac Vasc Anesth 1995;9:168-173.

87. Wong BI, McLean RF, Fremes SE, et al: Aprotinin and tranexamic acid for high transfusion risk cardiac surgery. Ann Thorac Surg 2000;69:808-816.

88. Levy JH, Pifarre R, Schaff HV, et al: A multicenter, double-blind, placebo-controlled trial of aprotinin for reducing blood loss and the requirement for donor-blood transfusion in patients undergoing repeat coronary artery bypass grafting. Circulation 1995;92:2236-2244.

89. Levi M, Cromheecke ME, de Jonge E, et al: Pharmacological strategies to decrease excessive blood loss in cardiac surgery: A meta-analysis of clinically relevant endpoints. Lancet 1999;354:1940-1947.

90. Mangano DT, Tudor IC, Dietzel C: The risk associated with aprotinin in cardiac surgery. N Engl J Med 2006;354:353-365.

91. Karkouti K, Beattie WS, Dattilo KM, et al: A propensity score case-control comparison of aprotinin and tranexamic acid in high-transfusion-risk cardiac surgery. Transfusion 2006;46:327-338.

92. Mazer D, Fergusson D, Hebert P, et al: Incidence of massive bleeding in a blinded randomized controlled trial of antifibrinolytic drugs in high risk cardiac surgery. Anesth Analg 2006;102:SCA95.

93. Nuttall GA, Oliver WC, Ereth MH, et al: Comparison of blood-conservation strategies in cardiac surgery patients at high risk for bleeding. Anesthesiology 2000;92:674-682.

94. Huet C, Salmi LR, Fergusson D, et al: A meta-analysis of the effectiveness of cell salvage to minimize perioperative allogeneic blood transfusion in cardiac and orthopedic surgery. International Study of Perioperative Transfusion (ISPOT) Investigators. Anesth Analg 1999;89:861-869.

95. Body SC, Birmingham J, Parks R, et al: Safety and efficacy of shed mediastinal blood transfusion after cardiac surgery: A multicenter

observational study. Multicenter Study of Perioperative Ischemia Research Group. J Cardiothorac Vasc Anesth 1999;13:410-416.

96. Steiner ME, Key NS, Levy JH: Activated recombinant factor VII in cardiac surgery. Curr Opin Anaesthesiol 2005;18:89-92.

97. Welsby IJ, Monroe DM, Lawson JH, Hoffmann M: Recombinant activated factor VII and the anaesthetist. Anaesthesia 2005;60: 1203-1212.

98. Sellman M, Intonti MA, Ivert T: Reoperations for bleeding after coronary artery bypass procedures during 25 years. Eur J Cardiothorac Surg 1997;11:521-527.

99. Munoz JJ, Birkmeyer NJ, Dacey LJ, et al: Trends in rates of reexploration for hemorrhage after coronary artery bypass surgery. Northern New England Cardiovascular Disease Study Group. Ann Thorac Surg 1999;68:1321-1325.

100. Durbin CG Jr, Kopel RF: Optimal atrioventricular (AV) pacing interval during temporary AV sequential pacing after cardiac surgery. J Cardiothorac Vasc Anesth 1993;7:316-320.

101. Jaeger FJ, Trohman RG, Brener S, Loop F: Permanent pacing following repeat cardiac valve surgery. Am J Cardiol 1994;74:505-507.

102. Brodell GK, Cosgrove D, Schiavone W, et al: Cardiac rhythm and conduction disturbances in patients undergoing mitral valve surgery. Cleve Clin J Med 1991;58:397-399.

103. Grant SC, Khan MA, Faragher EB, et al: Atrial arrhythmias and pacing after orthotopic heart transplantation: Bicaval versus standard atrial anastomosis. Br Heart J 1995;74:149-153.

104. Haught WH, Bertolet BD, Conti JB, et al: Theophylline reverses high-grade atrioventricular block resulting from cardiac transplant rejection. Am Heart J 1994;128:1255-1257.

105. Mathew JP, Fontes ML, Tudor IC, et al: A multicenter risk index for atrial fibrillation after cardiac surgery. JAMA 2004;291:1720-1729.

106. Mathew JP, Parks R, Savino JS, et al: Atrial fibrillation following coronary artery bypass graft surgery: Predictors, outcomes, and resource utilization. MultiCenter Study of Perioperative Ischemia Research Group. JAMA 1996;276:300-306.

107. Almassi GH, Schowalter T, Nicolosi AC, et al: Atrial fibrillation after cardiac surgery: A major morbid event? Ann Surg 1997;226:501-511; discussion 511-513.

108. Stanley TO, Mackensen GB, Grocott HP, et al: The impact of postoperative atrial fibrillation on neurocognitive outcome after coronary artery bypass graft surgery. Anesth Analg 2002;94:290-295.

109. Podgoreanu MV, Mathew JP: Prophylaxis against postoperative atrial fibrillation: Current progress and future directions. JAMA 2005;294: 3140-3142.

110. Hogue CW Jr, Creswell LL, Gutterman DD, Fleisher LA: Epidemiology, mechanisms, and risks: American College of Chest Physicians guidelines for the prevention and management of postoperative atrial fibrillation after cardiac surgery. Chest 2005;128:9S-16.

111. Waldo AL, MacLean WA, Cooper TB, et al: Use of temporarily placed epicardial atrial wire electrodes for the diagnosis and treatment of cardiac arrhythmias following open-heart surgery. J Thorac Cardiovasc Surg 1978;76:500-505.

112. Tebbenjohanns J, Niehaus M, Korte T, Drexler H: Noninvasive diagnosis in patients with undocumented tachycardias: Value of the adenosine test to predict AV nodal reentrant tachycardia. J Cardiovasc Electrophysiol 1999;10:916-923.

113. England MR, Gordon G, Salem M, Chernow B: Magnesium administration and dysrhythmias after cardiac surgery: A placebo-controlled, double-blind, randomized trial. JAMA 1992;268:2395-2402.

114. Kowey PR, Taylor JE, Rials SJ, Marinchak RA: Meta-analysis of the effectiveness of prophylactic drug therapy in preventing supraventricular arrhythmia early after coronary artery bypass grafting. Am J Cardiol 1992;69:963-965.

115. Fuster V, Ryden LE, Asinger RW, et al: ACC/AHA/ESC guidelines for the management of patients with atrial fibrillation: Executive summary. A Report of the American College of Cardiology/American Heart Association Task Force on Practice Guidelines and the European Society of Cardiology Committee for Practice Guidelines and Policy Conferences (Committee to Develop Guidelines for the Management of Patients with Atrial Fibrillation): Developed in collaboration with the North American Society of Pacing and Electrophysiology. J Am Coll Cardiol 2001;38:1231-1266.

116. Fuster V, Ryden LE, Cannom DS, et al: ACC/AHA/ESC 2006 Guidelines for the Management of Patients with Atrial Fibrillation: A report of the American College of Cardiology/American Heart Association Task Force on Practice Guidelines and the European Society of Cardiology Committee for Practice Guidelines (Writing Committee to Revise the 2001 Guidelines for the Management of Patients with Atrial Fibrillation): Developed in collaboration with the European Heart Rhythm Association and the Heart Rhythm Society. Circulation 2006;114:e257-354.

117. Mitchell LB, Exner DV, Wyse DG, et al: Prophylactic oral amiodarone for the prevention of arrhythmias that begin early after revascularization, valve replacement, or repair: PAPABEAR: A randomized controlled trial. JAMA 2005;294:3093-3100.

118. Huikuri HV, Yli-Mayry S, Korhonen UR, et al: Prevalence and prognostic significance of complex ventricular arrhythmias after coronary arterial bypass graft surgery. Int J Cardiol 1990;27:333-339.

119. Tam SK, Miller JM, Edmunds LH Jr: Unexpected, sustained ventricular tachyarrhythmia after cardiac operations. J Thorac Cardiovasc Surg 1991;102:883-889.

120. Kaul TK, Fields BL, Riggins LS, et al: Ventricular arrhythmia following successful myocardial revascularization: Incidence, predictors and prevention. Eur J Cardiothorac Surg 1998;13:629-636.

121. Topol EJ, Lerman BB, Baughman KL, et al: De novo refractory ventricular tachyarrhythmias after coronary revascularization. Am J Cardiol 1986;57:57-59.

122. A comparison of antiarrhythmic-drug therapy with implantable defibrillators in patients resuscitated from near-fatal ventricular arrhythmias. The Antiarrhythmics versus Implantable Defibrillators (AVID) Investigators. N Engl J Med 1997;337:1576-1583.

123. Bommer WJ, Follette D, Pollock M, et al: Tamponade in patients undergoing cardiac surgery: A clinical-echocardiographic diagnosis. Am Heart J 1995;130:1216-1223.

124. Tsang TS, Oh JK, Seward JB: Diagnosis and management of cardiac tamponade in the era of echocardiography. Clin Cardiol 1999;22: 446-452.

125. Meurin P, Weber H, Renaud N, et al: Evolution of the postoperative pericardial effusion after day 15: The problem of the late tamponade. Chest 2004;125:2182-2187.

126. Ramsay J, Shernan S, Fitch J, et al: Increased creatine kinase MB level predicts postoperative mortality after cardiac surgery independent of new Q waves. J Thorac Cardiovasc Surg 2005;129:300-306.

127. Klatte K, Chaitman BR, Theroux P, et al: Increased mortality after coronary artery bypass graft surgery is associated with increased levels of postoperative creatine kinase-myocardial band isoenzyme release: Results from the GUARDIAN trial. J Am Coll Cardiol 2001;38:1070-1077.

128. Januzzi JL, Lewandrowski K, MacGillivray TE, et al: A comparison of cardiac troponin T and creatine kinase-MB for patient evaluation after cardiac surgery. J Am Coll Cardiol 2002;39:1518-1523.

129. Benoit MO, Paris M, Silleran J, et al: Cardiac troponin I: Its contribution to the diagnosis of perioperative myocardial infarction and various complications of cardiac surgery. Crit Care Med 2001;29: 1880-1886.

130. Hou SH, Bushinsky DA, Wish JB, et al: Hospital-acquired renal insufficiency: A prospective study. Am J Med 1983;74:243-248.

131. Nash K, Hafeez A, Hou S: Hospital-acquired renal insufficiency. Am J Kidney Dis 2002;39:930-936.

132. Clermont G, Acker CG, Angus DC, et al: Renal failure in the ICU: Comparison of the impact of acute renal failure and end-stage renal disease on ICU outcomes. Kidney Int 2002;62:986-996.

133. Conlon PJ, Little MA, Pieper K, Mark DB: Severity of renal vascular disease predicts mortality in patients undergoing coronary angiography. Kidney Int 2001;60:1490-1497.

134. Conlon PJ, Stafford-Smith M, White WD, et al: Acute renal failure following cardiac surgery. Nephrol Dial Transplant 1999;14: 1158-1162.

135. Chertow GM, Levy EM, Hammermeister KE, et al: Independent association between acute renal failure and mortality following cardiac surgery. Am J Med 1998;104:343-348.

136. Mangano CM, Diamondstone LS, Ramsay JG, et al: Renal dysfunction after myocardial revascularization: Risk factors, adverse outcomes, and hospital resource utilization. The Multicenter Study of

Perioperative Ischemia Research Group. Ann Intern Med 1998;128:194-203.

137. van den Berghe G, Wouters P, Weekers F, et al: Intensive insulin therapy in the critically ill patients. N Engl J Med 2001;345: 1359-1367.

138. Denton MD, Chertow GM, Brady HR: "Renal-dose" dopamine for the treatment of acute renal failure: Scientific rationale, experimental studies and clinical trials. Kidney Int 1996;50:4-14.

139. Argalious M, Motta P, Khandwala F, et al: "Renal dose" dopamine is associated with the risk of new-onset atrial fibrillation after cardiac surgery. Crit Care Med 2005;33:1327-1332.

140. Caimmi PP, Pagani L, Micalizzi E, et al: Fenoldopam for renal protection in patients undergoing cardiopulmonary bypass. J Cardiothorac Vasc Anesth 2003;17:491-494.

141. Renton MC, Snowden CP: Dopexamine and its role in the protection of hepatosplanchnic and renal perfusion in high-risk surgical and critically ill patients. Br J Anaesth 2005;94:459-467.

142. Alpert RA, Roizen MF, Hamilton WK, et al: Intraoperative urinary output does not predict postoperative renal function in patients undergoing abdominal aortic revascularization. Surgery 1984;95:707-711.

143. Roach GW, Kanchuger M, Mangano CM, et al: Adverse cerebral outcomes after coronary bypass surgery. Multicenter Study of Perioperative Ischemia Research Group and the Ischemia Research and Education Foundation Investigators. N Engl J Med 1996;335:1857-1863.

144. Wolman RL, Nussmeier NA, Aggarwal A, et al: Cerebral injury after cardiac surgery: Identification of a group at extraordinary risk. Multicenter Study of Perioperative Ischemia Research Group (McSPI) and the Ischemia Research Education Foundation (IREF) Investigators. Stroke 1999;30:514-522.

145. Selnes OA, Goldsborough MA, Borowicz LM, McKhann GM: Neurobehavioural sequelae of cardiopulmonary bypass. Lancet 1999;353:1601-1606.

146. Selnes OA, McKhann GM: Neurocognitive complications after coronary artery bypass surgery. Ann Neurol 2005;57:615-621.

147. Newman MF, Kirchner JL, Phillips-Bute B, et al: Longitudinal assessment of neurocognitive function after coronary-artery bypass surgery. N Engl J Med 2001;344:395-402.

148. Newman MF, Wolman R, Kanchuger M, et al: Multicenter preoperative stroke risk index for patients undergoing coronary artery bypass graft surgery. Multicenter Study of Perioperative Ischemia (McSPI) Research Group. Circulation 1996;94:II74-80.

149. Aantaa R, Jalonen J: Perioperative use of alpha2-adrenoceptor agonists and the cardiac patient. Eur J Anaesthesiol 2006;23:361-372.

150. Floyd TF, Cheung AT, Stecker MM: Postoperative neurologic assessment and management of the cardiac surgical patient. Semin Thorac Cardiovasc Surg 2000;12:337-348.

151. Dyer CB, Ashton CM, Teasdale TA: Postoperative delirium: A review of 80 primary data-collection studies. Arch Intern Med 1995;155:461-465.

152. Rudolph JL, Babikian VL, Birjiniuk V, et al: Atherosclerosis is associated with delirium after coronary artery bypass graft surgery. J Am Geriatr Soc 2005;53:462-466.

153. Baddour LM, Kluge RM: Infections in open heart surgery. Asepsis 1989;11:10-17.

154. Kluge RM, Calia FM, McLaughlin JS, Hornick RB: Sources of contamination in open heart surgery. JAMA 1974;230:1415-1418.

155. Roy MC: Surgical-site infections after coronary artery bypass graft surgery: Discriminating site-specific risk factors to improve prevention efforts. Infect Control Hosp Epidemiol 1998;19:229-233.

156. National Nosocomial Infections Surveillance (NNIS) System Report, Data Summary from January 1992–June 2001, issued August 2001. Am J Infect Control 2001;29:404-421.

157. Haas JP, Evans AM, Preston KE, Larson EL: Risk factors for surgical site infection after cardiac surgery: The role of endogenous flora. Heart Lung 2005;34:108-114.

158. Furnary AP, Zerr KJ, Grunkemeier GL, Starr A: Continuous intravenous insulin infusion reduces the incidence of deep sternal wound infection in diabetic patients after cardiac surgical procedures. Ann Thorac Surg 1999;67:352-360; discussion 360-362.

159. Kreuzer E, Kaab S, Pilz G, Werdan K: Early prediction of septic complications after cardiac surgery by APACHE II score. Eur J Cardiothorac Surg 1992;6:524-528; discussion 529.

160. Toumpoulis IK, Anagnostopoulos CE, Swistel DG, DeRose JJ Jr: Does EuroSCORE predict length of stay and specific postoperative complications after cardiac surgery? Eur J Cardiothorac Surg 2005;27:128-133.

161. Aouifi A, Piriou V, Bastien O, et al: Usefulness of procalcitonin for diagnosis of infection in cardiac surgical patients. Crit Care Med 2000;28:3171-3176.

162. Grocott HP, Mackensen GB, Grigore AM, et al: Postoperative hyperthermia is associated with cognitive dysfunction after coronary artery bypass graft surgery. Stroke 2002;33:537-541.

163. Kollef MH, Sharpless L, Vlasnik J, et al: The impact of nosocomial infections on patient outcomes following cardiac surgery. Chest 1997;112:666-675.

164. Hessel EA 2nd: Abdominal organ injury after cardiac surgery. Semin Cardiothorac Vasc Anesth 2004;8:243-263.

165. D'Ancona G, Baillot R, Poirier B, et al: Determinants of gastrointestinal complications in cardiac surgery. Tex Heart Inst J 2003;30:280-285.

166. Zehr KJ, Dawson PB, Yang SC, Heitmiller RF: Standardized clinical care pathways for major thoracic cases reduce hospital costs. Ann Thorac Surg 1998;66:914-919.

167. Aps C: Fast-tracking in cardiac surgery. Br J Hosp Med 1995;54:139-142.

168. Weintraub WS, Craver JM, Jones EL, et al: Improving cost and outcome of coronary surgery. Circulation 1998;98:II23-28.

169. Pronovost PJ, Jenckes MW, Dorman T, et al: Organizational characteristics of intensive care units related to outcomes of abdominal aortic surgery. JAMA 1999;281:1310-1317.

170. Cannon CP, Battler A, Brindis RG, et al: American College of Cardiology key data elements and definitions for measuring the clinical management and outcomes of patients with acute coronary syndromes: A report of the American College of Cardiology Task Force on Clinical Data Standards (Acute Coronary Syndromes Writing Committee). J Am Coll Cardiol 2001;38:2114-2130.

171. Silbert BS, Santamaria JD, O'Brien JL, et al: Early extubation following coronary artery bypass surgery: A prospective randomized controlled trial. The Fast Track Cardiac Care Team. Chest 1998;113:1481-1488.

172. Zarate E, Latham P, White PF, et al: Fast-track cardiac anesthesia: Use of remifentanil combined with intrathecal morphine as an alternative to sufentanil during desflurane anesthesia. Anesth Analg 2000;91:283-287.

173. Parlow JL, Steele RG, O'Reilly D: Low dose intrathecal morphine facilitates early extubation after cardiac surgery: Results of a retrospective continuous quality improvement audit. Can J Anaesth 2005;52:94-99.

174. Pastor MC, Sanchez MJ, Casas MA, et al: Thoracic epidural analgesia in coronary artery bypass graft surgery: Seven years' experience. J Cardiothorac Vasc Anesth 2003;17:154-159.

175. Cohen AJ, Katz MG, Frenkel G, et al: Morbid results of prolonged intubation after coronary artery bypass surgery. Chest 2000;118:1724-1731.

176. Calafiore AM, Scipioni G, Teodori G, et al: Day 0 intensive care unit discharge: Risk or benefit for the patient who undergoes myocardial revascularization? Eur J Cardiothorac Surg 2002;21:377-384.

177. Reyes A, Vega G, Blancas R, et al: Early vs conventional extubation after cardiac surgery with cardiopulmonary bypass. Chest 1997;112:193-201.

178. Epstein SK, Ciubotaru RL, Wong JB: Effect of failed extubation on the outcome of mechanical ventilation. Chest 1997;112:186-192.

179. Alexander WA, Cooper JR Jr: Preoperative risk stratification identifies low-risk candidates for early extubation after aortocoronary bypass grafting. Tex Heart Inst J 1996;23:267-269.

180. Wong DT, Cheng DC, Kustra R, et al: Risk factors of delayed extubation, prolonged length of stay in the intensive care unit, and mortality in patients undergoing coronary artery bypass graft with fast-track cardiac anesthesia: A new cardiac risk score. Anesthesiology 1999;91:936-944.

181. Becker RB, Zimmerman JE, Knaus WA, et al: The use of APACHE III to evaluate ICU length of stay, resource use, and mortality after coronary artery by-pass surgery. J Cardiovasc Surg (Torino) 1995;36:1-11.

182. Higgins TL, Estafanous FG, Loop FD, et al: ICU admission score for predicting morbidity and mortality risk after coronary artery bypass grafting. Ann Thorac Surg 1997;64:1050-1058.

183. Edgerton JR, Herbert MA, Prince SL, et al: Reduced atrial fibrillation in patients immediately extubated after off-pump coronary artery bypass grafting. Ann Thorac Surg 2006;81:2121-2126; discussion 2126-2127.

184. Horswell JL, Herbert MA, Prince SL, Mack MJ: Routine immediate extubation after off-pump coronary artery bypass surgery: 514 consecutive patients. J Cardiothorac Vasc Anesth 2005;19:282-287.

185. Glower DD, Landolfo KP, Clements F, et al: Mitral valve operation via port access versus median sternotomy. Eur J Cardiothorac Surg 1998;14(Suppl 1):S143-147.

186. Cohn LH, Adams DH, Couper GS, et al: Minimally invasive cardiac valve surgery improves patient satisfaction while reducing costs of cardiac valve replacement and repair. Ann Surg 1997;226:421-426; discussion 427-428.

187. Cosgrove DM 3rd, Sabik JF, Navia JL: Minimally invasive valve operations. Ann Thorac Surg 1998;65:1535-1538; discussion 1538-1539.

188. Hadjinikolaou L, Cohen A, Glenville B, Stanbridge RD: The effect of a "fast-track" unit on the performance of a cardiothoracic department. Ann R Coll Surg Engl 2000;82:53-58.

189. London MJ, Shroyer AL, Jernigan V, et al: Fast-track cardiac surgery in a Department of Veterans Affairs patient population. Ann Thorac Surg 1997;64:134-141.

190. Cheng DC, Wall C, Djaiani G, et al: Randomized assessment of resource use in fast-track cardiac surgery 1-year after hospital discharge. Anesthesiology 2003;98:651-657.

Chapter

32 General Thoracic Surgery

Todd W. Sarge and Alan Lisbon

At the conclusion of most general thoracic surgical procedures, patients can be extubated and sent to recover in the general postanesthesia care unit (PACU) before being sent to an inpatient ward. This concept was shown in a recent series of 500 patients who underwent thoracotomy and "fast-track pulmonary resections."[1] The authors concluded that most patients who undergo elective pulmonary resection could be extubated immediately after the operation, avoid the intensive care unit (ICU), be discharged on postoperative day 3 or 4, and have minimal morbidity and mortality with high satisfaction both at discharge and at the 2-week follow-up contact. Techniques that seem to help with this strategy include the use and removal of epidural catheters on postoperative day 2; early chest tube management, including immediate water seal and treatment of persistent air leaks with Heimlich valves; and daily reinforcement of the planned events for each day, including the date of discharge, with the patients and their families.[1]

Many exceptions occur that require ICU care and monitoring with and without mechanical ventilation. In this chapter, we will discuss the various issues with regard to the early postoperative management of the general thoracic surgery patient, with emphasis on specific complications encountered that require intensive care. We will discuss the various management strategies with an emphasis on evidence-based practice. Establishing criteria that determine whether a patient goes to the PACU or the ICU for recovery is not our intention, but rather to develop general guidelines based on current standards of care and common complications that will help an experienced clinician choose the best course.

■ GENERAL CARE

Patients arriving in either the ICU or the PACU from the operating room should be hemodynamically stable, comfortable, and breathing without difficulty if extubated. Otherwise, the patient should be sedated and mechanically ventilated until hemodynamic and respiratory functions are optimized. The decision to discontinue mechanical ventilatory support and extubate the patient is a team decision based on the combined experiences of the anesthesiologist and the surgeon, and it depends on the preoperative status of the patient, the intraoperative course, and the expected postoperative pulmonary status. Patients with marginal preoperative function and those with intraoperative complications (e.g., bleeding) need every advantage prior to extubation. Achieving this goal can require a short stay in the PACU

prior to extubation to resolve issues of residual anesthetics or sedatives and to optimize pain control.

Alternatively, if hemodynamic instability is a problem, admission to the ICU may be warranted. Double-lumen endotracheal tubes should be changed to standard single-lumen tubes unless there is a simple and quickly reversible need for remaining intubated (e.g., persistent effects of narcotics or muscle relaxants) or if intubation was exceedingly difficult with airway trauma. The double-lumen tubes can pose a danger to the patient in the PACU or the ICU when the nursing and respiratory staff members are unfamiliar with their use and design. Both the anesthesiologist and the surgeon should accompany the patient to the designated recovery area so that a complete and thorough sign-out from "both sides of the ether screen" can be given to the nursing and physician team responsible for the patient's recovery. Routine orders should include a postoperative chest radiograph, arterial blood gas measurement, a complete blood count and chemistry panel, chest tube care, fluid orders, pain control plan, and oxygen and ventilator settings, if necessary.

Monitoring

In the early postoperative period, patients are typically maintained on standard monitors, including five-lead electrocardiograph, pulse oximeter, and peripheral radial arterial line. Central venous pressure should be transduced and recorded if a central line is present. Pulmonary artery catheterization and monitoring are rarely used intraoperatively or in the immediate postoperative setting, as the values are unreliable intraoperatively and difficult to interpret in the lateral decubitus thoracotomy position because of alterations of normal pulmonary artery flow and the pressures that result. Furthermore, pulmonary artery catheterization has been shown in a recent large randomized controlled trial of high-risk surgical patients to be of no value in improving outcome and to have higher complication rates for those patients.[2] Peripheral arterial catheters are considered the standard of care for most procedures that involve any degree of lung resection. Their use is invaluable not only for hemodynamic monitoring but, more importantly, for obtaining arterial blood for blood gas measurements and other laboratory studies.

Radiography

Routine daily chest radiography has been a common practice in many institutions caring for postoperative thoracic patients, particularly for mechanically ventilated patients. This practice has recently faded for the general ICU population, but it might be considered more useful in the early postoperative care of the thoracic surgical patient. Even so, Graham and colleagues showed in a prospective observational study of 100 consecutive thoracotomy patients that routine chest radiographs altered management in only 43 of 769 studies (5.6%), which included 33 routine (4.5%) and 10 nonroutine (26.3%) studies.[3] The authors concluded that routine daily portable chest radiographic studies have minimal impact on management. Nonroutine radiography often alters management. The authors recommended that for major thoracic procedures, it is safe, efficacious, and cost effective to eliminate routine postoperative portable chest radiography and order nonroutine portable studies only when clinically indicated. Their conclusion included a cost savings analysis that showed that $286,000 could be saved annually with the elimination of all routine chest radiographs with the exception of one study in the immediate postoperative period.

Chest radiographs, whether ordered immediately postoperatively or as indicated, should be reviewed systematically to avoid missing important findings. Their assessment should include the following:

- Invasive devices: endotracheal tube, chest tubes, central venous or pulmonary artery catheters
- Lung fields: pneumothorax, atelectasis, effusions, infiltrates
- Mediastinum: heart size and location, trachea and carina position, mediastinal size and shift
- Diaphragm: position and elevation, gastric and bowel distention

The endotracheal tube should be positioned just inside the thoracic inlet and several centimeters above the carina. Central venous lines should be in the superior vena cava. Pulmonary artery catheters should be no more than 3 cm from midline. Chest tubes should be positioned with all ports inside the thoracic cavity and directed posterior-cephalad without evidence of kinks. The remaining lung fields should be well aerated, although discoid atelectasis is normal in the early postoperative period. Large segments with atelectasis require further investigation and recruitment. Small apical pneumothoraces are common; however, large pneumothoraces should be addressed with regard to chest tube position and suction. Large pneumothoraces may be a sign of bronchial stump leaks and need close observation. Furthermore, significant air leaks from lung parenchyma are best resolved with reexpansion of the atelectatic lung, and they often do not resolve until the lung meets the visceral pleura. Similarly, effusions and blood should be easily drained by the chest tubes, and their presence requires attention to the drainage system or the need for return to the operating room if they are the result of significant bleeding. The mediastinum should be midline and of normal width. Substantial mediastinal shifts need to be addressed, as they may be caused by an enlarging hemothorax, a pneumothorax, or a vacuum effect after pneumonectomy. Appropriate resolution depends on recognition of the underlying cause. The presence of gastric or small-intestinal distention determines whether there is a need for nasogastric tube suction. These findings are also indicative of the presence of postoperative ileus.

Drainage Tubes

Chest tubes are typically connected to underwater suction at 20 cm H_2O to facilitate drainage of blood and air while maintaining a constant low-pressure gradient to minimize fluctuations in wall suction. Chest tube drainage is a good indicator of postoperative bleeding, and although 200 mL/hr of drainage may be seen in the early postoperative period, drainage should decrease rapidly thereafter. Persistently high drainage beyond 4 hours should be cause for alarm and possible surgical exploration to find and correct the source of bleeding. However, a recent study looked at the efficacy of using suction for chest tube drains connected to an underwater seal in 239 patients undergoing various thoracic surgical procedures.[4] The conclusion was that applying suction to the underwater seal drains after lung surgery makes no difference in terms of air leak duration.

Perioperative Antibiotics

Perioperative antibiotic prophylaxis is commonly practiced, although the literature supporting this practice is less compelling for clean noncardiac thoracic surgery than for cardiac and vascular surgery. A randomized, double-blinded trial of 127 patients undergoing noncardiac thoracic surgery was conducted by Aznar and coworkers, who compared the use of a single dose cefazolin (1 g) versus placebo and found the relative risk of wound infection for the patients in the placebo group was 3.27 (95% CI, 1.5 to 11.5).[5] Furthermore, cefazolin significantly reduced ($P < .01$) the wound infection rate; there was one case (1.5%) in the cefazolin group but there were eight cases (14%) in the placebo group. Antibiotic prophylaxis did not decrease the incidence of postoperative pleural empyema; there were five cases in the antibiotic group (7%) versus eight cases (14%) in the placebo group. Antibiotic prophylaxis also did not change the incidence of nosocomial pneumonia: three cases (4%) versus five cases (9%). It was concluded that a single preoperative 1-g dose of cefazolin was effective for reducing the wound infection rate in noncardiac thoracic surgery.[5]

In a similar fashion, most antibiotic guidelines, including those offered by the American Academy of Family Practitioners (AAFP) recommend antibiotic prophylaxis for nearly all thoracic procedures but especially for those with complete or partial obstruction of the trachea and involvement of the esophagus.[6] However, the AAFP guidelines point out the lack of evidence, with the exception of two trials in patients undergoing pulmonary resections. The AAFP guidelines indicate that cefazolin is adequate in most instances. Bratzler and colleagues published an advisory statement from the National Surgical Infection Prevention Project, recommending prophylactic antimicrobials for cardiothoracic operations to include cefazolin or cefuroxime.[7] Also, for patients with serious allergy or adverse reaction to β-lactam antibiotics, vancomycin is appropriate, and clindamycin may be an acceptable alternative. The authors also commented that prophylactic antibiotics should continue no longer than 24 hours. This recommendation was made even though many cardiothoracic surgeons continue antibiotics postoperatively while drains remain in situ, and the Society of Thoracic Surgeons currently recommends antimicrobial prophylaxis be continued for 24 to 48 hours.

The prophylactic use of antibiotics for chest tube insertion has been more controversial. Most studies have been done in the setting of penetrating chest trauma. Gonzalez and Holevar showed that patients receiving antibiotics have a significantly reduced incidence of infectious complications and suggested that patients who undergo tube thoracostomy for chest trauma would benefit from administration of prophylactic antibiotics.[8] However, a more recent prospective, randomized, double-blind trial of 224 patients by Maxwell and colleagues compared the use of cefazolin for the duration of tube thoracostomy placement versus using it for 24 hours versus placebo and concluded that the incidence of empyema was low and the use of prophylactic antibiotics does not reduce the risk of empyema or pneumonia.[9] These authors showed that duration of tube placement and thoracic acute injury score were predictive of empyema ($P < .05$). Empyema tended to occur more frequently in patients with penetrating injuries ($P = .09$), whereas pneumonia occurred significantly more frequently in blunt than in penetrating injuries ($P < .05$). Another study by Demetriades and coworkers reached a similar finding and concluded that single-dose prophylaxis in penetrating chest trauma is as effective as prolonged prophylaxis.[10]

■ CARDIAC COMPLICATIONS

Arrhythmias

Cardiac complications are extremely common in the postoperative period after noncardiac thoracic surgery. Arrhythmias are the most common cardiac complication after thoracic surgery, and the most common of these is atrial fibrillation. Atrial fibrillation has a reported incidence of 20% after lobectomy and 40% after pneumonectomy.[11] This complication is considered significant because it is associated with higher rates of pneumonia, increased length of stay, and mortality.[12,13] The relation between atrial fibrillation and other complications remains controversial, as it is unclear whether poor outcome is the cause or effect of atrial fibrillation. Because perioperative atrial fibrillation has been linked with poor outcome and morbidity, extensive research has been done to both identify risk factors and provide prophylaxis against it. Amar and associates showed that age and a preoperative heart rate greater than 72 to 74 beats per minute are independently associated with the development of postoperative atrial fibrillation, and they developed a prediction rule based on these variables.[12,14] Recently, Vaporciyan and colleagues studied a larger population of 2588 patients and determined that age, male sex, intraoperative transfusions, peripheral vascular disease, history of arrhythmias, congestive heart failure, and increasing size of pulmonary resection (i.e., pneumonectomy greater than lobectomy) were all associated with a higher incidence of atrial fibrillation after noncardiac thoracic surgery.[15] Also, Amar and associates showed that increased right heart pressure, as estimated by the presence of a tricuspid regurgitant jet on the echocardiogram, but not fluid overload or right heart enlargement, predisposes to

clinically significant supraventricular tachycardia (SVT) after pulmonary resection.[16] Attempts to provide prophylaxis for patients deemed to be at high risk for development of perioperative atrial fibrillation have included the use of digitalis, beta-adrenergic blockade, calcium channel antagonists, and class 1 antiarrhythmics (e.g., flecainide). De Decker and colleagues recently reviewed these trials and concluded the following[11]:

- Prophylaxis with magnesium sulfate is supported by one clinical trial (Terzi and coworkers[17]) and is very attractive because of its benign side effect profile when compared with other antiarrhythmic treatment options. Caution is warranted in patients with renal failure.
- Beta-adrenergic blockade, particularly using metoprolol, has been shown in one small randomized trial of 30 patients to reduce the incidence of atrial fibrillation postoperatively[18] and should be used perioperatively for patients with known heart disease or significant risk factors.
- Prophylaxis with digitalis, although common practice in some centers, is not supported by clinical trials at this time.

Myocardial Ischemia and Heart Failure

Other cardiac complications that require vigilant monitoring and treatment are myocardial ischemia or infarction and right ventricular heart failure with concomitant left heart failure. Myocardial ischemia occurs in 0.13% of patients without known cardiac disease and 2.8% to 17% of patients with a cardiac history; mortality rates range from 2% to 21%.[11] Although large studies are lacking, there is no apparent association with anesthetic technique. Intensive monitoring for at least 72 hours has been advocated, during which time patients remain at risk for postoperative myocardial infarction. Right coronary artery (RCA) ischemia or infarction occurs more frequently in patients with chronic lung disease and right ventricular hypertrophy, and it carries a high mortality when associated with inferior myocardial infarction. Furthermore, right ventricular ischemia or infarction necessitates a higher preload to maintain adequate cardiac output. This necessity can pose a significant dilemma in the early postoperative care of patients who have undergone lung resection and whose fluid has been relatively restricted to avoid problems with pulmonary edema. Because the primary blood supply to both the sinoatrial and the atrioventricular nodes is in a right dominant system, RCA infarcts can also precipitate significant dysrhythmias and high-degree heart block, which may require urgent cardiac pacing.

New data from a prospective study of 240 diverse surgical patients recently correlated the maximal amplitude on thromboelastography (TEG) with thromboembolic complications, including perioperative myocardial infarction.[19] These data support other observations and suggest that this complication is less related to hemodynamic perturbations during or after surgery and more related to complex hematologic and coagulation factors. Although TEG is not used routinely at this time, further studies in this area are needed to determine the full potential of this test in assisting with prediction and possible treatment of patients at risk for perioperative thromboembolic events.

Right ventricular heart failure is usually caused by increased afterload with pulmonary hypertension, most likely as a result of alterations in the pulmonary circulation and excess intravascular volume. Pulmonary edema is a dangerous complication, with high mortality in patients who have undergone lung resection, and it is further discussed later in this chapter. Other causes of right ventricular failure include pulmonary embolism, RCA ischemia or infarction, and cardiac herniation.

Cardiac Herniation

Cardiac herniation is a very rare complication caused by a combination of a pericardial defect and abnormal intrathoracic pressures after lung resection. This complication rate is associated with a high morality (>50%).[20,21] The signs and symptoms can be a dramatic loss of cardiac output and blood pressure as venous return is compromised. This diagnosis must be added to the differential diagnosis for pulseless electrical activity after pneumonectomy with tumor resection that involves the pericardium. However, the signs and symptoms may be less obvious, including dysrhythmias, ischemic changes on the electrocardiogram, and protrusion of the heart into the thorax on the chest radiograph. The radiographic finding may be particularly striking with right-sided herniation. Treatment is operative and patients should be transported to the operating room immediately for reduction of the heart and repair of the pericardium. In preparation for surgery, chest tubes should be removed from suction, positive ventilation pressures minimized, and the patient positioned in such a way that the force of gravity limits further herniation.

■ PULMONARY COMPLICATIONS

Postoperative pulmonary complications (PPCs) are still a leading cause of morbidity and mortality after noncardiac thoracic surgery[22] and have been associated with increased hospital and ICU lengths of stay and with poor outcomes.[23-30] PPCs have been defined in various ways but can include any pulmonary insult or dysfunction leading to increased morbidity or mortality in the postoperative period. Common PPCs include the following: prolonged ventilator dependence, atelectasis, aspiration pneumonitis, nosocomial and ventilator-associated pneumonia, bronchospasm, pleural effusions, pneumothorax, bronchopleural fistula, postintubation membranous tracheal rupture or laceration, postpneumonectomy pulmonary edema (PPE), and acute lung injury (ALI) or acute respiratory distress syndrome (ARDS).

In general, the pathophysiology of many of these complications begins with the alteration of normal respiratory mechanics that is observed in postoperative thoracic surgery patients—specifically, a decrease in functional residual capacity in the presence of an unchanged closing volume, leading to atelectasis and premature airway closure during tidal breathing.[31] Postoperatively, pulmonary function is further complicated by pain, sedation, and narcosis, leading

to inadequate cough, shallow breathing, and immobility. All of these issues contribute to worsening atelectasis and difficulty in clearing secretions.

Adequate pain control can positively attenuate the altered pulmonary mechanics after thoracotomy and reduce the overall incidence of respiratory complications. Also, the surgical approach can affect early postoperative pulmonary function. For example video-assisted thoracoscopic surgery (VATS) is associated with improved pulmonary function in the early postoperative period.[32] Preoperative chest physiotherapy and pulmonary exercise have been shown to improve postoperative pulmonary function and reduce respiratory complications. A recent article by Takaoka and colleagues states that pulmonary rehabilitation is a cost-effective, benign intervention with no adverse effects and should remain an essential component of patient management before any elective thoracic surgical procedure.[33]

In an attempt to predict and risk stratify patients presenting for thoracic surgery, a myriad of studies have addressed the preoperative risk factors for developing PPCs. Most of these studies have been derived from retrospective or prospective observational data collections. These studies are limited by a lack of consensus with regard to defining and diagnosing PPCs, and many are limited by inadequate numbers to perform multivariate regression to determine the independent risk factors. Consequently, dozens of risk factors have been reported in the literature, and there is confusion and controversy about risk stratification.

For example, many studies have demonstrated a correlation with preoperative pulmonary function (particularly, forced expiratory volume in 1 second, or FEV_1), whereas a recent prospective data collection of 193 pneumonectomies by Licker and associates demonstrated that advanced age, right-sided procedures, and preoperative pulmonary function testing did not accurately predict the incidence of PPCs.[26] It should be noted, however, that Licker and colleagues excluded patients with FEV_1 less than 40% and maximal oxygen uptake less than 50%.[26] Therefore, the definition of risk factors may be a moving target as best practice changes in response to work in prior studies. Also of interest, Licker and associates noted that patients with American Society of Anesthesia (ASA) classification of III and IV, extended resections, and those unable to receive epidural anesthesia had significantly higher rates of PPCs.

A larger retrospective study by Algar and colleagues of 242 patients undergoing pneumonectomy used a multiple logistic regression model to determine the independent risk factors for respiratory complications and concluded that the following parameters were important: anesthetic time, FEV_1, heart disease, lack of previous chest physiotherapy, and chronic obstructive pulmonary disease (COPD).[23] Stephan and colleagues[27] conducted a retrospective study of patients who underwent lung resection and determined the following independent risk factors for PPCs: ASA score of III or more, an operating time greater than 80 minutes, and the need for postoperative mechanical ventilation for greater than 48 minutes. These authors also concluded that preoperative pulmonary function tests did not appear to contribute to the identification of high-risk patients.[27]

Wang and coworkers conducted several studies looking at diffusion capacity of carbon monoxide (DLCO) to assess the risk for postoperative pulmonary complications. In a retrospective study of 193 pneumonectomy patients, Wang determined that a DLCO of 70% of the predicted value was the best functional predictor of postoperative complications.[29] There was a complication rate of 94% in patients with a DLCO of less than 70% of predicted, compared with a 27% complication rate in patients with a DLCO of 70% or greater of predicted (sensitivity, 62%; specificity, 96%). In a prospective study of 40 patients undergoing any lung resection, Wang and colleagues again concluded that DLCO predicts the likelihood of pulmonary complications after major lung resection.[28]

With regard to VATS, a recent retrospective study by Haraguchi and associates determined that the most sensitive risk factor for development of respiratory complications was duration of surgery.[34] These authors concluded that VATS procedures should be limited to less than 5 hours or converted to a muscle-sparing open technique.

Atelectasis

Postoperative atelectasis is a uniform complication after major surgery of the upper abdomen and thorax. The clinical significance is often minimal, but in patients with poor preoperative pulmonary function, it may assume clinical significance because of the development of hypoxemia and respiratory distress. Preventive measures, including incentive spirometry and chest physiotherapy, have been advocated as useful, and their use remains widespread. Although there is some evidence in favor of chest physiotherapy for diseases such as cystic fibrosis and COPD, the studies evaluating its use in the postoperative setting are much less decisive. A review by Stiller and Munday concluded that chest physiotherapy was useful for reducing pulmonary complications via unknown mechanisms.[35] On the other hand, a recent and thorough critique of the available literature on incentive spirometry by Overend and associates concluded that the evidence does not support its use for decreasing the incidence of PPCs after cardiac or upper abdominal surgery.[36] Similarly, Pasquina and colleagues reviewed the literature for prophylactic respiratory physiotherapy (including physical therapy, incentive spirometry, continuous positive airway pressure, and intermittent positive airway pressure) in patients after cardiac surgery and concluded that the usefulness of respiratory physiotherapy for the prevention of pulmonary complications after cardiac surgery remains unproven.[37] Patients with symptomatic atelectasis may require bronchoscopy for therapeutic suctioning and removal of mucus plugs.

Nosocomial Pneumonia and Ventilator-Associated Pneumonia

Nosocomial pneumonia and ventilator-associated pneumonia (VAP) are defined as pneumonia developing in patients after 48 hours from hospitalization or the start of mechanical ventilation, respectively. Common risk factors include chronic lung disease, prior use of antibiotics, thoracic surgery, large-volume aspiration, histamine (H_2)-blocker therapy, presence of nasogastric tubes, and head of bed at less than 30 degrees for mechanically ventilated patients. The diagnosis is made by finding bacterial growth (>10,000 colony-forming units) via bronchoalveolar lavage or blind bronchial suctioning in the presence of fever, elevated white blood cell count, and definitive infiltrate on chest radiography. Treatment should include broad-spectrum antibiotics directed at typical pathogens including gram-negative bacteria (particularly *Pseudomonas aeruginosa*) and *Staphylococcus aureus*. Also, knowledge of common institutional pathogens and sensitivities should factor into initial therapy. Broad-spectrum antibiotics should be de-escalated once definitive speciation of bacteria with sensitivity analysis has been reported by the microbiology laboratory.

Aspiration Pneumonitis

Aspiration pneumonitis is a common perioperative complication that is of particular concern in thoracic surgery patients with preoperative lung dysfunction. Aspiration pneumonitis refers to the passage of gastric and oral secretions into the tracheobronchial system, with resultant chemical irritation and inflammation. This chemical injury may be of little significance or may result in infection, aspiration pneumonia, or ARDS. When aspiration occurs, treatment involves turning the patient to the lateral decubitus position while suctioning the airway and monitoring for desaturation, tachycardia, respiratory distress, and bronchospasm. Intubation should be contemplated if large volumes of gastric contents have been aspirated in the presence of significant desaturation. Although antibiotics were formerly used to treat acute aspiration pneumonitis, they may in fact be harmful if they allow colonization and subsequent superinfection. However, if aspiration pneumonitis does progress to pneumonia, antibiotics targeted at the specific pathogens are warranted.

Pleural Effusions

Pleural effusions that persist and worsen after thoracic surgery are worrisome because they may represent infection or empyema and chylous effusion from thoracic duct disruption. Infections should be suspected with worsening poorly draining effusions in the presence of fever, leukocytosis, and other clinical findings associated with sepsis syndrome. Management of empyema requires broad-spectrum antibiotics, attempted tube drainage, and often surgical drainage, often with VATS. The use of fibrinolytics has recently been criticized because of a large randomized trial of patients diagnosed with pleural infections, who had a higher adverse-event profile without improvement in mortality, rate of surgery, or length of hospital stay.[38] Chylous effusions are more common with left-sided procedures, and they are usually sterile and can be easily managed conservatively. Surgery is required only if the effusion fails to resolve after several weeks of chest tube drainage. Congestive heart failure, paraneoplastic effusions, and malnutrition are separate causes of chronic effusions and are managed as they would be in the nonsurgical patient.

Bronchospasm

Bronchospasm is common in postoperative thoracic surgery patients, as it is preoperatively. Most thoracic patients are continued on bronchodilator therapy, including beta-adrenergic agonists as well as anticholinergics. However, endotracheal intubation with frequent suctioning in the setting of increased secretions may exacerbate bronchoconstriction, necessitating the need for systemic and inhaled steroids in severe cases.

Pneumothorax

Small pneumothoraces are common in the immediate postoperative period, but resolution can be prolonged and hampered by positive pressure ventilation. Persistence or worsening with onset of signs and symptoms of increased tension (hypotension, tracheal deviation, dyspnea) require the presence of a definitive closed chest tube system. Indwelling chest tubes should be evaluated for patency and should be repositioned or replaced as necessary.

Postintubation Tracheal Rupture

Postintubation tracheal rupture is a very rare complication after intubation, and no large randomized controlled trials have been performed to study its treatment. However, a number of case series have been reported with acceptable outcomes achieved by both surgical and conservative treatment strategies. Typical risk factors include difficult intubation and intubation of short women. This complication may be more frequent after thoracic surgery with double-lumen endotracheal tube placement, but this notion is not proven. Furthermore, a recent series by Carbognani and colleagues demonstrated that a tear was caused by insertion of a double-lumen tube in only three of 13 patients.[39]

The diagnosis is typically made by tracheobronchoscopy performed because of symptoms, such as dyspnea, subcutaneous emphysema, and hemoptysis, that are all nonspecific in postoperative thoracic surgery patients. Another sign that should arouse suspicion is unexplained pneumomediastinum on chest radiograph. Carbognani and associates advocate a very reasonable treatment plan of conservative nonsurgical treatment with prophylactic antibiotics and observation of uncomplicated tears less than 2 cm in length; otherwise, surgical repair via thoracotomy or a transcervical approach is warranted.

Bronchopleural Fistula

Bronchopleural fistula with persistent air leak is also a relatively uncommon but serious complication following lung resection and pneumonectomy. The incidence varies between 2% and 5%, and the complication carries a mortality rate as high as 27%.[40-42] Typical signs include increased air leaks, hemoptysis, and worsening pneumothorax on chest radiography. Typical causes of stump leaks and fistula formation include infection, inadequate tumor resection, ischemia, preoperative radiation therapy, severe malnutrition, postoperative mechanical ventilation, right-sided pneumonectomy, and large stump diameter.[40-44] Because of its relatively small incidence, there are no large randomized trials comparing treatments of bronchopleural fistula. Management strategies can

be conservative or surgical, depending on the severity and overall status of the patient. Management can be especially difficult in patients requiring prolonged positive pressure ventilatory support because of ALI/ARDS and higher ventilator pressures, including positive end-expiratory pressure (PEEP). The goals in mechanically ventilated patients are to prevent persistent pneumothoraces and to minimize flow across the stump, thereby facilitating healing. In general, these goals can be accomplished in lobectomy patients with stump leaks via prolonged chest tube drainage with or without suction. Ventilation strategies include high-frequency ventilation, lung isolation with double-lumen endotracheal tubes, and decreasing PEEP, when tolerated. Pneumonectomy patients who develop stump leaks will need more aggressive surgical management.

Postpneumonectomy Pulmonary Edema and Acute Respiratory Distress Syndrome

One of the most feared postoperative complications after any lung resection, but more often after pneumonectomy, is the development of noncardiogenic pulmonary edema, or postpneumonectomy pulmonary edema (PPE). PPE is now considered a subset of ALI that carries a high mortality similar to that of ALI and ARDS seen in other critically ill patients.[45] The pathophysiology underlying this complication appears to be a combination of increased filtration gradient across the pulmonary microcirculation, together with hyperpermeability.[46] PPE usually occurs within postoperative days 0 to 3, although it can occur later in the postoperative course, but then it is more often associated with pneumonia and aspiration (more typical causes of ARDS).

The incidence of "early PPE" is generally reported to be 4% to 5% after pneumonectomy; right-sided procedures carry a slightly higher risk than left-sided ones.[47-49] Other major risk factors originally described by Zeldin and colleagues[50] and confirmed by others include excessive perioperative fluid administration and high postoperative urine output.[47,48] Further studies on perioperative risk for PPE have shown even more potential risk factors. Parquin and associates demonstrated in a retrospective analysis of 146 consecutive postpneumonectomy patients that previous treatment with radiotherapy, resection of well-perfused lung parenchyma (i.e., remaining lung perfusion scan of 55% or less), and excessive fluid load (at least 2000 mL intraoperatively) are high risk factors for the development of noncardiogenic pulmonary edema in the postoperative period.[51] Van der Werff and colleagues also conducted a retrospective study of 197 patients, which demonstrated that the risk of PPE was increased by administration of fresh frozen plasma transfusions and higher mechanical ventilation pressures during surgery.[52] More recently, Licker and associates retrospectively studied a cohort of 897 consecutive patients undergoing pulmonary resection and found that early ALI was associated with preoperative alcohol consumption, pneumonectomy, high intraoperative pressure index, and excessive fluid intake over the first 24 hours.[53]

In addition to these effects of mechanical ventilation and fluid management, other therapies used in the treatment of PPE include perioperative steroids, inhaled nitric oxide, and extracorporeal membrane oxygenation (ECMO). However, the success of these therapies has been limited to case reports and small nonrandomized case-control studies.[54-58] Inhaled nitric oxide has been used in broader ALI/ARDS populations as well, but despite the early excitement from case reports and case series of patients with ALI/ARDS, benefits were not realized in larger randomized control trials. As a result, pharmacologic therapies such as these have been relegated to being rescue therapies. Therefore, relying on the presumption that the pathophysiology of PPE is similar to that of ARDS, it would be best to consider these therapies as being reserved for rare cases of PPE as well. However, carefully constructed randomized control trials would settle the issue, as it is certainly possible that this subset of ALI/ARDS (in which decreased lung perfusion scans and pulmonary hypertension place patients at increased risk) may in fact derive mortality benefit from the ability of inhaled nitric oxide to improve ventilation–perfusion mismatch and thus oxygenation via pulmonary vasodilation.

Although large randomized control trials studying this complication are still lacking, ample evidence supports some basic general management strategies that have been advocated by others, including Slinger[59]:

- Careful preoperative assessment with consideration given to preoperative pulmonary function and radiation history
- Judicious perioperative fluid administration with limitation of intravenous volume (about 2 L) in the first 24 hours while accepting urine outputs of 0.5 mL/kg/hr
- Avoidance of hyperinflation both intraoperatively and postoperatively by using a lung protection ventilation strategy including low tidal volumes of 4 to 6 mL/kg
- Using a reasonable PEEP to avoid atelectasis while maintaining peak plateau pressures below 30 cm H_2O

■ PAIN CONTROL

Pain control must not be overlooked when caring for postoperative thoracic surgical patients. Good pain control can ameliorate the adverse pulmonary function changes observed in the early postoperative period after thoracic surgery, whereas poor pain control can exacerbate them. This aspect of the patient's care is usually determined preoperatively (preemptive analgesia), and the prevention of central sensitization is the current trend in most perioperative pain management strategies. This approach is believed to reduce both the absolute requirement for pain medication and the incidence of chronic pain syndromes, such as post-thoracotomy pain syndrome.[60,61] Furthermore, pain control should always be reevaluated and monitored as all other vital signs are in the postoperative period. This point cannot be emphasized enough, as inadequate pain control impacts nearly every aspect of the early postoperative care of the general thoracic surgery patient. Clearly, the approach used for pain control is a function of the surgery performed. That is, lateral limited muscle-sparing thoracotomy, or mini-thoracotomy, and VATS have been shown to reduce postoperative analgesic

medication requirements when compared with traditional thoracotomy.[62,63]

Postoperative pain control can be accomplished by systemic, neuraxial, and regional techniques. Systemic pain medication, regardless of the route of administration, is largely dominated by opiates and nonsteroidal anti-inflammatory drugs (NSAIDs). Systemic opiates (especially with patient-controlled analgesia devices) are effective for treating postoperative pain, but they are limited by their notorious side effects, such as nausea, vomiting, ileus, respiratory suppression, and excessive sedation. NSAIDs also have a host of side effects including platelet dysfunction, hypertension, and kidney dysfunction. Furthermore, a recent animal study demonstrated decreased quality of mechanical pleurodesis after administration of NSAIDs.[64] Neuraxial analgesia typically includes epidural infusion of local anesthetics with or without opioids, but it can also include intrathecal opioid administration. Regional pain control techniques include intercostal nerve blocks, paravertebral injections, and intrapleural administration of local anesthetics. The advantages of neuraxial and regional techniques over systemic opioids are numerous. The most important is the decreased total dose of opioids,[65] leading to fewer side effects.[66] The one exception seems to be intrapleural administration of local anesthetics, which seems to be much less efficacious and less feasible in clinical trials and a recent meta-analysis.[67,68]

Epidural analgesia is the most common and well-accepted choice for post-thoracotomy analgesia. This technique has been proven in randomized controlled trials dating back to 1984 when Shulman and associates demonstrated its superior analgesia when compared to systemic medications.[69] Furthermore, a recent meta-analysis by Ballantyne and colleagues demonstrated improvement in pulmonary mechanics with fewer pulmonary complications after thoracotomy in those patients who received epidural analgesia compared with those who did not.[70] A similar meta-analysis of 55 studies by Richardson and associates demonstrated that regional and neuraxial techniques (particularly paravertebral, epidural, and intercostal nerve blocks) attenuate post-thoracotomy pulmonary dysfunction.[67] Richardson and colleagues also suggested that providing effective analgesia without regard to maintaining pulmonary function is inadequate, and that improvements in outcome might be realized if pulmonary function were made the standard outcome measure for adequate analgesia rather than pain scores and rescue pain medications.[71] This hypothesis remains to be tested in a randomized trial with morbidity and mortality as primary endpoints.

■ REFERENCES

1. Cerfolio RJ, Pickens A, Bass C, Katholi C: Fast-tracking pulmonary resections. J Thorac Cardiovasc Surg 2001;122:318-324.
2. Sandham JD, Hull RD, Brant RF, et al: A randomized, controlled trial of the use of pulmonary-artery catheters in high-risk surgical patients. N Engl J Med 2003;348:5-14.
3. Graham RJ, Meziane MA, Rice TW, et al: Postoperative portable chest radiographs: Optimum use in thoracic surgery. J Thorac Cardiovasc Surg 1998;115:45-50; discussion 50-52.

4. Alphonso N, Tan C, Utley M, et al: A prospective randomized controlled trial of suction versus non-suction to the under-water seal drains following lung resection. Eur J Cardiothorac Surg 2005;27:391-394.

5. Aznar R, Mateu M, Miro JM, et al: Antibiotic prophylaxis in noncardiac thoracic surgery: Cefazolin versus placebo. Eur J Cardiothorac Surg 1991;5:515-518.

6. Woods RK, Dellinger EP: Current guidelines for antibiotic prophylaxis of surgical wounds. Am Fam Physician 1998;57:2731-2740.

7. Bratzler DW, Houck PM, Richards C, et al: Use of antimicrobial prophylaxis for major surgery: Baseline results from the National Surgical Infection Prevention Project. Arch Surg 2005;140:174-182.

8. Gonzalez RP, Holevar MR: Role of prophylactic antibiotics for tube thoracostomy in chest trauma. Am Surg 1998;64:617-620; discussion 620-621.

9. Maxwell RA, Campbell DJ, Fabian TC, et al: Use of presumptive antibiotics following tube thoracostomy for traumatic hemopneumothorax in the prevention of empyema and pneumonia: A multi-center trial. J Trauma 2004;57:742-748; discussion 748-749.

10. Demetriades D, Breckon V, Breckon C, et al: Antibiotic prophylaxis in penetrating injuries of the chest. Ann R Coll Surg Engl 1991;73:348-351.

11. De Decker K, Jorens PG, Van Schil P: Cardiac complications after noncardiac thoracic surgery: An evidence-based current review. Ann Thorac Surg 2003;75:1340-1348.

12. Amar D, Zhang H, Leung DH, etal: Older age is the strongest predictor of postoperative atrial fibrillation. Anesthesiology 2002;96:352-356.

13. Brathwaite D, Weissman C: The new onset of atrial arrhythmias following major noncardiothoracic surgery is associated with increased mortality. Chest 1998;114:462-468.

14. Passman RS, Gingold DS, Amar D, et al: Prediction rule for atrial fibrillation after major noncardiac thoracic surgery. Ann Thorac Surg 2005;79:1698-1703.

15. Vaporciyan AA, Correa AM, Rice DC, et al: Risk factors associated with atrial fibrillation after noncardiac thoracic surgery: Analysis of 2588 patients. J Thorac Cardiovasc Surg 2004;127:779-786.

16. Amar D, Roistacher N, Burt M, et al: Clinical and echocardiographic correlates of symptomatic tachydysrhythmias after noncardiac thoracic surgery. Chest 1995;108:349-354.

17. Terzi A, Furlan G, Chiavacci P, et al: Prevention of atrial tachyarrhythmias after non-cardiac thoracic surgery by infusion of magnesium sulfate. Thorac Cardiovasc Surg 1996;44:300-303.

18. Jakobsen CJ, Bille S, Ahlburg P, et al: Perioperative metoprolol reduces the frequency of atrial fibrillation after thoracotomy for lung resection. J Cardiothorac Vasc Anesth 1997;11:746-751.

19. McCrath DJ, Cerboni E, Frumento RJ, et al: Thromboelastography maximum amplitude predicts postoperative thrombotic complications including myocardial infarction. Anesth Analg 2005;100:1576-1583.

20. Groh J, Sunder-Plassmann L: [Heart dislocation following extensive lung resection with partial pericardial resection.] Anaesthesist 1987;36:182-184.

21. Asamura H: Early complications: Cardiac complications. Chest Surg Clin N Am 1999;9:527-541, vii-viii.

22. Brooks-Brunn JA: Postoperative atelectasis and pneumonia. Heart Lung 1995;24:94-115.

23. Algar FJ, Alvarez A, Salvatierra A, et al: Predicting pulmonary complications after pneumonectomy for lung cancer. Eur J Cardiothorac Surg 2003;23:201-208.

24. Busch E, Verazin G, Antkowiak JG, et al: Pulmonary complications in patients undergoing thoracotomy for lung carcinoma. Chest 1994;105:760-766.

25. Licker M, de Perrot M, Hohn L, et al: Perioperative mortality and major cardio-pulmonary complications after lung surgery for non-small cell carcinoma. Eur J Cardiothorac Surg 1999;15:314-319.

26. Licker M, Spiliopoulos A, Frey JG, et al: Risk factors for early mortality and major complications following pneumonectomy for non-small cell carcinoma of the lung. Chest 2002;121:1890-1897.

27. Stephan F, Boucheseiche S, Hollande J, et al: Pulmonary complications following lung resection: A comprehensive analysis of incidence and possible risk factors. Chest 2000;118:1263-1270.

28. Wang J, Olak J, Ultmann RE, Ferguson MK: Assessment of pulmonary complications after lung resection. Ann Thorac Surg 1999;67:1444-1447.

29. Wang JS: Relationship of carbon monoxide pulmonary diffusing capacity to postoperative cardiopulmonary complications in patients undergoing pneumonectomy. Kaohsiung J Med Sci 2003;19:437-446.

30. Zwischenberger JB, Alpard SK, Bidani A: Early complications: Respiratory failure. Chest Surg Clin N Am 1999;9:543-564, viii.

31. Sabanathan S, Eng J, Mearns AJ: Alterations in respiratory mechanics following thoracotomy. J R Coll Surg Edinb 1990;35:144-150.

32. Kaseda S, Aoki T, Hangai N, Shimizu K: Better pulmonary function and prognosis with video-assisted thoracic surgery than with thoracotomy. Ann Thorac Surg 2000;70:1644-1646.

33. Takaoka ST, Weinacker AB: The value of preoperative pulmonary rehabilitation. Thorac Surg Clin 2005;15:203-211.

34. Haraguchi S, Koizumi K, Hatori N, et al: Postoperative respiratory complications of video-assisted thoracic surgery for lung cancer. J Nippon Med Sch 2004;71:30-34.

35. Stiller KR, Munday RM: Chest physiotherapy for the surgical patient. Br J Surg 1992;79:745-749.

36. Overend TJ, Anderson CM, Lucy SD, et al: The effect of incentive spirometry on postoperative pulmonary complications: A systematic review. Chest 2001;120:971-978.

37. Pasquina P, Tramer MR, Walder B: Prophylactic respiratory physiotherapy after cardiac surgery: Systematic review. BMJ 2003;327:1379.

38. Maskell NA, Davies CW, Nunn AJ, et al: U.K. controlled trial of intrapleural streptokinase for pleural infection. N Engl J Med 2005;352:865-874.

39. Carbognani P, Bobbio A, Cattelani L, et al: Management of postintubation membranous tracheal rupture. Ann Thorac Surg 2004;77:406-409.

40. Javadpour H, Sidhu P, Luke DA: Bronchopleural fistula after pneumonectomy. Ir J Med Sci 2003;172:13-15.

41. Algar FJ, Alvarez A, Aranda JL, et al: Prediction of early bronchopleural fistula after pneumonectomy: A multivariate analysis. Ann Thorac Surg 2001;72:1662-1667.

42. Sirbu H, Busch T, Aleksic I, et al: Bronchopleural fistula in the surgery of non-small cell lung cancer: Incidence, risk factors, and management. Ann Thorac Cardiovasc Surg 2001;7:330-336.

43. Hollaus PH, Setinek U, Lax F, Pridun NS: Risk factors for bronchopleural fistula after pneumonectomy: Stump size does matter. Thorac Cardiovasc Surg 2003;51:1626.

44. Gall SA Jr, Wolfe WG: Management of microfistula following pulmonary resection. Chest Surg Clin N Am 1996;6:543-565.

45. Turnage WS, Lunn JJ: Postpneumonectomy pulmonary edema: A retrospective analysis of associated variables. Chest 1993;103:1646-1650.

46. Shapira OM, Shahian DM: Postpneumonectomy pulmonary edema. Ann Thorac Surg 1993;56:190-195.

47. Waller DA, Gebitekin C, Saunders NR, Walker DR: Noncardiogenic pulmonary edema complicating lung resection. Ann Thorac Surg 1993;55:140-143.

48. Verheijen-Breemhaar L, Bogaard JM, van den Berg B, Hilvering C: Postpneumonectomy pulmonary oedema. Thorax 1988;43:323-326.

49. Turnage WS, Lunn JJ: Postpneumonectomy pulmonary edema. What's the cause? Chest 1994;106:320-321.

50. Zeldin RA, Normandin D, Landtwing D, Peters RM: Postpneumonectomy pulmonary edema. J Thorac Cardiovasc Surg 1984;87:359-365.

51. Parquin F, Marchal M, Mehiri S, et al: Post-pneumonectomy pulmonary edema: Analysis and risk factors. Eur J Cardiothorac Surg 1996;10:929-932; discussion 933.

52. van der Werff YD, van der Houwen HK, Heijmans PJ, et al: Postpneumonectomy pulmonary edema: A retrospective analysis of incidence and possible risk factors. Chest 1997;111:1278-1284.

53. Licker M, de Perrot M, Spiliopoulos A, et al: Risk factors for acute lung injury after thoracic surgery for lung cancer. Anesth Analg 2003;97:1558-1565.

54. Della Rocca G, Coccia C: Nitric oxide in thoracic surgery. Minerva Anestesiol 2005;71:313-318.

55. Cerfolio RJ, Bryant AS, Thurber JS, et al: Intraoperative Solumedrol helps prevent postpneumonectomy pulmonary edema. Ann Thorac Surg 2003;76:1029-1035; discussion 1033-1035.

56. Rabkin DG, Sladen RN, DeMango A, et al: Nitric oxide for the treatment of postpneumonectomy pulmonary edema. Ann Thorac Surg 2001;72:272-274.

57. Verhelst H, Vranken J, Muysoms F, et al: The use of extracorporeal membrane oxygenation in postpneumonectomy pulmonary oedema. Acta Chir Belg 1998;98:269-272.

58. Mathisen DJ, Kuo EY, Hahn C, et al: Inhaled nitric oxide for adult respiratory distress syndrome after pulmonary resection. Ann Thorac Surg 1998;66:1894-1902.

59. Slinger PD: Perioperative fluid management for thoracic surgery: The puzzle of postpneumonectomy pulmonary edema. J Cardiothorac Vasc Anesth 1995;9:442-451.

60. Peeters-Asdourian C, Gupta S: Choices in pain management following thoracotomy. Chest 1999;115(5 Suppl):122S-124.

61. Yegin A, Erdogan A, Kayacan N, Karsli B: Early postoperative pain management after thoracic surgery—Pre- and postoperative versus postoperative epidural analgesia: A randomised study. Eur J Cardiothorac Surg 2003;24:420-424.

62. Landreneau RJ, Wiechmann RJ, Hazelrigg SR, et al: Effect of minimally invasive thoracic surgical approaches on acute and chronic postoperative pain. Chest Surg Clin N Am 1998;8:891-906.

63. Sedrakyan A, van der Meulen J, Lewsey J, Treasure T: Video assisted thoracic surgery for treatment of pneumothorax and lung resections: Systematic review of randomised clinical trials. BMJ 2004;329:1008.

64. Lardinois D, Vogt P, Yang L, et al: Non-steroidal anti-inflammatory drugs decrease the quality of pleurodesis after mechanical pleural abrasion. Eur J Cardiothorac Surg 2004;25:865-871.

65. Carretta A, Zannini P, Chiesa G, et al: Efficacy of ketorolac tromethamine and extrapleural intercostal nerve block on post-thoracotomy pain: A prospective, randomized study. Int Surg 1996;81:224-228.

66. Carli F, Trudel JL, Belliveau P: The effect of intraoperative thoracic epidural anesthesia and postoperative analgesia on bowel function after colorectal surgery: A prospective, randomized trial. Dis Colon Rectum 2001;44:1083-1089.

67. Richardson J, Sabanathan S, Shah R: Post-thoracotomy spirometric lung function: The effect of analgesia—A review. J Cardiovasc Surg (Torino) 1999;40:445-456.

68. Miguel R, Hubbell D: Pain management and spirometry following thoracotomy: A prospective, randomized study of four techniques. J Cardiothorac Vasc Anesth 1993;7:529-534.

69. Shulman M, Sandler AN, Bradley JW, et l: Postthoracotomy pain and pulmonary function following epidural and systemic morphine. Anesthesiology 1984;61:569-575.

70. Ballantyne JC, Carr DB, deFerranti S, et al: The comparative effects of postoperative analgesic therapies on pulmonary outcome: Cumulative meta-analyses of randomized, controlled trials. Anesth Analg 1998;86:598-612.

71. Richardson J, Sabanathan S, Jones J, et al: A prospective, randomized comparison of preoperative and continuous balanced epidural or paravertebral bupivacaine on post-thoracotomy pain, pulmonary function and stress responses. Br J Anaesth 1999;83:387-392.

33 Major Abdominal Surgery

Patrick J. Neligan and Jacob Gutsche

Major abdominal surgery refers to operations performed on the upper and lower GI tracts, diaphragm, hepatobiliary system, abdominal wall, and genitourinary tract. Although abdominal aortic aneurysm repair is a major abdominal procedure, it is considered a vascular operation and is covered elsewhere in this text. The majority of patients undergoing procedures within the abdominal cavity or pelvis are of advanced age, often presenting with cancer and with multiple confounding medical disorders. Such patients are at elevated risk for a large number of perioperative complications, both medical and surgical. Surgical complications are usually localized to the surgical site. Complications may be early or late, depending on the nature of the surgical procedure. Early complications include bleeding, wound hematoma, anastomotic leakage, and paralytic ileus. Later complications include surgical site infection, wound infection, wound dehiscence, and intestinal obstruction. Medical complications are less specific, involve many organ systems, and usually occur early after surgery. These include respiratory failure, pulmonary edema, deep venous thrombosis, pulmonary embolism, cardiac arrhythmias, acute renal failure, and delirium.

In many ways, the distinction between medical and surgical complications is artificial and unnecessary. Patients at elevated risk of developing surgical complications are at similar risk for medical complications. This elevated risk results from the problem of a significant surgical stress response in an older adult patient with minimal functional, or physiologic, reserve.

The stress response is an organism-wide response to surgery or injury characterized by changes in metabolism and neurohormonal function. It is characterized by enhanced release of pituitary hormones, increased sympathoadrenal activity, pancreatic hypersecretion, and the activation of inflammation. There is a dramatic increase in protein turnover, anabolism is postponed, fluid accumulates in the extravascular space, and there is a dramatic increase in oxygen delivery to the tissues.

The ability of the body to deal with stress is known as physiologic, or functional, reserve. Physiologic reserve is the excess capacity that exists in organ systems to deal with injury; it allows the body to restore homeostasis. The cardiovascular system, lungs, kidneys, and liver have enormous functional reserve. Aging and chronic illness deplete physiologic reserve. Critical illness is a state in which physiologic reserve is inadequate to maintain life and exogenous organ support is required.

In this chapter we will explore several areas of perioperative risk associated with major surgery of the abdomen and pelvis (Fig. 33-1). Key to the understanding of these complications is the patient population involved, the nature of the underlying pathology, and the type of surgery involved. We will revisit the stress response several times and explore how the balance between stress and functional organ response is a critical aspect of the development of perioperative complications. Later, we will address prevention of pulmonary complications, fluid management strategies, nutrition, prevention and treatment of delirium, surgical site infections, and deep venous thrombosis.

■ REDUCING POSTOPERATIVE PULMONARY COMPLICATIONS

Patients undergoing major abdominal surgery, in particular to the upper abdomen, are at elevated risk of developing pulmonary complications. These include hypoxemia during induction of anesthesia and atelectasis after extubation. Morbidly obese patients undergoing surgery are at additional risk as a result of airway obstruction consequent to narcosis, hypercarbia, and obstructive sleep apnea/hypopnea. As this cohort represents the extreme end of the risk spectrum for perioperative pulmonary complications, this part of the chapter will focus on the bariatric patient as a model for perioperative risk reduction.

Preoxygenation, Positive Pressure, and Induction of Anesthesia

The administration of sedative hypnotic drugs and neuromuscular blockers is generally referred to as induction of general anesthesia. For major abdominal surgery, the principal purpose of induction is to secure the airway through translaryngeal placement of a cuffed plastic (endotracheal) tube. The major early complications of this process include aspiration of gastric contents, hypoxemia, and failure to obtain an adequate airway. Preoxygenation is widely used to reduce the risk for hypoxemia as a result of airway complications.

The hypothesis behind preoxygenation is that replacement of the nitrogen content of the lungs with oxygen increases apneic time (i.e., the time between administration of drugs that halt respiration and the restoration of ventilation). A high concentration of oxygen (100% is preferable but rarely achieved) is delivered to the airway for 3 minutes. Alternatively, the patient may take eight vital capacity

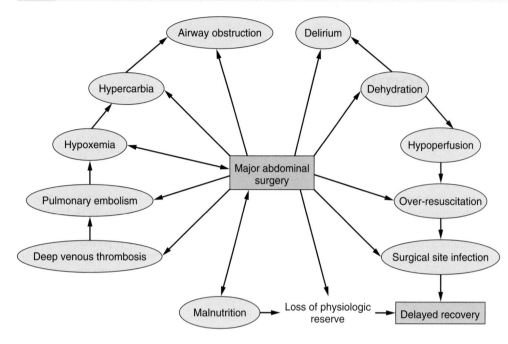

Figure 33-1 ■ Overview of the risk profile of patients undergoing major abdominal surgery.

breaths.[1,2] The vital capacity now becomes a reservoir for oxygenation.

There are several potential problems with induction of anesthesia. Both neuromuscular blockade and anesthesia induced by sedative hypnotic agents cause significant reduction (16% to 20% in the supine position) in functional residual capacity (FRC).[3] FRC falls immediately after induction and reaches its final value within the first few minutes. The reduction in FRC is correlated with age and chest wall elastance.[4] This leads to airway closure, reduced compliance, and ventilation-perfusion mismatch. High inspired oxygen tension (FIO_2) causes atelectasis (absorption atelectasis).[5] This results from the presence of a large oxygen gradient between the alveolus and the mixed venous blood; nitrogen washout removes the normal buttress for alveolar stability. Oxygen flows rapidly along the concentration gradient, and alveoli destabilize and collapse. Atelectasis also results from compression of pulmonary tissue, particularly the left lower lobe (compressed by the heart)[6] and the juxtadiaphragmatic region.[7] The combination of loss of FRC, leading to airway closure, diaphragmatic repositioning, and compressive and absorptive atelectasis commonly results in postintubation hypoxemia and increased airway pressures.[8] Apneic oxygenation (the time from onset of apnea until hypoxemia develops) may be considerably shorter than expected.[9] Patients most vulnerable to this include the morbidly obese, those with increased intra-abdominal pressures (including pregnancy), and those with extrapulmonary acute respiratory distress syndrome (ARDS). The combination of hypoxemia and low respiratory system compliance is an indication for recruitment maneuvers: the use of high transalveolar pressures to reexpand collapsed lung tissue. Unfortunately, the combination of the vasodilatory properties of sedative hypnotic drugs, loss of adrenergic tone (caused by all anesthetic agents—none is cardiovascularly neutral), relative and abso-

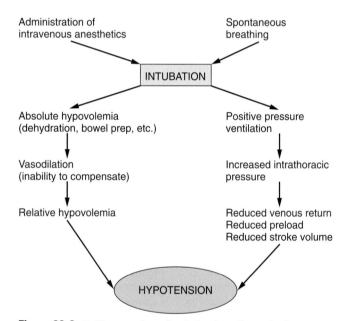

Figure 33-2 ■ Hypotension after induction of anesthesia.

lute hypovolemia (particularly if the patient has received a bowel preparation), and the institution of positive-pressure ventilation (leading to increased intrathoracic pressure, reduced preload, increased right ventricular afterload) frequently results in hypotension (Fig. 33-2).

Clearly, any method that will prolong apneic oxygenation and prevent atelectasis on induction of anesthesia, without accompanying adverse effects, would be beneficial. Perioperative patients with a high risk profile include pregnant women and the morbidly obese, and these have been studied. The earliest published data came from Berthoud and associates in 1991.[10] They looked at time taken for the oxygen saturation (SpO_2) to decrease to 90% after preoxygenation in six morbidly obese patients and six matched controls of normal weight. During apnea, the obese patients maintained an SpO_2 of greater than 90% for 196 (standard deviation [SD], 80) seconds (range, 55 to 208 sec), compared with 595 (SD, 142) seconds (range, 430 to 825 sec) in the control group ($P < .001$). Thus preoxygenation did not significantly increase apneic oxygenation time in morbidly obese patients. "Normal controls" infers, in this case, absence of lung and airway pathology. There is evidence that patient positioning may have a significant impact on the apneic duration in this patient group.

Lane and colleagues investigated whether positioning patients who were undergoing general anesthesia for cholecystectomy in a 20-degree head-up position, as opposed to supine, improved the efficacy of 3 minutes of standard preoxygenation via a circle breathing system.[11] After preoxygenation, patients received a standard induction of anesthesia and the apnea time (from administration of rocuronium to the arterial oxygen saturation to fall to 95%) was recorded. Mean apnea time was 386 seconds (95% confidence interval [CI], 343-429) in the 20-degree head-up position ($n = 17$) versus 283 seconds (95% CI, 243-322) in the supine position ($n = 18$; $P = .002$).

Baraka and colleagues investigated the influence of preoxygenation in the supine ($n = 10$) versus the 45-degree head-up ($n = 10$) position in 20 women undergoing elective cesarean section at term of pregnancy.[12] The duration of apnea leading to a decrease in SpO_2 to 95%, as monitored by pulse oximetry, was investigated. The results were compared with those obtained in a control group of 20 nonpregnant women. In the supine position, the average time to desaturation to 95% was significantly shorter in the pregnant group (173 ± 4.8 sec [mean $\pm$ SD]) than in the control group of nonpregnant women (243 ± 7.4 sec). Using the head-up position resulted in an increase in the apneic oxygenation time in the nonpregnant group (331 ± 7.2 sec) but had no significant effect in the pregnant group (156 ± 2.8 sec).

Dixon and coworkers explored preoxygenation in the 25-degree head-up position during induction of anesthesia in 42 consecutive, morbidly obese (body mass index [BMI] >40 kg/m^2) patients (male-to-female ratio, 13 : 29).[13] Patients were randomly assigned to the supine position or the 25-degree head-up position. Serial arterial blood gases were taken before and after preoxygenation and 90 seconds after induction. After induction, ventilation was delayed until blood oxygen saturation reached 92%, and this desaturation safety period was recorded. The group randomly assigned to the 25-degree head-up position achieved higher preinduction oxygen tensions (442 ± 104 versus 360 ± 99 mm Hg; $P = .012$) and took longer to reach an oxygen saturation of 92% (201 ± 55 versus 155 ± 69 sec; $P = .023$). There was a strong positive correlation between the induction oxygen tension achieved and the time to reach an oxygen saturation of 92% ($r = 0.51$, $P = .001$).

Altermatt and colleagues studied 40 morbidly obese patients (BMI ≥ 35 kg/m^2) undergoing surgery with general anesthesia and randomly assigned them to induction of

anesthesia in the sitting or the supine position.[14] Preoxygenation was achieved with eight deep breaths within 60 seconds and an oxygen flow of 10 L/min. After rapid-sequence induction, the trachea was intubated and the patient was left apneic and disconnected from the anesthesia circuit until SpO_2 decreased to 90%, and the time taken for this to occur was recorded. The mean time to desaturation to 90% was significantly longer in the sitting group than in the supine group (mean, 214 [SD, 28] versus 162 sec [SD, 38]; $P < .05$).

There is emerging evidence that nursing and transport of the critically ill patient in the semirecumbent position is associated with a lower incidence of nosocomial pneumonia.[15-18] Furthermore, data indicate improved lung mechanics and prolonged apneic oxygenation with head elevation, reverse Trendelenburg positioning (RTP), or seated positioning. Therefore, we recommend that, unless contraindicated, the majority of patients be intubated (in emergency or high-risk circumstances) with the head elevated, or in reverse Trendelenburg position, at 30 degrees.

Postoperative atelectasis with associated hypoxemia and increased pulmonary workload is a significant problem for morbidly obese patients Morbid obesity is associated with dramatic reductions in total respiratory system compliance.[19] Induction of anesthesia is associated with widespread atelectasis that worsens over 24 hours (Fig. 33-3).[20] During general anesthesia, there is a significant reduction in total respiratory system compliance.[21] This leads to significantly lower lung volumes and ventilation–perfusion mismatch.[19] In addition, morbidly obese patients had significantly higher airway resistance than normal.[21] Changes in lung mechanics associated with obesity are positive end-expiratory pressure (PEEP)

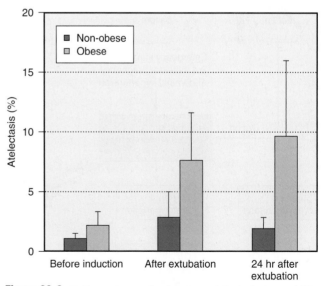

Figure 33-3 ■ Percentages of pulmonary atelectasis in morbidly obese compared with non-obese patients, shown at three stages: before anesthesia induction, after extubation, and 24 hr later. *(Redrawn from Eichenberger A, Proietti S, Wicky S, et al: Morbid obesity and postoperative pulmonary atelectasis: An underestimated problem. Anesth Analg 2002;95:1788-1792.)*

sensitive,[22,23] although PEEP requirements are higher than in normal patients.[24] These patients also respond to RTP.[25,26]

Morbidly obese patients have significantly more atelectasis than non-obese patients before induction (2.1% of total lung area versus 1.0%, $P < .01$), after tracheal extubation (7.6% versus 2.8%, $P < .05$), and 24 hours after laparoscopic surgery (9.7% versus 1.9%, $P < .01$).[20] This occurred despite the application of 6 cm H_2O PEEP to both groups intraoperatively. This leads to significantly increased perioperative risk in terms of primary and secondary respiratory failure. Vital capacity and a loss of FRC falls after extubation. This relationship varies linearly with BMI.[27] Atelectasis increases the workload of breathing. Hence, in the recovery room, the combination of partial neuromuscular blockade, opioids, and segmental lung collapse may lead to acute respiratory distress requiring reintubation. Of more concern is the progressive increase in atelectasis that occurs over the first 24 hours, at which stage the patients are often less supervised on the ward. Atelectasis and hypoventilation, secondary to opioids and leading to hypercapnia-induced somnolence, may lead to airway obstruction and respiratory arrest.

Loss of FRC, lung de-recruitment, and airway obstruction predispose patients to hypoxemia.[10] High inspired concentrations of oxygen increase the extent of absorption atelectasis and reduce FRC further.[28] These competing problems can be offset by the application of continuous positive airway pressure (CPAP) during preoxygenation.[29-31]

Coussa and colleagues randomly assigned 23 patients with a BMI of greater than 35, to one of two groups.[31] The treatment group was preoxygenated with 100% oxygen and CPAP of 10 cm H_2O, which was continued after intubation.

There was a significantly higher incidence of hypoxemia and atelectasis, as evidenced by computed tomography (CT), in the control group that did not receive CPAP. It is unclear whether hypoxemia on induction is associated with unfavorable outcomes or whether recruitment maneuvers, after induction, have an effect similar to that of CPAP.[32]

Gander and coworkers[9] randomized 30 morbidly obese patient undergoing bariatric surgery to preoxygenation with 100% O_2 plus 10 cm H_2O CPAP for 5 minutes before induction and then pressure control ventilation plus 10 cm H_2O PEEP for 5 minutes until the trachea was intubated. The control group received neither CPAP before induction nor PEEP subsequently. No positive pressure was applied to the airway after intubation, until the patient was desaturated below 92%. Then a recruitment breath was given and positive-pressure ventilation commenced. Nonhypoxic apnea duration was longer in the PEEP group than in the control group (188 ± 46 versus 127 ± 43 sec; $P = .002$). PaO_2 was higher before apnea in the PEEP group ($P = .038$). Thus, application of positive airway pressure during induction of general anesthesia in morbidly obese patients increases nonhypoxic apnea duration by 50% (Fig. 33-4). This may significantly increase patient safety.

Intraoperative PEEP and Positioning and Postoperative Respiratory Complications

Pelosi and colleagues investigated respiratory system mechanics in morbidly obese patients versus non-obese controls during anesthesia and neuromuscular blockade.[24] With no PEEP, morbidly obese patients had significantly lower lung

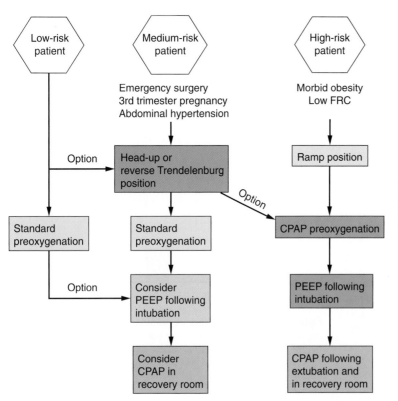

Figure 33-4 ■ Preoxygenation for prevention of atelectasis. CPAP, continuous positive airway pressure; FRC, functional residual capacity; PEEP, positive end-expiratory pressure.

volumes, lower total respiratory system compliance, lower chest wall compliance, higher intra-abdominal pressure, an increased alveolar-arterial PO_2 gradient, and a higher $PaCO_2$. Adding PEEP of 10 cm H_2O significantly improved lung and chest wall compliance in morbidly obese patients, but not in patients with a normal BMI. There was a significant improvement in oxygenation in the morbidly obese group. In both overweight and obese patients, the application of PEEP improved oxygenation at 30 and 90 minutes after extubation.[22]

Although PEEP appears to improve oxygenation and pulmonary mechanics in morbidly obese patients perioperatively, some evidence indicates that the amount of PEEP applied is important. Tusman and colleagues studied 90 patients who were either normal weight or obese.[23] Obese patients were treated with PEEP 5 cm H_2O (obese 5) or 10 cm H_2O (obese 10) intraoperatively. All patients received recruitment maneuvers. The oxygenation in the "obese 10" group was similar to that in the control group, and this was significantly better than in the "obese 5" group.

If possible, 30-degree RTP should be used for morbidly obese anesthetized patients, as this appears to be the optimal position with respect to oxygenation.[25,33] However, it is unclear whether this is of equal value when chest wall and lung compliance diminish during CO_2 pneumoperitoneum.[34] An alternative is to use 25- to 45-degree RTP for preoxygenation, which appears to significantly prolong apneic time before desaturation in morbidly obese patients.[12-14] Lung compliance and oxygenation improve by turning the patient prone.[35] RTP and PEEP may improve oxygenation equally, and both increase total respiratory system compliance.[26]

There is some evidence that postoperative noninvasive positive-pressure ventilation (NIPPV), begun in the recovery room, may reduce postoperative pulmonary complications. Squadrone and colleagues studied 209 consecutive patients who had undergone elective major abdominal surgery.[36] The patients were randomized to receive either oxygen or oxygen plus CPAP (delivered through a helmet) in the recovery room. Patients who received oxygen plus CPAP had a lower reintubation rate (1% versus 10%; $P = .005$; relative risk [RR], 0.099; 95% CI, 0.01-0.76) and had lower occurrence rates of pneumonia (2% versus 10%; RR, 0.19; 95% CI, 0.04-0.88; $P = .02$), infection (3% versus 10%; RR, 0.27; 95% CI, 0.07-0.94; $P = .03$), and sepsis (2% versus 9%; RR, 0.22; 95% CI, 0.04-0.99; $P = .03$) than patients treated with oxygen alone. Kindgen-Milles and associates studied 56 patients who underwent thoracoabdominal aortic aneurysm repair and were randomized to noninvasive ventilation (CPAP) for 12 to 24 hours after extubation or to standard oxygen therapy.[37] The application of CPAP was associated with fewer pulmonary complications compared with the control group (7 of 25 patients versus 24 of 25 subjects, respectively; $P = .019$). Patients in the CPAP group remained in the hospital for fewer days (22 ± 2 versus 34 ± 5 days, respectively; $P = .048$) and had better oxygenation without hemodynamic complications.

NIPPV is a prophylactic therapy in this circumstance. In the presence of postoperative respiratory distress, NIPPV does not improve outcomes.[38]

Obstructive Sleep Apnea/Hypopnea Syndrome and Perioperative Outcomes

Obstructive sleep apnea (OSA)/hypopnea syndrome (OSAHS) occurs in up to 70% of morbidly obese patients undergoing bariatric surgery.[39] It is characterized by five or more episodes of apnea or hypopnea per hour with daytime somnolence, or 15 episodes without somnolence. Hypopnea is a 30% reduction in airflow for 10 seconds or longer together with at least a 4% reduction in oxygen saturation. There is no direct relationship between OSA and BMI,[40] although there is a correlation with central (truncal) obesity. OSA is caused by narrowing of the upper airway due to fat in the pharyngeal wall (at the level of the soft palate and submental area) with loss of pharyngeal dilator activity during sleep. In addition, there is an abnormality of central control of breathing.

Obstructive sleep apnea is quantified by performing sleep studies (polysomnography). This generates either an apnea-hypopnea index (AHI) or a respiratory disturbance index (RDI). An AHI or RDI of greater than 30 signifies severe OSA.

The treatment for OSA is continuous positive airway pressure (CPAP), with or without inspiratory pressure support (biphasic positive airway pressure [BiPAP]). Although CPAP is probably beneficial to postoperative patients with a history of OSA, evidence that this intervention improves outcomes is lacking. The incidence and severity of OSA significantly diminish after gastric bypass surgery.[41]

There appears to be a relationship between the presence of OSA and difficult tracheal intubation.[42] In a case-matched study of 15 patients, difficult intubation and AHI were significantly related.[43] Using ultrasound of the soft tissue of the neck, Ezri and colleagues showed that obese patients who are difficult to intubate have more paratracheal soft tissue.[42] This may be of more importance in predicting difficult intubation than BMI.

There is little doubt that obesity–hypoventilation syndrome results in worse intermediate-term outcomes in morbid obesity (Fig. 33-5).[44] Although it is universally accepted that the presence of OSA increases perioperative risk, particularly in terms of postoperative airway problems (e.g., narcotic-induced obstruction of the airway), the data to support this contention are limited.[45] The American Society of Anesthesiologists (ASA) has approved guidelines for the perioperative management of these patients.[46]

The risk for postoperative respiratory failure and airway obstruction in patients with OSA (in particular, those with an AHI >30) cannot be overemphasized. Although anesthesiologists typically worry about airway problems during induction of anesthesia, they are more likely to encounter problems immediately after extubation. All patients should be nursed in the semirecumbent or reverse Trendelenburg position for the duration of hospitalization. Early mobilization leads to lung recruitment and should be encouraged. All patients with a diagnosis of OSA should receive CPAP or BiPAP in the recovery room (this is titrated to response) and at night while they sleep. If patient-controlled analgesia (PCA) is used, continuous (basal) infusions should be

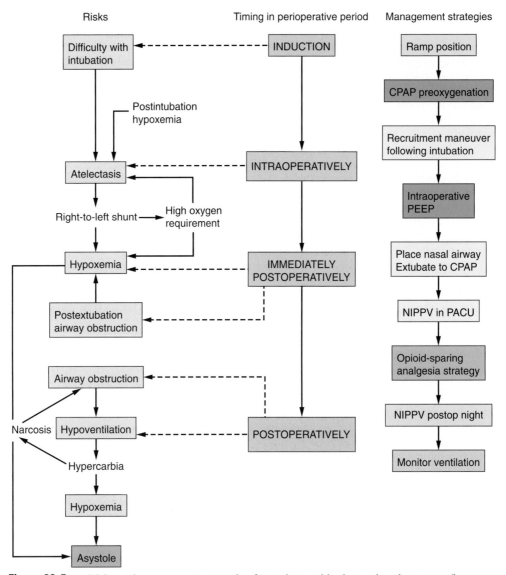

Figure 33-5 ■ Risks and management strategies for patients with obstructive sleep apnea/hypopnea syndrome (OSAHS) or morbid obesity undergoing major surgery. CPAP, continuous positive airway pressure; NIPPV, noninvasive positive-pressure ventilation; PACU, postanesthesia care unit; PEEP, positive end-expiratory pressure.

avoided. In patients with severe sleep apnea and obesity hypoventilation syndrome, prophylactic tracheostomy may be considered.

■ FLUID MANAGEMENT AND POSTOPERATIVE COMPLICATIONS

Perioperative care is characterized by dramatic changes in fluid and electrolyte content and distribution in the various fluid spaces in the body. These changes are predictable and follow a characteristic pattern described by Cuthbertson and Tilstone[47] and Moore,[48,49] widely known as the stress response. An understanding of this process is central to understanding the dynamics of fluid and electrolyte flux in the perioperative period and is helpful in deciding therapy.

The Surgical Stress Response

The stress response has traditionally been considered a biphasic ebb-and-flow phenomenon. Initially, after an injury or a surgical incision, there is significant peripheral vasoconstriction, a shunting of blood from the periphery to the midline (to preserve vital organs), and a drop in body temperature. Simultaneously, the capillary hydrostatic pressure falls, promoting a rapid shift of protein-free fluid from the interstitium into the capillaries.[50] This is known as transcapillary refill and it includes mobilization of fluid from the splanchnic circulation, in particular the splanchnic veins.[51]

This induces a state of absolute hypovolemia in the extracellular space. There is a dramatic increase in the release of vasopressin (antidiuretic hormone) and activation of the renin-angiotensin-aldosterone axis to conserve salt and water.

The second phase, the hypermetabolic (or flow) phase, occurs within hours and is characterized by a dramatic increase in cardiac output, driven by catecholamines, vasodilation, increased capillary permeability, and an increase in temperature. A generalized catabolic state ensues, characterized by insulin resistance, hypercortisolism, and protein breakdown. Thus the patient develops tachycardia, leukocytosis, hyperthermia, hyperglycemia, and tissue edema. The magnitude of this response is proportionate to the degree of injury or extent of surgery. Significant intracellular fluid deficit may be incurred to maintain circulating volume. A period of fluid sequestration occurs because of the extravasation of fluid that follows widespread capillary leak; urinary output falls and tissue edema may become evident. Vasodilation and relative intravascular hypovolemia occur. During this period, patients typically require administration of resuscitation fluids to maintain blood pressure and circulating volume. Weight gain ensues.

Eventually, a state of equilibrium arrives, usually day 2 postoperatively, when active sequestration stops. This is followed by a phase of diuresis during which the patient mobilizes fluid and recovers. Initially, there is a precipitous drop in serum albumin. Restoration of albumin levels is associated with recovery. Moreover, intracellular fluid volume returns to normal. Inward shift of fluid from the extracellular to the intracellular space is associated with intracellular movement of ions such as potassium, magnesium, and phosphate. Hypophosphatemia, hypomagnesemia, and, in particular, hypokalemia are usually evident on a serum chemistry panel at this time.

The clinician must be aware of the stages of the stress response when deciding whether to administer fluid and electrolytes. For example, early in the flow phase, significant intracellular and interstitial fluid depletion may exist, despite the appearance of normal cardiovascular measurements (blood pressure, cardiac output, stroke volume). This requires repletion with free water and isotonic crystalloid. During the vasodilatory, hypermetabolic phase, the circulating volume requires support, taking into account the large volume of distribution of administered crystalloid. During the equilibrium phase, the administration of intravenous fluid is dependent on the objective of the clinician. The clinician may choose to continue fluid administration to keep organs well hydrated, or to stop administering fluid, preventing the development of further tissue edema. During the diuretic phase, the major objective of the clinician is to allow the patient to return to baseline bodyweight and to aggressively replete electrolytes.

It can be argued that the administration of anesthesia significantly reduces the ebb or shock phase. Nevertheless, patients undergoing surgery are usually dehydrated secondary to fasting, bowel lavage, or their primary disease (e.g., esophageal cancer). Consequently, the perioperative period should be viewed as follows: (1) dehydration phase, (2) shock phase, (3) relative and absolute hypovolemic phase (due to vasodilation, fluid sequestration, and blood loss), (4) equilibrium phase, and (5) diuresis phase. Certain operations are associated with greater blood loss because of overt or microvascular bleeding (vascular surgery); other operations are associated with greater tissue injury because of, for example, bowel handling. Thus, within this paradigm, a one-formula-fits-all approach is neither scientific nor effective. Where extensive fluid shifts are to be expected in the perioperative period, it is worthwhile to obtain a preoperative weight to have a baseline goal for the patient's postoperative diuresis.

Traditional approaches to perioperative fluid management have focused on rigorous calculation of fluid deficits, the administration of maintenance fluids (calculated on the basis of bodyweight and metabolic activity), repletion of insensible losses and third-space losses (dependent on the anatomic region of the surgery), and replacement of blood loss with crystalloid (in a 1 : 3 ratio) or colloid (in a 1 : 1 ratio). Of the many limitations to this approach, the main one is the potential for significant weight gain and fluid overload. Additionally, the importance of third-space fluid loss has been questioned.[52]

Preoperative Fluid Deficits and Risk

In adults undergoing elective surgery, despite guidelines that water is permissible up to 2 hours preoperatively,[53] oral intake is usually restricted for up to 12 hours before the procedure. This period of restricted oral intake may be considerably longer when surgery is scheduled late in the day. The resulting fluid deficit is primarily the result of water loss.

A series of studies have addressed whether perioperative patients should receive preoperative rehydration. Yogendran and colleagues studied 200 ambulatory surgical patients, ASA grades I to III, randomized into two groups to receive high (20 mL/kg) or low (2 mL/kg) volumes of infusions of balanced salt solution (Plasmalyte 148) over 30 minutes preoperatively.[54] A minimal amount of fluid was given during the intraoperative and postoperative periods. Adverse outcomes were assessed by an investigator blinded to the fluid treatment group. The incidence of thirst, drowsiness, and dizziness was significantly lower in the high-infusion group at 30 and 60 minutes after surgery, on the first postoperative day, and at discharge.

Maharaj and colleagues studied 80 patients (ASA grades I to III) presenting for gynecologic laparoscopy who were randomized to receive large (2 mL/kg per hour fasting) or small (3 mL/kg) volumes of infusions of lactated Ringer's solution over 20 minutes preoperatively.[55] The incidence and severity of postoperative nausea and vomiting (PONV) were significantly reduced in the large-volume infusion group at 0.5, 1, and 4 hours postoperatively (absolute risk reduction [ARR], 28%; number needed to treat [NNT], 3.5; $P < .05$). The large-volume infusion group also had decreased postoperative pain scores and required less supplemental analgesia.

Bennet and colleagues studied 77 patients who were undergoing dental surgery, randomized to a high volume (16 to 17 mL/kg) or a low volume (1 to 2 mL/kg) of balanced salt solution.[56] Subjective feelings of well-being were greater for patients who received the larger volume of intravenous fluid.

Magner and colleagues randomized 141 (ASA I) female patients undergoing elective gynecologic laparoscopy, to receive either 10 mL/kg lactated Ringer's (LR) or 30 mL/kg LR, started in the preoperative area and completed by the end of surgery.[57] The incidence of PONV and antiemetic use was significantly lower in the group that received 30 mL/kg LR.

Ali and colleagues randomized 80 patients undergoing laparoscopic cholecystectomy or gynecologic surgery to receive 2 mL/kg or 15 mL/kg LR before induction of anesthesia.[58] There was a significantly lower incidence of PONV in the patients treated with 15 mL/kg.

Many clinicians suggest that caloric supplementation with dextrose may reduce postoperative nausea and vomiting and pain. This was refuted in a prospective double-blind trial of 120 ASA I female patients undergoing elective gynecologic laparoscopy who were randomized to no intravenous fluid, 1.5 mL/kg/hr fasting of LR, or 1.5 mL/kg/hr fasting of combined LR and dextrose 5%.[59] Patients treated with dextrose had greater postoperative thirst, more pain requiring opioids, and a higher incidence of PONV compared with those treated with LR alone.

In summary, rehydration of patients with either 30 mL/kg or 2 mL/kg/hour fasting significantly reduces the incidence of PONV and improves patients' subjective sense of well-being after ambulatory surgery (Fig. 33-6). Why is rehydration successful in these patients? Klein and colleagues studied 48 patients undergoing coronary artery bypass graft surgery and randomized them to a preoperative of LR, at 1.5 mL/kg/hr, or no preoperative intravenous fluid.[60] Patients in the intravenous hydration group had significantly greater hepatosplanchnic blood flow (as identified by clearance after injection of indocyanine green) than in the control group. This is consistent with previous studies that have associated reduced splanchnic blood flow with PONV.[61]

Additional preoperative deficits may also occur. The most common is volume loss through the bowel as a consequence of preoperative administration of purgatives ("bowel preps"). This leads to an absolute deficit of water and electrolytes, principally sodium and potassium but also chloride because of renal compensatory loss. This requires replacement with balanced salt solution. There is no clear published guideline for the absolute volume that must be replaced to overcome bowel prep losses, but the majority of anesthesiologists estimate this at 1000 to 2000 mL. Other preoperative causes of absolute hypovolemia with associated electrolyte loss include vomiting, gastric suction, diarrhea, and ostomy output. Upper gastrointestinal (GI) losses should be repleted with chloride-rich solutions, preferably 0.9% saline. Lower GI losses should be repleted with balanced salt solutions.

Perioperative Fluid Losses

Internal losses are volume deficits that cannot be easily quantified, as they represent redistribution of fluid within the body. Traditionally, these are considered "relocation" losses into cavities and third spaces, but they also represent expansion of the extracellular fluid (ECF) space secondary to capillary leak. The cavitary losses (e.g., pleural, ascitic, and pericardial fluid) are simple transudates of plasma that often

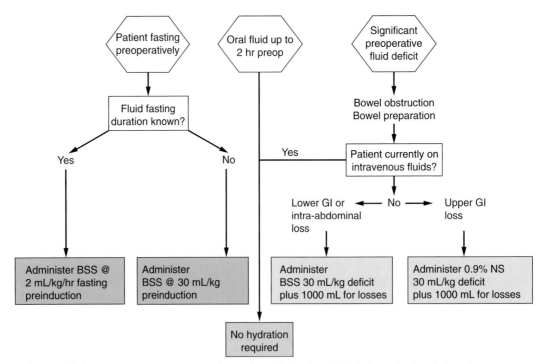

Figure 33-6 ■ Replacing dehydration losses by prehydration. BSS, balanced salt solution; GI, gastrointestinal; NS, normal saline.

require a relatively prolonged period to accumulate in significant quantities. The impact on the ECF volume is therefore generally minor, as there is usually some degree of compensation for this redistribution of vascular fluid. Although significant cavitary fluid accumulation does occur in hypervolemic states, the most important variant of this genre is ascites. Ascitic fluid, secondary to cirrhosis, ovarian cancer, or carcinomatosis, once drained, inevitably reaccumulates, leading to massive fluid shifts and the potential for significant intravascular dehydration.

There are many other causes of fluid redistribution losses in perioperative medicine. They usually involve significant edema in conjunction with injured tissue (as may occur with obstructed, ischemic, or dead bowel), in particular when compartment syndromes occur and when secretory fluid becomes trapped in obstructed bowel. These third-space and cavitary losses create a new ECF pool that is sequestered and essentially nonfunctional.

Internal blood loss also diminishes the ECF volume. Such losses may be significant when associated with retroperitoneal hematoma, leaking aneurysm, pseudoaneurysm or vascular anastomosis, pelvic or femoral fracture, or splenic rupture. Depending on the acuteness of the hemorrhage, some degree of compensation may have occurred. Typically, this involves transcapillary refill, the movement of extracellular fluid into the vascular space to maintain perfusion of fight-or-flight organs (midline structures and skeletal muscle). This may lead to a small drop in the hemoglobin concentration, but in situations of acute isovolemic blood loss, hemoglobin concentration remains essentially unchanged even when blood loss is massive. This may lead to false reassurance, particularly in young patients, who have tremendous compensatory capacity via tachycardia and intense vasoconstriction.

Clearly, estimation of fluid deficits and ongoing fluid losses differs depending on the individual patient and the type of surgery. Emergency procedures are often associated with significant fluid shifts that must be accounted for.

Fluid used to replace pure volume losses should be nearly isotonic with respect to plasma, and should also contain sodium and chloride. In general, a polyvalent, balanced salt solution (e.g., mildly hypotonic, lactated Ringer's solution) is used. Ideally, both internal and external preoperative fluid deficits are totally corrected before the administration of an anesthetic. However, an urgent need for surgery may preclude replacement of the entire deficit. Relatively small volume deficits (i.e., less than 20% of the blood volume) can often be replaced with an isotonic or balanced salt solution administered over a period of 15 minutes or less. Most patients will tolerate this amount of acute intravascular volume expansion, but care must be taken in patients with a history of hypertension or diastolic dysfunction. In this case, rapid volume administration may precipitate acute pulmonary edema. Importantly, 40% to 60% of the infused solution will redistribute to the extracellular compartment within 15 to 30 minutes, and 80% will redistribute by 1 hour. If the patient has significant extracellular fluid deficit, this is an effective method of resuscitating that space. However, if blood loss is the problem, significant tissue edema will result

from large-volume crystalloid resuscitation to maintain hemodynamic goals.

Intraoperative Fluid Losses

Intraoperative fluid losses (like preoperative losses) can be categorized as either internal or external. Traditional approaches to intraoperative fluid management involve estimation of distribution volume deficits and repletion of this apparent ECF volume loss with isotonic fluids. Significant volume is lost or sequestered into "third" spaces. It is assumed that the volume of fluid sequestered is proportional to the amount of surgical trauma. Thus, major orthopedic procedures, surgery within the chest cavity, bowel resections, and hysterectomies are examples in which a significant quantity of third spacing occurs (i.e., perhaps 4% to 5% of bodyweight). The exact quantity of sequestered fluid is impossible to ascertain, and replacement of these third-space losses is an approximation.

Conservative approaches to third-space fluid replacement, based on the amount of tissue exposure and degree of tissue trauma, are as follows: minimal trauma, 2 to 4 mL/kg/hr; moderate trauma, 4 to 6 mL/kg/hr; extensive trauma, 6 to 12 mL/kg/hr. This volume replacement is in addition to maintenance fluids and repletion of preoperative losses.

External fluid losses during surgery are predominantly caused by insensible or evaporative losses and blood loss. Significant evaporative losses may occur when either the peritoneal or the pleural surfaces are exposed to ambient conditions, depending on the relative humidity of the air in the operating room and the rate of exchange of air within the room. This is free water loss, which is also almost impossible to quantify. Traditional approaches involve the administration of 1 to 4 mL/kg/hr fluid to replete these losses, with higher volumes administered depending on the cavity or tissue surface exposed. Patients with extensive burns have massive insensible volume losses, and volume repletion is formula driven, based on the surface area burned.

Intraoperative blood loss may lead to significant tissue hypoperfusion and organ injury. It is, however, difficult to quantify because of accumulation in, for example, drains, drapes, suction canisters, and administration of lavage fluid. The estimated blood loss almost always underestimates true blood loss. Administration of crystalloid or colloid to fixed hemodynamic goals progressively depletes the hemoglobin concentration, providing a useful index of blood loss. However, under-resuscitation of the patient is often associated with a falsely reassuring hemoglobin concentration.

Traditional approaches to blood replacement have identified a 3:1 ratio of crystalloid to blood loss. This is, however, incorrect.[62] With increasing volumes of crystalloid administration, the extracellular space becomes progressively more compliant, with the result that transcapillary leakage of fluid increases geometrically, and volume replacement for blood loss parallels this.[63] This process is known as cytopempsis and reflects, principally, progressive hypoalbuminemia associated with volume replacement.[64] In his original animal study, Moss described a 5:1 ratio of crystalloid replacement to blood loss when losses reached 35% of blood volume, reaching an inflection point at this level, with subsequent ratios increasing geometrically. At 75% blood loss, the ratio reaches 16 : 1.[64] Consequently, consideration should be given to replete blood losses with colloid solutions or blood component therapy.

Limitations of Crystalloid Resuscitation

Traditional approaches to perioperative fluid management, as described previously, have been formulaic, centered on crystalloid resuscitation in the belief that dehydration and excessive third-space loss lead to adverse outcomes. However, an emerging movement questions these assumptions.[65] Advocates of aggressive crystalloid resuscitation have tended to ignore the impact of this fluid on tissue compartments (a dramatic increase in interstitial fluid volume), water dissociation (acid–base balance), electrolyte composition, colloid balance, and coagulation.

Resuscitation with crystalloid fluids may actually reduce oxygen delivery and tissue perfusion. Funk and colleagues[66] undertook a laboratory experiment of isovolemic hemodilution of awake Syrian golden hamsters. The hamsters were given either lactated Ringer's solution or dextran 60 to replace blood loss. Four times the volume of blood loss was replaced with lactated Ringer's to maintain mean arterial pressure, central venous pressure, and heart rate. Tissue perfusion and PaO_2 were unchanged in the colloid group, but they were reduced by 62% and 58%, respectively, in the crystalloid group. Lang, Boldt, and associates investigated the impact of colloid fluid replacement compared with crystalloid therapy on tissue oxygen tension in major abdominal surgery.[67] Forty-two patients were randomized to receive 6% hydroxyethyl starch (HES) plus lactated Ringer's or lactated Ringer's solution alone for 24 hours, targeted to a central venous pressure (CVP) of 8 to 12 mm Hg. The investigators measured tissue oxygen tension in the deltoid muscle by using a LICOX CMP monitoring device placed after induction of anesthesia. Patients in the crystalloid group had received significantly more fluid by the end of surgery (5940 mL ± 1910 mL versus 3920 mL ± 1350 mL, $P < .05$) and at the end of 24 hours (11,740 ± 2630 mL versus 5950 mL ± 800 mL, $P < .05$). The patients in the combined crystalloid–colloid group had significantly greater tissue perfusion (oxygen tension increased from baseline) compared with the crystalloid-only group (oxygen tension reduced from baseline).

An ideal resuscitative fluid would maintain intravascular volume without expanding the interstitial space. Ernest and colleagues investigated the volume of distribution of NaCl 0.9% versus albumin in 55 cardiac surgical patients.[68] Plasma and extracellular fluid volumes were measured by dilution of radiolabeled albumin and sodium. Administration of isotonic saline increased plasma volume by 9% ± 23% of the volume infused. Administration of 5% albumin increased plasma volume by 52% ± 84% of the volume infused. Albumin increased the cardiac index significantly more than saline, and it had an equal impact on hemoglobin dilution. In the saline treatment group, the mean net fluid balance (fluid infusion + fluid losses) was approximately double the mean increase in ECF volume, which on average was distributed equally between the plasma volume (PV) and interstitial fluid volume (ISFV). In contrast, in the albumin treatment group,

the net fluid balance approximated the mean increase in extracellular fluid volume, which approximated the mean increase in PV.

Normal saline (NS) is an equimolar solution of sodium (154 mEq/L) and chloride (154 mEq/L). The solution has an osmolality of 308 mOsm, slightly hypertonic to plasma, and a strong ion difference (SID) of 0. Consequently, administration of moderate to large quantities of NS is associated with mild hypernatremia, progressive hyperchloremia, and metabolic acidosis.[69]

What is the relevance of hyperchloremic acidosis? Metabolic acidosis, regardless of origin, can depress myocardial contractility, and it can reduce cardiac output and tissue perfusion. Acidosis inactivates membrane calcium channels and inhibits the release of norepinephrine from sympathetic nerve fibers leading to vasodilation and maldistribution of blood flow. Additionally, metabolic acidosis is associated with an increased incidence of postoperative nausea and emesis.[70]

Saline continues to be widely used in hospital practice, particularly in neurosurgery, where it is a component of osmotic therapy. The widely accepted use of this solution in patients with renal failure has been questioned. Traditionally, balanced salt solutions were avoided in this patient population because of concerns about accumulation of potassium in renal failure. However, a study by O'Malley and colleagues demonstrated a 20% absolute risk increase (NNT, 5) for hyperkalemia in patients undergoing renal transplantation who were administered saline rather than lactated Ringer's solution.[71] Moreover, there was a 30% incidence of metabolic acidosis, requiring treatment, in the saline group, versus 0% in the lactated Ringer's group.

Although not widely recognized, chloride ion excretion is one of the primary roles of the kidney, as sodium and chloride are absorbed in roughly equimolar concentrations in the diet. A net excretion of chloride over sodium is necessary. Chloride is involved with regulation of renal vascular tone. Hansen has demonstrated that K^+-induced contraction of smooth muscle cells in the afferent arteriole is highly sensitive to chloride.[72] Thus, chloride is functionally a renal vasoconstrictor.

Hyperchloremia can reduce renal blood flow and glomerular filtration rate (GFR),[73] and it reduces splanchnic blood flow.[61] In a study of healthy volunteers, normal saline was associated with reduced urinary output compared with lactated Ringer's.[74] Hyperchloremia has been shown to produce dosage-dependent renal vasoconstriction and a reduction in GFR.[73,75] Finally, in a study of fluid prehydration to prevent contrast nephropathy, the use of sodium bicarbonate was associated with an 11.9% absolute reduction in the risk for renal injury (defined as a 25% increase in creatinine).[76]

Wilkes and colleagues studied saline-based intravenous fluids (crystalloid and HES) versus balanced salt solution (BSS)–based fluids (crystalloid and HES) on acid–base status and gut perfusion, estimated using gastric tonometry.[61] Patients who received saline were significantly more acidotic and had a lower gastric mucosal pH (indicative of gut perfusion), compared with the patients receiving BSS. This was strongly related to increases in serum chloride. Williams and associates randomizes healthy volunteers to 0.9% saline or an equal volume of lactated Ringer's solution. Saline administration was associated with lower pH and longer time to first urination.[74] This tendency toward fluid retention may result from the higher chloride content or the higher osmolality of the solution, which sends the erroneous message to the midbrain that the patient is dehydrated, which in turn induces inappropriate ADH secretion.[74]

Crystalloid solutions of any type enhance coagulation as measured by thromboelastography analysis and routine coagulation studies.[77,78] When patients were hemodiluted up to 30% with saline, coagulation parameters increased.[77,79] The most likely mechanism is an imbalance between the naturally occurring anticoagulants and activated procoagulants, with a reduction in antithrombin III probably being the most important.[80] This effect lowers the threshold above which positive feedback into the intrinsic coagulation pathway occurs, leading to the enhanced coagulation. Although it has been suggested that resuscitation with 0.9% saline (as opposed to BSS) is associated with an increased risk for bleeding,[81] the human data to support this claim are minimal. One study of 0.9% saline versus lactated Ringer's solution in aortic aneurysm surgery showed no difference in outcome variables, but there was a higher perioperative blood loss in the saline group.[82]

Animal data indicate that intravenous fluids may have indigenous proinflammatory and anti-inflammatory properties. In a pig model of volume-controlled hemorrhagic shock, Rhee and colleagues demonstrated a significant increase in neutrophil activation and oxidative burst activity associated with the administration of lactated Ringer's solution.[83] This solution activated inflammation regardless of whether blood was shed or not. This did not occur when volume was replaced with whole blood or 7.5% hypertonic saline. Similar findings were reported with isotonic saline, dextran, and HES, but not with albumin (5% or 25%), blood, or anesthesia.[84]

Lactated Ringer's solution administration was associated with expression of adhesion molecules that were increased in lung and spleen whether or not hemorrhage took place. This was not seen if the animal was not resuscitated or was resuscitated with fresh blood.[85] However, when preceded by shock,

LR resuscitation was associated with histologic evidence of pulmonary edema and inflammation.[85]

Ketone-buffered intravenous fluids such as ethyl pyruvate (EP) may have opposite anti-inflammatory effects. In a rat model, the use of EP resulted in significantly less pulmonary cellular apoptosis than lactated Ringer's.[84]

Flow- or Goal-Directed Volume Resuscitation

Because of significant limitations regarding formulaic approaches to fluid resuscitation, concerns about over-resuscitation, and the need for a scientific approach based on the dynamics of the stress response, a body of evidence is emerging that supports the use of goal-directed volume resuscitation (GDVR), which combines crystalloid and colloid in perioperative medicine and critical illness. Proponents of this system use dynamic flow-directed physiologic endpoints that emphasize timing rather than total volume, for fluid administration. The modern approach to GDVR involves the use of specific "normal" endpoints of blood flow and tissue perfusion.[86]

The goal-directed approach involves the use of specific monitors that measure input (fluid loading), tissue blood flow, and response. Arterial and central lines are placed and goals for resuscitation are set. These include a central venous pressure of 8 to 12 cm H_2O, a mean arterial pressure (MAP) of greater than 65 mm Hg, and, if the appropriate device is placed, a mixed venous oxygen saturation of greater than 70% (Fig. 33-7) and a stroke volume of between 0.7 and 1.0 mL/kg (ideal bodyweight) (Fig. 33-8). The purpose of stroke volume monitoring is to construct Starling curves, using one of a variety of surrogates of end-diastolic volume as an index of cardiac preload. These include CVP, pulmonary artery occlusion pressure, or pulmonary artery diastolic pressure. Changes in stroke volume are more sensitive to changes in circulating volume than changes in cardiac output or cardiac index.[64]

A variety of other devices that measure surrogates of stroke volume or cardiac output are available. These include esophageal Doppler monitoring (EDM), lithium dilution cardiac output, Fick principle CO_2 rebreathing cardiac output (noninvasive cardiac output [NICO]), bioimpedance cardiac

Figure 33-7 ■ Central venous pressure versus mixed venous oxygen saturation. There is great interpatient variability in central venous pressure, but the normal range *(B)* for mixed venous oxygen saturation is between 70% and 80%. Lower levels *(A)* suggest inadequate tissue blood flow, and higher levels *(C)* suggest excessive tissue blood flow.

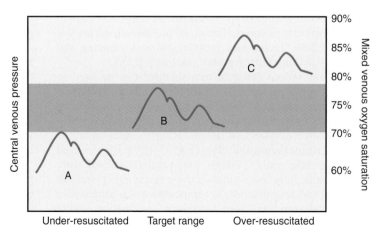

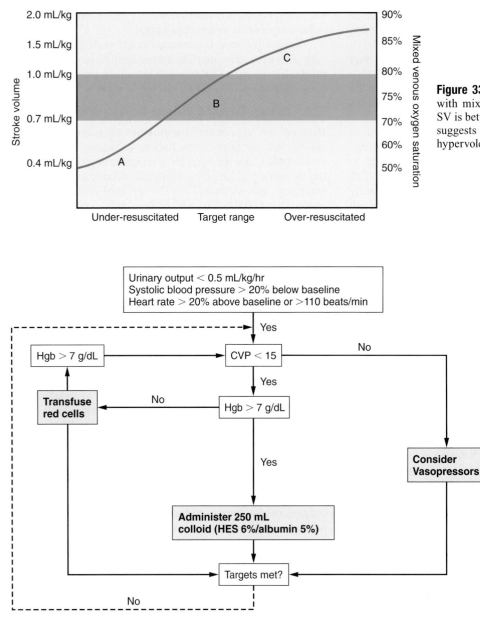

Figure 33-8 ■ Stroke volume (SV) compared with mixed venous oxygen saturation. Normal SV is between 0.7 and 1.0 mL/kg *(B)*. Lower SV suggests hypovolemia *(A)*. Higher SV suggests hypervolemia *(C)*.

Figure 33-9 ■ Central venous pressure (CVP) approach to goal-directed resuscitation. HES, hydroxyethyl starch; Hgb, hemoglobin.

output, and echocardiography. Alternative approaches are to directly measure tissue perfusion, or to measure surrogates of blood flow. Techniques include gastric tonometry and tissue oxygen monitoring probes, such as LICOX.

Central venous pressure measurement can be used to ensure precise perioperative hydration. Moretti and colleagues randomized 90 patients undergoing major elective (noncardiac) surgery to receive either 6% hetastarch (in NS), 6% hetastarch (in BSS), or lactated Ringer's solution on the basis of a resuscitation algorithm (Fig. 33-9).[87] CVP was used for therapeutic goals. Patients who received colloid were given significantly less fluid than those receiving crystalloid alone and had a significantly lower incidence of postoperative nausea and vomiting, need for rescue antiemetics, severe pain, periorbital edema, and double vision.

A number of studies have used EDM stroke volume to guide perioperative fluid administration. Mythen and Webb studied 60 patients undergoing cardiac surgery, randomly assigned to a protocol that included 200-mL boluses of colloid throughout to specified stroke volume using EDM or control.[88] The volume administration approach in the control group was at the anesthesiologist's discretion. Patients in the EDM group had higher splanchnic perfusion at the end of surgery, fewer major complications, and shorter intensive care and hospital stays.

Gan and colleagues studied 100 patients undergoing major elective surgery with anticipated blood loss of greater than 500 mL, randomly assigned to a control or protocol group.[89] The protocol included EDM-guided plasma volume expansion (with colloid) to maximize stroke volume. The protocol group had a significantly shorter duration of hospital stay, tolerated solid oral food earlier, and had significantly less postoperative nausea and vomiting.

Venn and colleagues randomized 90 patients into three groups, one that received conventional fluid management (CVM, based on formulas), one that received colloid fluid challenges with a CVP line, and a third that received colloid fluid challenges with EDM.[90] Patients were deemed medically fit for discharge more rapidly in the EDM group than in the CVP group, and in the CVP group than in the CVM group.

Sinclair and coworkers randomized 40 patients undergoing repair of proximal femoral fracture to receive CVM versus EDM and colloid fluid challenges, again, to a specific stroke volume goal.[91] Patients in the EDM group were deemed medically fit for discharge earlier than those in the conventional therapy group.

Wakeling and associates randomized 128 consecutive patients undergoing colorectal surgery to EDM-guided or CVP-based (conventional) intraoperative fluid management.[92] The CVP-guided protocol aimed at a CVP of 12 to 15 mm Hg. There was a significant reduction in postoperative stay, shorter time to resuming full diet, and lower incidence of GI morbidity in the patients randomized to EDM-guided therapy.

Noblett and colleagues recruited 108 patients undergoing elective colorectal resection and inserted EDMs into all.[93] The patients were randomized into fluid therapy (that was at the discretion of the anesthesiologist) or a fluid therapy protocol that included colloid boluses. The intervention group had a reduced postoperative hospital stay, had fewer intermediate or major postoperative complications, and tolerated diet earlier. In addition, there was a reduced rise in perioperative level of the cytokine interleukin-6 in the intervention group.

An alternative approach to flow monitoring, derived from the seminal work of Shoemaker, is to use oxygen consumption (or its surrogate, mixed venous oxygen saturation [SvO_2]) to determine tissue oxygen flow.[86,94] Low SvO_2 is indicative of excessive extraction per unit volume, strongly suggestive of hypovolemia. Rivers and associates studied early goal-directed therapy in sepsis, in 263 patients randomized to "standard" therapy versus aggressive goal-directed therapy that included the use of an oximetric CVP line (Fig. 33-10).[95] This measured SvO_2 in the superior vena cava distribution. The patients in the study group received significantly more fluid than the control group in the first 6 hours, more red cell transfusions overall, and an equivalent volume of intravenous fluid over the first 72 hours. There was a 16% decrease in 28-day mortality (NNT, 6). The implication of this study is that early aggressive volume resuscitation ensures tissue blood flow. Once goals are met, further resuscitation is not helpful and may be harmful.

Taking these data together, it appears that perioperative patients undergoing major nonvascular surgery require early aggressive goal-targeted volume resuscitation. Stroke volume monitoring appears to be more effective than CVP, which appears to be more effective than the use of standard formulaic approaches (Fig. 33-11). Patients appear to do better if

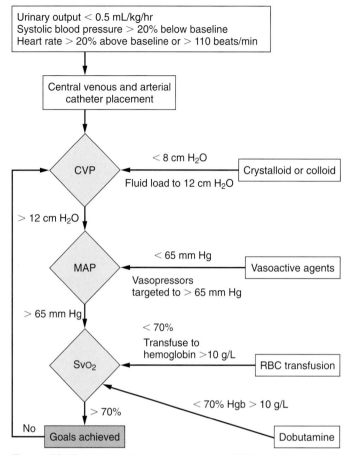

Figure 33-10 ■ Central venous pressure (CVP) and venous oxygen saturation (SvO₂) approach to goal-directed volume resuscitation. Hgb, hemoglobin; MAP, mean arterial pressure; RBC, red blood cell.

resuscitated on the day of surgery, and if colloids are administered to achieve volume goals.

Fluid Restriction

One of the questions that arise from these data is whether the convention of administering postoperative maintenance fluids to patients who have undergone major abdominal surgery is helpful or hurtful. Brandstrup and colleagues performed a randomized observer-blinded multicenter trial (eight Danish Hospitals) that included 172 patients randomized to a restrictive or a standard perioperative fluid regimen (Fig. 33-12).[96] All of the patients underwent colorectal surgery. The restrictive therapy group received no volume preloading, no adjustment for third-space loss, and hetastarch or blood to replace blood losses. Postoperative fluid management was adjusted to prevent weight gain of more than 1 kg. The standard therapy group received formula-driven volume replacement. There was a significant reduction in postoperative (including cardiopulmonary and wound healing) complications in the restrictive therapy group.

In another study, 152 patients with an ASA physical status of I to III who were undergoing elective intra-abdominal surgery were randomized to receive intraoperatively

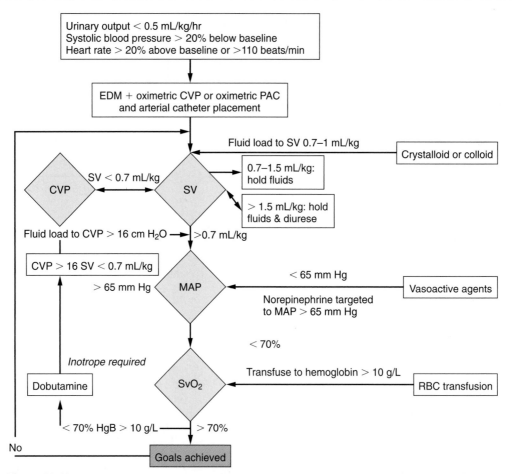

Figure 33-11 ■ Central venous pressure (CVP), venous oxygen saturation (SvO₂), and stroke volume (SV) approach to goal-directed volume resuscitation. EDM, esophageal Doppler monitoring; Hgb, hemoglobin; MAP, mean arterial pressure; PAC, pulmonary artery catheter; RBC, red blood cell.

either liberal or restrictive amounts of lactated Ringer's solution.[97] The liberal protocol group received a bolus of 10 mL/kg, followed by 12 mL/kg/hr. The restrictive protocol group received 4 mL/kg/hr and no bolus. The majority of patients underwent lower GI surgery. The median volume of fluid administered to the restrictive group was 1230 mL, versus 3670 mL in the liberal group. The number of complications was lower in the restrictive protocol group. Return of bowel function was later in the liberal (fluid) group and their hospital stay was longer.

Lobo and colleagues randomized 10 patients, undergoing surgery for colonic cancer, to receive liberal postoperative fluids (3 L water and 154 mmol sodium per day) and 10 to receive a restricted intake (2 L water and 77 mmol sodium per day).[73,75] Patients who had a weight gain of less than 3 kg had earlier return of GI function and a shorter hospital stay. A similar study by Tambyraja and colleagues demonstrated a significant relationship between postoperative sodium and water gain and complications after colonic surgery.[98]

Summary and Recommendations

Perioperative fluid management is a complex process involving the patient's preexisting disease, preoperative volume status, physiologic reserve, degree of perioperative stress, and perioperative fluid losses.

For the majority of patients, prehydration with 2 mL/kg/hr fasting or 30 mL/kg crystalloid, before or at the time of induction, reduces postoperative nausea, vomiting, pain, and lightheadedness. For patients undergoing minor surgery or ambulatory surgery without appreciable blood loss, this is all the intravenous fluid that is required.[99]

A formula-based approach to perioperative fluid management appears reasonable for low-risk patients undergoing moderately traumatic surgery (e.g., laparoscopic operations, peripheral vascular surgery, neurosurgery). However, management of patients undergoing extensive or high-risk surgery requires a more elegant approach. Patients undergoing bowel resection appear to have worse outcomes when over-resuscitated with crystalloid. Patients undergoing major vascular surgery, hip surgery, or extensive upper abdominal surgeries appear to benefit from a dynamic flow-based goal-directed approach to volume resuscitation. This can be achieved using (in increasing order of invasiveness): central venous pressure (CVP) and mixed venous oxygen saturation or stroke volume (SV) and mixed venous oxygen saturation (dynamic volume responsiveness and tissue flow). In the

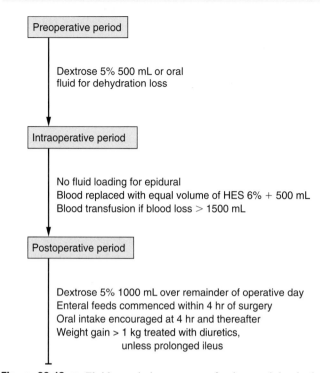

Preoperative period

Dextrose 5% 500 mL or oral
fluid for dehydration loss

Intraoperative period

No fluid loading for epidural
Blood replaced with equal volume of HES 6% + 500 mL
Blood transfusion if blood loss > 1500 mL

Postoperative period

Dextrose 5% 1000 mL over remainder of operative day
Enteral feeds commenced within 4 hr of surgery
Oral intake encouraged at 4 hr and thereafter
Weight gain > 1 kg treated with diuretics,
    unless prolonged ileus

Figure 33-12 ■ Fluid restriction strategy for lower abdominal surgery. *(From Brandstrup B, Tonnesen H, Beier-Holgersen R, et al: Ann Surg 2003;238:641-648.)*

latter approach, SV is targeted to 0.7 to 1 mL per kilogram of ideal bodyweight. A stroke volume in excess of 1.0 mL/kg is indicative of over-resuscitation, and fluids are withheld until the SV drifts back into normal range (see Fig. 33-8). If the SV exceeds 1.5 mL/kg, serious consideration is given to the administration of diuretics (see Fig. 33-11). Respiratory pulse pressure variation is gaining popularity and may emerge as a simple surrogate for stroke volume.[100] Intraoperative blood loss should be replaced 1 : 1 with blood or colloid, or 4 : 1 with crystalloid; crystalloid requirements to replace blood increase geometrically as blood loss continues. Patient outcomes appear to be optimal when the patient is resuscitated fully on the day of surgery or injury and the resuscitation efforts rapidly decelerate.

Postoperative fluid management remains a controversial area. Although transcompartmental fluid sequestration continues for a day or two after surgery or injury (longer if a septic source remains uncontrolled), continued administration of crystalloid leads to increasing tissue edema and weight gain. On the other hand, intravascular dehydration may lead to hypoperfusion organ injury, particularly to the kidney. A prudent approach to postoperative fluid administration is recommended. Maintenance fluids are probably unnecessary unless the period of fasting is prolonged. Evidence of tissue hypoperfusion, as evidenced by low urinary output, low SvO_2, or low stroke volume, should be treated with fluid boluses; keeping in mind that lower volumes of colloid are required to achieve the same hemodynamic goals. Once spontaneous diuresis commences, continuous fluid infusions

should be discontinued and attention directed toward repletion of intracellular ions, potassium, magnesium, and phosphate. A reasonable goal for perioperative fluid management is restoration of normal bodyweight by day 7 postoperatively.

■ FEEDING THE POSTOPERATIVE PATIENT

During the stress response, the demand for substrate to fuel tissue repair and leukocyte activity results in increased energy expenditure (evident as an increase in oxygen consumption and CO_2 production), increased substrate turnover with protein catabolism, and enhanced glycogenolysis and gluconeogenesis to provide energy for the process. Substrate delivery is enhanced by peripheral vasodilation with increased blood flow to damaged tissue, the liver (the site of glucose elaboration), and skeletal muscle (the source of amino acids for protein elaboration, tissue repair, and gluconeogenesis). The anabolic effects of hyperinsulinemia are antagonized by the actions of leukocyte-derived cytokines and counter-regulatory hormones such as epinephrine, glucagons, and cortisol. There is a global increase in temperature and cardiac output. The patient is hypercatabolic, glucose and lipid undergo apparent futile recycling, and visceral and skeletal protein is used as a major fuel source. The stress response distinctly contrasts with starvation, which is characterized by low levels of metabolic activity, lipid oxidation, reduced reliance on glucose, and an ability to respond to exogenous substrate.

The hypermetabolic state characteristic of the perioperative period can lead to depletion of functional reserve. Lean body or cell mass diminishes and, in severe cases, complications can follow. For example, the development of GI mucosal atrophy, abnormal gut permeability, and immune dysfunction is associated with an increased risk for infection and delayed wound healing.[101]

Strategies that have been proposed to modulate the inflammatory response include tight glycemic control, epidural analgesia, and nutritional support. Perioperative malnutrition is reported to impair wound healing and anastomotic strength and believed to increase infectious risk. It is logical to postulate that perioperative nutrition will offset the risk for these complications.

Nutrition Assessment and Goals

The four basic goals of perioperative nutritional therapy include provision of metabolic substrate, retardation of the loss of lean body mass and physiologic reserve, improvement in wound healing and immune function, and prevention of fluid and electrolyte disturbances.

Methods for determining an individual's nutritional requirement vary from simple estimates (e.g., energy requirement = 25 kcal/kg [of lean body mass] per day) to empirically derived, weighted polynomial equations (e.g., the Harris-Benedict equation, with or without stress factors, a prognostic nutritional index, and so on) to indirect calorimetry using a portable metabolic cart. The use of these techniques depends on the availability of support staff. Serum levels of albumin, prealbumin, retinol-binding protein, and transferrin are often used to assess the state of nutrition, but they become unreliable in the perioperative period,[102] reflecting reprioritization of hepatic production, extravasation, hemodilution, and increased consumption. Thus, in acute illness, hypoalbuminemia reflects severity of illness,[102] but for elective surgical patients, failure of nutritional support to increase albumin levels before surgery is a harbinger of poor outcome.[103] Currently, no single measure is universally accepted as an indicator of nutritional status in the perioperative period.

One key characteristic of the stress response is a reprioritization of substrate utilization. In this catabolic state, glucose, and occasionally lipid, is not used efficiently. Therefore, there is a reliance on amino acids to function as substrate not only for protein synthesis but also for energy, with glucogenic amino acids entering the Krebs cycle. It often is not possible, despite aggressive nutritional support, to make perioperative patients anabolic.[104] Indeed, there is evidence that administration of excessive calorie load is associated with worse outcomes.[105] Overfeeding is associated with increased risk for infections due to hyperglycemia and impaired macrophage and neutrophil function. There is increased lipogenesis, hepatic steatosis, and increased carbon dioxide production, leading to increased respiratory work. To address this, a permissive underfeeding strategy has been developed. The use of hypocaloric, hyperproteinic feeds have been proposed to minimize hyperglycemia and spare lean body mass. It is believed that isocaloric feeds increase energy expenditure, thermogenesis, and blood glucose and fail to reduce protein breakdown. Hypocaloric feeds reduce length of stay, possibly by reducing infectious complications secondary to hyperglycemia. The clinical benefit of this strategy remains unproven.[106]

Nutrition Routes

Total parenteral nutrition (TPN) is a widely used technique in perioperative medicine. However, its use is associated with a significant number of technical, metabolic, and infectious complications.[107] Therefore, although metabolic support is clearly desirable, it has been difficult to prove that the use of TPN improves outcome. Muller and colleagues demonstrated a fourfold decrease in mortality in patients treated with TPN as compared with controls in a small series of perioperative patients with GI cancer.[108] On the other hand, a larger Department of Veterans Affairs study of 395 malnourished patients undergoing abdominal or thoracic surgery demonstrated the tradeoff between metabolic support and complications.[109] In this study, only severely malnourished patients benefited from hyperalimentation, in part because the complication risk offset the benefits offered by TPN. Other studies have confirmed these findings. Likewise systematic reviews of parenteral nutrition versus fasting in perioperative medicine and critical care have failed to demonstrate improved outcomes.[110]

The concern with all of these studies is that it is unclear whether TPN, as provided, was sufficient to meet nutritional goals. A study by Starker and colleagues highlights the problem.[103] In three groups of patients treated with TPN before surgery, there was a marked reduction (4.3% to 12.5% rate of complications versus 45%, $P < .05$) in morbidity and mortality in patients whose surgery was delayed until nutritional status was demonstrably improved.

The enteral route is effective and may provide a substantial cost savings when therapy can be successfully initiated and maintained. Of concern, however, is that numerous studies have reported that achieving target levels of enteral feeds is difficult, and that delay is the rule rather than the exception. Various studies indicate that the enteral route is preferable to the intravenous approach. In a randomized prospective trial of perioperative enteral versus parenteral (TPN) feeding of patients with GI cancer, patients fed enterally had significantly fewer complications (34% versus 49%, $P = .005$) and a shorter length of stay (13.4 versus 15 days, $P = .009$).[111] There was a higher incidence of adverse effects such as vomiting in the enterally fed group. Moore and colleagues compared enteral versus parenteral nutrition in trauma patients. Enterally fed patients had significantly improved nutritional markers and reduced infectious complications (17% versus 37%).[112]

Early Enteral Nutrition

Traditionally, after abdominal surgery, patients have been treated with intravenous fluids, nasogastric suctioning, and nothing by mouth (NPO). Oral and enteral feeding is withheld until bowel sounds are heard, flatus passed, and clear fluids tolerated. This approach is based on a number of assumptions that may be incorrect. These involve the physician's understanding of ileus, the risk for anastomotic dehiscence, and the likely intolerance of food or tube feeds compared with clear fluids.

Gastric and colonic ileus, which commonly follows abdominal surgery, is attributed to inhibitory sympathetic reflexes, various neurotransmitters and inflammatory mediators, anesthetic agents, and opioid analgesics.[113] The result is absence of bowel sounds (air leaving the stomach) and flatus. However, small bowel function returns very soon after surgery.[114] Consequently, postpyloric feeding is commonly used in the first 24 hours after surgery. There is little or no evidence of benefit for the use of routine nasogastric suctioning. Nor does it appear that clear fluids are safer or better tolerated than standard enteral feeds. Furthermore, not only is it unlikely that anastomoses are jeopardized by the proximal administration of feeds[115] but also experimental evidence suggests that enteral feeding strengthens wound sites.[116]

Postoperative Complications

No study has demonstrated a mortality benefit from enteral nutrition, either early or otherwise (Table 33-1). Three studies of standard enteral feeding formulas demonstrated reduced infectious complications.[117-119] Beier-Holgersen and Boesby[117] studied 60 patients undergoing GI surgery (two thirds had cancer, 87% had colon resections). Patients were randomized to either enteral feed or water through a nasoduodenal tube. There were significantly fewer infectious complications (2 versus 14) in the study group. These were principally wound infections (Buzby II to IV in 10 of 14 in the placebo group). Rayes and colleagues studied a similar group of patients undergoing abdominal surgery.[118] In this study, 60 patients received nasojejunal enteral feed (half of which contained

| 33-1 | **Studies of Early Enteral Nutrition** |

First Author	Type	Patients (N)	Route (Intervention)	Route (Control)	Outcomes*
Aiko[125]	UGI	24	Jej	TPN	Improved immunologic markers
Beier-Holgersen[117]	LGI, UGI	60	ND	Fluid placebo	Reduced infectious complications
Binderlow[132]	LGI	64	Oral	IVF	No difference in outcomes
Bozzetti[111]	GI	317	Jej	TPN	Decreased complications, decreased LOS, increased GI intolerance
Braga[134]	UGI	257	Jej	TPN	No difference in outcomes
Carr[121]	GI	28	Jej	IVF	Decreased complications, improved nutritional and immunologic parameters
Harrison[120]	UGI	29	Jej	IVF	Improved protein energy kinetics
Hartsell[131]	LGI	58	Oral	IVF	No difference in outcomes
Hedberg[128]	GI, LGI	225	Jej	IVF	Cost savings
Hochwald[312]	UGI	29	Jej	IVF	Improved nutritional parameters
Hoover[122]	UGI	48	Jej	IVF	Improved nutritional parameters
MacMillan[135]	GYN	139	Oral	IVF	No difference in outcomes, GI intolerance
Ortiz[130]	LGI	190	Oral	IVF	No difference in outcomes, GI intolerance
Rayes[118]	UGI, HB	90	NJ	TPN	Reduced infectious complications
Reissman[313]	LGI	161	Oral	IVF	No difference in outcomes
Ryan[124]	LGI	14	Jej	IVF	Improved nutritional parameters
Sagar[129]	LGI, UGI	30	NJ	IVF	Decreased LOS, Improved nutritional parameters
Sand[133]	UGI	29	NJ	TPN	No difference in outcomes
Schilder[126]	GYN	96	Oral	IVF	Reduced LOS, GI intolerance
Schroeder[116]	GI	32	Jej	IVF	Improved wound healing
Siedmon[123]	URO	32	NJ	IVF	Improved nutritional parameters
Singh[119]	LGI	43	Jej	IVF	Reduced infectious complications
Steed[127]	GYN	96	Oral	IVF	Decreased LOS
Stewart[152]	LGI	80	Oral	IVF	Decreased LOS
Watters[136]	UGI, HB	28	Jej	IVF	Impaired pulmonary mechanics, increased fatigue in study group

*Outcomes favor intervention unless otherwise stated.
General: GI, gastrointestinal; LOS, length of stay; No., total number of patients enrolled.
Type of surgery: GI, unspecified GI; GYN, gynecologic; HB, hepatobiliary; LGI, lower GI; UGI, upper GI; URO, urologic.
Route (intervention), route of feeding in intervention group: Jej, feeding jejunostomy; NJ, nasojejunal feeding tube; ND, nasoduodenal feeding tube.
Route (control), route of feeding in control group: IVF, intravenous fluids; TPN, total parenteral nutrition.

active *Lactobacillus*), and 30 control patients received TPN. Significantly fewer infectious complications (principally pneumonia) occurred in the study population (10% versus 30%, $P < .01$). The addition of *Lactobacillus* was associated with less antibiotic usage but no specific outcome improvements. Singh and colleagues[119] studied 43 patients who had surgery after intestinal perforation. Of the 43 patients, 21 received early enteral nutrition (EEN) through a feeding jejunostomy within 12 hours of surgery, and 22 patients were controls, managed conservatively with intravenous fluids. Although the EEN group had a slightly higher severity of illness, as determined by a sepsis score, they had significantly fewer infectious complications (8 versus 22), and more rapid restoration of anabolism (as evidenced by positive nitrogen balance by study day 3). The control group remained catabolic throughout the 7-day study period.

A number of studies have demonstrated improvements in nutritional and immunologic markers associated with EEN. Harrison and associates studied 29 patients who had surgery for upper GI cancer.[120] The 12 study patients who were given EEN via jejunostomy had improved protein

energy kinetics compared with the 17 controls treated with intravenous fluids. Measured increases in amino acid flux and respiratory quotient at postoperative day 5 are suggestive of greater anabolic activity in the study group. Carr and coworkers[121] studied 30 patients undergoing laparotomy for benign GI disease. Fourteen patients were fed immediately via nasojejunal tube; the control group received intravenous fluids. Urinary nitrogen balance was positive in all patients in the treatment group on the first postoperative day. In addition, evidence of increased intestinal permeability in the control group was absent in the study group.

Hoover and colleagues demonstrated significantly less weight loss and better nitrogen balance in patients fed early and through jejunostomy after upper GI surgery.[122] A study of 32 urologic patients, 21 of whom received EEN via nasojejunal tube, reported a positive nitrogen balance, in the study group, on postoperative day 4.[123] Weight loss was significantly reduced in a study of 14 patients (seven received elemental feed via jejunostomy) after lower GI surgery.[124] Schroeder and colleagues studied muscle strength and wound healing (using subcutaneously implanted Gortex grafts) in 32 patients, randomized to EEF via jejunostomy (16 patients) or to intravenous fluids (16 patients).[115] There was evidence of improved wound healing but not muscle function in the study group. Aiko and colleagues proposed a potential immunologic benefit of EEN in a group of 24 patients after esophageal surgery.[125] Patients in the study group had earlier recovery of lymphocyte count, lower bilirubin, and lower C-reactive protein levels than the control group. However, the controls received TPN, which has been associated with a higher incidence of infection (compared with no nutrition) and cholestasis.[108,110]

Hospital Length of Stay

Early enteral feeding may be associated with reduced length of stay after surgery. Schilder and colleagues[126] studied a group of 96 gynecologic patients, half of whom received oral feeding on the day of surgery, provided that they had tolerated 500 mL of fluid. These patients passed flatus and were discharged earlier (3.12 days versus 4.02 days, $P < .008$) than controls (treated with intravenous fluid and fed only if they had bowel sounds, bowel motion, or flatus, or if they complained of hunger). These results were confirmed in a similar study of 96 gynecologic patients by Steed and coworkers,[127] who reported a 30% reduction in length of stay (4 days versus 6 days, $P < .001$) for patients fed orally compared with controls. This reduced length of stay may translate to significant cost savings.[128] Similar reduction in length of stay was also reported by Sagar and associates in a group of 30 patients after (predominantly) lower GI surgery.[129]

Bozzetti and colleagues compared early enteral feeding to TPN in 317 malnourished patients after GI surgery for cancer (approximately 55% had had surgery to the upper GI tract or hepatobiliary system).[111] Malnutrition was defined as weight loss of 10% or more over the previous 6 months. This patient population is known to benefit from perioperative nutrition.[111] There were significantly fewer complications (34% versus 49%, $P < .05$, ARR 15%) and shorter length of hospital stay (13.4 days versus 15 days, $P < .009$) in the enterally fed patients. Complications were defined as major (respiratory failure, shock, renal failure, peritonitis, re-laparotomy, intra-abdominal abscess) and minor (infection, pleural effusions, systemic inflammatory response syndrome [SIRS], deep vein thrombosis, bleeding). Outcome differences resulted from a lower incidence of infectious and noninfectious minor complications in the enterally fed group. It is notable that this study provided isocaloric and isonitrogenous feeds to both groups; none of the patients received preoperative nutrition, and significant hyperglycemia was absent. It is unclear whether the improved outcomes in the enterally fed group simply represented a reduction in complications associated with TPN. The authors cite ethical concerns for the absence of a no-intervention control group.[111] Moreover, it is unclear whether these results apply outside the malnourished patient population.

A number of other studies comparing EEN to conservative therapy[130-132] or TPN[133] have failed to demonstrate a difference in outcome or hospital length of stay. In general, these were small and underpowered studies, but a larger study ($N = 257$) by Braga and colleagues,[134] which compared EEF to TPN, returned similar results. This contrasts with the positive outcomes described by Bozzetti and colleagues,[111] favoring enteral feeding, suggesting that Braga's study, in spite of its size, was also underpowered.

Adverse Outcomes with Enteral Feeding

As expected, many of the studies reported a higher incidence of GI symptoms, such as nausea, vomiting, and diarrhea, in patients fed enterally.[111,119,126,130,135] None of the studies classified these symptoms as complications in outcome compilations. Nevertheless, such symptoms must be considered treatment failure. For example, Hoover and colleagues reported a 34% incidence of diarrhea in their study group.[122] Their "positive" outcome was improved nitrogen balance and reduced weight loss. Singh reported four cases of abdominal distention, requiring temporary halting of enteral feeds,[119] and four patients with diarrhea. Ortiz and colleagues reported a 21% incidence of vomiting in their cohort of patients fed orally.[130] There were no other differences in outcomes. MacMillan and colleagues reported a 10% increase in the incidence of nausea (23% versus 13%, $P < .04$) in their orally fed patients compared with controls.[135] Again, there were no other differences in postoperative outcomes. One study that looked at 28 patients after esophagectomy or pancreatoduodenectomy described worse pulmonary outcomes in the patients fed immediately postoperatively.[136] Patients were randomized to receive immediate postoperative enteral feeding via jejunostomy ($N = 13$), or no enteral feeding during the first 6 postoperative days ($N = 15$). Patients in the treatment group had significantly worse pulmonary function tests, increased fatigue, and decreased mobility compared with controls.

The onus of proof lies on the intervention rather than the control. Studies asserting the safety of enteral feeds versus controls, without clinically significant outcome benefits,[130] tend to minimize the importance of the GI complications, and each should be considered a negative study. Modern multimodal strategies in the management of pain, nausea, and ileus may significantly reduce such symptoms.[113] These include opioid-sparing (multimodal) analgesia, thoracic epidurals, peripheral opioid antagonists, prophylactic antiemetics, and early mobilization.[113]

Early Enteral Immunonutrition

It has been proposed that loss of gut barrier function may predispose to the development of postoperative complications and organ failure. Although this association has never been convincingly demonstrated in patients, the loss of barrier function represents a form of organ dysfunction. EEN may enhance gut barrier function.[121] In addition, a number of "pharmaconutrients" have been proposed as useful additives to boost the immune system during stressed states.

Arginine enhances T-cell–mediated immune function and modulates nitrogen balance and protein synthesis. Omega-3 fatty acids have potent anti-inflammatory properties. Glutamine nourishes the gut mucosa, reduces protein loss and muscle wasting, and enhances the phagocytic activity of monocytes and neutrophils. Glycine appears to have anti-ischemia and anti-inflammatory properties.[137]

Nucleotides may become essential in the perioperative period and during critical illness because of enhanced turnover. They are essential components of cell function and may enhance hepatic and gut function.[137] Omega-6 fatty acids have immune-stimulating effects, whereas omega-3 fatty acids have immune-suppressive effects.

Braga and colleagues studied 196 malnourished patients undergoing surgery for GI malignancy.[138] The study compared immunonutrition with standard EEN in 150 patients randomized into three groups of 50 each. Group 1 (the preoperative group) received preoperative immunonutrition, 1 L/day orally for 7 consecutive days, of a liquid diet enriched with arginine, omega-3 fatty acids, and RNA; patients were fed a standard enteral feed early postoperatively (within 12 hours of surgery). Group 2 (the perioperative group), received the immunonutrition regimen both preoperatively and early postoperatively. Group 3 (the control group) received standard EEN. There were significantly fewer complications in the perioperative group than in the control group (9 versus 24, $P = .02$), and a shorter length of hospital stay in both the preoperative and perioperative group than in the control group (13 and 12 versus 15.3 days, $P < .01$). Complications were defined as major and minor, as in the study by Bozzetti and associates described earlier.[111] Statistical significance was achieved only through compilation of major and minor complications. A similar study by the same group compared 104 patients receiving preoperative and postoperative immune-enriched enteral feed, with 102 patients receiving standard enteral feeds, all administered early postoperatively.[111] There was a significant reduction in postoperative infectious complications (principally pneumonia) (14 versus 31, $P = .009$) and length of hospital stay (11.1 versus 12.9 days, $P < .01$) in the patients receiving immunonutrition.

Senkal and coworkers[139] studied preoperative and postoperative immunonutrition in 154 patients undergoing surgery for GI cancer. Patients were randomized to 1000 mL/day of either an enriched diet ($n = 78$) or an isocaloric and isonitrogenous control diet ($n = 76$) for 5 days before surgery, in addition to the usual hospital diet. After surgery, the same diet was administered via either a catheter jejunostomy or a nasoenteric feeding tube. As with the majority of studies, enteral feeds were gradually advanced over 3 to 5 days. Significantly fewer infections occurred in the immunonutrition group (14 versus 27, $P = .05$). The number of patients with complications (infections and anastomotic leaks) was significantly lower in the supplemented diet group after postoperative day 3 (7 versus 16, $P = .04$). Immunonutrition appeared to be more cost effective than standard therapy, principally because of the lower cost of treating infectious complications.

It is unclear whether the apparent benefit of immunonutrition in these studies arises from early postoperative feeding with enriched formulae or from improved preoperative nutrition.[140,141] Gianotti and colleagues tested this hypothesis on 305 malnourished patients undergoing GI surgery for malignancy.[142] Patients were randomized into three groups. Group 1 received oral supplementation for 5 days before surgery with 1 L/day of immune-enhanced enteral feeds, with no nutritional support given after surgery (preoperative group,

$n = 102$). Group 2 received the same preoperative treatment plus postoperative jejunal infusion with the same enriched formula (perioperative group, $n = 101$). Group 3 received no artificial nutrition before or after surgery (conventional group, $n = 102$). Intention-to-treat analysis showed a 13.7% incidence of postoperative infections in the preoperative group, 15.8% in the perioperative group, and 30.4% in the conventional group ($P = .006$ compared with preoperative; $P = .02$ compared with perioperative). Length of hospital stay was 11.6 ± 4.7 days in the preoperative group, 12.2 ± 4.1 days in the perioperative group, and 14.0 ± 7.7 days in the conventional group ($P = .008$ compared with preoperative and $P = .03$ compared with perioperative). Interestingly, there was no significant difference in outcomes between patients fed only preoperatively and those fed only postoperatively with enhanced formulas.

Di Carlo and colleagues[143] and Gianotti and colleagues[144] compared postoperative immune-enhanced early enteral feeds (IEEF) with standard EEF and TPN in 100 patients undergoing pancreatic surgery and 260 patients undergoing pancreatic or gastric surgery, respectively. Di Carlo and coworkers[143] reported significantly fewer infections, lower severity of infectious complications, and shorter lengths of stay (16.3 versus 17.8 versus 19.3 days, respectively; $P < .05$, IEEF versus TPN) in patients receiving IEEF compared with EEN and TPN. Gianotti and associates[144] reported a significant reduction in length of stay in their IEEF group (16.1 days IEEF, 19.2 days EEF [$P < .01$], and 21.6 days TPN [$P < .004$ versus IEEF]). In addition, interleukin-6 levels were lower and prealbumin levels higher in the IEEF group on day 8, suggesting more rapid resolution of the inflammatory response in this group. Daly and colleagues studied IEEF in comparison with EEF in 60 patients undergoing surgery for upper GI cancer.[145] Infectious or wound complications occurred in 10% of the IEEF group compared with 43% of the EEF group ($P < .05$); mean length of hospital stay was 16 versus 22 ($P < .05$) days, respectively. Senkal and colleagues[141] also studied IEEF versus EEF in 154 patients after upper GI surgery. Enhanced feeding was associated with fewer late infectious complications (after day 5), although they were relatively small in number (5 versus 13, $P < .05$).

Kemen and colleagues[146] studied 42 patients after surgery for upper GI malignancy. Again patients were randomized to an immunonutrition diet or standard enteral feeds. There were significant differences in select markers of immune function between the two groups. For example, the number of T lymphocytes and their subsets, helper T cells (CD4) and activated T cells (CD3, HLA-DR), were significantly higher in the IEEF group on postoperative days 10 and 16 ($P < .05$); mean immunoglobulin M concentrations were significantly higher on postoperative day 10 and mean immunoglobulin G concentrations were higher on postoperative day 16 ($P < .05$); and B-lymphocyte indices were significantly higher in the IEEF group on postoperative days 7 and 10 ($P < .05$).

Although the data comparing IEEF and EEF appear to support using enhanced feeds for patients undergoing abdominal surgery, data comparing IEEF and no nutrition are conspicuously light. Heslin and colleagues[147] randomized 195 patients undergoing upper GI surgery to either early IEEF, via jejunostomy, or intravenous fluids. There was no difference in outcomes, including complications, infections, mortality, and length of stay between the two groups.

Summary and Recommendations

Perioperative feeding is an established standard for malnourished patients undergoing major surgery (Fig. 33-13). These patients benefit significantly from preoperative nutrition.[147] Although previous studies have suggested TPN as the route of choice,[148,149] data are accumulating that enteral feeds, particularly if enhanced with arginine, omega-3 fatty acids, and nucleotides, may be an effective, less costly approach.[138,140,142] Postoperative early enteral feeding is superior to total parenteral nutrition.[111,118,133,140,142,150] The benefit of early enteral

feeding in well-nourished patients remains unclear. No study has shown a mortality benefit. Early enteral nutrition is apparently safe and associated with better nutritional markers postoperatively. Early enteral feeding appears to reduce the risk for infection, general complications, and length of hospital stay compared with conservative therapy (see Table 33-1). However, studies have been underpowered, unblinded, and heterogeneous. GI complications of enteral feeds, commonly reported in the literature, are regarded neither as treatment failure nor as complications. The logic of this position is questionable, and it significantly weakens many studies.[130] Furthermore, when complications have been described as outcome measures, they are often compiled to reach statistical significance.[138] Within this group, complications, ranging

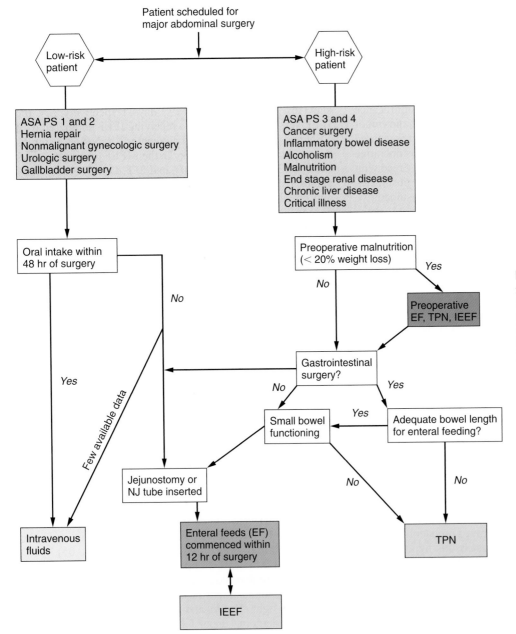

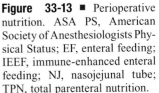

Figure 33-13 ■ Perioperative nutrition. ASA PS, American Society of Anesthesiologists Physical Status; EF, enteral feeding; IEEF, immune-enhanced enteral feeding; NJ, nasojejunal tube; TPN, total parenteral nutrition.

from acute lung injury to shock to wound infections to delayed gastric emptying, are given equal weight.

When immune-enhanced feeds have been studied in comparison with standard feeds, additional benefit appears to be derived in patients undergoing major abdominal surgery (Table 33-2).[140,141,143,145,150] This is because of a reduction in infectious complications. However, the mechanism of diagnosis of infection is unclear in many reports. Nosocomial pneumonia, for example, is notoriously difficult to diagnose.[151]

Outcomes in studies in which oral feeding was started in the first postoperative day have been particularly disappointing (see Table 33-2). Among eight published studies, the only benefit demonstrated was shorter duration of hospital stay, and this in only three.[152] Oral feeding appears to be associated with a higher incidence of GI complications.[126,135,153]

■ PREVENTING POSTOPERATIVE DELIRIUM

Delirium is a complex neuropsychiatric syndrome with an acute onset and a fluctuating course. It is known by a number of terms—"sundowning," acute confusional state, acute cerebral insufficiency, postoperative psychosis, ICU psychosis, and acute or integrative brain failure. It commonly occurs early in the postoperative period, as a result of the negative effects of aging, the stress response, and chronic illness on cognitive function. Delirium significantly increases the cost of hospitalization and length of hospital stay, and it is associated with poorer long-term outcomes.

Functional Reserve and the Aging Brain

Perioperative care strategies require modification for patients with low levels of cardiovascular, pulmonary, and renal reserve.[154] The extent of reserve can be quantified, for example, by exercise or dobutamine stress echocardiography, pulmonary function tests, and creatinine clearance, for these systems, respectively. Likewise, acute loss of reserve presents with devastating symptoms and signs: shock, respiratory failure, and uremia. Unfortunately, many physicians fail to appreciate that similar problems affect many other organ systems in the body, whose function is more difficult to quantify, and whose failure may not appear life-threatening. Chief among these organs is the brain, which frequently malfunctions during the stress or systemic inflammatory response. *Delirium,* the term used to describe this phenomenon, is a synonym for acute/integrative brain failure.[155]

The majority of patients undergoing major abdominal surgery are advanced in age. Aging is associated with progressive deterioration in neurologic function. There is loss of sensory sensitivity because of depletion in the quantity and quality of afferent neurons, neurotransmitters, brain cells, and interconnections. Brain mass reduces with age; there is a 20% drop by age 80, with a significant increase in cerebrospinal fluid volume.[156] This principally affects gray matter, metabolically active and specialized tissue.[157] Consequently, crystallized memory—language, personality, long-term memory, and general knowledge—is maintained, whereas fluid memory—short-term memory, reaction time, new learning, and visual–spatial coordination—declines.[156] There is also significant neuronal loss and demyelination of

33-2	**Studies of Immune-Enhanced Early Enteral Nutrition (IEEN)**						
First Author	**Type**	**No.**	**IG1**	**IG2**	**Control**	**Outcomes***
Braga[138]	UGI, LGI	196	Preop and postop IEEF	Preop IEEF Postop EEN	Postop EEF	Reduced complications, reduced LOS IG1 vs control
Braga[140]	UGI, LGI	206	Preop and postop IEEF	—	Postop EEF	Reduced complications, Reduced LOS IG1 vs control
Di Carlo[143]	Pancreatic	100	IEEF	EEF	TPN	Reduced complications, Reduced LOS IG1 vs control
Daly[145]	UGI	60	IEEF	—	EEF	Reduced complications, reduced LOS vs control
Gianotti[142]	UGI, LGI	305	Preop IEEF	Preop and Postop IEEN	IVF	Reduced complications & LOS IG1+2 vs control
Gianotti[144]	UGI, LGI	260	IEEF	EEF	TPN	Reduced LOS IG1 vs IG2 & control
Heslin[147]	UGI	195	IEEF	—	IVF	No difference in outcomes
Kemen[146]	UGI	42	IEEF	—	EEF	Improved immunologic markers
Senkal[139]	UGI	154	Pre and postop IEEF	—	Pre- and postop EEF	Reduced complications, reduced infections
Senkal[141]	UGI	154	IEEF	—	EEF	Reduced late complications
Soliani[150]	UGI, LGI, URO	171	IEEF	EEF	TPN	Reduced infections IG1 vs control Reduced LOS IG1 & IG2 vs control

*Outcomes favor intervention group 1 unless otherwise stated. Preoperative IEEF was oral. All postoperative enteral feeds were by jejunostomy or nasojejunal tube.
General: LOS, length of stay; No., total number of patients enrolled.
Type of surgery: LGI, lower GI; UGI, upper GI; URO, urologic.
Intervention groups: IG1, group 1; IG2, group 2.
Nutrition routes: EEF, early enteral feeding; IEEF, immune-enhanced early enteral feeding; IVF, intravenous fluids; TPN, total parenteral nutrition.

the spinal cord, leading principally to loss of proprioception. Furthermore, there is decline in visual and auditory function, leading to difficulty in understanding and processing sensorimotor information. Despite this, there is increased sensitivity to pain, with lower neuronal firing thresholds.[158]

The aging brain, with its low functional reserve, is vulnerable to a variety of insults and injuries. These include, but are not limited to, perioperative cognitive dysfunction and delirium.

The aging nervous system responds differently to anesthetic agents. Alterations in drug behavior are principally pharmacodynamic.[159] There is increased sensitivity to intravenous and inhalational agents. The dosage requirement drops by 30% by age 80 years.[160] There does not appear to be any change in the effectiveness of local anesthetics or neuromuscular blockers.[159] However, pharmacokinetically, reduced hepatic and renal function leads to prolongation of the effects of almost all anesthetic agents.[160] Older patients are more sensitive to neuraxial local anesthetics, requiring lower dosage for subarachnoid and epidural blockade.[161]

Definition of Delirium

Delirium is an acute disturbance of consciousness (reduced clarity of awareness of the environment) and cognition, leading to reduced ability to focus, sustain, or shift attention (Box 33-1).[162] It characteristically comes on rapidly and fluctuates in severity during the day. There is memory deficit, disorientation, or language disturbance. There is abnormal attention, which represents a global failure to focus motivation and perform cogent and sustained tasks.[163]

Perioperative delirium usually presents on the first or second postoperative day, with symptoms worse at night (Table 33-3).[164] Often the patient may appear a "poor historian" being overattentive, underattentive, or both.[163] Disturbed perception results in illusions or hallucinations.[165] The majority of patients are disoriented to time. In more severe forms, there is disorientation to place and person.[165]

33-1	**Diagnostic and Statistical Manual of Mental Disorders (DSM) IV Classification of Delirium**

1. Disturbance of consciousness (i.e., reduced clarity of awareness of the environment) with reduced ability to focus, sustain, or shift attention
2. A change in cognition (e.g., memory deficit, disorientation, language disturbance) or the development of a perceptual disturbance that is not accounted for better by a preexisting, established, or evolving dementia
3. The disturbance develops during a short period (usually hours to days) and tends to fluctuate during the course of the day
4. There is evidence from the history, physical examination, or laboratory findings that the disturbance is caused by the direct physiologic consequences of a general medical condition

From American Psychiatric Association: Diagnostic and Statistical Manual of Mental Disorders, ed 4. Washington, DC, APA Press, 1994.

To diagnose delirium, knowledge of the patient's baseline mental status is essential. A collateral history should be obtained from a family member. Often, the patient is described as "not herself" or "acting strangely" or "fine a few minutes ago, now completely confused." Clinicians are often called to a previously placid patient who has suddenly turned "wild" and is presenting a physical threat to the nursing staff. Frequently, several caregivers are required to restrain the patient. Although the hyperactive or belligerent patient frequently gets the most attention, this type of delirium probably only represents 15% to 20% of all patients with this disorder.[166] The majority of patients fluctuate between hypoactive and hyperactive.[166] Many patients who appear normal (because they stay quietly in their beds and do not interact) have hypoactive delirium, leading to dehydration, malnutrition, and sleep deficit.[166]

Epidemiology of Delirium

There appears to be a reciprocal relationship between the magnitude of the injury or injuries and the vulnerability of the patient to developing delirium. If baseline vulnerability is low, patients are resistant to delirium, even in the presence of multiple precipitating factors. On the other hand, if vulnerability is high, minor insults can cause delirium (Fig. 33-14 and see Table 33-3).[167,168]

Francis and colleagues studied the prevalence, risk factors, and outcomes of delirium in 229 advanced-age patients,[169] of whom 50 (22%) met criteria for delirium. Abnormal sodium levels, illness severity, dementia, fever or hypothermia, psychoactive drug use, and azotemia were associated with delirium. Patients with three or more risk factors had a 60% incidence of delirium. Delirious patients stayed 12.1 days in the hospital (compared with 7.2 days for controls) and were more likely to die (8% versus 1%) or be institutionalized (16% versus 3%). This increase in the risk for death reflected severity of illness in this patient population.

In a study of 153 patients undergoing major vascular surgery, 39.2% of whom developed delirium, Bohner and colleagues determined that the major predictors of postoperative delirium were age greater than 65, height less than 170 cm, history of major amputation, preoperative psychiatric problems, and significant intraoperative blood loss.[170] In another cohort of patients undergoing vascular surgery, the incidence of postoperative delirium was 38.9% after peripheral arterial surgery, and 30.9% after aortic surgery.[171]

In a study of 541 patients after hip fracture, the incidence of delirium was 16%.[172] Risk factors included heart failure, abnormalities of blood pressure, and cognitive impairment. Inadequate analgesia (opioids) was associated with increased incidence of delirium (in cognitively intact patients), as was the use of meperidine. After elective orthopedic surgery, the incidence of delirium was 26%, and it was associated with the use of propranolol, benzodiazepines, and scopolamine.[173] Patients affected suffered increased postoperative complications.

Among patients undergoing cataract surgery, the incidence of delirium was reported as 4.4%.[174] Litaker and colleagues prospectively followed 500 patients undergoing

33-3	**Studies on the Incidence of Delirium in Postoperative Patients**				
First Author	**Year**	**Surgery**	**Patients (N)**	**Age Group**	**Incidence of Delirium (%)**
Adunsky[187]	2003	Hip fracture surgery	281	>65	31
Aldemir[185]	2001	General surgery	808	Variable	11
Bohner[170]	2003	Vascular surgery	153	Variable	39.2
Bohner[171]	2000	Vascular surgery	54	Variable	Arterial surgery, 38.9 Aortic surgery, 30.9
Dai[178]	2000	Mixed	710	>65	5.1
Diaz[189]	2001	Hip fracture surgery	46	>70	17.4
Duppils[179]	2000	Hip surgery	225	>65	Hip fracture surgery, 24.3 Hip replacement surgery, 11.7
Edlund[190]	2001	Hip fracture surgery	101	>65	29.7 preoperatively + 18.8 postoperatively
Edlund[164]	1999	Hip fracture surgery	54	>70	27.8
Gokgoz[314]	1997	Cardiac surgery	50	Variable	12
Kaneko[177]	1997	Gastrointestinal surgery	36	>70	17
Litaker[175]	2001	Mixed	500	Variable	11.4
Marcantonio[184]	1994	General (noncardiac) surgery	1341	>50	9
Milstein[174]	2002	Cataract surgery	296	Variable	4.4
Rogers[173]	1989	Elective orthopedics	46	Variable	26
Rolfson[315]	1999	Cardiac surgery	71	>65	32
Sasajima[182]	2000	Vascular surgery	110	>60	42.3
Schneider[181]	2002	Vascular surgery	47	Variable	36
Schor[316]	1992	General medical surgery	291	>65	31
Seymour[176]	1989	General surgery	288	>65	7
Van der Mast[317]	1999	Cardiac surgery	296	Variable	13.5
Williams-Russo[188]	1992	Elective orthopedics	60	>65 (variable)	41

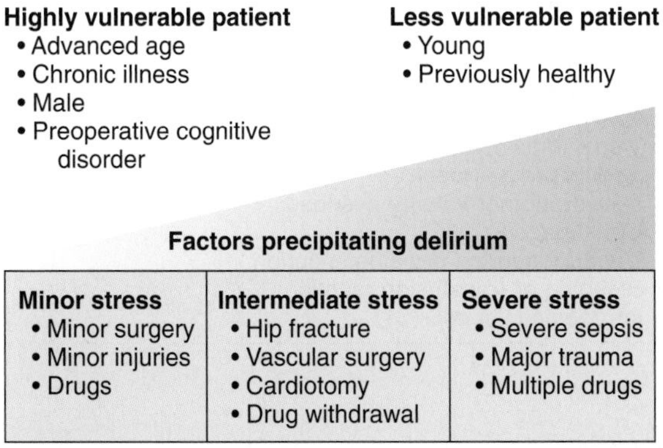

Highly vulnerable patient
- Advanced age
- Chronic illness
- Male
- Preoperative cognitive disorder

Less vulnerable patient
- Young
- Previously healthy

Factors precipitating delirium

Minor stress	Intermediate stress	Severe stress
• Minor surgery • Minor injuries • Drugs	• Hip fracture • Vascular surgery • Cardiotomy • Drug withdrawal	• Severe sepsis • Major trauma • Multiple drugs

Figure 33-14 ■ Risk assessment for the perioperative development of delirium. The tendency toward the development of delirium is determined by patient factors and precipitating factors. The more vulnerable the patient (e.g., advanced age, chronic illness), and the greater the severity of the injury, the more likely it is that delirium will develop.

elective surgery.[175] The incidence of delirium was 11.4% overall, with increased risk associated with age greater than 70 years and preexisting cognitive impairment. A prospective study of 288 older adult general surgical patients revealed a 7% incidence of delirium.[176] In a group of Japanese patients undergoing GI surgery, the incidence of delirium was 17%.[177] Cognitive dysfunction and older age were associated with delirium.[178]

A difference in the incidence of delirium after hip surgery depended on whether the reason for surgery was trauma. In a series of 225 patients, Duppils and Wikblad reported the incidence of delirium to be 24.3% in patients with fractured hips, versus 11.7% in patients undergoing hip replacement surgery.[179] This may be explained by a higher incidence of postoperative hypoxemia in the hip-fractured patients.[180] Administration of supplemental oxygen may reduce the frequency and severity of delirium in this patient population.[164] These data are presumably applicable to patients undergoing surgery for intra-abdominal trauma.

Schneider and colleagues reported a 36% incidence of delirium in postoperative vascular surgery patients.[181] In a similar group of older adult patients admitted with chronic lower limb ischemia, the incidence of delirium was 42.3%.[182] There was an association between delirium and age greater than 70 years, low serum albumin, and surgery longer than 7 hours.

A 1995 systematic review of 80 primary data-collecting studies, of which 54 were eliminated for methodological reasons, revealed a 36.8% mean published incidence of postoperative delirium.[183] Significant risk factors were age, preoperative cognitive dysfunction, and the use of anticholinergic drugs. Marcantonio and colleagues studied 1341 patients undergoing general, orthopedic, or gynecologic surgery.[184] They included all consenting patients over 50 years of age. The incidence of delirium was 9%, increasing with age, preoperative cognitive dysfunction, alcoholism, electrolyte disorders, hyperglycemia, and thoracic and aortic surgery.

Aldemir and colleagues studied 808 general surgical patients. The incidence of delirium was 11%, significantly more common in men and older patients.[185] More of the delirious patients had been admitted as emergencies. In addition, delirious patients remained in the intensive care unit (ICU) and hospital longer than nondelirious patients. Certain factors predicted delirium: respiratory disease, sepsis, fever/SIRS, anemia, hypotension, hypocalcemia, hyponatremia, renal dysfunction, liver dysfunction, and metabolic acidosis. Thus, delirium occurs as part of the SIRS–multiorgan dysfunction (MODS) paradigm. In addition to surgical stress, postoperative pain scores also demonstrate a strong correlation with delirium.[186]

The wide variation in the prevalence of delirium in perioperative patients, varying between 5% and 40%, can be explained on the basis of study methodology (see Table 33-3). Studies that focused primarily on advanced-age patients[164,187,188] and studies following patients with hip fractures or undergoing vascular surgery[164,174,182,189,190] reported high incidences of delirium. Furthermore, there is wide variability in the tools used to diagnose this problem, and they have different sensitivities and specificities.

It is important to emphasize that the cause of delirium usually cannot be ascribed to a single agent or incident. The majority of cases are multifactorial, with between two to six causative factors involved.[191]

Pathogenesis of Delirium

Although delirium is a neurologic condition, the major factors responsible are typically found outside the central nervous system (CNS) (Box 33-2).[163] Delirium has been classified as (1) being caused by a general medical condition, (2) being substance induced, (3) having multiple etiologies, and (4) having unknown causes.[162,192] In general, in perioperative patients, delirium is caused by a combination of the stress response, drugs, or toxins (including drug withdrawal—Table 33-4) and patient vulnerability (low cerebral reserve).

The areas of the brain associated with delirium are the prefrontal cortex, the right parietal lobe, and the subcortical nuclei. Within these anatomic structures are alterations in neurotransmission affecting the cholinergic, dopaminergic, serotonergic, and γ-aminobutyric acid (GABA)-ergic systems. Most attention has been focused on the development of delirium associated with depletion of acetylcholine and abundance of dopamine. This is based on experimental data in which delirium may be produced by anticholinergic drug administration and reversed by cholinergic (anticholinesterases) agents. For example, Greene, with physostigmine, successfully reversed atropine- or scopolamine-induced delirium in 30 patients in the postanesthesia recovery room.[193] The

33-2	**Risk Factors for Postoperative Delirium**

- Age >65, males > females
- Alcohol or benzodiazepine abuse
- Low baseline cognitive status
- Hypoxia
- Hypotension
- Type of surgery
  - Orthopedic trauma
  - Noncardiac thoracic surgery
  - Major vascular surgery
- Drugs
  - Anticholinergics
  - Benzodiazepines
  - Propranolol
  - H_2 antagonists
  - Selective serotonin reuptake inhibitors (SSRIs)
  - Narcotics
  - Antiemetics
  - >Six medications total[168]
  - >Three medications added[168]
- Admission to intensive care unit (ICU) or high dependency unit (HDU)
- Infection
- Pain
- Visual impairment
- Auditory impairment
- Dehydration or volume overload
- Constipation
- Urinary retention or catheterization
- Bleeding or transfusion reactions
- Iatrogenic injuries

33-4	**Substances That Can Cause Delirium by Intoxication or Withdrawal**

Drugs of Abuse	**Medications**	**Toxins**
Alcohol	Anesthetics	Anticholinesterases
Cannabis	Opioid analgesics, tramadol	Organophosphate poisoning
Cocaine	Antiasthmatic drugs	Carbon monoxide
Hallucinogens	Anticonvulsants	Carbon dioxide
Inhalants (glue, petroleum)	Antihistamines	Volatile substances (e.g., fuel)
Opioids	Antihypertensives and cardiovascular drugs	Organic solvents
Phencyclidine	Antimicrobials	
Benzodiazepines	Antiparkinsonian medications	
Barbiturates	Corticosteroids	
	H_2-receptor antagonists	
	Muscle relaxants	
	Immunosuppressives	
	Lithium and antipsychotics	
	Medications with cholinergic properties	

From American Psychiatric Association: Am J Psychiatry 1999;156:1-20.

same agent has been reported to reverse delirium caused by ranitidine, homatropine eye drops, benztropine, and meperidine.[192] Delirium is associated with intoxication from dopaminergic drugs and opioids and with hypoxemia, both of which are associated with increased dopamine release.[194] Serotonergic mechanisms have also been hypothesized for delirium, although the relationship is less clear.[194] Bayindir and colleagues reported a significant improvement in the mental status of delirious patients treated with ondansetron, a serotonin type 3 (5-HT$_3$) receptor antagonist, after cardiac surgery.[195] On the other hand, the selective serotonin reuptake inhibitor paroxetine has been implicated as a potential cause of delirium.[196,197] GABA is involved with episodes of delirium associated with alcohol and drug withdrawal.

Medications have been implicated in 20% to 40% of cases of delirium[167] (see Table 33-4). Benzodiazepines, opioids, and other psychoactive drugs are associated with a 3- to 11-fold increase in the relative risk of developing delirium.[198] Anticholinergic agents, which include atropine, scopolamine, glycopyrrolate, and phenothiazines, are a common cause of delirium. Often physicians are unaware that the drugs they prescribe have anticholinergic properties.[199] Because delirium is a multisystem disorder more frequently caused by drugs than relieved by them, physicians should rationalize patient medications after admission and avoid polypharmacy when possible. This is particularly important in critical care, where multiple consultants may be prescribing simultaneously.

Studies of delirium in the hospitalized patients have suggested that this problem is associated with an increased risk for death, institutionalization, and readmission.[200] On the other hand, it is known that delirium occurring in perioperative patients is more easily treated and is associated with better outcomes than that occurring with intercurrent illness or spontaneously.[200,201] This suggests that the operative stress response's effect on reserve is preventable and reversible and may lead to better outcomes.[200,202]

Although anesthesia has been associated with delirium, the anesthesia technique appears to be less a causative factor than the nature of the surgery and the associated stress response. For example, Kamitani and colleagues,[203] in a study of 40 older adult patients with femoral neck fracture, were unable to show a difference in the incidence of delirium between general and spinal anesthesia.

There is a strong relationship between sleep deprivation and delirium. The perioperative stress response interferes significantly with normal sleep architecture. Melatonin, which is produced in the pineal gland, is involved in circadian rhythms and the sleep–wake cycle. There has been some suggestion that abnormal perioperative melatonin secretion is associated with disordered sleep, triggering delirium.[204] Analgesic and sedative agents may also cause sleep fragmentation. There is a striking inverse relationship between nocturnal morphine dosage and time spent in rapid eye movement (REM) sleep.[205] Likewise, lorazepam and other intermediate- to long-acting benzodiazepines are associated with atypical sleep patterns. It is likely that perioperative sleep dysfunction arises from multiple etiologies; pain, surgery, stress response, sedatives, noise, unfamiliar environment, and facilitation of sleep require environmental change in patient care areas[206] (Fig. 33-15).

Diagnosis of Delirium

Unexplained delirium is a medical emergency and requires immediate investigation.[163] Delirium is a physical sign implying the development of significant systemic upset, and this may precede the development of more commonly recognized indicators, such as tachycardia, pyrexia, and hypotension. Unfortunately, many physicians are aware of neither the significance of delirium nor the diagnostic criteria. This is best illustrated in two studies of older adult patients presenting to the emergency department. Naughton and colleagues diagnosed delirium in 24% of older adult patients in the emergency department.[207] An additional 15% had other alterations in mental status. In a study of 385 patients, Lewis and colleagues diagnosed delirium in 10% of patients.[208] However, emergency department physicians noted delirium to be present in only 17% of this group, of whom 46% were discharged home and half had subsequent problems. Similar underdiagnosis has been reported in inpatients. Gustafson and colleagues reported on delirium in elderly patients after femoral neck fracture; a very high risk group.[209] The presence of an acute confusional state was recorded correctly by a nurse in 43.9% of cases, and by a physician in 8.1% of cases. This and other studies[210] suggest that delirium is significantly under-recognized and under-reported by physicians and nurses.

The Confusion Assessment Method (CAM), developed specifically to diagnose delirium,[211] has the dual benefit of simplicity and rapidity. The CAM instrument consists of four diagnostic criteria: acute onset and fluctuating course, inattention, disorganized thinking, and altered level of consciousness (Box 33-3). The CAM algorithm for diagnosis of delirium requires the presence of both the first and the second criteria and either the third or the fourth criterion.

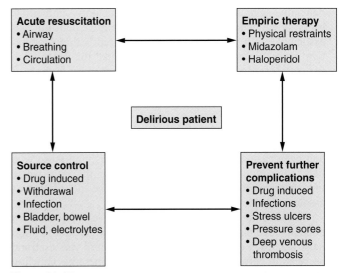

Figure 33-15 ■ The four pillars of medical therapy for the delirious patient.

33-3 | **The Confusion Assessment Method for Diagnosing Delirium**

The diagnosis requires the presence of features 1, 2, and 3, and either 4 or 5.

1. Acute changes in mental status
   Is there evidence of an acute change in cognition from the patient's baseline?
2. Fluctuating symptoms
   Does the abnormal behavior fluctuate during the day (i.e., tend to come and go, or increase or decrease in severity)?
3. Inattention
   Does the patient have difficulty focusing attention?
4. Disorganized thinking
   Is the patient disorganized or incoherent?
5. Altered level of consciousness
   Is the patient hyperalert-agitated, lethargic, stuporous, or comatose?

From Inouye SK, van Dyck CH, Alessi CA, et al: Ann Intern Med 1990;113:941-948.

33-4 | **Preventing Perioperative Delirium**

1. Identify preoperative risk factors
   a. Preexisting cognitive deficit
   b. History of alcohol or benzodiazepine abuse
   c. Assessment of medical problems (risk is increased with history of chronic medical disease)
2. Preoperative preparation
   a. Optimal control of blood pressure, hypertension, and diabetes
   b. Intravenous rehydration during and after bowel preparation
   c. Correction of preexisting electrolyte imbalance
   d. Mental preparation (orientation and communication)
3. Intraoperative care
   a. Multimodal analgesia strategy
   b. Avoidance of intravenous agents with prolonged effects (thiopental)
   c. Avoidance of atropine, scopolamine, and H_2-antagonists
4. Postoperative care
   a. Reorientation and environmental support
   b. Facilitate sleep—avoiding narcotics and sedatives when possible
   c. Continue multimodal analgesia regimen
   d. Avoidance of dehydration, constipation, and urinary retention
   e. Avoidance or early detection and treatment of infections
   f. Minimization of medications, particularly with CNS activity
5. Early mobilization

The CAM method was subsequently modified for use in critically ill patients, for whom verbal communication may be difficult.[212] CAM-ICU has been fully validated in a study of 111 consecutive mechanically ventilated patients. Using this method, the investigators were able to demonstrate an 83.3% incidence of delirium in this patient population.[212] As delirium is not routinely monitored in ICUs, these results suggest that intensivists are missing a significant sign of organ dysfunction.

Outcomes from Delirium

Outcome data on patients incurring perioperative delirium is restricted to orthopedic trauma patients. It is unclear whether these data can be applied to patients undergoing major abdominal surgery. Adunsky and colleagues retrospectively studied 281 older adult patients with hip fractures undergoing surgical fixation.[187] The incidence of delirium was 31%. Interestingly, 53% of those patients developed preoperative delirium, suggesting that this is a particularly vulnerable group of patients (see Fig. 33-14). Preoperative delirium was associated with poorer outcomes compared with postoperative cases. Edlund and associates studied 101 older adult patients before and after surgery for femoral neck fracture.[190] The incidence of delirium was 29.7% preoperatively, and an additional 18.8%, postoperatively. Preoperative delirium persisted into the postoperative period. There was a significant difference between the groups—perioperative delirium occurred principally in patients with dementia, patients who had been treated with anticholinergic drugs, and those who had fallen indoors. These patients had significantly worse intermediate-term outcomes. Postoperative delirium was associated with hypotension and sepsis.

Lundstrom and colleagues prospectively followed 78 nondemented patients (age >65) who had surgery for femoral neck fractures over a 5-year period.[213] There was a strong correlation between the incidence of postoperative delirium and the presence of dementia at 5 years (69% of delirious patients developed dementia compared with 20% of nondelirious patients—absolute risk increase, 49%). Furthermore, the 5-year mortality rate was significantly higher in the delirious patients (72.4% versus 34.7%, absolute risk increase, 37.7%). This suggests that the development of delirium is indicative of low cerebral and systemic functional reserve and is an independent predictor of poor long-term outcomes.

Prevention of Delirium

Risk stratification involves identifying patients who are vulnerable and addressing the nature of the insult or injury facing them. The more vulnerable the patient, the lower the magnitude of insult required to cause delirium (see Fig. 33-14). Hence, a young cerebrally robust patient may become delirious only under the stress of critical illness; whereas an older patient may become delirious after minor surgery. Advanced-age patients with a history of chronic illness, dementia, or preoperative cognitive dysfunction, who are undergoing major surgery or admitted to intensive or high-dependency care, are those most at risk.

Key preventative mechanisms involve reducing the stressors applied to the patient, avoiding drugs or interventions known to precipitate delirium, and environmental manipulation (Box 33-4).

Marcantonio and colleagues looked at the use of perioperative geriatric consultation in older adult patients undergoing hip surgery.[214] In the study group, a geriatrician rounded daily for the duration of the patient's hospitalization and made targeted recommendations based on a structured protocol. This resulted in an absolute risk reduction of delirium of 18% (NNT, 5.5) (32% versus 50%, $P = .04$). This suggests that meticulous attention to homeostasis may prevent the development of delirium.

Inouye and colleagues prospectively studied 852 patients, 70 years or older, admitted to a general medicine service, and randomized them to either aggressive preventative intervention or control.[206] The intervention consisted of standardized protocols for the management of six risk factors for delirium: cognitive impairment, sleep deprivation, immobility, visual impairment, hearing impairment, and dehydration. These interventions resulted in an absolute risk reduction for delirium of 5.1% (from 15.0% to 9.9%; 95% CI, 0.39-0.92; NNT, 19.6). There were associated reductions in the total number of days with delirium and the total number of episodes in the intervention group. This provides good evidence that primary prevention of delirium is possible.

A prospective nurse-led intervention study aimed to prevent delirium in patients who underwent surgery for hip fracture.[215] This involved education of nursing staff, systematic cognitive screening, consultative services by a specialist, and use of a scheduled pain protocol. The incidence of delirium was similar in both groups, 23% in the control group and 20% in the intervention (not significant). Delirium was significantly shorter, and less severe, in the intervention group. The low incidence of delirium as opposed to in historic controls (see Table 33-3) suggests Hawthorne effects in the control group.

Management of Delirium

Acute delirium is a medical emergency. It is frequently the earliest overt manifestation of malevolent underlying pathology. The patient requires immediate medical workup to investigate and treat the precipitating problem, in addition to treating the symptoms of delirium. It is imperative that life-threatening causes of delirium—hypoxemia, hypotension, or fulminant sepsis—are excluded or treated.

Workup for the delirious patient requires investigation of the patient's history and collateral history, in particular looking for evidence of preoperative cognitive disorders, chronic illness, alcohol, or benzodiazepine abuse. Withdrawal syndromes should be strongly suspected in each case. The patient's medication list should be queried for drugs known to precipitate delirium, particularly those with anticholinergic properties (see Table 33-4). The patient should undergo a full physical examination, from head to toe, front and back, for evidence of infection. This should include, in addition to routine physical examination, looking for dental abscess, ischiorectal abscess, prostatitis, pelvic inflammatory disease, line infections, and endocarditis. A number of studies can assist in the diagnosis process: complete blood count including differential count, electrolytes including urea, creatinine, liver function tests, serum amylase and lipase, calcium and phosphorous, chest radiograph, urinalysis. If raised temperature is present, blood cultures should be sent. Intravenous lines should be removed and replaced. In general, CT and lumbar puncture are of low yield in this patient population. In the absence of focal neurologic signs or significant antecedent risk, stroke is unlikely to present in this way.

Acute control of delirium requires a four-part approach—protecting the airway and maintaining oxygenation and tissue perfusion, empiric therapy, source control (treating the inciting cause), and prevention of further complications (see Fig. 33-15). In the critically ill patient, acute delirium may be associated with patient–ventilation dyssynchrony, and traumatic removal of endotracheal tubes, tracheostomy, or lines. Restraints are essential, both physical and pharmacologic. The treatment of choice is haloperidol.

Acute episodes of delirium are usually multifactorial in origin, but the individual precipitating factor must be identified: a drug, infection, bleeding, urinary retention, constipation, dehydration, or electrolyte imbalance. The source should be sought out and controlled. The savvy clinician will rapidly recognize an acute deterioration in mental status as a red flag for a significant underlying problem. After source control, which may vary from bladder decompression to secondary surgery, meticulous attention should be paid to preventing further complications. Environmental adjustment (Fig. 33-16) is essential to modulate the current delirious episode. Sedative and opioid analgesic agents should be discontinued, electrolyte balance corrected, and central lines and urinary catheters removed. These patients are at increased risk for stress ulceration, deep venous thrombosis, nosocomial infections, and pressure sores. Management modalities for the delirious or potentially delirious patient are (1) environmental therapy, (2) medical optimization, and (3) pharmacotherapy.

Environmental therapy involves optimizing the area in which the patient is being cared for to treat and prevent delirium. This involves cognitive–emotional support and sensory optimization (see Fig. 33-16). Patients with minimal mental reserve may benefit greatly from the presence of

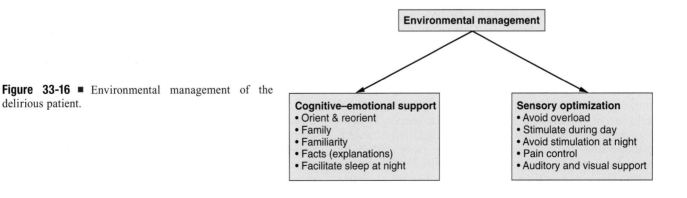

Figure 33-16 ■ Environmental management of the delirious patient.

Environmental management

Cognitive–emotional support
- Orient & reorient
- Family
- Familiarity
- Facts (explanations)
- Facilitate sleep at night

Sensory optimization
- Avoid overload
- Stimulate during day
- Avoid stimulation at night
- Pain control
- Auditory and visual support

friendly recognizable faces and voices. This is achieved by involving the patient's family in the care, and in continuity of caregiver assignments. The patient must be oriented in time and place continuously, by the family and by nursing and medical staff. Furthermore, each intervention or test requires explanation. If a confusional state exists, both the patient and the family require reassurance that this is temporary, and common. An organized sleep–wake cycle is imperative, with minimal light, noise, and nursing interruption during the night. Pain control is essential. If the patient needs glasses or a hearing aid, these should be worn.

It is essential that the patient experiences neither sensory deprivation nor overload. Thus the number of visitors at any time should be restricted and televisions and radios, useful for orientation and communication during the day, shut off at night. Pagers, alarms, and public address systems can significantly add to the "white noise" of critical care units. Mechanisms to develop quiet times for sleep in such units have been promoted.[206]

Secondary complications frequently cause acute depletion of physiologic reserve and delirium. Thus rigorous screening for, and treatment of, infection is essential, as is rehydration, correction of electrolyte imbalance, and avoidance of constipation. Patients being treated with opioids should also receive purgatives. Order sets should be interrogated daily for unnecessary medications. A minimalist approach to prescribing should be adopted.[206]

A variety of neuroleptic and psychotropic agents have been used in the acute treatment of delirium. Haloperidol remains the agent of choice in acutely delirious patients.[216] The dosage in older adult patients is 0.5 to 2 mg intravenously every 20 to 30 minutes until symptoms are controlled, then 25% of the loading dose every 6 hours. Although it is a neuroleptic, haloperidol has fewer active metabolites and anticholinergic activity than phenothiazines. Benzodiazepines appear to be useful only in withdrawal syndromes. Other agents that have been used include pimozide, risperidone, olanzapine, trazodone and mianserin (both 5-HT$_2$ receptor antagonists), and donezepil. Piracetam, a nootropic agent, which may protect neurons from hypoxia, ischemia, and intoxication, reduced the incidence of delirium in a number of studies in Germany.[217] Many clinicians now prescribe risperidone to treat agitated delirium. The dosage is 0.25 to 0.5 mg twice a day.[218]

A number of investigators have suggested that sleep deprivation is a significant precipitating factor for delirium. Use of a protocol that facilitated sleep reduced the incidence of delirium from 35% to 5% (ARR, 30%).[219] Melatonin has been successfully used therapeutically to facilitate sleep in perioperative patients.[220]

The optimal analgesia method for the prevention of delirium is unclear. Williams-Russo and colleagues failed to demonstrate that the use of epidural analgesia (compared with intravenous analgesia) significantly reduced the incidence of delirium in patients after knee replacement surgery.[188] Multimodal analgesia strategies have been suggested to reduce postoperative complications, particularly those caused by high-dose opioids, known to induce delirium and disrupt sleep. This involves the use of multiple different analgesic agents in an individual patient: local or regional anesthesia, nonsteroidal anti-inflammatory agents, acetaminophen, and low-dose narcotics.[221] This approach significantly reduces postoperative opioid requirements, with consequent reduction in related complications—constipation, immobilization, dysphoria, nausea, and vomiting.[222]

Summary and Recommendations

Delirium is a medical emergency that is indicative of acute loss of functional reserve and, frequently, a harbinger of a devastating underlying process. The development of delirium in a hospitalized patient requires an urgent medical workup, empiric therapy, source control, and modification of the environment. This involves cognitive–emotional support and sensory optimization.

Awareness, prevention, and management of delirium must become a priority in postoperative clinical units. It is unlikely that this can occur without significant multidisciplinary cultural change and the development of clinical practice guidelines (Fig. 33-17).

■ PERIOPERATIVE ANTIMICROBIAL THERAPY AND INFECTION

Surgical site infections (SSIs) are the second most common cause of nosocomial infection.[223] Up to 20% of patients undergoing major abdominal surgery will develop an SSI. The Centers for Disease Control and Prevention (CDC) estimate that approximately 500,000 SSIs occur annually in the United States.[224] Patients who develop SSIs have longer and costlier hospitalizations than patients who do not develop such infections. They are twice as likely to die, 60% more likely to spend time in an ICU, and more than five times more likely to be readmitted to the hospital.[225] This translates to significant increases in health-care costs. Programs that reduce the incidence of SSIs can substantially decrease morbidity and mortality and reduce the economic burden for patients and hospitals.

Risk for Surgical Site Infection

Increased risk for SSI occurs with increasing degree of wound contamination, regardless of other risk factors, and also as the number of risk factors increases (Box 33-5).[226] The CDC has developed guidelines for prevention of SSIs, and Box 33-6 shows the four classes of surgical wounds: class I (clean), class II (clean-contaminated), class III (contaminated), and class IV (dirty-infected).

Patients undergoing procedures that entail entry into a hollow viscus under controlled conditions should receive antimicrobial prophylaxis. Bowel preparation to decrease the number of bacteria in the GI tract is also indicated for certain clean-contaminated procedures such as elective bowel resection. Thus, antibiotic prophylaxis is indicated for most clean-contaminated and contaminated (or potentially contaminated) operations. An example of a clean-contaminated operation is elective cholecystectomy. The majority of patients that undergo laparoscopic cholecystectomy do not require antibiotic prophylaxis; older, diabetic patients or those undergoing

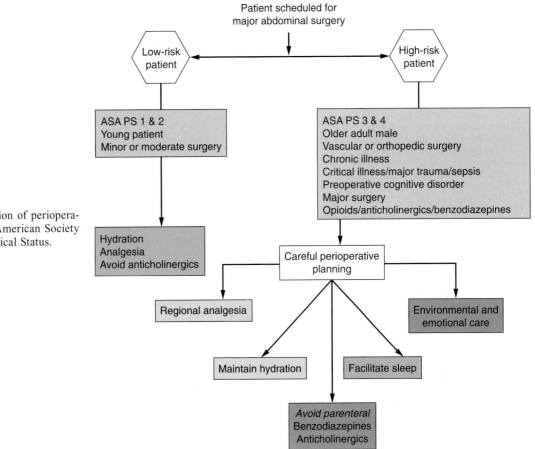

Figure 33-17 ■ Prevention of perioperative delirium. ASA PS, American Society of Anesthesiologists Physical Status.

33-5	Risk Factors for the Development of Surgical Site Infections

Patient Factors

- Ascites
- Chronic inflammation
- Corticosteroid therapy (controversial)
- Obesity
- Diabetes
- Extremes of age
- Hypocholesterolemia
- Hypoxemia
- Peripheral vascular disease (especially for lower extremity surgery)
- Postoperative anemia
- Prior site irradiation
- Recent operation
- Remote infection
- Skin carriage of staphylococci
- Skin disease in the area of infection (e.g., psoriasis)
- Undernutrition

Environmental Factors

- Contaminated medications
- Inadequate disinfection/sterilization
- Inadequate skin antisepsis
- Inadequate ventilation

Treatment Factors

- Drains
- Emergency procedure
- Hypothermia
- Inadequate antibiotic prophylaxis
- Oxygenation (controversial)
- Prolonged preoperative hospitalization
- Prolonged operative time

Data from National Nosocomial Infections Surveillance (NNIS) System Report: Am J Infect Control 2001;29:404-421.

33-6	**Surgical Wound Classification**

Class I/Clean: An uninfected operative wound in which no inflammation is encountered and the respiratory, alimentary, genital, or uninfected urinary tract is not entered. In addition, clean wounds are primarily closed and, if necessary, drained with closed drainage. Operative incisional wounds that follow nonpenetrating (blunt) trauma should be included in this category if they meet the criteria.

Class II/Clean-Contaminated: An operative wound in which the respiratory, alimentary, genital, or urinary tracts are entered under controlled conditions and without unusual contamination. Specifically, operations involving the biliary tract, appendix, vagina, and oropharynx are included in this category, provided no evidence of infection or major break in technique is encountered.

Class III/Contaminated: Open, fresh, accidental wounds. In addition, operations with major breaks in sterile technique (e.g., open cardiac massage) or gross spillage from the gastrointestinal tract, and incisions in which acute, nonpurulent inflammation is encountered are included in this category.

Class IV/Dirty-Infected: Old traumatic wounds with retained devitalized tissue and those that involve existing clinical infection or perforated viscera. This definition suggests that the organisms causing postoperative infection were present in the operative field before the operation.

From Mangram AJ, Horan TC, Pearson ML, et al: Infect Control Hosp Epidemiol 1999;20:250-278, available at http://www.cdc.gov/ncidod/dhqp/pdf/guidelines/SSI.pdf.

biliary instrumentation (such as stenting) should be administered antibiotics.

Antibiotic prophylaxis of clean surgery is controversial. Where bone is incised (e.g., craniotomy, sternotomy) or a prosthesis is inserted, antibiotic prophylaxis is generally indicated. The utility of antibiotics in cases of clean surgery of soft tissues (e.g., breast, hernia) is unclear. In two situations, antimicrobial prophylaxis has traditionally been given for class I wounds. These are operations in which prosthetic material is placed intravascularly (e.g., aortic aneurysm repair with graft placement) or into a joint (e.g., total hip arthroplasty), or any surgery after which infection of the incision or organ or space would be clinically devastating (e.g., cardiac surgery, neurosurgical procedures).

Patients undergoing class IV (dirty-infected) operations should not receive antimicrobial prophylaxis. They should receive therapeutic antimicrobials directed at anticipated organisms based on the anatomic location and clinical situation surrounding the injury. In such scenarios, therapeutic agents are started at the time of injury or suspected infection, often before the patient presents to the operating room.

Antimicrobial Prophylaxis

Antimicrobial prophylaxis is directed against the most likely infecting organism (Fig. 33-18 and Table 33-5). Prophylaxis does not have to cover every potential pathogen. Skin organisms such as staphylococci and streptococci are the most likely pathogens in surgeries that do not enter a chronically colonized body cavity. Cephalosporins are effective against many gram-positive and gram-negative bacteria. Cefazolin is generally viewed as the antimicrobial of first choice in

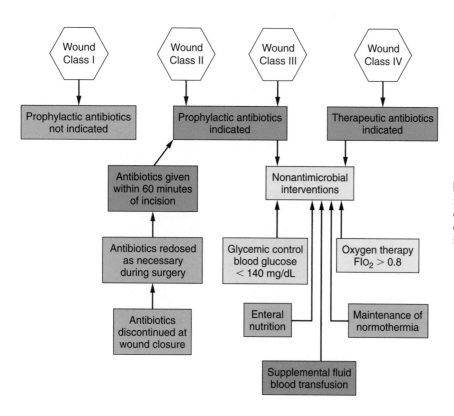

Figure 33-18 ■ Preventing surgical site infections in major abdominal surgery. Wound class I (clean), class II (clean-contaminated), class III (contaminated), and class IV (dirty-infected). FIO₂, inspired oxygen tension.

clean operations. A full therapeutic dose of cefazolin (1 to 2 g depending on volume of distribution) should be given to adult patients no more than 30 minutes before skin incision. Prophylaxis for operations involving the lower GI tract should include coverage against gram-negative enteric bacteria and bowel anaerobes, particularly *Bacteroides fragilis.*

Most SSIs are caused by gram-positive cocci (see Table 33-5).[227] The most common etiologic agent causing SSI after clean surgery is *Staphylococcus aureus,* followed by *Staphylococcus epidermidis. Enterococcus faecalis, Escherichia coli,* and *B. fragilis* are common pathogens in SSI after clean-contaminated surgery. The antibiotic chosen should be directed primarily against staphylococci for clean cases and high-risk clean-contaminated elective surgery of the biliary and upper GI tracts. A first-generation cephalosporin is the preferred agent for most patients, with clindamycin preferred for patients with a history of anaphylaxis to penicillin (Table 33-6).

When should parenteral antibiotics be given for optimal effect? The best time to give cephalosporin prophylaxis is within 1 hour before the time of incision (Table 33-7).[228] The goal is to obtain blood and tissue drug levels that exceed the minimum inhibitory concentration of the organisms likely to be encountered. Antibiotics are less effective if given earlier or after incision has been made. Incorrect timing of surgical prophylaxis is associated with increases by a factor of two to six in the rates of SSI for operative procedures in which prophylaxis is generally recommended (Box 33-7).[228,229] In a New York State study published in 1996, there was failure to administer the first dose of antibiotic within the 2-hour window before incision in 27% to 54% of all patients selected.[230] Antibiotics with short half-lives (<2 hours—e.g., cefazolin, cefoxitin) should be re-dosed every 3 to 4 hours during surgery for longer operations or if there is significant blood loss (Table 33-8). Antibiotics should not be administered for more than 24 hours (more than one dose is probably unnecessary). Antibiotics should not be administered to cover indwelling drains or catheters.

Antimicrobial prophylaxis after wound closure is unnecessary.[224] Prolonged administration is associated with the emergence of resistant bacterial strains and other complications, including catheter-related bloodstream infections, pneumonia, multidrug-resistant organisms, and antibiotic-associated colitis. *Clostridium difficile* colitis is increasing in frequency and severity.[231] Disruption of the normal balance of gut flora results in overgrowth of the enterotoxin-

---

33-5	Bacterial Pathogens in Surgical Site Infections	

Pathogen	Prevalence (% of Isolates)
Staphylococcus	19
Coagulase-negative *Staphylococcus*	14
Enterococcus species	12
Escherichia coli	8
Pseudomonas aeruginosa	8
Miscellaneous aerobic gram-negative bacilli	8
Enterobacter species	7
Streptococcus species	6
Klebsiella species	4
Miscellaneous anaerobic bacteria	3
Miscellaneous aerobic gram-positive bacteria	2

Data from Emori TG, Gaynes RP: Clin Microbiol Rev 1993;6:428-442.

33-6	Antibiotic Prophylaxis for Abdominal and Pelvic Surgery		

Surgery

Gastrointestinal Surgery	Bacteria	Antimicrobial	Dosage
Esophageal gastroduodenal	Enteric gram-negative bacilli, gram-positive cocci	High-risk only: cefazolin	1-2 g IV
Biliary tract	Enteric gram-negative bacilli, enterococci, clostridia	High-risk only: cefazolin	1-2 g IV
Colorectal	Enteric gram-negative bacilli, anaerobes, enterococci	Oral: neomycin + erythromycin	neomycin: 1g; erythromycin: 1 g × 3 doses prior to surgery
		Parenteral: cefoxitin	1-2 g IV
		OR cefotetan	1-2 g IV
		OR cefazolin + metronidazole	1-2 g IV
			0.5 g IV
Appendectomy, nonperforated	Enteric gram-negative bacilli, anaerobes, enterococci	Cefoxitin	1-2 g IV
		OR cefotetan	1-2 g IV
Genitourinary Surgery			
	Enteric gram-negative bacilli, enterococci	High-risk only: ciprofloxacin	500 mg PO or 400 mg IV
Gynecologic and Obstetric Surgery			
Vaginal or abdominal hysterectomy	Enteric gram-negative anaerobes, group B streptococci, enterococci	Cefazolin	1-2 g IV
		OR cefotetan	1-2 g IV
		OR cefoxitin	1 g IV
Cesarean section	Same as for hysterectomy	High-risk only: cefazolin	1 g IV after cord-clamping

IV, intravenously; PO, by mouth.

33-7	Risk of Development of Surgical Site Infection Relative to Timing of Antibiotic Prophylaxis				
Timing*	Patients (N)	No. (%) Infections	RR (95% CI)	OR (95% CI)	
Early	369	14 (3.80)	6.7[†] (2.9-14.7)	4.3[†] (1.8-10.4)	
Preoperative	1708	10 (0.59)	1.0	—	
Perioperative	282	4 (1.40)	2.4 (0.9-7.9)	2.1 (0.6-7.4)	
Postoperative	488	16 (3.30)	5.8[†] (2.6-12.3)	5.8[†] (2.4-13.8)	
All	2847	44 (1.5)	—	—	

*Early, administration more than 2 hr before skin incision; preoperative, administration during the recommended interval (≤2 hr before skin incision); perioperative, administration within 2 hr after skin incision; postoperative, administration more than 2 hr after the skin incision.

[†]$P < .0001$ when compared with preoperative group.

CI, confidence interval; OR, odds ratio; RR, relative risk.

Data from Classen DC, Evans RS, Pestotnik SL, et al: N Engl J Med 1992;326:281-286.

33-7	Recommendations for Perioperative Antimicrobial Treatment
Antibiotic timing	Infusion of the first antimicrobial dose should begin within 60 minutes before the surgical incision is made.
Duration of prophylaxis	Prophylactic antimicrobials should be discontinued within 24 hours of the end of surgery.
Screening for β-lactam allergy	For operations in which the cephalosporins represent the most appropriate antimicrobials for prophylaxis, the medical history should be adequate to determine whether the patient has a history of allergy or has had a serious adverse antibiotic reaction. Alternative testing strategies (e.g., skin testing) may be useful in patients with reported allergy.
Antimicrobial dosing	The initial antimicrobial dose should be adequate for the patient's weight, adjusted dosing weight, or body mass index. An additional dose of antimicrobial should be given intraoperatively if the surgery is still continuing two half-lives after the initial dose.

From Bratzler DW, Houck PM, Richards C, et al: Arch Surg 2005;140:174-182.

producing *C. difficile*. Therefore, antimicrobial prophylaxis should be discontinued within 24 hours of the end of surgery (see Table 33-7).

Nonantibiotic Therapies to Prevent Surgical Site Infection

Figure 33-18 also shows some nonantibiotic therapies.

Glycemic Control

A key part of the surgical stress response is the presence of white cells in the damaged tissues. These cells phagocytize cellular debris, secrete growth factors, and catalyze the synthesis of collagen. As part of this response, there is a dramatic increase in blood glucose levels, resulting from enhanced glycogenolysis and gluconeogenesis. This homeostatic mech-

anism mobilizes substrate, principally from the liver and skeletal muscle, to restore function, fight infection, and repair damaged tissue. White cells are obligate glucose users. Hyperglycemia is facilitated by a dramatic increase in the secretion of cortisol, growth hormone, epinephrine, and glucagon. Epinephrine induces glycogenolysis, lipolysis, and increased lactate production, independent of cellular redox state.[232] This is termed aerobic glycolysis. A simultaneous increase in insulin production leads to increased peripheral glucose uptake.[233]

There appears to be a glycemic concentration ceiling above which hyperglycemia is associated with adverse outcomes, which leads to an interest in the benefits of tight glycemic control.[234,235] Hyperglycemia can induce immune dysfunction by promoting inflammation, associated with abnormalities of white cell function.[236,237] These include granulocyte adhesion, chemotaxis, phagocytosis, respiratory burst and superoxide formation, and intracellular killing.[238] Importantly, hyperglycemia negatively affects wound healing[239] and may predispose the patient to surgical wound site infection. A caveat about these claims is that the studies were performed in diabetic patients, not those with stress hyperglycemia; thus, immune suppression may result from the disease—one of absolute or relative insulin deficiency—rather than the glucose.

Animal models of stroke demonstrated that hyperglycemia in the presence of cerebral ischemia may be detrimental.[240] Hyperglycemia may worsen prognosis as a result of increased brain tissue acidosis, accumulation of extracellular glutamate, increased blood–brain barrier permeability, and increased formation of cerebral edema. A consensus exists that hyperglycemia leads to localized tissues acidosis,[241] and this in turn may increase the risk for ischemia in the penumbra.[241] Consequently, clinicians have used observational data, animal studies,[240] and human studies in different fields[242,243] to justify tight glycemic control, using insulin, in perioperative patients.

Insulin has significant anti-inflammatory properties and antioxidant activity, and it reduces the quantity of circulating cytokines.[244] Obese patients with insulin-resistant type 2 diabetes have larger infarcts than nondiabetics. In a rat model of myocardial ischemia, the introduction of insulin into the reperfusion fluid reduced infarct size by 50%.[245] A similar effect was seen in humans given insulin, tissue-plasminogen activator (TPA), and heparin.[246]

33-8   Suggested Dosage Schedules for Antimicrobials for Surgical Prophylaxis

Antimicrobial	Half-Life, Normal Renal Function (hr)	Half-Life, End-Stage Renal Disease (hr)	Recommended Infusion Time (min)	Standard Intravenous Dosage	Weight-Based Dosage Recommendation*	Recommended Redosage Interval† (hr)
Aztreonam	1.5-2	6	3-5‡	1-2 g	Maximum, 2 g (adults)	3-5
Ciprofloxacin	3.5-5	5-9	60	400 mg	400 mg	4-10
Cefazolin	1.2-2.5	40-70	3-5‡ 15-60§	1-2 g	20-30 mg/kg <80 kg, 1 g ≥80 kg, 2 g	2-5
Cefuroxime	1-2	15-22	3-5‡ 15-60§	1.5 g	50 mg/kg	3-4
Cefamandole	0.5-2.1	12.3-18¶	3-5‡ 15-60§	1 g		3-4
Cefoxitin	0.5-1.1	6.5-23	3-5‡ 15-60§	1-2 g	20-40 mg/kg	2-3
Cefotetan	2.8-4.6	13-25	3-5‡ 20-60§	1-2 g	20-40 mg/kg	3-6
Clindamycin	2-5.1	3.5-5.0¶	10-60 (Do not exceed 30 mg/min)	600-900 mg	<10 kg: at least 37.5 mg ≥10 kg: 3-6 mg/kg	3-6
Erythromycin base	0.8-3	5-6	NA	1 g orally: 19, 18, 9 hr before surgery	9-13 mg/kg	NA
Gentamicin	2-3	50-70	30-60	1.5 mg/kg**	See footnote**	3-6
Neomycin	2-3 (3% absorbed under normal gastrointestinal conditions)	12-≥24	NA	1 g orally: 19, 18, 9 hr before surgery	20 mg/kg	NA
Metronidazole	6-14	7-21 no change	30-60	0.5-1 g	15 mg/kg (adult), 7.5 mg/kg on subsequent doses	6-8
Vancomycin	4-6	44.1-406.4 (Cl$_{cr}$ <10 mL/min)	1 g in ≥60 min (use longer infusion time if dose <1 g)	1.0 g	10-15 mg/kg (adult)	6-12

*Weight-based dosages are primarily from published pediatric recommendations.

†For procedures of long duration, antimicrobials should be re-administered at intervals of 1 to 2 times the half-life of the drug. The intervals in the table were calculated for patients with normal renal function.

‡Dose injected directly into vein or running intravenous fluids.

§Intermittent intravenous infusion.

¶In patients with a serum creatinine level of 5 to 9 mg/dL.

¶The half-life of clindamycin is the same or slightly increased in patients with end-stage renal disease compared with patients with normal renal function.

**If the patient's weight is 30% higher than ideal bodyweight, dosage weight can be determined as follows: dosage weight = ideal bodyweight + 0.4 × (total bodyweight – ideal bodyweight).

Cl$_{cr}$, creatinine clearance.

Data from Bratzler DW, Houck PM, Richards C, et al: Arch Surg 2005;140:174-182.

Zerr, Furnary, and colleagues demonstrated that meticulous control of blood glucose significantly reduces the incidence of deep sternal wound infections and perioperative mortality in diabetic patients undergoing cardiac surgery.[247-249]

Insulin appears to be cardioprotective in the presence of ischemia.[245] Insulin therapy in perioperative and, in particular, cardiothoracic surgical patients was associated with a significant reduction in the risk for death.[242] Enthusiasm for insulin therapy, rather than glycemic control, must be tempered by the knowledge that increased insulin administration is positively associated with death in the ICU regardless of the prevailing blood glucose level.[250]

A prospective randomized unblinded clinical trial randomized 1548 surgical ICU patients into two groups. The first group received a conventional therapy of an insulin drip adjusted to maintain a blood glucose level of 180 to 200 mg/dL.[251] The second group received "intensive insulin therapy": an insulin drip was started if the blood glucose level exceeded 100 mg/dL, and the drip was adjusted to maintain blood glucose between 80 and 100 mg/dL. Overall, intensive insulin therapy resulted in an absolute risk reduction of death of

3.4%. Subgroup analysis suggested that this mortality difference accrued principally to patients who were critically ill rather than to those who underwent a standard perioperative stress response. Given the small number of abdominal or pelvic surgical patients recruited, it is unlikely that this study is applicable to that patient population. It was also concluded that glycemic control was more important than insulin dosage.[251,252] Indeed, increasing insulin dosage was related to increased incidence of renal failure in this study.[251] Finney and associates showed that increased insulin administration is positively associated with death in the ICU regardless of the prevailing blood glucose level.[250]

A single-center cohort study of intensive insulin therapy versus recent historic controls found a significant reduction in hospital mortality, ICU length of stay, and blood transfusion.[253]

The Leuven group (in Belgium) followed their initial report with a study of intensive insulin therapy in the medical ICU.[254] Twelve hundred patients were enrolled into the study. There was no statistical significant difference in mortality outcomes—37.3% in the intensive insulin therapy group versus 40.0% in the conventional therapy group ($P = .33$). Subgroup analysis suggested that patients who stayed in the ICU for more than 3 days benefited from insulin therapy, although it is difficult to interpret the usefulness of these data.

The issue of hypoglycemia cannot be ignored. A German multicenter study of intensive insulin therapy in patients with severe sepsis was stopped early because of a significantly excess risk for severe hypoglycemia without any evidence of improved survival (see www.clinicaltrials.gov/show/NCT00135473). The brain depends on glucose as its main source of energy, and a significant glucose gradient from the blood to the brain is required. Vespa and colleagues have shown by cerebral microdialysis that a glucose level of 0.2 mmol/L or less during intensive glucose control is an independent predictor of bad outcome in a patient with traumatic brain injury.[255] Hence, care must be taken to avoid hypoglycemia in patients with traumatic brain injury who are receiving intravenous insulin. The margin of safety between beneficial and detrimental effects appears to be narrow.

In conclusion, we cannot recommend intensive insulin therapy, at this time, for the perioperative care of patients undergoing major abdominal or pelvic surgery. However, some degree of glycemic control appears to be beneficial. A glycemic target of 140 to 160 mg/dL or less is recommended.

Temperature Control

Mild perioperative hypothermia (a core body temperature 34° to 36° C) is commonly observed in surgical patients, and this may have an impact on SSIs. Hypothermia leads to cutaneous vasoconstriction. Hopf and colleagues studied 130 general surgical patients to determine whether subcutaneous (SC) wound oxygen tension (PsqO$_2$) predicted SSIs.[256] In patients with a PsqO$_2$ greater than 90 mm Hg, there were no infections, whereas patients with a PsqO$_2$ of 40 to 50 mm Hg had an infection rate of 43%. Leukocyte bacteria-killing capacity is significantly impaired at low oxygen tensions.[257]

Hypothermia decreases perfusion and thus oxygen supply to the wound, and it also reduces the production of superoxide radicals for any given oxygen tension. In addition, mild hypothermia may be associated with an unfavorable cytokine profile.[258]

Kurz and colleagues studied 200 patients undergoing colorectal surgery, randomly assigned to routine intraoperative thermal care (the hypothermia group) or additional warming (the normothermia group).[259] The patients' anesthetic care and antimicrobial therapy were standardized (antibiotics were administered on induction of anesthesia and for 4 days postoperatively). Their wounds were evaluated daily until discharge from the hospital, and in the clinic after 2 weeks; wounds containing culture-positive pus were considered infected. The mean (±SD) final intraoperative core temperature was $34.7° ± 0.6°$ C in the hypothermia group and $36.6° ± 0.5°$ C in the normothermia group ($P < .001$). The presence of hypothermia was associated with a 13% absolute risk increase of 13% (NNT 7; $P = .009$). In addition, the duration of hospitalization was prolonged by 2.6 days (approximately 20%) in hypothermia group ($P = .01$). There was a nonsignificantly greater incidence of blood transfusion in the hypothermia group, leading to the suggestion that blood transfusion, a known risk factor, rather than hypothermia was responsible for the outcome differences.

To address this, Flores-Maldonado and colleagues reported on wound infections in a series (blood transfusion was an exclusion criterion) of 290 consecutive cholecystectomy patients with a 30-day follow-up.[260] The average temperature in their hypothermic group was $35.4° ± 0.4°$ C, and it was $36.2° ± 0.2°$ C in the normothermic group, based on tympanic membrane measurement immediately postoperatively. The incidence of SSI was 11.5% in the hypothermic group and 2% in the normothermic group, an absolute risk increase of 9% (NNT, 12; $P = .004$). This study was limited by lack of standardization of anesthesia and by incomplete follow-up.

A retrospective cohort study of 1472 patients who had undergone bowel surgery over a 3 month period in 2002 in 31 academic medical centers in the United States, addressed risk factors for perioperative wound infection.[261] Surprisingly, the authors demonstrated that lower intraoperative temperatures were associated with fewer infectious wound complications. Conclusions based on this study are limited by variability of practice, retrospective analysis, and absence of randomization.

Melling and colleagues studied 421 patients undergoing clean surgery, randomizing them to preoperative warming for 30 minutes before surgery or to routine care.[262] There were 19 wound infections in 139 nonwarmed patients (14%) but only 13 in 277 who received warming (5%; $P = .001$), an ARR of 9% (NNT, 11) associated with warming.

In summary, available data appear to favor the maintenance of normothermia in the operating room as a method of reducing SSIs.

Oxygen Therapy

If low oxygen tension in the tissues is associated with poor wound healing and infection, is oxygen therapy beneficial?

Some data support the concept of oxygen as a bactericidal agent[263] and as a positive factor in the promotion of wound healing.[264] The formation of scars requires hydroxylation of proline and lysine residues. The propyl and lysyl hydroxylases that catalyze this reaction require oxygen as a substrate. In the presence of infection, available local oxygen is reduced and wound healing is impaired.[265] In a study of 500 patients undergoing elective colorectal surgery, administration of 80% oxygen (versus 30% oxygen) during surgery and for 2 hours thereafter decreased the incidence of SSI by more than 50% (5.2% versus 11.2%).[265] On the other hand, Pryor and colleagues studied the utility of 80% versus 35% oxygen administered to 165 patients undergoing major intra-abdominal procedures and found that the infection rate was twice as high (25.0% versus 11.3%) after 80% oxygen.[266] This study, at 300 patients, may have been underpowered. The patients in the 80% group weighed more (they were more than twice as likely to be obese). They also had longer operations, lost significantly more blood, required significantly more fluid replacement, and were more likely to require postoperative intubation.

In summary, it is unclear whether supplemental oxygen promotes wound healing and reduces wound complications.

Fluid Resuscitation

Based on the hypothesis that hypoperfusion and vasoconstriction increase the risk for wound infection, it has been proposed that aggressive perioperative fluid administration may reduce such complications. Although supplemental fluid appears to increase tissue oxygen tension,[267] this has not translated into reduced risk for wound complications.[268] Indeed, there is emerging evidence that large-volume fluid resuscitation may worsen wound healing outcomes.[96,97]

Allogeneic blood transfusion would be expected to increase oxygen delivery and wound perfusion. However, transfusion is known to have an immunosuppressive effect. In the previously described study by Walz and colleagues,[261] perioperative transfusion was associated with a significant increase in the risk of developing SSIs. No prospective study has associated blood transfusion with increased or reduced infectious risk in patients undergoing abdominal surgery.

In summary, supplemental fluid and blood transfusion cannot be recommended for the prevention of surgical wound infections.

■ DEEP VENOUS THROMBOSIS AND PULMONARY EMBOLISM

One of the most feared complications of surgery is pulmonary embolus (PE) syndrome. This represents the extreme end of a spectrum of diseases characterized by the deposition and embolization of venous clot and referred to as venous thromboembolic disease (VTE). The core clinical problem in VTE is deep venous thrombosis (DVT). This involves clots that form in large veins in the extremities, inferior vena cava, pelvis, or renal veins. They are often painless and asymptomatic. Edema forms proximal to the obstruction, because of raised venous pressure. Subsequent morbidity depends on the degree of occlusiveness and the extent of recanalization. The

sequelae of deep vein thrombosis vary from complete resolution of the clot without any ill effects, to death due to pulmonary embolism. Morbidity due to deep vein thrombosis includes post-thrombotic syndrome, encompassing chronic venous hypertension causing limb pain, swelling, hyperpigmentation, dermatitis, ulcers, venous gangrene, and lipodermatosclerosis.

In the perioperative realm, this disorder is clinically relevant for three reasons: (1) Patients who have a history of VTE are at risk for recurrent events. (2) Patients with active VTE, treated with anticoagulants, may present for surgery. (3) VTE may develop postoperatively and is associated with risk for cardiopulmonary failure and chronic venous disease.

Pathogenesis of Venous Thromboembolism

The majority of clinicians cite Virchow's classic triad of risk factors for DVT, which include venous stasis, damage to the vessel wall, and hypercoagulability. Although purportedly described in 1860, and widely accepted today, Virchow described neither hypercoagulability nor stasis in his description of thrombosis and embolism.[269] Nevertheless, hypercoagulability is seen in perioperative and critically injured patients.[270,271] Whether this contributes to or causes DVT is unclear.

In the surgical patient, impaired venous pulsation occurs on induction of anesthesia because of the vasodilatory effects of anesthetic agents, positive pressure ventilation, and immobilization of the extremities (Box 33-8).[269] Loss of venous pulsatility, endothelial hypoxemia, and mechanical disruption of flow and venous turbulence, particularly adjacent to venous valve pockets, create the platform for clot formation within deep veins. Clots in pelvic and iliac veins are particularly vulnerable to embolization to the pulmonary circulation.

Most venous thrombi exist in two regions: One is composed predominantly of fibrin and trapped erythrocytes (red thrombi), and the other is composed mainly of aggregated platelets (white thrombi). In the fibrin-rich region, the thrombi are attached to the vessel wall, whereas in the platelet-rich region, the thrombi are located distant from the attachment site. These findings suggest that activation of the coagulation system precedes platelet activation and aggregation during the formation of venous thrombi.[272]

Certain illnesses, age profiles, and physiologic states predispose patients to a higher risk of developing VTE (see Box 33-8). These include malignancy, obesity, trauma, immobilization, and advanced age.

Incidence of Venous Thromboembolism

The incidence of spontaneous VTE in the general population is estimated to be 117 per 100,000. Intraoperative thromboembolic pulmonary embolism is rare. Usually it occurs in the postoperative period, often after hospital discharge.[273] Perioperative VTE risk is determined by underlying pathophysiology and the type of surgery (Table 33-9). For example, major pelvic and orthopedic surgeries are high risk, whereas thyroid surgery is low risk. One large study examined the California Patient Discharge Data Set to estimate the

33-8	Risk Factors for Venous Thromboembolism

Advanced age
Obesity
Previous venous thromboembolism
Surgery
Trauma
Neoplasm
Acute medical illnesses
Respiratory failure
Infection
Inflammatory bowel disease
Antiphospholipid syndrome
Dyslipoproteinemia
Nephrotic syndrome
Paroxysmal nocturnal hemoglobinuria
Myeloproliferative diseases
Behçet's syndrome
Varicose veins
Superficial vein thrombosis
Congenital venous malformation
Immobilization (including long-distance travel, bedrest)
Limb paresis
Chronic care facility stay
Pregnancy/puerperium
Heparin-induced thrombocytopenia
Central venous catheter
Vena cava filter
Intravenous drug abuse
Medications (tamoxifen, chemotherapy, antipsychotics, oral contraceptives, hormone replacement)

Data from Kyrle PA, Eichinger S: Lancet 2005;365:1163-1174.

33-9	Risk of Venous Thromboembolism (VTE) in Surgical Procedures

Surgical Procedure	VTE Incidence (%)	Incidence with Malignancy (%)
Gastrointestinal		
Splenectomy	1.6	1.6
Excision of small bowel	1.5	2.1
Exploratory laparotomy	0.7	2.4
Urologic		
Nephrectomy	0.4	2.0
Gynecologic		
Total abdominal hysterectomy	0.3	1.2

Data from White RH, Zhou H, Romano PS: Thromb Haemost 2003;90:446.

incidence of VTE in patients undergoing specific types of surgery.[273] In major abdominal surgery, the incidence ranged from a low of 0.3% in total abdominal hysterectomy to 1.6% for splenectomy. This study did not analyze thromboprophylaxis practice and excluded patients with a previous diagnosis of VTE. About 90% of pulmonary emboli emanate from deep vein thromboses in the extremities. The other 10% arise from pelvic veins, renal veins, and the inferior vena cava.

33-10	Pretest Probability* of Deep Venous Thrombosis (DVT)

Clinical Feature[†]	Points
Active cancer	1
Paralysis, paresis, or recent cast immobilization of the lower extremities	1
Bedridden >3 days, or major surgery within 4 weeks	1
Tenderness localized to the distribution of the deep veins	1
Entire leg swollen	1
Calf swelling >3 cm, compared with asymptomatic leg (measured 10 cm below tibial tuberosity)	1
Pitting edema	1
Collateral superficial veins (not varicose)	1
Previously documented DVT	1
Alternative diagnosis as likely or greater than that of DVT	−2

*Adding the scores gives a number that yields the probability of a DVT: ≥2 = DVT likely, <2 = DVT unlikely.
[†]If both legs are symptomatic, use the more symptomatic leg.
Data from Wells PS, Anderson DR, Rodger M, et al: N Engl J Med 2003;349:1227-1235.

Upper extremity venous thrombosis accounts for about 10% of deep venous thrombosis and is associated with indwelling central venous catheters and malignancy. Patients present with swelling, erythema, and pain in the arm affected by the clot. Treatment for upper extremity DVT includes removal of the thrombogenic source (usually a catheter) and systemic anticoagulation when possible.

Diagnosing Deep Venous Thrombosis

The diagnosis of DVT results from either clinical suspicion or meticulous screening. Patients with DVT may have extremity swelling, pain, and erythema. Physical examination may reveal edema, venous congestion, or perhaps a palpable thrombosed vein in the affected extremity. This constellation of symptoms leads to the diagnosis of one third of all DVTs.[274] Nonetheless, these cases require investigative confirmation, and undiagnosed cases require screening.

D-dimers are the degradation products of fibrinolysis that are produced in the presence of ongoing clotting and lysis. Although useful as outpatient screening tools, D-dimer tests are nonspecific in the perioperative period because of acute phase production.

Contrast venography remains the gold standard in the diagnosis of DVT. This procedure is infrequently performed because of its expense, invasiveness, and inconvenience. It has been widely replaced by compression ultrasonography (CUS), which is less expensive, noninvasive, and can easily be performed at the bedside. Also, it has been shown to correlate very well with contrast venography in diagnosing or excluding DVT.[275] CUS is widely used to screen for the presence or absence of DVT, especially in trauma patients. Several algorithms have been developed using history and physical examination to give a pretest probability score to increase the usefulness of CUS for diagnosing DVT. A commonly used algorithm is the Wells Score (Table 33-10).[276]

Diagnosing Pulmonary Embolism

The signs and symptoms of PE are nonspecific, and diagnosis of the disease is notoriously difficult. The majority of cases of PE detected postmortem had not been diagnosed (or treated) prior to death.[277] The sensitivity of the clinical recognition of PE could be as low as 25%.[278] One reason the clinical diagnosis is inaccurate is that PE can present as four different syndromes—pulmonary infarction, acute cor pulmonale, acute unexplained dyspnea, and acute respiratory distress syndrome.

Symptoms include dyspnea, chest pain, cough, and blood-tinged sputum. Signs include fever, tachycardia, tachypnea, and coarse breath sounds, and auscultation may yield a new fourth heart sound or accentuation of the pulmonic component of the second heart sound. Electrocardiography may reveal evidence of right heart strain, tachycardia, or atrial fibrillation.

Imaging Studies

The presence or absence of PE is confirmed or excluded by radiologic imaging studies. Chest radiography is neither sensitive nor specific. Currently, two modalities are widely used for the diagnosis of PE: perfusion lung scans and CT-pulmonary angiography.

Ventilation–perfusion lung scans (V/Q scans) have been available since the mid 1960s. Their purpose is to detect the presence of perfusion defects in the patients' pulmonary circulation. These involve the injection of radionucleotide agents, followed by sequential scans. The major advantage of this approach is the avoidance of potentially nephrotoxic radiographic contrast. In the PIOPED study, 755 patients underwent V/Q scans and selective pulmonary angiography within 24 hours of the occurrence of symptoms that suggested PE.[279] Of these patients, 251 (33%) had angiographic evidence of pulmonary embolism. Almost all patients with PE (98%) had abnormal V/Q scan findings. Thus, V/Q scans are highly sensitive for acute PE, but are they specific? Unfortunately, although pulmonary embolism was documented by angiography in 88%, only 41% of the patients with PE had a high-probability scan. The majority of patients with pulmonary embolism (57%) had an intermediate-probability or low-probability scan. For postoperative patients who have significant atelectasis, consolidation, or PE, the negative predictive value is low.

High-resolution multidetector CT (MDCT) has replaced the V/Q scan as the study of choice in many hospitals for PE evaluation. CT scanning is widely available, can be performed rapidly, provides clear anatomic and pathologic lung images (so that the clinician often obtains a diagnosis despite a negative angiographic examination), and has the ability to concurrently evaluate potential embolic sources in the legs or pelvis. The results of studies that have evaluated CT pulmonary angiography have shown sensitivities up to 90% with single-detector CT scans.[280] With developing technology, in particular the availability of multidetector units, the accuracy of these scans is improving. Four-slice MDCT scans have an increased sensitivity for subsegmental PE. In two studies of approximately 100 patients, sensitivities for the detection of

PE with four-slice CT angiography have been reported to be 96%[281] and 100%,[282] with respective specificities of 98% and 89%. The combination of arterial-phase and venous-phase CT angiography appears more sensitive (90%) and specific (96%) than arterial-phase alone.[283] For nonoperative patients, the combination of a negative CT pulmonary angiogram and negative D-dimers effectively excludes PE.[284,285] However, D-dimers are neither sensitive nor specific in the perioperative period. Postoperative patients with high clinical suspicion of PE and a negative MDCT scan should undergo lower extremity ultrasonography.[286]

Prevention of Deep Venous Thrombosis

Given the significant morbidity and mortality associated with VTE, perioperative preventative measures are essential (Fig. 33-19).[278] Prevention usually involves the combination of venous compression devices and systemic anticoagulation. Therapy should be begun before induction of anesthesia (Box 33-9).

External compression devices (ECDs) intermittently and sequentially compress the calf and thigh, accelerating deep venous flow and preventing pooling. These devices are known to enhance blood fibrinolytic activity. Hills demonstrated that 12% of patients treated with ECD developed DVT, compared with 30% of the untreated control subjects, an ARR of 18% (NNT, 5.5; $P < .05$).[287] Studying orthopedic patients, Hull and colleagues also compared ECD to no therapy.[288] The incidence of postoperative DVT as assessed by venography was 49% in 158 control patients compared with 24% of 152 patients treated with external pneumatic compression (EPC) (ARR, 25%; NNT, 4; $P = .00001$). Proximal DVT was detected in 27% of the control subjects, compared with 14% of patients treated with EPC ($P = .008$).

33-9	**General Surgery DVT Prophylaxis Recommendations**
Low-dose unfractionated heparin	Start 1-2 hr before surgery, continue every 8-12 hr after surgery
Adjusted-dose heparin	Heparin SC given every 8 hr, starting at about 3500 units and adjusting dose (±500 units) to maintain a mid-interval aPTT at high normal
General surgery: moderate risk	*Enoxaparin:* 20 mg SC 1-2 hr before surgery and then once daily after surgery *Tinzaparin:* 3500 units SC 2 hr before surgery and then once daily after surgery
General surgery: high risk	*Danaparoid:* 750 units SC 1-4 hr before surgery and then every 12 hr after surgery *Enoxaparin:* 40 mg SC 1-2 hr before surgery and then once daily after surgery

aPTT, activated partial thromboplastin time; SC, subcutaneously.
Adapted from Geerts WH, Heit JA, Clagett GP, et al: Chest 2001;119: 132S-175.

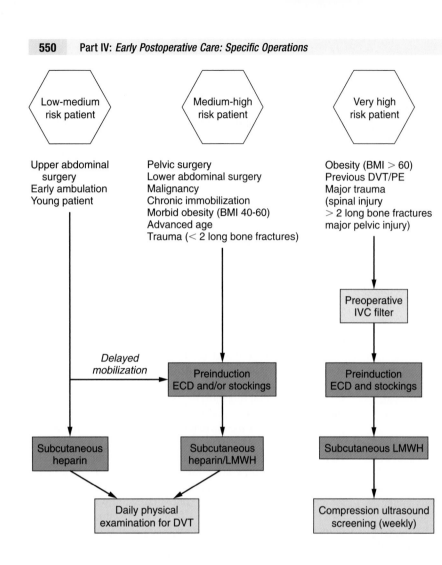

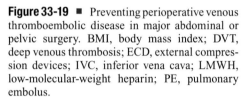

Figure 33-19 ■ Preventing perioperative venous thromboembolic disease in major abdominal or pelvic surgery. BMI, body mass index; DVT, deep venous thrombosis; ECD, external compression devices; IVC, inferior vena cava; LMWH, low-molecular-weight heparin; PE, pulmonary embolus.

Elastic compression stockings (ECS) are widely used to prevent DVT in the perioperative period. Allan and colleagues randomized 200 patients undergoing abdominal surgery, to receive ECS (both legs) or no intervention.[289] The incidence of postoperative DVT was 35.9% in control subjects, compared with 15.5% in the group with stockings (ARR, 20%; NNT, 5; P < .025). Wells and colleagues performed a meta-analysis of 12 studies of elastic stockings in moderate-risk surgery (abdominal, gynecologic, and neurosurgery).[290] The relative risk reduction associated with the wearing of the stockings was 68% (P < .0001; odds ratio, 0.28).

Turpie and colleagues compared ECS alone, ECS plus ECDs, and no treatment, in a group of neurosurgical patients. The use of ECS with or without ECDs reduced the DVT rate by 50%, but there was no difference between the combination therapy and ECS alone.[291]

Low-dose subcutaneous unfractionated heparin (ScUFH) has been used as a prophylactic measure in the prevention of DVT and PE since the results of several major trials in the 1970s. In 1972, Kakkar and associates compared low-dose ScUFH to no treatment in patients undergoing major surgery. They reported a decrease in DVT from 42% in control subjects to 8% in treated subjects (ARR, 36%; NNT, 3; P < .001).[292] Nicolaides and colleagues reported a 23% ARR in

patients treated with SC heparin (ScH) compared with no treatment.[293] Ballard and coworkers similarly demonstrated a 17% ARR (25% versus 8%) for DVT and PE in gynecologic patients randomized to subcutaneous heparin or no therapy. A large trial published in 1975 randomized 4121 patients to either no prophylaxis or (ScH). Among patients investigated for DVT, there was an ARR of 17% (NNT, 5.5) in the group receiving ScH.

Low-molecular-weight heparin (LMWH) and heparinoids are produced by either chemical or enzymatic depolymerization of heparin and have a mean molecular weight of 4000 to 6500 Da and a chain length of 13 to 22 sugars. They have greater bioavailability than standard unfractionated heparin and more predicable activity, and they require no laboratory monitoring.

Turpie and colleagues demonstrated an ARR of 30% in high-risk patients undergoing hip surgery and treated with LMWH (compared with placebo), without increasing the risk for bleeding.[294] Although theoretically the favorable pharmacology of these agents gives them an advantage over UFH in perioperative abdominal surgery patients, comparative data are scant in this patient population. LMWH is significantly more expensive than UFH in the United States. Hence, its use is reserved for patients deemed to be at higher risk.

The Cochrane collaboration has evaluated perioperative DVT prophylaxis in a variety of clinical situations. The combination of graduated compression stockings and perioperative low-dose heparin (or LMWH) is supported.[295]

The American College of Chest Physicians (ACCP) has published evidence-based guidelines for perioperative DVT and PE prophylaxis.[296] Patients are stratified into several categories. Moderate-risk general surgery patients are those patients undergoing a non-major procedure and who are between the ages of 40 and 60 years or have additional risk factors, or they are undergoing major operations and are less than 40 years of age with no additional risk factors. Recommended prophylaxis is either low-dose unfractionated heparin (LDUFH), 5000 units twice a day, or LMWH, 3400 units once daily (both grade 1A). Higher-risk general surgery patients are those undergoing nonmajor surgery and who are older than 60 years or have additional risk factors, or patients undergoing major surgery who are older than 40 years or have additional risk factors.

Recommend thromboprophylaxis is ScUFH (5000 units three times a day) or LMWH (>3400 units daily) (both grade 1A). In high-risk general surgery patients with multiple risk factors, anticoagulants (i.e., ScUFH, three times a day, or LMWH, >3400 units daily) should be combined with the use of compression devices or elasticized stockings (grade 1C+). For patients undergoing major, open urologic procedures, recommended routine prophylaxis involves ScUFH twice or three times daily (grade 1A). Acceptable alternatives include prophylaxis with compression devices (grade 1B) or LMWH (grade 1C+). For patients undergoing major gynecologic surgery for benign disease, without additional risk factors, recommended therapy is ScUFH, 5000 units twice a day (grade 1A). Alternatives include once-daily prophylaxis with LMWH, 3400 units/day (grade 1C+), or compression devices started just before surgery and used continuously while the patient is not ambulating (grade 1B). For patients undergoing extensive surgery for gynecologic malignancy, and for patients with additional VTE risk factors, recommended prophylaxis is ScUFH, 5000 unit three times a day (grade 1A), or higher doses of LMWH (e.g., >3400 units/day) (grade 1A) plus mechanical compression devices (all grade 1C).

Implementation

Prevention of DVT usually begins in the preoperative period. Lower extremity compression devices should be applied before induction of anesthesia. In addition, fractionated and unfractionated heparin may be started before surgery for higher-risk patients, in particular the morbidly obese and those patients undergoing surgery to the hip and pelvis. Patients at significant risk for bleeding should be treated with compression devices alone. Pre-incision anticoagulation may increase bleeding complications. Care must be taken to ensure that the dosage of heparin and heparinoids is appropriate for weight. For the majority of advanced-age patients undergoing major abdominal or pelvic surgery, the combination of anticoagulation and sequential or graduated mechanical compression is recommended.

Treatment of Deep Venous Thrombosis

Anticoagulation

Anticoagulation is the therapy of choice for acute DVT. The objectives of anticoagulant therapy include prevention of thrombus extension, prevention of pulmonary embolism, and avoidance of recurrence of DVT (Table 33-11 and Fig. 33-20). Surprisingly, the evidence to support this intervention is based on a single study published in 1960.[297] Untreated patients had a high mortality rate after PE. Subsequent uncontrolled studies confirmed both high mortality without anticoagulation and reduced mortality with heparin.[298,299] Hence, clinicians universally recommend immediate treatment of DVT with heparin. Likewise, when there is significant clinical suspicion, therapy should be begun before confirmation of the diagnosis and discontinued if the diagnosis is not confirmed.

The three options available for the initial treatment of DVT are (1) bodyweight-adjusted LMWH administered subcutaneously without monitoring, (2) intravenous UFH, and (3) ScUFH administered with monitoring, and subsequent dosage adjustments. Thrombolysis has no role in the management of DVT in patients after major abdominal surgery.

The ACCP consensus document provides a useful therapeutic guideline.[300] For patients with objectively confirmed DVT, short-term treatment with SC LMWH or intravenous (IV) UFH or ScUFH (all grade 1A) is recommended. Subcutaneous administration of UFH is as effective and as safe as intravenous UFH. This approach has been extensively studied and its efficacy proven.[301] The key to this approach is to ensure that an adequate starting dose is administered and that dosages are adjusted to maintain an appropriate activated partial thromboplastin time (aPTT). The usual regimen includes an initial IV bolus of 5000 units followed by a SC dose of 17,500 units twice on the first day. When patients are receiving SC heparin, the aPTT should be drawn 6 hours

33-11	Anticoagulant Treatment for Acute Deep Venous Thrombosis	
Medication	**Dosage**	**Dosage Adjustment**
Unfractionated heparin, IV	80-unit (U) bolus, and 18-U/kg/hr infusion	Maintain aPTT corresponding to plasma heparin levels of 0.3-0.7 IU/mL
Unfractionated heparin, SC	5000-U IV bolus followed by 17,500 U bid	
Low-molecular-weight heparin	Specific to agent	Unnecessary in most patients. May use anti-Xa assay in renal failure and for pregnant patients.

aPTT, activated partial thromboplastin time; bid, twice a day; IV, intravenous; SC, subcutaneous.
Data from Buller HR, Agnelli G, Hull RD, et al: Chest 2004;126:401S-428.

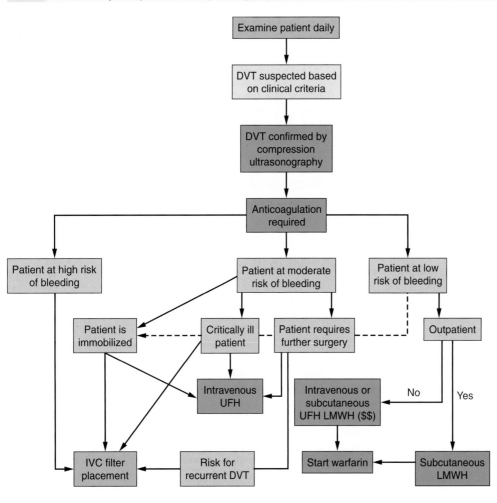

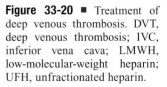

Figure 33-20 ■ Treatment of deep venous thrombosis. DVT, deep venous thrombosis; IVC, inferior vena cava; LMWH, low-molecular-weight heparin; UFH, unfractionated heparin.

after the morning administration and the dosage of UFH adjusted to achieve a 1.5 to 2.5 prolongation.

If patients require large daily doses of UFH and do not achieve a therapeutic aPTT, the ACCP recommends the measurement of the anti-Xa level for dosage guidance (grade 1B).[300]

LMWH has more predictable pharmacokinetics and a greater bioavailability than UFH. Because of these pharmacologic features, bodyweight-adjusted doses of LMWH can be administered SC once or twice daily without laboratory monitoring in the majority of patients. However, in certain clinical situations, such as severe renal failure or pregnancy, dosage adjustment might be required and can be achieved by monitoring plasma anti-Xa level. Anti-Xa assay should be performed 4 hours after the SC administration of a weight-adjusted dose of LMWH.[300,301]

Dolovich and colleagues meta-analyzed 13 randomized studies comparing IV heparin and LMWHs for the initial treatment of acute DVT.[302] There was no statistically significant difference in risk between UFH and LMWHs for recurrent VTE (RR, 0.85; 95% CI, 0.65-1.12), pulmonary embolism (RR, 1.02; 95% CI, 0.64-1.62), major bleeding (RR, 0.63; 95% CI, 0.37-1.05), minor bleeding (RR, 1.18; 95% CI, 0.87-1.61), or thrombocytopenia (RR, 0.85; 95% CI, 0.45-1.62).

There was a statistically significant difference for risk for total mortality (RR, 0.76; 95% CI, 0.59-0.98) in favor of LMWHs. The survival benefit was essentially accounted for by patients with malignancy. No apparent differences were observed in efficacy and safety among the different LMWHs. Where applicable, and if cost effective, LMWH should be used as an alternative to UFH, as there is no requirement to measure anticoagulation. The dosage of these agents must be adjusted in patients with acute renal failure.

Inferior Vena Cava Filters

Inferior vena cava (IVC) filters interrupt transmission of emboli to the pulmonary circulation. They may be inserted through either the femoral or the internal jugular vein, they are fluoroscopically placed, and they may be permanent or removable. Proximal lower extremity DVTs (above the knee) have a high likelihood of embolization to the pulmonary circulation. For this reason, patients who develop a proximal lower extremity DVT should be considered for therapeutic anticoagulation. If the patient cannot be anticoagulated because of recent surgery or continued bleeding, insertion of an IVC filter should be considered. Recently, many patients have had IVC filters placed preemptively in select patient groups with high risk for VTE, such as the morbidly obese or trauma patients with multiple long-bone fractures.[303] Outcome data are sparse that support this approach in the majority of patients undergoing major abdominal surgery.

Treatment of Pulmonary Embolism

Therapeutic options for DVT and PE are similar, as they are manifestations of the same disease processes. Without treatment, mortality from PE approaches 30%.[287] The majority of patients with proximal DVT also have PE, and vice versa.[300] In patients treated for PE, the overall mortality decreases to 15%.[304] The treatment of PE in the postoperative patient is complicated by the inherent potential for bleeding with therapeutic anticoagulation and thrombolytics (Fig. 33-21).

For acute PE, the options for treatment include therapeutic anticoagulation, IVC filter placement to prevent continued embolization from the lower extremities, clot thrombolysis, and surgical embolectomy. Hemodynamically stable patients diagnosed with a PE should receive therapeutic anticoagulation with IV unfractionated heparin or SC low-molecular-weight heparin. Meta-analyses have shown that LMWH treatment, adjusted to bodyweight, is at least as effective and safe as dosage-adjusted UFH.[302] However, in postoperative and critically ill patients, and patients in whom epidural catheter have been placed, the shorter half-life and reversibility of IV UFH provides a safety buffer over LMWH. Hence, when there is a risk for clinically significant bleeding, UFH is preferred. Treatment should be begun before confirmation of the diagnosis if there is clinical suspicion of PE.[300] As discussed, heparin should be adjusted to a target aPTT, and anti-Xa levels should be checked if the patient is requires large dosages of UFH without achieving therapeutic aPTT.

Patients who cannot be anticoagulated (e.g., those with intracranial bleeding) should have an IVC filter placed as soon as possible to prevent further embolization.

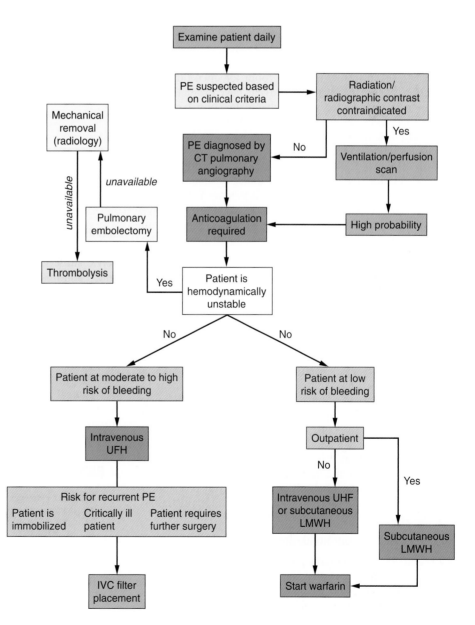

Figure 33-21 ■ Treatment of pulmonary embolism in the postoperative patient. CT, computed tomography; IVC, inferior vena cava; LMWH, low-molecular-weight heparin; PE, pulmonary embolus; UFH, unfractionated heparin.

After the success of thrombolytics in the management of acute myocardial infarction, thrombolysis has been proposed as therapy for massive PE. Thrombolytic agents currently available for use in the United States include tissue-plasminogen activator, streptokinase, and urokinase. These agents all convert plasminogen to plasmin, which in turn breaks down fibrin and promotes clot lysis. The International Cooperative Pulmonary Embolism Registry (ICOPER) reported on 108 patients with massive PE.[305] Thrombolysis did not improve 90-day outcomes in the 33 patients treated. This is consistent with an earlier systematic review that failed to demonstrate outcome improvement between thrombolysis and IV heparin.[306] In the absence of supportive data, and with evidence of increased risk for intracranial hemorrhage and bleeding from the wound site, thrombolysis cannot be recommended for postoperative patients who have undergone major abdominal or pelvic surgery.

Pulmonary embolectomy has been performed in patients who have had a massive PE, are hemodynamically unstable despite heparin and fluid resuscitation, and are not candidates for thrombolysis. Patients with life-threatening PE may be placed on extracorporeal membrane oxygenation for stabilization and taken to the operating room for open thrombus extraction. No prospective clinical trials have evaluated outcomes from embolectomy; available data consist of case reports and case series. The largest series of pulmonary embolectomies at one institution was reported by Meyer and colleagues in Paris in 1991.[307] During a 20-year period from 1968 to 1988, 96 of 3000 patients (3%) with confirmed PE underwent pulmonary embolectomy under cardiopulmonary bypass. The overall hospital mortality was 37.5%. Two factors were associated with an increased mortality: preoperative cardiac arrest and preoperative shock. Mortality in patients in shock was 42%, as compared with 17% in those without shock. In general, embolectomy is considered a therapy of last resort and should not be considered for the majority of patients with PE.[308]

The most common cause of death after pulmonary embolectomy is recurrent PE. Hence concurrent interruption of the IVC (such as with a filter) is recommended.[307]

Regional Anesthesia and DVT

Epidural anesthesia has been shown to lower the incidence of intraoperative VTE.[309,310] However, it does not appear to lower the incidence of postoperative VTE. When considering the use of epidural or spinal anesthesia, current and future anticoagulant therapy must be considered. Patients who are anticoagulated when a neuraxial (spinal or epidural) procedure is initiated are at risk for peri-spinal hematoma. This is particularly troublesome in patients treated with LMWH.[311] Consequently, timing of insertion and removal of epidural catheters must be coordinated with timing of administration of prophylactic anticoagulants (Table 33-12).

Summary and Recommendations

DVT and PE are common postoperative complications of surgery. It is important that the perioperative clinician be aware of the risks to the patient and the benefit of prophylactic therapy. Prophylaxis should be begun before induction of

33-12	Discontinuation Times for Anticoagulants before Neuraxial Anesthesia
Anticoagulant	**Timing of Discontinuation**
Antiplatelet medication	NSAIDs—No contraindication. Discontinue ticlopidine 14 days before. Discontinue clopidogrel 7 days before. Discontinue glycoprotein (GP) IIb/IIIa inhibitors 8-48 hours before needle or catheter placement.
Subcutaneous heparin	No contraindication for neuraxial procedure. In case of anticipated difficult placement of needle or catheter, can delay until neuraxial procedure finished.
Intravenous heparin	Start 1 hr after neuraxial procedure is completed. Catheter to be removed 2-4 hr after stopping infusion.
Low-molecular-weight heparin	Discontinue 10-12 hr before neuraxial procedure. Once-daily dosing—start 4 hr after neuraxial procedure. Twice-daily dosing—start 24 hr after neuraxial procedure.
Warfarin	Check for normal INR before initiating neuraxial procedure; INR ≤1.5 before removing catheter.

INR, International Normalized Ratio; NSAIDs, nonsteroidal anti-inflammatory drugs.

Data from Horlocker TT, Wedel DJ, Benzon H, et al: Reg Anesth Pain Med 2003;28:172-197.

anesthesia and continued until the patient is ambulating. For the majority of patients undergoing major abdominal or pelvic surgery, this involves the combination of anticoagulants, administered subcutaneously, and leg compression devices or elasticized stockings. Therapy for established DVT is targeted at prevention of further clot accumulation, using IV or SC anticoagulants. PE is a potentially devastating process that has many guises and may be difficult to diagnose clinically. The emergence of CT pulmonary angiography has significantly advanced our diagnostic capabilities. The development of a massive pulmonary embolus represents a difficult clinical conundrum in the postsurgical patient. The risk for bleeding appears to outweigh any potential benefit from thrombolysis. Thus, mechanical removal, extracorporeal life support, or pulmonary embolectomy may be preferred.

■ REFERENCES

1. Pandit JJ, Duncan T, Robbins PA: Total oxygen uptake with two maximal breathing techniques and the tidal volume breathing technique: A physiologic study of preoxygenation. Anesthesiology 2003;99:841-846.
2. Drummond GB, Park GR: Arterial oxygen-saturation before intubation of the trachea: An assessment of oxygenation techniques. Br J Anaesth 1984;56:987-993.
3. Hedenstierna G, Edmark L: The effects of anesthesia and muscle paralysis on the respiratory system. Intensive Care Med 2005;31: 1327-1335.

4. Reber A, Engberg G, Sporre B, et al: Volumetric analysis of aeration in the lungs during general anaesthesia. Br J Anaesth 1996;76:760-766.

5. Rothen HU, Sporre B, Engberg G, et al: Reexpansion of atelectasis during general anaesthesia may have a prolonged effect. Acta Anaesthesiol Scand 1995;39:118-125.

6. Malbouisson LM, Busch CJ, Puybasset L, et al: Role of the heart in the loss of aeration characterizing lower lobes in acute respiratory distress syndrome. The CT Scan ARDS Study Group. Am J Respir Crit Care Med 2000;161:2005-2012.

7. Hedenstierna G: Atelectasis and its prevention during anaesthesia. Eur J Anaesthesiol 1998;15:387-390.

8. Rothen HU, Sporre B, Engberg G, et al: Airway closure, atelectasis and gas exchange during anaesthesia. Br J Anaesth 1998;81:681-686.

9. Gander S, Frascarolo P, Suter M, et al: Positive end-expiratory pressure during induction of general anesthesia increases duration of non-hypoxic apnea in morbidly obese patients. Anesth Analg 2005;100:580-584.

10. Berthoud MC, Peacock JE, Reilly CS: Effectiveness of preoxygenation in morbidly obese patients. Br J Anaesth 1991;67:464-466.

11. Lane S, Saunders D, Schofield A, et al: A prospective, randomised controlled trial comparing the efficacy of pre-oxygenation in the 20 degrees head-up vs supine position. Anaesthesia 2005;60:1064-1067.

12. Baraka AS, Hanna MT, Jabbour SI, et al: Preoxygenation of pregnant and nonpregnant women in the head-up versus supine position. Anesth Analg 1992;75:757-759.

13. Dixon BJ, Dixon JB, Carden JR, et al: Preoxygenation is more effective in the 25 degrees head-up position than in the supine position in severely obese patients: A randomized controlled study. Anesthesiology 2005;102:1110-1115.

14. Altermatt FR, Munoz HR, Delfino AE, Cortinez LI: Pre-oxygenation in the obese patient: Effects of position on tolerance to apnoea. Br J Anaesth 2005;95:706-709.

15. Torres A, Serra-Batlles J, Ros E, et al: Pulmonary aspiration of gastric contents in patients receiving mechanical ventilation: The effect of body position. Ann Intern Med 1992;116:540-543.

16. Orozco-Levi M, Torres A, Ferrer M, et al: Semirecumbent position protects from pulmonary aspiration but not completely from gastroesophageal reflux in mechanically ventilated patients. Am J Respir Crit Care Med 1995;152:1387-1390.

17. Drakulovic MB, Torres A, Bauer TT, et al: Supine body position as a risk factor for nosocomial pneumonia in mechanically ventilated patients: A randomised trial. Lancet 1999;354:1851-1858.

18. Bercault N, Wolf M, Runge I, et al: Intrahospital transport of critically ill ventilated patients: A risk factor for ventilator-associated pneumonia: A matched cohort study. Crit Care Med 2005;33:2471-2478.

19. Pelosi P, Croci M, Ravagnan I, et al: The effects of body mass on lung volumes, respiratory mechanics, and gas exchange during general anesthesia. Anesth Analg 1998;87:654-660.

20. Eichenberger A, Proietti S, Wicky S, et al: Morbid obesity and postoperative pulmonary atelectasis: An underestimated problem. Anesth Analg 2002;95:1788-1792.

21. Auler JO Jr, Miyoshi E, Fernandes CR, et al: The effects of abdominal opening on respiratory mechanics during general anesthesia in normal and morbidly obese patients: A comparative study. Anesth Analg 2002;94:741-748.

22. Yoshino J, Akata T, Takahashi S: Intraoperative changes in arterial oxygenation during volume-controlled mechanical ventilation in modestly obese patients undergoing laparotomies with general anesthesia. Acta Anaesthesiol Scand 2003;47:742-750.

23. Tusman G, Bohm SH, Melkun F, et al: [Effects of the alveolar recruitment manoeuver and PEEP on arterial oxygenation in anesthetized obese patients.] Rev Esp Anestesiol Reanim 2002;49:177-183.

24. Pelosi P, Ravagnan I, Giurati G, et al: Positive end-expiratory pressure improves respiratory function in obese but not in normal subjects during anesthesia and paralysis. Anesthesiology 1999;91:1221-1231.

25. Perilli V, Sollazzi L, Bozza P, et al: The effects of the reverse Trendelenburg position on respiratory mechanics and blood gases in morbidly obese patients during bariatric surgery. Anesth Analg 2000;91:1520-1525.

26. Perilli V, Sollazzi L, Modesti C, et al: Comparison of positive end-expiratory pressure with reverse Trendelenburg position in morbidly obese patients undergoing bariatric surgery: Effects on hemodynamics and pulmonary gas exchange. Obes Surg 2003;13:605-609.

27. Ungern-Sternberg BS, Regli A, Schneider MC, et al: Effect of obesity and site of surgery on perioperative lung volumes. Br J Anaesth 2004;92:202-207.

28. Edmark L, Kostova-Aherdan K, Enlund M, Hedenstierna G: Optimal oxygen concentration during induction of general anesthesia. Anesthesiology 2003;98:28-33.

29. Rusca M, Proietti S, Schnyder P, et al: Prevention of atelectasis formation during induction of general anesthesia. Anesth Analg 2003;97:1835-1839.

30. Herriger A, Frascarolo P, Spahn DR, Magnusson L: The effect of positive airway pressure during pre-oxygenation and induction of anaesthesia upon duration of non-hypoxic apnoea. Anaesthesia 2004;59:243-247.

31. Coussa M, Proietti S, Schnyder P, et al: Prevention of atelectasis formation during the induction of general anesthesia in morbidly obese patients. Anesth Analg 2004;98:1491-1495.

32. Hedenstierna G, Rothen HU: Atelectasis formation during anesthesia: Causes and measures to prevent it. J Clin Monit Comput 2000;16:329-335.

33. Boyce JR, Ness T, Castroman P, Gleysteen JJ: A preliminary study of the optimal anesthesia positioning for the morbidly obese patient. Obes Surg 2003;13:4-9.

34. Casati A, Comotti L, Tommasino C, et al: Effects of pneumoperitoneum and reverse Trendelenburg position on cardiopulmonary function in morbidly obese patients receiving laparoscopic gastric banding. Eur J Anaesthesiol 2000;17:300-305.

35. Pelosi P, Croci M, Calappi E, et al: Prone positioning improves pulmonary function in obese patients during general anesthesia. Anesth Analg 1996;83:578-583.

36. Squadrone V, Coha M, Cerutti E, et al, for the Piedmont Intensive Care Units Network: Continuous positive airway pressure for treatment of postoperative hypoxemia: A randomized controlled trial. JAMA 2005;293:589-595.

37. Kindgen-Milles D, Muller E, Buhl R, et al: Nasal-continuous positive airway pressure reduces pulmonary morbidity and length of hospital stay following thoracoabdominal aortic surgery. Chest 2005;128:821-828.

38. Keenan SP, Powers C, McCormack DG, Block G: Noninvasive positive-pressure ventilation for postextubation respiratory distress: A randomized controlled trial. JAMA 2002;287:3238-3244.

39. Frey WC, Pilcher J: Obstructive sleep-related breathing disorders in patients evaluated for bariatric surgery. Obes Surg 2003;13:676-683.

40. O'Keeffe T, Patterson EJ: Evidence supporting routine polysomnography before bariatric surgery. Obes Surg 2004;14:23-26.

41. Guardiano SA, Scott JA, Ware JC, Schechner SA: The long-term results of gastric bypass on indexes of sleep apnea. Chest 2003;124:1615-1619.

42. Ezri T, Gewurtz G, Sessler DI, et al: Prediction of difficult laryngoscopy in obese patients by ultrasound quantification of anterior neck soft tissue. Anaesthesia 2003;58:1111-1114.

43. Hiremath AS, Hillman DR, James AL, et al: Relationship between difficult tracheal intubation and obstructive sleep apnoea. Br J Anaesth 1998;80:606-611.

44. Nowbar S, Burkart KM, Gonzales R, et al: Obesity-associated hypoventilation in hospitalized patients: Prevalence, effects, and outcome. Am J Med 2004;116:1-7.

45. Meoli AL, Rosen CL, Kristo D, et al: Upper airway management of the adult patient with obstructive sleep apnea in the perioperative period: Avoiding complications. Sleep 2003;26:1060-1065.

46. Practice guidelines for the perioperative management of patients with obstructive sleep apnea: A report by the American Society of Anesthesiologists Task Force on Perioperative Management of Patients with Obstructive Sleep Apnea. Anesthesiology 2006;104:1081-1093.

47. Cuthbertson D, Tilstone WJ: Metabolism during the postinjury period. Adv Clin Chem 1969;12:1-55.

48. Moore FD: Some observations on the metabolic requirement in surgical patients. Bull New Engl Med Cent 1949;11:193-201.

49. Moore FD: Common patterns of water and electrolyte change in injury, surgery and disease. N Engl J Med 1958;258:277-285.

50. Drucker WR, Chadwick CD, Gann DS: Transcapillary refill in hemorrhage and shock. Arch Surg 1981;116:1344-1353.

51. Marty AT, Zweifach BW: Splanchnic contribution to transcapillary refill after hemorrhagic shock. Ann Surg 1971;174:131-136.

52. Brandstrup B, Svensen C, Engquist A: Hemorrhage and operation cause a contraction of the extracellular space needing replacement: Evidence and implications? A systematic review. Surgery 2006;139: 419-432.

53. Practice guidelines for preoperative fasting and the use of pharmacologic agents to reduce the risk of pulmonary aspiration: Application to healthy patients undergoing elective procedures: A report by the American Society of Anesthesiologist Task Force on Preoperative Fasting. Anesthesiology 1999;90:896-905.

54. Yogendran S, Asokumar B, Cheng DC, Chung F: A prospective randomized double-blinded study of the effect of intravenous fluid therapy on adverse outcomes on outpatient surgery. Anesth Analg 1995;80:682-686.

55. Maharaj CH, Kallam SR, Malik A, et al: Preoperative intravenous fluid therapy decreases postoperative nausea and pain in high risk patients. Anesth Analg 2005;100:675-682.

56. Bennett J, McDonald T, Lieblich S, Piecuch J: Perioperative rehydration in ambulatory anesthesia for dentoalveolar surgery. Oral Surg Oral Med Oral Pathol Oral Radiol Endod 1999;88:279-284.

57. Magner JJ, McCaul C, Carton E, et al: Effect of intraoperative intravenous crystalloid infusion on postoperative nausea and vomiting after gynaecological laparoscopy: Comparison of 30 and 10 ml kg(-1). Br J Anaesth 2004;93:381-385.

58. Ali SZ, Taguchi A, Holtmann B, Kurz A: Effect of supplemental preoperative fluid on postoperative nausea and vomiting. Anaesthesia 2003;58:780-784.

59. McCaul C, Moran C, O'Cronin D, et al: Intravenous fluid loading with or without supplementary dextrose does not prevent nausea, vomiting and pain after laparoscopy. Can J Anaesth 2003;50:440-444.

60. Klein TF, Osmer C, Muller M, et al: The effect of a pre-operative infusion of Ringer's solution on splanchnic perfusion in patients undergoing coronary artery bypass grafting. Anaesthesia 2002;57: 756-760.

61. Wilkes NJ, Woolf R, Mutch M, et al: The effects of balanced versus saline-based hetastarch and crystalloid solutions on acid-base and electrolyte status and gastric mucosal perfusion in elderly surgical patients. Anesth Analg 2001;93:811-816.

62. Dillon J, Lynch LJ Jr, Myers R, Butcher HR Jr: The treatment of hemorrhagic shock. Surg Gynecol Obstet 1966;122:967-978.

63. Skillman JJ, Awwad HK, Moore FD: Plasma protein kinetics of the early transcapillary refill after hemorrhage in man. Surg Gynecol Obstet 1967;125:983-996.

64. Moss G: Fluid distribution in prevention of hypovolemic shock. Arch Surg 1969;98:281-286.

65. Holte K, Sharrock NE, Kehlet H: Pathophysiology and clinical implications of perioperative fluid excess. Br J Anaesth 2002;89: 622-632.

66. Funk W, Baldinger V: Microcirculatory perfusion during volume therapy: A comparative study using crystalloid or colloid in awake animals. Anesthesiology 1995;82:975-982.

67. Lang K, Boldt J, Suttner S, Haisch G: Colloids versus crystalloids and tissue oxygen tension in patients undergoing major abdominal surgery. Anesth Analg 2001;93:405-409.

68. Ernest D, Belzberg AS, Dodek PM: Distribution of normal saline and 5% albumin infusions in septic patients. Crit Care Med 1999;27: 46-50.

69. Scheingraber S, Rehm M, Sehmisch C, Finsterer U: Rapid saline infusion produces hyperchloremic acidosis in patients undergoing gynecologic surgery. Anesthesiology 1999;90:1265-1270.

70. Tournadre JP, Allaouchiche B, Malbert CH, Chassard D: Metabolic acidosis and respiratory acidosis impair gastro-pyloric motility in anesthetized pigs. Anesth Analg 2000;90:74-79.

71. O'Malley CM, Frumento RJ, Hardy MA, et al: A randomized, double-blind comparison of lactated Ringer's solution and 0.9% NaCl during renal transplantation. Anesth Analg 2005;100:1518-1524.

72. Hansen PB, Jensen BL, Skott O: Chloride regulates afferent arteriolar contraction in response to depolarization. Hypertension 1998;32: 1066-1070.

73. Wilcox CS: Regulation of renal blood flow by plasma chloride. J Clin Invest 1983;71:726-735.

74. Williams EL, Hildebrand KL, McCormick SA, Bedel MJ: The effect of intravenous lactated Ringer's solution versus 0.9% sodium chloride solution on serum osmolality in human volunteers. Anesth Analg 1999;88:999-1003.

75. Lobo DN, Bostock KA, Neal KR, et al: Effect of salt and water balance on recovery of gastrointestinal function after elective colonic resection: A randomised controlled trial. Lancet 2002;359: 1812-1818.

76. Merten GJ, Burgess WP, Gray LV, et al: Prevention of contrast-induced nephropathy with sodium bicarbonate: A randomized controlled trial. JAMA 2004;291:2328-2334.

77. Ruttmann TG, James MF, Finlayson J: Effects on coagulation of intravenous crystalloid or colloid in patients undergoing peripheral vascular surgery. Br J Anaesth 2002;89:226-230.

78. Boldt J: New light on intravascular volume replacement regimens: What did we learn from the past three years? Anesth Analg 2003;97:1595-1604.

79. Ng KF, Lam CC, Chan LC: In vivo effect of haemodilution with saline on coagulation: A randomized controlled trial. Br J Anaesth 2002; 88:475-480.

80. Ruttmann TG, Jamest MF, Lombard EH: Haemodilution-induced enhancement of coagulation is attenuated in vitro by restoring antithrombin III to pre-dilution concentrations. Anaesth Intensive Care 2001;29:489-493.

81. Healey MA, Davis RE, Liu FC, et al: Lactated Ringer's is superior to normal saline in a model of massive hemorrhage and resuscitation. J Trauma 1998;45:894-899.

82. Waters JH, Gottlieb A, Schoenwald P, et al: Normal saline versus lactated Ringer's solution for intraoperative fluid management in patients undergoing abdominal aortic aneurysm repair: An outcome study. Anesth Analg 2001;93:817-822.

83. Rhee P, Burris D, Kaufmann C, et al: Lactated Ringer's solution resuscitation causes neutrophil activation after hemorrhagic shock. J Trauma 1998;44:313-319.

84. Alam HB, Stanton K, Koustova E, et al: Effect of different resuscitation strategies on neutrophil activation in a swine model of hemorrhagic shock. Resuscitation 2004;60:91-99.

85. Deb S, Martin B, Sun L, et al: Resuscitation with lactated Ringer's solution in rats with hemorrhagic shock induces immediate apoptosis. J Trauma 1999;46:582-588.

86. Shoemaker WC, Montgomery ES, Kaplan E, Elwyn DH: Physiologic patterns in surviving and nonsurviving shock patients: Use of sequential cardiorespiratory variables in defining criteria for therapeutic goals and early warning of death. Arch Surg 1973;106: 630-636.

87. Moretti EW, Robertson KM, el Moalem H, Gan TJ: Intraoperative colloid administration reduces postoperative nausea and vomiting and improves postoperative outcomes compared with crystalloid administration. Anesth Analg 2003;96:611-617.

88. Mythen MG, Webb AR: Perioperative plasma volume expansion reduces the incidence of gut mucosal hypoperfusion during cardiac surgery. Arch Surg 1995;130:423-429.

89. Gan TJ, Soppitt A, Maroof M, et al: Goal-directed intraoperative fluid administration reduces length of hospital stay after major surgery. Anesthesiology 2002;97:820-826.

90. Venn R, Steele A, Richardson P, et al: Randomized controlled trial to investigate influence of the fluid challenge on duration of hospital stay and perioperative morbidity in patients with hip fractures. Br J Anaesth 2002;88:65-71.

91. Sinclair S, James S, Singer M: Intraoperative intravascular volume optimisation and length of hospital stay after repair of proximal femoral fracture: Randomised controlled trial. BMJ 1997;315: 909-912.

92. Wakeling HG, McFall MR, Jenkins CS, et al: Intraoperative oesophageal Doppler guided fluid management shortens postoperative hospital stay after major bowel surgery. Br J Anaesth 2005;95:634-642.

93. Noblett SE, Snowden CP, Shenton BK, Horgan AF: Randomized clinical trial assessing the effect of Doppler-optimized fluid management on outcome after elective colorectal resection. Br J Surg 2006;93: 1069-1076.

94. Shoemaker WC, Appel PL, Kram HB, et al: Prospective trial of supranormal values of survivors as therapeutic goals in high-risk surgical patients. Chest 1988;94:1176-1186.

95. Rivers E, Nguyen B, Havstad S, et al: Early goal-directed therapy in the treatment of severe sepsis and septic shock. N Engl J Med 2001;345:1368-1377.

96. Brandstrup B, Tonnesen H, Beier-Holgersen R, et al: Effects of intravenous fluid restriction on postoperative complications: Comparison of two perioperative fluid regimens—A randomized assessor-blinded multicenter trial. Ann Surg 2003;238:641-648.

97. Nisanevich V, Felsenstein I, Almogy G, et al: Effect of intraoperative fluid management on outcome after intraabdominal surgery. Anesthesiology 2005;103:25-32.

98. Tambyraja AL, Sengupta F, MacGregor AB, et al: Patterns and clinical outcomes associated with routine intravenous sodium and fluid administration after colorectal resection. World J Surg 2004;28:1046-1051.

99. Holte K, Hahn RG, Ravn L, et al: Influence of "liberal" versus "restrictive" intraoperative fluid administration on elimination of a postoperative fluid load. Anesthesiology 2007;106:75-79.

100. Solus-Biguenet H, Fleyfel M, Tavernier B, et al: Non-invasive prediction of fluid responsiveness during major hepatic surgery. Br J Anaesth 2006;97:808-816.

101. Hernandez G, Velasco N, Wainstein C, et al: Gut mucosal atrophy after a short enteral fasting period in critically ill patients. J Crit Care 1999;14:73-77.

102. McClave SA, Mitoraj TE, Thielmeier KA, Greenburg RA: Differentiating subtypes (hypoalbuminemic vs marasmic) of protein-calorie malnutrition: Incidence and clinical significance in a university hospital setting. JPEN J Parenter Enteral Nutr 1992;16:337-342.

103. Starker PM, LaSala PA, Askanazi J, et al: The influence of preoperative total parenteral nutrition upon morbidity and mortality. Surg Gynecol Obstet 1986;162:569-574.

104. Streat SJ, Beddoe AH, Hill GL: Aggressive nutritional support does not prevent protein loss despite fat gain in septic intensive care patients. J Trauma 1987;27.

105. Klein CJ, Stanek GS, Wiles CE III: Overfeeding macronutrients to critically ill adults: Metabolic complications. J Am Diet Assoc 1998;98:795-806.

106. Dickerson RN, Boschert KJ, Kudsk KA, Brown RO: Hypocaloric enteral tube feeding in critically ill obese patients. Nutrition 2002;18:241-246.

107. Ochoa JB, Caba D: Advances in surgical nutrition. Surg Clin North Am 2006;86:1483-1493.

108. Muller JM, Brenner U, Dienst C, Pichlmaier H: Preoperative parenteral feeding in patients with gastrointestinal carcinoma. Lancet 1982;1:68-71.

109. Perioperative total parenteral nutrition in surgical patients. The Veterans Affairs Total Parenteral Nutrition Cooperative Study Group. N Engl J Med 1991;325:525-532.

110. Heyland DK, Montalvo M, MacDonald S, et al: Total parenteral nutrition in the surgical patient: A meta-analysis. Can J Surg 2001;44:102-111.

111. Bozzetti F, Braga M, Gianotti L, et al: Postoperative enteral versus parenteral nutrition in malnourished patients with gastrointestinal cancer: A randomised multicentre trial. Lancet 2001;358:1487-1492.

112. Moore FA, Moore EE, Jones TN, et al: TEN versus TPN following major abdominal trauma: Reduced septic morbidity. J Trauma 1989;29:916-922.

113. Holte K, Kehlet H: Postoperative ileus: A preventable event. Br J Surg 2000;87:1480-1493.

114. Catchpole BN: Smooth muscle and the surgeon. Aust N Z J Surg 1989;59:199-208.

115. Lewis SJ, Egger M, Sylvester PA, Thomas S: Early enteral feeding versus "nil by mouth" after gastrointestinal surgery: Systematic review and meta-analysis of controlled trials. BMJ 2001;323:773-776.

116. Schroeder D, Gillanders L, Mahr K, Hill GL: Effects of immediate postoperative enteral nutrition on body composition, muscle function, and wound healing. JPEN J Parenter Enteral Nutr 1991;15:376-383.

117. Beier-Holgersen R, Boesby S: Influence of postoperative enteral nutrition on postsurgical infections. Gut 1996;39:833-835.

118. Rayes N, Hansen S, Seehofer D, et al: Early enteral supply of fiber and Lactobacilli versus conventional nutrition: A controlled trial in patients with major abdominal surgery. Nutrition 2002;18:609-615.

119. Singh G, Ram RP, Khanna SK: Early postoperative enteral feeding in patients with nontraumatic intestinal perforation and peritonitis. J Am Coll Surg 1998;187:142-146.

120. Harrison LE, Hochwald SN, Heslin MJ, et al: Early postoperative enteral nutrition improves peripheral protein kinetics in upper gastrointestinal cancer patients undergoing complete resection: A randomized trial. JPEN J Parenter Enteral Nutr 1997;21:202-207.

121. Carr CS, Ling KD, Boulos P, Singer M: Randomised trial of safety and efficacy of immediate postoperative enteral feeding in patients undergoing gastrointestinal resection. BMJ 1996;312:869-871.

122. Hoover HC Jr, Ryan JA, Anderson EJ, Fischer JE: Nutritional benefits of immediate postoperative jejunal feeding of an elemental diet. Am J Surg 1980;139:153-159.

123. Seidmon EJ, Pizzimenti KV, Blumenstock FA, et al: Immediate postoperative feeding in urological surgery. J Urol 1984;131:1113-1118.

124. Ryan JA Jr, Page CP, Babcock L: Early postoperative jejunal feeding of elemental diet in gastrointestinal surgery. Am Surg 1981;47:393-403.

125. Aiko S, Yoshizumi Y, Sugiura Y, et al: Beneficial effects of immediate enteral nutrition after esophageal cancer surgery. Surg Today 2001;31:971-978.

126. Schilder JM, Hurteau JA, Look KY, et al: A prospective controlled trial of early postoperative oral intake following major abdominal gynecologic surgery. Gynecol Oncol 1997;67:235-240.

127. Steed HL, Capstick V, Flood C, et al: A randomized controlled trial of early versus "traditional" postoperative oral intake after major abdominal gynecologic surgery. Am J Obstet Gynecol 2002;186:861-865.

128. Hedberg AM, Lairson DR, Aday LA, et al: Economic implications of an early postoperative enteral feeding protocol. J Am Diet Assoc 1999;99:802-807.

129. Sagar S, Harland P, Shields R: Early postoperative feeding with elemental diet. Br Med J 1979;1:293-295.

130. Ortiz H, Armendariz P, Yarnoz C: Early postoperative feeding after elective colorectal surgery is not a benefit unique to laparoscopy-assisted procedures. Int J Colorectal Dis 1996;11:246-249.

131. Hartsell PA, Frazee RC, Harrison JB, Smith RW: Early postoperative feeding after elective colorectal surgery. Arch Surg 1997;132:518-520.

132. Binderow SR, Cohen SM, Wexner SD, Nogueras JJ: Must early postoperative oral intake be limited to laparoscopy? Dis Colon Rectum 1994;37:584-589.

133. Sand J, Luostarinen M, Matikainen M: Enteral or parenteral feeding after total gastrectomy: Prospective randomised pilot study. Eur J Surg 1997;163:761-766.

134. Braga M, Gianotti L, Gentilini O, et al: Early postoperative enteral nutrition improves gut oxygenation and reduces costs compared with total parenteral nutrition. Crit Care Med 2001;29:242-248.

135. MacMillan SL, Kammerer-Doak D, Rogers RG, Parker KM: Early feeding and the incidence of gastrointestinal symptoms after major gynecologic surgery. Obstet Gynecol 2000;96:604-608.

136. Watters JM, Kirkpatrick SM, Norris SB, et al: Immediate postoperative enteral feeding results in impaired respiratory mechanics and decreased mobility. Ann Surg 1997;226:369-377.

137. Wyncoll D, Beale R: Immunologically enhanced enteral nutrition: Current status. Curr Opin Crit Care 2001;7:128-132.

138. Braga M, Gianotti L, Nespoli L, et al: Nutritional approach in malnourished surgical patients: A prospective randomized study. Arch Surg 2002;137:174-180.

139. Senkal M, Zumtobel V, Bauer KH, et al: Outcome and cost-effectiveness of perioperative enteral immunonutrition in patients undergoing elective upper gastrointestinal tract surgery: A prospective randomized study. Arch Surg 1999;134:1309-1316.

140. Braga M, Gianotti L, Radaelli G, et al: Perioperative immunonutrition in patients undergoing cancer surgery: Results of a randomized double-blind phase 3 trial. Arch Surg 1999;134:428-433.

141. Senkal M, Mumme A, Eickhoff U, et al: Early postoperative enteral immunonutrition: Clinical outcome and cost-comparison analysis in surgical patients. Crit Care Med 1997;25:1489-1496.

142. Gianotti L, Braga M, Nespoli L, et al: A randomized controlled trial of preoperative oral supplementation with a specialized diet in patients with gastrointestinal cancer. Gastroenterology 2002;122: 1763-1770.

143. Di Carlo V, Gianotti L, Balzano G, et al: Complications of pancreatic surgery and the role of perioperative nutrition. Dig Surg 1999;16: 320-326.

144. Gianotti L, Braga M, Vignali A, et al: Effect of route of delivery and formulation of postoperative nutritional support in patients undergoing major operations for malignant neoplasms. Arch Surg 1997;132: 1222-1229.

145. Daly JM, Weintraub FN, Shou J, et al: Enteral nutrition during multimodality therapy in upper gastrointestinal cancer patients. Ann Surg 1995;221:327-338.

146. Kemen M, Senkal M, Homann HH, et al: Early postoperative enteral nutrition with arginine-omega-3 fatty acids and ribonucleic acid-supplemented diet versus placebo in cancer patients: An immunologic evaluation of impact. Crit Care Med 1995;23:652-659.

147. Heslin MJ, Latkany L, Leung D, et al: A prospective, randomized trial of early enteral feeding after resection of upper gastrointestinal malignancy. Ann Surg 1997;226:567-577.

148. Bozzetti F, Gavazzi C, Miceli R, et al: Perioperative total parenteral nutrition in malnourished, gastrointestinal cancer patients: A randomized, clinical trial. JPEN J Parenter Enteral Nutr 2000;24:7-14.

149. Starker PM, LaSala PA, Forse RA, et al: Response to total parenteral nutrition in the extremely malnourished patient. JPEN J Parenter Enteral Nutr 1985;9:300-302.

150. Soliani P, Dell'Abate P, Del Rio P, et al: [Early enteral nutrition in patients treated with major surgery of the abdomen and the pelvis.] Chir Ital 2001;53:619-632.

151. Hubmayr RD, Burchardi H, Elliot M, et al: Statement of the 4th International Consensus Conference in Critical Care on ICU-Acquired Pneumonia—Chicago, Illinois, May 2002. Intensive Care Med 2002;28:1521-1536.

152. Stewart BT, Woods RJ, Collopy BT, et al: Early feeding after elective open colorectal resections: A prospective randomized trial. Aust N Z J Surg 1998;68:125-128.

153. Ortiz H, Armendariz P, Yarnoz C: Is early postoperative feeding feasible in elective colon and rectal surgery? Int J Colorectal Dis 1996;11:119-121.

154. Liu LL, Wiener-Kronish JP: Perioperative anesthesia issues in the elderly. Crit Care Clin 2003;19:641-656.

155. Coffey CE, Saxton JA, Ratcliff G, et al: Relation of education to brain size in normal aging: Implications for the reserve hypothesis. Neurology 1999;53:189-196.

156. Oskvig RM: Special problems in the elderly. Chest 1999;115: 158S-164.

157. Morrison JH, Hof PR: Life and death of neurons in the aging brain. Science 1997;278:412-419.

158. Cook DJ, Rooke GA: Priorities in perioperative geriatrics. Anesth Analg 2003;96:1823-1836.

159. Vuyk J: Pharmacodynamics in the elderly. Best Pract Res Clin Anaesthesiol 2003;17:207-218.

160. Muravchick S: The effects of aging on anesthetic pharmacology. Acta Anaesthesiol Belg 1998;49:79-84.

161. Sharrock NE: Epidural anesthetic dose responses in patients 20 to 80 years old. Anesthesiology 1978;49:425-428.

162. American Psychiatric Association: Diagnostic and Statistical Manual, ed 4. Washington, DC, APA Press, 1994.

163. Flacker JM, Marcantonio ER: Delirium in the elderly: Optimal management. Drugs Aging 1998;13:119-130.

164. Edlund A, Lundstrom M, Lundstrom G, et al: Clinical profile of delirium in patients treated for femoral neck fractures. Dement Geriatr Cogn Disord 1999;10:325-329.

165. Parikh SS, Chung F: Postoperative delirium in the elderly. Anesth Analg 1995;80:1223-1232.

166. Liptzin B, Levkoff SE: An empirical study of delirium subtypes. Br J Psychiatry 1992;161:843-845.

167. Meagher DJ: Delirium: Optimising management. BMJ 2001;322: 144-149.

168. Inouye SK, Charpentier PA: Precipitating factors for delirium in hospitalized elderly persons: Predictive model and interrelationship with baseline vulnerability. JAMA 1996;275:852-857.

169. Francis J, Martin D, Kapoor WN: A prospective study of delirium in hospitalized elderly. JAMA 1990;263:1097-1101.

170. Bohner H, Hummel TC, Habel U, et al: Predicting delirium after vascular surgery: A model based on pre- and intraoperative data. Ann Surg 2003;238:149-156.

171. Bohner H, Schneider F, Stierstorfer A, et al: [Delirium after vascular surgery interventions. Intermediate-term results of a prospective study.] Chirurg 2000;71:215-221.

172. Morrison RS, Magaziner J, Gilbert M, et al: Relationship between pain and opioid analgesics on the development of delirium following hip fracture. J Gerontol A Biol Sci Med Sci 2003;58:76-81.

173. Rogers MP, Liang MH, Daltroy LH, et al: Delirium after elective orthopedic surgery: Risk factors and natural history. Int J Psychiatry Med 1989;19:109-121.

174. Milstein A, Pollack A, Kleinman G, Barak Y: Confusion/delirium following cataract surgery: An incidence study of 1-year duration. Int Psychogeriatr 2002;14:301-306.

175. Litaker D, Locala J, Franco K, et al: Preoperative risk factors for postoperative delirium. Gen Hosp Psychiatry 2001;23:84-89.

176. Seymour DG, Vaz FG: A prospective study of elderly general surgical patients: II. Post-operative complications. Age Ageing 1989;18: 316-326.

177. Kaneko T, Takahashi S, Naka T, et al: Postoperative delirium following gastrointestinal surgery in elderly patients. Surg Today 1997;27: 107-111.

178. Dai YT, Lou MF, Yip PK, Huang GS: Risk factors and incidence of postoperative delirium in elderly Chinese patients. Gerontology 2000;46:28-35.

179. Duppils GS, Wikblad K: Acute confusional states in patients undergoing hip surgery: A prospective observation study. Gerontology 2000;46:36-43.

180. Clayer M, Bruckner J: Occult hypoxia after femoral neck fracture and elective hip surgery. Clin Orthop Relat Res 2000;270:265-271.

181. Schneider F, Bohner H, Habel U, et al: Risk factors for postoperative delirium in vascular surgery. Gen Hosp Psychiatry 2002;24:28-34.

182. Sasajima Y, Sasajima T, Uchida H, et al: Postoperative delirium in patients with chronic lower limb ischaemia: What are the specific markers? Eur J Vasc Endovasc Surg 2000;20:132-137.

183. Dyer CB, Ashton CM, Teasdale TA: Postoperative delirium: A review of 80 primary data-collection studies. Arch Intern Med 1995;155: 461-465.

184. Marcantonio ER, Goldman L, Mangione CM, et al: A clinical prediction rule for delirium after elective noncardiac surgery. JAMA 1994;271:134-139.

185. Aldemir M, Ozen S, Kara IH, et al: Predisposing factors for delirium in the surgical intensive care unit. Crit Care 2001;5:265-270.

186. Lynch EP, Lazor MA, Gellis JE, et al: The impact of postoperative pain on the development of postoperative delirium. Anesth Analg 1998;86:781-785.

187. Adunsky A, Levy R, Heim M, et al: The unfavorable nature of preoperative delirium in elderly hip fractured patients. Arch Gerontol Geriatr 2003;36:67-74.

188. Williams-Russo P, Urquhart BL, Sharrock NE, Charlson ME: Postoperative delirium: Predictors and prognosis in elderly orthopedic patients. J Am Geriatr Soc 1992;40:759-767.

189. Diaz V, Rodriguez J, Barrientos P, et al: [Use of procholinergics in the prevention of postoperative delirium in hip fracture surgery in the elderly: A randomized controlled trial.] Rev Neurol 2001;33: 716-719.

190. Edlund A, Lundstrom M, Brannstrom B, et al: Delirium before and after operation for femoral neck fracture. J Am Geriatr Soc 2001;49:1335-1340.

191. Rudberg MA, Pompei P, Foreman MD, et al: The natural history of delirium in older hospitalized patients: A syndrome of heterogeneity. Age Ageing 1997;26:169-174.

192. American Psychiatric Association: Practice guideline for the treatment of patients with delirium. Am J Psychiatry 1999;156:1-20.

193. Greene LT: Physostigmine treatment of anticholinergic-drug depression in postoperative patients. Anesth Analg 1971;50:222-226.

194. Trzepacz PT: Delirium: Advances in diagnosis, pathophysiology, and treatment. Psychiatr Clin North Am 1996;19:429-448.

195. Bayindir O, Akpinar B, Can E, et al: The use of the 5-HT3-receptor antagonist ondansetron for the treatment of postcardiotomy delirium. J Cardiothorac Vasc Anesth 2000;14:288-292.

196. Palmer JL: Postoperative delirium indicating an adverse drug interaction involving the selective serotonin reuptake inhibitor, paroxetine? J Psychopharmacol 2000;14:186-188.

197. Stanford BJ, Stanford SC: Postoperative delirium indicating an adverse drug interaction involving the selective serotonin reuptake inhibitor, paroxetine? J Psychopharmacol 1999;13:313-317.

198. Inouye SK, Schlesinger MJ, Lydon TJ: Delirium: A symptom of how hospital care is failing older persons and a window to improve quality of hospital care. Am J Med 1999;106:565-573.

199. Tune LE, Damlouji NF, Holland A, et al: Association of postoperative delirium with raised serum levels of anticholinergic drugs. Lancet 1981;2:651-653.

200. George J, Bleasdale S, Singleton SJ: Causes and prognosis of delirium in elderly patients admitted to a district general hospital. Age Ageing 1997;26:423-427.

201. Cole MG, Primeau FJ, Elie LM: Delirium: Prevention, treatment, and outcome studies. J Geriatr Psychiatry Neurol 1998;11:126-137.

202. Kesler SR, Adams HF, Blasey CM, Bigler ED: Premorbid intellectual functioning, education, and brain size in traumatic brain injury: An investigation of the cognitive reserve hypothesis. Appl Neuropsychol 2003;10:153-162.

203. Kamitani K, Higuchi A, Asahi T, Yoshida H: [Postoperative delirium after general anesthesia vs. spinal anesthesia in geriatric patients.] Masui 2003;52:972-975.

204. Shigeta H, Yasui A, Nimura Y, et al: Postoperative delirium and melatonin levels in elderly patients. Am J Surg 2001;182:449-454.

205. Knill RL, Moote CA, Skinner MI, Rose EA: Anesthesia with abdominal surgery leads to intense REM sleep during the first postoperative week. Anesthesiology 1990;73:52-61.

206. Inouye SK, Bogardus ST Jr, Charpentier PA, et al: A multicomponent intervention to prevent delirium in hospitalized older patients. N Engl J Med 1999;340:669-676.

207. Naughton BJ, Moran MB, Kadah H, et al: Delirium and other cognitive impairment in older adults in an emergency department. Ann Emerg Med 1995;25:751-755.

208. Lewis LM, Miller DK, Morley JE, et al: Unrecognized delirium in ED geriatric patients. Am J Emerg Med 1995;13:142-145.

209. Gustafson Y, Brannstrom B, Norberg A, et al: Underdiagnosis and poor documentation of acute confusional states in elderly hip fracture patients. J Am Geriatr Soc 1991;39:760-765.

210. Milisen K, Foreman MD, Wouters B, et al: Documentation of delirium in elderly patients with hip fracture. J Gerontol Nurs 2002;28:23-29.

211. Inouye SK, van Dyck CH, Alessi CA, et al: Clarifying confusion: The confusion assessment method—A new method for detection of delirium. Ann Intern Med 1990;113:941-948.

212. Ely EW, Margolin R, Francis J, et al: Evaluation of delirium in critically ill patients: validation of the Confusion Assessment Method for the Intensive Care Unit (CAM-ICU). Crit Care Med 2001;29:1370-1379.

213. Lundstrom M, Edlund A, Bucht G, et al: Dementia after delirium in patients with femoral neck fractures. J Am Geriatr Soc 2003;51:1002-1006.

214. Marcantonio ER, Flacker JM, Wright RJ, Resnick NM: Reducing delirium after hip fracture: A randomized trial. J Am Geriatr Soc 2001;49:516-522.

215. Milisen K, Foreman MD, Abraham IL, et al: A nurse-led interdisciplinary intervention program for delirium in elderly hip-fracture patients. J Am Geriatr Soc 2001;49:523-532.

216. Lacasse H, Perreault MM, Williamson DR: Systematic review of antipsychotics for the treatment of hospital-associated delirium in medically or surgically ill patients. Ann Pharmacother 2006;40:1966-1973.

217. Gallinat J, Moller HJ, Hegerl U: [Piracetam in anesthesia for prevention of postoperative delirium.] Anasthesiol Intensivmed Notfallmed Schmerzther 1999;34:520-527.

218. Horikawa N, Yamazaki T, Miyamoto K, et al: Treatment for delirium with risperidone: Results of a prospective open trial with 10 patients. Gen Hosp Psychiatry 2003;25:289-292.

219. Aizawa K, Kanai T, Saikawa Y, et al: A novel approach to the prevention of postoperative delirium in the elderly after gastrointestinal surgery. Surg Today 2002;32:310-314.

220. Hanania M, Kitain E: Melatonin for treatment and prevention of postoperative delirium. Anesth Analg 2002;94:338-339.

221. Kehlet H, Wilmore DW: Multimodal strategies to improve surgical outcome. Am J Surg 2002;183:630-641.

222. Basse L, Raskov HH, Hjort JD, et al: Accelerated postoperative recovery programme after colonic resection improves physical performance, pulmonary function and body composition. Br J Surg 2002;89:446-453.

223. Burke JP: Infection control: A problem for patient safety. N Engl J Med 2003;348:651-656.

224. Bratzler DW, Houck PM, Richards C, et al: Use of antimicrobial prophylaxis for major surgery: Baseline results from the National Surgical Infection Prevention Project. Arch Surg 2005;140:174-182.

225. Kirkland KB, Briggs JP, Trivette SL, et al: The impact of surgical-site infections in the 1990s: Attributable mortality, excess length of hospitalization, and extra costs. Infect Control Hosp Epidemiol 1999;20:725-730.

226. National Nosocomial Infections Surveillance (NNIS) System Report: Data summary from January 1992-June 2001, issued August 2001. Am J Infect Control 2001;29:404-421.

227. Emori TG, Gaynes RP: An overview of nosocomial infections, including the role of the microbiology laboratory. Clin Microbiol Rev 1993;6:428-442.

228. Classen DC, Evans RS, Pestotnik SL, et al: The timing of prophylactic administration of antibiotics and the risk of surgical-wound infection. N Engl J Med 1992;326:281-286.

229. Mangram AJ, Horan TC, Pearson ML, et al: Guideline for prevention of surgical site infection, 1999. Hospital Infection Control Practices Advisory Committee. Infect Control Hosp Epidemiol 1999;20:250-278.

230. Silver A, Eichorn A, Kral J, et al: Timeliness and use of antibiotic prophylaxis in selected inpatient surgical procedures. The Antibiotic Prophylaxis Study Group. Am J Surg 1996;171:548-552.

231. Morris AM, Jobe BA, Stoney M, et al: *Clostridium difficile* colitis: An increasingly aggressive iatrogenic disease? Arch Surg 2002;137:1096-1100.

232. Gladden LB: Lactate metabolism: A new paradigm for the third millennium. J Physiol Online 2004;558:5-30.

233. Lang CH, Obih JC, Bagby GJ, et al: Increased glucose uptake by intestinal mucosa and muscularis in hypermetabolic sepsis. Am J Physiol 1991;261:G287-294.

234. Langouche L, Van den Berghe G: Glucose metabolism and insulin therapy. Crit Care Clin 2006;22:119-129, vii.

235. Gropper MA: Evidence-based management of critically ill patients: Analysis and implementation. Anesth Analg 2004;99:566-572.

236. Guha M, Bai W, Nadler JL, Natarajan R: Molecular mechanisms of tumor necrosis factor alpha gene expression in monocytic cells via hyperglycemia-induced oxidant stress-dependent and -independent pathways. J Biol Chem 2000;275:17728-17739.

237. Sampson MJ, Davies IR, Brown JC, et al: Monocyte and neutrophil adhesion molecule expression during acute hyperglycemia and after antioxidant treatment in type 2 diabetes and control patients. Arterioscler Thromb Vasc Biol 2002;22:1187-1193.

238. Montori VM, Bistrian BR, McMahon MM: Hyperglycemia in acutely ill patients. JAMA 2002;288:2167-2169.

239. Lin LH, Hopf HW: Paradigm of the injury-repair continuum during critical illness. Crit Care Med 2003;31:S493-495.

240. Garg R, Chaudhuri A, Munschauer F, Dandona P: Hyperglycemia, insulin, and acute ischemic stroke: A mechanistic justification for a trial of insulin infusion therapy. Stroke 2006;37:267-273.

241. Wagner KR, Kleinholz M, de Courten-Myers GM, Myers RE: Hyperglycemic versus normoglycemic stroke: Topography of brain

metabolites, intracellular pH, and infarct size. J Cereb Blood Flow Metab 1992;12:213-222.

242. Van den Berghe G, Wouters P, Weekers F, et al: Intensive insulin therapy in the surgical intensive care unit. N Engl J Med 2001;345: 1359-1367.

243. Malmberg K, Ryden L, Efendic S, et al: Randomized trial of insulin-glucose infusion followed by subcutaneous insulin treatment in diabetic patients with acute myocardial infarction (DIGAMI study): Effects on mortality at 1 year. J Am Coll Cardiol 1995;26:57-65.

244. Jeschke MG, Einspanier R, Klein D, Jauch KW: Insulin attenuates the systemic inflammatory response to thermal trauma. Mol Med 2002;8:443-450.

245. Jonassen AK, Sack MN, Mjos OD, Yellon DM: Myocardial protection by insulin at reperfusion requires early administration and is mediated via Akt and p70s6 kinase cell-survival signaling. Circ Res 2001;89:1191-1198.

246. Chaudhuri A, Janicke D, Wilson MF, et al: Anti-inflammatory and profibrinolytic effect of insulin in acute ST-segment-elevation myocardial infarction. Circulation 2004;109:849-854.

247. Zerr KJ, Furnary AP, Grunkemeier GL, et al: Glucose control lowers the risk of wound infection in diabetics after open heart operations. Ann Thorac Surg 1997;63:356-361.

248. Furnary AP, Zerr KJ, Grunkemeier GL, Starr A: Continuous intravenous insulin infusion reduces the incidence of deep sternal wound infection in diabetic patients after cardiac surgical procedures. Ann Thorac Surg 1999;67:352-360.

249. Furnary AP, Gao G, Grunkemeier GL, et al: Continuous insulin infusion reduces mortality in patients with diabetes undergoing coronary artery bypass grafting. J Thorac Cardiovasc Surg 2003;125: 1007-1021.

250. Finney SJ, Zekveld C, Elia A, Evans TW: Glucose control and mortality in critically ill patients. JAMA 2003;290:2041-2047.

251. Van den Berghe G, Wouters PJ, Bouillon R, et al: Outcome benefit of intensive insulin therapy in the critically ill: Insulin dose versus glycemic control. Crit Care Med 2003;31:359-366.

252. Van den Berghe G: How does blood glucose control with insulin save lives in intensive care? J Clin Invest 2004;114:1187-1195.

253. Krinsley JS: Effect of an intensive glucose management protocol on the mortality of critically ill adult patients. Mayo Clin Proc 2004;79:992-1000.

254. Van den Berghe G, Wilmer A, Hermans G, et al: Intensive insulin therapy in the medical ICU. N Engl J Med 2006;354:449-461.

255. Vespa P, Boonyaputthikul R, McArthur DL, et al: Intensive insulin therapy reduces microdialysis glucose values without altering glucose utilization or improving the lactate/pyruvate ratio after traumatic brain injury. Crit Care Med 2006;34:850-856.

256. Hopf HW, Hunt TK, West JM, et al: Wound tissue oxygen tension predicts the risk of wound infection in surgical patients. Arch Surg 1997;132:997-1004.

257. Allen DB, Maguire JJ, Mahdavian M, et al: Wound hypoxia and acidosis limit neutrophil bacterial killing mechanisms. Arch Surg 1997;132:991-996.

258. Mauermann WJ, Nemergut EC: The anesthesiologist's role in the prevention of surgical site infections. Anesthesiology 2006;105: 413-421.

259. Kurz A, Sessler DI, Lenhardt R: Perioperative normothermia to reduce the incidence of surgical-wound infection and shorten hospitalization. The Study of Wound Infection and Temperature Group. N Engl J Med 1996;334:1209-1215.

260. Flores-Maldonado A, Medina-Escobedo CE, Rios-Rodriguez HM, Fernandez-Dominguez R: Mild perioperative hypothermia and the risk of wound infection. Arch Med Res 2001;32:227-231.

261. Walz JM, Paterson CA, Seligowski JM, Heard SO: Surgical site infection following bowel surgery: A retrospective analysis of 1446 patients. Arch Surg 2006;141:1014-1018.

262. Melling AC, Ali B, Scott EM, Leaper DJ: Effects of preoperative warming on the incidence of wound infection after clean surgery: A randomised controlled trial. Lancet 2001;358:876-880.

263. Knighton DR, Halliday B, Hunt TK: Oxygen as an antibiotic: A comparison of the effects of inspired oxygen concentration and antibiotic administration on in vivo bacterial clearance. Arch Surg 1986;121:191-195.

264. Gottrup F: Oxygen in wound healing and infection. World J Surg 2004;28:312-315.

265. Greif R, Akca O, Horn EP, et al: Supplemental perioperative oxygen to reduce the incidence of surgical-wound infection. Outcomes Research Group. N Engl J Med 2000;342:161-167.

266. Pryor KO, Fahey TJ III, Lien CA, Goldstein PA: Surgical site infection and the routine use of perioperative hyperoxia in a general surgical population: A randomized controlled trial. JAMA 2004;291:79-87.

267. Arkilic CF, Taguchi A, Sharma N, et al: Supplemental perioperative fluid administration increases tissue oxygen pressure. Surgery 2003;133:49-55.

268. Kabon B, Akca O, Taguchi A, et al: Supplemental intravenous crystalloid administration does not reduce the risk of surgical wound infection. Anesth Analg 2005;101:1546-1553.

269. Malone PC, Agutter PS: The aetiology of deep venous thrombosis. QJM 2006;99:581-593.

270. Schietroma M, Carlei F, Mownah A, et al: Changes in the blood coagulation, fibrinolysis, and cytokine profile during laparoscopic and open cholecystectomy. Surg Endosc 2004;18:1090-1096.

271. Engelman DT, Gabram SG, Allen L, et al: Hypercoagulability following multiple trauma. World J Surg 1996;20:5-10.

272. Sevitt S: The structure and growth of valve-pocket thrombi in femoral veins. J Clin Pathol 1974;27:517-528.

273. White RH, Zhou H, Romano PS: Incidence of symptomatic venous thromboembolism after different elective or urgent surgical procedures. Thromb Haemost 2003;90:446-455.

274. Huisman MV, Buller HR, ten Cate JW, Vreeken J: Serial impedance plethysmography for suspected deep venous thrombosis in outpatients. The Amsterdam General Practitioner Study. N Engl J Med 1986;314:823-828.

275. Lensing AW, Prandoni P, Brandjes D, et al: Detection of deep-vein thrombosis by real-time B-mode ultrasonography. N Engl J Med 1989;320:342-345.

276. Wells PS, Anderson DR, Bormanis J, et al: Value of assessment of pretest probability of deep-vein thrombosis in clinical management. Lancet 1997;350:1795-1798.

277. Uhland H, Goldburg LM: Pulmonary embolism: A commonly missed clinical entity. Dis Chest 1964;45:533-536.

278. Dalen JE: Pulmonary embolism: What have we learned since Virchow? Natural history, pathophysiology, and diagnosis. Chest 2002;122:1440-1456.

279. Value of the ventilation/perfusion scan in acute pulmonary embolism: Results of the prospective investigation of pulmonary embolism diagnosis (PIOPED). The PIOPED Investigators. JAMA 1990;263: 2753-2759.

280. Mullins MD, Becker DM, Hagspiel KD, Philbrick JT: The role of spiral volumetric computed tomography in the diagnosis of pulmonary embolism. Arch Intern Med 2000;160:293-298.

281. Coche E, Verschuren F, Keyeux A, et al: Diagnosis of acute pulmonary embolism in outpatients: Comparison of thin-collimation multidetector row spiral CT and planar ventilation-perfusion scintigraphy. Radiology 2003;229:757-765.

282. Winer-Muram HT, Rydberg J, Johnson MS, et al: Suspected acute pulmonary embolism: Evaluation with multi-detector row CT versus digital subtraction pulmonary arteriography. Radiology 2004;233: 806-815.

283. Stein PD, Fowler SE, Goodman LR, Gottschalk A, et al, PIOPED II Investigators: Multidetector computed tomography for acute pulmonary embolism. N Engl J Med 2006;354:2317-2327.

284. Perrier A, Roy PM, Sanchez O, et al: Multidetector-row computed tomography in suspected pulmonary embolism. N Engl J Med 2005;352:1760-1768.

285. Writing Group for the Christopher Study Investigators: Effectiveness of managing suspected pulmonary embolism using an algorithm combining clinical probability, D-dimer testing, and computed tomography. JAMA 2006;295:172-179.

286. Stein PD, Woodard PK, Weg JG, et al: Diagnostic pathways in acute pulmonary embolism: Recommendations of the PIOPED II Investigators. Radiology 2007;242:15-21.

287. Hills NH, Pflug JJ, Jeyasingh K, et al: Prevention of deep vein thrombosis by intermittent pneumatic compression of calf. Br Med J 1972;1:131-135.

288. Hull RD, Raskob GE, Gent M, et al: Effectiveness of intermittent pneumatic leg compression for preventing deep vein thrombosis after total hip replacement. JAMA 1990;263:2313-2317.

289. Allan A, Williams JT, Bolton JP, Le Quesne LP: The use of graduated compression stockings in the prevention of postoperative deep vein thrombosis. Br J Surg 1983;70:172-174.

290. Wells PS, Lensing AW, Hirsh J: Graduated compression stockings in the prevention of postoperative venous thromboembolism: A meta-analysis. Arch Intern Med 1994;154:67-72.

291. Turpie AG, Hirsh J, Gent M, et al: Prevention of deep vein thrombosis in potential neurosurgical patients: A randomized trial comparing graduated compression stockings alone or graduated compression stockings plus intermittent pneumatic compression with control. Arch Intern Med 1989;149:679-681.

292. Kakkar VV, Corrigan T, Spindler J, et al: Efficacy of low doses of heparin in prevention of deep-vein thrombosis after major surgery: A double-blind, randomised trial. Lancet 1972;2:101-106.

293. Nicolaides AN, Dupont PA, Desai S, et al: Small doses of subcutaneous sodium heparin in preventing deep venous thrombosis after major surgery. Lancet 1972;2:890-893.

294. Turpie AG, Levine MN, Hirsh J, et al: A randomized controlled trial of a low-molecular-weight heparin (enoxaparin) to prevent deep-vein thrombosis in patients undergoing elective hip surgery. N Engl J Med 1986;315:925-929.

295. Wille-Jorgensen P, Rasmussen MS, Andersen BR, Borly L: Heparins and mechanical methods for thromboprophylaxis in colorectal surgery. Cochrane Database Syst Rev 2003;CD001217.

296. Geerts WH, Pineo GF, Heit JA, et al: Prevention of venous thromboembolism: The seventh ACCP Conference on Antithrombotic and Thrombolytic Therapy. Chest 2004;126:338S-400.

297. Barritt DW, Jordan SC: Anticoagulant drugs in the treatment of pulmonary embolism: A controlled trial. Lancet 1960;1:1309-1312.

298. Alpert JS, Smith R, Carlson J, et al: Mortality in patients treated for pulmonary embolism. JAMA 1976;236:1477-1480.

299. Kernohan RJ, Todd C: Heparin therapy in thromboembolic disease. Lancet 1966;1:621-623.

300. Buller HR, Agnelli G, Hull RD, et al: Antithrombotic therapy for venous thromboembolic disease: The seventh ACCP Conference on Antithrombotic and Thrombolytic Therapy. Chest 2004;126:401S-428.

301. Hommes DW, Bura A, Mazzolai L, et al: Subcutaneous heparin compared with continuous intravenous heparin administration in the initial treatment of deep vein thrombosis: A meta-analysis. Ann Intern Med 1992;116:279-284.

302. Dolovich LR, Ginsberg JS, Douketis JD, et al: A meta-analysis comparing low-molecular-weight heparins with unfractionated heparin in the treatment of venous thromboembolism: Examining some unanswered questions regarding location of treatment, product type, and dosing frequency. Arch Intern Med 2000;160:181-188.

303. Giannoudis PV, Pountos I, Pape HC, Patel JV: Safety and efficacy of vena cava filters in trauma patients. Injury 2007;38:7-18.

304. Goldhaber SZ, Visani L, DeRosa M: Acute pulmonary embolism: Clinical outcomes in the International Cooperative Pulmonary Embolism Registry (ICOPER). Lancet 1999;353:1386-1389.

305. Kucher N, Rossi E, De Rosa M, Goldhaber SZ: Massive pulmonary embolism. Circulation 2006;113:577-582.

306. Anderson DR, Levine MN: Thrombolytic therapy for the treatment of acute pulmonary embolism. CMAJ 1992;146:1317-1324.

307. Meyer G, Tamisier D, Sors H, et al: Pulmonary embolectomy: A 20-year experience at one center. Ann Thorac Surg 1991;51:232-236.

308. Meneveau N, Seronde MF, Blonde MC, et al: Management of unsuccessful thrombolysis in acute massive pulmonary embolism. Chest 2006;129:1043-1050.

309. Christopherson R, Beattie C, Frank SM, et al: Perioperative morbidity in patients randomized to epidural or general anesthesia for lower extremity vascular surgery. Perioperative Ischemia Randomized Anesthesia Trial Study Group. Anesthesiology 1993;79:422-434.

310. Rosenfeld BA, Beattie C, Christopherson R, et al: The effects of different anesthetic regimens on fibrinolysis and the development of postoperative arterial thrombosis. Perioperative Ischemia Randomized Anesthesia Trial Study Group. Anesthesiology 1993;79:435-443.

311. Horlocker TT, Wedel DJ, Benzon H, et al: Regional anesthesia in the anticoagulated patient: Defining the risks. Second ASRA Consensus Conference on Neuraxial Anesthesia and Anticoagulation. Reg Anesth Pain Med 2003;28:172-197.

312. Hochwald SN, Harrison LE, Heslin MJ, et al: Early postoperative enteral feeding improves whole body protein kinetics in upper gastrointestinal cancer patients. Am J Surg 1997;174:325-330.

313. Reissman P, Teoh TA, Cohen SM, et al: Is early oral feeding safe after elective colorectal surgery? A prospective randomized trial. Ann Surg 1995;222:73-77.

314. Gokgoz L, Gunaydin S, Sinci V, et al: Psychiatric complications of cardiac surgery postoperative delirium syndrome. Scand Cardiovasc J 1997;31:217-222.

315. Rolfson DB, McElhaney JE, Rockwood K, et al: Incidence and risk factors for delirium and other adverse outcomes in older adults after coronary artery bypass graft surgery. Can J Cardiol 1999;15:771-776.

316. Schor JD, Levkoff SE, Lipsitz LA, et al: Risk factors for delirium in hospitalized elderly. JAMA 1992;267:827-831.

317. van der Mast RC, van den Broek WW, Fekkes D, et al: Incidence of and preoperative predictors for delirium after cardiac surgery. J Psychosom Res 1999;46:479-483.

Chapter

34 Major Orthopedic Surgery

Babak Sarani, David T. Huang, and Robin West

The number of Americans aged 65 and older is projected to double over the next 3 decades, from less than 13% of the population now to 20% in 2030.[1] This means that an increasing portion of health-care resources will be used by the "baby boomer" generation. In the United States, approximately 440,000 hip and knee replacement procedures were performed in the year 2000.[2] It is expected that an increasing number of both elective and urgent orthopedic procedures, such as joint replacement and complex fracture repair, will be required in older adult patients with complex comorbid conditions. Therefore, the number of orthopedic patients who may require postoperative critical care management is expected to increase. The critical care provider must be familiar with issues unique to these patients.

Several factors have been shown to impact morbidity and mortality in orthopedic patients. For hip replacement surgery, age has been found to be the most important determinant of mortality, although it is not known if this is a function of increasing age alone or the comorbidities associated with advanced age. Patients 66 to 69 years old undergoing elective total hip arthroplasty have a less than 0.5% perioperative mortality, whereas those older than 85 years have a 2% to 6% mortality.[3-5] As expected, those undergoing urgent surgery as a result of fracture and those with pre-existing pulmonary or cardiac conditions, hypertension, renal insufficiency, or diabetes mellitus also have higher morbidity.[3,4] Finally, patients undergoing spine operations have the potential for unique postoperative complications; these will be discussed separately.

Although many studies have documented the utility and benefits of joint replacement and spine surgery, there is a paucity of large randomized clinical trial data on interventions to minimize postoperative complications. The recommendations in this chapter are based mostly on small case series, meta-analyses, and retrospective reviews. This chapter will focus on the care of patients undergoing total joint or spine surgery and will not discuss care of the multiply injured trauma patient.

■ CARE AFTER TOTAL JOINT ARTHROPLASTY

Several issues are unique to patients after total joint arthroplasty. These include venous thromboembolic disease prophylaxis, fat embolism, and complications related to the intraoperative use of cement.

Venous Thromboembolic Disease

Deep venous thrombosis (DVT) and pulmonary embolism (PE) are generally considered to be a single clinical entity referred to as venous thromboembolic disease (VTED). It is estimated that 80% to 90% of pulmonary emboli originate as lower extremity, pelvic, or caval DVT. Total joint arthroplasty is associated with a very high rate of DVT.[6-8] The reasons for this are most likely related to extensive soft tissue dissection, inflammatory reaction in proximity to major blood vessels, and the extremity immobility required after such procedures. The incidence of asymptomatic, venographically evident DVT in postoperative total joint arthroplasty patients is 50% to 80% without prophylaxis, but the majority of these thrombi resolve spontaneously with no clinical sequelae.[7,9] Although there are no studies with sufficient follow-up and number of patients to precisely know the incidence, prevalence, or time course for the development of symptoms, those undergoing total knee replacement have a much higher risk of symptomatic DVT (10% to 15%) than those undergoing total hip replacement (3% to 4%).[10,11] Symptoms of DVT include edema, pain, erythema, or, less commonly, ulceration. Asymptomatic DVT refers to thrombi that are evident only by screening venography or duplex ultrasound. The risk of fatal PE is the same whether patients have symptomatic or asymptomatic DVT (<1%).

Although medical society guidelines have been written,[6] there is no clear definition of adequate prophylaxis for patients undergoing elective joint replacement operations. This standard is absent mainly because of the lack of adequately powered, randomized, blinded, controlled studies comparing one modality against another for the prevention of VTED. Most studies evaluating the efficacy of one agent against another for the prevention of DVT have been unblinded or nonrandomized. Studies evaluating various agents for the prevention of PE would be difficult to carry out because of the low incidence of fatal PE. For example, a randomized prospective trial with an 80% power to demonstrate a 5% difference in efficacy of mechanical versus pharmacologic prophylaxis for prevention of PE would require 45,000 patients.[12]

Total Hip Arthroplasty

Studies evaluating the efficacy of pharmacologic versus mechanical (e.g., foot pumps or sequential compression devices) prophylaxis against DVT after elective hip surgery have yielded conflicting findings. Small studies have shown that mechanical devices alone are efficacious in preventing asymptomatic DVT, but compliance with the use of these devices is highly variable.[6,8,13-15] Other studies have shown that pharmacologic prophylaxis is superior to mechanical prophylaxis for the prevention of asymptomatic DVT,[16] but most studies have been either unblinded or nonrandomized.

Two meta-analyses showed very little difference in efficacy between low-molecular-weight heparin (LMWH) and warfarin (INR target 2 to 3) for prevention of asymptomatic DVT after total hip replacement.[16,17] However, a separate meta-analysis showed a significantly higher rate of bleeding associated with the use of LMWH.[18] Most recently, fondaparinux, a pentasaccharide and selective factor X inhibitor, has been approved for thromboprophylaxis after major orthopedic surgery. In blinded, randomized trials, fondaparinux was shown to be superior to enoxaparin in preventing asymptomatic DVT, although there was no difference between the rates of symptomatic DVT and PE.[19,20]

Although the rates of asymptomatic DVT are similar for patients with a hip fracture and those undergoing elective joint surgery, patients with a hip fracture have a significantly higher rate of fatal PE (4% to 10%).[6,21] The reason for this difference is unknown, and the exact site of the fracture (subcapital versus intertrochanteric) does not affect the rate of VTED.[21] No studies have compared mechanical prophylaxis alone to pharmacologic agents in preventing VTED in this patient population, but pharmacologic intervention has been shown to be far superior to placebo alone.[22] Low-dose unfractionated heparin has been shown to be efficacious in preventing VTED in small uncontrolled studies.[23,24] Similarly, LMWH and warfarin have also been shown to be effective in larger studies.[24-28] There are no studies directly comparing these regimens or the associated bleeding risks. As with elective hip surgery, fondaparinux has been shown to have higher efficacy than enoxaparin for the prevention of DVT, although the incidence of PE remains unchanged.[29] A Cochrane review of various modalities to prevent DVT after hip fracture concluded that "unfractionated and LMW heparins protect against lower limb DVT. There is insufficient evidence to confirm either protection against pulmonary embolism or an overall benefit, or to distinguish between various applications of heparin. Foot and calf pumping devices appear to prevent DVT, may protect against pulmonary embolism, and reduce mortality, but patient compliance is problematic."[30] This review was published prior to the availability of fondaparinux.

Total Knee Arthroplasty

As is the case for total hip arthroplasty, there are conflicting data regarding the various prophylactic regimens after total knee replacement. It is generally accepted that mechanical devices are less efficacious than pharmacologic agents in preventing asymptomatic DVT after knee arthroplasty.[6,15,31] There are no randomized studies comparing LMWH to warfarin or unfractionated heparin for prevention of DVT after total knee replacement. In a meta-analysis of the various pharmacologic agents used to prevent DVT, Brookenthal and colleagues found that warfarin, low-dose heparin, and LMWH are equally efficacious in preventing DVT.[32] In a randomized, blinded study, Bauer and coworkers showed that fondaparinux is superior to enoxaparin for the prevention of DVT.[33] They also noted a significantly higher risk of bleeding with fondaparinux if the patient received a dose less than 6 hours after surgery. As with previous studies, there were no

differences between the rates of symptomatic DVT and fatal PE, most likely because the study was not adequately powered to detect such a difference.

Recommendations for Prophylaxis against VTED

Prophylaxis against VTED is currently based more on the danger of PE than on prevention of DVT. Previous studies from the 1970s cited the incidence of fatal PE after joint replacement surgery to be higher than 2% to 3% despite some form of prophylactic anticoagulation.[34,35] Based on these papers, such operations were considered to have high risk for VTED, and either mechanical or pharmacologic prophylaxis was encouraged. However, more recent studies have documented an incidence of fatal PE of only 0.05% to 0.2%, regardless of whether prophylaxis of any modality is used.[7,9,12] Possible reasons for the significant decrease in the rate of fatal PE include improved surgical and anesthetic techniques with shorter operative times, faster discharge of patients from the hospital (resulting in earlier mobility), and improved rehabilitation techniques.

Because the incidence of fatal PE is extremely low, some have suggested that pharmacologic prophylaxis is not warranted. They argue that the incidence of fatal PE is nearly equal to the incidence of complications from therapy (e.g., bleeding), and that pharmacologic intervention has not been shown to be more efficacious than mechanical measures alone in preventing symptomatic DVT or PE.[36] Furthermore, the vast majority of deep venous thromboses resolve spontaneously, and thus the risk of bleeding associated with pharmacologic intervention may not be justified. Others, however, note that nonfatal PE and DVT carry substantial morbidity, such as heart strain, respiratory embarrassment, and thrombophlebitis, and thus the risk associated with pharmacologic prophylaxis is justified.

Patients in the intensive care unit (ICU) have limited opportunity for movement because of either the nature of their critical illness or the need for continuous monitoring. Thus, it is possible that these patients will have a higher rate of fatal PE, and strong consideration should be given to providing both mechanical and pharmacologic prophylaxis against VTED. Three out of four randomized, blinded trials and a meta-analysis have shown that fondaparinux is superior to enoxaparin for the prevention of DVT, and that the risk of bleeding can be minimized by administering the drug no less than 6 hours after surgery.[20,29,33,37,38] At this time, fondaparinux appears to be the best agent to prevent VTED after major orthopedic surgery; however, more studies are needed to define its role in orthopedic patients in the ICU.

The current guidelines from the College of Chest Physicians Consensus Conference on Antithrombotic Therapy also recommend pharmacologic prophylaxis to guard against VTED after total joint replacement surgery.[6] Their recommendations, which were published prior to studies evaluating fondaparinux, are based mainly on case series, retrospective reviews, and meta-analyses. These recommendations and level of evidence to support them are summarized in Box 34-1 and Figure 34-1.

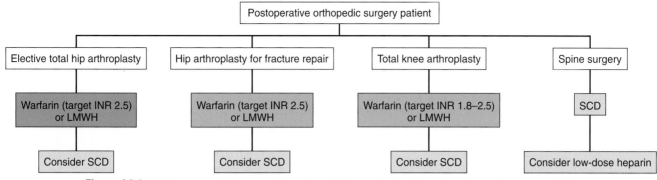

Figure 34-1 ■ Recommended venous thromboembolic prophylaxis based on type of surgery. INR, International Normalized Ratio; LMWH, low-molecular-weight heparin; SCD, sequential compression device.

34-1	**Recommendations of the Sixth American College of Chest Physicians Consensus Conference on Antithrombotic Therapy**

- *Elective total hip arthroplasty:* Prophylaxis using either warfarin (target International Normalized Ratio [INR]. 2.5) or low-molecular-weight heparin (level A evidence, based on meta-analyses)
- *Hip fracture surgery:* Prophylaxis using either warfarin (target INR, 2.5) or low-molecular-weight heparin (level B evidence, based on pooled evidence from various studies)
- *Elective total knee replacement:* Prophylaxis using either low-molecular-weight heparin or warfarin (level B evidence, based on pooled evidence from various studies). Addition of pneumatic compression devices for those with added risk factors for deep venous thrombosis (level C evidence, based on expert opinion)

From Geerts WH, Heit JA, Clagett GP, et al: Chest 2001;119(1 Suppl):132S-175.

Fat Embolism Syndrome

Fat embolism must be distinguished by the critical care provider from fat embolism syndrome (FES). Fat embolism occurs in almost all patients who have suffered multiple trauma or have had major orthopedic surgery, it is rarely symptomatic, and it is most often diagnosed incidentally on postmortem examination.[39,40] On the other hand, FES has a distinct triad of signs and symptoms with a variable disease course.

Von Bergmann first described FES in 1873 while treating a patient with a femur fracture.[41] In the orthopedic population, it occurs most often after joint replacement surgery (1% to 3% incidence) and in those with multiple long bone fractures (5% to 10% incidence).[42] It is much more commonly seen in adults than in children because olein, a lipid that is more abundant in the marrow of adults, is more likely to produce emboli than palmitin and stearin, which are found mainly in younger individuals.[43] Prolonged bedrest or delayed definitive fracture repair (greater than 48 hours) has been shown to increase the incidence of FES. The overall mortality rate has improved since the mid 20th century but remains at 5% to 15%, although this figure may be an underestimation of the true incidence of death due to FES.[40,44]

Fat embolism syndrome is classically characterized by pulmonary, cerebral, and cutaneous or retinal findings. The most severe manifestations of FES are usually noted after trauma; it is unusual to have severe multiorgan dysfunction due to FES after joint replacement surgery. Signs and symptoms tend to occur 12 to 24 hours after injury or operation and to worsen from 72 to 96 hours after the initial insult. Nearly all patients have some degree of pulmonary impairment, tachypnea often being the first sign. Later findings are hypoxemia and increasing requirements for supplemental oxygen. Cerebral findings are present in 80% of patients and can manifest as headache, agitation, confusion, or seizure.[45] Finally, a petechial rash localized to nondependent regions and the oral mucosa and possible retinal edema or hemorrhage occur in 40% of patients after 24 to 48 hours.[46] The rash tends to resolve after 1 week. Other nonspecific findings may include tachycardia and fever. Mortality is most often related to severe pulmonary dysfunction, whereas morbidity is most often the result of cerebral complications.

The exact pathophysiology underlying FES remains unknown. The two leading theories are mechanical and biochemical, and it is possible that the actual cause is a combination of both proposed mechanisms. The mechanical theory states that intramedullary pressure exceeds venous pressure and causes embolization of fat globules, which then lodge in pulmonary capillaries. The resulting pulmonary hypertension causes opening of the foramen ovale (if not already patent) and allows for arterial embolization of other globules, which lodge in cerebral, retinal, and dermal arterioles.[42,47] Because there is a 12- to 24-hour latency in the development of symptoms and there is not a direct relationship between the amount of embolized fat and pulmonary distress, the biochemical theory states that the embolized fat globules initiate an inflammatory cascade in the lung leading to respiratory impairment and noncardiogenic pulmonary edema.[40,42] Cerebral impairment is postulated to be caused by a similar mechanism.

Although scoring systems have been described,[40,48] FES remains mostly a clinical diagnosis, as no test is sensitive or specific enough to be of use. The critical care provider must have a high index of suspicion to accurately make this diagnosis. A near ubiquitous finding is hypoxemia. Many patients have PAO_2 values less than 50 mm Hg on room air within 72 hours. Accordingly, arterial blood gas analysis is the only uniformly helpful test, although the results do not differentiate FES from other causes of hypoxemia. Most patients have a normal electrocardiogram. The chest radiograph is often normal initially and lags behind clinical findings, much as is noted for acute respiratory distress syndrome (ARDS). There are only isolated case reports and small series on the use of high-resolution computed tomography for the diagnosis of FES. These reports consistently show bilateral ground-glass opacities and thickening of the interlobular septa in nondependent regions of the lungs, but these findings are not specific to FES.[49,50] Other tests, such as urinalysis or evaluation of cerebrospinal fluid or blood for fat cells or eosinophils, are too sensitive to be helpful. For patients with respiratory embarrassment, bronchoalveolar lavage (BAL) showing fat cells might allow FES to be differentiated from other causes, but the role of BAL has not been studied in large, prospective trials.[51]

The treatment of FES is centered on definitive fixation of all fractures, and on respiratory support to maintain adequate oxygenation. Studies evaluating therapies such as alcohol and dextran have not shown them to be of benefit.[40,42,52] Additionally, reports on the usefulness of corticosteroids are conflicting. Corticosteroids were first used in the 1960s and their use today remains controversial, with some studies suggesting that they may be harmful.[42] It is thought that corticosteroids may help by inhibiting the inflammatory reaction seen with FES and by decreasing the rise in plasma free fatty acids by inhibiting pulmonary lipase activity. Currently, there is no consensus or recommendation on whether corticosteroids should be prescribed, or on the dosage regimen to be used. Suggested doses of methylprednisolone have ranged from 1.5 mg/kg every 8 hours for four doses, to 30 mg/kg every 2 hours for two doses, to 7.5 mg/kg every 6 hours for twelve doses.[40]

The overall approach to the patient with FES should be based on ensuring adequate oxygen delivery to the peripheral tissues. Management involves restoring euvolemia, correcting severe anemia, monitoring indices of perfusion, and utilizing mechanical ventilation as necessary. On the basis of current knowledge, the use of corticosteroids or other medical therapies cannot be recommended.

Complications Relating to the Use of Intramedullary Cement

Traditionally, polymethylmethacrylate has been used to fix prostheses implanted during total hip replacement surgery. Reports of severe transient hypotension or hypoxemia related to the use of cement first appeared in 1970, but the incidence has decreased from greater than 50% to 5%.[44] The reason for this significant decrease in incidence remains speculative because the cause of cement-related hypotension has never been determined. The decrease may be the result of improve-

ment in anesthetic technique, such as maintaining euvolemia and oxygenation, and also the result of better prostheses, which decrease the incidence of cement or fat (bone marrow) emboli. Cement-related hypotension may be related to systemic release of polymethylmethacrylate with resulting systemic inflammation, vasodilation, and cardiac depression.[44] Hypoxemia may result from air and fat emboli caused by forceful instillation of cement into the medullary cavity of the femur. Intraoperative transesophageal echocardiography has demonstrated numerous emboli traveling through the right heart during cement and component insertion, but relatively few patients manifest symptoms of pulmonary embolism.[53]

It is not known what predisposes some patients to become hypotensive or hypoxemic while most remain asymptomatic. Patients at high risk for developing cement-related complications include older adults with cancer, patients with preexisting cardiopulmonary conditions, patients undergoing operations with a long-stem femoral component, and patients with hypovolemia.[54] Unfortunately, the factors that have been shown to decrease the incidence of cement-related complications are outside of the direct control of the intensivist and include maintenance of euvolemia intraoperatively, lavage of the femoral canal, and placement of a vent hole in the prosthesis.

Patients who develop complications related to the use of cement most commonly present with isolated hypoxemia that can last 30 minutes to 48 hours.[44,55] Most often, these patients have a normal chest radiograph. The need for mechanical ventilation depends on the patient's preexisting cardiopulmonary reserve, the severity of the reaction to the cement, and other insults that may have occurred intraoperatively (such as excessive bleeding, long operative time, or inadequate resuscitation). Ries and colleagues showed a 28% increase in the pulmonary shunt fraction after instillation of cement and further demonstrated that it took up to 48 hours for the shunt fraction to return to normal.[55] These authors recommended evaluating patients' pulmonary function when use of cement is planned during total hip replacement surgery. Significant hypotension is noted in only 5% of patients and is usually much more transient, often lasting less than 30 minutes. All in all, cement-related complications should be considered a diagnosis of exclusion, and physicians caring for such patients postoperatively must exclude other causes of persistent hypotension, such as myocardial infarction or hypovolemia, even in patients who are at risk for cement-related complications. Therapy is mainly supportive and centers on ensuring adequate oxygen delivery.

■ CARE AFTER SPINE SURGERY

The types of procedures performed on the spine are varied and becoming increasingly common. Lumbar fusion rates doubled from 1979 to 1990, and the highest rise was seen in those greater than 60 years old.[56] The planned surgery may involve single or multiple levels of vertebrae using an anterior or posterior approach and may or may not require instrumentation. The indications for and physiologic consequences of each approach will be discussed.

Although the various operations have a low morbidity and mortality, the need for a postoperative ICU stay is increased for patients older than 60 years, when there is extensive decompression and fusion, with greater than 60 degrees in curvature of the spine (e.g., severe scoliosis), for an anterior approach to the thoracic or lumbar spine, and in the presence of other comorbidities.[57] Comorbidities that are associated with the need for postoperative ICU care include preexisting myelopathy, pulmonary disease, cardiac or coronary artery disease, renal impairment, and diabetes mellitus. Preexisting myelopathy and severe scoliosis can lead to impaired pulmonary mechanics, significant pulmonary hypertension, and right ventricular failure in those older than 40 years.[44] Furthermore, myelopathy often requires more extensive surgical repair, resulting in increased operative time, increased blood loss, and multilevel fusion.

It is not known whether an anterior or posterior spine fusion is more physiologically taxing to the patient. However, studies suggest that complications are more common and severe after a posterior approach than with an anterior approach.[58-60] Nonetheless, patients may require ICU care after an anterior approach because of the volume shifts and possible respiratory dysfunction associated with violation of the thoracic or peritoneal cavity. An anterior approach may result in transiently worsening pulmonary function, whereas a posterior approach is often better tolerated from a cardio-respiratory standpoint.[61] Complications of a posterior approach to spinal fusion include bleeding, dural tear, neurologic injury, or prolonged operative time; complications of an anterior approach include ileus, deep venous thrombosis, or respiratory impairment (in cases involving the thoracic vertebrae). The main advantage of the posterior approach is the ability to visualize the posterior spinal elements (lamina, intervertebral disks, and spinal cord) without opening a body cavity. The main disadvantage of this approach is the limited operative field provided to the surgeon, which can make instrumentation and multilevel fusion more difficult. Thus, most patients requiring multilevel fusion or tumor resection undergo an anterior approach. In this circumstance, the exposure can involve retroperitoneal dissection only, or it can be much more invasive, involving a thoracoabdominal approach. A combined anterior–posterior approach is used most often when a large correction is necessary (e.g., for scoliosis) or when an anterior approach alone is insufficient to allow multilevel fusion (e.g., for osteoporosis).

Unique Issues after Spine Surgery

Patients undergoing spine surgery, like other surgical patients, are at risk for developing congestive heart failure, arrhythmia, bleeding, and other common postoperative complications. However, spine surgery patients have a particularly increased risk for cardiopulmonary dysfunction, infection, and certain unusual complications, such as syndrome of inappropriate antidiuretic hormone (SIADH) release, injury during intubation, and recurrent laryngeal nerve injury.

Cardiopulmonary Dysfunction

Patients are at increased risk for hypoventilation after surgery involving the thoracic or lumbar spine. Surgery involving the thorax is associated with a marked decline in the 1-second forced expiratory volume (FEV_1), forced vital capacity, and total lung volume.[62] Severe atelectasis is noted in 5% to 15% of patients, and 3% to 4% develop pneumonia.[56] Thoracoabdominal procedures are associated with significant pain, which, if not treated appropriately, can lead to hypoventilation. The severe pain can last as long as 4 days,[62] so many patients may benefit from either epidural or patient-controlled analgesia (PCA) postoperatively. Rarely, patients who have undergone a thoracoabdominal approach may have phrenic nerve injury, which may be transient (due to traction) or permanent. Unilateral phrenic nerve injury manifests radiographically as elevation of the ipsilateral hemidiaphragm and is often well tolerated in individuals with only mild to moderate preoperative pulmonary impairment. The rate of symptomatic DVT after spine surgery is 0.5% in patients receiving either mechanical or pharmacologic prophylaxis,[63] and Dearborn and colleagues found a 2% incidence of PE in such patients.[64] PE is rarely the cause of hypoxemia in patients who have undergone spine surgery and have received VTED prophylaxis. Critical care providers must expeditiously exclude other causes of hypoxemia in these patients.

Patients with severe scoliosis are at high risk of cardiac or pulmonary failure in the perioperative period.[44] The severe angulation of the spine results in a restrictive pattern of ventilation, with resultant hypercapnia, hypoxemia, and pulmonary hypertension, especially in those older than 40 years.[62] Accordingly, pulmonary or right ventricular function may deteriorate acutely in the perioperative period, particularly after aggressive fluid resuscitation. These patients may benefit from cardiac performance monitoring and may require pharmacologic support to maintain adequate right ventricular function.

Many patients with scoliosis have muscular dystrophy or cerebral palsy. A majority of these patients have a cardiac abnormality of some nature. Dysrhythmias and cardiac conduction defects also have been reported in up to 50% of these patients.[62] Such patients require telemetry postoperatively. In addition, many patients with muscular dystrophy have involvement of the bulbar muscles and so are at risk for aspiration postoperatively.

Infection

Patients undergoing thoracic or lumbar surgery have a higher risk of infection than other surgical patients undergoing clean operations. Clean operations are nontraumatic cases that do not involve violation of hollow viscera or infected fields. Whereas discectomy with antibiotic prophylaxis is associated with a 1% risk of infection, fusion with instrumentation is associated with a 3% to 8% risk, depending on the number of levels fused and amount of instrumentation needed.[44] It is thought that the higher risk of infection seen with increasing levels of fusion is the result of greater dissection, operative time, and blood loss. Other contributing factors include malnutrition, chronic steroid use, and preexisting distant infections (e.g., of the urinary tract).

Syndrome of Inappropriate Antidiuretic Hormone

Approximately 5% of patients undergoing spinal fusion develop SIADH postoperatively.[65] Risk factors for developing this complication include severe blood loss, intraoperative hypotension, and rapid correction of the spine. The cause remains uncertain and therapy is directed at maintenance of normal serum sodium through water restriction. Most often, the disorder is self-limiting. Partly because of the very long operative time needed for single-stage correction, most patients with severe scoliosis are corrected in a two-stage procedure. Depending on the operation planned, the first stage can involve exposure and decompression of the cord from either an anterior or a posterior approach. The second stage, which is usually performed 5 to 7 days after the first, may involve instrumentation and can also be approached from either side. Dividing the operation into two stages might protect against the development of SIADH because blood loss and operative time for each operation are minimized. However, many studies have shown that two-stage procedures are actually associated with more net blood loss, longer net operative time, and longer duration of hospitalization.[66-69] In conclusion, the intensive care physician needs to maintain a high index of suspicion for SIADH in the patient who has undergone spine surgery and presents with hyponatremia and high urinary sodium. Patients undergoing two-stage procedures may require more ICU care than those undergoing a single-stage operation.

Injury during Intubation

Caution should be exercised in intubating patients for cervical spine surgery. For several reasons, these patients should be considered as if they had high-risk injuries during intubation. They may have a very limited range of motion because of chronic degenerative disease, or they may have cervical spine instability due to acute traumatic injury. Rarely, such patients develop pulmonary complications requiring mechanical ventilation before they have cervical spine surgery, especially in the trauma population at risk for aspiration or pulmonary contusion. Awake fiberoptic intubation is preferred to minimize complications. If time or lack of equipment or expertise precludes fiberoptic intubation, a two-person technique (one person stabilizes the head and neck while the other intubates the patient) is strongly recommended.

Recurrent Laryngeal Nerve Injury

Finally, those who have undergone cervical spine surgery may have edema of the airway or recurrent laryngeal nerve damage.[44] Damage to the recurrent laryngeal nerve may be transient or permanent, depending on the underlying cause. Patients with unilateral damage to the recurrent laryngeal nerve present with hoarseness resulting from paralysis of the ipsilateral vocal cord. Patients with bilateral nerve injury present with occlusion of the airway requiring emergent cricothyroidotomy.

■ CONCLUSIONS

In summary, the number of patients older than 65 years who require elective or urgent orthopedic surgery is expected to increase. Often, these patients have significant comorbidities that need to be addressed in the perioperative period, and they may require ICU care. In addition to the routine care of the postoperative patient, those undergoing major orthopedic surgery have unique issues related to their propensity for thromboembolic disease or cardiopulmonary failure, and to their need for pain management. Similarly, those undergoing spine operations are at risk for atypical postoperative complications. The astute critical care provider should be aware of these possible complications to minimize morbidity and length of stay in this patient population.

■ REFERENCES

1. Claliff R: Developing Chronic Disease Therapies. Health Affairs 2004;23:77-88.
2. Kim S, Koebel S, Duffy R: Cost burden of hip and knee replacements in Ohio: Estimates from the National Hospital Discharge Survey, 2000. Manag Care Interface 2004;17:22-25.
3. Parvizi J, Ereth MH, Lewallen DG: Thirty-day mortality following hip arthroplasty for acute fracture. J Bone Joint Surg Am 2004;86A: 1983-1988.
4. Parvizi J, Johnson BG, Rowland C, et al: Thirty-day mortality after elective total hip arthroplasty. J Bone Joint Surg Am 2001;83-A: 1524-1528.
5. Whittle J, Steinberg EP, Anderson GF, et al: Mortality after elective total hip arthroplasty in elderly Americans: Age, gender, and indication for surgery predict survival. Clin Orthop 1993:119-126.
6. Geerts WH, Heit JA, Clagett GP, et al: Prevention of venous thromboembolism. Chest 2001;119(1 Suppl):132S-175.
7. Pierson JL, Tavel ME: Thromboembolic prophylaxis in total joint replacement. Chest 2001;120:302-304.
8. Warwick D: Postoperative thromboprophylaxis: An orthopedic surgeon's view—Is it a valid concept in today's practice? Curr Hematol Rep 2003;2:411-416.
9. Murray DW, Britton AR, Bulstrode CJ: Thromboprophylaxis and death after total hip replacement. J Bone Joint Surg Br 1996;78:863-870.
10. Warwick D, Williams MH, Bannister GC: Death and thromboembolic disease after total hip replacement: A series of 1162 cases with no routine chemical prophylaxis. J Bone Joint Surg Br 1995;77:6-10.
11. Warwick DJ, Whitehouse S: Symptomatic venous thromboembolism after total knee replacement. J Bone Joint Surg Br 1997;79:780-786.
12. Fender D, Harper WM, Thompson JR, Gregg PJ: Mortality and fatal pulmonary embolism after primary total hip replacement: Results from a regional hip register. J Bone Joint Surg Br 1997;79:896-899.
13. Hooker JA, Lachiewicz PF, Kelley SS: Efficacy of prophylaxis against thromboembolism with intermittent pneumatic compression after primary and revision total hip arthroplasty. J Bone Joint Surg Am 1999;81:690-696.
14. Woolson ST, Watt JM: Intermittent pneumatic compression to prevent proximal deep venous thrombosis during and after total hip replacement: A prospective, randomized study of compression alone, compression and aspirin, and compression and low-dose warfarin. J Bone Joint Surg Am 1991;73:507-512.
15. Kaempffe FA, Lifeso RM, Meinking C: Intermittent pneumatic compression versus Coumadin: Prevention of deep vein thrombosis in lower-extremity total joint arthroplasty. Clin Orthop 1991;(269): 89-97.
16. Imperiale TF, Speroff T: A meta-analysis of methods to prevent venous thromboembolism following total hip replacement. JAMA 1994;271: 1780-1785.
17. Mohr DN, Silverstein MD, Murtaugh PA, Harrison JM: Prophylactic agents for venous thrombosis in elective hip surgery: Meta-analysis of studies using venographic assessment. Arch Intern Med 1993;153: 2221-2228.
18. Freedman KB, Brookenthal KR, Fitzgerald RH Jr, et al: A meta-analysis of thromboembolic prophylaxis following elective total hip arthroplasty. J Bone Joint Surg Am 2000;82A:929-938.

19. Turpie AG, Bauer KA, Eriksson BI, Lassen MR: Postoperative fondaparinux versus postoperative enoxaparin for prevention of venous thromboembolism after elective hip-replacement surgery: A randomised double-blind trial. Lancet 2002;359:1721-1726.

20. Lassen MR, Bauer KA, Eriksson BI, Turpie AG: Postoperative fondaparinux versus preoperative enoxaparin for prevention of venous thromboembolism in elective hip-replacement surgery: A randomised double-blind comparison. Lancet 2002;359:1715-1720.

21. Perez JV, Warwick DJ, Case CP, Bannister GC: Death after proximal femoral fracture: An autopsy study. Injury 1995;26:237-240.

22. Todd CJ, Palmer C, Camilleri-Ferrante C, et al: Differences in mortality after fracture of hip. BMJ 1995;311:1025.

23. Moskovitz PA, Ellenberg SS, Feffer HL, et al: Low-dose heparin for prevention of venous thromboembolism in total hip arthroplasty and surgical repair of hip fractures. J Bone Joint Surg Am 1978;60:1065-1070.

24. Monreal M, Lafoz E, Navarro A, et al: A prospective double-blind trial of a low molecular weight heparin once daily compared with conventional low-dose heparin three times daily to prevent pulmonary embolism and venous thrombosis in patients with hip fracture. J Trauma 1989;29:873-875.

25. Borgstroem S, Greitz T, Van Der Linden W, et al: Anticoagulant prophylaxis of venous thrombosis in patients with fractured neck of the femur: A controlled clinical trial using venous phlebography. Acta Chir Scand 1965;129:500-508.

26. Hamilton HW, Crawford JS, Gardiner JH, Wiley AM: Venous thrombosis in patients with fracture of the upper end of the femur: A phlebographic study of the effect of prophylactic anticoagulation. J Bone Joint Surg Br 1970;52:268-289.

27. Powers PJ, Gent M, Jay RM, et al: A randomized trial of less intense postoperative warfarin or aspirin therapy in the prevention of venous thromboembolism after surgery for fractured hip. Arch Intern Med 1989;149:771-774.

28. Barsotti J, Gruel Y, Rosset P, et al: Comparative double-blind study of two dosage regimens of low-molecular weight heparin in elderly patients with a fracture of the neck of the femur. J Orthop Trauma 1990;4:371-375.

29. Eriksson BI, Bauer KA, Lassen MR, Turpie AG: Fondaparinux compared with enoxaparin for the prevention of venous thromboembolism after hip-fracture surgery. N Engl J Med 2001;345:1298-1304.

30. Handoll HH, Farrar MJ, McBirnie J, et al: Heparin, low molecular weight heparin and physical methods for preventing deep vein thrombosis and pulmonary embolism following surgery for hip fractures. Cochrane Database Syst Rev 2002:CD000305.

31. Levine MN, Gent M, Hirsh J, et al: Ardeparin (low-molecular-weight heparin) vs graduated compression stockings for the prevention of venous thromboembolism: A randomized trial in patients undergoing knee surgery. Arch Intern Med 1996;156:851-856.

32. Brookenthal KR, Freedman KB, Lotke PA, et al: A meta-analysis of thromboembolic prophylaxis in total knee arthroplasty. J Arthroplasty 2001;16:293-300.

33. Bauer KA, Eriksson BI, Lassen MR, Turpie AG: Fondaparinux compared with enoxaparin for the prevention of venous thromboembolism after elective major knee surgery. N Engl J Med 2001;345:1305-1310.

34. Coventry M, Nolan D, Beckenbaugh R: Delayed prophylactic anticoagulation: A study of results and complications in 2012 total hip arthroplasties. J Bone Joint Surg Am 1973;55A:1487-1492.

35. Johnson R, Green J, Charnley J: Pulmonary embolism and its prophylaxis following the Charnley total hip replacement. Clin Orthop 1977;127:123-132.

36. Unwin AJ, Jones JR, Harries WJ: Current UK opinion on thromboprophylaxis in orthopaedic surgery: Its use in routine total hip and knee arthroplasty. Ann R Coll Surg Engl 1995;77:351-354.

37. Turpie AG, Bauer KA, Eriksson BI, Lassen MR: Fondaparinux vs enoxaparin for the prevention of venous thromboembolism in major orthopedic surgery: A meta-analysis of 4 randomized double-blind studies. Arch Intern Med 2002;162:1833-1840.

38. Lobo BL: Emerging options for thromboprophylaxis after orthopedic surgery: A review of clinical data. Pharmacotherapy 2004;24(7 Pt 2):66S-72.

39. Palmovic V, McCarroll J: Fat embolism in trauma. Arch Pathol 1965;80:630.

40. Johnson MJ, Lucas GL: Fat embolism syndrome. Orthopedics 1996;19:41-48; discussion 48-49.

41. Von Bergmann E: Fall todlicher Fettembolie. Berl Klin Wochenschr 1873;10:385.

42. Levy D: The fat embolism syndrome: A review. Clin Orthop 1990;(261):281-286.

43. Gossling HR, Pellegrini VD Jr: Fat embolism syndrome: A review of the pathophysiology and physiological basis of treatment. Clin Orthop 1982;(165):68-82.

44. Nazon D, Abergel G, Hatem CM: Critical care in orthopedic and spine surgery. Crit Care Clin 2003;19:33-53.

45. Moylan J, Birnbaum M, Katz A, Everson M: Fat emboli syndrome. J Trauma 1976;16:341-347.

46. Gurd A, Wilson R: The fat embolism syndrome. J Bone Joint Surg 1974;56B:408-416.

47. Fabian TC: Unravelling the fat embolism syndrome. N Engl J Med 1993;329:961-963.

48. Gurd AR: Fat embolism: An aid to diagnosis. J Bone Joint Surg Br 1970;52:732-737.

49. Malagari K, Economopoulos N, Stoupis C, et al: High-resolution CT findings in mild pulmonary fat embolism. Chest 2003;123:1196-1201.

50. Choi JA, Oh YW, Kim HK, et al: Nontraumatic pulmonary fat embolism syndrome: Radiologic and pathologic correlations. J Thorac Imaging 2002;17:167-169.

51. Chastre J, Fagon JY, Soler P, et al: Bronchoalveolar lavage for rapid diagnosis of the fat embolism syndrome in trauma patients. Ann Intern Med 1990;113:583-588.

52. Peltier L: Fat embolism: A perspective. Clin Orthop 1988;232:263-270.

53. Lafont ND, Kostucki WM, Marchand PH, et al: Embolism detected by transoesophageal echocardiography during hip arthroplasty. Can J Anaesth 1994;41:850-853.

54. Patterson BM, Lieberman JR, Salvati EA: Intraoperative complications during total hip arthroplasty. Orthopedics 1995;18:1089-1095.

55. Ries MD, Lynch F, Rauscher LA, et al: Pulmonary function during and after total hip replacement: Findings in patients who have insertion of a femoral component with and without cement. J Bone Joint Surg Am 1993;75:581-587.

56. Fujita T, Kostuik JP, Huckell CB, Sieber AN: Complications of spinal fusion in adult patients more than 60 years of age. Orthop Clin North Am 1998;29:669-678.

57. Harris OA, Runnels JB, Matz PG: Clinical factors associated with unexpected critical care management and prolonged hospitalization after elective cervical spine surgery. Crit Care Med 2001;29:1898-1902.

58. Pradhan BB, Nassar JA, Delamarter RB, Wang JC: Single-level lumbar spine fusion: A comparison of anterior and posterior approaches. J Spinal Disord Tech 2002;15:355-361.

59. Humphreys SC, Hodges SD, Patwardhan AG, et al: Comparison of posterior and transforaminal approaches to lumbar interbody fusion. Spine 2001;26:567-571.

60. Scaduto AA, Gamradt SC, Yu WD, et al: Perioperative complications of threaded cylindrical lumbar interbody fusion devices: Anterior versus posterior approach. J Spinal Disord Tech 2003;16:502-507.

61. Vedantam R, Lenke LG, Bridwell KH, et al: A prospective evaluation of pulmonary function in patients with adolescent idiopathic scoliosis relative to the surgical approach used for spinal arthrodesis. Spine 2000;25:82-90.

62. Raw DA, Beattie JK, Hunter JM: Anaesthesia for spinal surgery in adults. Br J Anaesth 2003;91:886-904.

63. Rokito SE, Schwartz MC, Neuwirth MG: Deep vein thrombosis after major reconstructive spinal surgery. Spine 1996;21:853-858; discussion 859.

64. Dearborn JT, Hu SS, Tribus CB, Bradford DS: Thromboembolic complications after major thoracolumbar spine surgery. Spine 1999;24:1471-1476.

65. Elster AD: Hyponatremia after spinal fusion caused by inappropriate secretion of antidiuretic hormone (SIADH). Clin Orthop Relat Res 1985;(194):136-141.

66. Shufflebarger HL, Grimm JO, Bui V, Thomson JD: Anterior and posterior spinal fusion: Staged versus same-day surgery. Spine 1991;16: 930-933.

67. Dick J, Boachie-Adjei O, Wilson M: One-stage versus two-stage anterior and posterior spinal reconstruction in adults: Comparison of outcomes including nutritional status, complications rates, hospital costs, and other factors. Spine 1992;17(8 Suppl):S310-316.

68. Viviani GR, Raducan V, Bednar DA, Grandwilewski W: Anterior and posterior spinal fusion: Comparison of one-stage and two-stage procedures. Can J Surg 1993;36:468-473.

69. Powell ET, Krengel WF 3rd, King HA, Lagrone MO: Comparison of same-day sequential anterior and posterior spinal fusion with delayed two-stage anterior and posterior spinal fusion. Spine 1994;19:1256-1259.

Chapter

35 Solid Organ Transplantation

David C. Kaufman and Carolyn E. Jones

This chapter focuses on liver, kidney, pancreas, heart, and lung transplants. Before organ transplantation can be considered, there must be failure of the native organ. Each organ failure is associated with specific morbidities, and there is also an association with death that is either direct (i.e., after complete failure) or indirect (from complications). To support the failing kidney, pancreas, heart, and lung, we have machines that are advanced from a technological vantage point, but biologically they are primitive and rudimentary. These machines can maintain life, but the quality of life is never optimal, so transplantation is often the best therapy. The risks of supportive therapy should be weighed against the risks of surgery and immunosuppression. Ideally, patients would have a choice and transplant physicians would be able to guide them in their decision. However, the demand for all organs outstrips the supply, engaging the transplant physician in a complicated ethical dialogue on a daily basis as patients wait on candidate lists. Each specialty has its own formula for determining who should receive the next available organ, but all struggle with the shortage of organs.

The organ shortage means that organ support is the only option for many individuals awaiting transplantation. Xenotransplantation as a bridge remains a concept, not a reality. Patients with chronic renal failure may spend years on hemodialysis or peritoneal dialysis as they await transplantation. People with diabetes mellitus from endocrine pancreatic insufficiency receive insulin replacement. Patients with heart failure may be connected to ventricular assist devices as they await their new heart. For respiratory failure, support may culminate in noninvasive or invasive mechanical ventilation, but it often starts with supplemental oxygen therapy. Artificial liver support remains experimental. Patients with fulminant hepatic failure are more likely than patients with chronic liver disease to benefit from liver replacement therapy. The vast majority of patients with liver disease, however, have chronic liver disease and develop acute-on-chronic liver failure. Complications such as intractable ascites and variceal hemorrhage are caused by portal hypertension and are not corrected by treatment with an artificial liver or a liver dialysis machine. Hepatic encephalopathy before or after a transjugular intrahepatic portosystemic shunt (TIPS) may be amenable to artificial liver support, but it is very unlikely that this therapy would ever replace pharmacologic management with lactulose and oral antibiotics.

To manage a patient after a transplant, the medical history before the organ replacement must be known, as well as the quality of the organ transplanted. Organs come from both dead and living donors. Donors may have been pronounced dead by brain criteria or by cardiorespiratory criteria. The practice of pronouncing someone dead because of absent brainstem function is accepted in many cultures. The concept of brain death was created during the infancy of transplantation. The brain-dead individual is ideal for organ recovery because organs are removed under controlled circumstances. This limits warm ischemia time, which is when organs undergo the greatest injury. Cold ischemia time is the time after removal of the organ when it is cooled and perfused with preservation solution.

Presently, most organs recovered for transplantation come from brain-dead donors.[1] The first heart and liver donors were people pronounced dead by cardiorespiratory criteria, a method of retrieving organs for transplantation that is becoming popular again. When organs are recovered from these donors, sometimes called non–heart-beating donors, there is always a period of warm ischemia, rendering the organs less desirable for transplantation. Because the supply of organs is limited, however, donor organs that are more marginal than desired are being transplanted into patients. These organs, classified as expanded-criteria organs, have specific donor or graft characteristics that increase the probability of poor graft function postoperatively and that are ultimately associated with poor graft or patient survival.[2] Recipients must consent to these marginal organs, but this may be the only choice for many on a waiting list.

Many transplant experts believe that the only meaningful answer to the organ shortage will come from increasing the number of living donors. In 1993, 37% of the organs transplanted were from live donors. The national Organ Procurement and Transplantation Network (OPTN) database reveals that a decade later, in 2003, 51% of the organs transplanted were from live donors.[3]

■ LIVER TRANSPLANTATION

Thomas Starzl attempted the first human liver transplant in 1963 after experimenting for 7 years with dogs. The recipient was a child with biliary atresia, who died intraoperatively because of massive hemorrhage.[4] More than 20 years later, bleeding remains the first major concern after the operation. The management of postoperative bleeding after hepatic transplantation is similar to the management of postoperative bleeding after any surgical procedure. The first priority is to determine whether the bleeding is surgical or nonsurgical. There is a heightened urgency after liver transplantation, because survival of the graft or the patient may be impacted by ischemic damage sustained in these early hours. It must be rapidly determined whether there is any surgical bleeding that would require reexploration. A negative reexploration is likely to do less harm than graft injury from poor perfusion. If the recipient is bleeding, plasma and platelets should be given to raise the platelet count and correct the coagulopathy. Procoagulant-like substances including ε-aminocaproic acid, desmopressin (aqueous vasopressin), and recombinant activated factor VII may be given, although data are lacking to support the routine use of these agents. During this time, the recipient must be monitored closely for the possible development of abdominal compartment syndrome. Elevated peak airway pressures may be the first clue to this diagnosis. If this possibility seems likely before the transplant operation is complete, it may be worthwhile to initially leave the fascia open and close the skin. Later, the fascia can be closed in a second operation.

A careful record should be made of the operation, with specific details of the events during reperfusion of the allograft, such as the clearance of lactate, the appearance and production of bile, and the need for epinephrine. Because lactate is converted to pyruvate in the liver, early clearance of lactate is evidence of graft function, even if bile production is not observed. As liver function improves, clearance of lactate increases. The more common scenario of overproduction of lactate in a critically ill patient, as pyruvate is shunted to lactate because of tissue hypoxia, may also be present in the post-transplant patient. Circulating lactate concentrations in liver transplant recipients may represent either end of this metabolic spectrum.

Another marker of early liver function after transplantation is the quality and quantity of bile measured through an externalized biliary drain. An intraoperative epinephrine infusion is often necessary during allograft reperfusion, and it is usually weaned within several hours postoperatively. An ongoing requirement for an epinephrine infusion to maintain hemodynamic stability often implies graft dysfunction.

Circulating transaminase levels typically peak approximately 24 hours after operation. The release of these enzymes is a manifestation of ischemic liver injury as well as of reperfusion injury. If the transaminase levels continue to rise after 24 hours, or if encephalopathy does not clear or a nonsurgical coagulopathy develops, the patient may have primary nonfunction of the allograft and need retransplant urgently. Risks for primary allograft nonfunction include preoperative steatosis in the donor organ and a need for administration of vasopressors to maintain hemodynamic stability. This diagnosis is one of exclusion, however, and hepatic artery and portal venous thrombosis must be ruled out by duplex ultrasonography first. Postoperative management has little or no impact on this devastating complication.[4]

The most common and devastating early vascular complication is hepatic artery thrombosis. Routine ultrasound should be performed to screen for this problem. If hepatic artery thrombosis is suspected, then the diagnosis should be confirmed angiographically. Unfortunately, this condition is usually not amenable to surgical correction, and retransplantation is often necessary. Concern is heightened if the resistive index (RI) is high, even if there is flow. The RI is calculated according to the following equation:

$$RI = (PS - ED)/PS$$

where PS is the peak systolic velocity and ED is the end-diastolic velocity. The normal range is 0.6 to 0.9. A low RI value is consistent with hepatic artery thrombosis.[4]

The liver has a dual blood supply. Flow to the bile canaliculi is dependent on the hepatic artery and not the portal vein. Collaterals from the diaphragm that traverse the bare area of the liver offer a second circulation route to the bile canaliculi. These vessels are transected during the transplantation. This phenomenon appears to be the reason that hepatic artery occlusion is better tolerated in the nontransplant patient than in the transplanted patient. When patients sustain hepatic artery thrombosis, biliary complications are likely to occur in the future. These complications can include biliary strictures and the biliary cast syndrome. Post-transplant portal venous thrombosis is an even less common complication. This diagnosis can be made on the basis of routine postoperative duplex ultrasonography.

The liver is a forgiving organ for acute cellular rejection in the immediate postoperative period, and when rejection does occur, it is usually easily managed with corticosteroids. Low-grade fever and elevated transaminase levels are often clues, but a high index of suspicion and confirmation of the diagnosis with a liver biopsy are frequently required.[5]

In recipients who receive an ABO-compatible but nonidentical liver, there is the possibility of developing passenger lymphocyte syndrome. In this scenario, a group O organ is transplanted to a non–group O recipient, or a group A or B organ is transplanted to a group AB recipient. In this syndrome, the transplanted donor lymphocytes promote hemolysis. Biochemical features of this syndrome include indirect hyperbilirubinemia and an elevated serum lactate dehydrogenase concentration. The circulating haptoglobin concentration may be low, but because haptoglobin is synthesized by the liver, this test is unreliable in these circumstances. The direct antiglobulin test is positive. Hemolysis resolves over the course of weeks to months.[6]

Many cirrhotic patients have renal dysfunction preoperatively and postoperatively. Recovery of renal function may depend as much on preexisting renal function as on any other factor, but the course of the operation and the quality of the donor liver also are important factors. Hepatorenal syndrome usually resolves postoperatively, but patients with preoperative renal dysfunction have a greater chance of chronic renal failure postoperatively. Hepatorenal syndrome can also evolve into acute tubular necrosis, and the line between the two disorders is not always distinct. The pathogenesis of hepatorenal syndrome is not well delineated and is most likely multifactorial. The end result is splanchnic vasodilatation and intrarenal vasoconstriction. Patients with hepatorenal syndrome have low urine sodium concentration but do not respond to intravascular volume expansion.

Early renal replacement therapy with ultrafiltration may help the liver transplant patient who is suffering from encephalopathy and fluid overload. However, encephalopathy is rarely caused simply by azotemia. If the liver transplant patient is fluid overloaded with normal arterial and central venous blood pressures, further volume resuscitation is usually not effective in reversing oliguria.

KIDNEY TRANSPLANTATION

Although the scientific story of transplantation began when Alexis Carrel attempted transplantation of various organs in animals, the clinical story began in 1954, when Joseph Murray transplanted a kidney from one identical twin into the other. Originally, it was believed that renal transplantation would confer only lifestyle benefits associated with freedom from dialysis, but it is now clear that there is a survival advantage as well. Younger white patients without diabetes mellitus seem to benefit the most in this regard.[7]

The major postoperative complication associated with kidney transplantation is delayed graft function. Primary nonfunction can occur as it does for livers after liver transplantation and may necessitate transplant nephrectomy (i.e., removal of the transplanted organ). Both oliguria and increasing plasma creatinine concentration are signs that indicate delayed graft function. The classic categorization of renal dysfunction as prerenal failure, intrarenal failure, and postrenal failure remains useful for classifying the etiology of delayed graft function.

Prerenal delayed graft function can be caused by intravascular volume contraction. The nephrotoxic effects of cyclosporine or tacrolimus also can contribute to delayed graft function. These immunosuppressive agents cause renal arteriolar vasoconstriction that can be distinguished from the effect of intravascular volume contraction by the lack of response to a volume challenge. An additional area of concern is the vascular anastomoses. Postoperatively, both the arterial and venous anastomoses may develop thromboses, a vascular emergency that requires urgent ultrasound evaluation, leading to surgical reexploration as appropriate. Venous thrombosis is more common than arterial thrombosis, but either can endanger the survival of the allograft.

Although there is often not a single and distinctive cause of intrarenal delayed graft function, it is most commonly caused by acute tubular necrosis or early cell-mediated rejection. Hyperacute (humoral) rejection and accelerated acute (humoral and cellular) rejection are less common today than in the past because of sensitive cross-matching techniques. Early cell-mediated rejection is the most common form of rejection in the postoperative period. However, it must be differentiated from acute tubular necrosis, and a renal biopsy is the only definitive way to do this. If the cause of delayed graft function is early cell-mediated rejection, it is necessary to adjust and augment the immunosuppressive regimen, and the most common strategy is to increase the dose of corticosteroids and antilymphocyte antibody. Delayed graft function increases the risk of cell-mediated rejection.[8] Additionally, delayed graft function is more likely to lead to allograft failure in patients with a 0-antigen match than in those with a 6-antigen match.[9]

Acute tubular necrosis is a common cause of renal dysfunction among hospitalized patients, including renal transplant recipients. The incidence of acute tubular necrosis after renal transplant is higher when the organ came from a cadaveric donor rather than from a living donor. Indeed, when expanded-criteria donors are used, it may be appropriate to increase the renal mass and give one patient both of the donor's kidneys. The logic of this approach has been well documented in an animal model of renal transplantation.[10]

Postrenal causes of delayed graft function are often related to the creation of a ureteroneocystostomy, which may become evident because of leaks or obstruction. Although stenting can be attempted to remediate these problems, reexploration is often necessary. A leak may be first noted because of delayed graft function, but it is sometimes diagnosed by the presence of fluid from a drain or the wound that has a higher concentration of creatinine than is present in plasma.

Lymphoceles may also develop and, if significant in size, require drainage to prevent external compression to the allograft's vascular supply. Drainage can be approached percutaneously or surgically by open or laparoscopic techniques.

PANCREAS TRANSPLANTATION

Pancreas transplantation may be carried out as an isolated procedure, simultaneously with kidney transplantation, or after kidney transplantation. The exocrine pancreas can be anastomosed with a segment of donor duodenum to the recipient's jejunum or bladder. The major postoperative complications are related to graft failure and include vascular and duodenal anastomotic leaks, rejection, and pancreatitis. Islet cell transplantation is another strategy for treating diabetes, but its success is often limited by the smaller β-cell mass transplanted compared with whole organ transplantation.[11]

Pancreatic function is difficult to monitor. Increasing circulating glucose concentration is the best clinical marker of pancreatic dysfunction. If dysfunction is suspected in the first 2 weeks after transplantation, arterial thrombosis must be in the differential diagnosis. Doppler ultrasonography should be completed urgently. The presence of a necrotic pancreas can lead to systemic inflammatory response syndrome and secondary acute respiratory distress syndrome. It is often wise to perform a transplant pancreatectomy rather than risk the morbidity and mortality associated with these serious complications.

If a duodenal leak is suspected, computed tomography should be performed to look for extraluminal contrast or air. Surgical repair is necessary. Further therapy is dictated by the means used to achieve drainage of the exocrine pancreas (i.e., enteric or bladder). Revision of the duodenojejunostomy to a Roux-en-Y anastomosis is a common approach to deal with an anastomotic leak with an enteral drainage system. These leaks may result in peritonitis from contamination of the peritoneal cavity with gastrointestinal contents. For bladder drainage, decompression with a Foley catheter is usually sufficient. A follow-up cystogram should be obtained when the patient is better.

All patients develop some degree of pancreatitis after transplantation, but this should peak and begin to decline in the first several postoperative days. Cell-mediated rejection must be gauged in the first weeks, and a pancreatic biopsy may become necessary. The possibility of cytomegalovirus infection can be investigated at that time and treated with antiviral therapy as necessary. Rejection requires enhancement of steroids and the administration of antilymphocyte thymoglobulin.

■ HEART TRANSPLANTATION

Caring for a heart transplant recipient postoperatively is more complex than caring for any other postcardiotomy patient. Most important, the preoperative condition of the recipient determines the potential risks for complications. As the number of cardiac transplant candidates grows without a corresponding increase in the number of organs available, patients wait longer to undergo the procedure, making the care of these patients even more complex. Advances in medical technology, such as ventricular assist devices (VADs), now permit patients with class IV heart failure to survive for extended periods. VADs can provide support for the right or left ventricle, or both, stabilizing patients with congestive heart failure and supporting perfusion of the lungs, kidneys, and liver. However, prolonged use of these devices places the transplant candidate at risk for developing other complications such as infection, hemolysis, or thrombosis, and the device may malfunction. Placement of a VAD also creates technical problems related to the need for a repeat sternotomy, concern for damage to the VAD cannulas, and added difficulties in placing the patient on cardiopulmonary bypass (CPB).

Recipient

The majority of heart transplant candidates are patients with class III or IV heart failure due to ischemic cardiomyopathy from coronary artery disease. Idiopathic and hypertrophic cardiomyopathies can also be treated with transplantation. Valvular disease leading to left ventricle failure, and congenital heart disease are less common indications for transplantation. Metabolic or immunologic disorders such as sarcoidosis and amyloidosis are rare causes of end-stage cardiac failure leading to transplantation.[12]

Regardless of the underlying etiology of heart failure, patients who meet criteria for transplantation must be refractory to the best medical therapies (angiotensin-converting enzyme inhibitors, beta-adrenergic receptor blockers, diuretics, inotropes) and without significant end-organ dysfunction.

Pulmonary vascular resistance (PVR) is a predictor of the function of the transplanted organ. PVR is a determinant of the right heart function of the donor organ. If the PVR index is greater than 6 to 8 Wood units per square meter or is unresponsive to treatment with a pulmonary vasodilator, then the patient should not be considered a transplant candidate.[13] Patients who perform poorly on metabolic stress testing with maximum peak oxygen consumption (VO_{2max}) less than 14 mL/kg/min have less than a 50% survival at 1 year and are considered candidates for heart transplantation.[14]

Donor

The adequacy of myocardial preservation and the length of ischemic time during recovery and transplantation of the donor heart are critical factors that influence the risk for postoperative complications for the recipient. Both myocardial preservation and ischemic time affect overall ventricular (especially right ventricular) function after completion of the transplant. The right ventricular myocardium is jeopardized more than the left ventricular myocardium by inadequate preservation. Injury to the right ventricle leads to right heart failure, which becomes evident as the recipient is weaned off CPB.

Postoperative Management

Postoperative care is determined in part by the medical state of the recipient and in part by the quality of the donor organ. Thus, the care of heart transplant recipients is dictated by their hemodynamic status and degree of end-organ dysfunction.

Postoperative bleeding can be more of a concern in cardiac transplant patients than in typical postcardiotomy patients for several reasons. Transplant recipients may have been therapeutically anticoagulated preoperatively, and this treatment may not have been reversed adequately prior to sternotomy. Need for reoperation or prolonged time in the operating room and on CPB can increase the risk for coagulopathy. Treatment of bleeding due to coagulopathy consists of administration of blood products and clotting factors.

The goal of hemodynamic support is to maintain systemic perfusion with an appropriate cardiac output (CO) while preventing right heart failure or overload. Appropriate management requires the use of a pulmonary artery catheter to evaluate CO and central venous and pulmonary artery pressures.

Inotropic support with the use of vasoactive drugs is often necessary to maintain the balance of end-organ perfusion, systemic arterial artery pressure, and PVR. Medications include milrinone, epinephrine, phenylephrine, and vasopressin, or combinations of these. Increased PVR can be treated with inhaled nitric oxide (NO) or epoprostenol. Persistently elevated PVR, leading to right heart failure and distention, may require short-term VAD support. Placement of an intra-aortic balloon pump may support right ventricular function by improving perfusion to the right ventricular myocardium.

In a normally innervated heart, a decrease in cardiac output results in an increase in heart rate. However, after transplantation, the recipient's new heart lacks parasympathetic and sympathetic innervation. Therefore, heart rate needs to be maintained by infusing chronotropic drugs and temporary epicardial pacing. The surgical procedure, whereby the donor heart is anastomosed to the recipient's remaining atrial tissue, results in two independent sets of contracting atria. Because of the surgical anastomosis, the recipient's sinus node electrical activity does not communicate or synchronize with the donor's atria. This results in an electrocardiogram with two sets of P-waves, but, more importantly, also leads to the loss of the normal atrial contribution to stroke volume. Over time (usually 1 to 2 weeks) the recipient becomes less dependent on external chronotropic support and can increase heart rate and stroke volume as needed based on the effects of endogenous circulating catecholamines. The patient also maintains a resting heart rate that is mildly elevated (90 to 120 beats/min) because of loss of vagal innervation.

Rejection of the transplanted heart peaks in the first month afer surgery. Symptoms and clinical signs are often nonspecific. Surveillance biopsies should be obtained every 1 to 2 weeks for several months. Thereafter, the frequency of this monitoring can be gradually decreased. Cardiac biopsies aid in the prompt recognition and treatment of rejection with intensified immunosuppression. Exact timing and frequency schedules depend on the specific transplant program.

Early graft failure, defined as cardiac dysfunction occurring within the first 30 days, may be caused in part by both donor and recipient parameters. Donor risk factors include older-age donors, long ischemic time, abnormal donor echocardiogram, and size discrepancy (small donor into large recipient). Although not a complication in the early postoperative period, cardiac allograft vasculopathy affects up to 50% of heart transplant recipients within 5 years of surgery. This problem accelerates diffuse obliterative atherosclerosis of the intramyocardial or epicardial coronary arteries and veins. This diffuse vascular intimal thickening obstructs blood flow and causes myocardial ischemia.[15]

■ LUNG TRANSPLANTATION

The focus in the following paragraphs is on the underlying disease processes of patients being evaluated for lung or heart-lung transplantation because the baseline pulmonary disease plays a significant role in postoperative management. The decision to do a single or double lung transplant will affect the treatment strategy for both the native and the transplanted lungs. Also, surgical approaches, with their intricacies, will alter management and pose different problems.

Allocation of donor lungs is determined more by waiting-list time than by geographic area and blood compatibility issues. As a result, patients are often listed early in their course and if necessary can become inactive on the list without losing their previous place in line. Patients in their 40s, 50s, and 60s account for the majority of transplant recipients. The largest cohort (between 50 to 64 years old) represents nearly 56%.[16]

The major primary diagnoses are emphysema, idiopathic pulmonary fibrosis, cystic fibrosis, α_1-antitrypsin deficiency, and primary pulmonary hypertension. In 2002, emphysema accounted for 39% of the lung transplants performed. The majority of recipients are not hospitalized at the time of transplantation. Recipients (from 2002 cohorts) in the intensive care unit (ICU) immediately prior to transplantation had significantly lower graft survival rates at all time points, compared with hospitalized and nonhospitalized cohorts.[16]

One-year adjusted graft survival (2001) was 77% and has been essentially unchanged over the past 9 years (75% graft survival in 1993). Patient survival was only slightly higher than graft survival. Retransplantation is rare (2% in

2002). One- and 5-year patient survivals were 78% and 45%, respectively.[16]

Living-donor lungs account for a very small number of transplants. Interestingly, the majority of living-donor lung recipients are in the ranges of 11 to 17 years and 18 to 34 years, consistent with recipients having a diagnosis of cystic fibrosis.[16]

Recipient

Candidates for lung transplantation have end-stage lung disease with a life expectancy of less than 2 years. Medical management has not been able to help these individuals. Exclusionary criteria include coexisting diseases that would adversely affect survival after transplantation, such as significant cardiac disease, cirrhosis, and malignancy.

Patients with emphysema should be considered for transplantation when the postbronchodilator forced expiratory volume in 1 second (FEV_1) is less than or equal to 25% of predicted. Single lung transplantation is most commonly performed, although sequential double lung transplantation is offered at some centers. Native lung hyperinflation may occur in the immediate postoperative period, which can be difficult to manage especially when the patient is on mechanical ventilation. For this reason, patients with significant bullous disease are often offered double lung transplants. Another option is lung volume reduction surgery on the native lung to control the underlying disease.[17]

Single lung transplantation is effective treatment for idiopathic pulmonary fibrosis. Decreases in lung compliance and perfusion of the native lung helps to maintain ventilation–perfusion (V/Q) matching of the transplanted lung.

Primary pulmonary hypertension can be treated with both single and double lung transplantation and, at times, heart-lung transplant. Centers that advocate double lung transplants argue that there is greater recovery of right ventricular function because of maximal reduction in PVR.[15]

Timing a transplantation for patients with cystic fibrosis is difficult. Malnutrition and colonization with resistant bacteria and fungi complicate decisions about the timing, the choice of single or double lung transplantation, and postoperative management.

The recipient operation can be done without the use of CPB, but CPB is scheduled when the patient has pulmonary hypertension and right heart failure. Single lung procedures are done via thoracotomy with exposure of the left atrium, transection of the bronchus and vascular structures, and then anastomosis of the donor bronchus, left atrium, and pulmonary artery. Double lung transplantation has evolved into sequential single lung procedures via a sternotomy with bilateral subcostal incisions.

Donor

Proper selection of the donor organ is crucial when evaluating lung donors. Most cadaveric donors have undergone a traumatic or other stressful situation that has resulted in extensive resuscitation and mechanical ventilation. Trauma patients could have sustained direct injury to the lung. Therefore, many potential donors are excluded from donating lungs because of pulmonary edema, pneumonia, contusions, or adult respiratory distress syndrome (ARDS).

Harvesting of the lungs is accomplished via median sternotomy with preservation of the organs with a cold pulmoplegia solution via the main pulmonary artery with simultaneous cardioplegic harvest of the heart.

Postoperative Management

The goals of postoperative care are the same as for any patient: appropriate ventilatory wean and extubation, early mobilization and nutrition, and prevention of infection by limiting the use of invasive lines and unnecessary antibiotics.

The goals of respiratory management are no different from those of any ICU patient: ventilatory support to maintain adequate oxygenation and ventilation without causing barotrauma or oxygen toxicity.

As discussed earlier, single lung transplantation for patients with emphysema results in differential compliance and V/Q mismatch. The native lung is more compliant than the donor lung, resulting in air trapping and hyperinflation. Overexpansion of the native lung shifts the lung toward the mediastinum, further decreasing compliance to the allograft. This phenomenon is more likely to occur when the allograft is placed on the left side, because the native organ (in the right thorax) is restricted from expanding in the caudal direction because of the liver. Reperfusion injury to the donor lung may further compromise compliance to the allograft. Therapies to combat such a V/Q mismatch include placement of a double-lumen tube and independent ventilation of the two lungs with lower tidal volumes and prolonged expiratory times to the native lung. Positioning the donor with the lung side upward may aid in improved ventilation to the allograft. With resolution of pulmonary edema from reperfusion injury to the allograft, single-lumen tube placement and unified ventilation can be successful and ventilatory weaning can be initiated.[18]

Differential perfusion to both organs can also occur with single lung transplantation for primary pulmonary hypertension. The donor lung in this situation has lower pulmonary pressures resulting in preferential blood flow to the transplanted organ. The increase in circulating blood volume, in turn, results in pulmonary edema to the allograft, further contributing to a potentially edematous lung from reperfusion injury. As with severe compliance differences, significant perfusion mismatch may need to be managed by independent ventilation of the two lungs with higher positive expiratory pressures to the allograft. Increases in intra-alveolar pressure will reduce the pressure gradient across the capillary bed and help to control pulmonary edema.[18]

Patients who undergo double lung transplants usually do not have significant issues with V/Q mismatch unless there is a difference in ischemia or the preservation of one of the two allografts. However, pulmonary edema from reperfusion injury can occur in both lungs. This would manifest as hypoxia and decreased compliance. The mechanisms of reperfusion injury are believed to be caused by long ischemia time, poor organ preservation, or immune-mediated injury. Long CPB times, large-volume resuscitation, and extensive use of blood products can add to edema of the lungs. In managing this condition, it is reasonable to employ the same maneuvers used to support patients with ARDS. All of these patients should be ventilated with low tidal volume ventilation (6 mL/kg of patient's ideal bodyweight).[19]

All lung transplant patients require aggressive pulmonary care including frequent suctioning, bronchodilators, deep coughing, postural drainage, and incentive spirometry. Ventilated patients may require daily bronchoscopy to maintain good pulmonary toilet.

Lung transplant patients are kept in a state of relative hypovolemia with judicial use of fluids, blood products, and inotropic support. These therapies are maintained while minimizing prerenal azotemia and maintaining adequate end-organ perfusion.

Aspiration can be a deadly complication and needs to be avoided at all costs. Aspiration precautions and swallowing evaluations are part of general care. Patients receiving enteral feedings should be maintained with head of bed elevation at 30 degrees and have feedings stopped well in advance of planned extubations.[12]

Anastomotic complications can have severe consequences to the lung transplant patient in the early postoperative period. These can be described as partial or full-thickness injuries ranging from necrosis and dehiscence to ulceration and formation of granulation tissue. Delayed complications include stricture formation and bronchomalacia.

The etiology of anastomotic complications is believed to involve ischemia. Bronchial arteries, which are fed by the aorta and intercostal arteries, are transected with procurement of the lung and are not reestablished with surgical implantation. The bronchial and tracheal anastomosis relies on retrograde flow through the pulmonary artery to collaterals from the bronchial arteries.[15]

A lung donor bronchial stump adds to the vulnerability of the anastomosis. Dissection and devascularization of the recipient's main bronchus up to the level of the carina further compromises anastomotic blood flow. Poor perfusion can be accentuated by hypotension, use of high-dose vasopressors, hypovolemia, poor organ preservation, long ischemia time, infection, and immunosuppression.

Necrosis and dehiscence typically occurs in the first few weeks after transplantation. Circumferential and large dehiscence must be treated as a surgical emergency, with debridement and reanastomosis of the bronchus. Coverage of the anastomosis with viable tissue and extensive drainage to treat pleural and mediastinal contamination is necessary. Localized areas of necrosis and dehiscence without pleural communication can be treated conservatively. A removable stent can be placed to act as scaffolding for secondary healing.

Weeks to months later, stricture formation may result from a healed necrotic or dehiscent area. Strictures are managed by dilation or laser resection. Stenting with wire or Silastic stents may be a necessary adjunct for the treatment of strictures. Airway obstruction caused by granulation tissue is usually remedied by laser ablation with stent placement, if there are recurrent and chronic problems. Bronchomalacia is characterized by airway collapse with obstruction on expiration. It can also be controlled with stent placement to support the involved area of the airway.[15]

Airway complications are reported to occur in 5% to 12% of cases at experienced transplant centers. The sequela of ischemia to the bronchial anastomosis is preemptively treated by the surgical management of the anastomosis at the time of implantation. Specifically, shortening of the donor bronchus to two or fewer cartilaginous rings proximal to the upper lobe take-off minimizes the watershed area of ischemia. Reinforcing the anastomosis with a vascularized flap (omentum, pericardium, or intercostal muscle) also aids in preventing anastomotic leaks. An intussuscepting anastomotic technique is performed at some transplant centers to help to accommodate size mismatch between the donor and recipient airway and to help to avoid extensive devascularization of the bronchus.[15]

Phrenic nerve injury is a potential intraoperative complication of lung transplantation. This is especially true in cases of repeat thoracotomy due to extensive pleural adhesions. Bilateral lung transplantation increases the risk of nerve damage. Nerve damage may be temporary or permanent and can be caused by stretching, crushing, thermal damage, or transection of the phrenic nerve. Phrenic nerve paralysis is a devastating complication that interferes with good pulmonary hygiene and may prevent independence from the ventilator.

Rejection as discussed here relates to the early postoperative period. Hyperacute rejection occurs immediately on reperfusion and is caused by preexisting antibodies to donor tissue. It is a rare event because of the routine screening of recipients and ABO matching.

Acute rejection is a cell-mediated process and can occur during the first 30 days after transplantation. It is diagnosed by both clinical and histologic criteria. In the early postoperative period, the histologic criteria are not very distinct and are difficult to separate from infection or from reperfusion injury. Therefore, the clinical presentation becomes crucial in the diagnosis. Symptoms of acute rejection include dyspnea, fatigue, dry cough, low-grade fever, malaise, and pulmonary infiltrates without evidence of infection.

Chronic rejection is manifested by obliterative bronchiolitis. This complication is caused by a fibroproliferative process that causes obliteration of tubular structures of the transplanted lung, similar to coronary artery vasculopathy seen in the transplanted heart.

■ IMMUNOSUPPRESSION

The goal of immunosuppressive therapy in solid organ transplant patients is to prevent rejection while limiting the adverse effects of the drugs, which include direct drug effects and secondary effects of immunosuppression (e.g., infection and cancer).

The major classes of immunosuppressive drugs are corticosteroids, antimetabolites, specific lymphocyte-signaling inhibitors, and antibodies. Combination therapy decreases the likelihood of adverse effects. Despite 4 decades of transplantation experience, achieving the delicate balance required to maintain enough immunosuppression to prevent rejection

of the transplanted organ and enough immunocompetence so that infections and cancer are held at bay remains a naive science. During the course of transplantation, different immunosuppressant medications are used in different amounts and at appropriate times. More immunosuppressant medication is needed during the induction phase (when there are more cellular and cytokine mechanisms that may lead to rejection) than later during the maintenance phase. During episodes of rejection, higher dosages of some of the same drugs may be used, or other drugs may be used, or both. Corticosteroids indiscriminately downregulate the immune system. In particular, expression and secretion of many proinflammatory cytokines are downregulated. It is ironic and telling that this drug class, which has the least specificity for the immune system, remains part of the scaffolding for all transplant regimens. Corticosteroids are given in high dosages, followed by a taper for a first episode of acute cellular rejection.

Azathioprine, a prodrug that is converted to mercaptopurine, is an antimetabolite. It is nonspecific and affects all rapidly dividing cells. Because lymphocytes are rapidly dividing cells, they are preferentially affected, which decreases the immune response. Intestinal cells divide rapidly and are injured by azathioprine, leading to the adverse side effect of diarrhea. The more tailored antimetabolites are mycophenolic acid and its prodrug mycophenolate mofetil, which has greater bioavailability. These drugs enzymatically inhibit the formation of the nucleoside guanosine, preferentially in T and B cells, avoiding some of the side effects of the azathioprine.

The calcineurin inhibitors cyclosporine and tacrolimus are the mainstays of immunosuppression. They work by inhibiting the lymphocyte signaling pathways that lead to interleukin-2 (IL-2) transcription. Cyclosporine and tacrolimus traverse the cell membrane and combine with cytoplasmic cyclophilin and FK binding protein (FKBP), respectively. Either one of these complexes inactivates calcineurin, an essential component of the enzyme complex that dephosphorylates nuclear factor for activated T cells (NFAT). NFAT traverses the nuclear membrane and ultimately prevents the transcription of IL-2. The major adverse effects in the early postoperative period include both neurotoxicity and nephrotoxicity. Both tacrolimus and cyclosporine cause a renal arteriolar vasoconstriction that may be reversible with low-dose intravenous nicardipine.

A newer drug, sirolimus (also called rapamycin), works through different cellular mechanisms. It, like tacrolimus, also binds to FKBP, and this complex then combines with mTOR (which stands for *molecular target of rapamycin*) and prevents protein translation from mRNA. Calcineurin is not involved in this reaction. Sirolimus does not have the neurotoxicity and nephrotoxicity seen with the calcineurin inhibitors.

A polyclonal antibody called antithymocyte globulin is prepared by injecting rabbits with human thymocytes. The antibody then attacks human T cells. It is used as rescue therapy in renal transplants when cellular rejection develops. It can cause the release of cytokines, and patients need to be monitored closely.

◼ INFECTIONS

Many infections can develop in the solid organ transplant patient after weeks to months on immunosuppression. In the immediate postoperative period, however, it is imperative to watch for the usual bacterial pathogens. Many of these patients were very sick preoperatively and now are susceptible to nosocomial infections, especially hospital-acquired pneumonia, ventilator-associated pneumonia, catheter-associated urinary tract infections, and catheter-related bloodstream infection. Catheters and tubes of all types should always be removed from patients as soon as possible. Indeed, these necessary tubes may be more responsible for the high incidence of postoperative infection than early immunosuppression.

Two organs deserve special mention in regard to bacterial infection. First, the liver is prone to biliary infections, particularly after hepatic artery thrombosis. Abscesses may require drainage. If the infection is confined to the liver, retransplantation is a viable option. Second, pneumonia in a transplanted lung could have disastrous consequences, so these patients must be observed closely for any signs and symptoms of pulmonary infection.

◼ CONCLUSION

The solid organ transplant recipient requires unique postoperative care. The quality of the organ is determined by the health of the donor and by postmortem factors such as warm and cold ischemia time and events at the surgery, including but not limited to, reperfusion. The preexisting health of the recipient also plays a role postoperatively. For patients with diabetes mellitus and renal failure, comorbid conditions include coronary artery disease. For the patient with cirrhosis, years of muscle wasting may leave the patient profoundly weak. Postoperative decisions that would be appropriate for nontransplant patients may be inappropriate for transplant patients. For example, transient hypoxemia or hypotension might be tolerated in other patients, but these problems can lead to early damage to the graft in transplant recipients. It is easy to ignore these issues in the early postoperative period but they are essential to the long-term outcome of the graft and, of course, the patient.

◼ REFERENCES

1. Port FK, Dykstra DM, Merion RM, Wolfe RA: Organ donation and transplantation trends in the USA, 2003. Am J Transplant 2004;4(Suppl 9):7-12.
2. Saggi BH, Farmer DG, Yersiz H, Busuttil RW: Surgical advances in liver and bowel transplantation. Anesthesiol Clin North America 2004;11:713-740.
3. Schulak JA: What's new in general surgery: Transplantation. J Am Coll Surg 2005;200:409-417.
4. Killenberg PG, Clavien PA: Medical Care of the Liver Transplant Patient, ed 2. Boston, Blackwell Science, 2001, pp 105-122.
5. Molmenti EP, Klintmalm GB: Atlas of Liver Transplantation. Philadelphia, Saunders, 2002, pp 135-177.
6. Jacobs LB, Shirey RS, Ness PN: Hemolysis due to the simultaneous occurrence of passenger lymphocyte syndrome and delayed hemolytic transfusion reaction in a liver transplant patient. Arch Pathol Lab Med 1996;120:684-686.
7. Wolfe RA: Comparison of mortality in all patients on dialysis, patients on dialysis awaiting transplantation, and recipients of a first cadaveric transplant. N Engl J Med 1999;341:1725-1730.
8. Shoskes DA, Cecka JM: Deleterious effects of delayed graft function in cadaveric renal transplant recipients independent of acute rejection. Transplantation 1998;66:1697-1701.
9. Shoskes DA, Hodge EE, Goormastic M, et al: HLA matching determines susceptibility to harmful effects of delayed graft function in renal transplant recipients. Transplant Proc 1995;27:1068-1069.
10. Mackenzie HS, Azuma H, Rennke H, et al: Renal mass as a determinant of late allograft outcome: Insights from experimental studies in rats. Kidney Int 1995;48:S38-42.
11. Sutherland DER, Gruessner R, Kandswamy R, et al: Beta-cell replacement therapy (pancreas and islet transplantation) for treatment of diabetes mellitus: An integrated approach. Transplant Proc 2004;36: 1697-1699.
12. Goudarzi BM, Bonvino S: Critical care issues in lung and heart transplantation. Crit Care Clin 2003;19:209-231.
13. Chanewise J: Cardiac transplantation. Anesthesiol Clin North America 2004;22:753-765.
14. Massad MG: Current trends in heart transplantation. Cardiology 2004;101:79-92.
15. Kuo PC, Schroeder RA, Johnson LB: Clinical Management of the Transplant Patient. London, Arnold, 2001, pp 74-103.
16. Pierson RN, Barr ML, McCullough KP, et al: Thoracic organ transplantation. Am J Transplant 2004;4(Supp 9):93-105.
17. Nathan SD: Lung transplantation: Disease-specific considerations for referral. Chest 2005;127:1006-1016.
18. Rosenberg AL, Rao M, Benedict PE: Anesthetic implications for lung transplantation. Anesthesiol Clin North America 2004;22:767-788.
19. Brower RG, Lanken PN, MacIntyre N, et al: National Heart, Lung, and Blood Institute ARDS Clinical Trials Network. Higher versus lower positive end-expiratory pressures in patients with the acute respiratory distress syndrome. N Engl J Med. 2004;351: 327-336.

Chapter

36 | Multisystem Trauma

Patrick K. Kim and Patrick M. Reilly

Care of the patient with multisystem trauma is challenging. Although well-defined constellations of injury exist, ultimately each patient is unique in preinjury health, injury complex, and postinjury management. Because many injuries are managed nonoperatively, many patients have no postoperative phase per se. However, some injured patients require multiple operations, and the distinction between postoperative care and preoperative care is blurred: the fundamental principles of care of the injured patient are similar to those of the postsurgical patient. The trauma patient's stress response is a function of the severity of injury. The postoperative or postinjury course of the trauma patient should be assessed with this paradigm in mind.

Initial evaluation of the injured patient typically follows guidelines set forth by the American College of Surgeons Advanced Trauma Life Support (ATLS) program. The ATLS paradigm of primary, secondary, and tertiary surveys prioritizes the ABCs—airway, breathing, and circulation—and ensures that the most immediately life-threatening injuries are diagnosed and treated before moving on to other injuries. The trauma evaluation is rapid and comprehensive, utilizing physical examination, vital signs, radiographs, and, increasingly, ultrasound. The patient's subsequent disposition—to the operating room, interventional radiology suite, computed tomography suite, intensive care unit (ICU), or general care floor—is based on the findings of the primary and secondary survey.

■ RESUSCITATION

Choice of Resuscitation Fluid

The fluid of choice for resuscitation after hemorrhage control in critically ill and injured patients is still controversial. Crystalloid solutions are less expensive but are theoretically less effective for maintaining intravascular volume. Although colloid solutions are more expensive, they theoretically remain longer in the intravascular space (at least for longer than crystalloid), and thus smaller volumes are required for infusion. Studies have not consistently shown one to be superior to the other for ICU resuscitation. The largest prospective randomized trial to address this issue is the Saline versus Albumin Fluid Evaluation (SAFE) trial,[1] which compared normal saline to 4% albumin for resuscitation in ICU patients. This trial showed no benefit of albumin over saline in a large cohort of ICU patients. In fact, post hoc subgroup analysis suggested that trauma patients in the albumin resuscitation group may have fared worse than those in the saline resuscitation group, but this was not conclusive.

Although the issue of crystalloid versus colloid has not been settled definitively, it is clear that over-resuscitation can occur with any fluid and lead to a variety of complications, both immediate and delayed (see later). Thus the choice of resuscitation fluid is probably less important than the timing and volume of resuscitation.

Transfusion Triggers

The concept of transfusion threshold should be applied very carefully in the trauma population: Any threshold for transfusion presupposes control of hemorrhage. Stated more bluntly, transfusion thresholds do not apply to patients who are still bleeding.

Not surprisingly, anemia is common in the postinjury period, especially among injured patients admitted to the ICU.[2] Enthusiasm for transfusion of blood and blood products is diminishing. When other factors are controlled for, blood transfusion correlates with organ dysfunction, mortality, and ICU length of stay.[3,4] Studies in trauma patients have suggested that blood transfusion is an independent predictor of worsened outcomes in patients with solid organ injuries.[5] Large controlled trials in critically ill patients have suggested that restrictive blood transfusion practices (e.g., a hemoglobin transfusion trigger of 7 g/dL) are equal or superior in mortality to more liberal transfusion practices (e.g., a transfusion trigger of 10 g/dL).[6] A smaller body of literature suggests the same is true in the injured population. Post hoc analysis of the Transfusion Requirements in Critical Care (TRICC) trial confirmed the safety of restrictive transfusion practices in trauma patients.[7] Both protocols are similar in terms of mortality and incidence of multiple organ dysfunction. A postinjury practice management guideline is safe and cost effective.[8] Although the transfusion trigger for patients with active cardiac ischemia and patients with head injury is not known, it is likely that most other injured patients with hemorrhage control will not benefit from liberal transfusion strategies.

Massive Transfusion and Its Alternatives

Many centers have established trauma exsanguination ("massive transfusion") protocols that permit hospital blood banks to rapidly release standard quantities of uncrossmatched type O-negative blood, plasma, and platelets at regular intervals until hemorrhage is controlled (Fig. 36-1). Despite being a strain on hospital blood banks, such protocols appear to be justified by studies showing reasonable survival rates—30% to 60%—among patients who underwent massive transfusions (sometimes >60 units).[9-12]

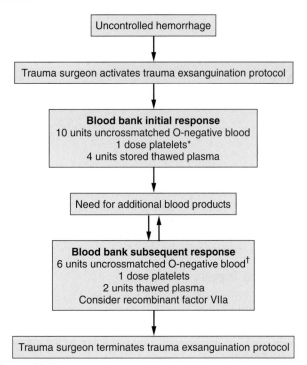

Figure 36-1 ■ Example of a trauma exsanguination protocol. *Equivalent to one "6-pack" of platelets. †Crossmatched blood when available.

Tradeoffs include risks of transfusion reaction, transmission of blood-borne diseases, and infectious and immune complications.

Allogeneic blood transfusion is still the mainstay for restoring the circulating volume of the exsanguinating patient. Blood substitutes such as hemoglobin-based oxygen carriers (HBOCs) have been studied extensively in animal and human trials. HBOCs have been shown to safely decrease the total amount of allogeneic blood transfusion in injured patients.[13,14] Studies may confirm the utility of HBOCs as a primary prehospital resuscitative fluid.[15]

Human recombinant factor VIIa has emerged as a viable option for control of hemorrhage. Mirroring the factor VIIa experience in hemophiliacs and patients with hepatic failure, many case reports and small case series have suggested rapid arrest of exsanguinating hemorrhage after trauma. Furthermore, factor VIIa administration causes complete correction of prothrombin time. This correction is a laboratory phenomenon, however, and not necessarily indicative of hemorrhage control. Also relevant to the exsanguinating trauma patient, recombinant factor VIIa has decreased activity below pH 7.10. Recombinant factor VIIa may decrease total transfusion volume after severe blunt injury but has not yet demonstrated improvement in survival.[16-18] Thrombotic events do not seem to be inordinate in the few studies that have placebo comparison. Until more data are available, factor VIIa may be best employed in trauma exsanguination policies as a second-line adjunct *after* adequate administration of blood components and only with adequate pH control (Box 36-1).

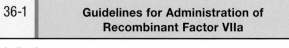

| 36-1 | Guidelines for Administration of Recombinant Factor VIIa |

Indications

- Transfusion requirement after >10 units of packed ed blood cells are transfused

Contraindications

- Known or suspected severe coronary artery disease or peripheral vascular disease
- Presence of surgical bleeding

Dosage

- 90 μg/kg rounded up to the nearest 1.2 mg. May repeat dose after 2 hr.
- Additional doses in consultation with hematology clinician

Requisites for optimal activity of recombinant factor VIIa

- pH >7.10
- Platelets >100,000/mm^3
- International Normalized Ratio <1.5
- Fibrinogen >100 mg/dL

| 36-2 | Endpoints of Resuscitation* |

Clinical

- Warm distal extremities
- Palpable distal pulses
- Brisk capillary refill
- Normal mentation
- Temperature >97°F
- Heart rate <100 (excluding patients on beta blockade)
- Systolic blood pressure >90 mm Hg
- Urine output >0.5 mL/kg bodyweight

Laboratory

- Stable hemoglobin ≥7.0 mg/dL (consider ≥9.0 mg/dL for head-injured patients)
- Base deficit <5 mmol/L in absolute value
- Serum lactic acid <2.0 mmol/L
- International Normalized Ratio <1.5

Monitoring

- Mean arterial pressure >65 mm Hg
- Central venous pressure 6 to 12 mm Hg
- Central venous O$_2$ saturation >65%
- Cardiac index 2.0 L/min/m^2
- Stroke volume 0.5 to 1.0 mL/kg
- Intracranial pressure <20 mm Hg
- Cerebral perfusion pressure >60 mm Hg
- Brain tissue O$_2$ partial pressure >20 mm Hg
- Abdominal compartment pressure <20 mm Hg

*General guidelines are presented here. Specific endpoints vary by patient and injury pattern.

Endpoints of Resuscitation

Judgment is an essential component of multisystem trauma resuscitation. Not all endpoints are applicable to all patients, and a global perspective of the patient's status is as important as attention to minute details. Endpoints can be classified as clinical, laboratory, or monitoring (Box 36-2).

The initial assessment of the trauma patient began with evaluating and treating the ABCs, and the ongoing care should ensure that the ABCs remain intact. Changes in hemodynamics or oxygenation should prompt reassessment of airway, breathing, and circulation, especially confirming proper position and function of endotracheal tube, chest tubes, catheters, monitors, and surgical drains. In the early postinjury period, hypotension should be assumed to be caused by hemorrhage until proven otherwise.

The traditional clinical indicators—blood pressure, heart rate, urine output, distal perfusion, and mentation—should be used as a starting point for assessing resuscitation. Abnormalities of these basic signs should prompt thorough physical examination and close monitoring of interventions (fluid challenge, analgesia, sedation). Several caveats relevant to the injured patient should be mentioned: Tachycardia is nonspecific and may represent hypovolemia, pain, agitation, presence of illicit substances, or myocardial injury. On the other hand, tachycardia may be absent or blunted in patients who were receiving beta-blocker therapy before the injury. Regarding blood pressure, essential hypertension is widely prevalent, and "normal" blood pressure may in fact be *relative* hypotension, and possibly indicative of hypovolemia. Finally, mental status may be altered by hypoperfusion, brain injury, or the presence of illicit substances.

Laboratory studies are useful for assessing endpoints of resuscitation. Postinjury acidosis, as manifested by persistently elevated lactic acid or by base deficit (or persistently low serum bicarbonate), suggests occult hypoperfusion or devitalized tissue. Although the initial value (i.e., immediately on arrival to the trauma center) has correlation to outcome,[19] the trend over hours is more useful for assessing treatments and predicting mortality.[20] Persistent acidosis is a grave sign. Failure to normalize serum lactic acid level by 24 hours after injury is associated with worse outcome in injured patients.[20] Similarly, persistent base deficit correlates with worse outcomes.[21]

Trauma patients who suffer deterioration of these indicators should be presumed to have ongoing or uncontrolled hemorrhage in the thorax, abdomen, retroperitoneum, and extremities. After physical examination, chest radiograph and focused abdominal sonography for trauma (FAST) may help triage the chest and abdominal cavities by diagnosing or excluding recurrent hemothorax or new hemoperitoneum. Hemorrhage in the thorax, abdomen, or extremities that is brisk enough to result in hypotension or acidosis often requires control in the operating room. However, hemorrhage from hepatic lacerations, pelvic fractures, or retroperitoneal injury is difficult to control in the operating room and instead may require interventional radiology—angiography for diagnosis and embolization for treatment.

Despite the vast cumulative experience with central venous pressure (CVP) monitoring, the amount of objective data available to guide clinicians in deciding which injured patients to monitor is limited. CVP monitoring is probably indicated for patients who have hemorrhage control but have not responded appropriately to initial volume resuscitation, or for patients with chronic cardiac and pulmonary disease and low physiologic reserve. The endpoints are similar to that of postsurgical patients.

The pulmonary artery (PA) catheter remains controversial in trauma patients. Although PA catheterization is theoretically attractive and commonly used, retrospective and prospective studies of critically ill patients have not consistently demonstrated that it has a mortality benefit compared with central venous monitoring.[22,23] Furthermore, these studies typically have relatively small numbers of injured patients, making results more difficult to apply to the trauma patient. It is likely that the benefit of the PA catheter is not in its presence or absence, but in how the clinician uses the data that are available. Ultimately, the usefulness of the PA catheter may lie in optimizing ventricular preload and overall cardiac efficiency[24,25] and in preventing *over*-resuscitation.

Many methods of assessing regional visceral perfusion have been proposed as adjuncts to clinical examination, laboratory studies, and central monitoring. Gastric tonometry demonstrates good correlation with other indices of global perfusion,[26] but it has not found widespread clinical acceptance. Sublingual capnometry may also prove to be a useful, noninvasive marker of perfusion.[27,28] Esophageal Doppler and surface ultrasound techniques have been investigated as noninvasive means of assessing cardiac output and preload, respectively.[29] Further studies will clarify their roles in achieving adequate resuscitation of the injured patient.

■ SPECIAL CONSIDERATIONS IN TRAUMA

Damage Control

Damage control has become widely employed in the care of the severely injured patient.[30-32] The paradigm involves rapid control of exsanguinating hemorrhage and gastrointestinal contamination (phase I), followed by resuscitation in the surgical ICU (phase II), then a return to the operating room for thorough identification and definitive treatment of injuries (phase III). Sometimes, multiple cycles between surgical ICU and OR are necessary, depending on the extent of injury and physiologic stability. Some patients have insufficient fascia in the abdominal domain after prolonged periods of damage control and require skin graft closure of the abdomen (phase IV) (Fig. 36-2). Originally described for abdominal injuries, damage control concepts have been extended to the thorax, extremities, neck, and even the cranium.

Successful implementation of damage control requires the coordinated efforts of the surgical team, anesthesiology team, and surgical intensivist team. In the trauma bay, the patient is rapidly evaluated by the trauma team using ATLS guidelines. Large-bore intravenous access is obtained, and a combined crystalloid and colloid resuscitation is initiated. The airway is secured by rapid-sequence intubation. Based on examination findings, vital signs, and initial imaging studies—typically chest and pelvic radiographs and FAST—the patient is transported to the operating room. Additional uncrossmatched blood is quickly released from the blood bank, usually via a trauma exsanguination protocol, while the crossmatch is performed. The surgical team begins lapa-

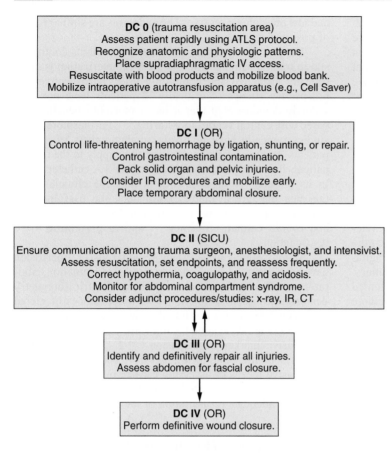

Figure 36-2 ■ The phases of damage control. ATLS, Advanced Trauma Life Support; CT, computed tomography; DC, damage control; IR, interventional radiology; OR, operating room; SICU, surgical intensive care unit.

rotomy and quickly packs all quadrants of the abdominal cavity. Meanwhile, the anesthesiology team begins aggressive resuscitation of the patient with blood and blood products. The surgical team systematically explores the abdominal cavity. The goal of the initial operation is rapid control of life-threatening hemorrhage and massive gastrointestinal contamination. Injuries to major arteries are shunted; injuries to smaller arteries and most veins (except suprarenal inferior vena cava) are ligated; gastrointestinal injuries are quickly closed primarily or resected with staplers without reestablishing continuity; and liver injuries are packed; splenic and renal injuries are treated by splenectomy or nephrectomy, respectively. The abdominal fascia is not closed. Rather, temporary abdominal closure is performed, for which many methods have been described. Patients with hepatic or pelvic injuries identified at the initial operation may require diagnostic arteriography and embolization immediately postoperatively. Among patients with hepatic injuries, the therapeutic yield of interventional radiology is high.[33]

Phase II is the surgical ICU phase of damage control. With cavitary hemorrhage and gastrointestinal contamination temporarily controlled by the trauma team, the intensivist team is charged with attaining physiologic "capture" of the patient. The goal of phase II is to prevent or reverse the lethal triad of hypothermia, coagulopathy, and acidosis.

Several measures are available to prevent and treat hypothermia. Straightforward measures decrease heat loss and allow rewarming, albeit slowly, by increasing the tempera-

ture of the room and using blankets, warming lights, and forced-air warming blankets. An intravenous fluid warmer should be used. The ventilator circuit should have warmed air. Warming pads, placed against the torso and extremities, are highly effective for rewarming. Warmed fluid is circulated through tubes in the pads. Although cavitary lavage with warmed fluid is described, it is unclear that the rate of rewarming is better than other, less invasive methods. The most rapid and invasive method of rewarming is venovenous bypass, but its primary disadvantage is the requirement for full systemic heparinization.

Coagulopathy is multifactorial, resulting from blood loss, consumption and dilution of platelets and clotting factors, accelerated fibrinolysis, impaired function of blood components, hypothermia, and hypocalcemia.[34] ProTime (PT) and activated partial thromboplastin time (aPTT) are usually performed at $37°C$. Thus in the normothermic patient, abnormalities of PT and aPTT indicate clotting factor deficiency. However, in the hypothermic patient, these studies fail to assess the qualitative deficiency of coagulation and thus *underestimate* coagulopathy. Similarly, infusion of crystalloid, colloid, and red blood cells after hemorrhage contributes to thrombocytopenia, which further worsens coagulation in the hypothermic patient with quantitative and qualitative clotting factor deficiencies. As is true for coagulation factors, the contribution of platelets to hemostasis is dependent on both platelet number and relative function. Given the importance of coagulation in trauma, there is little consensus for replacement of blood components in coagulopathic patients. Guidelines are largely based on expert opinion. Both prophylactic and objective approaches have been proposed. Objective approaches suggest plasma transfusion when PT or aPTT is greater than 1.5 times normal, cryoprecipitate transfusion when fibrinogen is less than 100 mg/dL, or platelet transfusion when platelet count is less than 50,000/mm[3].[34] The ranges of recommended ratios of fresh-frozen plasma to red blood cells (RBCs) or of platelets to RBCs in prophylactic transfusions vary too widely to make an evidence-based recommendation, but transfusion to restore whole blood may be reasonable.[35]

Acidosis is primarily caused by hypoperfusion and hypothermia and so should correct when normothermia and circulating volume are restored. Acidosis per se should not be treated with bicarbonate solutions except to treat myocardial irritability (i.e., pH <7.2).

Intra-abdominal Hypertension and the Abdominal Compartment Syndrome

Intra-abdominal hypertension (IAH) and the abdominal compartment syndrome (ACS) are well-recognized complications of critically ill trauma patients. Injury, hemorrhage, ischemia, reperfusion, and resuscitation all contribute to these complications. IAH exists when the pressure in the abdomen is elevated without evidence of organ dysfunction. ACS exists when abdominal hypertension causes organ dysfunction or failure. Typically, the bladder pressure is used as a surrogate for intra-abdominal pressure. The bladder is filled with 50 mL sterile saline, and the bladder catheter tubing is clamped. The pressure of the system is transduced. The normal intra-abdominal pressure is between 5 and 10 mm Hg. Mild IAH exists between 10 and 20 mm Hg. Severe IAH exists at greater than 25 mm Hg, and ACS is likely when intra-abdominal pressures exceed 35 mm Hg. IAH is heralded by a rising central venous pressure (CVP), by high peak airway pressures or difficulty generating tidal volume, by oliguria or worsening renal function, or by worsening or new onset of lactic acidosis. Immediate decompressive laparotomy is indicated to relieve the pressure and restore perfusion. Risk factors for ACS include large crystalloid infusions, and blood transfusion of greater than 10 units.[36] After decompressive laparotomy, the abdominal fascia is left open, and a temporary abdominal closure is fashioned to cover the viscera without exerting tension on the closure. Even so, recurrent ACS in the open abdomen has been described.[37] Even when treated, ACS is associated with increased morbidity and mortality.[38] There is growing appreciation for the iatrogenic component of IAH and ACS,[39] highlighting the importance of reaching—but not exceeding—resuscitation endpoints.[40]

Other Compartment Syndromes

Both blunt and penetrating mechanisms put tissue at risk for compartment syndromes. Extremities—not only calves but also thighs, buttocks, and upper extremities—should be examined carefully for increases in tenseness. Extremities with increased tenseness should be immediately evaluated by a surgeon. The presence of a distal pulse that can be detected by Doppler ultrasonography or palpated does not rule out compartment syndrome. New onset of pain should alert the physician, but pain is often already present, and its absence does not rule out compartment syndrome. Other neurologic findings, such as motor or sensory deficits, should prompt immediate surgical evaluation. Invasive monitoring of compartment pressures may help establish the diagnosis, but normal pressures may lead to a false sense of security. In general, it is safer to act on a strong clinical suspicion than to allow compartment syndrome to go untreated. Wide fasciotomies should be performed immediately if compartment syndrome is diagnosed or clinically suspected.

Management of Patients with Brain Injury

Resuscitation of brain-injured patients deserves special mention. Although clinical signs and laboratory studies are useful for global perfusion, head-injured patients with severe head injury (Glasgow Coma score [GCS] ≤8) benefit from more direct assessment of brain perfusion. Outcome after head injury is markedly dependent on cerebral perfusion. Hypotension and hypoxemia are to be avoided at all costs. Even one brief episode of hypotension (systolic blood pressure [BP] <90 mm Hg) or hypoxemia (PaO$_2$ ≤60 mm Hg) is detrimental to long-term outcome after head injury.[41] The clinically relevant index of brain perfusion is cerebral perfusion pressure (CPP), defined as the difference between mean arterial pressure (MAP) and intracranial pressure (ICP). Retrospective studies suggest that failure to maintain CPP above 60 mm Hg is associated with worse outcome.[42,43] ICP monitors can guide medical therapies (e.g., fluids and/or pressors to increase CPP; osmotic diuretic to decrease ICP). Maintaining ICP consistently at less than 20 mm Hg probably improved outcome after brain injury.[44] The Brain Trauma Foundation recommends ICP monitoring in the following situations:

- Severe head injury (defined as GCS 3 to 8) with abnormal computed tomography (CT) of the head at admission (e.g., CT demonstrates hematoma, contusion, edema, or compressed basal cisterns)
- Severe head injury with normal CT of the head at admission and two or more of the following at admission: age greater than 40 years, unilateral or bilateral motor posturing, systolic BP less than 90 mm Hg
- At the physician's discretion among conscious patients with traumatic mass lesions

Furthermore, the ICP transducer may have a ventriculostomy catheter to allow drainage of cerebrospinal fluid (CSF) and thereby decrease the ICP. CPP is increased by increasing MAP (volume resuscitation, then vasopressor if necessary) and/or by decreasing ICP (by an osmotic diuretic agent such as mannitol, or by drainage of CSF). The ideal transfusion trigger for brain-injured patients is not known. The traditional trigger is 10 g/dL, but this has recently been challenged. Until more definitive studies are completed, it is prudent to be more liberal in RBC transfusion when caring for brain-injured patients. Hypertonic saline is a safe and effective component of brain trauma resuscitation[45] and should be considered after colloid resuscitation. Deliberate hyperventilation is indicated for acute control of ICP, but it has no benefit as a sustained ICU therapy, because the ICP control by hyperventilation is based on decreased cerebral blood flow.

Cerebral cortical oxygenation is being investigated as an adjunct to ICP monitoring.[46] These devices alert the clinician to occult brain tissue hypoxia (partial pressure of oxygen (PO_2) <15 to 20 mm Hg)—that is, ischemic brain tissue despite adequate CPP. Further studies will clarify its role in brain resuscitation.

Venous Thromboembolism

Injured patients are at markedly higher risk for deep venous thrombosis (DVT) and pulmonary embolism (PE) than either uninjured patients or other groups of hospitalized patients. Meta-analysis reveals an overall DVT rate of 11.8% and a PE rate of 1.5% among all injured patients.[47]

Despite the frequency of thromboembolic complications, there is significant controversy and variability in current practice. Most trauma centers have developed standardized approaches to prophylaxis for venous thromboembolic events (Box 36-3). Patients who have any risk factor should undergo surveillance duplex within 3 to 5 days of admission. Early mobilization is the simplest prophylactic measure of all. However, many patients are limited by their injuries or mental status. Many single-center studies have demonstrated efficacy of one or more of the three most common prophylaxis measures—mechanical prophylaxis with sequential compression devices (SCD), low-dose unfractionated subcutaneous heparin (SQH), and subcutaneous low-molecular-weight heparin (LMWH). When subjected to meta-analysis, none of the measures was statistically more effective than no prophylaxis at all,[47] but this meta-analysis was insufficiently powered to exclude a true benefit of any of the therapies. Among SCD, SQH, and LMWH, LMWH is probably the best choice for DVT prophylaxis in injured patients who are not at excessive risk for bleeding.[48] LMWH is more effective than SQH in prevention of DVT with no increased risk for bleeding complications. Contraindications to LMWH include renal insufficiency or renal failure, or the presence of an epidural analgesia catheter. In these situations, unfractionated heparin and intermittent compression devices are acceptable alternatives.

The groups at highest risk for thromboembolic events are those with immobility from spinal cord injury, combined long-bone and posterior element pelvic fractures, multiple (more than three) long-bone fractures, or combined long-bone fracture and serious head or neck injury. Patients in the highest risk category for DVT and PE in whom hemorrhage would be fatal (e.g., with intracranial injury, posterior element pelvic fracture) should receive inferior vena cava (IVC) filter as thromboembolic prophylaxis. For patients at high risk for thromboembolic events who cannot undergo anticoagulation or tolerate additional bleeding (e.g., patients with intracranial hemorrhage, pelvic hematoma, ocular injury with hemorrhage, or injury to liver, spleen, or kidney), pro-

36-3	**Venous Thromboembolism Prophylaxis Risk Stratification**

Low risk

- Absence of all standard, high, and very high factors

Standard risk

- Age >40 yr
- Immobilization
- Minor pelvis fracture
- Foot, ankle, or fibula fracture
- Extensive soft tissue trauma
- Surgical procedure >2-hr duration
- Injury Severity Score (ISS) >9
- Pregnancy
- Estrogen therapy
- History of deep venous thrombosis or pulmonary embolism
- Malignancy
- Hypercoagulable state (e.g., antithrombin III deficiency)
- Blood transfusion
- Congestive heart failure

High risk

- Age >50 years
- Glasgow Coma Scale score (GCS) <8
- Complex pelvic fracture
- Femur or tibia fracture
- ISS >16
- Abbreviated Injury Score (AIS) >3 (any body region)
- Femoral venous catheter
- Venous injury

Very high risk

- Spinal cord injury
- AIS head/neck >3 **and** any long-bone fracture
- Severe pelvic fracture (e.g., posterior element) **and** any long-bone fracture
- Three or more long-bone fractures

Management

	Early Mobilization	SCD or LMWH	Surveillance Duplex	Prophylactic IVC Filter
Low risk	X			
Standard risk	X	X		
High risk	X	X	X	
Very high risk	X	X	X	Consider

IVC, inferior vena cava; LMWH, low-molecular-weight (fractionated) heparin; SCD, sequential compression device.

Contraindications to Anticoagulation

- Intracranial injury
- Epidural analgesia catheter
- Posterior element pelvic fracture (relative)
- Solid organ injury (relative)

phylactic placement of an IVC filter has been advocated. The long-term sequelae of IVC filters are not known. A variety of removable IVC filters exist, and they should be considered in patients who are expected to regain mobility with rehabilitation.

■ OTHER POSTINJURY CONSIDERATIONS

Stress Ulcer Prophylaxis

Injured patients have an increased risk for stress ulcers, and prophylaxis is indicated for patients with coagulopathy, mechanical ventilation for longer than 48 hours, or a history of upper gastrointestinal bleeding. Furthermore, prophylaxis should be considered for patients with central nervous system injury, corticosteroid therapy, vasopressor therapy, burns, cirrhosis or hepatic failure, and a history of peptic ulcer disease (Box 36-4). A variety of treatment options exist (sucralfate, ranitidine, and proton-pump inhibitors [PPIs]). Sucralfate and histamine-2 receptor antagonists (H_2RAs) have been studied extensively in critically ill patients, and experience with PPIs for prophylaxis in the ICU is increasing. Among mechanically ventilated patients, sucralfate and H_2RAs are effective for prevention of bleeding, with H_2RAs possibly slightly more effective.[49] Some studies suggest that sucralfate is associated with a lower rate of nosocomial pneumonia,[50] but others have been unable to show a difference.[51,52] PPIs appear to be at least as effective a prophylactic agent as sucralfate and H_2RAs,[53,54] and they have a favorable side-effect profile. The relative risk for nosocomial pneumonia with PPI therapy compared with sucralfate and H_2RAs is not known.

Nutrition Support

Nutrition support is of utmost importance in the injured patient once acute hemodynamic issues have been addressed. Injured patients are catabolic and have nutritional requirements up to 40% higher than in the preinjury state (the notable exception is spinal cord injury patients, who may have lower nutritional needs). Both enteral nutrition and parenteral nutrition have roles in postinjury care. The enteral route is preferred. Among critically ill patients, especially those with abdominal injury, enteral nutrition is associated with a lower rate of septic complications (pneumonia, intra-abdominal abscess, line sepsis) than the parenteral route.[55-58] Enteral nutrition is ideally initiated in the hemodynamically stable patient within 3 days of injury. Although technically feasible, it is not clear that "early" enteral nutrition (i.e., initiated within 24 hours of injury) is more beneficial than enteral nutrition initiated 72 hours after injury. About half of all patients cannot tolerate goal enteral nutrition at 1 week postinjury. Parenteral nutrition should be considered in patients who do not achieve at least 50% of goal enteral nutrition by postinjury day 7.

Enteral nutrition can be delivered by the intragastric or postpyloric route. Neither route has been proven superior in trauma patients. Because intragastric feeding is typically simpler, it should be the first choice. Postpyloric feeds should be considered for patients with high gastric residuals, especially patients with head injury, in whom gastroparesis is common. Definitions of high gastric residuals vary, but generally the residual should be less than half of the volume administered when checked 30 minutes after administration. Enteral formulas with various supplements (e.g., arginine, glutamine, fish oils) have been studied in critical care populations, including trauma patients, but no specific enteral formulation has demonstrated consistently superior outcomes. Based on systematic review, guidelines have not formally recommended enhanced enteral nutrition formulas but simply suggest considering them.[59] Rather, it appears that simply avoiding starvation is the key to reducing septic morbidity in the critically ill.

Glycemic Control

Intensive glycemic control has been shown to decrease complications and mortality in surgical patients.[60] Hyperglycemia in trauma patients is associated with increased infectious complications and mortality.[61-64] Injured patients with a serum glucose level of greater than 200 mg/dL have consistently demonstrated worsened outcomes: increased ICU length of stay (and thus increased hospital length of stay), longer duration of mechanical ventilation, higher rates of infection, and higher mortality. However, milder hyperglycemia—serum glucose between 110 and 200 mg/dL—has not consistently shown harm in injured patients. In one study, there was no significant correlation between hyperglycemia and mortality when hyperglycemia was defined as a serum glucose level greater than 110 mg/dL or greater than 150 mg/dL,[62] whereas another study suggested that harm occurs at a serum glucose level of greater than 135 mg/dL.[61] At present, serum glucose should certainly be maintained below 200 mg/dL, with a target somewhere between normoglycemia and mild hyperglycemia, avoiding hypoglycemia.

Infectious Complications

Trauma patients often have gastric contents present at the time of injury, placing them at higher risk for aspiration pneumonitis and aspiration pneumonia, either from inability

---

36-4	**Stress Ulcer Prophylaxis**

Risk Stratification

Absolute risk factors

- Coagulopathy
- Mechanical ventilation >48 hr
- History of gastrointestinal bleeding

Relative risk factors

- Multisystem organ failure
- Cirrhosis or hepatic failure
- Central nervous system injury
- Burns
- Steroid therapy
- Vasopressor therapy
- History of peptic ulcer disease

Management

	No Prophylaxis	Sucralfate PO or Ranitidine IV*
Risk factors absent	X	
Risk factors present		X

*Sucralfate PO if access to stomach is present; ranitidine otherwise.

IV, intravenously; PO, by mouth.

to protect the airway or from rapid-sequence intubation. "Ventilator bundles," designed to reduce the risk for ventilator-associated pneumonia (VAP), are commonplace in the ICU. Within limits of the patient's injuries and treatments, mechanically ventilated trauma patients should receive all such therapies to decrease the incidence of VAP. Intubated trauma patients should have the head of the bed at 45 degrees after thoracic and lumbar spine clearance. Until then, or if spine injury is present, the patient should be placed in reverse Trendelenburg position.

With respect to penetrating abdominal trauma, there is strong evidence for limiting postoperative antibiotics to 24 hours postoperatively.[65] Longer courses of antibiotics do not decrease rates of infection and abscess formation.

Analgesia

Numerous studies have documented a strong relationship between rib fractures and either respiratory complications or mortality.[66-68] Although rib fractures are debilitating to all patients, older adult patients with rib fractures are particularly susceptible. Some studies have suggested that epidural analgesia is superior to patient-controlled analgesia in patients with rib fractures,[68,69] but others have found no benefit.[67,70]

■ SUMMARY

Multisystem trauma patients are heterogeneous in preinjury status, injury pattern, and postinjury management. Some injured patients require no operative intervention, whereas others require multiple operations. Thus, for many multiply-injured patients, the early postoperative phase is an aggregate of the early postinjury phase and a preoperative phase. In all patients, resuscitation, treatments, and interventions should be rapidly implemented and frequently reassessed. Judgment is required to select among the many endpoints of resuscitation. The rapid arrival at a resuscitation goal should not give way to iatrogenic over-resuscitation, which has its own consequences. Damage-control techniques have improved outcomes from severe trauma, underscoring the importance of collaboration among trauma surgeons, anesthesiologists, and intensivists. Many evidence-based practices in postsurgical care and critical care have been applied successfully to postinjury care. Ideally, all such practices are evaluated to further improve the care of patients with multisystem trauma.

■ REFERENCES

1. Finfer S, Bellomo R, Boyce N, et al, and SAFE Study Investigators: A comparison of albumin and saline for fluid resuscitation in the intensive care unit. N Engl J Med 2004;350:2247-2256.
2. Shapiro MJ, Gettinger A, Corwin HL, et al: Anemia and blood transfusion in trauma patients admitted to the intensive care unit. J Trauma 2003;55:269-273.
3. Dunne JR, Malone DL, Tracy JK, Napolitano LM: Allogenic blood transfusion in the first 24 hours after trauma is associated with increased systemic inflammatory response syndrome (SIRS) and death. Surg Infect (Larchmt) 2004;5:395-404.
4. Malone DL, Dunne J, Tracy JK, et al: Blood transfusion, independent of shock severity, is associated with worse outcome in trauma. J Trauma 2003;54:898-905.
5. Robinson WP 3rd, Ahn J, Stiffler A, et al: Blood transfusion is an independent predictor of increased mortality in nonoperatively managed blunt hepatic and splenic injuries. J Trauma 2005;58:437-444.
6. Hebert PC, Wells G, Blajchman MA, et al: A multicenter, randomized, controlled clinical trial of transfusion requirements in critical care: Transfusion requirements in critical care investigators. Canadian Critical Care Trials Group. N Engl J Med 1999;340:409-417.
7. McIntyre L, Hebert PC, Wells G, et al, and Canadian Critical Care Trials Group: Is a restrictive transfusion strategy safe for resuscitated and critically ill trauma patients? J Trauma 2004;57:563-568.
8. Earley AS, Gracias VH, Haut E, et al: Anemia management program reduces transfusion volumes, incidence of ventilator-associated pneumonia, and cost in trauma patients. J Trauma 2006;61:1-5.
9. Vaslef SN, Knudsen NW, Neligan PJ, Sebastian MW: Massive transfusion exceeding 50 units of blood products in trauma patients. J Trauma 2002;53:291-295.
10. Cinat ME, Wallace WC, Nastanski F, et al: Improved survival following massive transfusion in patients who have undergone trauma. Arch Surg 1999;134:964-968.
11. Criddle LM, Eldredge DH, Walker J: Variables predicting trauma patient survival following massive transfusion. J Emerg Nurs 2005;31:236-242.
12. Velmahos GC, Chan L, Chan M, et al: Is there a limit to massive blood transfusion after severe trauma? Arch Surg 1998;133:947-952.
13. Gould SA, Moore EE, Moore FA, et al: Clinical utility of human polymerized hemoglobin as a blood substitute after acute trauma and urgent surgery. J Trauma 1997;43:325-331.
14. Gould SA, Moore EE, Hoyt DB, et al: The first randomized trial of human polymerized hemoglobin as a blood substitute in acute trauma and emergent surgery. J Am Coll Surg 1998;187:113-120.
15. Moore EE, Johnson JL, Cheng AM, et al: Insights from studies of blood substitutes in trauma. Shock 2005;24:197-205.
16. Boffard KD, Riou B, Warren B, et al, and NovoSeven Trauma Study Group: Recombinant factor VIIa as adjunctive therapy for bleeding control in severely injured trauma patients: Two parallel randomized, placebo-controlled, double-blind clinical trials. J Trauma 2005;59:8-15.
17. Holcomb JB: Use of recombinant activated factor VII to treat the acquired coagulopathy of trauma. J Trauma 2005;58:1298-1303.
18. Khan AZ, Parry JM, Crowley WF, et al: Recombinant factor VIIa for the treatment of severe postoperative and traumatic hemorrhage. Am J Surg 2005;189:331-334.
19. Rutherford EJ, Morris JA Jr, Reed GW, Hall KS: Base deficit stratifies mortality and determines therapy. J Trauma 1992;33:417-423.
20. Husain FA, Martin MJ, Mullenix PS, et al: Serum lactate and base deficit as predictors of mortality and morbidity. Am J Surg 2003;185:485-491.
21. Kincaid EH, Miller PR, Meredith JW, et al: Elevated arterial base deficit in trauma patients: A marker of impaired oxygen utilization. J Am Coll Surg 1998;187:384-392.
22. Richard C, Warszawski J, Anguel N, et al: Early use of the pulmonary artery catheter and outcomes in patients with shock and acute respiratory distress syndrome: A randomized controlled trial. JAMA 2003;290:2713-2720.
23. Shah MR, Hasselblad V, Stevenson LW, et al: Impact of the pulmonary artery catheter in critically ill patients: Meta-analysis of randomized clinical trials. JAMA 2005;294:1664-1670.
24. Chang MC, Meredith JW: Cardiac preload, splanchnic perfusion, and their relationship during resuscitation in trauma patients. J Trauma 1997;42:577-582.
25. Cheatham ML, Nelson LD, Chang MC, Safcsak K: Right ventricular end-diastolic volume index as a predictor of preload status in patients on positive end-expiratory pressure. Crit Care Med 1998;26:1801-1806.
26. Ivatury RR, Simon RJ, Islam S, et al: A prospective randomized study of end points of resuscitation after major trauma: Global oxygen transport indices versus organ-specific gastric mucosal pH. J Am Coll Surg 1996;183:145-154.
27. Weil MH, Nakagawa Y, Tang W, et al: Sublingual capnometry: A new noninvasive measurement for diagnosis and quantitation of severity of circulatory shock. Crit Care Med 1999;27:1225-1229.

28. Baron BJ, Sinert R, Zehtabchi S, et al: Diagnostic utility of sublingual PCO$_2$ for detecting hemorrhage in penetrating trauma patients. J Trauma 2004;57:69-74.

29. Madan AK, UyBarreta VV, Aliabadi-Wahle S, et al: Esophageal Doppler ultrasound monitor versus pulmonary artery catheter in the hemodynamic management of critically ill surgical patients. J Trauma 1999;46:607-611.

30. Rotondo MF, Schwab CW, McGonigal MD, et al: "Damage control": An approach for improved survival in exsanguinating penetrating abdominal injury. J Trauma 1993;35:375-382.

31. Rotondo MF, Zonies DH: The damage control sequence and underlying logic. Surg Clin North Am 1997;77:761-777.

32. Johnson JW, Gracias VH, Schwab CW, et al: Evolution in damage control for exsanguinating penetrating abdominal injury. J Trauma 2001;51:261-269.

33. Johnson JW, Gracias VH, Gupta R, et al: Hepatic angiography in patients undergoing damage control laparotomy. J Trauma 2002;52:1102-1106.

34. Spahn DR, Rossaint R: Coagulopathy and blood component transfusion in trauma. Br J Anaesth 2005;95:130-139.

35. Ho AM, Karmakar MK, Dion PW: Are we giving enough coagulation factors during major trauma resuscitation? Am J Surg 2005;190:479-484.

36. Shafi S, Kauder DR: Fluid resuscitation and blood replacement in patients with polytrauma. Clin Orthop Relat Res 2004;422:37-42.

37. Gracias VH, Braslow B, Johnson J, et al: Abdominal compartment syndrome in the open abdomen. Arch Surg 2002;137:1298-1300.

38. Balogh Z, McKinley BA, Holcomb JB, et al: Both primary and secondary abdominal compartment syndrome can be predicted early and are harbingers of multiple organ failure. J Trauma 2003;54:848-859.

39. Balogh Z, McKinley BA, Cocanour CS, et al: Supranormal trauma resuscitation causes more cases of abdominal compartment syndrome. Arch Surg 2003;138:637-642.

40. Bilkovski RN, Rivers EP, Horst HM: Targeted resuscitation strategies after injury. Curr Opin Crit Care 2004;10:529-538.

41. Stocchetti N, Furlan A, Volta F: Hypoxemia and arterial hypotension at the accident scene in head injury. J Trauma 1996;40:764-767.

42. Chesnut RM, Marshall LF, Klauber MR, et al: The role of secondary brain injury in determining outcome from severe head injury. J Trauma 1993;34:216-222.

43. Fearnside MR, Cook RJ, McDougall P, McNeil RJ: The Westmead head injury project outcome in severe head injury: A comparative analysis of pre-hospital, clinical and CT variables. Br J Neurosurg 1993;7:267-279.

44. Narayan RK, Kishore PR, Becker DP, et al: Intracranial pressure: To monitor or not to monitor? A review of our experience with severe head injury. J Neurosurg 1982;56:650-659.

45. Hartl R, Ghajar J, Hochleuthner H, Mauritz W: Hypertonic/hyperoncotic saline reliably reduces ICP in severely head-injured patients with intracranial hypertension. Acta Neurochir Suppl 1997;70:126-129.

46. Gracias VH, Guillamondegui OD, Stiefel MF, et al: Cerebral cortical oxygenation: A pilot study. J Trauma 2004;56:469-472.

47. Velmahos GC, Kern J, Chan LS, et al: Prevention of venous thromboembolism after injury: An evidence-based report—Part I. Analysis of risk factors and evaluation of the role of vena cava filters. J Trauma 2000;49:132-139.

48. Geerts WH, Jay RM, Code KI, et al: A comparison of low-dose heparin with low-molecular-weight heparin as prophylaxis against venous thromboembolism after major trauma. N Engl J Med 1996;335:701-707.

49. Cook D, Guyatt G, Marshall J, and Canadian Critical Care Trials Group: A comparison of sucralfate and ranitidine for the prevention of upper gastrointestinal bleeding in patients requiring mechanical ventilation. N Engl J Med 1998;338:791-797.

50. Cook DJ: Stress ulcer prophylaxis: Gastrointestinal bleeding and nosocomial pneumonia. Best evidence synthesis. Scand J Gastroenterol Suppl 1995;210:48-52.

51. Pickworth KK, Falcone RE, Hoogeboom JE, Santanello SA: Occurrence of nosocomial pneumonia in mechanically ventilated trauma patients: A comparison of sucralfate and ranitidine. Crit Care Med 1993;21:1856-1862.

52. Thomason MH, Payseur ES, Hakenewerth AM, et al: Nosocomial pneumonia in ventilated trauma patients during stress ulcer prophylaxis with sucralfate, antacid, and ranitidine. J Trauma 1996;41:503-508.

53. Spirt MJ: Acid suppression in critically ill patients: What does the evidence support? Pharmacotherapy 2003;23:87S-93.

54. Stollman N, Metz DC: Pathophysiology and prophylaxis of stress ulcer in intensive care unit patients. J Crit Care 2005;20:35-45.

55. Moore FA, Moore EE, Jones TN, et al: TEN versus TPN following major abdominal trauma-reduced septic morbidity. J Trauma 1989;29:916-922.

56. Moore FA, Feliciano DV, Andrassy RJ, et al: Early enteral feeding, compared with parenteral, reduces postoperative septic complications: The results of a meta-analysis. Ann Surg 1992;216:172-183.

57. Peter JV, Moran JL, Phillips-Hughes J: A metaanalysis of treatment outcomes of early versus late parenteral nutrition in hospitalized patients. Crit Care Med 2005;33:213-220.

58. Kudsk KA, Croce MA, Fabian TC, et al: Enteral versus parenteral feeding: Effects on septic morbidity after blunt and penetrating abdominal trauma. Ann Surg 1992;215:503-511.

59. Heyland DK, Dhaliwal R, Drover JW, et al, Canadian Critical Care Clinical Practice Guidelines Committee: Canadian clinical practice guidelines for nutrition support in the adult critically ill patient. JPEN J Parenter Enteral Nutr 2003;27:355-373.

60. van den Berghe G, Wouters P, Weekers F, et al: Intensive insulin therapy in critically ill patients. N Engl J Med 2001;345:1359-1367.

61. Yendamuri S, Fulda GJ, Tinkoff GH: Admission hyperglycemia as a prognostic indicator in trauma. J Trauma 2003;55:33-38.

62. Laird AM, Miller PR, Kilgo PD, et al: Relationship of early hyperglycemia to mortality in trauma patients. J Trauma 2004;56:1058-1062.

63. Sung J, Bochicchio GV, Joshi M, et al: Admission hyperglycemia is predictive of outcome in critically ill trauma patients. J Trauma 2005;59:80-83.

64. Bochicchio GV, Sung J, Joshi M, et al: Persistent hyperglycemia is predictive of outcome in critically ill trauma patients. J Trauma 2005;58:921-924.

65. Velmahos GC, Toutouzas KG, Sarkisyan G, et al: Severe trauma is not an excuse for prolonged antibiotic prophylaxis. Arch Surg 2002;137:537-541.

66. Bulger EM, Arneson MA, Mock CN, Jurkovich GJ: Rib fractures in the elderly. J Trauma 2000;48:1040-1046.

67. Holcomb JB, McMullin NR, Kozar RA, et al: Morbidity from rib fractures increases after age 45. J Am Coll Surg 2003;196:549-555.

68. Flagel BT, Luchette FA, Reed RL, et al: Half-a-dozen ribs: The breakpoint for mortality. Surgery 2005;138:717-723.

69. Bulger EM, Edwards T, Klotz P, Jurkovich GGJ: Epidural analgesia improves outcome after multiple rib fractures. Surgery 2004;136:426-430.

70. Kieninger AN, Bair HA, Bendick PJ, Howells GA: Epidural versus intravenous pain control in elderly patients with rib fractures. Am J Surg 2005;19:327-330.

Chapter

37 Neurosurgery

Michael L. James and Cecil O. Borel

After an uncomplicated neurosurgical procedure, a patient is admitted to an intensive care unit (ICU) for close observation. In the large majority of cases, this level of care is warranted as a means to carefully monitor for changes in the patient's neurologic function, and to expedite appropriate intervention if necessary. Observation and evaluation of postoperative neurosurgical patients is, of course, complicated by the residual effects of the prior anesthetic and an ongoing need for analgesia and sedation.

The Leapfrog Group has shown that the implementation of basic intensive care practices can vastly improve patient safety. One of these practices is choosing a hospital with ICUs that are staffed at least 8 hours daily by specially trained critical care physicians.[1,2] Mirski and colleagues[3] showed that treatment in a dedicated specialty neurologic-neurosurgical ICU (NSICU) improved mortality and disposition at discharge for patients with intracerebral hemorrhage, compared with a similar cohort treated 2 years earlier in a general ICU setting. Furthermore, critically ill postoperative neurosurgical and neurologic patients who are treated in the NSICU had shorter hospital stays and lower total costs of care than a national benchmark. The data suggest that a neuroscience specialty ICU staffed by specialty-trained intensivists and nurses is beneficial.[3] Only a small fraction of patients require prolonged ICU stay after craniotomy for tumor resection. A patient's risk of prolonged stay can be predicted by certain radiologic findings, large intraoperative blood loss, fluid requirements, and the decision to keep the patient intubated at the end of surgery.[4] For those patients requiring ICU resources beyond the first 4 hours, the interventions can be critical. It is, therefore, crucial to have appropriate skills and resources readily available.

In this chapter, we describe the methods we have implemented in our NSICU to improve outcome after neurosurgical procedures (Fig. 37-1). In basic terms, most improvement in postoperative outcome is attained by recognizing acute reversible neurologic injury and distinguishing it from expanding intracompartmental mass lesions or edema, and by preventing secondary neurologic insults from decreased ventilation or cerebral hypoperfusion. We summarize the care given to postoperative patients who have undergone major neurosurgical procedures that carry a higher risk for neurologic impairment.

■ NEUROLOGIC SUPPORT

Focused Neurologic Examination

Postoperative neurosurgical patients require rapid initial neurologic assessment. The Glasgow Coma Scale (GCS) score is the most widely recognized assessment of cortical function, consisting of motor, verbal, and eye opening (arousal) responses (Box 37-1) The GCS offers simplicity and reproducibility, but it is affected by other factors causing cortical impairment such as sedatives, narcotics, temperature, glucose levels, and electrolyte imbalances, and it lacks compensatory scores for intubated or aphasic patients.[5] Regardless of a patient's level of consciousness, an examiner must evaluate cranial nerve and brainstem reflexes, including pupil size and light reflex, eye deviation and extraocular muscle movements, oculovestibular and oculocochlear reflexes, facial symmetry/movement, gag reflex, and midline tongue protrusion (see Box 37-1).

Spinal cord function can be assessed using reflexes, muscle strength, and peripheral sensation. Triceps, biceps, brachioradialis, patellar, and ankle reflexes are graded and compared to the contralateral side. The standardized motor strength grading is based on a scale of 1 to 5. Typically, flexor and extensor muscle groups in the proximal and distal portion of each extremity are tested as an initial screen, with further and more detailed testing of individual muscles as warranted by the history or initial screen. If a patient is unable to fully comply with the motor examination because of an alteration in level of consciousness, an examiner may still observe some measure of muscle strength based on spontaneous movement or withdrawal from stimuli. Passively flexing and extending the extremities can be used to assess the patient's muscle tone.

A screening examination consists of light touch and pain sensation attained proximally and distally in each extremity, as well as proprioceptive sense in the thumbs and great toes. Stimulating the lateral sole assesses plantar responses. Testing finger-to-nose and heel-to-shin maneuvers is used to assess cerebellar function.

The results of the focused neurologic examination are used as the basis for further monitoring, which requires coordination between examiners as they assess neurologic recovery. With the exception of some simple reflexes (which are

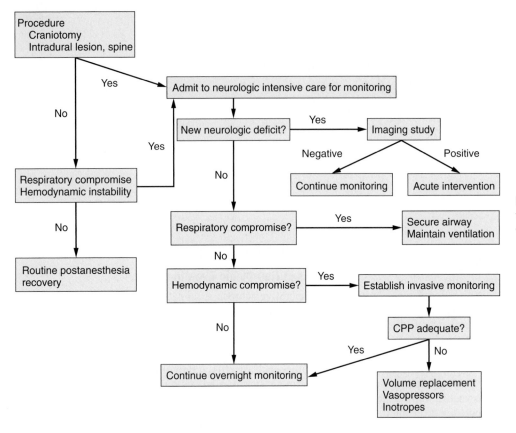

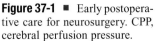

Figure 37-1 ■ Early postoperative care for neurosurgery. CPP, cerebral perfusion pressure.

either present or not present), the neurologic examination is subjective, and variability can be expected to exist between examiners; however, repeated examinations by the same health-care professional are consistent, and this consistency is bolstered by knowledge of the clinical history.[6] In sum, the intensive and intermediate nursing care of postoperative neurosurgical patients is based on the repeated observations of responses to the neurologic examination.

Postoperative Imaging

Central nervous system imaging studies are often an extension of the neurologic examination, as they can be used to assess anatomic lesions, which may then be related to neurologic dysfunction uncovered by the examination. In the postoperative neurosurgical population, imaging is useful for any of three reasons: (1) because the patient is unable to arouse fully in a reasonable amount of time after anesthesia, (2) because a neurologic deficit is seen postoperatively that was not seen preoperatively, or (3) because a preexisting deficit is worse postoperatively than it was preoperatively.

Computed tomography (CT) scanning, which provides fast, detailed images by computerized analysis of circumferential radiographs, is the mainstay for urgent or emergent evaluation of ventricular size, edema, hemorrhage, and bony structures. The main advantage of CT is the speed with which the scans can be obtained, as patient compliance may be limited in this population. Spiral CT scans provide three-dimensional (3-D) images (especially useful in examining

vascular anatomy and cerebrospinal fluid [CSF] flow), and perfusion CT scanning may give some measure of regional cerebral blood flow.

Magnetic resonance imaging (MRI) may be used in addition to or instead of CT to provide the highest anatomic detail available. MRI uses pulse sequences of magnetic radio waves to orient cellular nuclei in a particular direction; computer analysis then converts the differences in radio energy imparted by the subsequent relaxation of these nuclei into excellent images that provide information on gray and white matter structures, edema, CSF, hemorrhage, blood–brain barrier integrity (with the use of gadolinium contrast), and tumors. Newer pulse sequences allow 3-D images of intracranial vasculature and perfusion studies. The main disadvantage of MRI is the length of time it takes to perform a study: complete imaging of the brain takes up to 1 hour. Also, acquiring the images can be difficult in the noncompliant or critically ill patient. Another disadvantage is that the noise and closeness of the MRI machine result in many patients' needing to be sedated because of claustrophobia and anxiety. For these reasons, MRI is usually reserved for situations in which CT is inadequate (e.g., for imaging in the posterior fossa), for nonemergent detailed imaging after intracranial tumor surgery, and for spinal cord imaging.

Finally, conventional angiography remains the gold standard for vascular imaging. In the postoperative period, it is mainly reserved for use after intracranial vascular surgery when MR angiography or CT angiography is contraindicated or of questionable efficacy.

37-1	**Focused Postoperative Neurologic Examination**

Cortical Function: Glasgow Coma Score

Eye opening
  Spontaneous   4
  Speech   3
  Pain   2
  None   1
Motor response
  Obeys commands   6
  Localizes   5
  Withdraws   4
  Flexes   3
  Extends   2
  No response   1
Verbal response
  Oriented   5
  Confused   4
  Inappropriate words 3
  Incomprehensible sounds 2
  No response   1

Brainstem Function

Reflexes
  Pupillary light reflex
  Ocular movements
  Corneal reflex
  Facial grimace
  Gag
  Cough

Spinal Cord Function

Deep tendon reflexes
  Brachial
  Achilles
Motor response
  Hands
  Toes
Sensory
  Light touch

Postoperative Intracranial Pressure Monitoring

Because the central nervous system is relatively incompressible, postoperative intracranial pressure (ICP) may be directly related to mean arterial pressure (MAP) after compensatory mechanisms have been exhausted. Cerebral perfusion pressure (CPP) equals MAP minus the highest downstream pressure, usually the ICP. If cortical function is normal, CPP may be approximated by measuring MAP when ICP is unknown. However, the central nervous system is somewhat compartmentalized because of the separation of the cerebral hemispheres and posterior fossa by the dural reflections, and thus raising or lowering the MAP may not directly raise or lower ICP in a linear manner. Therefore, it is often necessary to monitor the ICP invasively.

ICP should be monitored directly when its manipulation involves prolonged attempts or when a degree of hydrocephalus might result in depressed neurologic function. Historically, this has been done by ventriculostomy or cranial bolt placement. However, newer ICP monitors can evaluate regional oxygenation, temperature, and pressure.[7] These catheters may be used to guide management of intracranial pressure, oxygenation, and cerebral metabolic rate (CMR) but are largely not validated with outcome data.[8-10]

Management of Postoperative Complications

Immediately after a neurosurgical procedure, complications include cerebral edema, hematoma, and seizures. Global cerebral edema, as seen after head trauma, with associated increases in ICP has been shown to have a high mortality rate, thought to be largely the result of decreased cerebral blood flow (CBF).[11] Although the regional edema seen at the surgical site is not associated with the same risks or mortality, postsurgical edema with neurologic compromise may be caused by local or diffuse decrements in CBF and thus may benefit from ICP management. The goals are to supply the metabolic demands of the brain by maintaining perfusion, oxygenation, and glucose. The treatment for elevated ICP is first directed at the cause, which in this patient population is typically postsurgical edema, but it may include intracerebral hemorrhage, cerebral venous occlusion, focal ischemia or infarction, infection, or unresected tumor.

Management of ICP begins with supporting the viable neuronal tissue until definitive therapy for the underlying cause can be achieved. Maneuvers intended to decrease ICP in the setting of cerebral edema range from hyperventilation to calvarium removal; however, in the immediate postoperative period, most interventions are meant to reduce the volume of CSF or blood in the cranial vault.

Hyperventilation, routinely used to reduce CBF via cerebral vasoconstriction, can be achieved through increases in either tidal volume or respiratory rate, or in both. Its disadvantages include reducing CBF in concurrently ischemic brain, presumably because of associated vasoconstriction, decreasing seizure threshold, rebound increase in ICP, and CSF acidosis after cessation.[12-15] Mannitol may be given intravenously to reduce ICP via osmotic diuresis; however, it could also diffuse into areas of brain where the blood–brain barrier is no longer intact and theoretically could cause worsening of regional edema.[16] Intravenous corticosteroids can be used to actively treat the cause of cerebral vasogenic edema, as seen in malignancies. High dosages may be necessary, and it may be difficult to wean quickly.[17] Finally, barbiturates have been used to decrease ICP through lowering of CBF and CMR.[18] In general, high dosages are required to induce burst-suppression patterns on the electroencephalogram. Therefore, blood pressure may need pharmacologic augmentation with inotropes and/or vasoconstrictors.

Postoperative hematoma formation is another major concern. The location of surgery best dictates the manner in which to monitor the patient for this. Epidural hematoma formation occurring after spinal surgery is usually indicated by new and progressive neurologic symptoms in the extremities and demands immediate diagnosis with MRI and treatment with surgical evacuation and decompression. Although the postoperative development of intracerebral or epidural hemorrhages is not unheard of, subdural hematoma formation is more common after intracranial procedures and may be signified by alteration in mental status, unilateral neurologic signs, or failing to fully recover from anesthesia. Again, immediate imaging with CT and consideration of evacuation is indicated.

Finally, seizures may complicate the early postoperative course. The largest incidence study suggests that early postoperative seizures may occur in as many as 17% of cases, allowing for wide variation between inciting pathologies.[19] Previous research found differing results of prophylactic treatment with antiepileptics, usually phenytoin or carbamazepine,[20] but recent studies have been performed with newer agents, including zonisamide, lamotrigine, and topiramate. Patients with low risk or no prior seizures generally do not benefit from preoperative antiepileptic dosing,[21] and no data suggest that continuation of antiepileptics beyond 6 postoperative months is of any benefit unless a patient develops seizures during that time. Current recommendations include the use of perioperative antiepileptics in patients with a history of seizures or considerable preoperative cerebral damage; these drugs should be continued indefinitely if postoperative seizures occur, or for several months if they do not. There are no recommendations about drug selection, and the use of each medication should be weighed against its side-effect profile and the patient's comorbidities.

■ RESPIRATORY SUPPORT

Airway and breathing are the initial concern in preventing secondary neurologic injury and therefore should be integral to the initial assessment of any postoperative patient. In the neurosurgical patient, control of both oxygen and carbon dioxide is critical.

Hypoxia and Hypercarbia in Brain Injury

Hypoxia can be detrimental by two mechanisms. First, in areas of the brain with cerebrovascular compromise, hypoxemia may be poorly tolerated, with subsequent neuronal infarction if not corrected. Second, hypoxemia may exacerbate intracranial hypertension. The normal compensatory mechanism for hypoxia in the brain is vasodilation. This seems to be a regional phenomenon[22] and may be controlled by regional factors.[23,24] Therefore, it is reasonable to assume that areas of maximal vasodilatation and decremental blood flow will not tolerate additional hypoxemia, as there may be few, if any, further compensatory mechanisms available to the neuronal tissue. If further vasodilatation is possible, however, subsequent cellular damage may occur because of increases in intracranial pressure, with consequent decrease in regional or global blood flow and altered cellular structure, leading to further edema and increases in ICP. Hyperoxia, on the other hand, is also theoretically detrimental because of the abundance of free radicals created as a result of ischemia and reperfusion.[25,26] However, with the data available, it still seems most reasonable to err on the side of too much oxygen rather than too little.

Carbon dioxide has an even more profound effect on cerebral vasculature. CBF is linearly related to $PaCO_2$ when it is between 20 and 60 mm Hg.[15] Therefore, decrements or increments in $PaCO_2$ will either decrease or increase CBF, respectively. This change in CBF has a direct effect on blood volume and therefore on ICP. It would then seem that when an increased ICP was detrimental, a lower $PaCO_2$ would be beneficial, as it would directly lower the ICP; however, the lower ICP is at the direct expense of blood flow, which is exactly the parameter that the clinician is attempting to maintain. The relation between ICP and $PaCO_2$ is even more complicated in the injured brain. When injured, the cerebral vasculature loses autoregulation, and increased $PaCO_2$ may not increase blood flow to injured areas, as arterioles in that area may be maximally dilated. There is also the theoretical issue of steal, as noninjured areas may increase their blood flow with increases in $PaCO_2$ at the expense of maximally dilated areas of injured brain. On the other hand, lowering ICP through decreases in $PaCO_2$ may cause hyperperfusion of injured areas, as vasoconstriction does not occur as readily there as it does in areas of normal brain.

Airway Assessment and Management

Decreased Level of Consciousness. Reduced level of consciousness (GCS < 10) correlates with the need to protect the airway by endotracheal intubation to prevent passive aspiration and intermittent airway obstruction. This was demonstrated in studies that used ICP monitoring after acute hemispheric stroke, in which the development of decreased level of consciousness was not correlated with a rise in ICP but was more closely correlated with edema and tissue shifts.[27,28]

Raised Intracranial Pressure. Patients presenting with acutely raised ICP often require control of the airway as the initial therapeutic intervention.[29] Preventing hypoxemia, hypercarbia, and acidosis can minimize secondary neurologic damage from raised ICP. A decreased level of consciousness (GCS < 9) is associated with a decreased ability to protect the airway and suggests additional potential benefit from mechanical hyperventilation to control raised ICP.[30] Potential cerebral herniation is associated with raised intracranial pressure and brainstem injury, which impairs airway reflexes, coughing, and ventilatory drive.[31,32] Laryngoscopy, hypoventilation, struggling, and the use of succinylcholine without using a small dose of nondepolarizing muscle relaxant to prevent muscle fasciculation[33] have been shown to raise ICP.

Brainstem Lesions. Brainstem disease may lead to several well-defined disorders of breathing and require endotracheal intubation. Patients with basilar artery infarction may suffer from obstructive or mixed apnea or impaired airway reflexes, which lead to positional airway obstruction or repeated aspiration. The dorsolateral medulla is primarily responsible for the integration of effective rhythmic breathing, and as long as this area, which includes the nucleus ambiguous and solitarius, is not affected by the ischemic infarct, central respiratory control may be relatively normal. Thus, even locked-in patients with rostral brainstem infarction may be left with a relatively normal respiratory drive if infarction spares the dorsal lateral medulla.[34] Disruption of automatic breathing may result from damage to the lateral medulla and pontine tegmentum caudal to trigeminal outflow. Lateral medullary stroke is most commonly the result of occlusion of the distal vertebral or posterior inferior cerebellar artery, and large infarcts involving the dorsolateral medulla may be associated with fatal apnea.[35] These patients may suffer from mild hypoventilation while awake, which can be reversed voluntarily. Respirations may cease entirely during sleep.

Spinal Cord Lesions. Priority is given to simultaneous airway assessment and management. Immobilization of the spine must be ensured until definitive radiographic studies are obtained. Listening for stridor caused by partial airway obstruction and feeling for air movement can determine adequacy of the airway. Patients who can speak without stridor or hoarseness usually have unobstructed airways. Some patients who demonstrate airway obstruction will respond to a jaw-thrust maneuver; however, during this process, spine manipulation must be avoided. Many patients with cervical cord lesions will require at least temporary endotracheal intubation. A significant proportion of spinal cord injured patients have associated head injuries and depressed levels of consciousness. Patients who are stuporous or unconscious are at increased risk of developing aspiration pneumonitis. In the patient with spinal cord injury, this risk is compounded by gastrointestinal paresis that develops soon after the injury.[36] Patients with significant chance for regurgitation and aspiration require intubation or tracheotomy to protect their airway. Gastric atony should be suspected and managed with nasogastric tube suction until it resolves.[37]

Sedation Strategies

Once a decision has been made to reintubate or to continue mechanical ventilation, the role of sedation becomes an issue, because agitation, increased physiologic stress, and inadvertent airway extubation may impair neurologic recovery. However, sedation hinders the neurologic examination and impairs functional monitoring. The perfect sedative would allow complete cooperation from an alert, awake, yet passive patient, would take effect immediately, and would dissipate immediately when infusion is stopped. The oldest agents are the barbiturates such as thiopental. Although thiopental's efficacy is limited because tissue redistribution causes prolonged sedation after cessation of drug infusion, it has cerebral-protective properties by lowering metabolic rate and decreasing ICP.[18]

Benzodiazepines (such as midazolam) are commonly used. These gamma-aminobutyric acid (GABA)ergic drugs cause sedation and amnesia. They retain some antiepileptic properties, decrease cerebral metabolic rate, and can be relatively short acting.[38] They have the added benefit of being reversible with flumazenil but at the expense of potentially lowering the seizure threshold. The main disadvantages are that benzodiazepine use is associated with delirium and hypotension.

Short-acting opioids (such as fentanyl, alfentanil, or remifentanil) may also be used for their sedative properties. They have the added bonus of conveying analgesia (they do not, however, consistently confer amnesia) and are also reversible with naloxone. Patients remain fairly cardiostable after dosing, and opioids blunt respiratory responses such as dyspnea, coughing, or gagging in ventilated patients. These drugs become more problematic with lengthier infusion, as all have context-sensitive half-lives (except remifentanil). Remifentanil, however, is very expensive, which may limit its use in the setting of prolonged postoperative sedation. There is also suggestion that opioids are less than beneficial in the ischemic brain.[39]

Newer agents include propofol and dexmedetomidine. Propofol is another GABAergic agent with both a very short half-life and sedative-hypnotic properties. Its main benefit is quick arousal times even with prolonged infusions. It may, however, have detrimental hemodynamic effects and can be rather expensive. Finally, dexmedetomidine, an alpha-2 agonist, grants both sedative and analgesic properties with minimal amnesia. Some hemodynamic depression may be seen (especially with bolus loading). It also has a relatively long half-life when compared with propofol, but, unlike the other sedatives, it allows patients to be aroused from sedation with minimal stimulation and there is little to no respiratory depression.[40-42]

■ CARDIOVASCULAR SUPPORT

Cerebral Perfusion and Arterial Blood Pressure

Under normal circumstances, cerebral blood flow is tightly autoregulated on the basis of regional tissue oxygenation, arterial carbon dioxide, and metabolism (i.e., glucose requirements), so oxygen and glucose delivery and carbon dioxide elimination are maintained despite wide changes in arterial pressure. However, after neuronal or vascular injury, as seen in postsurgical changes, cerebral perfusion may be uncoupled from autoregulatory mechanisms and, therefore, will be tied directly to arterial blood pressure. In these circumstances, the arterial–intracranial pressure curve will change to reflect linear increases in ICP as arterial pressure increases until compensatory mechanisms are overwhelmed, at which point ICP increases exponentially. For these reasons, increased systemic arterial pressure may exacerbate, or even cause, cerebral edema or hemorrhage and decreased systemic pressure may worsen ischemia. It may be necessary, then, to control systemic arterial pressure within tightly defined parameters until neuronal or vascular repair has been accomplished sufficiently to reestablish cerebral blood flow autoregulation.

Hypertension and Brain Injury

Postoperative neurosurgical patients often display varying degrees of hypertension as they recover from anesthesia and postsurgical changes to the brain. The essential question is whether the elevated systemic arterial pressure is detrimental to (or, on the contrary, sustains) cerebral perfusion. When the brain undergoes periods of relative hypoperfusion, systemic arterial pressure may be elevated to maintain adequate cerebral perfusion pressure. At some point along this perfusion–pressure curve, additional systemic pressure no longer increases cerebral perfusion but instead begins to reduce blood flow because the surrounding cranium is not compressible. It is often very difficult to determine immediately and empirically where along the pressure–perfusion curve any individual patient is lying. Therefore, it may be necessary to judiciously manipulate the systemic arterial pressure while vigilantly monitoring the patient for neurologic changes and for indications of improvement or deterioration. Additionally, an estimation of the potential for postsurgical complications (e.g., hemorrhage, edema) should be made to determine whether to lower or to increase a patient's arterial blood pressure. These factors can make blood pressure manipulation precarious, and clinical decisions are best made for individual patients after considering all significant patient and surgical factors.

Inotropes and Vasodilators

A variety of pharmacologic agents are at the disposal of the intensivist who chooses to manipulate systemic arterial pressure in an attempt to maximize cerebral perfusion. Inotropes include agents, such as epinephrine, norepinephrine, dopamine, dobutamine, milrinone, and phenylephrine, that demonstrate varying degrees of alpha- and/or beta-adrenergic agonism. The selection of an agent is best made in the specific clinical context in which it is to be used while weighing the drug's intended benefits and its expected side effects. A discussion of the properties of each inotrope is beyond the scope of this paper. General considerations include the patient's comorbidities, including cardiac and renal function, and whether the patient's arterial pressure and cardiac output are best maintained or enhanced through alpha (i.e., peripheral) or beta (i.e., cardiac) effects.

When induced hypotension is required, the clinician can choose from vasodilators, angiotensin-converting enzyme (ACE) inhibitors, and sympatholytics. The vasodilators include nitroglycerin, sodium nitroprusside, hydralazine, and nicardipine, but in general, nitroglycerin and nitroprusside are avoided for the postoperative neurosurgical patient because of their tendency to dilate cerebral vasculature, which can raise intracranial pressure and thus decrease cerebral blood flow. Nicardipine, a newer calcium channel blocker, can theoretically worsen intracranial pressure, but it has been found to reliably decrease systemic arterial pressure without clinically significant intracranial pressure changes, and it has the additional benefit of potential cerebral protective properties.[43]

ACE inhibitors have also been shown to decrease systemic blood pressure and have additional benefits in patients with cardiac comorbidities. The sympatholytics include beta-adrenergic blockers (i.e., labetalol and metoprolol) and centrally acting alpha-2 agonists (i.e., clonidine). The beta-blockers slow heart rate and decrease the contractility of the heart, among other effects. Clonidine is not routinely used in the immediate postoperative phase because of its long-acting and sedative effects. However, it has potential uses in patients with refractory or poorly controlled hypertension, ongoing drug abuse, or signs and symptoms of narcotic withdrawal.[44,45]

■ FLUID AND ELECTROLYTE SUPPORT

Hypovolemia and Cerebral Perfusion

Hypovolemia may lead to hypotension and thereby worsen ischemia because of decreased perfusion of organs. This is

also true in the brain. With regional brain injury and ischemia, cerebral blood vessels may be maximally dilated in an attempt to maintain perfusion and lose autoregulation, which ties perfusion directly to mean arterial pressure. In states of hypovolemia, hypotension may be induced despite compensatory mechanisms (decreased blood flow to peripheral tissues and nonessential organs, increased movement of water intravascularly), thereby worsening ischemia in poorly perfused neuronal tissue. Therefore, patients with hypovolemia, whatever its cause, warrant aggressive fluid resuscitation.

In the immediate postoperative period, hypovolemia is most likely related to blood loss, intraoperative diuresis with mannitol and/or furosemide, or inadequate resuscitation. Blood loss, whether it occurred intraoperatively or is ongoing postoperatively, should be replaced with crystalloid until a lowest limit of allowable hemoglobin is reached (see later), at which point blood transfusion should begin. Intraoperative fluid manipulation to decrease brain water generally consists of osmotic diuresis with mannitol and/or loop diuresis with furosemide. Use of either of these agents can result in depleted total body water in the postoperative patient and potentially hypovolemia with resultant hypotension. It then becomes necessary to replace body water without worsening cerebral edema. In general, this is done through the use of iso-osmolar fluid solutions, such as normal saline, and 5% albumin.

The use of hyperosmolar saline solutions has been evaluated during resuscitation. These solutions expand intravascular volume with the benefit of a favorable osmotic pressure gradient in the cerebral vasculature.[46,47] Their disadvantage is the propensity to cause hypernatremia with even modest amounts of volume.[48]

Finally, colloids have long been used to increase intravascular volume while attempting to avoid third-space loss. Natural colloids include fractionated plasma protein, albumin, and blood products. Synthetic colloids continue to be developed but currently in this country are largely limited to Hespan and Hextend. Although there is no evidence in neurosurgical patients, the synthetic colloids are largely avoided because of antiplatelet effects in vivo and concerns about clinical bleeding.[49,50] In general, we use plasma protein colloids when there is concern about excessive crystalloid use without indication for the use of blood products.[51,52]

Hyponatremia, Edema, and Seizures

Hyponatremia has been associated with delirium, cerebral edema, and seizures. Usually, sodium levels below 120 mEq/L are required for hyponatremia alone to cause a significant decline in neurologic status. However, all cases of hyponatremia merit attention and being evaluated for a cause. The three major reasons for the development of new-onset hyponatremia in the postoperative neurosurgical patient are syndrome of inappropriate antidiuretic hormone (SIADH), cerebral salt wasting, and inappropriate free water administration.[53]

It is helpful to describe hyponatremia as it relates to intravascular volume. SIADH most commonly falls in the hypervolemia category, cerebral salt wasting in the hypovolemic category, and dilutional in the euvolemic category. An assessment of volume status should be made from change in weight, the fluid balance record, or measurement of ventricular filling pressure with central venous or pulmonary capillary wedge pressure. It may also be helpful to check the osmolarity of both serum and urine, and to check the urine sodium to make a distinction between the causes. Both SIADH and cerebral salt wasting increase urine sodium, differentiating them from dilutional causes. SIADH has high (often very high) urine osmolarity, which is typically normal in cerebral salt wasting.

It is, of course, important to rule out other causes of hyponatremia (e.g., medication; renal failure; excess loss from fever, diarrhea, or vomiting; or endocrine disorder such as hypothyroidism or cortisol deficiency), as the treatment is dictated by the cause. If free water is being given, the practitioner should switch the intravenous fluid to an iso-osmolar or a hyperosmolar salt solution, depending on the degree of hyponatremia. SIADH is generally treated by fluid restriction; however, this may be inappropriate in the hemodynamically unstable patient. In this case, administration of hyperosmolar saline or the addition of extra sodium to the patient's diet may be more desirable. Cerebral salt wasting is treated by replacing urine sodium lost with normal or hypertonic saline. It is important to begin therapy before reaching critically low serum sodium levels, as correction of hyponatremia should be performed gradually to avoid the complication of central pontine myelinolysis.[54] Usually, correction of 1 to 2 mEq/L/hr is recommended, up to 12 mEq/L/day.

Routine Fluid Management

Unlike other tissues, which respond to both hydrostatic and oncotic pressures, the brain's water content is regulated most by serum osmolarity, in large part because of the blood–brain barrier.[55] Therefore, to avoid the possibility of producing or worsening cerebral edema, it is important to avoid hypo-osmolarity in the serum. This is accomplished by the administration of an isotonic intravenous fluid such as normal saline or a balanced salt solution such as Normosol. The use of colloid solutions is not recommended, as oncotic pressure is not as useful in regulating brain water. Maintenance of euvolemia is imperative in the typical postoperative neurosurgical patient, as both hypovolemia and hypervolemia may have detrimental side effects. Hypovolemia can lead to hypotension and, therefore, hypoperfusion. Hypervolemia may increase intracranial pressure, leading to hypertension or an edematous state. Finally, dextrose-containing fluids are not recommended for routine use, as the presence of hyperglycemia has been shown to worsen outcomes in cerebral injury, and in general they add to the amount of hypo-osmolar fluid administered.[56]

Management of Diabetes Insipidus

Diabetes insipidus results from dysfunction of the pituitary gland through primary causes or, more likely in the postoperative neurosurgical patient, ischemia, tumor, or surgical manipulation. It should be suspected when urine output is higher than expected and serum sodium appears to be rising. It is the most common cause, behind iatrogenic causes, of hypernatremia in the neurosurgical patient.[57] The diagnosis

is suggested by a large hypotonic urine volume in the presence of hyperosmolar hypernatremia leading to hypovolemic states. Treatment is aimed at replacing total body water with hypo-osmolar salt solutions. This deficit should be replaced over 24 hours at a rate no faster than 2 mEq/L/hr, as too-rapid correction may result in seizures, delirium, or cerebral edema, presumably from what the brain perceives to be a hyponatremic state.[58] Ultralow dosages of arginine vasopressin given by continuous infusion are very effective in correcting both hypovolemia and hyponatremia in patients with diabetes insipidus,[59] brain-injured patients,[60] and children.[61] These protocols involve administering 1 or 2 IU/L of arginine vasopressin in hyponatremic fluid, at hourly urine output rates plus 10%, to gradually correct hypovolemia and hyponatremia.

■ HEMATOLOGIC SUPPORT

Role of Anemia in Cerebral Ischemia

Normovolemic anemia has been shown to increase cerebral blood flow[62] by increasing cardiac output and cerebral vasodilation to ensure an adequate oxygen supply to the brain. Decreased blood viscosity may also contribute to the increase in cerebral blood flow. The compensatory increase cerebral hemodynamics may be impaired by hypovolemia associated with perioperative blood loss. However, if adequate intravascular volume is maintained through the use of intravenous crystalloids, even moderate anemia has little effect on cerebral ischemia.[63] In fact, it has not been shown that even severe anemia (hemoglobin level <6 g/dL) can cause long-term or permanent cerebral injury alone. Higher hemoglobin levels may, in fact, be detrimental in some pathologic processes, as in subarachnoid hemorrhage–induced vasospasm and diffuse axonal injury.[26,64] It is also possible, at least in theory, that normovolemic anemia may cause detrimental increases in cerebral blood flow in patients with raised intracranial pressure, but this has not been studied. Finally, only one human study has demonstrated any adverse effects of severe anemia (hemoglobin level <6 g/dL), consisting of mild cognitive changes in healthy volunteers that was readily reversible by increasing the amount of inspired oxygen.[65]

The American Society of Anesthesiologists has published guidelines for the administration of blood products. They recommend first maintaining normovolemia by the use of crystalloids and colloids. Red blood cell transfusions are recommended for hemoglobin levels of less than 6 g/dL and for physiologic signs of inadequate oxygenation such as hemodynamic instability, oxygen extraction greater than 50%, and myocardial ischemia (new ST-segment depressions >0.1 mV, new ST-segment elevations >0.2 mV, or new wall motion abnormalities in transesophageal echocardiography). Fresh-frozen plasma transfusions are recommended for urgent reversal of anticoagulation, known coagulation factor deficiencies, microvascular bleeding in the presence of elevated (>1.5 times normal) prothrombin time (PT) or partial thromboplastin time (PTT), and microvascular bleeding after the replacement of more than one blood volume when PT or PTT cannot be obtained. Platelet transfusions are recommended (1) before major operations for patients with platelet counts of less than 50,000/μL, (2) intraoperatively when there is microvascular bleeding and platelet counts are less than 50,000/μL, and (3) for patients with platelet counts in the range of 50,000 to 100,0000/μL after cardiopulmonary bypass and when undergoing surgery where minimal bleeding may cause major damage, such as in neurosurgery.[66,67] There are no specific guidelines for the transfusion of blood products in neurosurgical patients. In our own practice, we aggressively correct any clotting abnormalities in actively bleeding patients with fresh-frozen plasma, platelets, and/or cryoprecipitate, as indicated by coagulant studies.

Thrombophlebitis

Deep venous thrombosis (DVT) has three classic antecedents: venous injury, stasis, and hypercoagulability. The postoperative neurosurgical patient is prone to many risk factors for development of DVT, including trauma, immobilization, tumors, acute stroke, estrogen use, obesity, age greater than 40 years, and acquired coagulopathy.[68] Several methods are used to prevent the development of DVT. Pneumatic compression devices and compression stockings have almost no contraindications and have proven efficacy after a number of types of surgery, including neurosurgery.[69] Enoxaparin decreases the incidence of DVT compared with compression stockings alone, and it does not increase the risk of major bleeding.[70] Low-dose anticoagulants such as minidose heparin have also proven efficacious against the formation of DVT[71]; however, there is at least a theoretical concern that intracranial hemorrhage may occur or worsen, although no data suggest this. Other strategies include ambulation and passive motion exercises for the nonambulatory. It is our practice to use pneumatic compression devices with elastic compression stockings in every patient not on subcutaneous heparin. Heparin is used in those patients with minimal to no risk of intracranial hemorrhage formation. Physical therapy and ambulation is encouraged in every patient.

■ GASTROINTESTINAL AND ENDOCRINE SUPPORT

Glucose and Cerebral Injury

Glucose is the main substrate of the brain and is actively transported across the blood–brain barrier by a carrier-mediated mechanism as well as by diffusional mechanisms that can be affected by blood glucose levels. Hypoglycemia is disadvantageous to ischemic brain. Hyperglycemia also worsens cerebral ischemia and neuronal damage after both head trauma and stroke.[56,72] It is less clear how, or at what level of hyperglycemia, global cerebral ischemia becomes worse, and the data are even less clear when applied to focal injury.[73,74] It is thought that organic acid accumulation in nonischemic areas may lead to cellular injury.[75] Another theory is that lactate production from anaerobic metabolism in areas of ischemia worsens existing damage.[76] Some data suggest that any amount of hyperglycemia (serum glucose greater than 120 mg/dL) may be detrimental.[77] It is not clear that maintenance of normal glucose levels through insulin therapy improves outcome, neurologic or otherwise. However,

it is common practice to keep serum glucose below 200 mg/dL in patients with known, or at risk for, cerebral ischemia. It is not uncommon to attempt to keep blood glucose in the range of normal or less than 140 mg/dL, usually by sliding-scale regular insulin injections or regular insulin infusion protocols.

Management of Diabetes Mellitus

Patients with premorbid diabetes mellitus may have serum glucose levels that are quite difficult to control. These patients are very likely to benefit most from tight glycemic control in the setting of cerebral ischemia, but studies suggesting how to maintain the serum glucose, and to what level, are scant. In our own practice, we routinely check every patient's serum glucose level every 6 hours after admission for at least the first 24 hours, and patients are placed in an insulin infusion nomogram after two consecutive blood glucose readings greater than 200 mg/dL. It has also become our practice to check glucose levels every 3 hours for the first 24 hours after admission or after beginning feeding for patients who are thought to be at high risk for glucose intolerance.

Nutrition

Neuronal tissue undergoes very high rates of oxidative metabolism with little or no stored energy, relying almost solely on blood-delivered glucose. Glucose undergoes active transport from the capillaries in areas with an intact blood–brain barrier. Throughout the brain, glucose also enters neuronal tissue through diffusion mechanisms. Areas of brain where the blood–brain barrier has been disrupted (e.g., by ischemia) may be totally reliant on diffusion mechanisms for their glucose supply. It is critical that nutritional demands be continually met in the critically ill. In the immediate postoperative period, nearly all neurosurgical patients receive nothing by mouth until they have been fully assessed and allowed to recover from the effects of anesthesia and post-surgical changes. If they are then able to self-feed, they are allowed a trial period, during which it is determined whether their nutritional demands can be adequately met. If self-feeding is not feasible, nasogastric tube feedings are initiated, and a determination is made about the long-term prognosis for adequate self-nutrition. If enteral nutrition is not successful, (i.e., if there are persistent large residual volumes after feeding or continuing lack of bowel sounds), parenteral nutrition via central venous catheters should be considered.

Postoperative Nausea and Vomiting

It is common for neurosurgical patients, especially those who underwent intracranial surgery, to have significant nausea and vomiting. This may result from the effects of anesthesia centrally or peripherally or from central effects of the surgery itself. Nausea can be uncomfortable for the patient, and vomiting can be catastrophic in cases of craniotomy. Nearly all antiemetics, including promethazine, corticosteroids, droperidol, and serotonergic drugs (e.g., ondansetron), have some effect on postoperative nausea and vomiting.[78] Ondansetron has been shown to be particularly efficacious in respect to postoperative craniotomy if given as a prophylactic.[79]

■ INFECTIOUS DISEASE

Infectious Risks of Neuraxial Devices

Several neuraxial catheters may be encountered in the post-operative neurosurgical patient, the most common of which is placed via a ventriculostomy. The major concern of the externalized neuraxial device is infection. The literature suggests that infection rates rise quickly at approximately 1 week after placement.[80] A number of different strategies have been used to combat this, including intrathecal antibiotic infusion, tunneling of the catheter, and changing the catheter weekly.[81] Rebuck found that administration of antibiotics to patients before or at the time of ventriculostomy placement did not decrease the incidence of CSF infection.[82] A greater risk for infection was attributable to duration greater than 5 days, use of a ventricular catheter, CSF leak, concurrent systemic infection, or serial ventricular devices. There are limited data to suggest that any method actually improves infection rates or patient morbidity or mortality, and each approach has its disadvantages, including microbial resistance and the risk of having to repeat the procedure.

■ REFERENCES

1. Manthous CA: Leapfrog and critical care: Evidence- and reality-based intensive care for the 21st century. Am J Med 2004;116:188-193.
2. Young MP, Birkmeyer JD: Potential reduction in mortality rates using an intensivist model to manage intensive care units. Eff Clin Pract 2000;3:284-289.
3. Mirski MA, Chang CW, Cowan R: Impact of a neuroscience intensive care unit on neurosurgical patient outcomes and cost of care: Evidence-based support for an intensivist-directed specialty ICU model of care. J Neurosurg Anesthesiol 2001;13:83-92.
4. Ziai WC, Varelas PN, Zeger SL, et al: Neurologic intensive care resource use after brain tumor surgery: An analysis of indications and alternative strategies. Crit Care Med 2003;31:2782-2787.
5. Clifton GL, Hayes RL, Levin HS, et al: Outcome measures for clinical trials involving traumatically brain-injured patients: Report of a conference. Neurosurgery 1992;31:975-978.
6. Vogel HP: Influence of additional information on interrater reliability in the neurologic examination. Neurology 1992;42:2076-2081.
7. Jaeger M, Soehle M, Schuhmann MU, et al: Correlation of continuously monitored regional cerebral blood flow and brain tissue oxygen. Acta Neurochir (Wien) 2005;147:51-56; discussion 56.
8. Stevens WJ: Multimodal monitoring: Head injury management using SjvO2 and LICOX. J Neurosci Nurs 2004;36:332-339.
9. Sarrafzadeh AS, Kiening KL, Callsen TA, Unterberg AW: Metabolic changes during impending and manifest cerebral hypoxia in traumatic brain injury. Br J Neurosurg 2003;17:340-346.
10. Sarrafzadeh AS, Sakowitz OW, Callsen TA, et al: Detection of secondary insults by brain tissue pO_2 and bedside microdialysis in severe head injury. Acta Neurochir Suppl 2002;81:319-321.
11. Nortje J, Menon DK: Traumatic brain injury: Physiology, mechanisms, and outcome. Curr Opin Neurol 2004;17:711-718.
12. Yundt KD, Diringer MN: The use of hyperventilation and its impact on cerebral ischemia in the treatment of traumatic brain injury. Crit Care Clin 1997;13:163-184.
13. Xi W, Sun L, Yao J, et al: Relationship between hyperventilation and intracranial pressure in patients with severe head injury. Chin J Traumatol 2001;4:190-192.
14. Stocchetti N, Maas AI, Chieregato A, van der Plas AA: Hyperventilation in head injury: A review. Chest 2005;127:1812-1827.
15. Bao Y, Jiang J, Zhu C, et al: Effect of hyperventilation on brain tissue oxygen pressure, carbon dioxide pressure, pH value and intracranial pressure during intracranial hypertension in pigs. Chin J Traumatol 2000;3:210-213.
16. Roberts PA, Pollay M, Engles C, et al: Effect on intracranial pressure of furosemide combined with varying doses and administration rates of mannitol. J Neurosurg 1987;66:440-446.
17. Kaal EC, Vecht CJ: The management of brain edema in brain tumors. Curr Opin Oncol 2004;16:593-600.
18. Roberts I: Barbiturates for acute traumatic brain injury. Cochrane Database Syst Rev 2000:CD000033.
19. Kuijlen JM, Teernstra OP, Kessels AG, et al: Effectiveness of anti-epileptic prophylaxis used with supratentorial craniotomies: A meta-analysis. Seizure 1996;5:291-298.
20. Manaka S, Ishijima B, Mayanagi Y: Postoperative seizures: Epidemiology, pathology, and prophylaxis. Neurol Med Chir (Tokyo) 2003;43:589-600; discussion 600.
21. Keranen T, Tapaninaho A, Hernesniemi J, Vapalahti M: Late epilepsy after aneurysm operations. Neurosurgery 1985;17:897-900.
22. Johnston AJ, Steiner LA, Gupta AK, Menon DK: Cerebral oxygen vasoreactivity and cerebral tissue oxygen reactivity. Br J Anaesth 2003;90:774-786.
23. Eintrei C, Lund N: Effects of increases in the inspired oxygen fraction on brain surface oxygen pressure fields in pig and man. Acta Anaesthesiol Scand 1986;30:194-198.
24. Schmetterer L, Findl O, Strenn K, et al: Role of NO in the O_2 and CO_2 responsiveness of cerebral and ocular circulation in humans. Am J Physiol 1997;273:R2005-2012.
25. Sjoberg F, Gustafsson U, Eintrei C: Specific blood flow reducing effects of hyperoxaemia on high flow capillaries in the pig brain. Acta Physiol Scand 1999;165:33-38.
26. Smielewski P, Czosnyka M, Kirkpatrick P, Pickard JD: Evaluation of the transient hyperemic response test in head-injured patients. J Neurosurg 1997;86:773-778.
27. Schwab S, Aschoff A, Spranger M, et al: The value of intracranial pressure monitoring in acute hemispheric stroke. Neurology 1996;47:393-398.
28. Frank J: Large hemispheric infarction, deterioration, and intracranial pressure. Neurology 1995;45:1286-1290.
29. O'Brien MJ, Van Eykern LA, Oetomo SB, Van Vught HA: Transcutaneous respiratory electromyographic monitoring. Crit Care Clin 1987;15:294-299.
30. Gildenberg P, Frost E: Respiratory care in head trauma. In Becker D, Povlishock J (eds): Central Nervous System Trauma. Bethesda, Md NINCDS National Institutes of Health, 1985, pp 161-176.
31. Silvestri S, Aronson S: Severe head injury: Prehospital and emergency department management. Mt Sinai J Med 1997;64:329-338.
32. Ampel L, Hott KA, Sielaff GW, Sloan TB: An approach to airway management in the acutely head-injured. J Emerg Med 1988;6:1-7.
33. Stirt JA, Grosslight KR, Bedford RF, Vollmer D: Defasciculation with metocurine prevents succinylcholine-induced increases in intracranial pressure. Anesthesiology 1987;67:50-53.
34. Feldman M: Physiological observations in a chronic case of "locked in" syndrome. Neurology 1971;21:459.
35. Devereaux M, Keane J, Davis R: Automatic respiratory failure associated with infarction in the medulla. Arch Neurol 1973;29:46.
36. Gore R, Mintzer R, Calenoff L: Gastrointestinal complications of spinal cord injury. Spine 1981;6:538-544.
37. Sutton RA, Macphail I, Bentley R, Nandy MK: Acute gastric dilatation as a relatively late complication of tetraplegia due to very high cervical cord injury. Paraplegia 1981;19:17-19.
38. Shafer A: Complications of sedation with midazolam in the intensive care unit and a comparison with other sedative regimens. Crit Care Med 1998;26:947-56.
39. Warner DS: Experience with remifentanil in neurosurgical patients. Anesth Analg 1999;89(4 Suppl):S33-39.
40. Bekker AY, Kaufman B, Samir H, Doyle W: The use of dexmedetomidine infusion for awake craniotomy. Anesth Analg 2001;92:1251-1253.
41. Gehlbach BK, Kress JP: Sedation in the intensive care unit. Curr Opin Crit Care 2002;8:290-298.
42. Citerio G, Cormio M: Sedation in neurointensive care: Advances in understanding and practice. Curr Opin Crit Care 2003;9:120-126.
43. Rose JC, Mayer SA: Optimizing blood pressure in neurological emergencies. Neurocrit Care 2004;1:287-300.

44. Haas CE, LeBlanc JM: Acute postoperative hypertension: A review of therapeutic options. Am J Health Syst Pharm 2004;61:1661-1673; quiz 1674-1675.

45. Szabo B: Imidazoline antihypertensive drugs: A critical review on their mechanism of action. Pharmacol Ther 2002;93:1-35.

46. Smith, JE, Hall MJ: Hypertonic saline. J R Army Med Corps 2004;150:239-243.

47. Bhardwaj A, Ulatowski JA: Hypertonic saline solutions in brain injury. Curr Opin Crit Care 2004;10:126-131.

48. Ducey JP, Mozingo DW, Lamiell JM: A comparison of the cerebral and cardiovascular effects of complete resuscitation with isotonic and hypertonic saline, hetastarch, and whole blood following hemorrhage. J Trauma 1989;29:1510-1518.

49. Niemi TT, Kuitunen AH: Artificial colloids impair haemostasis: An in vitro study using thromboelastometry coagulation analysis. Acta Anaesthesiol Scand 2005;49:373-378.

50. Scharbert G, Deusch E, Kress HG, et al: Inhibition of platelet function by hydroxyethyl starch solutions in chronic pain patients undergoing peridural anesthesia. Anesth Analg 2004;99:823-827.

51. Stump DC, Strauss RG, Henriksen RA: Effects of hydroxyethyl starch on blood coagulation, particularly factor VIII. Transfusion 1985;25: 349-354.

52. Zhuang J, Shackford SR, Schmoker JD, Pietropaoli JA Jr: Colloid infusion after brain injury: Effect on intracranial pressure, cerebral blood flow, and oxygen delivery. Crit Care Med 1995;23:140-148.

53. Rabinstein AA, Wijdicks EF: Hyponatremia in critically ill neurological patients. Neurologist 2003;9:290-300.

54. Sterns RH, Riggs JE, Schochet SS Jr: Osmotic demyelination syndrome following correction of hyponatremia. N Engl J Med 1986;314: 1535-1542.

55. Pollay M, Roberts PA: Blood-brain barrier: A definition of normal and altered function. Neurosurgery 1980;6:675-685.

56. Lanier WL, Stangland KJ, Scheithauer BW: The effect of dextrose infusion and head position on neurological outcomes after complete cerebral ischemia in primates. Anesthesiology 1987;66:39-48.

57. Ciric I, Ragin A, Baumgartner C, Pierce D: Complications of transsphenoidal surgery: Results of a national survey, review of the literature, and personal experience. Neurosurgery 1997;40:225-236; discussion 236-237.

58. Zornow MH, Todd MM, Moore SS: The acute cerebral effects of changes in plasma osmolality and oncotic pressure. Anesthesiology 1987;67:936-941.

59. Chanson P, Jedynak CP, Dabrowski G, et al: Ultralow doses of vasopressin in the management of diabetes insipidus. Crit Care Med 1987;15:44-46.

60. Lee YJ, Shen EY, Huang FY, et al: Continuous infusion of vasopressin in comatose children with neurogenic diabetes insipidus. J Pediatr Endocrinol Metab 1995;8:257-262.

61. Wise-Faberowski L, Soriano SG, Ferrari L, et al: Perioperative management of diabetes insipidus in children (corrected). J Neurosurg Anesthesiol 2004;16:14-19.

62. Tu YK, Liu HM: Effects of isovolemic hemodilution on hemodynamics, cerebral perfusion, and cerebral vascular reactivity. Stroke 1996;27: 441-445.

63. Hebert PC, Van der Linden P, Biro G, Hu LQ: Physiologic aspects of anemia. Crit Care Clin 2004;20:187-212.

64. Kudo T, Suzuki S, Iwabuchi T: Importance of monitoring the circulating blood volume in patients with cerebral vasospasm after subarachnoid hemorrhage. Neurosurgery 1981;9:514-520.

65. Weiskopf RB, Kramer JH, Viele M, et al: Acute severe isovolemic anemia impairs cognitive function and memory in humans. Anesthesiology 2000;92:1646-1652.

66. Spahn DR: Strategies for transfusion therapy. Best Pract Res Clin Anaesthesiol 2004;18:661-673.

67. Drews RE: Critical issues in hematology: Anemia, thrombocytopenia, coagulopathy, and blood product transfusions in critically ill patients. Clin Chest Med 2003;24:607-622.

68. Kroegel C, Reissig A: Principle mechanisms underlying venous thromboembolism: Epidemiology, risk factors, pathophysiology and pathogenesis. Respiration 2003;70:7-30.

69. Epstein NE: A review of the risks and benefits of differing prophylaxis regimens for the treatment of deep venous thrombosis and pulmonary embolism in neurosurgery. Surg Neurol 2005;64:295-301; discussion 302.

70. Agnelli G, Piovella F, Buoncristiani P, et al: Enoxaparin plus compression stockings compared with compression stockings alone in the prevention of venous thromboembolism after elective neurosurgery. N Engl J Med 1998;339:80-85.

71. Browd SR, Ragel BT, Davis GE, et al: Prophylaxis for deep venous thrombosis in neurosurgery: A review of the literature. Neurosurg Focus 2004;17:E1.

72. Welsh FA, Ginsberg MD, Rieder W, Budd WW: Deleterious effects of glucose pre-treatment on recovery from diffuse cerebral ischemia in the cat. Stroke 1980;11:355-363.

73. de Courten-Myers G, Myers RE, Schoolfield L: Hyperglycemia enlarges infarct size in cerebrovascular occlusion in cats. Stroke 1988;19:623-630.

74. Zasslow MA, Pearl RG, Shuer LM, et al: Hyperglycemia decreases acute neuronal ischemic changes after middle cerebral artery occlusion in cats. Stroke 1989;20:519-523.

75. Zygun DA, Steiner LA, Johnston AJ, et al: Hyperglycemia and brain tissue pH after traumatic brain injury. Neurosurgery 2004;55:877-881; discussion 882.

76. Makimattila S, Malmberg-Ceder K, Hakkinen AM, et al: Brain metabolic alterations in patients with type I diabetes and hyperglycemia-induced injury. J Cereb Blood Flow Metab 2004;24:1393-1399.

77. Wass CT, Lanier WL: Glucose modulation of ischemic brain injury: Review and clinical recommendations. Mayo Clin Proc 1996;71:801-812.

78. Fabling JM, Gan TJ, El-Moalem HE, et al: A randomized, double-blinded comparison of ondansetron, droperidol, and placebo for prevention of postoperative nausea and vomiting after supratentorial craniotomy. Anesth Analg 2000;91:358-361.

79. Fabling JM, Gan TJ, El-Moalem HE, et al: A randomized, double-blind comparison of ondansetron versus placebo for prevention of nausea and vomiting after infratentorial craniotomy. J Neurosurg Anesthesiol 2002;14:102-107.

80. Holloway KL, Barnes T, Choi S, et al: Ventriculostomy infections: The effect of monitoring duration and catheter exchange in 584 patients. J Neurosurg 1996;85:419-424.

81. Arabi Y, Memish ZA, Balkhy HH, et al: Ventriculostomy-associated infections: Incidence and risk factors. Am J Infect Control 2005;33: 137-143.

82. Rebuck JA, Murry KR, Rhoney DH, et al: Infection related to intracranial pressure monitors in adults: Analysis of risk factors and antibiotic prophylaxis. J Neurol Neurosurg Psychiatry 2000;69:381-384.

Specific Problems

Chapter

38 Sepsis and Septic Shock

Michael D. Malinzak and Laura E. Niklason

Severe sepsis and septic shock remain among the most serious conditions threatening patients during the postoperative period. Over the past 15 years, advances in knowledge of supportive care and the advent of direct therapy have allowed significant reductions in the mortality of this disease state. In light of recent developments, the Surviving Sepsis Campaign international advisory committee published guidelines with regard to the standard of care for the management of severe sepsis and septic shock in 2004. This chapter provides an overview of the pathogenesis and burden of sepsis and then thoroughly explores current consensus recommendations and supporting scientific rationale for the treatment of adult sepsis.

Sepsis is a physiologic state representing a systemic inflammatory response to a delocalized infection (Box 38-1). Often, this represents a blood-borne bacterial or fungal infection, but sepsis and septicemia are not synonymous. A full 30% of blood cultures taken from patients who are clinically septic remain negative.[1] Although the terms *sepsis, severe sepsis,* and *septic shock* were once used almost interchangeably, a consensus definition was reached in 1992, and *sepsis* is now defined as infection accompanied by two or more of the following signs of systemic inflammation: hypothermia or hyperthermia, tachycardia, tachypnea, or elevated or depressed leukocyte count.[1,2] Whereas severe sepsis requires only the additional presence of organ system failure or hypoperfusion, septic shock is defined as hypotension with organ system dysfunction that is not correctable by intravenous fluid resuscitation.[1-3]

■ DIAGNOSIS, PATHOGENESIS, AND EPIDEMIOLOGY

In clinical practice, early signs of severe sepsis (i.e., organ hypoperfusion) include hypotension, oliguria, mottled skin, confusion, delayed capillary refill, and elevated serum lactate. Given the elevated metabolic demands of sepsis and the direct effects of systemic inflammation on the lungs, respira-

tory decompensation is an almost universal event and frequently necessitates mechanical ventilation. Mild elevations in serum aminotransferases and bilirubin are common, and ileus is frequently present for 24 to 48 hours after restoration of normal splanchnic perfusion.[4] Endocrine abnormalities are also observed, with serum cortisol and glucose elevations appearing early in the course of illness. Other underlying noninfectious causes of shock must be ruled out, especially in the setting of recent trauma or burns and in cases where pancreatitis, cardiac pathology, or chemical intoxication is suspected. When infection is deemed unlikely, the diagnosis of aseptic shock is ultimately a clinical decision. Obtaining a serum procalcitonin concentration of less than 0.25 mg/L can lend support for this diagnosis.[1]

The pathophysiology of sepsis is complex and incompletely understood. In response to an overwhelming infection, leukocytes and endothelial cells are activated and upregulate expression of inflammatory surface moieties such as intercellular adhesion marker (ICAM)-1. In addition, soluble factors such as tumor necrosis factor (TNF)-α, interferon-γ, interleukin (IL)-1, IL-6, and IL-8 are elevated. These changes in expression are mediated by a number of transcription factors, the most intensely studied of which is nuclear factor kappa B (NFκB). Indeed, most pharmacologic agents that have progressed to phase 3 clinical trials for the direct treatment of sepsis have functioned by inhibiting NFκB in either endothelial cells or leukocytes.

Cytokines and bacterial endotoxin drive the leukocyte inflammatory response and promote tissue factor expression by monocytes and endothelial cells.[1] Abnormal activation of coagulation factors is initially offset by the presence of endogenous anticoagulants, such as activated protein C and antithrombin (previously, antithrombin III). As these endogenous anticoagulants are depleted, systemic activation of the coagulation pathway leads to diffuse thrombin-mediated endothelial damage.[5] Additionally, vascular permeability increases, facilitating leukocyte extravasation and promoting

38-1	**Definitions of Sepsis**

Sepsis (Both A and B)

A. Infection
  • Common sources include the lung, abdomen, urinary tract, primary bloodstream infection, vascular access devices, and surgical wounds.
  • Unusual sources include cellulitis, sinusitis, and toxic shock syndrome.
  • Risk factors include chronic organ failure, immunodeficiency, and underlying malignancy.
B. Systemic inflammation (two or more of the following):
  • Hypothermia or hyperthermia
  • Tachycardia
  • Tachypnea
  • Leukocytosis or leukopenia

Severe Sepsis

A. Sepsis, as defined above, plus one of the following:
B. Generalized hypoperfusion
  • Signs include hypotension, delayed capillary refill, mottled skin, mental status changes.
  • Laboratory tests may reveal elevated serum lactate.
C. Organ failure in at least one organ system
  • Signs include oliguria and ileus.
  • Laboratory tests may demonstrate elevated liver function tests and bilirubin.

Septic Shock

A. Sepsis, as defined above, plus hypotension and organ system dysfunction that prove refractory to intravenous fluid resuscitation.

---

capillary leak. Cyclooxygenase activity is also upregulated in sepsis, resulting in increased plasma levels of the arachidonic acid metabolites thromboxane A2, prostacyclin, and prostaglandin E_2 (PGE_2), which are believed to be directly responsible for the clinical picture of tachycardia, tachypnea, ventilation–perfusion mismatch, and lactic acidosis.[4] The combined results of resultant intravascular depletion, vasodilation, and myocardial depression produce discrepancies between tissue metabolic demands and oxygen delivery, leading to global hypoxia and organ failure.[6]

Severe sepsis, septic shock, and the infections that initiate these conditions are frequently sequelae of other underlying illnesses. Indeed, patients with immunodeficiency, cancer, and chronic organ failure are all highly predisposed to becoming septic. Epidemiologic studies have demonstrated that the primary site of infection is most frequently the lung, followed by the abdomen and urogenital tract.[2,4] These nidi, taken together with primary bloodstream infections, are thought to be responsible for more than 80% of all sepsis cases.[1] In clinical practice, however, no definite infection can be identified in 20% to 30% of all patients with sepsis.[2,4] When caring for postoperative patients, the possibility of wound infection must be thoroughly assessed, especially in the setting of recent abdominal surgery. Other causative pathologies that are easily overlooked include cellulitis, toxic shock syndrome, and infections of the pleural cavities, peritoneal cavity, and paranasal sinuses.[4] In all cases, diagnostic aspirates or purulent discharge must be retained for culture and sensitivity screening. Therapeutic evacuation or debridement should be performed whenever not immediately contraindicated.

The incidence of sepsis is increasing annually by 1.5% to 9% in the United States and Europe and currently accounts for an estimated 2% of all hospital admissions and 7.0% to 9.7% of all intensive care unit (ICU) admissions.[1,2,7] Given that the peak incidence of sepsis is during the 6th decade of life, it is likely that this trend will continue as the demographics of the West become increasingly top-heavy.[1,7] An observational cohort study of the 192,980 patients with sepsis cared for in seven states in 1995 estimated the national annual incidence to be 3.0 per 1000.[7] The average cost per case of sepsis in this analysis was $22,100, with an estimated yearly national cost of $16.7 billion.[7]

As the disease progresses, approximately 9% of patients with sepsis advance to severe sepsis, and 3% go on to develop septic shock.[1] During the course of severe sepsis, a median of two organ systems display signs of failure.[4] The proportion of polymicrobial and resistant bacterial infections, especially those caused by *Pseudomonas aeruginosa* and methicillin-resistant *Staphylococcus aureus,* increased significantly between 1993 and 2000.[2] Most organ dysfunction is believed to resolve within weeks to months in patients who survive acute illness.

Sepsis-associated mortality has decreased significantly over the past 2 decades, largely as a result of advances in treatment. Still, septicemia is among the leading causes of death in the United States, accounting for 9.3% of all mortality in 1995.[2] Pediatric sepsis (which is beyond the scope of treatment recommendations for this chapter) is the second leading cause of pediatric mortality in the United States and remains among the foremost global health challenges.[8,9] In terms of outcome, a study of 100,554 European ICU admissions found that the mortality of adult severe sepsis decreased from 62.1% in 1993 to 55.9% in 2000.[2] The increased risk of mortality attributable to sepsis as compared with matched nonseptic ICU patients was 25.7%.[1,2] Current mortality estimates in U.S. hospitals range from about 30% to 70%.[2,4] A variety of patient subgroups display differential mortalities, but poorer outcomes are associated with male sex, older age, and the existence of underlying life-shortening illness or immunosuppression. One study found that prognosis could be stratified by the number of organ systems that failed on the first day of severe sepsis presentation. Significantly, 20% mortality was observed for patients with less than three organ system failures, whereas greater than three organ system failures was associated with 70% mortality.[10]

■ SUPPORTIVE THERAPY AND PROPHYLACTIC CONSIDERATIONS

Hemodynamic Optimization

Early and aggressive fluid resuscitation is perhaps the most critical intervention for reducing all-cause mortality after a patient is found to be septic (Fig. 38-1). A landmark clinical trial randomized 263 patients presenting to the emergency department with severe sepsis and septic shock (i.e., systolic

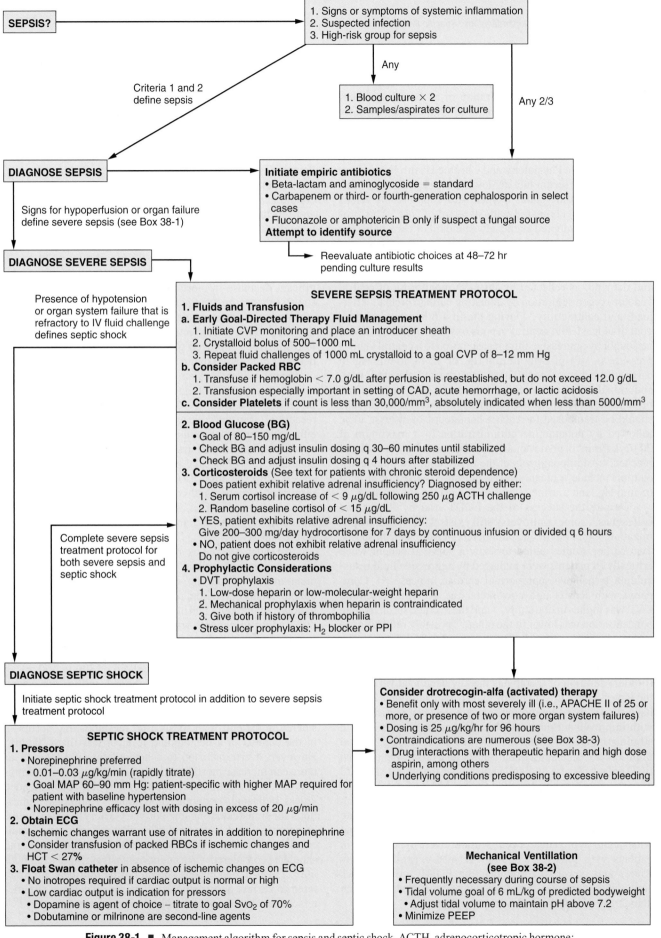

Figure 38-1 ■ Management algorithm for sepsis and septic shock. ACTH, adrenocorticotropic hormone; CAD, coronary artery disease; CVP, central venous pressure; DVT, deep vein thrombosis; ECG, electrocardiography; HCT, hematocrit; IV, intravenous; MAP, mean arterial pressure; PEEP, positive end-expiratory pressure; PPI, proton-pump inhibitor; q, every; RBC, red blood cell.

blood pressure <90 mm Hg after an initial 20- to 30-mL/kg fluid bolus, or serum lactate >4 mmol/L) to be treated with an early goal-directed therapy (EGDT) resuscitation protocol or standard of care.[6] Administration of an EGDT for the 6 hours prior to ICU transfer reduced in-hospital mortality from 46.5% to 30.5% (P = .009) as compared with the standard of care.[6,11] During the 7- to 72-hour interval following initial treatment, patients treated with EGDT had lower APACHE (Acute Physiology and Chronic Health Evaluation) II scores, lower serum lactate, lower base deficit, higher pH, and higher central venous oxygen saturation (70.4% versus 65.3%, P < .02) compared with standard of care.[6] This protocol has been adopted as the new standard of care and is the basis of the fluid resuscitation guidelines put forth by the Surviving Sepsis Campaign.[12]

The goal of EGDT is to better balance oxygen delivery and demand, as reflected by invasive monitoring of central venous oxygen saturation by adjusting cardiac preload, afterload, and contractility.[6] During the first 6 hours, a primary goal of at least 70% central venous oxygen saturation should be sought by aggressive fluid resuscitation to a central venous pressure (CVP) of 8 to 12 mm Hg, or 12 to 15 mm Hg in cases of mechanical ventilation or suspected elevated intra-abdominal pressure.[6,11,12] Should the target oxygen saturation be unachievable at these pressures, packed red blood cells should be transfused to reach a hematocrit of at least 30%, followed by dobutamine administration to a maximum of 20 µg/kg/min if goal venous oxygen saturation is still not reached.[12] Additional goals of the first 6 hours of fluid resuscitation include a mean arterial pressure (MAP) of at least 65 mm Hg, and a urine output of at least 0.5 mL/kg/hr.[6,11,12]

Despite the success of the EGDT trial by Rivers and colleagues,[13] some controversy still exists with regard to optimization of hemodynamic parameters in patients with sepsis. Two earlier studies failed to show a survival benefit when critically ill patients were managed by aggressive fluid resuscitation to achieve supranormal cardiac indices.[13a,13b] Compared with Rivers and coworkers, the average presenting CVP was higher in one study,[13a] and the average serum lactate concentration was lower in the other,[13b] possibly reflecting the inclusion of more severely ill patients in the EGDT trial.[6] The consensus opinion with regard to reconciling these discrepancies has focused on the earlier initiation and shorter (6-hour) duration of therapy as the key beneficial variants in the Rivers trial.[6] In support of EGDT, two additional studies have shown that supranormal oxygen delivery is associated with improved surgical outcome, suggesting that early fluid administration and attention to oxygen delivery are of critical importance.[12] In a subsequent subset analysis of the original EGDT data, Rivers and colleagues note that those standard of care patients who presented with a MAP of greater than 100 mm Hg but a serum lactate concentration of greater than 4 mmol/L suffered an impressive 40% higher mortality rate than matched EGDT enrollees.[13] This finding suggests that widespread hypoxia can occur without overt hypotension in patients with sepsis, a condition termed *cryptic shock* by Rivers and coworkers, and that the EGDT protocol does confer an important survival advantage by increasing oxygen delivery in patients with severe sepsis.[13]

Intraoperative fluid management also impacts recovery time and postoperative complications including infections. Thus, intraoperative anesthetic care may well affect rates of postoperative sepsis. The first of two salient studies employed esophageal Doppler ultrasound during surgery and found that repeated colloid fluid challenge to optimize stroke volume reduced length of hospital stay by 39% as compared with matched standard of care control.[14] A larger trial randomized surgical patients into three groups that received conventional intraoperative fluid management, repeated colloid challenge guided by esophageal Doppler ultrasound, and repeated colloid challenge guided by CVP to optimize hemodynamic parameters.[15] The invasively guided management strategies were found comparable, and they significantly reduced the time until discharge—from 14 to 10 days—as compared with conventional therapy, with no significant decrease in mortality.[15] Taken together, these trials suggest that more stringent monitoring and management of intraoperative intravascular volume can improve postoperative recovery. These effects are thought, as seen with EGDT, to result from improved global perfusion and prevention of perioperative tissue hypoxia.[14,15]

Some evidence exists for the use of supplemental perioperative oxygen to reduce rates of postoperative wound infection. In a trial of 500 patients undergoing colorectal resection, Grief and colleagues randomized patients to receive either 80% or 30% FIO$_2$ during surgery and for 2 hours postoperatively and found associated wound infection rates of 28% and 13% (P = .01), respectively.[16] In cases of existing sepsis, however, high FIO$_2$ can potentially cause increased respiratory damage and contribute to acute respiratory distress syndrome (ARDS). Accordingly, no recommendations exist with regard to supranormal FIO$_2$ administration during severe sepsis.

An older debate has stirred for years over the merits of resuscitation with colloid versus crystalloid fluids. A large meta-analysis found no evidence for preferential use of colloid versus crystalloid resuscitation using general surgery patient populations, and it seems reasonable to extrapolate this finding to patients with sepsis.[12] The Surviving Sepsis Campaign notes only that more crystalloid must be given than colloid because of the greater volume of distribution, and that 500 to 1000 mL of crystalloid or 300 to 500 mL of colloid is appropriate for the initial bolus and for subsequent fluid challenges until hemodynamic goals are reached.[12]

Transfusion of packed red blood cells should be considered in patients with sepsis after reestablishing perfusion in the context of a hemoglobin level of less than 7.0 g/dL. However, overtransfusion to a hemoglobin of 12.0 g/dL or more can increase mortality in critically ill patients.[17] Administration of exogenous erythropoietin is not recommended unless indicated by another condition.[12] Additional indications for transfusion include coronary artery disease, active hemorrhage, and lactic acidosis.[12] Platelet infusion is indicated for all patients with counts of less than 5000/mm^3 and should be considered when counts range from 5000 to 30,000/mm^3. Fresh-frozen plasma should not be routinely administered to correct perturbations in laboratory clotting parameters in the absence of acute bleeding or planned surgery.[12]

Ventilatory Support

Sepsis places increased demand on the lungs through the respiratory requirements of systemic inflammation. The inflammatory milieu also promotes the development of acute lung injury (ALI) and ARDS. ARDS is an inflammatory condition defined by the appearance of bilateral pulmonary infiltrates on chest radiograph, decreased lung compliance, and resultant hypoxemia.[18] The confounding result of ARDS in sepsis is a requirement for high minute ventilation concomitant with low lung compliance, impaired alveolar diffusion, and reduced respiratory muscle efficiency.[4] Consequently, tachypnea is almost ubiquitous in sepsis, and a sustained respiratory rate of greater than 30 breaths/min, even in the setting of a normal arterial partial pressure of oxygen (PaO_2), should be interpreted as a sign of potential ventilatory decompensation.[4] Mechanical ventilation is required for 1 to 2 weeks in 81% to 85% of patients with severe sepsis, and approximately 50% develop ARDS.[2,4] ARDS often develops with mechanical ventilation even when the primary indication for intubation was not respiratory distress.[11]

Arguably the most important development in ventilatory care of patients with sepsis came when Brower and coworkers,[19] under the auspices of the ARDS Network, reported decreased mortality in ARDS patients ventilated with lower rather than higher tidal volumes. In this randomized trial, 861 patients with ALI and ARDS were ventilated with goals of either 6 mL/kg of predicted bodyweight and a plateau pressure of 30 cm H_2O or less, or 12 mL/kg of predicted bodyweight and a plateau pressure of 50 cm H_2O or less.[19] The trial was terminated early because mortality in the lower tidal volume group was 31.0%, versus 39.8% in the higher tidal volume group ($P = .007$).[20] Serum IL-6 concentrations were also significantly lower in the lower tidal volume group.[19] Lower tidal volume patients required higher positive end-expiratory pressure (PEEP) and FIO_2.[19] Predicted bodyweight was calculated for men—$50 + 0.91 \times$ (height in centimeters − 152.4)—and for women—$45.5 + 0.91 \times$ (height in centimeters − 152.4).[19] An uncontrolled study of the implementation of the ARDS Net tidal volume recommendations revealed similar decreases in mortality.[21] Importantly, ventilation at 6 mL/kg of predicted bodyweight remains the current recommendation for severe sepsis and associated ARDS (Box 38-2), but debate over the mechanism of reduced mortality continues.[12]

The cause of the striking 22% relative reduction in mortality conferred by lower ventilatory tidal volume has been controversial. Brower and colleagues suggested that lower tidal volume may reduce the traumatic mechanical ventilatory component of systemic inflammation.[19] In support of this hypothesis, a study of serum cytokines in ARDS Net patients found that lower tidal volumes were associated with 26% and 12% reductions in IL-6 and IL-8, respectively, and that higher IL-6, IL-8, and IL-10 serum concentrations were each associated with increased mortality.[22] It has been speculated that lower tidal volumes, in addition to reducing the release of inflammatory cytokines, may also produce a protective hypercarbia via the inhibitory effects of lower serum pH on

38-2	Mechanical Ventilation Guidelines during Severe Sepsis

Tidal Volume

- Goal tidal volume is 6 mL/kg predicted bodyweight.
- Initial tidal volumes up to 12 mL/kg are acceptable.
  - Reduce to goal by stepwise reductions of 1 mL/kg over 1 to 2 hours.

End-Inspiratory Plateau Pressure

- Goal plateau pressure is 30 to 35 cm H_2O or less.

Significance of pH

- Adjust ventilator rate to maintain normal pH.
- Modest hypercapnia, to a pH of approximately 7.2, should be tolerated to achieve tidal volume and plateau pressure goals.
- Bicarbonate infusion provides no hemodynamic improvement and is not indicated in lactic acidemia, even when pH is less than 7.15.

Positive End-Expiratory Pressure (PEEP)

- Employ minimal PEEP necessary to prevent lung collapse.
- Titrate PEEP on basis of severity of oxygen deficit.

Positioning

- Semirecumbent positioning with head at 45-degree angle reduces risk of ventilator-associated pneumonia.
- Patients should be laid flat during episodes of hypotension to ensure central nervous system perfusion.

Extubation Criteria

- Low PEEP requirements of 5 cm H_2O or less
- FIO_2 requirement safely deliverable by face mask or nasal canula
- Hemodynamic stability (i.e., vasopressors discontinued)
- Consider extubation after spontaneous breathing trial

Adapted from Shapiro N, Howell M, Talmor D: Acad Emerg Med 2005;12:352-359; Dellinger R, Carlet J, Masur H, et al: Crit Care Med 2004;32:858-873; and Brower R, Matthay M, Morris A, et al: N Engl J Med 2000;342:1301-1308.

cytokine activity.[22] Because alveolar involvement is heterogeneous in ARDS, it has long been suspected that lower plateau pressures, such as those used in the low tidal volume group, may reduce lung trauma by lessening overstretching of those alveoli that retain baseline compliance.[4] Interestingly, rates of gross barotrauma (e.g., in pneumothorax) did not differ significantly between the high and low tidal volume groups, thus calling into question whether the reduction in plateau pressure was significant enough to prevent overstretch-related microanatomic and biochemical changes.[19] One study randomized 44 ICU patients to receive either 11.1 mL/kg tidal volume with 6.5 cm H_2O PEEP or 7.6 mL/kg tidal volume with 14.8 cm H_2O PEEP.[23] The lower tidal volume, higher PEEP group yielded significantly lower serum concentrations of IL-6, and bronchoalveolar lavage samples with less IL-1, TNF-α, IL-8, and IL-6 and lower neutrophil counts.[23] In this trial, however, lower tidal volume was not associated with a reduction in mortality; this discrepancy from the ARDS Net trial may derive from the smaller patient population, a smaller difference between tidal volume groups, and the lower average respiratory rates used by Ranieri and associates.[18,19]

The benefits of low tidal volume ventilation may stem more directly from increased exogenous PEEP, and the high ventilatory rates necessitated by low tidal volumes also produce elevated intrinsic PEEP by means of dynamic hyperinflation.[11] Indeed, Durante and coworkers demonstrated that ventilating ARDS patients with tidal volumes 6 mL/kg versus 12 mL/kg was associated with average total PEEPs of 16.3 and 11.7 cm H_2O, as well as average intrinsic PEEPs of 5.8 and 1.4 cm H_2O, respectively.[24] Accordingly, the ARDS Net study group led a subsequent study in which 549 patients with ALI and ARDS received a goal tidal volume of 6 mL/kg of predicted bodyweight and a plateau pressure of less than 30 cm H_2O with either 8.3 ± 3.2 cm H_2O PEEP or 13.2 ± 3.5 cm H_2O PEEP; no significant differences in mortality or 28-day ventilator-free period were observed between the groups.[20] In conclusion, minimizing tidal volume and plateau pressure, but not PEEP, improves outcome in patients with ventilated ARDS and severe sepsis.

Normothermia

Although not addressed in the recommendations of the Surviving Sepsis Campaign, there is evidence that avoiding hypothermia may reduce infection and sepsis-related mortality in the perioperative period. One study of 200 patients who had colorectal surgery found that intraoperative use of forced-air body warmers and warmed intravenous fluids yielded an average core temperature of 36.6° C as compared with the 34.7° C that was achieved with standard of care.[25] Compared with control, intraoperative warming was associated with a reduction in wound infection rate from 19% to 6%, and a 20% decrease in average length of hospital stay.[25] Perioperative normothermia is thought to reduce wound infections by preventing cutaneous vasoconstriction and thus improving leukocyte delivery and oxidative killing at sites prone to bacterial colonization. There may be other hemodynamic benefits to normothermia as reflected by the positive association that exists between mild hypothermia during abdominal aortic aneurysm repair, mortality, and increased requirements for transfusions, pressors, and inotropic agents.[26]

With regard to established sepsis, one study found that presenting core temperatures of 35.6° C and lower and of 38.3° C and higher were associated with a 66% and a 41% 28-day mortality, respectively.[27] This finding is further supported in animal models of sepsis, which have shown that postoperative external warming is associated with improved survival.[28] Interestingly, investigators have been unable to demonstrate significant differences in plasma cytokine profiles between hypothermic and hyperthermic septic patient populations, and thus fever regulation is thought to be centrally mediated at the hypothalamic level in sepsis.[27] Attempts to control fever in sepsis using external cooling and acetaminophen have not been successful.[29] No consensus recommendations exist with regard to temperature control during the course of severe sepsis.

Adjunctive Therapy and Prophylactic Considerations

Hypoperfusion with the associated renal dysfunction leads to the requirement for renal replacement therapy in 25.2% of patients with severe sepsis.[2] The Surviving Sepsis Campaign guidelines stress the equivalence of venovenous hemofiltration and intermittent hemodialysis, with the caveat that the former may be superior in terms of ease of fluid management when patients are particularly unstable.[12]

Deep vein thrombosis (DVT) prophylaxis should always be a priority in incapacitated patients and is of increased importance in the coagulopathic septic population. The Surviving Sepsis Campaign recommends low-dose unfractionated heparin or low-molecular-weight heparin as the first line of treatment, but it notes that mechanical compression devices are an appropriate substitute in cases of severe underlying coagulopathy, thrombocytopenia, or recent hemorrhage.[12] Both pharmacologic and mechanical prophylaxis should be used in patients with a prior history of thrombophilia.[12]

As with other ICU patients, stress ulcer prophylaxis is indicated for patients with sepsis. Dellinger and colleagues suggest that proton-pump inhibitors have not been rigorously tested in this setting and that histamine receptor (H_2R) antagonists are thus the treatment of choice.[12] Other gastrointestinal considerations include provisions for nutritional support in the common setting of ileus and sepsis. Some sources emphasize that nutrition can be withheld until after hemodynamic stabilization (i.e., 1 to 2 days), and enteric feeding is preferable after that time unless otherwise contraindicated by recent gastrointestinal surgery.[4]

■ PHARMACOLOGIC INTERVENTIONS

Antibiotics

Early empirical treatment with broad-spectrum parenteral antibiotics is the mainstay of therapy in the hours following the diagnosis of sepsis. At least two blood cultures, preferably one taken percutaneously and another from a vascular access port, should be performed before initiation of antibiotics. Vascular access devices can be the source of infection, and any port producing positive cultures 2 or more hours sooner than other draws, or any existing port when a primary source cannot be identified, should be removed as soon as another vascular access is present.[12] Imaging studies should also be performed early in the course of sepsis, and attempts at source control by debridement or drainage should be delayed only until fluid resuscitation renders hemodynamics permissible. Culture and sensitivity should be obtained for all aspirates or suspicious discharges.

Several analyses emphasize the importance of early and appropriate antibiotic coverage. In one retrospective study of 18,209 Medicare patients presenting with community-acquired pneumonia, initiation of empiric antibiotic therapy within 4 hours of arrival yielded 6.8% in-hospital mortality, 11.6% 30-day mortality, and a 0.4-day reduced hospital stay as compared with 7.4% in-hospital mortality and 12.7% 30-day mortality in patients who received antibiotics later.[30] In another retrospective study of empirical therapy, patients with sepsis were grouped on the basis of having received either appropriate ($n = 2158$) or inappropriate ($n = 1255$) initial antibiotics by final culture results. Appropriate empiric treatment was associated with 20% mortality and a 9-day average survivor hospital stay as opposed 34% mortality and an 11-day stay among inappropriately treated patients ($P <$ .05 for all comparisons).[31] Even more striking, initial appropriate antibiotics versus inappropriate coverage can reduce mortality to 28% from 49% in cases of gram-negative sepsis.[11]

The suspected class of causative organism, which in most cases is bacterial, should govern the initial choice of antibiotics. In otherwise uncomplicated septic patients, empiric therapy to cover both gram-positive and gram-negative infection is sufficient. Classically, this regimen consisted of a β-lactam and an aminoglycoside. Recent reviews, however, conclude that use of empiric monotherapy consisting of carbapenem or a third- or fourth-generation cephalosporin is as effective as the combination of a β-lactam and an aminoglycoside when treating non-neutropenic patients with severe sepsis.[32,33] Although less highly recommended, an extended-spectrum carboxypenicillin or ureidopenicillin combined with a β-lactamase inhibitor may be also used as initial therapy.[33] Empiric treatment with a glycopeptide antibiotic (e.g., vancomycin or teicoplanin), an oxazolidinone (e.g., linezolid), or a streptogramin (e.g., quinupristin/dalfopristin) is appropriate in patients with allergies to other drug classes or when antibiotic-resistant gram-positive infections are suspected.[32,33] Antibiotic penetration to the suspected site of initial infection should also be confirmed.[12]

Empiric treatment with antifungals is not recommended for routine practice. Should candidemia be suspected, treatment with an azole (e.g., fluconazole) or echinocandin is thought to produce equivalent outcomes with less toxicity than seen with amphotericin B.[32,33]

In all cases, empiric therapy should be initiated within 1 hour of septic diagnosis, preceded only by initiation of fluid resuscitation and collection of blood cultures.[11,12,33] A loading dose should be employed, and renal function, hepatic function, and altered volume of distribution after fluid resuscitation should be considered.[12] Most sources recommend reassessment of antibiotic regimen at 48 to 72 hours once culture and sensitivity data are available.[11,33] The therapy with the narrowest spectrum appropriate should be employed once the organism is identified, to reduce toxicity and the development of resistance or superinfection. The decision to discontinue antibiotics is ultimately a clinical one, but in general it to can be made safely at 7 to 10 days; neutropenic patients are an important exception for whom antibiotic combination therapy should be continued until neutrophil counts improve.[12]

Pressors and Inotropes

Judicious use of pressors is recommended when hemodynamic instability is refractory to appropriate fluid resuscitation, as is the case in as many as 85% of cases of severe sepsis.[2] Specifically, should fluid resuscitation to a goal CVP (8 to 12 or 10 to 15 mm Hg in ventilated patients) fail to correct hypotension or signs of organ hypoperfusion, or

should hypotension become life-threatening before the fluid challenge is complete, infusion of norepinephrine or dopamine through a central catheter is the treatment of choice.[1,12] Dopamine may be preferred when systolic dysfunction is prominent because of its inotropic and chronotropic effects, whereas norepinephrine is a more potent vasoconstrictor with fewer cardiac side effects and may be more appropriate for the most severe cases of hypotension.[12] Multiple studies have failed to demonstrate any renal-protective effects of dopamine in severe sepsis, and administration of low-dose dopamine for renal protection is not indicated.[4,12] Second-line choices include epinephrine and phenylephrine, which can have the unwanted effects of impairing splanchnic circulation and stroke volume, respectively.[12] Guidelines for pressor administration recommend titration to a MAP of 60 to 90 mm Hg, with goals for baseline hypertensive patients toward the higher end of this range.[1]

Septic shock that is refractory to high-dose vasopressors may warrant treatment with 0.02 to 0.04 units/min of vasopressin, although this therapy yields little in most patients.[12] Importantly, vasopressin is contraindicated in patients with significant coronary artery disease because of the risk of myocardial ischemia.

Clinically, cardiac output may be depressed despite adequate fluid resuscitation and pressor administration to support left ventricular end-diastolic pressure and MAP.[12] Although intraoperative use of inotropes to ensure appropriate tissue oxygenation decreases subsequent mortality and complication rates, two randomized trials have failed to show benefit from inotropically induced supranormal oxygen delivery.[12,34,35] Accordingly, inotropic support should be given with the goal of balancing oxygen consumption and delivery at physiologic baseline as indicated by a low serum lactate and a venous oxygen saturation (SvO_2) of approximately 70%.

Pharmacologic Advances toward Direct Intervention

A number of directly acting pharmacologic agents have been used in clinical practice or have unsuccessfully undergone phase 3 clinical trials. Most centered on controlling the inflammatory response to ameliorate hypoperfusion and cytokine-induced organ injury. For many years, high-dose corticosteroid therapy was used to treat sepsis, but controlled studies in the 1980s demonstrated no survival benefit with such nonspecific anti-inflammatory agents.[1] The observation that cyclooxygenase metabolites are elevated during sepsis led to promising work in which ibuprofen was shown to decrease mortality and complications in animal models of sepsis.[36] Unfortunately, a clinical trial of ibuprofen in 455 patients with sepsis failed to significantly reduce mortality, severity of hypotension, or ARDS.[36]

In the mid 1990s, attention shifted toward the use of engineered proteins to combat severe sepsis. A tumor necrosis factor receptor and an immunoglobulin G1 (IgG_1) Fc fusion protein showed promise in animal studies but actually had a detrimental impact on mortality during phase 3 clinical trials.[37] Most recently, research has focused on the infusion of recombinant forms of endogenous anticoagulants and fibrinolytic agents. Antithrombin (AT) and tissue factor pathway inhibitor (TFPI) both yielded encouraging phase 2 clinical trial results but failed to produce favorable outcomes because of a risk of bleeding in phase 3 testing.[5,12] AT was a candidate of particular interest because it was found to directly inhibit activation of NFκB in activated endothelial cells in vitro. A large clinical trial of AT in severe sepsis, however, yielded a 28-day mortality 38.9%, compared with 38.7% for placebo ($P = .94$).[38] Importantly, this trial design was confounded by the co-administration of therapeutic doses of heparin in some patients, which was later found to abrogate the anti-inflammatory actions of AT on cultured endothelial cells and to prevent reductions in mortality and associated inflammatory markers in a rat model of sepsis.[39] Subgroup analysis demonstrated that AT and concomitant heparin significantly increased the risk of bleeding compared with AT alone (23.8% versus 13.5%), and the patients who received AT without heparin actually had a significantly lower 90-day mortality (44.9% versus 52.5%) with placebo despite a lack of improvement at 28 days.[38] The study of yet another endogenous factor, activated protein C, has led to the approval of a novel treatment for severe sepsis.

Drotrecogin-Alfa (Activated)

Drotrecogin-alfa (activated) (droAA), or recombinant human activated protein C, is currently the only pharmacologic agent approved by the U.S. Food and Drug Administration (FDA) to reduce mortality in severe sepsis. Endogenous protein C is activated in the setting of thrombin formation after being cleaved by the thrombomodulin–thrombin complex. Activated protein C inhibits the activity of factors Va, VIIIa, plasminogen activator inhibitor-1, and thrombin-activatable fibrinolysis inhibitor, thus preventing excess coagulation and promoting fibrinolysis in the microvasculature.[5] Additionally, activated protein C inhibits NFκB nuclear translocation and downregulates inflammatory expression patterns in endothelial cells.[40] DroAA is thus thought to produce survival benefit in sepsis through both anticoagulant effects and direct modulation of the systemic inflammatory state.

An international phase 3 clinical trial of droAA, known as the PROWESS study, was performed to assess efficacy and safety in 1690 patients with severe sepsis.[41] DroAA infused at 24 µg/kg/hr for 96 hours provided a significant reduction in 28-day mortality from 32% to 25% compared with placebo.[1,41] Analyses for all subgroups demonstrated significant reductions in mortality at the time of PROWESS. Surgical patients composed 28% of the PROWESS cases, and a later subgroup analysis found absolute mortality reductions of 3.2% for this population as a whole and 9.1% for abdominal surgery patients.[42] Similarly, another subgroup analysis determined that 35.6% of PROWESS patients were afflicted with severe community-acquired pneumonia and that this population also experienced significant reductions in 28- and 90-day mortality compared with placebo.[43] Further evidence supporting droAA treatment came with the ENHANCE US study, which collected more 28-day mortality and safety data on 273 patients with severe sepsis who were treated with droAA following the PROWESS protocol.[44] Compared with the placebo arm of PROWESS, ENHANCE US demonstrated

a 26.4% relative risk reduction in 28-day mortality, which is comparable to the results of PROWESS.[44]

The PROWESS study also recorded APACHE II scores for enrollees, and a post hoc subgroup analysis demonstrated significantly greater mortality risk reduction (13% absolute reduction) in patients with APACHE II scores of 25 or greater as compared with less seriously ill patients.[11] The FDA subsequently mandated an investigation of droAA treatment in patients with severe sepsis and APACHE II scores of less than 25, and the trial was halted because of lack of apparent efficacy.[1,11] In addition to differential subgroup efficacy, the high cost of droAA complicates the decision to treat. An economic analysis of droAA treatment for severe sepsis lends support for increased benefit when treating more seriously ill patients. Although the cost per life-year gained in all patients treated with droAA was estimated at $27,936, this study found that treating patients with an APACHE II of 25 or more yielded $24,484 per life-year gained, compared with $575,054 per life-year gained in patients with lower scores.[45] In short, a number of studies following PROWESS suggest that droAA confers the most survival benefit to the more critically ill population of patients with severe sepsis.

The risks of droAA treatment stem almost entirely from its anticoagulant and fibrinolytic effects. In the PROWESS population, the relative risk of a bleeding event with droAA treatment compared with placebo was 1.41.[41] There was no significant increase in overall bleeding events in patients with overt disseminated intravascular coagulation (DIC) or patients less than 30 days postoperative compared with matched placebos in the PROWESS trial.[41] Serious bleeding occurred in 4.0% of PROWESS patients treated with droAA and a comparable 2.8% of patients in the ENHANCE US trial.[44] In all safety trials, rates of serious bleeding events were comparable between the surgical and nonsurgical populations, thus emphasizing the safety of droAA treatment when treating perioperative severe sepsis.[41,42]

A number of conditions can increase the risk of bleeding associated with droAA treatment. Accordingly, PROWESS excluded certain high-risk patient populations on the basis of safety considerations. When deciding whether to treat with droAA, the PROWESS exclusion criteria should be weighed against the likelihood of benefit for the individual patient (Box 38-3). The effects of droAA in pregnancy and in mothers who are breastfeeding have not been established.[46] Additionally, it is worth noting that no dosage alterations are necessary in cases of acute renal failure, chronic renal insufficiency, or mild hepatic enzyme abnormalities, which occur commonly in sepsis.[46]

In addition to considering underlying conditions, the clinician must also be mindful of pharmacologic interactions that can increase the risk of a serious bleed when treating with droAA. Although use of low-dose heparin (i.e., 15,000 units/day or less) or low-molecular-weight heparin is recommended for DVT prophylaxis, higher doses of either agent should not be given within 8 and 12 hours of droAA treatment, respectively.[1,46] Thrombolytic administration and aspirin at dosages greater than 650 mg/day within the past 3 days, as well as antithrombin (>10,000 units) within the preceding 12 hours were also PROWESS exclusion criteria.[1,46]

<table>
<tr><td>38-3</td><td>Comorbidities Posing Safety Concerns with Drotrecogin-Alfa (Activated) (droAA) Treatment</td></tr>
</table>

Recent Traumatic or Invasive Interventional Events

- Major surgery within the past 12 hours, active postoperative bleeding, or planned surgery during the infusion period
- Presence of epidural catheter, or anticipated placement during infusion period

Central Nervous System (CNS) Considerations

- Severe head trauma, intracranial surgery, or stroke within the past 3 months
- Intracerebral arteriovenous malformation, cerebral aneurysm, or CNS mass lesion

Hematologic Abnormalities

- Heritable bleeding diatheses
- Thrombocytopenia with platelet count of <30,000/mm^3 before droAA initiation
  - Note: patients with recent-onset thrombocytopenia (i.e., decreases of 50% or more in platelet count in the previous 3 days) were not excluded from PROWESS.
- Hypercoagulability disorders may produce rebound thrombophilia after droAA treatment.
  - Hereditary protein C deficiency, protein S deficiency, or antithrombin deficiency
  - Acquired anticardiolipin antibody, antiphospholipid antibody, lupus anticoagulant, or homocystinemia
  - Documented or highly suspected deep vein thrombosis or pulmonary embolism in past 3 months

Gastrointestinal (GI) and Hepatic Pathologies

- Significant GI bleeding within past 6 weeks
- Cirrhosis, chronic jaundice, or chronic ascites (pharmacokinetic concerns)
- Known portal hypertension or esophageal varices
- Pancreatitis

Renal Pathology

- Chronic renal failure requiring peritoneal dialysis or hemodialysis

Immunosuppression

- Human immunodeficiency virus (HIV)-positive patients with a CD4 count of 50/μL or less
- Immunosuppressed patients after bone marrow, lung, liver, pancreas, or small bowel transplant

Adapted from Rivers E, Nguyen B, Havstad S, et al: N Engl J Med 2001;345:1368-1377; Morris P, Light R, Garber G: Am J Surg 2002;184: S19-24; and Ely W, Laterre P, Angus D, et al: Crit Care Med 2003;31:12-19.

Similarly, patients who had received warfarin and glycoprotein IIb/IIIa antagonists within the past 7 days were excluded.[46]

Should a patient's condition necessitate an invasive intervention during the course of droAA treatment, droAA infusion should be discontinued 2 hours before any invasive procedure and restarted 12 hours after a major procedure or immediately after a minor uncomplicated invasive procedure, provided that adequate hemostasis has been achieved.[44] Invasive manipulation of major vessels or highly vascular organs should be avoided whenever possible.[47]

In summary, many factors must be weighed when deciding which patients with severe sepsis would best benefit from droAA therapy. A number of relative contraindications exist, and the decision to treat is ultimately a clinical one. Unfortunately, the APACHE II score is cumbersome to calculate and not a widely used tool in practice. Based on analysis of the PROWESS trial data, patients with severe sepsis who are at a high risk of death from multiple organ failure, shock, or ARDS, and thus are likely to correspond to an APACHE II score of 25 or more, are the best candidates for droAA infusion, provided that relative contraindications with regard to risk of bleeding do not outweigh the potential benefit.[11]

■ ENDOCRINE AND METABOLIC CONSIDERATIONS

Glycemic Control

Stress hyperglycemia and peripheral insulin resistance are nearly universal occurrences in sepsis. In one large clinical study of ventilated surgical ICU (SICU) patients, 97.5% had at least one recorded blood glucose level greater than 110 mg/dL, 74.5% had a baseline glucose of 110 mg/dL or more, and 12% had a baseline glucose of more than 200 mg/dL.[48,49] Interestingly, the degree of hyperglycemia during sepsis appears to correlate with baseline glycemic control, and stress hyperglycemia tends to be more severe in patients with higher-normal hemoglobin A$_1$c (HbA$_1$c) levels than in patients with lower HbA$_1$c levels.[50] Both proinflammatory cytokines and counter-regulatory hormones contribute to hyperglycemia. TNF-α and IL-1 inhibit pancreatic insulin secretion, whereas increased release of cortisol via the hypothalamic-pituitary-adrenal (HPA) axis stress response blocks translocation of the glucose transporter 4 (GLUT4) receptor to skeletal myocyte plasma membranes.[49] High levels of endogenous and exogenous epinephrine and norepinephrine, as well as increased circulating glucagon and growth hormone, all serve to further bolster blood glucose.[5,49] Calorimetric analysis of metabolism in patients with sepsis versus healthy volunteers demonstrates decreased glucose uptake, storage, and oxidation, which are all correctable by high levels of circulating insulin.[51] Additionally, glucose appears to have proinflammatory effects of its own, in that oral glucose loading is associated with increased strength of neutrophil respiratory burst and increased circulating levels of IL-8 in healthy volunteers.[49]

In a landmark study by Van den Berghe and coworkers, 1548 adult ventilated SICU patients were randomized to receive either intensive insulin therapy to maintain blood glucose levels between 80 and 110 mg/dL, or standard of care as defined by maintenance of blood glucose levels between 180 and 200 mg/dL and infusion of insulin only when hyperglycemia exceeded 215 mg/dL.[48] Intensive insulin therapy was associated with a 12-month total mortality reduction from 8.0% to 4.6% ($P < .04$) and yielded an even more pronounced reduction in mortality from 20.2% to 10.6% ($P = .005$) in the subgroup of patients who resided in the SICU for 5 days or longer.[48] Furthermore, the greatest reduction in mortality was observed in patients with severe sepsis and multiorgan failure. Overall, the incidence of bloodstream infections was reduced by 46%, onset of acute renal failure requiring renal replacement therapy was decreased by 41%, and the times to extubation and SICU discharge were also significantly improved with intensive insulin therapy.[5,10,48] The impressive results of this trial raised the question of whether the benefits resulted directly from normoglycemia or from increased circulating insulin, which is known to have a number of anti-inflammatory effects. In a subsequent multivariant logistic regression analysis of the same data, Van den Berghe and colleagues determined that the reduction in blood glucose was responsible for the improvements observed, with the exception of decreased acute renal failure, for which elevated insulin was an independent determinant.[11,52] A similar analysis performed on a separate population of 523 ICU patients found that maintenance of blood glucose level between 111 and 144 mg/dL yielded a significant survival benefit that was attributable to reduced hyperglycemia as opposed to hyperinsulinemia.[53]

With regard to clinical management, the Surviving Sepsis Campaign guidelines recommend that blood glucose should be maintained below 150 mg/dL and that blood glucose checks and insulin dosage adjustments occur every 30 to 60 minutes until glycemic stabilization, and every 4 hours thereafter.[12] Although the Van den Berghe and coworkers trial recommended maintenance between 80 and 110 mg/dL, a post hoc analysis demonstrated benefit when glucose was kept below 150 mg/dL, a goal more easily attained in clinical practice without inducing hypoglycemia.[12,53] Van den Berghe and colleagues initiated insulin infusion at 2 or 4 international units (IU) per hour, depending on whether blood glucose was above 110 mg/dL or 220 mg/dL.[52] Insulin infusion was titrated by increasing 1 to 2 IU/hr for greater than 140 mg/dL, 0.5 IU/hr for 110 to 140 mg/dL, and decreasing dosage only when glucose dropped below 80 mg/dL, or below 60 mg/dL at which time insulin was discontinued.[52] Glucose substrate should be given at the same time as insulin, initially in the form of 5% or 10% dextrose intravenously and later by transition to enteral feeding as soon as is practical.[12,48]

The Role of Corticosteroids

Although high-dose corticosteroid therapy is no longer indicated as a direct therapy for severe sepsis, corticosteroid replacement confers benefit in patients experiencing relative adrenal insufficiency. Not surprisingly, corticosteroids have pleiotropic effects in the physiology of sepsis. In response to septic stresses of fever, pain, and hypovolemia, the HPA axis increases adrenocorticotropic hormone (ACTH) stimulation of corticosteroid secretion.[54] Corticosteroids, in turn, have immunomodulatory functions as well as direct supportive roles in maintenance of vascular tone, vascular impermeability, endothelial integrity, and the potentiation of catecholamine-induced vasoconstriction.[54]

Corticotropin-stimulation testing should yield an increase in serum cortisol of at least 18 µg/dL above baseline, 30 to 60 minutes after administration of 250 µg cosyntropin in a healthy volunteer.[54] Physiologic stress, such as that endured during laparotomy, results in maximal secretion of 200 to 300 µg of cortisol during the first 24 hours and an average cortisol increase of 84% above baseline by 48 hours postoperatively.[54,55] A state of relative corticosteroid insufficiency occurs during sepsis and is thought to be mediated by cytokine inhibition of adrenal function in addition to development of cellular steroid resistance in the presence of maximal stress-induced adrenal stimulation.[56]

Corticosteroid supplementation should be considered for three groups of patients in the setting of severe sepsis: those with baseline primary adrenal insufficiency, those with underlying secondary adrenal insufficiency, and those experiencing relative adrenal insufficiency as a sequela of sepsis. Chronic primary adrenal insufficiency, or Addison's disease, ensues from an underlying HPA pathology (e.g., autoimmune cortical damage, tuberculosis, adrenal metastases, human immunodeficiency virus [HIV]-related pathology, adrenal hemorrhage, or ketoconazole therapy) and results in chronic dependence on exogenous corticosteroids.[54,55] These patients will require continuation of baseline steroid maintenance dosing as well as supplemental steroids in the range of 100 to 150 mg/day of hydrocortisone (continuous infusion) on the first day they present with sepsis.[55]

Secondary adrenal insufficiency can result from hypopituitarism or, more commonly, from chronic corticosteroid therapy for autoimmune disease. A thorough history including dosage and duration of steroid treatment should be obtained, but unfortunately these factors have poor predictive value for determining the rate and extent of adrenal recovery within 1 year of steroid discontinuation.[54,55] Accordingly, these patients should receive a corticotropin-stimulation test to determine the presence and severity of adrenal suppression in sepsis. Those patients receiving chronic immunomodulatory corticosteroid treatment via intranasal or inhalation delivery rarely develop adrenal suppression.[55]

The concept of relative adrenal insufficiency in severe sepsis stemmed from a prospective cohort study of 189 ICU patients with sepsis, in whom baseline cortisol levels and response to corticotropin stimulation testing were found to have predictive value for 28-day mortality.[57] Patients with a baseline cortisol of less than 34 µg/dL and greater than 9 µg/dL maximal cortisol increase (at 30 or 60 minutes after corticotropin test) had the best prognosis, with 26% mortality.[57] An intermediate-prognosis group carried an associated mortality of 67%, and a third group of patients defined by a cortisol baseline of greater than 34 µg/dL and less than 9 µg/dL maximal increase was associated with 82% mortality and impaired responsiveness to norepinephrine.[57] Thus, those patients with sepsis who had high basal cortisol levels and minimal ability to increase secretion in response ACTH were deemed to have relative adrenal insufficiency. Clinically, relative adrenal insufficiency can be defined as pressor-dependent septic shock that responds to steroid supplementation and that can be accompanied by unexplained eosinophilia, hypothermia, hyperpigmentation, hyperkalemia, hyponatremia, or vomiting.[55]

A subsequent clinical trial randomized 300 ICU patients with severe sepsis to receive either 50 mg hydrocortisone intravenous boluses every 6 hours and 50 μg fludrocortisone daily or matching placebos for 7 days.[58] All patients received corticotropin stimulation tests prior to therapy and were stratified as responders or nonresponders, depending on whether or not an increase in serum cortisol of at least 9 μg/dL was achieved, respectively.[58] Given this definition, between 50% and 67% of patients with severe sepsis can be classified as exhibiting relative adrenal insufficiency.[5,56] Nonresponders receiving steroids exhibited 53% mortality, compared with the significantly greater 63% mortality in the nonresponder placebo group; no significant difference was observed in mortality rates between the treatment and placebo arms of the responder group.[58] A number of related studies have demonstrated that low-dose steroids (i.e., in the range of 300 mg hydrocortisone for 5 days) can shorten the duration of shock, restore the vasoconstrictive response to catecholamines, and increase the median time until death in patients with pressor-dependent shock, but no benefit has been observed for crude mortality except for patients with relative adrenal insufficiency.[1,56,59]

Accordingly, current treatment recommendations for corticosteroid therapy in severe sepsis are limited to those patients with relative adrenal insufficiency. A corticotropin-stimulation test should be performed on all patients with severe sepsis. Patients who do not respond with an increase in serum cortisol of at least 9 μg/dL after administration of 250 μg ACTH, or who have baseline random cortisol levels below 15 μg/dL, should be considered to exhibit relative adrenal insufficiency.[1,12] These cutoff points should be adjusted when albumin concentrations are less than 2.5 g/dL, such that relative adrenal insufficiency is defined by a cortisol increase of 3.1 μg/dL or less after ACTH stimulation or a baseline random cortisol of 2 μg/dL or less.[1]

Corticosteroid therapy should be initiated only if ACTH stimulation results are consistent with nonresponder status.[12,56,58] The recommended regimen for patients with relative adrenal insufficiency is 200 to 300 mg of hydrocortisone per day for 7 days, divided into three to four doses daily or administered via continuous infusion.[12,58] Some choose to add fludrocortisone (50 μg) daily for additional mineralocorticoid supplementation, but this intervention is entirely at the discretion of the clinician.

CONCLUSIONS

Management strategies for the treatment of sepsis are rapidly evolving. The greatest reductions in mortality have been achieved through optimization of supportive care parameters—namely, early goal-directed fluid resuscitation, low tidal volume mechanical ventilation, and improved glycemic control. Early and appropriate empiric antibiotic therapy is invaluable. Recent definition of the relative adrenal insufficiency syndrome has conferred additional survival benefit by identifying those patients who may benefit from low-dose corticosteroid therapy, and direct pharmacologic intervention with drotrecogin-alfa (activated) is indicated in a substantial subset of severe sepsis patients.

REFERENCES

1. Annane D, Bellissant E, Cavaillon J: Septic shock. Lancet 2005;365:63-78.
2. Annane D, Aegerter P, Jars-Guincestre M, Guidet B: Current epidemiology of septic shock. CUB-Rea Network. Am J Respir Crit Care Med 2003;168:165-172.
3. Bone R, Balk R, Cerra F, et al: Definitions for sepsis and organ failure and guidelines for the use of innovative therapies in sepsis. The ACCP/SCCM Consensus Conference Committee. American College of Chest Physicians/Society of Critical Care Medicine. Chest 1992;101: 1644-1655.
4. Wheeler AP, Bernard GR: Treating patients with severe sepsis. N Engl J Med 1999;340:207-214.
5. Gropper M: Evidence-based management of critically ill patients: Analysis and implementation. Anesth Analg 2004;99:566-572.
6. Rivers E, Nguyen B, Havstad S, et al: Early goal-directed therapy in the treatment of severe sepsis and septic shock. Early Goal-Directed Therapy Collaborative Group. N Engl J Med 2001;345:1368-1377.
7. Angus D, Linde-Zwirble W, Lidicker J, et al: Epidemiology of severe sepsis in the United States: Analysis of incidence, outcome, and associated costs of care. Crit Care Med 2001;29:1303-1310.
8. Carcillo J: Reducing the global burden of sepsis in infants and children: A clinical practice research agenda. Pediatr Crit Care Med 2005;6: S157-164.
9. Watson RS, Carcillo JA: Scope and epidemiology of pediatric sepsis. Pediatr Crit Care Med 2005;6:S3-5.
10. Herbert P, Drummond A, Singer J, et al: A simple multiple system organ failure scoring system predicts mortality of patients who have sepsis syndrome. Chest 1993;103:230-235.
11. Shapiro N, Howell M, Talmor D: A blueprint for a sepsis protocol. Acad Emerg Med 2005;12:352-359.
12. Dellinger R, Carlet J, Masur H, et al: Surviving Sepsis Campaign guidelines for management of severe sepsis and septic shock. Surviving Sepsis Campaign Management Guidelines Committee. Crit Care Med 2004;32:858-873.
13. Rivers E, Nguyen B, Huang D, Donnino M: Early goal-directed therapy. Crit Care Med 2004;32:314-315.
13a. Gattioni L, Brazzi L, Pelosi P, et al: A trial of goal-oriented hemodynamic therapy in critically ill patients. N Engl J Med 1995;333: 1025-1034.
13b. Hayes MA, Timmins AC, Yau EHS, et al: Elevation of systemic oxygen delivery in the treatment of critically ill patients. N Engl J Med 1994;330:1717-1722.
14. Sinclair S, James S, Singer M: Intraoperative intravascular volume optimisation and length of hospital stay after repair of proximal femoral fracture: Randomised controlled trial. BMJ 1997;315:909-912.
15. Venn R, Steele A, Richardson P, et al: Randomized controlled trial to investigate influence of the fluid challenge on duration of hospital stay and perioperative morbidity in patients with hip fractures. Br J Anesth 2002;88:65-71.
16. Greif R, Akca O, Horn E, et al: Supplemental perioperative oxygen to reduce the incidence of surgical-wound infection. Outcomes Research Group. N Engl J Med 2000;342:161-167.
17. Hebert PC, Wells G, Blajchman MA, et al: A multicenter, randomized, controlled clinical trial of transfusion requirements in critical care. N Engl J Med 1999;340:409-417.
18. Slutsky A, Ranieri V: Mechanical ventilation: Lessons from the ARDSNet trial. Respir Res 2000;1:73-77.
19. Brower R, Matthay M, Morris A, et al: Ventilation with lower tidal volumes as compared with traditional tidal volumes for acute lung injury and the acute respiratory distress syndrome. The Acute Respiratory Distress Syndrome Network. N Engl J Med 2000;342:1301-1308.
20. Brower R, Lanken P, MacIntyre N, et al: Higher versus lower positive end-expiratory pressures in patients with the acute respiratory distress syndrome. The National Heart, Lung, and Blood Institute ARDS Clinical Trials Network. N Engl J Med 2004;351:327-336.
21. Kallet R, Jasmer R, Pittet J, et al: Clinical implementation of the ARDS Network protocol is associated with reduced hospital

mortality compared with historical controls. Crit Care Med 2005;33: 925-929.

22. Parsons P, Eisner M, Thompson T, et al: Lower tidal volume ventilation and plasma cytokine markers of inflammation in patients with acute lung injury. NHLBI Acute Respiratory Distress Syndrome Clinical Trials Network. Crit Care Med 2005;33:1-6.

23. Ranieri V, Suter P, Tortorella C, et al: Effect of mechanical ventilation on inflammatory mediators in patients with acute respiratory distress syndrome. JAMA 1999;282:54-61.

24. Durante G, del Turco M, Rustichini L, et al: ARDSNet lower tidal volume ventilatory strategy may generate intrinsic positive end-expiratory pressure in patients with acute respiratory distress syndrome. Am J Respir Crit Care Med 2002;165:1271-1274.

25. Kurz A, Sessler D, Lenhardt R: Perioperative normothermia to reduce the incidence of surgical-wound infection and shorten hospitalization. N Engl J Med 1996;334:1209-1215.

26. Mortensen N: Colorectal surgery comes in from the cold. N Engl J Med 1996;334:1263-1264.

27. Marik P, Zaloga G: Hypothermia and cytokines in septic shock. Norasept II Study Investigators. Intensive Care Med 2000;26:716-721.

28. Xiao H, Remick D: Correction of perioperative hypothermia decreases experimental sepsis mortality by modulating the inflammatory response. Crit Care Med 2005;33:161-167.

29. Su F, Nguyen N, Wang Z, et al: Fever control in septic shock: Beneficial or harmful? Shock 2005;23:516-520.

30. Houck P, Bratzler D, Nsa W, et al: Timing of antibiotic administration and outcomes for medicare patients hospitalized with community-acquired pneumonia. Arch Intern Med 2004;164:637-644.

31. Leibovici L, Shraga I, Drucker M, et al: The benefit of appropriate empirical antibiotic treatment in patients with bloodstream infection. J Intern Med 1998;244:379-386.

32. Bochud P, Glauser M, Calandra T: Antibiotics in sepsis. Intensive Care Med 2001;27:S33-48.

33. Bochud P, Bonten M, Marchetti O, Calandra T: Antimicrobial therapy for patients with severe sepsis and septic shock: An evidence-based review. Crit Care Med 2004;32(11 Suppl):S495-512.

34. Boyd O, Grounds R, Bennet E: A randomized clinical trial of the effect of deliberate perioperative increase of oxygen delivery on mortality in high-risk surgical patients. JAMA 1993;270:2699-2707.

35. Wilson J, Woods I, Fawcett J, et al: Reducing the risk of major elective surgery: Randomised controlled trial of preoperative optimisation of oxygen delivery. BMJ 1999;318:1099-1103.

36. Bernard G, Wheeler A, Russell J, et al: The effects of ibuprofen on the physiology and survival of patients with sepsis. Ibuprofen in Sepsis Study Group. N Engl J Med 1997;336:912-918.

37. Fisher C, Agosti J, Opal S, et al: Treatment of septic shock with the tumor necrosis factor Receptor:Fc fusion protein. Soluble TNF Receptor Sepsis Study Group. N Engl J Med 1996;334:1697-1702.

38. Warren B, Eid A, Singer P, et al: High-dose antithrombin III in severe sepsis. KyberSept Trial Study Group. JAMA 2001;286:1869-1878.

39. Pulletz S, Lehmann C, Volk T, et al: Influence of heparin and hirudin on endothelial binding of antithrombin in experimental thrombinemia. Crit Care Med 2000;28:2881-2886.

40. Joyce DE, Grinnell BW: Recombinant human activated protein C attenuates the inflammatory response in endothelium and monocytes by modulating nuclear factor kappa B. Crit Care Med 2002;30: S288-293.

41. Ely W, Laterre P, Angus D, et al: Drotrecogin alfa (activated) administration across clinically important subgroups of patients with severe sepsis. PROWESS Investigators. Crit Care Med 2003;31:12-19.

42. Barie P, Williams M, McCollam J, et al: Benefit/risk profile of drotrecogin alfa (activated) in surgical patients with severe sepsis. PROWESS Surgical Evaluation Committee. Am J Surg 2004;188: 212-220.

43. Laterre P, Garber F, Levy H, et al: Severe community-acquired pneumonia as a cause of severe sepsis: Data from the PROWESS study. PROWESS Clinical Evaluation Committee. Crit Care Med 2005;33: 952-961.

44. Bernard G, Margolis B, Shanies H, et al: Extended evaluation of recombinant activated protein C, United States trial (ENHANCE US): A single-arm, phase 3B, multicenter study of drotrecogin alfa (activated) in severe sepsis. Extended Evaluation of Recombinant Human Activated Protein C United States Investigators. Chest 2004;125: 2206-2216.

45. Manns B, Lee H, Doig C, et al: An economic evaluation of activated protein C treatment for severe sepsis. N Engl J Med 2002;347:993-1000.

46. Morris P, Light R, Garber G: Identifying patients with severe sepsis who should not be treated with drotrecogin alfa (activated). Am J Surg 2002;184:S19-24.

47. McCoy C: Safety of drotrecogin alfa (activated) in the treatment of patients with severe sepsis. Expert Opin Drug Saf 2004;3:625-637.

48. Van den Berghe G, Wouters P, Weekers F, et al: Intensive insulin therapy in critically ill patients. N Engl J Med 2001;345:1359-1367.

49. Marik P, Raghavan M: Stress-hyperglycemia, insulin and immuno-modulation in sepsis. Intensive Care Med 2004;30:748-756.

50. Cely C, Pratheep A, Quartin A, et al: Relationship of baseline glucose homeostasis to hyperglycemia during medical critical illness. Chest 2004;126:879-887.

51. Rusavy Z, Sramek V, Lacigova S, et al: Influence of insulin on glucose metabolism and energy expenditure in septic patients. Crit Care 2004;8: R213-220.

52. Van den Berghe G, Wouters P, Bouillon R, et al: Outcome benefit of intensive insulin therapy in the critically ill: Insulin dose versus glycemic control. Crit Care Med 2003;31:359-366.

53. Finney S, Zekveld C, Elia A, Evans T: Glucose control and mortality in critically ill patients. JAMA 2003;290:2041-2047.

54. Lamberts SW, Bruining HA, de Jong FH: Corticosteroid therapy in severe illness. N Engl J Med 1997;337:1285-1292.

55. Shenker Y, Skatrud J: Adrenal insufficiency in critically ill patients. Am J Respir Crit Care Med 2001;163:1520-1523.

56. Annane D, Bellissant E, Bollaert P, et al: Corticosteroids for severe sepsis and septic shock: A systematic review and meta-analysis. BMJ 2004;329:480.

57. Annane D, Sebille V, Troche G, et al: A 3-level prognostic classification in septic shock based on cortisol levels and cortisol response to corticotropin. JAMA 2000;283:1038-1045.

58. Annane D, Sebille V, Charpentier C, et al: Effect of treatment with low doses of hydrocortisone and fludrocortisone on mortality in patients with septic shock. JAMA 2002;288:862-871.

59. Luce J: Physicians should administer low-dose corticosteroids selectively to septic patients until an ongoing trial is completed. Ann Intern Med 2004;141:70-72.

39 | Acute Respiratory Failure

S. Rob Todd, Gary A. Vercruysse, and Frederick A. Moore

Respiratory failure in the postoperative patient can be alarming, confusing, and at times deadly. At a minimum, postoperative respiratory complications delay discharge, and at worst they lead to rapid death.[1] Every physician should strive to minimize these complications. Perioperative respiratory failure can be broken down into three categories: preoperative, intraoperative, and postoperative. Each has its own unique characteristics.

Preoperative respiratory failure is usually secondary to an underlying disease process or the cause for surgery. It occurs almost exclusively in nonelective surgery patients with early sepsis, peritonitis, or ileus with abdominal distention. Clinical signs include respiratory difficulty, tachypnea, and hypoxia. Chest radiography often demonstrates progressive pulmonary infiltrates. The treatment for this condition is multifaceted and includes aggressive resuscitation, elective endotracheal intubation, and source identification and control (i.e., surgery).

Intraoperative respiratory failure is frequently seen in patients who are undergoing an emergent surgical procedure. There are multiple etiologies, including massive blood transfusion, aspiration, and systemic inflammatory response syndrome (SIRS).[2,3] The septic patient undergoing emergency surgery often develops intraoperative hypoxia secondary to resuscitation (worsened pulmonary edema) and anesthetic agents (loss of hypoxic pulmonary vasoconstriction).

Postoperative acute respiratory failure is far more common than either preoperative or intraoperative respiratory failure and is the primary focus of this chapter, in which we discuss the pathophysiology of postoperative acute respiratory failure, the approach to the hypoxic patient, predictors of postoperative acute respiratory failure, and the clinical manifestations, diagnosis, and treatment strategies for the most common causes of postoperative acute respiratory failure.

■ PATHOPHYSIOLOGY

Respiratory failure can be divided into three types based on the arterial blood gas (ABG) analysis: type I or oxygenation failure, type II or ventilatory failure, and type III or combined oxygenation and ventilatory failure. The parameters that define acute respiratory failure are shown in Table 39-1.[4]

Type I Respiratory Failure (Oxygenation Failure; Arterial Hypoxemia)

Type I respiratory failure occurs as a result of inadequate oxygenation.[5,6] It is defined by an arterial partial pressure of oxygen (PaO_2) less than 60 mm Hg. In addition, there will be an increase in the gradient from the alveolar partial pressure of oxygen (PAO_2) minus the PaO_2 (the A-a gradient), the venous admixture or shunt fraction (Q_S/Q_T), and the ratio of the dead space to the tidal volume (V_D/V_T).[5,6]

The A-a gradient describes the relationship between the PAO_2 and the PaO_2 and represents the oxygen gradient across the alveolar capillary membrane. It is generally used as an indirect measurement of ventilation–perfusion (V/Q) abnormalities.[7] The normal A-a gradient is approximately 10 to 25 mm Hg. An increased A-a gradient implicates a parenchymal lung process as the etiology of the arterial hypoxemia.[7]

The pulmonary shunt fraction (Q_S/Q_T) is defined as the fraction of the cardiac output (Q_T) that perfuses unventilated alveoli (Q_S).[4] It represents the intrapulmonary shunt and is used to quantify the extent of impaired oxygenation. The normal Q_S/Q_T is 3% to 5%. Between 10% and 19%, the Q_S/Q_T rarely requires support; however, a Q_S/Q_T of 20% or more is clinically significant and requires treatment.[7,8] Shunt fraction is also known as pulmonary venous admixture.

The P/F ratio is another way to quantify impaired oxygenation. P representing PaO_2 is divided by F, the fraction of inspired oxygen (FIO_2) as a decimal. It is a simple calculation and correlates well with Q_S/Q_T. A P/F ratio of less than 200 is equivalent to a Q_S/Q_T of greater than 20%.[8]

The fraction of the tidal volume (V_T) that is not engaged in gas exchange with the pulmonary blood flow is referred to as the physiologic dead space (V_D). It is composed of anatomic dead space and alveolar dead space. Anatomic dead space represents the conducting airways and usually measures 150 mL in the normal human. Alveolar dead space represents alveoli that are ventilated but not perfused. The ratio of dead space to tidal volume (V_D/V_T) is normally 0.2 to 0.3.[4]

The mechanisms responsible for type I respiratory failure include inadequate PAO_2, V/Q mismatch, shunt, and diffusion abnormality. Of these, V/Q mismatch is the most frequently encountered.[9,10] Most of these abnormalities improve with supplemental oxygenation, except for a shunt. A "true shunt" develops when portions of the lung are perfused in total absence of ventilation. The most frequent causes of a shunt in the postoperative patient are consolidated pneumonia, lobar atelectasis, and the later phases of the acute respiratory distress syndrome (ARDS).[5,11] Other causes of type I respiratory failure in the postoperative population include asthma, pulmonary edema, chronic obstructive pulmonary disease (COPD), pneumothorax, pulmonary embolism, and pulmonary hypertension.[5]

39-1   Parameters that Define Acute Respiratory Failure

Parameter	Abbreviation	Normal Range
Arterial partial pressure of oxygen	PaO_2	80-95 mm Hg*
Arterial partial pressure of carbon dioxide	$PaCO_2$	35-45 mm Hg
Alveolar partial pressure of oxygen	PAO_2	95-110 mm Hg
Ventilation–perfusion abnormality	V/Q	—
Alveolar minus arterial PO_2 gradient	A-a gradient	10-25 mm Hg
Shunt fraction (venous admixture)	Q_S/Q_T	3%-5%
Ratio of dead space to tidal volume	V_D/V_T	0.2-0.3
Myocardial oxygen consumption	MvO_2	9 mL/100 g/min

*Varies with age and altitude.

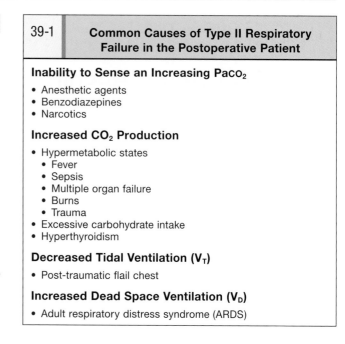

39-1   Common Causes of Type II Respiratory Failure in the Postoperative Patient

Inability to Sense an Increasing $PaCO_2$
- Anesthetic agents
- Benzodiazepines
- Narcotics

Increased CO_2 Production
- Hypermetabolic states
  - Fever
  - Sepsis
  - Multiple organ failure
  - Burns
  - Trauma
- Excessive carbohydrate intake
- Hyperthyroidism

Decreased Tidal Ventilation (V_T)
- Post-traumatic flail chest

Increased Dead Space Ventilation (V_D)
- Adult respiratory distress syndrome (ARDS)

Type II Respiratory Failure (Ventilatory Failure, Arterial Hypercapnia)

Type II respiratory failure refers to inadequate ventilation. It is characterized by an arterial partial pressure of carbon dioxide ($PaCO_2$) greater than 50 mm Hg in the presence of acute respiratory acidemia. There is a concurrent decrease in the PAO_2 and PaO_2; therefore, the A-a gradient remains unchanged. The four basic mechanisms underlying type II respiratory failure are inability to sense an increasing $PaCO_2$, increased CO_2 production, decreased V_T, and increased V_D. The common causes of each in the postoperative patient are listed in Box 39-1.[5,6,10]

Type III Respiratory Failure (Combined Oxygenation and Ventilatory Failure)

Type III respiratory failure is defined by both a PaO_2 of less than 60 mm Hg and a $PaCO_2$ of greater than 50 mm Hg. Like type I respiratory failure, there is also an increase in the A-a gradient, Q_S/Q_T, and V_D/V_T. Theoretically, any process that causes type I or type II respiratory failure can result in type III respiratory failure.[6]

■ THE APPROACH TO THE HYPOXIC PATIENT

The most common clinical presentation of all three types of acute respiratory failure is acute hypoxia.[12] Early identification and appropriate management are critical in limiting adverse outcomes. In the nonintubated patient, evaluation includes a physical examination, a review of recent events, an inspection of any supplemental oxygen equipment, an ABG analysis, a portable anteroposterior chest radiograph, and an electrocardiogram (selectively). Following this, management should be as indicated (see Etiologies of Postoperative Acute Respiratory Failure, later).

In the intubated patient, the evaluation is more complex. An algorithm for the approach to the hypoxic intubated patient is found in Figure 39-1.[13] In this scenario, hypoxia is defined as a 5% decrease in continuous pulse oximetry (SpO_2) or a 10% decrease in mixed venous oximetry (SvO_2). After identification of hypoxia, the supplemental oxygen should be enhanced. The patient should be disconnected from the mechanical ventilator and hand ventilated. If there is a cuff leak, the tube should be repaired or replaced. If there is difficulty bagging the patient, an attempt at passing a suction catheter should be made. Inability to do so confirms obstruction. If this cannot be reversed by altering the patient's head position, checking the tube's position, or deflating the cuff, the tube should be replaced. If there is no evidence of obstruction, despite bagging difficulty, a tension pneumothorax should be ruled out. Assuming that the patient is hand ventilated easily, the mechanical ventilator and its circuitry should be inspected to exclude a mechanical flaw. Additional workup at this time should include a physical examination, review of recent events, an ABG analysis, a portable anteroposterior chest radiograph, and an electrocardiogram (selectively). Further diagnostic studies should be guided by the findings in the algorithm of Figure 39-1.

■ PREOPERATIVE PREDICTORS

Identification of risk factors for postoperative acute respiratory failure is helpful in that it identifies those patients most in need of preoperative optimization and postoperative vigilance. Many studies have been performed to identify predictors of postoperative acute respiratory failure and other pulmonary complications. These can be classified as patient related, procedure related, or surgical site related.[14]

The literature examining patient-related predictors is vast. Most recently, McAlister and colleagues examined risk factors in elective nonthoracic surgical procedures (Table 39-2).[15] In univariate analysis, the following were significant: age, extended smoking history, daily productive cough, positive cough test, forced expiratory time of 9 seconds or greater,

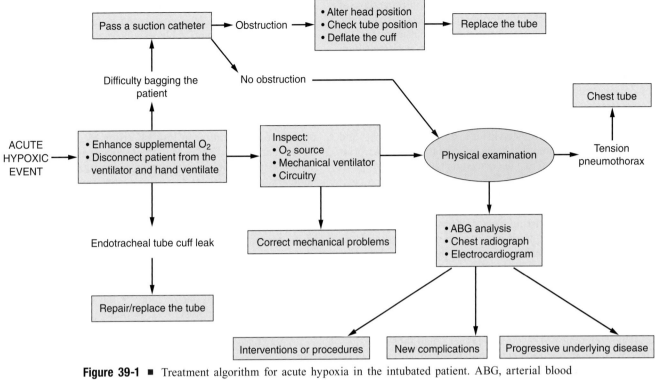

Figure 39-1 ■ Treatment algorithm for acute hypoxia in the intubated patient. ABG, arterial blood gas.

| **39-2** | **Association between Preoperative/Operative Variables and the Occurrence of Postoperative Pulmonary Complications** |

Variable* (N = 1055)	No. of Patients with Particular Finding (%)	Odds Ratio (95% CI)	P Value
Age ≥65 years	332 (31)	5.73 (2.49-13.15)	<.001
Male sex	531 (50)	1.54 (0.72-3.32)	.27
Ever smoked (vs. never)	630 (60)	2.06 (0.87-4.89)	.12
Current smoker (within 2 wk of operation)	218 (21)	0.83 (0.31-2.21)	.82
Smoked ≥40 pack-years	94 (9)	2.91 (1.15-7.37)	.03
Recent (within 2 wk) URI	90 (9)	1.82 (0.62-5.38)	.29
History of COPD	54 (5)	3.26 (1.09-9.74)	.05
History of asthma	104 (10)	2.03 (0.76-5.48)	.19
Daily productive cough	100 (9)	2.71 (1.07-6.84)	.04
Exercise capacity ≤2 blocks or 1 flight of stairs	126 (12)	0.88 (0.26-2.96)	1.00
Body mass index ≥30	339 (32)	0.57 (0.23-1.42)	.22
Positive cough test	74 (7)	3.84 (1.51-9.80)	.01
Positive wheeze test	40 (4)	0.94 (0.12-7.08)	1.00
Forced expiratory time ≥9 sec	31 (3)	4.28 (1.22-15.02)	.04
Maximum laryngeal height ≤4 cm	166 (16)	1.17 (0.44-3.12)	.79
Wheezing on standard auscultation	34 (3)	2.39 (0.54-10.51)	.23
Upper abdominal incision	92 (9)	4.49 (1.92-10.50)	.002
General anesthesia	931 (88)	1.11 (0.33-3.74)	1.00
Duration of operation ≥2.5 hr	321 (30)	5.07 (2.27-11.33)	<.001
Perioperative nasogastric tube	66 (6)	13.50 (6.08-29.96)	<.001
FEV_1 <1 L	14 (1)	6.51 (1.38-30.56)	.05
Chest radiograph abnormal	44 (4)	1.80 (0.41-7.85)	.33

*In the case of operative variables, referent groups were as follows: all other surgeries vs. upper abdominal incision, regional or spinal anesthesia vs. general anesthesia, and <2.5 hr vs. ≥2.5 hr.

CI, confidence interval; COPD, chronic obstructive pulmonary disease; FEV_1, forced expiratory volume in 1 sec; URI, upper respiratory tract infection.

Modified from McAlister FA, Bertsch K, Man, J, et al: Am J Respir Crit Care Med 2005;171:514-517.

upper abdominal incision, duration of surgical procedure of 2.5 hours or greater, and perioperative nasogastric tube placement. The multivariate regression analysis identified the following variables: age of 65 years or greater, positive cough test (meaning the patient continued to cough after taking a deep breath and providing a voluntary cough), perioperative nasogastric tube, and anesthesia lasting at least 2.5 hours. Some factors can be optimized before elective surgical procedures. Interestingly, although current smoking was not a significant variable in McAlister's analysis, Warner and coworkers documented that smoking cessation 8 weeks prior to elective surgery led to a decreased incidence of postoperative acute respiratory failure.[16]

Although age, obesity, and asthma did not emerge as independent predictors in McAlister's analysis, other studies have shown that preexisting comorbidities are important contributors.[17,18] However, their importance may be lessened by preoperative optimization. Likewise, patients with active pulmonary infections should not undergo elective surgery.

Several predictors are related to the surgical procedure. Patients undergoing longer procedures have a greater incidence of postoperative pulmonary complications.[18,19] Similarly, patients anesthetized with longer-acting paralytics have a greater incidence of residual weakness than those anesthetized with shorter-acting agents, potentially resulting in postoperative hypoxia and respiratory failure.[20] Epidural and spinal anesthesia is an alternative to general anesthesia. These modalities result in less postoperative respiratory compromise.[21]

A less frequent complication of general anesthesia is laryngospasm-induced negative-pressure pulmonary edema.[22] The primary pathologic event is negative intrapleural pressure. This increases venous return to the right side of the heart and decreases the output of the left ventricle, thereby increasing pulmonary blood volume and microvascular pressures, resulting in pulmonary edema. Negative-pressure pulmonary edema should be suspected in young patients during the immediate postoperative period. The pulmonary edema may develop up to 25 minutes after extubation.

The surgical site also affects the patients' postoperative respiratory status. Pulmonary resections pose an extreme example. Traditionally, those in need of lung resections are at high risk of respiratory compromise postoperatively. A forced expiratory volume in 1 second (FEV_1) of less than 800 mL classically has been a contraindication to resection. This chapter does not focus on pulmonary resections any further, but rather on how nonthoracic procedures affect pulmonary mechanics.

Many studies have examined how the choice of incision or the type of surgical procedure affects postoperative pulmonary mechanics.[13] In general, the farther an incision is from the diaphragm and the shorter is its length, the less it negatively affects postoperative pulmonary mechanics and overall respiratory status. Thoracic incisions are by far the most morbid incisions, followed by upper abdominal incisions, and then lower abdominal incisions. Surgical procedures unrelated to the torso generally pose minimal risks to postoperative pulmonary mechanics.[23] In general, laparoscopic procedures result in significantly less postoper-

ative acute respiratory failure. Several studies in the 1990s demonstrated less postoperative pulmonary morbidity in laparoscopic cholecystectomies than in open cholecystectomies.[24,25]

Numerous trials have determined predictors of postoperative pulmonary complications, including acute respiratory failure. Unfortunately, most of these studies are retrospective and too underpowered to detect statistically significant findings. In 2002, Fisher and colleagues conducted a systematic review of the literature in English, using MEDLINE (1966-2001), manual searches of identified articles, and contact with content experts.[26] Studies reporting independent and blinded comparisons of risk factors for postoperative respiratory complications were included. Seven studies met the inclusion criteria and were evaluated in the final analysis. All seven studies were, at a minimum, independent, blind comparisons of an appropriate spectrum of patients.[27] In this systematic review, postoperative pulmonary complications occurred in 2% to 19% of the patients. There were 16 predictors of postoperative pulmonary complications that were significant in univariate analysis in one or more of the studies. However, when multivariate analysis was accounted for, only 10 predictors were statistically significant (Box 39-2).

The Charlson Comorbidity score, based on 1-year mortality data from internal medicine patients admitted to an inpatient setting, is the most widely used comorbidity index in oncology. Note that the majority of the significant predictors are related to the patient's preoperative status. Thus, the key to the management of postoperative respiratory failure is prevention. Clearly, patients who have chronic obstructive pulmonary disease or symptoms of an acute respiratory illness should be optimized medically prior to emergent surgical procedures. Elective cases under similar circumstances should be delayed until the patient has recovered from the acute illness or has been optimized medically in the case of a preexisting pulmonary condition.

■ ETIOLOGIES OF POSTOPERATIVE ACUTE RESPIRATORY FAILURE

After surgery, all patients are at risk for acute respiratory failure. Some of the more common etiologies are atelectasis,

---

39-2	**Predictors of Postoperative Pulmonary Complications in Multivariate Analysis**

- Preexisting chronic obstructive pulmonary disease
- Preoperative sputum production
- American Society of Anesthesiologists score >2
- Nasogastric tube placement
- Abnormal pulmonary physical examination (e.g., decreased breath sounds, prolonged expiration, rales, rhonchi, or wheezes)
- Charlson Comorbidity score
- Goldman Cardiac Risk Index
- Abnormal chest radiograph (i.e., hyperinflation, pulmonary hypertension, vascular redistribution or edema, atelectasis, effusion, infiltrate, or other parenchymal abnormalities)
- Type of surgery
- Duration of anesthesia

39-3	Causes of Altered Mucociliary Clearance in the Mechanically Ventilated Patient

- Tracheostomy or endotracheal tubes bypass the upper airway and prevent secretion evacuation
- Cold and dry inspired gases
- High inspired fraction of oxygen (FIO_2)
- Mucociliary clearance blocked by cuffs of endotracheal or tracheostomy tubes
- Elevated insufflation pressure of the endotracheal or tracheostomy tubes' cuffs crushes the vibratile cilia and reverses the direction of their movement
- Supine positioning of the patient results in accumulation of secretions
- Repeated tracheal suctioning causes abrasions that damage the cilia
- Use of anesthetic agents and sedatives

39-4	Risk Factors for Atelectasis

- Very young age (infants and young children)
- Obesity
- Smoking
- Preexisting pulmonary disease
- Dehydration
- Anesthetic agents (see Box 39-3)
- Mechanical ventilation (see Box 39-3)
- Types of surgery
  - Cardiopulmonary bypass surgery
  - Thoracic surgery
  - Upper abdominal surgery
  - Midline incisions
  - Prolonged anesthesia

bronchospasm, pulmonary aspiration, anesthetic effects, pulmonary edema, pulmonary embolism, acute lung injury (ALI), and ARDS. Pulmonary edema, ALI, and ARDS are very broad topics that cannot be covered in this chapter. We will now discuss atelectasis, pulmonary aspiration, and pulmonary embolism in further detail.

Atelectasis

The term *atelectasis* is derived from the Greek words *ateles* and *ektasis,* which mean incomplete expansion. Atelectasis is defined as alveolar collapse with reduced intrapulmonary air. It is the most common postoperative respiratory complication, with radiographic evidence in up to 70% of patients undergoing a thoracotomy or a celiotomy.[28] If left untreated, it can result in pulmonary gas exchange alterations leading to severe hypoxemia and acute respiratory failure. The mechanisms leading to atelectasis are multifactorial and include alterations in ventilatory mechanics, changes in the mechanical properties of the thoracic wall, stagnation of bronchial secretions, and airway obstruction.[9]

The alterations in ventilatory mechanics seen postoperatively include diminished vital capacity (VC), diminished V_T, increased respiratory rate, and diminished functional residual capacity (FRC), resulting in atelectasis. The primary cause of these alterations is postoperative diaphragmatic dysfunction.[9,29] The second mechanism of atelectasis involves reduction of total lung compliance in the mechanically ventilated patient. This reduction is secondary to decreased elasticity. In spontaneously breathing postoperative patients, this same diminished pulmonary elasticity results in a decreased FRC and subsequent atelectasis. Stagnation of bronchial secretions is the third mechanism leading to atelectasis. This problem is normally prevented by mucociliary clearance and coughing. When these functions are inhibited, stagnation of bronchial secretions occurs, and atelectasis develops.[9]

Mucociliary clearance is significantly diminished during mechanical ventilation, via the mechanisms shown in Box 39-3.[9] Coughing may be suppressed secondary to mechanical ventilation, opioids, diaphragmatic dysfunction, pain, altered mental status, and airway obstruction. A final mechanism of atelectasis is airway obstruction. In this case, atelectasis is either passive or absorptive. Passive atelectasis is secondary to external or internal compression of a lung segment (e.g., pneumothorax, hemothorax, abdominal distention). Absorptive atelectasis occurs when the inhaled gas is rich in oxygen and poor in nitrogen. In this instance, oxygen diffuses rapidly into venous blood, leading to alveolar collapse.[9]

Risk factors for atelectasis are shown in Box 39-4.[9] The type of surgical procedure performed has tremendous influence on the occurrence of postoperative atelectasis. Thoracic and upper abdominal surgeries pose a greater risk for atelectasis than do other procedures. Several studies have documented progressive deterioration of pulmonary gas exchange during the course of thoracic and abdominal surgeries.[30,31] Likewise, cardiopulmonary bypass surgery increases the risk of atelectasis more than other surgeries (including noncardiac thoracic surgeries).[32-34] In addition, midline celiotomies have an increased risk of atelectasis relative to transverse or subcostal abdominal incisions.

Clinical Manifestations

Clinically, atelectasis ranges from asymptomatic to severe hypoxemia and acute respiratory failure. The variability in presentation depends on the rapidity of onset, the degree of lung involvement, and the presence of an underlying pulmonary infection. In the worst-case scenario with rapid onset, major pulmonary airway collapse, and underlying infection, atelectasis presents with sudden dyspnea, chest pain, cyanosis, tachycardia, and an elevated temperature. On physical examination, the patient often exhibits diminished chest wall excursion, dullness to percussion, and diminished or absent breath sounds. In the less severe presentations, elevated temperature on the first postoperative day may be the only manifestation of atelectasis.[35] Other manifestations of less severe atelectasis include diminished breath sounds and bronchial breathing.

Diagnosis

The diagnosis of atelectasis is generally made from radiographic findings of diminished lung volumes in the presence of the aforementioned clinical manifestations. On chest radiographs, findings indicative of atelectasis relate to volume loss and include displacement of the lobar fissure, retracted ribs, an elevated hemidiaphragm, mediastinal or tracheal deviation to the affected side, and overinflation of the unaffected lung. The exact radiographic findings depend on which portion of the lung is involved and to what degree, in addition to how the surrounding structures compensate for the volume loss. On ABG analysis, significant atelectasis results in hypoxemia. Atelectasis also may be identified by means of chest computed tomography (CT).[4,9,35]

Treatment

For postoperative atelectasis, prevention is the key.[36] Because tobacco use and underlying pulmonary disease processes are predictors of postoperative atelectasis, preoperative optimization is essential. Both smoking cessation and improved bronchial toilet preoperatively should be encouraged. During anesthesia induction, the use of positive end-expiratory pressure (PEEP) has been shown to be beneficial. Rusca and coworkers documented significantly decreased atelectasis and improved oxygenation by applying PEEP at 6 cm H_2O on induction.[37] In addition to this maneuver, long-acting anesthetics and those with significant postanesthesia narcosis should be limited.[9]

During the postoperative period, a number of measures can be taken to prevent atelectasis (Fig. 39-2). Control of postoperative pain is critical. Insufficient analgesia results in pleural and parietal pain, causing inadequate coughing and expectoration. However, narcotics depress the cough reflex, so overdosing should be avoided.[4,9,35] The traditional intermittent dosing of narcotics at 3- to 4-hour intervals is insufficient. The patient cycles from overdosing after administration (oversedation with resultant poor coughing and expectoration) to pain and anxiety before receiving the next dose. This cyclical pattern may be avoided by using patient-controlled analgesia (PCA). Another alternative is epidural analgesia, which is very effective. A recent meta-analysis supports the view that postoperative atelectasis is decreased when patients receive epidural opioids instead of systemic opioids.[38]

Just as pain control is critical, so is meticulous nursing care. In nonintubated patients, several steps should be taken

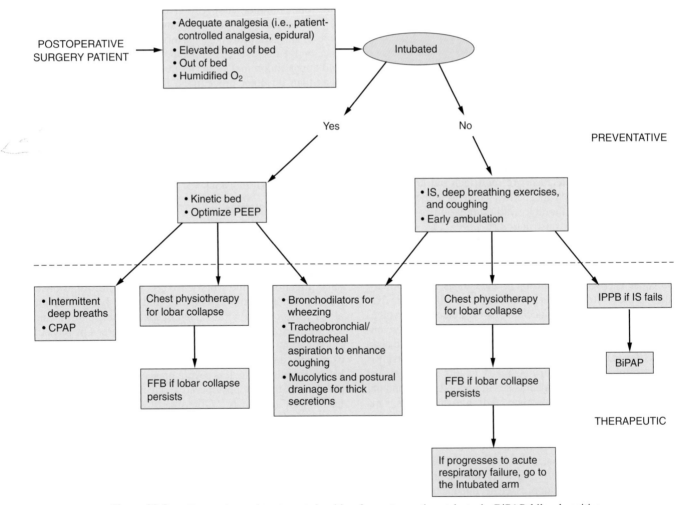

Figure 39-2 ■ Prevention and treatment algorithm for postoperative atelectasis. BiPAP, bilevel positive airway pressure; CPAP, continuous positive airway pressure; FFB, flexible fiberoptic bronchoscopy; IPPB, intermittent positive-pressure breathing; IS, incentive spirometry; PEEP, positive end-expiratory pressure.

to prevent atelectasis. Early ambulation and techniques that encourage deep breathing are important.[39-41] Incentive spirometry (IS) is the most widely used postoperative pulmonary therapy. Its purpose is to imitate the natural sighing or yawning that healthy individuals perform regularly. The simplicity of IS and its lack of required personnel account for its popularity. A meta-analysis suggests that IS, intermittent positive-pressure breathing (IPPB), and chest physiotherapy are all equally efficacious in decreasing postoperative pulmonary complications after upper abdominal surgery.[42] Chest physiotherapy encompasses deep breathing and coughing, postural drainage, and chest percussions. Because physiotherapy is labor intensive and effective for lobar collapse only, it is relatively unpopular. Additional physiotherapy regimens include bronchodilators, tracheobronchial aspiration, and mucolytic agents. If lobar collapse persists, flexible fiberoptic bronchoscopy should be performed to reexpand the collapsed segments.

Either bilevel positive airway pressure (BiPAP) or continuous positive airway pressure (CPAP) can be used as a last means in attempting to prevent intubation. In a recent randomized controlled trial, Squadrone and colleagues documented that CPAP decreases the incidence of postoperative complications (including endotracheal intubation) in patients who develop hypoxia after major elective abdominal surgery.[43] If these maneuvers are unsuccessful and the patient continues to progress to acute respiratory failure, the patient should be intubated.

In intubated patients, several modifications can be made to these maneuvers to prevent and treat atelectasis. In preventing atelectasis, a kinetic bed should be considered for selected patients (e.g., patients receiving paralytics). Likewise, the optimization of PEEP should be performed early. If these maneuvers are unsuccessful, treatment measures include intermittent deep breaths, CPAP, bronchodilators, endotracheal tube suctioning, mucolytic agents and postural drainage, and chest physiotherapy.[9] As in the nonintubated patient, if lobar collapse persists, flexible fiberoptic bronchoscopy should be performed to reexpand the collapsed segments.

Pulmonary Aspiration

Pulmonary aspiration of gastric contents is generally preventable with meticulous anesthesia technique and critical care. Despite this, the incidence varies from 1 in every 3900 elective surgical cases to 1 in every 895 emergent surgical cases. The number increases dramatically to 8% to 19% during emergent intubations without anesthesia.[9]

Aspiration of gastric contents results in chemical pneumonitis, which develops in four stages.[9] Initially, the aspirate causes mechanical obstruction of the airways, with distal collapse. Obstruction alters ventilatory mechanics, leading to increased shunt, loss of FRC, and increased work of breathing. In the second stage, chemical injury occurs in response to the acidity of the aspirate. The pattern of injury includes mucosal edema, bronchorrhea, and bronchoconstriction, all resulting in an increased risk of bacterial infection. The third stage in the pathophysiology of aspiration is the inflammatory response. The release of tumor necrosis factor, interleu-

kin 1, leukotrienes, and thromboxane A_2 contributes to mucosal edema and bronchoconstriction resulting in lung injury.[28] The final phase is progression to infection if appropriate interventions are not performed. Risk factors for pulmonary aspiration are shown in Table 39-3.[44-46]

Clinical Manifestations

Hypoxemia is the most consistent finding in aspiration. In addition, patients present with increased temperature, tachypnea, tachycardia or bradycardia, cyanosis, and altered mental status. On physical examination, the pulmonary findings include crackles, rales, decreased breath sounds, and a pleural friction rub. The extent of these manifestations depends on the degree of aspiration.[9,35]

The outcome of these clinical manifestations varies widely from asymptomatic to rapid death.[9] Fortunately, patients improve rapidly within several days without further treatment. A second subset of patients improves initially and then deteriorates over the following 2 to 5 days. These patients develop increased temperature, productive cough, and hypoxemia and progress from aspiration pneumonitis to aspiration pneumonia. The remaining patients do not improve from their initial pneumonitis but rapidly progress to diffuse pulmonary infiltrates, refractory hypoxemia, and ARDS.

Diagnosis

After a witnessed pulmonary aspiration, the diagnosis is clear. However, in other situations, the diagnosis of aspiration is based on the clinical symptoms and a high index of suspicion. On laboratory evaluation, significant aspiration results in hypoxemia and leukocytosis. Aspiration also may be identified by means of chest radiography. There are no pathognomonic radiologic features; however, infiltrates in gravity-dependent lung regions are the most consistent finding. The most common sites of infiltration are the superior segment of the right lower lobe and the right middle lobe.

39-3	Risk Factors for Pulmonary Aspiration	
Risk Factor	**Clarification/Examples**
Endotracheal intubation	The cuff does not prevent aspiration.
Decreased level of consciousness	GCS <9, alcohol or drug overdose/withdrawal, excessive analgesics or sedatives, chemical paralysis
Neuromuscular disease and structural abnormalities of the aerodigestive tract	Diabetic gastroparesis, Parkinson's disease, scleroderma, gastroesophageal reflux disease, esophageal cancer
Recent cerebrovascular accident	Within 4 to 6 wk
Major intra-abdominal surgery	Less than 5 days postoperative
Persistently high GRV	GRV >500 mL
Prolonged supine positioning	Spine fractures
Persistent hyperglycemia	Blood glucose >140 mg/dL

GCS, Glasgow coma scale; GRV, gastric residual volume.
Modified from Marr AB, McQuiggan MM, Kozar R, Moore FA: Nutr Clin Pract 2004;19:504-510.

However, depending on the aspirate volume and the patient's position during aspiration, left and bilobar aspiration is possible. Flexible fiberoptic bronchoscopy may also be used for diagnosing aspiration.[9,35]

Treatment

As in atelectasis, prevention is the key. An algorithm for the prevention and treatment of pulmonary aspiration is in Figure 39-3.[47] During the preoperative assessment by the anesthesiologist, patients at risk for aspiration need to be identified. These include patients requiring emergency procedures, patients with diabetes mellitus, and pregnant patients. In these instances, an experienced anesthesiologist is required. If feasible, regional anesthesia should be entertained. As for preoperative NPO (*non per os* or *nil per os*) orders, the American Society for Anesthesiologists (ASA) published more liberal preoperative fasting guidelines in 1999[48] (Table 39-4).

After the surgical procedure, meticulous nursing care is required.[9] The head of the bed should be elevated to 30

39-4	Preoperative Fasting Recommendations* of the American Society of Anesthesiologists

Liquid and Food Intake	Minimal Fasting Period (hr)
Clear liquids (e.g., water, clear tea, black coffee, carbonated beverages, and fruit juice without pulp)	2
Breast milk	4
Nonhuman milk, including infant formula	6
Light meal (e.g., toast and clear liquids)	6
Regular or heavy meal (e.g., may include fried or fatty food, meat)	8

*For healthy patients of all ages undergoing elective surgery (excluding women in labor).

Modified from American Society of Anesthesiologist Task Force on Preoperative Fasting: Anesthesiology 1999;90:896-905.

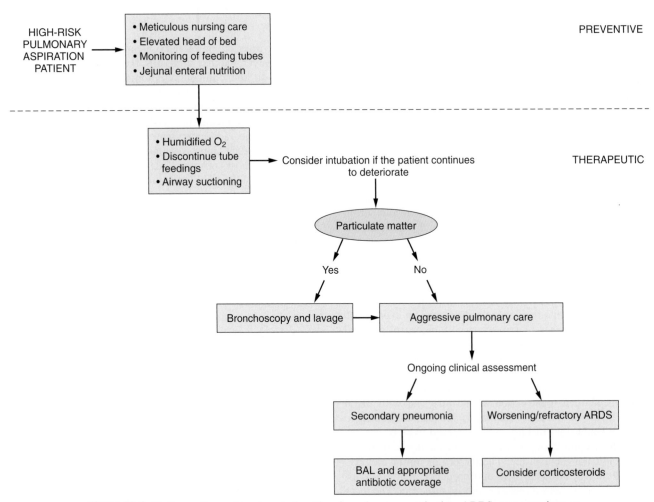

Figure 39-3 ■ Prevention and treatment algorithm for pulmonary aspiration. ARDS, acute respiratory distress syndrome; BAL, bronchoalveolar lavage.

degrees at a minimum; elevation to 45 degrees is better. In addition, particular attention should be paid to oral hygiene. Nasogastric and orogastric tubes should be monitored closely, as they may become displaced during the course of hospitalization. The placement of small-bore (3-mm) feeding tubes should be confirmed by radiography.

Gastric feeding is a major risk factor for pulmonary aspiration, and there appears to be no difference in risk between nasogastric/orogastric tubes and small-bore feeding tubes.[49] To avoid this problem, many clinicians advocate postpyloric feeding. However, randomized controlled trials comparing gastric to postpyloric feeding have produced conflicting results,[50-56] possibly because most postpyloric feeding tubes are too short to go beyond the ligament of Treitz. When the tube is too short, enteral nutrition is administered into the duodenum, and there is a high incidence of duodenogastric reflux in patients at risk for aspiration.[51] Heyland and coworkers documented an 80% rate of reflux into the stomach, 25% into the esophagus, and 4% into the lung when radioisotope-labeled enteral formulas were fed through postpyloric feeding tubes in mechanically ventilated patients in the intensive care unit.[54] In postoperative patients, Tournadre and colleagues demonstrated gastroparesis and rapid discoordinated duodenal contractions.[57] These studies provide compelling evidence that duodenogastric reflux is present in postoperative and critically ill patients. Thus, with regard to aspiration risk, we believe that feeding into the duodenum is not significantly different from feeding into the stomach in these patients. In addition to these findings, there appears to be no difference in the rate of pulmonary aspiration between patients with nasogastric feeding tubes and percutaneous endoscopic gastrostomy (PEG) tubes.[58] For all of these reasons, we advocate jejunal feeding when feasible.

Once the diagnosis of aspiration is entertained, the resultant hypoxemia should be addressed. Supplemental oxygen via a nasal cannula or a face mask should be administered while the diagnosis is confirmed. In severe cases, patients may require intubation and positive-pressure mechanical ventilation. If tube feeding is ongoing, it should be discontinued. Suctioning should be performed to clear the upper airway of any residual aspirate.

The role of bronchoscopy is limited to the retrieval of large particulate matter. The acidic aspirate is neutralized by pulmonary secretions within minutes of aspiration, so bronchoscopy and saline lavage are not required for the aspiration of nonparticulate matter. The use of empiric antibiotic coverage is not supported by current literature; however, if a subsequent aspiration pneumonia is identified, antibiotic coverage should be tailored according to the findings obtained by bronchoalveolar lavage (BAL). Not only are empiric antibiotics not indicated in aspiration but they often select for resistant organisms.[9] Likewise, corticosteroids have a limited role in pulmonary aspiration, although they may be indicated in the treatment of aspiration-induced refractory ARDS.[59-61]

Pulmonary Embolism

In 1856, Virchow described a triad of conditions associated with the development of venous thromboembolism (VTE): vessel intimal injury, venous stasis, and hypercoagulability.[62]

Today, VTE remains a significant source of morbidity and mortality after surgical procedures. The most common and clinically significant forms of VTE are deep vein thrombosis (DVT) and pulmonary embolism (PE).[63] PE is the most common preventable source of hospital mortality.[64]

Venous thromboembolic disorders vary in incidence depending on the type of surgical procedure being performed; the highest rates are reported in urologic and orthopedic procedures.[65] The goal of these paragraphs is to address VTE, and PE specifically, as a complication of general surgical procedures. Studies prior to 1984 documented a 15% to 30% rate of DVT, and a 0.2% to 0.9% rate of fatal PE among general surgical patients not treated with VTE prophylaxis.[66-68] The current risk of DVT and PE in general surgical procedures is unknown because trials devoid of prophylaxis are no longer ethical. The combination of individual predisposing factors and the specific type of surgery determine the risk of DVT and PE in surgical patients. Risk factors are shown in Box 39-5.[69-74]

Clinical Manifestations

The clinical manifestations of pulmonary embolism are quite variable, depending on the magnitude of the embolic event. The majority of emboli are asymptomatic. In those that are symptomatic, the most common complaint is dyspnea, which is sudden in onset. Additional findings include rales, pleuritic chest pain, and hemoptysis. Patients with massive pulmonary emboli often present with chest discomfort in addition to anxiety and a sense of impending doom. In the most severe form, massive embolic events involve complete circulatory collapse, characterized by shock and/or syncope.[75] The physical examination is often unremarkable, the most common finding being tachypnea. On cardiac examination, sinus tachycardia is the most common finding, followed in frequency by right-sided heart strain.[35]

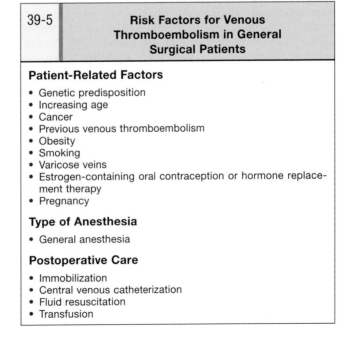

39-5	**Risk Factors for Venous Thromboembolism in General Surgical Patients**

Patient-Related Factors
- Genetic predisposition
- Increasing age
- Cancer
- Previous venous thromboembolism
- Obesity
- Smoking
- Varicose veins
- Estrogen-containing oral contraception or hormone replacement therapy
- Pregnancy

Type of Anesthesia
- General anesthesia

Postoperative Care
- Immobilization
- Central venous catheterization
- Fluid resuscitation
- Transfusion

Diagnosis

A high index of suspicion is critical for diagnosing a PE. A detailed history should be obtained specifically inquiring about a history of VTE, preexisting medical conditions, and other risk factors. On ABG analysis, most patients are hypoxemic; however, during the Urokinase-Streptokinase Pulmonary Embolism Trial, 10% of patients with a PE had a PaO_2 of greater than 80 mm Hg.[76] On the electrocardiogram, the most common finding is sinus tachycardia. Other common abnormalities are right-sided heart strain, nonspecific ST changes, and new-onset atrial fibrillation or right bundle branch block.[77] The chest radiograph is generally nondiagnostic; however, a wedge-shaped infiltrate (Hampton's hump) should heighten suspicion of a PE. Additional findings can include focal hyperlucency of the lung in the presence of diminished pulmonary vasculature markings (Westermark's sign) or an enlarged right descending pulmonary artery (Palla's sign).[35,78]

Recently, some experts have advocated measuring circulating D-dimer levels as an aid in diagnosing DVT and PE, but the role of this test remains unclear. In 2004, Stein and coworkers performed a systematic review of the current literature on measurements of D-dimer levels.[79] They concluded that the D-dimer enzyme-linked immunosorbent assay (ELISA) was superior to other assays. The D-dimer ELISA has negative likelihood ratios comparable to those of a normal or near-normal ventilation–perfusion (V-P) lung scan or a negative Doppler ultrasound for diagnosing PE or DVT respectively. The main problem with this test is that D-dimer levels are elevated in multiple medical conditions, including routine recovery from operations. As such, the specificity and positive likelihood ratios are of little clinical value in diagnosing DVT or PE. Despite these limitations, if the D-dimer ELISA is not elevated, the patient does not have a PE.

More definitive diagnostic tools for PE include V-P scans, helical CT scans, and selective pulmonary angiography. Pulmonary angiography remains the gold standard; however, it is invasive, costly, time consuming, and associated with real risks for morbidity and mortality.[80,81] The Prospective Investigation of Pulmonary Embolism Diagnosis (PIOPED) study reviewed V-P scanning as a diagnostic modality for PE.[82] Seventy-five percent of V-P scans are in the indeterminate category. Thus, V-P scanning alone is insufficient to either confirm or exclude the diagnosis of PE. The D-dimer test and Doppler ultrasound are useful adjuncts in this situation.[83,84]

Since the 1990s, helical CT scans have become a routine means of diagnosing PE. Advantages of the CT scan include its rapidity, widespread availability, and noninvasiveness. In 2005, Hayashino and colleagues performed a meta-analysis of the diagnostic performance of helical CT scanning in comparison to V-P scanning in suspected PE.[85] On the basis of a summary receiver operating characteristic (ROC) analysis, they determined that when the V-P scan is normal or near-normal, the CT scan is superior in the diagnosis of PE. However, in situations of high probability, the V-P scan is equivalent to CT scan for diagnosing PE. An algorithm for the diagnosis of postoperative PE is found in Figure 39-4.

Prophylaxis

Because of the inherent risk of DVT and PE in postoperative patients, numerous modalities have been developed for prophylaxis. Prophylactic measures are categorized by mechanism of action as pharmacologic or mechanical. The most commonly used pharmacologic measures are low-dose unfractionated heparin (LDUH) and low-molecular-weight heparin (LMWH).[86] In the past, LDUH was the pharmacologic standard of care for VTE prevention, but a number of disadvantages have made it unattractive as a prophylactic agent. These include, yet are not limited to, nonspecific binding, low bioavailability, anticoagulant and dose-response variability, resistance, and heparin-induced thrombocytopenia (HIT). LMWH overcomes the majority of these limitations, with the exception of HIT.[87]

Mechanical measures include thromboembolism-deterrent stockings (TEDS) and intermittent pneumatic compression (IPC) devices, such as venous foot pumps (VFP) and sequential compression devices (SCD). In 1986, the National Institutes of Health Consensus Development Conference on the Prevention of Venous Thrombosis and Pulmonary Embolism endorsed IPC devices as an effective prophylactic measure.[88] In addition to the device's efficacy, there are few associated complications. Only isolated case reports of pressure necrosis, peroneal nerve palsy, and compartment syndrome have been documented.[89,90] Mechanical measures should be considered in patients with a high bleeding potential. In addition, they should be considered in combination with chemical prophylaxis to improve efficacy in high-risk patients.[91]

The mechanism of action of intermittent pneumatic compression devices is twofold. The first is mechanical: the devices increase the velocity of venous return and decrease venous stasis. The second mechanism is the systemic activation of the fibrinolytic system. Compression results in the release of plasminogen activators, which are found in high concentrations in the vaso vasorum.

In multiple trauma patients, when neither chemical nor standard mechanical prophylaxis approaches are an option, placement of an inferior vena cava (IVC) filter should be considered.[92,93] Likewise, for high-risk morbidly obese patients (e.g., those with sleep apnea and pulmonary hypertension) undergoing bariatric surgery, prophylactic IVC filter placement should be considered.[94]

Routine use of VTE prophylaxis is recommended for at-risk surgical patients (see Box 39-5), specifically those older than 40 years or those undergoing major surgical procedures.[95] The Seventh American College of Chest Physicians Conference on Antithrombotic and Thrombolytic Therapy: Evidence-Based Guidelines for thromboprophylaxis in the general surgical population may be found in Table 39-5.[96]

Treatment

Once the diagnosis of PE is seriously entertained, the treatment is supportive. Treatment includes the administration of oxygen, fluid resuscitation, and anticoagulation. For medical patients, in whom the diagnostic certainty of PE is greater

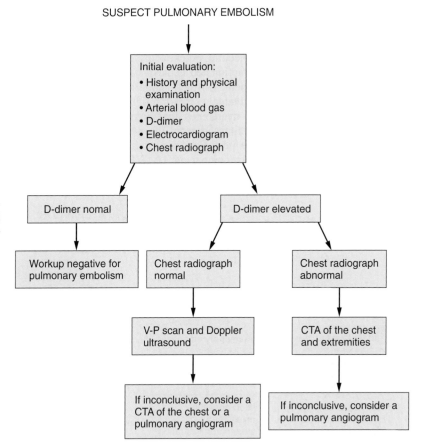

SUSPECT PULMONARY EMBOLISM

Initial evaluation:
- History and physical examination
- Arterial blood gas
- D-dimer
- Electrocardiogram
- Chest radiograph

D-dimer nomal

D-dimer elevated

Workup negative for pulmonary embolism

Chest radiograph normal

Chest radiograph abnormal

V-P scan and Doppler ultrasound

CTA of the chest and extremities

If inconclusive, consider a CTA of the chest or a pulmonary angiogram

If inconclusive, consider a pulmonary angiogram

Figure 39-4 ■ Algorithm for diagnosis of post-operative pulmonary embolism. CTA, computed tomographic angiography; V-P, ventilation–perfusion.

39-5	Venous Thromboembolism Prophylaxis: General Surgery Recommendations

Patient Characteristics and Risk Factors	Recommendations	Strength of Recommendation
Minor surgery, younger than 40 yr, no additional risk factors	Early and persistent mobilization	Strong recommendation; can apply to most patients in most circumstances
Not major surgery, 40 to 60 years of age or additional risk factors	LDUH 5000 U bid, or LMWH ≤3400 U daily	Strong recommendation; can apply to most patients in most circumstances without reservation
Major surgery, younger than 40 yr, no additional risk factors	LDUH 5000 U bid, or LMWH ≤3400 U daily	Strong recommendation; can apply to most patients in most circumstances without reservation
Not major surgery, older than 60 yr or additional risk factors	LDUH 5000 U tid, or LMWH >3400 U daily	Strong recommendation; can apply to most patients in most circumstances without reservation
Major surgery, older than 40 yr or additional risk factors	LDUH 5000 U tid, or LMWH >3400 U daily	Strong recommendation; can apply to most patients in most circumstances without reservation
Surgery, older than 40 yr, multiple risk factors, hip or knee arthroplasty, HFS, major trauma, SCI	LDUH 5000 U tid, or LMWH >3400 U daily in addition with TEDS and/or IPC devices	Strong recommendation; can apply to most patients in most circumstances
Patients with a high risk of bleeding	Mechanical prophylaxis (TEDS or IPC) initially, until the bleeding risk decreases	Strong recommendation; can apply to most patients in most circumstances without reservation
Selected high-risk patients, including those who have undergone major cancer surgery	Prophylaxis with LMWH after hospital discharge	Intermediate strength recommendation; best action may differ depending on circumstances

bid, twice a day; HFS, hip fracture surgery; IPC, intermittent pneumatic compression; LDUH, low-dose unfractionated heparin; LMWH, low-molecular-weight heparin; RCT, randomized controlled trial; SCI, spinal cord injury; TEDS, thromboembolic deterrent stockings; tid, three times a day; U, units.
Modified from Geerts WH, Pineo GF, Heit JA, et al: Chest 2004;126:338S-400.

(than in surgical patients), rapid anticoagulation before the definitive diagnosis is acceptable. However, this treatment strategy should be avoided in the surgical population, where the diagnostic uncertainty and bleeding potential are greater. Dose-adjusted intravenous unfractionated heparin has been the cornerstone of PE management. Unfractionated heparin for treatment has the same disadvantages as for prophylaxis. As previously stated, LMWH overcomes the majority of these limitations and offers an alternative for the treatment of PE.[87] Quinlan and coworkers performed a meta-analysis of randomized controlled trials comparing LMWH with intravenous unfractionated heparin in the treatment of PE.[97]

This meta-analysis revealed that fixed-dose LMWH is as effective and safe as intravenous unfractionated heparin for the treatment of nonmassive PE. In this study, the rate of bleeding, recurrent VTE, and mortality were not significantly different between the two treatment arms.

Other modalities of PE treatment include thrombolytic therapy and IVC filters. The literature on thrombolytic therapy documents varying results.[98-101] However, neither of two recent limited meta-analyses showed that thrombolytic therapy is clearly better than intravenous unfractionated heparin.[102,103] IVC filters should be limited to patients who are not candidates for anticoagulation.[104]

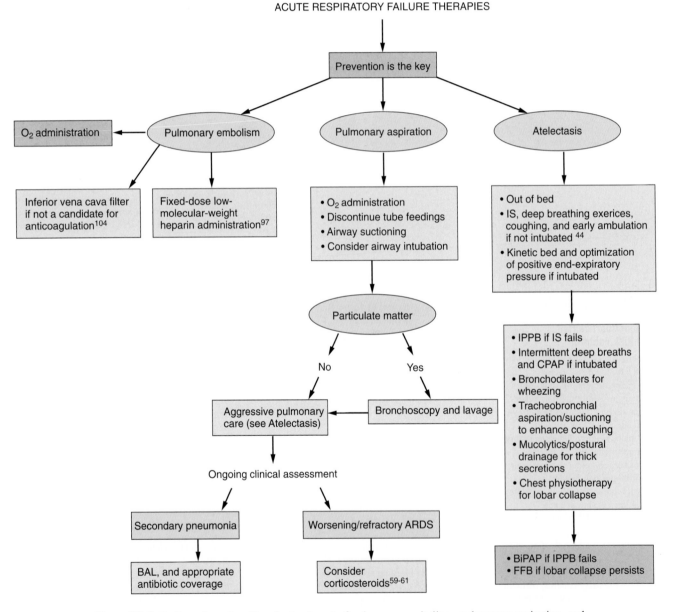

Figure 39-5 ■ Overview algorithm for treatment of pulmonary embolism, pulmonary aspiration, and atelectasis. ARDS, acute respiratory distress syndrome; BAL, bronchoalveolar lavage; BiPAP, bilevel positive airway pressure; CPAP, continuous positive airway pressure; FFB, flexible fiberoptic bronchoscopy; IS, incentive spirometry; IPPB, intermittent positive-pressure breathing.

■ SUMMARY

Throughout this chapter, we have focused on the clinically relevant issues regarding postoperative respiratory failure. Initially, we addressed the pathophysiology of the varying types of acute respiratory failure and the approach to the hypoxic patient. In addition, we identified the preoperative, intraoperative, and postoperative predictors of postoperative pulmonary complications including respiratory failure. We then took an in-depth look at the more common etiologies of acute respiratory failure: atelectasis, pulmonary aspiration, and pulmonary embolism. We proposed algorithms for their diagnosis, prevention, and treatment. The algorithm in Figure 39-5 is an overview of the treatments for these three etiologies.

■ REFERENCES

1. Lawrence VA, Hilsenbeck SG, Mulrow CD, et al: Incidence and hospital stay for cardiac and pulmonary complications after abdominal surgery. J Gen Intern Med 1995;10:671-678.
2. Moore EE, Feliciano DL, Mattox KL: Trauma, ed 5. New York, McGraw-Hill, 2005.
3. Mattox KL: Complications of Trauma, ed 1. New York, Churchill Livingstone, 1994.
4. Wilmore DW, Cheung LY, Harken AH, et al: American College of Surgeons ACS Surgery: Principles and Practice. New York, WebMD Corporation, 2002.
5. Tisi GM: Pulmonary Physiology in Clinical Medicine, ed 2. Baltimore, Williams & Wilkins, 1983.
6. Neema PK: Respiratory failure. Indian J Anaesth 2003;47:360-366.
7. Marino PL: The ICU Book, ed 2. Baltimore, Williams & Wilkins, 1998.
8. Bongard FS, Leighton TA: Continuous dual oximetry in surgical critical care. Ann Surg 1992;216:60-68.
9. Webb AR, Shapiro MJ, Singer M, Suter PM: Oxford Textbook of Critical Care. New York, Oxford University Press, 1999.
10. Parrillo JE, Dellinger RP: Critical Care Medicine: Principles of Diagnosis and Management in the Adult, ed 2. St Louis, Mosby, 2002.
11. Cameron JL: Current Surgical Therapy, ed 5. St Louis, Mosby, 1995.
12. Barcroft JT: Anoxemia. Lancet 1920;2:485-489.
13. Moore FA, Haenel JB, Moore EE, Abernathy CM: Hypoxic events in the surgical intensive care unit. Am J Surg 1990;160:647-651.
14. Smetana GW: Current concepts: Preoperative pulmonary evaluation. N Engl J Med 1999;340:937-944.
15. McAlister FA, Bertsch K, Man, J, et al: Incidence of and risk factors for pulmonary complications after nonthoracic surgery. Am J Respir Crit Care Med 2005;171:514-517.
16. Warner MA, Offord KP, Warner ME, et al: Role of preoperative cessation of smoking and other factors in postoperative pulmonary complications: A blinded prospective study of coronary artery bypass patients. Mayo Clin Proc 1989;64:609-616.
17. Moulton MJ, Creswell LL Mackey ME, et al: Obesity is not a risk factor for significant adverse outcomes after cardiac surgery. Circulation 1996;94(Suppl II):II87-92.
18. Pasulka PS, Bistrian BR, Benotti PN, Blackburn GL: The risks of surgery in obese patients. Ann Intern Med 1986;104:540-546.
19. Celli BR, Rodriguez KS, Snider GL: A controlled trial of intermittent positive pressure breathing, incentive spirometry, and deep breathing exercises in preventing pulmonary complications after abdominal surgery. Am Rev Respir Dis 1984;130:12-15.
20. Berg H, Viby-Morgensen J, Roed J, et al: Residual neuromuscular block is a risk factor for postoperative pulmonary complications: A prospective, randomized, and blinded study of postoperative pulmonary complications after atracurium, vecuronium, and pancuronium. Acta Anaesthesiol Scand 1997;41:1095-1103.
21. Tarhan S, Moffitt EA, Sessler AD, et al: Risk of anesthesia and surgery in patients with chronic bronchitis and chronic obstructive pulmonary disease. Surgery 1973;74:720-726.
22. Cascade PN, Alexander GD, Mackie DS: Negative-pressure pulmonary edema after endotracheal intubation. Radiology 1993;186: 671-675.
23. Brooks-Brunn JA: Predictors of postoperative pulmonary complications following abdominal surgery. Chest 1997;111:564-571.
24. Phillips EH, Carrol BJ, Fallas MJ, Pearlstein AR: Comparison of laparoscopic cholecystectomy in obese and non-obese patients. Am Surg 1994;60:316-321.
25. The Southern Surgeons Club: A prospective analysis of 1518 laparoscopic cholecystectomies. N Engl J Med 1991;324:1073-1078.
26. Fisher BW, Majumdar SR, McAlister FA: Predicting pulmonary complications after nonthoracic surgery: A systematic review of blinded studies. Am J Med 2002;112: 219-225.
27. McAlister FA, Straus SE, Sackett DL, et al: Why we need large simple studies of the clinical examination: The problem and a proposed solution. Lancet 1999;354:1721-1724.
28. Sabiston DC, Lyerly HK: Textbook of Surgery: The Biological Basis of Modern Surgical Practice, ed 15. Philadelphia, WB Saunders, 1997.
29. Duggan M, Kavanagh BP: Pulmonary atelectasis: A pathogenic perioperative entity. Anesthesiology 2005;102:838-854.
30. Lundh R, Hedenstierna G: Ventilation-perfusion relationships during anesthesia and abdominal surgery. Acta Anaesthesiol Scand 1983; 27:167-173.
31. Jonmarker C, Nordstrom L, Werner O: Changes in functional residual capacity during surgery. Br J Anaesth 1986;58:428-432.
32. Magnusson L, Zemgulis V, Wicky S, et al: Atelectasis is a major cause of hypoxemia and shunt after cardiopulmonary bypass: An experimental study. Anesthesiology 1997;87:1153-1163.
33. Tenling A, Hachenberg T, Tyden H, et al: Atelectasis and gas exchange after cardiac surgery. Anesthesiology 1998;89:371-378.
34. Macnaughton PD, Braude S, Hunter DN, et al: Changes in lung function and pulmonary capillary permeability after cardiopulmonary bypass. Crit Care Med 1992;20:1289-1294.
35. Beers MH, Berkow R: Merck Manual of Diagnosis and Therapy. Whitehouse Station, NJ, Merck, 2005.
36. Warner DO: Preventing postoperative pulmonary complications: The role of the anesthesiologist. Anesthesiology 2000;92:1467-1472.
37. Rusca M, Proietti S, Schnyder P, et al: Prevention of atelectasis formation during induction of general anesthesia. Anesth Analg 2003;97: 1835-1839.
38. Ballantyne JC, Carr DB, deFerranti S, et al: The comparative effects of postoperative analgesic therapies on pulmonary outcome: Cumulative meta-analysis of randomized, controlled trials. Anesth Analg 1998;86:598-612.
39. Dohi S, Gold MI: Comparison of two methods of postoperative respiratory care. Chest 1978;73:592-595.
40. Bartlett RH, Gazzaniga AB, Geraghty TR: Respiratory maneuvers to prevent postoperative pulmonary complications: A critical review. JAMA 1973;224:1017-1021.
41. Hedstrand U, Liw M, Rooth G, Ogren CH: Effect of respiratory physiotherapy on arterial oxygen tension. Acta Anaesthesiol Scand 1978;22:349-352.
42. Thomas JA, McIntosh JM: Are incentive spirometry, intermittent positive pressure breathing, and deep breathing exercises effective in the prevention of postoperative pulmonary complications after upper abdominal surgery? A systematic overview and meta-analysis. Phys Ther 1994;74:3-10.
43. Squadrone V, Coha M, Cerutti E, et al: Continuous positive airway pressure for treatment of postoperative hypoxia: A randomized controlled trial. JAMA 2005;293:589-595.
44. Marr AB, McQuiggan MM, Kozar R, Moore FA: Gastric feeding as an extension of an established enteral nutrition protocol. Nutr Clin Pract 2004;19:504-510.
45. McClave SA, DeMeo MT, DeLegge MH, et al: North American Summit on Aspiration in the Critically Ill Patient: Consensus statement. JPEN J Parenter Enteral Nutr 2002;26(6 Suppl):S80-85.
46. Metheny NA: Risk factors for aspiration. JPEN J Parenter Enteral Nutr 2002;26(6 Suppl):S26-31.

47. Moore FA: Treatment of aspiration in intensive care unit patients. JPEN J Parenter Enteral Nutr 2002;26:S69-74.

48. American Society of Anesthesiologist Task Force on Preoperative Fasting: Practice guidelines for preoperative fasting and the use of pharmacological agents to reduce the risk of pulmonary aspiration: Application to healthy patients undergoing elective procedures. Anesthesiology 1999;90:896-905.

49. Ferrer M, Bauer TT, Torres A, et al: Effect of nasogastric tube size on gastroesophageal reflux and microaspiration in intubated patients. Ann Intern Med 1999;130:991-994.

50. Kearns PJ, Chin D, Mueller L, et al: The incidence of ventilator-associated pneumonia and success in nutrient delivery with gastric versus small intestinal feeding: A randomized clinical trial. Crit Care Med 2000;28:1742-1746.

51. Kortbeek JB, Haigh PI, Doig C: Duodenal versus gastric feeding in ventilated blunt trauma patients: A randomized controlled trial. J Trauma 1999;46:992-996.

52. Montejo JC, Grau T, Acosta J, et al: Multicenter, prospective, randomized, single-blind study comparing the efficacy and gastrointestinal complications of early jejunal feeding with early gastric feeding in critically ill patients. Crit Care Med 2002;30:796-800.

53. Strong RM, Condon SC, Solinger MR, et al: Equal aspiration rates from postpylorus and intragastric-placed small-bore nasoenteric feeding tubes: A randomized, prospective study. JPEN J Parenter Enteral Nutr 1992;16:59-63.

54. Heyland DK, Drover JW, MacDonald S, et al: Effect of postpyloric feeding on gastroesophageal regurgitation and pulmonary microaspiration: Results of a randomized controlled trial. Crit Care Med 2001;29:1495-1500.

55. Davis AR, Froomes PRA, French CJ, et al: Randomized comparison of nasojejunal and nasogastric feeding in critically ill patients. Crit Care Med 2002;30:586-590.

56. Montecalvo MA, Steger KA, Farber HW, et al: Nutritional outcome and pneumonia in critical care patients randomized to gastric versus jejunal tube feedings: The Critical Care Research Team. Crit Care Med 1992;20:1377-1387.

57. Tournadre JP, Barclay M, Fraser R, et al: Small intestinal motor patterns in critically ill patients after major abdominal surgery. Am J Gastroenterol 2001;96:2418-2426.

58. Park RH, Allison MC, Lang J, et al: Randomised comparison of percutaneous endoscopic gastrostomy and nasogastric tube feeding in patients with persisting neurologic dysphagia. BMJ 1992;304:1406-1409.

59. Wolfe JE, Bone RC, Ruth WE: Effects of corticosteroids in the treatment of patients with gastric aspiration. Am J Med 1977;63:719-722.

60. Sukumaran M, Granada MJ, Berger HW, et al: Evaluation of corticosteroid treatment in aspiration of gastric contents: A controlled clinical trial. Mt Sinai J Med 1980;47:335-340.

61. Biffl WL, Moore FA, Moore EE, et al: Are corticosteroids salvage therapy for refractory acute respiratory distress syndrome? Am J Surg 1995;170:591-596.

62. Knudson MM, Lewis FR, Clinton A, et al: Prevention of venous thromboembolism in trauma patients. J Trauma 1994;37:480-487.

63. Bell WR, Simon TL: Current status of pulmonary thromboembolism disease: Pathophysiology, diagnosis, prevention, and treatment. Am Heart J 1982;103:239-262.

64. Anderson FA, Wheeler HB, Goldberg RJ, et al: A population-based perspective of the hospital incidence and case-fatality rates of deep vein thrombosis and pulmonary embolism: The Worcester DVT study. Arch Intern Med 1991;151:933-938.

65. Geerts WH, Pineo GF, Heit JA, et al: Prevention of venous thromboembolism: The Seventh ACCP Conference on Antithrombotic and Thrombolytic Therapy. Chest 2004;126:338S-400.

66. Mismetti P, Laporte S, Darmon JY, et al: Meta-analysis of low molecular weight heparin in the prevention of venous thromboembolism in general surgery. Br J Surg 2001;88:913-930.

67. Clagett GP, Reisch JS: Prevention of venous thromboembolism in general surgical patients: Results of a meta-analysis. Ann Surg 1988;208:227-240.

68. Pezzuoli G, Neri Serneri CG, Settembrini P, et al: Prophylaxis of fatal pulmonary embolism in general surgery using low-molecular-weight heparin Cy 216: A multicentre, double-blinded, randomized, con-

69. Goldhaber SZ: Medical progress: Pulmonary embolism. N Engl J Med 1998;339:93-104.

70. Nicolaides A, Irving D, Pretzell M, et al: The risk of deep-vein thrombosis in surgical patients. Br J Surg 1973;60:312.

71. Wille-Jorgensen P, Ott P: Predicting failure of low-dose heparin in general surgical procedures. Surg Gynecol Obstet 1990;171:126-130.

72. Huber O, Bounameaux H, Borst F, et al: Postoperative pulmonary embolism after hospital discharge: An underestimated risk. Arch Surg 1992;127:310-313.

73. Flordal PA, Berggvist D, Burmark US, et al: Risk factors for major thromboembolism and bleeding tendency after elective general surgical operations. Eur J Surg 1996;162:783-789.

74. Hendolin H, Mattila MAK, Poikolainen E: The effect of lumbar epidural analgesia on the development of deep vein thrombosis of the legs after open prostatectomy. Acta Chir Scand 1981;147:425-429.

75. Parrillo JE, Dellinger RP: Critical Care Medicine: Principles of Diagnosis and Management in the Adult, ed 2. St Louis, Mosby, 2002.

76. Sasahra AA, Bell WR, Simon TL, et al: The phase II Urokinase-Streptokinase Pulmonary Embolism Trial: A national cooperative study. Thromb Diath Haemorrh 1975;33:464-476.

77. Moser KM, Hull R, Saltzman HA, et al: Recent advances in diagnosis of pulmonary embolism and deep venous thrombosis. Am Rev Respir Dis 1988;138:1046-1047.

78. Palla A, Donnamaria V, Petruzzelli S, et al: Enlargement of the right descending pulmonary artery in pulmonary embolism. Am J Roentgenol 1983;141:513-517.

79. Stein PD, Russell DH, Kalpesh CP, et al: D-dimer for the exclusion of acute venous thrombosis and pulmonary embolism. Ann Intern Med 2004;140:589-602.

80. Mills SR, Jackson DC, Older RA, et al: The incidence, etiologies, and avoidance of complications of pulmonary angiography in a large series. Radiology 1980;136:295-299.

81. Stein PD, Athanasoulis C, Alavi A, et al: Complications and validity of pulmonary angiography in acute pulmonary embolism. Circulation 1992;85:462-468.

82. The PIOPED Investigators: Value of the ventilation/perfusion scan in acute pulmonary embolism: results of the prospective investigation of pulmonary embolism diagnosis (PIOPED). JAMA 1990;263:2753-2759.

83. Stein PD, Hull RD, Raskob GE: Withholding treatment in patients with acute pulmonary embolism who have a high risk of bleeding and negative serial noninvasive leg tests. Am J Med 2000;109:301-306.

84. Righini M, Goehring C, Bounameaux H, Perrier A: Effects of age on the performance of common diagnostic tests for pulmonary embolism. Am J Med 2000;109:357-361.

85. Hayashino Y, Goto M, Noguchi Y, Fukui T: Ventilation-perfusion scanning and helical CT in suspected pulmonary embolism: Meta-analysis of diagnostic performance. Radiology 2005;234:740-748.

86. Rogers FB: Venous thromboembolism in trauma patients. Surg Clin North Am 1995;75:279-291.

87. Fiorica JV: Prophylaxis and treatment of venous thromboembolism. Surgical Rounds 2001;S:6-9.

88. National Institutes of Health Consensus Development Conference: Prevention of venous thrombosis and pulmonary embolism. JAMA 1986;256:744-749.

89. Parra RO, Farber R, Feigel A: Pressure necrosis from intermittent pneumatic compression stockings. N Engl J Med 1989;321:1615

90. Pittman GR: Peroneal nerve palsy following sequential pneumatic compression. JAMA 1989;261:2201-2202.

91. Amaragiri SV, Lees TA: Elastic compression stockings for prevention of deep vein thrombosis. Cochrane Database Syst Rev 2000;(3):CD001484.

92. Gosin JS, Graham AM, Ciocca RG, Hammond JS: Efficacy of prophylactic vena cava filters in high-risk trauma patients. Ann Vasc Surg 1997;11:100-105.

93. Rosenthal D, Wellons ED, Levitt AB, et al: Role of prophylactic temporary inferior vena cava filters placed at the ICU bedside under intravascular ultrasound guidance in patients with multiple trauma. J Vasc Surg 2004;40:958-964.

trolled, clinical trial versus placebo (STEP). Int Surg 1989;74:205-210.

94. Sapala JA, Wood MH, Schuhknecht MP, Sapala MA: Fatal pulmonary embolism after bariatric operations for morbid obesity: A 24-year retrospective analysis. Obes Surg 2003;13:819-825.

95. Geerts WH, Heit JA, Clagett GP, et al: Prevention of venous thromboembolism. Chest 2001;119:132S-175.

96. Guyatt G, Schunemann HJ, Cook D, et al: Applying the grades of recommendations for antithrombotic and thrombolytic therapy: The Seventh ACCP Conference on Antithrombotic and Thrombolytic Therapy. Chest 2004;126:179S-187.

97. Quinlan DJ, McQuillan A, Eikelboom JW: Low-molecular-weight heparin compared with intravenous unfractionated heparin for the treatment of pulmonary embolism: A meta-analysis of randomized, controlled trials. Ann Intern Med 2004;140:175-183.

98. Arcasoy SM, Kreit JW: Thrombolytic therapy of pulmonary embolism: A comprehensive review of current evidence. Chest 1999;115:1695-1707.

99. Grifoni S, Olivotto I, Cecchini P, et al: Short-term clinical outcome of patients with acute pulmonary embolism, normal blood pressure, and echocardiographic right ventricular dysfunction. Circulation 2000;101:2817-2822.

100. Hamel E, Pacouret G, Vincentelli D, et al: Thrombolysis or heparin therapy in massive pulmonary embolism with right ventricular dilation: Results from a 128-patient monocenter registry. Chest 2001;120:120-125.

101. Krivec B, Voga G, Zuran I, et al: Diagnosis and treatment of shock due to massive pulmonary embolism: Approach with transesophageal echocardiography with intrapulmonary thrombolysis. Chest 1997;112:1310-1316.

102. Thabut G, Thabut D, Myers RP, et al: Thrombolytic therapy of pulmonary embolism: A meta-analysis. J Am Coll Cardiol 2002;40:1660-1667.

103. Agnelli G, Becattini C, Kirschstein T: Thrombolysis vs heparin in the treatment of pulmonary embolism: A clinical outcome-based meta-analysis. Arch Intern Med 2002;162:2537-2541.

104. Streiff MB: Vena cava filters: A review for intensive care specialists. J Intensive Care Med 2003;18:59-79.

40 | Endocrine and Electrolyte Disorders

Eugene W. Moretti and Duane J. Funk

The management of perioperative electrolyte and endocrine disorders involves anesthesiologists on a daily basis. With the rising incidence of diabetes and obesity, and their relationship to increased morbidity in the perioperative period, clinicians must be skilled in the management of these disorders. This chapter discusses the management of these conditions as well as other common endocrinologic problems, such as thyroid disease, and the controversy surrounding perioperative steroid supplementation. Finally, this chapter discusses the etiology and management of some of the more commonly encountered electrolyte disturbances.

■ ENDOCRINE DYSFUNCTION

Diabetes Mellitus

Diabetes mellitus is a metabolic disease characterized by an absolute or relative lack of insulin from the pancreas. Three types can be distinguished. Although it can occur at any age, type I diabetes usually occurs in adolescence. It is believed to result from the autoimmune destruction of insulin-producing cells in the pancreatic islets. There is an absolute deficiency in insulin production, and these patients are dependant on exogenous insulin administration for survival. Type II diabetes is caused by insulin resistance, which results in a relative deficiency of insulin. Its onset is typically in adulthood, although recent epidemiologic data suggest that the mean age of onset is decreasing. Type II diabetes has a heterogeneous group of causes, but it is usually associated with obesity and abnormal insulin levels. As is seen for many diseases, there may also be a genetic component.

Gestational diabetes is defined as carbohydrate intolerance beginning in or first recognized during pregnancy. It is believed to occur in 2% to 9% of all pregnancies, and it is associated with substantial rates of maternal and perinatal complications, such as shoulder dystocia, bone fractures, nerve palsies, and hypoglycemia. Long-term adverse health outcomes reported among these infants include sustained glucose intolerance, obesity, and impaired intellectual performance. Gestational diabetes is a strong risk factor for the subsequent development of diabetes in the mother.[1]

A recent study randomly assigned women with gestational diabetes whose gestation was between 24 and 34 weeks to receive dietary advice, blood glucose monitoring, and insulin therapy as needed, or routine care.[2] Primary outcomes were serious perinatal complications (defined as death, shoulder dystocia, bone fracture, and nerve palsy), admission to the neonatal nursery, jaundice requiring phototherapy,

induction of labor, caesarian birth, maternal anxiety, depression, and health status. When factors such as maternal age, race, and ethnic group were corrected for, the rate of serious perinatal complications was significantly lower among the infants in the intervention group than among the infants in the routine care group (1 versus 4%, 95% confidence interval [CI], 0.14-0.75; $P = .01$). Thus, it appears that treatment of gestational diabetes reduces serious perinatal morbidity.

Pathophysiology

Diabetes is marked by long-term complications involving the microvasculature and the macrovasculature. This vascular disease is made manifest by retinopathy, neuropathy, and nephropathy and constitutes a major risk factor for heart disease, stroke, kidney disease, blindness, and nontraumatic amputation. The etiology of these complications is multifactorial and includes glycosylation of proteins, and sorbitol synthesis as a result of glucose reduction, which functions as a tissue toxin.

Management and Outcome

Diabetes itself is not as important an issue as the degree of end-organ dysfunction that it causes and the degree of glycemic control in the perioperative period, including in the intensive care unit (ICU).[3-5] A few major trials (the Diabetes Control and Complications Trial, the UK Prospective Diabetes Study Group) have shown that tight glycemic control, tight blood pressure control, and regular physical activity can postpone the microvascular complications in both types of diabetic patients. In addition to benefiting critically ill patients, tight glycemic control in the perioperative period has been shown to benefit pregnant diabetic patients, diabetic patients undergoing cardiac surgery with cardiopulmonary bypass, and those with brain injury and global central nervous system (CNS) ischemia. There is little evidence to indicate that tight glycemic control may be of benefit to any other group.

Wound Healing and Postoperative Infection

There is increasing evidence that perioperative hyperglycemia impairs wound healing. Inadequate insulin action in the early postoperative period leads to impaired hydroxyproline incorporation into the structure of healing wounds.[6] Laboratory studies in diabetic animals have demonstrated that, in insulin-treated animals, repaired tissue could withstand up to three times the mechanical force that separated the incision in non–insulin-treated animals.[7] An additional study in a murine diabetic model revealed that blocking insulin activity inhibited DNA and protein synthesis in wounds, thus resulting in decreased fibroblast activation and collagen synthesis, and in reduction of capillary proliferation.[8] There is now greater recognition that glycemic control is crucial in maintaining healthy tissue repair and regeneration in the perioperative period.

Diabetic patients are also at higher risk for postoperative wound infections. High glucose levels hinder immune function by increasing neutrophil adhesiveness, decreasing phagocytic activity, and decreasing microbicidal function.[9] Glycemic control is vital in the immediate postoperative period when the patient is particularly vulnerable to infection. Rassias and associates prospectively studied diabetic patients undergoing cardiac surgery. These patients were randomized to an aggressive insulin infusion or standard therapy. Tight glucose control during cardiac surgery was found to significantly improve leukocyte function.[10]

Several clinical studies support short-term hyperglycemia and perioperative infection risk. One investigation involving diabetic patients undergoing major vascular surgery or major abdominal procedures revealed that diabetic patients had higher nosocomial infection rates when their serum glucose values exceeded 220 mg/dL. Zerr and colleagues found an association between infection risk and the mean concentration of blood glucose on the first postoperative day.[11] In that study, the incidence of postoperative wound infection was 1.3% among patients with glucose levels between 100 and 150 mg/dL, versus 6.7% among patients with glucose levels between 250 and 300 mg/dL. In a prospective cohort of diabetic patients undergoing coronary artery bypass graft (CABG) surgery, those patients with mean glucose concentrations in excess of 200 mg/dL within the first 36 postoperative hours were more likely to develop infectious complications, including infections of their leg and chest wounds. In a similar prospective study involving 2467 diabetic patients undergoing cardiac surgery, a continuous insulin infusion resulted in decreases in perioperative serum glucose levels to consistently less than 200 mg/dL, which led to a significant reduction in the incidence of wound infection.[12]

As a result, perioperative hyperglycemia is now recognized as an independent risk factor for the development of infectious complications in the perioperative period.[13] Based on these studies, the current recommendation is to maintain a perioperative glucose concentration of less than 200 mg/dL to reduce the risk of infection.

Tight Glycemic Control and Cardiac Surgery

Myocardial ischemia that precedes myocardial revascularization has been shown to be independently associated with the stress response of surgery. Numerous studies have shown that stress hyperglycemia is associated with an increased risk of a myocardial infarction (MI) and in-hospital mortality in both diabetic and nondiabetic patients.[14-18]

The Diabetes and Insulin-Glucose Infusion in Acute Myocardial Infarction (DIGAMI) study investigated predictive variables and the effect of conventional or aggressive treatment of hyperglycemia instituted within 24 hours of myocardial infarction on diabetic patients.[14] The 1-year mortality was reduced by 30% in the intensively treated group. After an average of 3.4 years, there was an 11% absolute mortality reduction among the intensively treated patients. Thus, this study revealed that the intensive insulin treatment during MI reduced the harmful effects of poor glycemic control and the subsequent risk of death. However, this study lacked the statistical power to offer a possible mechanism for the mortality reduction.[14]

Subsequent to this study, the DIGAMI 2 trial was carried out to explore the possible benefit of insulin-based management of diabetic patients with MI. The investigators hypothesized that early and continued insulin-based metabolic control was a key to mortality reduction. In this trial, patients with type 2 diabetes and suspected acute MI were randomly assigned to three groups: (1) insulin-glucose infusion followed by insulin-based long-term glucose control, (2) insulin-glucose infusion followed by standard glucose control, or (3) routine metabolic management according to local practice. The primary objective was to compare mortality between groups 1 and 2, and the secondary objective was to compare mortality between groups 2 and 3. The median study duration was 2.1 years. Hemoglobin A1c and initial glucose levels were similar in all groups. There was a significant reduction in blood glucose after 24 hours in all groups, more in groups 1 and 2 (9.1 mmol/L each) receiving insulin-glucose infusion than in group 3 (10.0 mmol/L). Mortality did not differ significantly between groups 1 and 2 or between 2 and 3. There were also no significant differences in morbidity (such as nonfatal reinfarctions and strokes) between the three groups. The investigators concluded that an acutely introduced, long-term insulin treatment failed to improve survival in type 2 diabetic patients following MI when compared with conventional management. Thus, the method of glycemic control is not as important as the control itself.[19]

During cardiac surgery involving cardiopulmonary bypass, intraoperative glycemic control presents major challenges to the anesthesiologist. Bypass alters glucose homeostasis by several mechanisms. Suppressed insulin release, stress-induced gluconeogenesis, renal tubular reabsorption of glucose, and insulin resistance all contribute to this perturbation.[20-22]

Accumulating evidence suggests that hyperglycemia is an independent risk factor for an increase in both short-term and long-term mortality after cardiovascular surgery. In an observational single-center study of 1175 CABG patients older than 75 years, postoperative plasma glucose greater than 300 mg/dL was one significant predictor of postoperative mortality.[23]

Most of the data on perioperative glycemic control and cardiovascular surgery center on the diabetic patient. This seems appropriate, as 20% to 30% of patients undergoing coronary artery bypass surgery have diabetes mellitus.[24] Furthermore, most studies have documented a 50% to 90% increase in long-term mortality in diabetic patients undergoing CABG surgery.[25,26] In an effort to define short-term mortality and morbidity in diabetic patients undergoing CABG surgery, Carson and colleagues performed a retrospective cohort study of 434 hospitals in North America.[24] This study included 146,786 patients undergoing CABG during 1997, of which 41,663 had diabetes. The primary outcome was 30-day mortality. Secondary outcomes included in-hospital morbidity, infections, and the composite outcome of mortality or morbidity and mortality or infection. The 30-day mortality was 3.7% in patients with diabetes mellitus and 2.7% in those without; after adjusting for baseline risk factors, the overall adjusted odds ratio (OR) for diabetic patients was 1.23. Patients on oral hypoglycemic medications had an adjusted OR of 1.13, whereas those on insulin had an adjusted OR of 1.39. Morbidity, infections, and the composite outcome occurred more commonly in diabetic patients and were associated with an adjusted risk approximately 35% higher in diabetic patients than in nondiabetic patients.

In an effort to assess the adequacy of perioperative glycemic control in cardiac surgery patients, McAlister and colleagues performed a retrospective cohort study in 291 diabetic patients who underwent CABG surgery and who survived at least 24 hours postoperatively.[27] Seventy-eight out of 291 patients suffered a nonfatal stroke, myocardial infarction, or septic complication, or died during their hospitalization. Glycemic control was considered to be suboptimal (average glucose on postoperative day 1 was 11.4 mmol/L) and was significantly associated with adverse outcomes after CABG. Patients whose mean blood glucose level on postoperative day 1 placed them in the highest quartile had a higher risk of adverse outcomes after the first postoperative day than those with glucose in the lowest quartile (OR, 2.5 [CI, 1.1-5.3]). Even after adjustment for other clinical and operative covariates, the average blood glucose level on the first postoperative day was significantly associated with subsequent adverse outcomes: for each 1 mmol/L increase in blood glucose above 6.1 mmol/L, risk increased by 17%.

Although it is now widely accepted that aggressive perioperative glucose control using intravenous insulin infusions is important for diabetic patients, the management of perioperative hyperglycemia in patients without a diagnosis of diabetes has not been extensively studied. Estrada and associates hypothesized that all patients undergoing CABG surgery with higher perioperative glucose levels would have worse outcomes than patients with lower glucose levels.[28] They reported on a historic cohort study of 1574 patients who had undergone CABG surgery, 34% of whom were diabetic. Outcomes were 30-day mortality, infection rates, and resource usage. After adjusting for calculated preoperative mortality, each 50 mg/dL blood glucose increase was not statistically associated with higher mortality or infection rate. However, each 50 mg/dL blood glucose increase was associated with a longer postoperative stay (by 0.76 day) and increased hospitalization cost (by $1769). In the unadjusted analysis, infections occurred more frequently in patients with diabetes (6.6% versus 4.1%). The authors concluded that perioperative hyperglycemia is associated with increased resource usage but not mortality in patients undergoing CABG surgery.

A few studies have sought to determine if the early beneficial effects of tight glycemic control would result in improved survival. Lazar and coworkers studied 141 diabetic patients undergoing CABG surgery and prospectively randomized them to tight glycemic control (serum glucose, 125 to 200 mg/dL) with a modified glucose-insulin-potassium solution (GIK) or standard therapy (serum glucose <250 mg/dL) using intermittent subcutaneous insulin beginning before anesthesia and continuing for 12 hours after surgery.[29] GIK patients had lower serum glucose levels, a lower incidence of atrial fibrillation (16.6% versus 42%), and a shorter postoperative length of stay (6.5 ± 0.1 versus 9.2 ± 0.3 days). GIK patients also showed a survival advantage 2 years after surgery, decreased episodes of recurrent ischemia (5% versus 19%; $P = .01$), and fewer wound infections (1% versus 10%). The authors concluded that tight glycemic control with GIK in diabetic CABG patients improves perioperative outcomes, enhances survival, and decreases the incidence of ischemic events and wound complications.

In a recently completed study, Ouattara and colleagues studied 200 consecutive diabetic patients undergoing cardiac surgery involving cardiopulmonary bypass.[30] Insulin therapy was initiated intraoperatively according to a predefined protocol as soon as the serum glucose level was about 180 mg/dL. Suboptimal glycemic control was defined as four consecutive blood glucose levels greater than 200 mg/dL without any decrease until the end of surgery. Blood glucose level was maintained postoperatively at less than 140 mg/dL. Perioperative data were prospectively collected, and a multivariate logistic regression analysis was performed to identify independent factors for severe in-hospital morbidity. Intraoperative insulin therapy was required in 36% of patients, 50% of whom exhibited poor glycemic control. In-hospital morbidity was significantly more frequent in patients experiencing poor intraoperative glycemic control: 37% versus 10% of those who did not have in-hospital morbidity ($P < .05$). A multivariate analysis identified five perioperative risk factors for severe morbidity: pulmonary hypertension greater than 50 mm Hg, poor intraoperative glycemic control, intraoperative erythrocyte transfusion, preoperative plasma creatinine, and increased cardiopulmonary bypass time.

For diabetic patients undergoing cardiac surgery with cardiopulmonary bypass, there are sufficient data to recommend maintaining a perioperative blood glucose level of less than 180 mg/dL. For nondiabetic patients, the data are not as compelling, and most anesthesiologists are satisfied with a serum glucose level of less than 200 mg/dL, especially in view of a study that revealed that nondiabetic patients experienced hypoglycemia after cardiopulmonary bypass when continuous insulin infusions were used intraoperatively to maintain normoglycemia.[31]

Glycemic Control and Noncardiac Surgery

Studies involving diabetic patients and outcomes after noncardiac surgery are sparse. No studies have examined glycemic control and either short- or long-term outcomes after noncardiac surgery. Mangano and colleagues have demonstrated a significant increase in long-term mortality among diabetic patients undergoing major noncardiac surgery.[32] However, diabetic patients represented a subgroup of that entire study population, and the investigators did not account for such risk factors as type of diabetes, duration of diabetes, and metabolic control.

Juul and associates retrospectively analyzed the long-term perioperative mortality of diabetic patients undergoing major noncardiac surgery.[33] They also sought to identify perioperative risk factors and possible causes of death. Their main outcome measure was postoperative mortality. Overall postoperative mortality was 24%. Ischemic heart disease diagnosed before the operation was associated with an overall postoperative mortality of 44%, which was significantly higher than in diabetic patients without known cardiovascular disease ($P < .03$). Unfortunately, the limitations of this study were noteworthy. It did not include a group of matched nondiabetic patients, and hence diabetes-related excess mortality could not be calculated. The authors were unable to obtain information about alcohol, tobacco habits, and known diabetic long-term complications. In addition, there was no information about perioperative hemodynamic perturbations and postoperative interventions. Finally, patients with poor perioperative metabolic control had statistically significant increased postoperative long-term mortality, but this significance disappeared when corrected for the presence of ischemic heart disease and urgency of surgery.

As stated earlier, preoperative hyperglycemia has been found to be an important predictor of late mortality in cardiac surgery, and perioperative tight metabolic control reduces morbidity after major cardiac surgery. Further studies are required to ascertain whether tight metabolic control in both diabetic and nondiabetic patients improves survival.

Perioperative Hyperglycemia and Neurologic Outcomes

Hyperglycemia in the presence of cerebral ischemia can increase neuronal damage and worsen the severity of neurologic injury. This is true for both global and focal ischemic events.[34] The contributing mechanisms include (1) an anaerobic metabolism resulting in intracellular lactic acidosis and microvascular dysregulation,[35] (2) hemorrhagic transformation of ischemic infarcts,[36] (3) endothelial swelling and microvascular plugging, resulting from decreased glutamine transport,[37] and (4) reduced blood–brain barrier transport and decreased regional cerebral blood flow.[38]

Hyperglycemia as a predictor of outcome has been studied in a variety of conditions. In the setting of global ischemia, hyperglycemia can affect outcome. Longstreth and Inui studied patients resuscitated after out-of-hospital cardiac arrest and found that mean blood glucose levels were higher in patients who failed to awaken (341 ± 13 mg/dL) than in those who regained consciousness (262 ± 7 mg/dL).[39] Among those who did regain consciousness but had persistent neurologic deficits, the mean blood glucose levels were higher (286 ± 15 mg/dL) than in those without deficits (251 ± 7 mg/dL).

In the setting of focal ischemia, hyperglycemia is just as influential on unfavorable outcomes. Bruno and coworkers investigated the relationship between acute blood glucose levels and outcome from ischemic stroke.[40] In patients presenting with acute ischemic stroke, a multivariate regression analysis revealed a strong correlation between high blood glucose and a worse clinical outcome in embolic stroke.

Hyperglycemia has been shown to worsen outcome in traumatic brain injury, where increased levels of circulating catecholamines result in an increase in intracranial pressure, a hyperdynamic circulation, increase in brain metabolic oxygen requirements, and increased blood glucose levels. Jeremitsky and coworkers performed a retrospective analysis in an ICU involving 77 patients with severe traumatic brain injury.[41] A hyperglycemia score (HS) was assigned to each patient, calculated on days 3 to 5 and assigning a value of 1 for each day the glucose exceeded 170 mg/dL. Outcomes included mortality, day 5 Glasgow Coma score (GCS), ICU length of stay, and hospital length of stay. Mortality was 31.2%, and nonsurvivors had higher glucose levels with a higher HS (2.4 versus 1.5).

A prospective study involving 267 head-injured patients (GCS score, 3 to 12) who were surgically treated for the evacuation of an intracranial hematoma and/or placement of a device for intracranial pressure monitoring revealed that patients with severe head injury had significantly higher serum glucose levels than those with moderate injury ($P < .001$).[42] A comparison of patients with a favorable outcome (good recovery or moderate disability) and those with an unfavorable outcome (severe disability, persistent vegetative state, death) revealed a significant difference in both admission and postoperative glucose values ($P < .001$). In the patients with severe head injury, admission and postoperative glucose levels greater than 200 mg/dL were associated with an unfavorable outcome ($P < .05$ and $P < .001$, respectively).

In cardiac surgery involving cardiopulmonary bypass, global and focal ischemic events are not uncommon. Global ischemia occurs when cerebral blood flow greatly decreases, such as during deep hypothermic circulatory arrest, whereas focal ischemia is commonly associated with cerebral embolization. In cardiac surgery involving cardiopulmonary bypass, hyperglycemia with glucose levels exceeding 250 mg/dL was significantly associated with poorer neurologic outcome in cases of global and focal ischemia.[43]

Most of the data reveal that in the setting of cerebral ischemia, glucose levels exceeding 200 mg/dL may have an unfavorable effect on perioperative outcome. Most agree that given the present evidence, diabetic and nondiabetic patients should have their blood glucose level maintained consistently below 200 mg/dL during surgery or an ICU stay that may involve periods of cerebral ischemia.

Glycemic Control in the Critically Ill

Hyperglycemia and insulin resistance are common in the critically ill patient. In a prospective randomized study, postoperative patients were assigned to either strict or traditional blood glucose control.[3] Traditional blood glucose control consisted of using insulin infusions only if the blood glucose exceeded 215 mg/dL (12 mmol/L), with the therapeutic endpoint being a blood glucose of 150 to 180 mg/dL (8.3 to 10 mmol/L). Among the patients that remained in the ICU for longer than 5 days, there was a significant improvement in overall hospital mortality in the tight control group. In addition, there was a significantly lower ICU mortality rate, a decrease in the development of renal failure, a decrease in bloodstream infection, fewer transfusions, shorter duration of mechanical ventilation, and a lower incidence of critical illness polyneuropathy. Of note, the incidence of hypoglycemia was low, only 5% in the tightly controlled group, and

0.7% in the control group, and there were no reported neuroglycopenic complications.[3]

What was left unclear in the preceding study was whether the benefits accrued from the metabolic effects of insulin or from the effects of normoglycemia. In a subsequent report on their database, the same investigators revealed that the main benefit was related to glycemic control and not the insulin alone.[44] A multivariate logistic regression analysis revealed that the lower blood glucose level rather than the insulin dose was related to reduced mortality ($P < .0001$), critical illness polyneuropathy ($P < .001$), bacteremia ($P = .02$), and inflammation ($P = .0006$), but not to prevention of acute renal failure, for which the insulin dose was an independent determinant ($P = .03$). As compared with normoglycemia, an intermediate blood glucose level (110 to 150 mg/dL) was associated with worse outcome.[44]

An overall management algorithm for the diabetic patient about to undergo either cardiac or noncardiac surgery is presented in Figure 40-1.

Medically Significant Obesity

Obesity is an abnormal accumulation of fat in proportion to body size. Overweight persons, although still technically obese, have a body-fat proportion that is intermediate between normal and obese. The most recently published U.S. data (1999 to 2002) reveal that approximately 65% of adults are above normal weight: about 30% are overweight (with a

body mass index [BMI] of 25 to 30), 30% are obese (BMI, 30 to 40), and 5% are extremely obese (BMI, ≥40).[45] Minority populations have seen a rise in the prevalence of obesity, with the highest rates found in Native Americans, Hispanics, and African Americans, and the lowest rates found in those of Asian ancestry. Prevalence rates for obesity are also highest in populations with less education and lower income levels. Internationally, obesity rates are generally lower than those in the United States, but even societies that traditionally had the lowest prevalence of obesity are starting to observe rates of weight gain that begin to meet or exceed those of Western societies.[46] Obesity has now become a major burden on our health-care system, as it has surpassed alcohol and tobacco abuse in terms of health-care costs and resource usage.[47]

Men aged 25 to 34 with extreme obesity have a 12-fold higher mortality rate, and men aged 35 to 44 with extreme obesity have a sixfold higher mortality rate than non-obese men in the same age group.[48] In addition, obese adults are at increased risk for other comorbidities, such as hypertension, diabetes mellitus, coronary artery disease, and a variety of neoplastic diseases.

Preoperative Evaluation

Obesity and its complications present major challenges for the anesthesiologist. For the morbidly obese patient, the main concern for the anesthesiologist is the airway and the

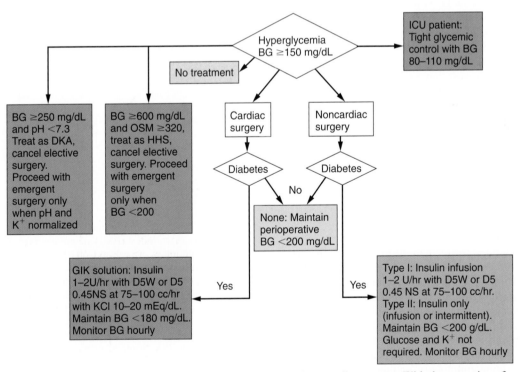

Figure 40-1 ■ Algorithm for glucose control in cardiac and noncardiac surgery. With the exception of cardiac surgery, most diabetic and nondiabetic patients need receive only insulin. Cardiac surgical patients and patients with type I diabetes require glucose and insulin. BG, blood glucose; D5W, 5% dextrose in water; DKA, diabetic ketoacidosis; HHS, hyperosmolar hyperglycemic state; ICU, intensive care unit; NS, normal saline; OSM, osmolarity. *(Algorithm developed using information found in references 14 to 27.)*

cardiopulmonary system. Abundant soft tissue in the upper airway makes the obese patient more susceptible to obstructive sleep apnea (OSA) and the development of hypoxemia and hypercapnia. Obesity also significantly increases the risk of a difficult tracheal intubation.[49,50]

Morbid obesity is the most common risk factor for OSA. Every two-unit increase in the BMI increases the likelihood of coexisting OSA by 4%.[51,52] The prevalence of OSA is 3% to 25% in morbidly obese men and 40% to 78% in morbidly obese women, as opposed to 2% in non-obese women and 4% in non-obese men in the general U.S. population.[53]

It is difficult to predict the presence of OSA solely on the basis of a clinical examination. The definitive diagnostic test for OSA is polysomnography. Sleep apnea is defined as five or more apneic events (cessation of airflow lasting 10 seconds or longer with continued respiratory effort) per hour, or 15 or more hypopneic events (decrease in airflow of 50% lasting 10 seconds or longer) during the course of a 7-hour sleep study.[51,54] The apnea-hypopnea index is the total number of apneic or hypopneic events or both that occur per hour during sleep. The severity of OSA is directly related to the magnitude of this index.[51]

A subgroup of obese patients are susceptible to the obesity-hypoventilation syndrome, which is characterized by chronic daytime hypoventilation and chronic daytime hypoxemia (PO_2 < 65 mm Hg) and easily detected by using room air pulse-oximetry. Sustained hypercapnia (PCO_2 > 45 mm Hg) in an obese patient without significant chronic obstructive pulmonary disease (COPD) is also diagnostic for this syndrome. These patients often have a BMI greater than 40 kg/m^2, and the likelihood of obesity-hypoventilation syndrome increases as the BMI increases. The underlying pathophysiology of this syndrome is unclear, and patients on the extreme end of this spectrum who have signs of cor pulmonale are called "Pickwickian." Pickwickian conditions are associated with increased perioperative morbidity and mortality, and these patients may require more extensive preoperative testing and postoperative management.[55]

Because most clinically severely obese patients do not undergo polysomnographic testing, the diagnosis and severity of OSA in a preoperative patient is most commonly gleaned from patient history. For example, reports of constant snoring, interrupted breathing during sleep, morning headache, and daytime somnolence may be indicative of OSA. Systemic hypertension, a BMI greater than 35, and a neck circumference greater than 40 to 42 cm at the cricoid cartilage are consistent with the diagnosis of OSA.[56] At present, polysomnographic testing is indicated in severely obese patients who continually snore, have daytime somnolence, or have observed periods of interrupted breathing during sleep. Unfortunately, there are no studies to suggest that this approach is correct. It should be noted that in the setting of morbid obesity and OSA without symptoms or signs of underlying pulmonary pathology, room air blood gases and pulmonary function tests have no predictive value in optimizing postoperative outcomes in severely obese patients.[57-60]

An algorithm for the preoperative evaluation of patients with morbid obesity is presented in Figure 40-2.

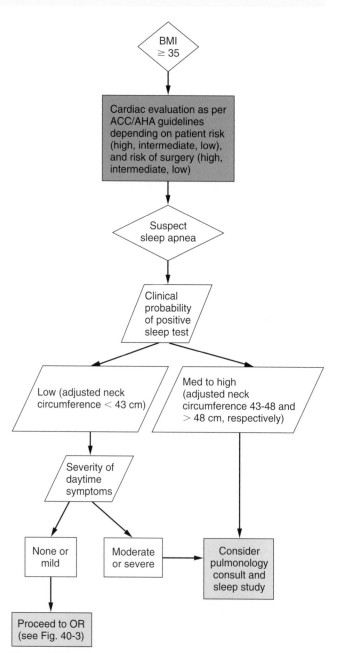

Figure 40-2 ■ Preoperative management algorithm for patients with a body mass index (BMI) of greater than 35. Preoperative testing should follow American College of Cardiology and American Heart Association (ACC/AHA) guidelines for cardiac disease. Decisions to consult a pulmonologist can be based on clinical symptoms and an adjusted neck circumference, which is calculated by measuring neck circumference in centimeters and adding 4 cm if the patient is hypertensive, and 3 cm for chronic snoring. BMI, body mass index; OR, operating room. *(Modified from Flemons WW, Whitelaw WA, Brant R, et al: Am J Respir Crit Care Med 1994;150[5 Pt 1]:1279-1285, and Eagle KA: J Am Coll Cardiol 2002;39:542-553.)*

Treatment with Noninvasive Ventilation

Continuous positive airway pressure (CPAP) can reduce or eliminate signs of sleep apnea. For CPAP to be successful, patient cooperation and experienced respiratory care practitioners are necessary. Thus, it is not surprising that use of CPAP results in failure postoperatively, because (1) it is often performed in sleepy and uncooperative patients who have not been formally diagnosed with OSA, and (2) it is often provided by practitioners who are not skilled in CPAP titration. Furthermore, patients require a period of adaptation to the mask and device, and not all patients can tolerate this treatment. The amount of airway pressure required varies depending on whether the sleep disorder involves rapid eye movement (REM) or non–rapid eye movement (NREM) sleep. For example, an airway pressure level that eliminates obstructive and hypoxic symptoms during naps may not be effective for night-time sleep when REM occurs. Unfortunately, compliance with CPAP is in the range of 50% to 80%, so the anesthesiologist must ask each patient on an individual basis regarding the use of their device.[61,62]

In the preoperative setting, it remains unclear whether surgery should be delayed to optimize airway status and oxygenation with CPAP therapy. One study failed to observe any major postoperative respiratory complications in 14 patients treated with nasal CPAP for a period of 3 weeks before surgery.[63] However, this study had a small sample size and lacked a control group, and it could not be determined if these complications would have occurred without the intervention. Other studies have shown that 3 weeks of CPAP therapy before bariatric surgery improved the left ventricular ejection fraction and afterload in patients with severe obesity and heart failure. Eight weeks of preoperative CPAP may be necessary to treat hypertension secondary to OSA.[64,65] In the postoperative setting, one study revealed that CPAP used on the first night after surgery failed to improve oxygenation.[66] Those authors believed that this may have been because REM rebound does not occur for several days after surgery.

Bilateral positive airway pressure (BiPAP) provides positive pressure to the airway during both inspiration and expiration. With this modality, spontaneous ventilation is further assisted with increases in airway pressure and flow. The best use of BiPAP may be in patients who require a significant amount of CPAP, or in those who have a severe underlying airway disease such as COPD. The effectiveness of BiPAP in the general sleep apnea population remains unknown.

Cardiovascular Complications of Obesity

Morbid obesity is associated with a higher frequency of cardiovascular disease, including essential hypertension, pulmonary hypertension, left ventricular hypertrophy, congestive heart failure, and ischemic heart disease. Therefore, many patients with morbid obesity require a thorough cardiac workup. Preoperative patients can be assigned to a risk group based primarily on history and physical examination and the extent of surgery as per the guidelines of the American College of Cardiology and the American Heart Association (ACC/AHA guidelines).[67]

Cardiac output must increase by 0.01 L/min to adequately perfuse each additional kilogram of adipose tissue. Not surprisingly, obese patients often have hypertension, which can lead to cardiomegaly and left ventricular failure. The mechanism for the development of hypertension may involve repeated episodes of desaturation and sleep arousals, resulting in the activation of the sympathetic nervous system. Although treatment of sleep apnea may result in improvement of hypertension, most often treatment cannot be initiated in time for the planned surgery. Treatment of hypertension should be based on current recommended guidelines for patients without sleep apnea.

The association between obesity, sleep apnea, and atherosclerotic cardiovascular disease remains incompletely understood.[68,69] Episodes of myocardial ischemia are not temporally related to apneic episodes despite sleep studies demonstrating myocardial ischemia in high-risk individuals. Myocardial ischemia in this setting could be caused by increased activation of the sympathetic nervous system, resulting in increased myocardial work and increased oxygen demand. Oxygen demand can easily outstrip delivery in this setting because of hemoglobin desaturation.[70] OSA also predisposes patients to congestive heart failure, arrhythmias, and diastolic heart dysfunction.[71-73]

Chronic daytime hypoxemia can also result in pulmonary hypertension, right ventricular hypertrophy, or right ventricular failure. Anesthesiologists should consider the use of echocardiography to evaluate right heart failure or pulmonary hypertension in selected patients with clinically severe obesity and OSA. However, data are lacking to support the widespread use of this modality at this time.

Deep Vein Thrombosis

Obesity is also an independent risk factor for deep vein thrombosis (DVT) and pulmonary embolus. The estimated incidences of DVT and pulmonary embolism in the postoperative period after bariatric surgery are 2.6% and 0.95%, respectively.[74,75] Migration of venous emboli to the pulmonary circulation is a significant contributor to the 30-day mortality rate of 1% to 2% after bariatric surgery. Most mortality in the 30-day period after bariatric surgery results from pulmonary embolism, and this cause of mortality is three times higher than anastomotic leak and subsequent sepsis. Unfractionated heparin in a dosage of 5000 units administered subcutaneously before surgery and then twice a day until the patient is ambulatory has been shown to reduce the risk of DVT.[76] Enoxaparin in a dosage of 40 mg given twice a day has also been shown to decrease the incidence of complications arising from postoperative DVT.[77]

Intraoperative Concerns

In the obese patient, the expiratory reserve volume (ERV) and functional residual capacity (FRC) are reduced to 60% and 80% of normal, respectively. ERV is the primary source of oxygen reserve during apnea. Decreased apneic reserve and the possibility of difficult mask ventilation has led some to suggest that awake intubation is the safest way to secure the airway in severely obese patients, indicating the potential for difficult intubation.[53] Because of the higher risk of aspiration in the severely obese patient, most practitioners perform a rapid-sequence induction to secure the airway, but the data to support this practice are limited.

It has been shown that drugs used for analgesia and neuromuscular blockade have an increased volume of distribution and prolonged elimination times in the severely obese patient. In one study involving eight obese patients (mean weight, 94 kg), the elimination half-life of sufentanil was 208 minutes, as opposed to 135 minutes for eight control patients (mean weight, 70 kg).[78] In a study examining twitch recovery times after vecuronium, the recovery of twitch response was 38.4 minutes in obese patients (mean weight, 93 kg) and 17.6 minutes for non-obese patients (mean weight, 61 kg).[79]

Postoperative Concerns

It is absolutely essential postoperatively that obese patients receive some form of continuous oxygen supplementation and be maintained in the semirecumbent or upright posture.[80] If oxygen therapy alone is insufficient to maintain adequate arterial oxygenation, it is recommended that CPAP or BiPAP therapy be instituted.

Recommendations

Data from well-designed randomized trials are lacking for the perioperative care of the morbidly obese patient. In particular, there are no data that suggest that outcomes are improved if coexisting conditions such as OSA are diagnosed and treated prior to surgery. In addition, there are no data that reveal whether the type of anesthetic administered has an impact on perioperative outcomes. We do recommend polysomnographic testing with CPAP titration in selected patients, and more extensive cardiac testing in some patients, prior to surgery. We also recommend that DVT prophylaxis begin prior to anesthetic induction, and early ambulation be encouraged in the postoperative period. In addition to oxygen supplementation, a low threshold for initiating noninvasive ventilation in the postoperative period is recommended for patients who are hypoxemic.

A generalized management algorithm for the intraoperative and postoperative care of the patient with OSA is presented in Figure 40-3.

Corticosteroid Supplementation

Since their introduction in 1949, corticosteroids have been used for a myriad of clinical purposes and have revolutionized the treatment of inflammatory diseases. In fact, it was not long after their initial use that Fraser and colleagues reported the first case of adrenal insufficiency secondary to withdrawal from glucocorticoid therapy.[81] The following paragraphs review (1) the normal physiologic secretion of glucocorticoids and the response to stress, (2) the alterations in the hypothalamic-pituitary-adrenal axis (HPA) with chronic steroid supplementation, (3) the incidence and diagnosis of adrenal insufficiency, and (4) current recommendations for identifying and treating patients who need perioperative steroid supplementation.

Normal Physiology

The zona fasciculata of the adrenal gland secretes approximately 5 mg/m^2 of cortisol per day. This is lower than the 12 to 15 mg/m^2 per day that was previously thought.[82] Glucocorticoid receptors are present on many different tissue types and play a key role in homeostasis. Specifically, glucocorticoids are necessary for lipid, carbohydrate, and protein metabolism. Glucocorticoids also facilitate catecholamine production and the maintenance of normal blood pressure, as well as having effects on cardiovascular homeostasis.[83] In healthy subjects, glucocorticoid secretion has a diurnal variation with peak levels occurring between 4 AM and 8 AM. The nadir of their secretion is between 2 AM and 4 AM. Interestingly, this diurnal variation is lost in critically ill patients.[84]

With stressors such as critical illness, trauma, and surgery, the normal physiologic response is an increase in the level of adrenocorticotrophic hormone (ACTH), which stimulates the adrenal gland to secrete cortisol. Still, there is considerable interindividual variation in the HPA response to these stresses. Some of the variation is thought to be the effect of anesthetics, endogenous and exogenous opioids, age, and sleep.[85] Furthermore, the amount of glucocorticoid secreted depends on the amount of surgical stress. Minor surgical procedures result in an adrenal secretion of approximately 50 mg of cortisol per day, whereas major surgical procedures produce between 75 and 150 mg of cortisol per day. To put these levels in perspective, patients with Cushing's syndrome secrete an average of 36 mg/day of cortisol.[82] The daily production of cortisol during periods of stress seldom exceeds 200 to 300 mg in normal subjects. This suggests that this is the maximum dosage that should be administered to patients thought to be at risk for postoperative adrenal insufficiency.

Effect of Chronic Steroid Supplementation on the HPA Axis

Adrenal insufficiency (AI) can be classified as either primary (resulting from the destruction of the adrenal gland by tumor, infection, or hemorrhage), secondary (resulting from pituitary dysfunction), or tertiary (resulting from the therapeutic administration of glucocorticoids). By far, the most common cause of AI is tertiary. Exogenous administration of glucocorticoids results in the inhibition of the hypothalamic and pituitary glands, which results in the atrophy of the adrenal gland over time. Precisely how long it takes for the adrenal gland to recover its function from the exogenous administration of glucocorticoids is the subject of much debate. Studies have shown that the adrenal gland can take as little as 2 to 5 days to recover its normal function, or as long as 9 months to a year.[86] Historically, clinicians thought that the duration of therapy and the maximum and cumulative dosages of corticosteroids could predict which patients were at risk for tertiary AI. Unfortunately, there is a lack of data to support these speculations. Thus, the clinician is forced to rely on biochemical testing of the integrity of the HPA axis in the preoperative patient to confirm the diagnosis of tertiary AI.

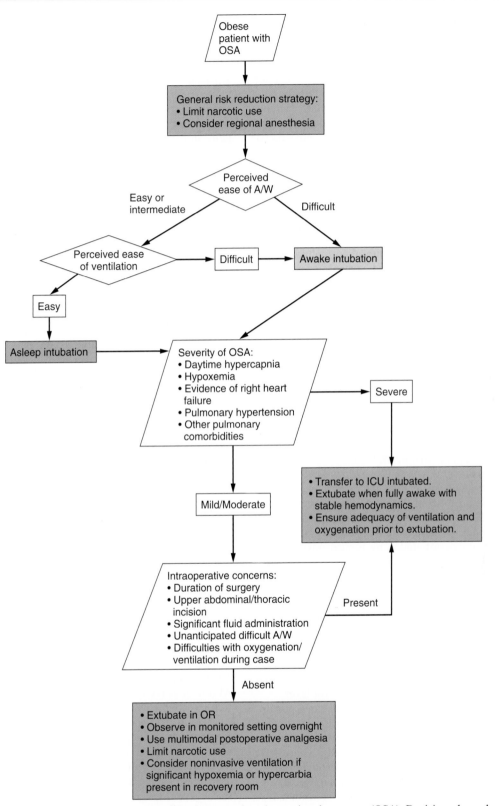

Figure 40-3 ■ Intraoperative algorithm for managing obstructive sleep apnea (OSA). Decisions depend on factors such as airway difficulty, severity of OSA, and intraoperative factors that might adversely affect gas exchange in the postoperative period. ICU, intensive care unit. *(Data from Benumof JL: J Clin Anesth 2001;13:144-156.)*

Incidence and Diagnosis of Adrenal Insufficiency

The reported incidence of tertiary AI in surgical patients ranges from 0.1 to 1 in 1000 patients.[85] Whether this represents an actual low incidence, or under-reporting, or poor recognition of this condition is unclear. Confounding the data on the incidence of this condition is that many patients undergo major surgical procedures without perioperative glucocorticoid coverage, or even without their baseline therapeutic dosage, without sequelae.[85] The likely explanation for this is that these patients had normal HPA axis function in response to stress. Bromberg and colleagues prospectively studied 40 renal transplant patients on long-term steroids for immunosuppression who required admission to the hospital for surgical procedures or acute illness.[87] An ACTH stimulation test was performed before discharge when the patients were not acutely ill. Despite abnormal results in 63% of patients, 97% of them had normal or increased urinary cortisol levels. There were 12 episodes of hyponatremia or hypotension that responded to therapy other than glucocorticoid administration and were explained by a process other than adrenal insufficiency. This suggests that circulating cortisol concentrations in these patients were sufficient to meet the patients' requirements during the times of physiologic stress. This study further enhances the argument that history alone is insufficient in diagnosing tertiary AI.

The diagnosis of tertiary AI in a postoperative patient is difficult and subject to error. Both clinical and physical examination findings need to be supplemented with biochemical testing to confirm the diagnosis.[88] The typical history of fatigue, anorexia, postural hypotension, and weight loss seen in adrenally insufficient patients in the outpatient setting is not relevant in the postoperative state. Surgical patients most often present with an Addisonian crisis that includes fever and hypotension unresponsive to fluid or vasopressor support. The diagnosis is thus confounded by typical postoperative mimics such as hypovolemic shock or sepsis.

Biochemically, the classic findings of adrenal insufficiency include hyponatremia and hyperkalemia. Hyponatremia might be masked by the administration of perioperative fluids. Hypokalemia is often not present because of intact mineralocorticoid secretion thanks to the renin-angiotensin-aldosterone system.[88] The limitations of the physical examination and baseline biochemical data therefore argue for a more focused interrogation of the HPA axis either with an ACTH stimulation test or with a random cortisol level.

Determining an adequate cortisol response in a postoperative patient suspected of having adrenal disease is made challenging by the previously mentioned interindividual and procedural variability in cortisol levels. Ideally, a threshold cortisol level could be defined, below which the diagnosis of adrenal insufficiency could be made with a high degree of certainty, and therapeutic replacement could be initiated. A random cortisol level of 15 µg/dL has been suggested as the threshold that best identifies patients who would benefit from steroid supplementation.[89] Patients whose cortisol level is above 34 µg/dL are unlikely to have AI and need not be treated.

Further testing of the HPA axis can be accomplished with the ACTH stimulation test. This involves the administration of 250 µg of intravenous cosyntropin (a synthetic ACTH analog) and the measurement of plasma cortisol levels at baseline and 30 minutes after administration. Failure to increase serum cortisol by greater than 9 µg/dL is usually accepted as an inadequate response to this supra-physiologic stimulation and has been associated with an increased mortality in patients with septic shock.[90]

Unfortunately, anesthesiologists often do not have the luxury of waiting for the results of specialized biochemical tests when faced with a hypotensive patient in the operating room or the recovery room who might have AI. One management option, should this situation arise, would be to administer 8 mg of dexamethasone to the patient, as this will adequately provide the "stress dose" required without interfering with any subsequent testing of the HPA axis. Concurrently, a random cortisol level should be drawn to check for the presence of AI.

Identifying Patients at Risk, and Perioperative Steroid Supplementation

As mentioned previously, identifying patients at risk of tertiary AI by history alone is fraught with difficulties. Nonetheless, focused questioning of patients with inflammatory conditions (such as rheumatoid arthritis or inflammatory bowel disease) for steroid use is simple, and the yield is potentially high. Clinicians should also inquire about any administration of epidural steroids in the past 90 days, as this has also been shown to suppress the adrenal axis.[91] Patients who take topical or inhaled steroids are at extremely low risk for developing tertiary AI.[86]

Further testing of the elective preoperative patient is not necessary for several reasons. First, there is a scarcity of cosyntropin in the United States, and obtaining this substance for testing is sometimes not possible. Furthermore, perioperative supplementation of steroids has not been associated with any untoward complications, providing rational doses are used. Finally, the time required to conduct the test and wait for the results, as well as its expense, make the ACTH stimulation test impractical in most situations.

Patients with a history of systemic steroid use within the past year or epidural steroid administration within the preceding 3 months should receive supplementation. The questions, however, are what dosage and by what route, and what duration of therapy is sufficient in patients at risk for tertiary AI. Previous recommendations of quadrupling the amount of steroid patients were receiving for stress are antiquated, are based only on case reports, and have the potential for increasing morbidity such as wound infections, gastrointestinal ulceration, altered glucose tolerance, and dysphoria.[85] A rational approach to supplementation takes into account the magnitude of the insult as well as the patient's baseline steroid dose.

The following recommendations can therefore be made, based on the magnitude of the stress and the known glucocorticoid production rate associated with it. For all procedures, patients should receive their daily dose of steroid preoperatively, either orally or parenterally. Patients who are receiving 5 mg of prednisone per day or less do not require steroid supplementation, as they continue to have an intact HPA axis. For minor surgical stresses (Box 40-1), based on daily cortisol secretion, a target of 25 mg hydrocortisone equivalent (Table 40-1) is sufficient to overcome the surgical stress.[92] If the postoperative course is uncomplicated, the patient may return to their usual steroid dose on postoperative day 1.

For moderate surgical stress, cortisol production rates suggest that a target of 50 to 75 mg/day of hydrocortisone or its equivalent should be administered for 1 to 2 days. After this period, patients may be put back on their usual oral regimen if they are tolerating and absorbing oral medications.

For major surgical stresses, 100 to 150 mg of hydrocortisone equivalent per day for 2 to 3 days is required to avoid tertiary AI. This amount can then be discontinued on postoperative day 3 with a return to the baseline regimen.

There are no data to support the contention that patients who are receiving maintenance doses of steroids that exceed the estimated stress requirements need higher perioperative doses. That is, a patient who is receiving a maintenance dose higher than the previously estimated stress requirement will not need extra coverage during the postoperative period.[84]

These recommended regimens do not require a long tapering, as there is little or no evidence to support the short-term (i.e., less than 48 hours) suppression of the adrenal gland.

A management algorithm for perioperative steroid supplementation is presented in Figure 40-4.

Thyroid Disease and Anesthesia

Anesthesiologists are frequently faced with patients who have preexisting hyperthyroidism or hypothyroidism. The treatment of these patients during elective surgery is straightforward and does not necessitate any change in anesthetic technique. Problems arise, however, when patients who are floridly hyperthyroid or hypothyroid present for surgery. Patients who are not in a euthyroid state should be operated on only for life-threatening illnesses. The postoperative complications that arise in patients who are not clinically euthyroid make elective surgery a dangerous adventure. The following paragraphs address some concerns related to anesthetizing the patient with untreated or uncontrolled thyroid disease. Unfortunately, evidence-based guidelines are not available because of the low incidence of patients with acute thyroid dysfunction presenting for surgery and the lack of controlled trials on management strategies.

Hypothyroidism

Hypothyroidism is a relatively common condition that occurs in 1% of all patients and in approximately 5% of those older than 50 years.[93] Women represent the vast majority of patients. The most common (noniatrogenic) cause of hypothyroidism is Hashimoto's thyroiditis, an autoimmune disorder caused by antibodies to thyroid tissue. Patients with this condition should be screened for other autoimmune diseases, which are often present. The diagnosis and treatment of these patients has been reviewed recently.[93]

Some of the manifestations of overt hypothyroidism of concern to the anesthesiologist are a decrease in the ventilatory response to hypercarbia and hypoxia, impaired gastric emptying, decrease in free-water clearance, altered ability to thermoregulate, and decreased cardiac output and bradycardia. These patients have a slightly decreased anesthetic requirement, so opiates, induction agents, and volatile anesthetic agents should be titrated accordingly.

Myxedema coma is the most extreme form of hypothyroidism, and anesthesiologists may encounter these patients in the perioperative setting. Common precipitants of myxedema coma include trauma, burns, stroke, sepsis, amiodarone, and the postoperative state. The mortality from myxedema coma is high (>60%), but fortunately this condition is exceedingly rare.

Clinical manifestations of this condition include a decreased level of consciousness, coma, decreased cardiac output, hyponatremia, hypoventilation, and hypothermia. Myxedema coma is an endocrinologic emergency and attention should be focused on securing the patient's airway, control of ventilation, and circulatory support, and these patients should be transferred to an ICU. Despite an increase in total body water, these patients are hypovolemic and subject to profound hypotension should they become vasodilated. Thus, external rewarming is ill advised, as the resultant

---

40-1	**Classification of Surgical Stresses**

Minor

- Inguinal hernia repair
- Colonoscopy
- Laparoscopic surgery

Moderate

- Open cholecystectomy
- Bowel resection
- Peripheral revascularization
- Joint replacement

Major

- Cardiopulmonary bypass
- Pancreaticoduodenectomy
- Esophagectomy
- Aortic surgery

From Salem M, Tainsh RE Jr, Bromberg J, et al. Ann Surg 1994;219: 416-425.

40-1	**Relative Potencies of Steroids**

Steroid	Relative Glucocorticoid Effect	Formulation
Hydrocortisone	1	PO, IV, IM
Prednisone	4	PO
Methylprednisolone	5	IV
Dexamethasone	30	PO, IV

IM, intramuscular; IV, intravenous; PO, by mouth.

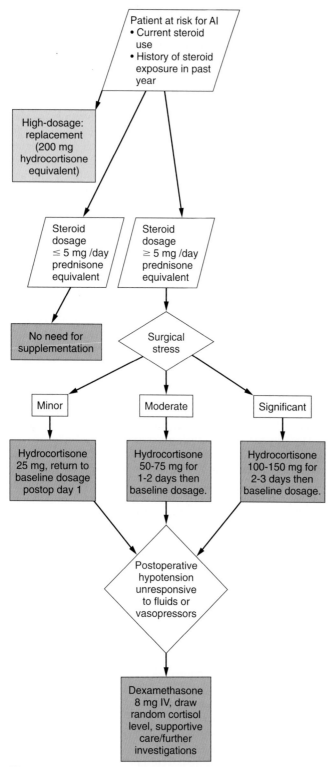

Figure 40-4 ■ Treatment algorithm for patients receiving perioperative steroids. Perioperative supplementation is based on the patient's baseline dosage and the perceived stress of the surgery. AI, adrenal insufficiency. A/W, airway. IV, intravenously. *(Data from Coursin DB, Wood KE: JAMA 2002;287:236-240.)*

vasodilation that occurs with rewarming could result in cardiovascular collapse. Normothermia is achieved with normalization of thyroid hormone levels. Hypotension should be treated with the administration of warmed intravenous fluids. Vasoactive agents should be used judiciously, as they may precipitate arrhythmias. Hypoglycemia, which is often present, responds well to glucose infusions. With the lack of a febrile response or leukocytosis, broad-spectrum antibiotics should be initiated in patients without an obvious precipitant for myxedema coma after appropriate cultures have been obtained.

Definitive management of myxedema coma relies on the administration of intravenous thyroid hormone. The proper initiation of thyroid hormone replacement is controversial with regard to the selection and dose of thyroid hormone (either thyroxine [T_4] or triiodothyronine [T_3]). In theory, T_3 is the logical choice, as it is the form of thyroid hormone active at the cellular level. Furthermore, T_4 is converted to the active T_3 by a deiodinase enzyme, levels of which are depressed in myxedema coma. This has led several investigators to suggest T_3 as the logical replacement choice. T_3, however, is expensive, is difficult to obtain, and may precipitate arrhythmias, and there are no controlled trials demonstrating improved outcome with T_3. Thus, most investigators recommend the use of intravenous T_4 as the sole replacement hormone. A loading dose of 200 to 500 μg intravenously (IV) followed by 50 to 100 μg IV per day afterward is suggested. Concomitant glucocorticoid therapy (hydrocortisone 50 mg IV every 6 hours) should also be initiated, as the presence of AI in these patients is high. Cortisol levels should be drawn prior to initiation of therapy, and if random levels greater than 25 μg/dL are found, glucocorticoid therapy can be discontinued.[93]

Hyperthyroidism

Graves' disease or thyrotoxicosis is the most common cause of hyperthyroidism and results from the presence of autoimmune antibodies directed against the thyroid hormone receptor. These autoantibodies cause stimulations of the thyroid-stimulating hormone (TSH) receptor and result in excessive production of thyroid hormone. Clinically, overt hyperthyroidism is manifested by tachycardia, tremor, diarrhea, ophthalmopathy, and goiter. The diarrhea might be severe enough to cause hypovolemia, acid–base abnormalities, and electrolyte disturbances. Anesthesiologists should pay particular attention to the size of the goiter, as it may be large enough to cause airway obstruction on induction of anesthesia. Historical features, such as shortness of breath with recumbent position, and supplemental tests, such as postural flow volume loops and computed tomography scans, should be evaluated prior to anesthesia. An awake intubation with an armored tube placed distal to the obstruction should be performed with a large goiter. Extubation should occur in the operating room or in the ICU with optimal circumstances (complete reversal of neuromuscular blockade and optimal level of consciousness). Postoperatively after thyroidectomy for a large goiter, the concern of tracheomalacia and tracheal collapse secondary to weakened tracheal rings warrants close observation.

The progression of thyrotoxicosis to thyroid storm is also a rare event. Most often, thyroid storm is caused by a thyroid event such as thyroid surgery, iodinated radiocontrast dye administration (Jod-Basedow effect), and withdrawal of anti-thyroid drugs. Other common precipitants include surgery, trauma, stroke, parturition, and severe infections.[93] Physical manifestations of thyroid storm result from sympathetic stimulation and include hyperthermia, altered mental status, tachycardia, high cardiac output (which might develop into heart failure), hypertension with a widened pulse pressure, and arrhythmias.

The treatment of thyroid storm mandates admission to an ICU and involves general support of the patient, blocking the peripheral effects of thyroid hormone, blocking synthesis of thyroid hormone, and treatment of precipitating causes. Initial management involves inhibition of iodine organification with the thiourea-type drug propylthiouracil (PTU) or methimazole. PTU has the added advantage of inhibiting the peripheral conversion of T_4 to T_3. PTU is administered in a 600- to 1000-mg loading dose, followed by 1200 mg/day in four divided doses. If the oral route is unavailable, PTU is also absorbed rectally. The next step is to inhibit the secretion of preformed thyroid hormone with iodine. PTU and methimazole inhibit the formation of new thyroid hormone only and have no effect on the release of preformed hormone. Several hours should elapse between the administration of the thiourea and iodine. If iodine is given before organification blockade, it may precipitate a substantial release of thyroid hormone (Jod-Basedow effect).[93] Stress-dose steroids (hydrocortisone, 100 mg IV three times daily) can also block the release of thyroid hormone.

At the same time that thyroid hormone release and synthesis are being inhibited, the peripheral effects of thyroid hormone should be antagonized with the use of beta-blockers. Propranolol has been the most commonly used beta-blocker for this, but other, more selective beta-blockers such as metoprolol and esmolol can also be used. Beta-blockers have the additional effect of blocking the peripheral conversion of T_4 to its active form T_3.

Thyroid Hormone and Cardiac Surgery

The effects of thyroid hormone on the heart have long been known. Furthermore, a low T_3 state occurs after cardiopulmonary bypass and results in a state of low cardiac output and high systemic vascular resistance. Studies that have shown thyroid hormone to be a positive inotrope and a vasodilator have led to clinical studies that assess its role in the treatment of this post-bypass abnormality.

In adults undergoing CABG surgery, T_3 levels decrease to between 50% and 75% of baseline levels and remain depressed for the first 1 to 4 postoperative days. The reason this occurs is not well known. Proposed mechanisms include hypothermia and increased interleukin (IL)-6 levels, both of which may cause decreased conversion of T_4 to T_3, or a decreased half-life of T_3.[94]

Initial clinical studies suggested that the administration of T_3 to patients undergoing CABG improved hemodynamics and overall outcome. These initial studies were small and based mostly on anecdotal experience, but they led to larger randomized placebo-controlled trials. Most of these showed a decrease in the need for inotropic support, but overall outcome was the same between groups. Interestingly, in some of the studies a lower incidence of atrial fibrillation was found, which is unusual because this is one of the more common dysrhythmias in patients with hyperthyroidism. Of note, none of the studies performed to date show an increased risk of adverse events in the treatment group. Despite the lack of clear outcome benefit, a potential role for thyroid hormone in CABG patients does exist and warrants further study.[94]

Alteration in the HPA axis resulting in hypothyroidism is also commonly present in organ donors who have suffered brain death. Studies where a protocol for hemodynamic support included replacement with thyroid hormone have shown a decreased need for vasopressors and a substantial increase in the number of organs transplanted. Thus, thyroid hormone replacement should be considered in any hemodynamically unstable donor patient who is receiving vasopressor therapy.[95]

■ ELECTROLYTE ABNORMALITIES

Sodium

Hyponatremia

Hyponatremia is defined as a serum sodium concentration less than 135 mEq/L, and it can occur in a hypotonic, hypertonic, or isotonic state. Hypertonic hyponatremia (increased plasma osmolality) is caused primarily by solutions such as glucose, or by mannitol, as seen in transurethral resection of the prostate (TURP).

The most common type of hyponatremia seen in the perioperative setting or in the critically ill is hypotonic hyponatremia, which can occur in the isovolemic, hypervolemic, or hypovolemic state (see Box 40-1). All three involve an impairment in the excretion of renal water along with continued intake of dilute fluid.

Isovolemic hyponatremia occurs with retention of water in the absence of sodium, and there are no clinical signs of edema. The most common postoperative cause of this condition is syndrome of inappropriate antidiuretic hormone (SIADH), which can be caused by pulmonary or cranial neoplasms or infections, postoperative pain (secondary to sympathetic activation), and drugs such as tricyclic antidepressants or diuretics.

Hypovolemic hyponatremia is commonly caused by gastrointestinal losses, third-space losses, or adrenal insufficiency.

Hypervolemic hyponatremia is characterized by edematous states such as congestive heart failure, cirrhosis, and renal failure. This state is characterized by sodium retention, with disproportionately larger amounts of water.

Management of Hyponatremia. When the serum sodium level remains greater than 125 mEq/L, patients are usually asymptomatic. Lower values usually result in symptoms, especially if the hyponatremia has developed quickly. Nausea, vomiting, visual disturbances, depressed level of consciousness, altered mental status, seizures, disordered reflexes, loss of thermoregulatory control, muscle cramps, and weakness can be seen. Cerebral edema begins to manifest at a sodium concentration of 123 mEq/L, and, if it progresses rapidly, it may lead to transtentorial herniation. Cardiac symptoms occur at levels of less than 100 mEq/L and can result in pulmonary edema, hypertension, and heart failure.

It is recommended that the rate of correction of asymptomatic hyponatremia be 0.6 to 1 mmol/L/hr until the sodium concentration is 125 mEq/L, using hypertonic saline. Then, one half of the deficit should be administered over 8 hours, and the remaining half over 1 to 3 days. Concurrent treatment with furosemide is also recommended to avoid volume overload. A further advantage to this combination is that furosemide treatment is equivalent to the administration of one-half normal saline and thus aids in the correction.[96] Patients who have symptomatic hyponatremia should have their serum sodium concentration raised by 3 to 7 mmol/L. Overly rapid correction of hyponatremia places patients at risk for osmotic demyelination. This usually occurs when serum sodium is increased by more than 12 mmol in a 24-hour period. The sodium dosage for deficit correction can be based on the following formula:

$$Dosage = (bodyweight \times 140 - [Na^+]) \times 0.6,$$

where dosage is in milliequivalents, the patient's bodyweight is in kilograms, and $[Na^+]$ is sodium concentration in milliequivalents per liter.

The treatment of hyponatremia involves two basic pathways: raising the low sodium levels and at the same time treating the underlying cause. Normal saline (308 mOsm/L) is usually sufficient in cases of hypovolemic hyponatremia, and fluid restriction works well in normovolemic or edematous cases. Severe coma or seizures are most effectively managed with hypertonic saline (513 mEq/L), fluid restriction, and furosemide.

Outcomes. For the anesthesiologist, the challenge of managing hyponatremia involves the presence of concomitant hepatic, renal, or cardiac disease. There is presently no level I evidence related to patient outcomes for the perioperative management of hyponatremia. Although acute hyponatremia is tolerated much better than chronic hyponatremia, it is not necessary to restore the serum sodium level to normal before surgery. Cerebral edema is usually absent at a level of 130 mEq/L. There are presently no data that show the level of serum sodium that might increase anesthetic risk. The lower sodium limit arbitrarily chosen by some authors is 131 mEq/L.

Hypernatremia

Hypernatremia is defined as a serum sodium concentration exceeding 145 mEq/L. The primary difference between hyponatremia and hypernatremia is that all patients with hypernatremia are by definition hyperosmolar. In addition, these patients are always free-water depleted. Total body water (TBW) is considered to be approximately 60% of the total bodyweight in kilograms.

The equation for an estimation of free-water deficit is as follows:

$$Free\ water\ deficit = [0.6 \times patient's\ weight\ (in\ kg) \times (patient's\ sodium\ level \div 140) - 1]$$

where the patient's bodyweight is in kilograms, and $[Na^+]$ is sodium concentration in milliequivalents per liter.

One of three circumstances must be present for hypernatremia to occur: water loss, decreased water ingestion, or overingestion of sodium.

Categories of water loss would include insensible losses such as sweating, burns, fever, gastrointestinal losses, and renal causes (central or nephrogenic diabetes insipidus). A major cause of increased sodium ingestion is usually iatrogenic, as might occur during the indiscriminate use of sodium bicarbonate during cardiopulmonary resuscitation.

Antidiuretic hormone (ADH) and thirst sensation as sensed by the hypothalamic osmoreceptors are the two basic mechanisms the body uses to combat the development of hypernatremia. The body's first response is to release ADH, which occurs when the plasma osmolality exceeds 275 to 285 mOsm/kg, but thirst is the more important regulator. Severe hypernatremia will not occur unless the patient is unable to ingest water or has a nonfunctional thirst reflex.

Diabetes insipidus results from the absence of ADH (central diabetes insipidus), or the inability of the renal tubules to respond to ADH (nephrogenic diabetes insipidus). Common etiologies of central diabetes insipidus include head trauma, neurosurgery, hypoxic/ischemic insults, and neoplasia. All these disorders are characterized by a lack of ADH. In nephrogenic diabetes insipidus, the production and secretion of ADH are normal, but renal responsiveness to it is not. The most common etiologies are lithium toxicity, hypercalcemia, and osmotic diuresis (seen in hyperglycemic hyperosmolar nonketotic syndrome). A urine osmolality of less than 300 mOsm/L and serum sodium greater than 150 mEq/L should make one suspect a diagnosis of diabetes insipidus.

Management of Hypernatremia. Regardless of the etiology of the hypernatremia, the symptoms are predominantly neurologic. Headache, weakness, dizziness, irritability, and, in severe cases, seizures and coma can be observed. In cases of a total body-water deficit, when dehydration is severe, hypotension, decreased central venous pressure, tachycardia, and oliguria become manifest. Glomerular filtration rate is decreased, and hence the blood urea nitrogen (BUN), and serum creatinine (Cr) are likely to increase. Peripheral edema is absent, indicating decreases in total body water are responsible for the hypernatremia. In cases of total body excess of sodium, hypertension and edema can be part of the clinical presentation.

Treatment of hypernatremia is directed at treating both the high sodium and the underlying disease. Patients with central diabetes insipidus should receive supplemental ADH in the form of desmopressin (DDAVP, a synthetic peptide with ADH activity). In cases of hypernatremia caused by a total body-water deficit, free water must be replaced judiciously. The sodium level should be lowered by 0.5 mEq/hr, or 12 mEq/day, to avoid the development of cerebral edema. The rate of free-water repletion should be half the total deficit administered in the first 12 to 24 hours, with slow correction thereafter.

Outcomes. For the anesthesiologist, managing hypernatremia centers on hypotension, and secondarily on dehydration and drug-induced hypovolemia. These can be made worse by positive pressure ventilation. These patients could theoretically experience an enhanced sensitivity to nondepolarizing neuromuscular blockers because they have a decreased volume of distribution for these drugs. When there is an excess of total body sodium, the anesthesiologist must be aware of an increased intravascular volume. There is presently no level I evidence related to patient outcomes for the perioperative management of hypernatremia. Although data are lacking that demonstrate a level of serum sodium above which anesthetic risk is increased, it is believed that all patients undergoing elective surgery should have a serum sodium concentration less than 150 mEq/L.

Potassium

Potassium differs greatly from sodium in terms of body distribution. Approximately 98% of the body's potassium stores are intracellular. Total body and serum potassium levels are under hormonal and renal regulation. Acute changes in serum potassium levels are less well tolerated than chronic changes, because chronic changes allow equilibration of serum and intracellular stores over time, which in turn allows the resting membrane potential of excitable cells (cardiac and CNS) to return to approximately normal levels.

Hypokalemia

Hypokalemia (potassium <3.5 mEq/L) can be seen with decreased intake, increased entry into cells (alkalosis, insulin and beta-2-adrenergic administration), increased gastrointestinal or urinary losses, and excessive sweating. Decreased serum potassium levels may reflect large changes in total-body potassium stores. A decrease in the serum potassium of 1 mEq/L may represent a total-body potassium deficit of 50 to 200 mEq. Hypokalemia can result in muscle weakness and paralysis, rhabdomyolysis (seen with serum levels <2.5 mEq/L), hyperglycemia, and renal dysfunction.

Ten percent to 50% of patients taking diuretic drugs become hypokalemic. However, many primary care providers are reluctant to prescribe oral potassium supplementation, even though patients taking diuretics experience some degree of hypokalemia.[97,98]

The most concerning manifestations of hypokalemia involve the cardiovascular system. These can range from autonomic neuropathy, decreased contractility, or disturbances in conduction that can result in serious life-threatening arrhythmias. Electrocardiographic (ECG) changes include ST segment abnormalities (usually depression), flattening or inversion of the T wave, and gradual increase in the U-wave amplitude.[99] These ECG changes are almost always manifest when the serum potassium level is less than 2.3 mEq/L.[100] The morphologic ECG changes do not correlate with the severity of potassium depletion. In addition, although U waves are not specific for hypokalemia, they are sensitive indicators of this condition. Cardiac ischemia, left ventricular

hypertrophy, and digitalis use all increase the risk of arrhythmias from hypokalemia.

Treatment. The main principles in the treatment of hypokalemia are that rapid administration of potassium is potentially harmful, and it should be administered only in life-threatening situations. The recommended replacement rate for a typical adult is 10 to 20 mEq/hr, with constant ECG monitoring.

Outcomes. There are no data revealing increased morbidity or mortality in patients undergoing anesthesia with a potassium level of at least 2.6 mEq/L. As a result, the decision to proceed with anesthesia or surgery in the face of hypokalemia is multifactorial.[101,102] The urgency of the operation, acid–base balance, medication history, onset, and degree of the abnormality must all be taken into consideration. Furthermore, retrospective data attribute considerable risk to potassium administration.[103] In one study involving a cohort of 16,048 hospitalized patients, 1910 of these patients were given oral potassium supplements. Hyperkalemia contributed to seven deaths, and the incidence of potassium therapy complications was 1 in 250.

Three separate studies examined the effects of modest hypokalemia by prospectively examining the incidence of arrhythmias in patients with varying levels of preoperative potassium.[102,104] Vitez and associates found no difference in the incidence of arrhythmias among moderately hypokalemic (K = 3 to 3.4 mEq/L), severely hypokalemic (K <2.9 mEq/L), or normokalemic patients (K >3.4 mEq/L).[102] Another study involving 2402 patients undergoing elective CABG reported that a serum potassium level of less than 3.5 mEq/L was predictive of serious perioperative arrhythmias, intraoperative arrhythmia, and postoperative atrial fibrillation/flutter.[104]

Although it is recommended that hypokalemic patients be given some form of potassium supplementation before elective surgery, the evidence for this is uncertain. One study administered 50 mg of hydrochlorothiazide to 21 patients twice a day for 4 weeks. These patients had become hypokalemic secondary to the diuretic therapy, and they had no history of demonstrable cardiac disease or other medication ingestion. Ambulatory ECG recordings revealed ventricular arrhythmias (ranging from premature ventricular contractions [PVCs] to ventricular tachycardia) in 33% of the patients. Potassium repletion decreased the average number of ventricular ectopic beats from 71.2 to 5.4 per hour.[105]

Patients have varying sensitivities to potassium depletion. Most studies have demonstrated complications that result from moderate and severe degrees.[97,105,106] However, even minor potassium depletion can result in ventricular ectopy. The Multiple Risk Factor Intervention Trial involved 361,662 patients, and more than 2000 were given diuretics for hypertension. The reduction in serum potassium was noted to be greater in those patients with PVCs.[97]

It is difficult to suggest a level of serum potassium below which elective surgery should be canceled. Some experts recommend postponing elective surgery if the level is less than 2.8 mEq/L. However, one must consider the etiology of the hypokalemia and the acuity of the hypokalemic state. This takes on greater importance as more data emerge on the safety of hypokalemia and the dangers of replacing potassium quickly in the hospital environment.

Hyperkalemia

Hyperkalemia (>5.5 mEq/L) occurs from three major processes: increased intake, decreased urinary excretion, and transcellular shifts (diabetic ketoacidosis [DKA], acidosis, beta-adrenergic blockade, succinylcholine administration, digitalis overdose). Of particular importance to the anesthesiologist is the reperfusion of a large vascular bed after a period of prolonged ischemia, as might occur during the reperfusion of a newly transplanted liver. The acidosis in the affected area causes an outflow of intracellular potassium, hence, on reperfusion, patients could receive a large bolus of potassium that cannot be redistributed quickly, which could result in fatal hyperkalemia. Factitious hyperkalemia can result from the lysis of cellular components, particularly blood products. Adrenal insufficiency is another potential cause of hyperkalemia (see later).

The most significant problem facing anesthesiologists in managing hyperkalemia involves abnormal cardiac function. Hyperkalemia lowers the resting membrane potential of cardiac conductive cells and decreases action potential duration and upstroke velocity. In severe states of hyperkalemia, this decreased rate of depolarization and repolarization in other areas of the myocardium produces a progressive widening of the QRS complex that merges with the T wave, resulting in a sine wave on the ECG.

The earliest manifestations of hyperkalemia are the narrowing and peaking of the T wave. These are not diagnostic of hyperkalemia, but T waves are almost always peaked when serum potassium levels are 7 to 9 mEq/L. When potassium levels exceed 6.7 mEq/L, the degree of hyperkalemia and duration of a QRS complex correlate closely. As serum potassium levels progress beyond 7 mEq/L, atrial conduction disturbances appear, such as a decrease in P-wave amplitude and an increase in the PR interval. As levels approach 10 to 12 mEq/L, progressive widening of the QRS complex to sine wave, ventricular fibrillation, or even asystole may occur.[100]

If significant ECG abnormalities are present, 5 to 10 mL of a 10% solution of calcium chloride should be administered intravenously over 3 to 5 minutes to stabilize the myocardial cell membrane. Calcium chloride's salutary effects on the myocardium last only 30 to 60 minutes. Other therapies for hyperkalemia that should be initiated are insulin (10 units of Reg IV), glucose (50 g of 50%), sodium bicarbonate (1 mmol/kg), and hyperventilation. Insulin, glucose, and bicarbonate lower serum potassium levels within 10 to 20 minutes, and the effects last for 4 to 6 hours. Outside of the operating room, dialysis, diuretics, beta-adrenergic agonists, and exchange resins are accepted therapies.

Acute hyperkalemia is more poorly tolerated than chronic hyperkalemia. The most common cause of chronic hyperkalemia is renal failure. It is recommended that any patient with a serum potassium level greater than 5.5 mEq/L should undergo ECG evaluation preoperatively. It is difficult to recommend a serum potassium level above which elective surgery should be canceled. Some experts recommend 5.9 mEq/L as a safe cutoff, because ECG changes start to become manifest at levels of 6.0 mEq/L or greater. It is important to consider dialytic therapy before elective surgery for potassium levels exceeding 6.0 mEq/L, although data are lacking here as well. Most clinicians agree that clinical presentation and ECG changes are the most important guides.

Magnesium

After potassium, magnesium is the second most abundant intracellular cation. Of total body magnesium, 99% is intracellular (primarily in the skeleton) and only 1% is extracellular. Of the total circulating magnesium (0.8 to 1.2 mmol/L [1.9 to 2.9 mg/dL]), 50% is free and physiologically active. Serum magnesium is regulated primarily by intrinsic renal mechanisms. Magnesium is an essential cofactor in more than 300 cellular reactions, including energy metabolism and maintenance of the Na^+,K^+-ATPase pump. Magnesium also modulates vascular tone, is an endogenous Ca^{2+} antagonist, and plays a role in nucleic acid and protein synthesis.

Hypomagnesemia

Hypomagnesemia (<1.5 mEq/L) arises primarily from three causes: intracellular serum shifts, gastrointestinal losses, and renal losses. Common causes of transcellular shifts include chelation by tissues during pancreatitis and rhabdomyolysis, or insulin therapy. Excessive gastrointestinal losses can result from malabsorption, diarrhea, nasogastric suction, or fistulas. Chronic alcohol ingestion leads to significant magnesium loss, and most hospitalized patients are hypomagnesemic. The most common cause of renal wasting is drug toxicity. Cyclosporine, amphotericin B, digitalis, aminoglycosides, and diuretics are frequently implicated.

Hypomagnesemia affects multiple organ systems, including the cardiovascular (arrhythmias, vasospasm, angina), neuromuscular (weakness, spasms, seizures, tetany), and gastrointestinal systems (anorexia, dysphagia, nausea).

Treatment of hypomagnesemia depends on the acuity or chronicity of the disorder. Acute hypomagnesemia should be treated intravenously with magnesium sulfate. Hypomagnesemia is often accompanied by hypokalemia, and potassium should be replenished as well. Treatment is generally with 1 to 2 mEq/kg of magnesium sulfate given over 8 to 12 hours, with careful periodic assessment of electrolyte levels. One concerning aspect of magnesium deficiency is that cardiac arrhythmias can be seen with deficient stores of magnesium that are not reflected in the serum levels. For acute life-threatening cardiac arrhythmias, 2 to 4 g of magnesium sulfate should be administered over 5 minutes, while blood pressure and heart rate are closely monitored. Arterial pressure, deep tendon reflexes, and serum magnesium concentration should be monitored during replacement for a symptomatic, life-threatening condition. In severe depletion without cardiac arrhythmias, the period of administration can be extended from 5 minutes to 3 hours. Chronic asymptomatic magnesium depletion is usually treated with oral magnesium.

Outcomes. The importance of magnesium deficiency, like that of most electrolyte abnormalities, relates to the underlying pathophysiologic process causing the deficiency. Clearly, associated conditions such as alcoholism and malnutrition contribute to anesthetic risk. There are no data related to how hypomagnesemia per se contributes to the risk of anesthesia and outcome.

There is a theoretical risk that low serum magnesium levels could lessen the effectiveness of neuromuscular blocking agents, but this possibility has never been investigated. Data on the management of patients in coronary care units show that magnesium infusion can reduce the incidence and severity of cardiac arrhythmias. In the perioperative setting, data show that magnesium may decrease the incidence of adrenergic-mediated arrhythmias, without interfering with the bronchodilating efficacy of beta-agonists, while at the same time contributing to the bronchiolar smooth muscle relaxation.[107]

The role of magnesium in the setting of an acute myocardial infarction has been studied extensively. The theoretical benefits of this electrolyte on the myocardium are extensive. First, magnesium plays a key role in the regulation of coronary vascular tone. Second, it helps to stabilize the myocardial membrane and reduce the incidence of dysrhythmias. Finally, magnesium has been shown to decrease platelet aggregation in vitro and in vivo. These properties have made magnesium an attractive therapy for patients presenting with myocardial ischemia.

Small preliminary studies showed a significant mortality decrease when patients were treated with magnesium. Subsequent larger studies, however, have failed to duplicate these early results. Thus, at present, magnesium replacement is not recommended in the setting of myocardial ischemia unless documented hypomagnesemia is present.[108]

Furthermore, although magnesium is used extensively in cardiac surgery to reduce the incidence of both atrial and ventricular dysrhythmias, there is some evidence that it might have an adverse effect on platelet function. Although this effect has been demonstrated in a recent study, no studies have shown that magnesium causes increased bleeding during the post-bypass period.[109] Thus, in the absence of data that show an increased risk of bleeding, the use of magnesium is still recommended based on its salutary effects on the myocardium in reducing dysrhythmias.

Hypermagnesemia

Hypermagnesemia (>2.5 mEq/L) is extremely uncommon in patients with normal renal function. It is commonly seen in patients with renal failure after ingestion of magnesium-containing antacids or laxatives. Lithium intoxication, hypothyroidism, and adrenal insufficiency are other causes. Importantly, clinical effects are not closely related to serum measurements of magnesium. Central and peripheral neuromuscular effects, the major complications of hypermagnesemia, include altered mental status, coma, decreased deep tendon reflexes, respiratory muscle weakness, and paralysis.

Electrocardiographic changes associated with hypermagnesemia do correspond to serum levels. At levels between 5 and 10 mg/dL, depressed cardiac conduction, widened QRS complexes, and prolonged PQ intervals appear. Seda-

tion, hypoventilation, decreased deep tendon reflexes, and muscle weakness appear at levels between 20 and 34 mg/dL, with hypotension, bradycardia, and diffuse vasodilation occurring between 24 and 48 mg/dL. Areflexia, coma, and respiratory paralysis occur at 48 to 72 mg/dL.

Treatment. The removal of magnesium can be accomplished with fluid loading followed by diuresis. In life-threatening cases, intravenous calcium can be administered to reverse neuromuscular and cardiac membrane instability while magnesium is removed via dialysis.

Outcomes. Of prime importance to the anesthesiologist is determining the underlying cause of hypermagnesemia. Euvolemia and the maintenance of acid–base homeostasis are of critical importance, as they both contribute to hypermagnesemia. Because hypermagnesemia potentiates the action of both depolarizing and nondepolarizing muscle relaxants, it may be necessary to decrease the initial doses of these drugs. Monitoring with a peripheral nerve stimulator is essential. Cardiac depression and vasodilation produced by anesthetic drugs could be accentuated in the presence of hypermagnesemia. The clinical significance of drug interactions between magnesium and anesthetic has never been investigated. Outcome data relating hypermagnesemia to postanesthetic outcomes are lacking.

Phosphorous

Phosphorous in the form of phosphate is distributed in equal concentrations throughout the intracellular and extracellular compartments. Of body phosphate, 85% is present in bone, 55% circulates as the free ion, 33% is in complexed form, and 12% is protein bound. Normal serum phosphate levels range from 1.3 to 8.0 mmol/L (12.3 to 7.6 mg/dL). Serum phosphate is under the control of both the parathyroid gland and the kidney. Phosphate plays an integral role in energy storage and is responsible for the high-energy phosphate bond in adenosine triphosphate and creatine phosphate. Phosphate is a major component of nucleic acids, phospholipids, and cellular membranes. It is also a part of vital second-messenger systems, including cyclic AMP and phosphatidylinositol. In addition, it plays a critically important role in the offloading of oxygen from hemoglobin, as part of the 2,3-diphosphoglycerate molecule.

Hypophosphatemia

Clinically significant hypophosphatemia occurs when serum levels fall below 2 mg/dL, and it is considered severe when serum phosphorous levels fall below 1.0 mg/dL. Major etiologies of hypophosphatemia include intracellular shifts, sepsis, alkalosis, alcoholism (it occurs in 50% of hospitalized alcoholics), diabetic ketoacidosis, and salicylate poisoning. Low levels of phosphorous, like low levels of magnesium and calcium, can have disastrous neuromuscular complications, including respiratory muscle paralysis, CNS changes, and skeletal myopathy. Hematologic manifestations (hemolysis and impaired platelet function) are seen less commonly.

The underlying etiology of hypophosphatemia, like that of all electrolyte disorders, should be clearly identified. This usually involves the sampling of arterial blood gases and the measurement of ionized calcium and magnesium and of serum and urinary phosphorus. A 24-hour urine phosphate level greater than 100 mg/dL when the serum phosphate level is less than 2 mg/dL is suggestive of renal disease. Treatment includes intravenous potassium phosphate (2.5 to 5.0 mg/kg every 6 hours). The rate of administration should not exceed 0.25 mmol/kg over 4 to 6 hours to avoid hypocalcemia and tissue damage. It is critically important to avoid hyperphosphatemia, because phosphorus and calcium bind together and hypocalcemia results. Calcium phosphate deposition can occur in the eyes, heart, lung, vasculature, and kidneys and is seen in long-term dialysis patients. For serum phosphorous levels greater than 2 mg/dL, an oral sodium phosphate solution can be used. This is usually limited to 30 mmol/day (1 g/day) because of severe diarrhea.

Data on the management of hypophosphatemia as it relates to anesthetic outcome are lacking.

Hyperphosphatemia

Hyperphosphatemia (serum phosphate level >4.5 mg/dL) can result from increased intestinal absorption, parenteral administration, renal dysfunction, frank renal failure, hyperthyroidism, or massive extracellular shifts, such as seen in sepsis, hypothermia or hyperthermia, rhabdomyolysis, or tumor lysis syndromes. Clinical manifestations are few, and usually symptoms of the underlying cause predominate. Hypoparathyroidism can cause hyperphosphatemia in the presence of normal renal function. A rapid rise in serum phosphate concentration can result in frank precipitation of calcium and phosphate and lead to severe hypocalcemia.

First-line therapy includes the administration of phosphate-binding antacids such as aluminum-containing antacids and sucralfate, calcium citrate, or calcium carbonate. High rates of intravenous fluids and acetazolamide are effective at increasing urine phosphate excretion. Phosphorous intake should be restricted to less than 200 mg/day. Dialysis is indicated in patients with renal failure.

Calcium

Calcium is a ubiquitous cation that is involved in many cellular functions, including the duration and strength of cardiac muscle contraction; smooth muscle contraction in blood vessels, airways, and the uterus; and apoptosis. It also has an effect on platelet aggregation and function.[110-114]

Calcium exists in the extracellular plasma in the free ionized state as well as bound to other molecules. The majority of bound calcium (80%) associates with albumin. Because mathematical formulas that are used to correct for changing albumin concentrations can be inaccurate, ionized calcium should be measured to ascertain accurate calcium concentrations.[115] Forty-five percent of the total calcium is biologically active and exists in the ionized form with a normal concentration of 4.5 to 5.0 mg/dL.

Ionized calcium concentrations are affected by the pH of the blood. An increase in one pH unit will decrease the ionized calcium concentration by 0.36 mmol/L; thus, it is not surprising that patients with a metabolic alkalosis are usually hypocalcemic.[116,117]

Calcium homeostasis is maintained through the actions of parathyroid hormone (PTH), calcitonin, and vitamin D acting primarily on the bone, kidney, and gastrointestinal tract.

Hypocalcemia

Hypocalcemia is defined as a decrease in serum calcium below 4.5 mg/dL. Its most common perioperative cause is hypoparathyroidism after thyroid surgery. Hypocalcemia can also arise from a variety of medical conditions, such as pancreatitis, vitamin D deficiency secondary to malnutrition, meningococcal sepsis, and critical illness in general. Hypocalcemia can also be caused by shifts in intravascular volume or by dialysis—for example, by sudden increases in anions that bind calcium (e.g., citrate and phosphate).

Clinical manifestations of hypocalcemia include perioral numbness, paresthesias, muscle cramps, and mental status changes such as irritability. As hypocalcemia increases in severity, there are neuromuscular and cardiac findings, including Chvostek's sign (spasm of facial muscles elicited by tapping the facial nerve anterior to the ear) and Trousseau's sign (carpal spasm produced by wrist pressure induced by blood pressure cuff inflation for 3 to 5 minutes or by tapping on the median nerve). Mental status changes, seizures, tetany, hypotension, and heart failure also may occur.[118,119]

Acutely, hypocalcemia decreases cardiac function by lengthening phase 2 of the cardiac action potential, resulting in prolongation of the ST segment and the QT interval on the ECG. This is significant, as QT lengthening is an independent risk factor for cardiac arrhythmias and sudden death. Often, patients who present to the hospital in cardiac arrest are hypocalcemic.[120,121] Hypocalcemia can lead to cardiac failure, and in patients with underlying heart disease who are on beta-blockers, hypocalcemia can precipitate severe cardiac failure.[122,123] Although patients with longstanding hypocalcemia may have normal cardiac function, it is desirable to keep their calcium concentrations in the normal range, especially in the setting of underlying heart disease. Other electrolyte abnormalities, such as alterations in magnesium concentration, may coexist with hypocalcemia.[124]

Successful management of hypocalcemia involves first correcting any underlying acid–base derangements. When plasma concentrations of calcium fall below 3.5 mg/dL or when symptoms of hypocalcemia (hypotension, tetany) manifest, treatment is recommended. Treatment consists of intravenous administration of a calcium salt, either calcium chloride (1.36 mEq/mL) or calcium gluconate (0.45 mEq/mL). Calcium chloride (2.5 mg/kg IV) or calcium gluconate (7.5 mg/kg IV) are equivalent in terms of their ability to increase the calcium concentration. Calcium is generally administered until serum calcium concentrations reach about 4 mEq/L or the ECG tracing returns to normal.[125]

Anesthetic Considerations and Outcomes. For the anesthesiologist, the goal in managing hypocalcemia is to identify its etiology, to prevent any further decreases in the serum calcium concentrations, and to treat its adverse cardiovascular effects.

In the setting of hypocalcemia, intraoperative hypotension may represent an exaggerated cardiac depression produced by anesthetic drugs, and responses to nondepolarizing muscle relaxants may be exaggerated. Coagulation abnormalities, skeletal muscle spasm, and laryngospasm may all accompany acute decreases in the serum calcium concentration.

Rapid infusion of blood (e.g., 500 mL every 5 to 10 minutes), decreased metabolism, elimination of citrate, cirrhosis of the liver, and renal dysfunction can all precipitate hypocalcemia. Data supporting the predisposition to citrate intoxication in the setting of hypocalcemia are limited.[126] ECG and blood pressure monitoring should be continuous in the perioperative period in all patients with hypocalcemia.

At present, there are no compelling data on the management of perioperative hypocalcemia and anesthetic outcome.

Hypercalcemia

Hypercalcemia is defined as a serum calcium concentration greater than 5.5 mEq/L. It is most commonly caused by hyperparathyroidism and malignant disorders that release PTH-related peptide (PTHrp) from tumor cells. Granulomatous diseases with pulmonary involvement (such as sarcoidosis), vitamin D intoxication, and immobilization are less common causes. In addition, drugs such as thiazide diuretics and lithium can cause hypercalcemia.[127,128]

The clinical manifestations of hypercalcemia arise primarily from the actions on the CNS, neuromuscular junction, heart, kidneys, and gastrointestinal tract. The earliest signs and symptoms involve sedation and emesis. Increased serum calcium concentrations (7 to 8 mEq/L) interfere with renal-concentrating ability, resulting in polyuria. Increased calcium concentrations can contribute to the formation of renal calculi, and eventually to oliguric renal failure. Serum concentrations exceeding 8 mEq/L result in cardiac conduction disturbances, such as prolonged PR interval, widened QRS complexes, and shortened QT intervals on the ECG tracing.

The cornerstone of treatment for hypercalcemia is hydration with 0.9% NaCl, at a rate of approximately 150 mL/hr.[129] This serves to lower calcium concentration by dilution, and sodium inhibits the renal tubular absorption of calcium. Combining saline resuscitation with furosemide diuresis every 4 hours decreases the risk of volume overload and aids in calcium excretion. A therapeutic goal should be a daily urine output of 3 to 5 L. It is important to ensure ambulation in this setting to decrease the calcium release from bone associated with immobilization. Hemodialysis and bisphosphonate therapy can be used in life-threatening cases of hypercalcemia to lower serum concentrations quickly. Calcitonin is effective for immediate lowering of the serum calcium concentration, but its effects are transient. Mithramycin is also effective to acutely lower calcium concentrations in the setting of malignancy, but thrombocytopenia, hepatotoxicity, and nephrotoxicity limit its use.

Anesthetic Considerations and Outcome. For the anesthesiologist, management of hypercalcemia includes saline resuscitation and diuresis, as mentioned. Continuous ECG monitoring perioperatively is necessary to watch for adverse effects of increased calcium on cardiac conduction. Maintenance of acid–base homeostasis is of prime importance, as

alkalosis could serve to lower the potassium concentration and leave the actions of calcium unopposed. The actions of nondepolarizing muscle relaxants are not well defined, but the presence of skeletal muscle weakness in a hyperkalemic patient may necessitate decreasing the dosages of these drugs.

At present, there are no compelling data on the management of hypercalcemia and anesthetic outcome.

Chloride

Chloride is the major anion in the extracellular fluid, and it is the major reabsorbable anion in the renal filtrate. Its relevance for the anesthesiologist involves two acid–base abnormalities.

Hypochloremia

Hypochloremia (blood chloride <96 mEq/L) results from excessive loss of chloride in gastric secretions or urine, resulting in hypochloremic alkalosis. Chloride depletion results in reduced delivery of chloride to the collecting tubules, resulting in limited bicarbonate excretion secondary to the interdependence of bicarbonate–chloride exchange. If less chloride is available for reabsorption, a greater amount of sodium must be reabsorbed with bicarbonate through increased proton secretion. Thus, metabolic alkalosis can generally be classified as chloride responsive or chloride resistant.

A chloride-responsive alkalosis (urinary chloride <15 mEq/L) constitutes the majority of cases of metabolic alkalosis in hospitalized patients. It results from gastric acid loss, diuretic therapy, volume depletion, or renal compensation for hypercapnia. Chloride replacement is the mainstay of management for this condition. Because volume depletion is a common etiology, 0.9% NaCl infusion is the most common means of chloride replacement.

A chloride-resistant alkalosis (urinary chloride >25 mEq/L) is rarely encountered by the anesthesiologist. It most commonly results from mineralocorticoid excess or potassium depletion. The mainstay of therapy is replacement of potassium in the form of potassium chloride.

Hyperchloremia

Hyperchloremic (>106 mEq/L) acidosis is frequently encountered by the anesthesiologist in the perioperative setting. It most commonly accompanies large-volume administration of 0.9% NaCl. It can also occur in the setting of acute normovolemic hemodilution with a 5% albumin solution or a 6% hetastarch solution.[130] Hyperchloremic acidosis is sometimes confused with dilutional acidosis.[131] In hyperchloremic acidosis, serum sodium should remain the same, or possibly increase because of chloride gain, most likely through NaCl. In dilutional acidosis, however, the serum sodium decreases because of the alteration of sodium and chloride in free water.

The clinical relevance of hyperchloremic acidosis is uncertain. One study revealed a significant difference in perioperative acidosis when patients undergoing aneurysm surgery were given normal saline in preference to lactated Ringer's solution.[132] However, there was no significant difference in outcomes. In a similar trial, acidosis associated with hyperchloremia was associated with significantly better outcomes than that associated with lactic acidosis or ketoacidosis.[133]

There are no compelling data relating serum chloride management and its attendant acid–base disorders to perioperative outcomes. However, it is the underlying problem that increases the patient's risk, not the acid–base disturbance itself.

■ CONCLUSION

Patients often go to the operating room with concomitant endocrinologic problems or electrolyte disorders. How the anesthesiologist manages these problems depends on their pathophysiology. Some disorders (such as hyperchloremia) require little more than observation. Other conditions (such as diabetes mellitus or thyroid storm) require aggressive treatment and diligent monitoring, as these disorders can impact perioperative morbidity and mortality.

Historically, perioperative steroid supplementation was used in supra-physiologic (stress-dose) dosages. More recent recommendations suggest a more conservative replacement strategy to obviate the side effects of these drugs.

■ REFERENCES

1. Kjos SL, Buchanan TA: Gestational diabetes mellitus. N Engl J Med 1999;341:1749-1756.
2. Crowther CA, Hiller JE, Moss JR, et al: Effect of treatment of gestational diabetes mellitus on pregnancy outcomes. N Engl J Med 2005;352:2477-2486.
3. van den Berghe G, Wouters P, Weekers F, et al: Intensive insulin therapy in the critically ill patients. N Engl J Med 2001;345:1359-1367.
4. Finney SJ, Zekveld C, Elia A, et al: Glucose control and mortality in critically ill patients. JAMA 2003;290:2041-2047.
5. Krinsley JS: Association between hyperglycemia and increased hospital mortality in a heterogeneous population of critically ill patients. Mayo Clin Proc 2003;78:1471-1478.
6. Goodson WH 3rd, Hung TK: Studies of wound healing in experimental diabetes mellitus. J Surg Res 1977;22:221-227.
7. Yue DK, Swanson B, McLennan S, et al: Abnormalities of granulation tissue and collagen formation in experimental diabetes, uraemia and malnutrition. Diabet Med 1986;3:221-225.
8. Weringer EJ, Kelso JM, Tamai IY, et al: Effects of insulin on wound healing in diabetic mice. Acta Endocrinol (Copenh) 1982;99:101-108.
9. Overett TK, Bistrian BR, Lowry SF, et al: Total parenteral nutrition in patients with insulin-requiring diabetes mellitus. J Am Coll Nutr 1986;5:79-89.
10. Rassias AJ, Marrin CA, Arruda J, et al: Insulin infusion improves neutrophil function in diabetic cardiac surgery patients. Anesth Analg 1999;88:1011-1016.
11. Zerr KJ, Furnary AP, Grunkemeier GL, et al: Glucose control lowers the risk of wound infection in diabetics after open heart operations. Ann Thorac Surg 1997;63:356-361.
12. Furnary AP, Zerr KJ, Grunkemeier GL, et al: Continuous intravenous insulin infusion reduces the incidence of deep sternal wound infection in diabetic patients after cardiac surgical procedures. Ann Thorac Surg 1999;67:352-360; discussion 360-362.
13. Golden SH, Peart-Vigilance C, Kao WH, et al: Perioperative glycemic control and the risk of infectious complications in a cohort of adults with diabetes. Diabetes Care 1999;22:1408-1414.
14. Malmberg K, Norhammar A, Wedel H, et al: Glycometabolic state at admission: Important risk marker of mortality in conventionally treated patients with diabetes mellitus and acute myocardial infarction—Long-term results from the Diabetes and Insulin-Glucose Infusion in Acute Myocardial Infarction (DIGAMI) study. Circulation 1999;99:2626-2632.
15. Capes SE, Hunt D, Malmberg K, et al: Stress hyperglycaemia and increased risk of death after myocardial infarction in patients with and without diabetes: A systematic overview. Lancet 2000;355:773-778.
16. Norhammar A, Malmberg K, Diderholm E, et al: Diabetes mellitus: The major risk factor in unstable coronary artery disease even after consideration of the extent of coronary artery disease and benefits of revascularization. J Am Coll Cardiol 2004;43:585-591.
17. Coutinho M, Gerstein HC, Wang Y, et al: The relationship between glucose and incident cardiovascular events: A metaregression analysis of published data from 20 studies of 95,783 individuals followed for 12.4 years. Diabetes Care 1999;22:233-240.
18. Imran SA, Malmberg K, Cox JL, et al: An overview of the role of insulin in the treatment of hyperglycemia during acute myocardial ischemia. Can J Cardiol 2004;20:1361-1365.
19. Malmberg K, Ryden L, Wedel H, et al: Intense metabolic control by means of insulin in patients with diabetes mellitus and acute myocardial infarction (DIGAMI 2): Effects on mortality and morbidity. Eur Heart J 2005;26:650-661.
20. Werb MR, Zinman B, Teasdale SJ, et al: Hormonal and metabolic responses during coronary artery bypass surgery: Role of infused glucose. J Clin Endocrinol Metab 1989;69:1010-1018.
21. Braden H, Cheema-Dhadli S, Mazer CD, et al: Hyperglycemia during normothermic cardiopulmonary bypass: The role of the kidney. Ann Thorac Surg 1998;65:1588-1593.
22. Svensson S, Ekroth R, Milocco I, et al: Glucose and lactate balances in heart and leg after coronary surgery: Influence of insulin infusion. Scand J Thorac Cardiovasc Surg 1989;23:145-150.
23. Rady MY, Ryan T, Starr NJ: Perioperative determinants of morbidity and mortality in elderly patients undergoing cardiac surgery. Crit Care Med 1998;26:225-235.
24. Carson JL, Scholz PM, Chen AY, et al: Diabetes mellitus increases short-term mortality and morbidity in patients undergoing coronary artery bypass graft surgery. J Am Coll Cardiol 2002;40:418-423.
25. Adler DS, Goldman L, O'Neil A, et al: Long-term survival of more than 2,000 patients after coronary artery bypass grafting. Am J Cardiol 1986;58:195-202.
26. Lawrie GM, Morris GC Jr, Glaeser DH: Influence of diabetes mellitus on the results of coronary bypass surgery: Follow-up of 212 diabetic patients ten to 15 years after surgery. JAMA 1986;256:2967-2971.
27. McAlister FA, Man J, Bistritz L, et al: Diabetes and coronary artery bypass surgery: An examination of perioperative glycemic control and outcomes. Diabetes Care 2003;26:1518-1524.
28. Estrada CA, Young JA, Nifong LW, et al: Outcomes and perioperative hyperglycemia in patients with or without diabetes mellitus undergoing coronary artery bypass grafting. Ann Thorac Surg 2003;75:1392-1399.
29. Lazar HL, Chipkin SR, Fitzgerald CA, et al: Tight glycemic control in diabetic coronary artery bypass graft patients improves perioperative outcomes and decreases recurrent ischemic events. Circulation 2004;109:1497-1502.
30. Ouattara A, Lecomte P, Le Manach Y, et al: Poor intraoperative blood glucose control is associated with a worsened hospital outcome after cardiac surgery in diabetic patients. Anesthesiology 2005;103:687-694.
31. Chaney MA, Nikolov MP, Blakeman BP, et al: Attempting to maintain normoglycemia during cardiopulmonary bypass with insulin may initiate postoperative hypoglycemia. Anesth Analg 1999;89:1091-1095.
32. Mangano DT, Layug EL, Wallace A, et al: Effect of atenolol on mortality and cardiovascular morbidity after noncardiac surgery. Multicenter Study of Perioperative Ischemia Research Group. N Engl J Med 1996;335:1713-1720.
33. Juul AB, Wetterslev J, Kofoed-Enevoldsen A: Long-term postoperative mortality in diabetic patients undergoing major non-cardiac surgery. Eur J Anaesthesiol 2004;21:523-529.

34. Wass CT, Lanier WL: Glucose modulation of ischemic brain injury: Review and clinical recommendations. Mayo Clin Proc 1996;71:801-812.
35. Davies MG, Hagen PO: Alterations in venous endothelial cell and smooth muscle cell relaxation induced by high glucose concentrations can be prevented by aminoguanidine. J Surg Res 1996;63:474-479.
36. Broderick JP, Hagen T, Brott T, et al: Hyperglycemia and hemorrhagic transformation of cerebral infarcts. Stroke 1995;26:484-487.
37. Kawai N, Stummer W, Ennis SR, et al: Blood-brain barrier glutamine transport during normoglycemic and hyperglycemic focal cerebral ischemia. J Cereb Blood Flow Metab 1999;19:79-86.
38. Kawai N, Keep RF, Betz AL, et al: Hyperglycemia induces progressive changes in the cerebral microvasculature and blood-brain barrier transport during focal cerebral ischemia. Acta Neurochir Suppl 1998;71:219-221.
39. Longstreth WT Jr, Inui TS: High blood glucose level on hospital admission and poor neurological recovery after cardiac arrest. Ann Neurol 1984;15:59-63.
40. Bruno A, Biller J, Adams HP Jr, et al: Acute blood glucose level and outcome from ischemic stroke. Trial of ORG 10172 in Acute Stroke Treatment (TOAST) Investigators. Neurology 1999;52:280-284.
41. Jeremitsky E, Omert LA, Dunham CM, et al: The impact of hyperglycemia on patients with severe brain injury. J Trauma 2005;58:47-50.
42. Rovlias A, Kotsou S: The influence of hyperglycemia on neurological outcome in patients with severe head injury. Neurosurgery 2000;46:335-342; discussion 342-343.
43. Ceriana P, Barzaghi N, Locatelli A, et al: Aortic arch surgery: Retrospective analysis of outcome and neuroprotective strategies. J Cardiovasc Surg (Torino) 1998;39:337-342.
44. Van den Berghe G, Wouters PJ, Bouillon R, et al: Outcome benefit of intensive insulin therapy in the critically ill: Insulin dose versus glycemic control. Crit Care Med 2003;31:359-366.
45. Hedley AA, Ogden CL, Johnson CL, et al: Prevalence of overweight and obesity among US children, adolescents, and adults, 1999-2002. JAMA 2004;291:2847-2850.
46. Seidell JC, Flegal KM: Assessing obesity: Classification and epidemiology. Br Med Bull 1997;53:238-252.
47. Sturm R: The effects of obesity, smoking, and drinking on medical problems and costs. Health Aff (Millwood) 2002;21:245-253.
48. Drenick EJ, Bale GS, Seltzer F, et al: Excessive mortality and causes of death in morbidly obese men. JAMA 1980;243:443-445.
49. Rocke DA, Murray WB, Rout CC, et al: Relative risk analysis of factors associated with difficult intubation in obstetric anesthesia. Anesthesiology 1992;77:67-73.
50. Wilson SL, Mantena NR, Halverson JD: Effects of atropine, glycopyrrolate, and cimetidine on gastric secretions in morbidly obese patients. Anesth Analg 1981;60:37-40.
51. Strollo PJ Jr, Rogers RM: Obstructive sleep apnea. N Engl J Med 1996;334:99-104.
52. Young T, Palta M, Dempsey J, et al: The occurrence of sleep-disordered breathing among middle-aged adults. N Engl J Med 1993;328:1230-1235.
53. Voyagis GS, Kyriakis KP, Dimitriou V, et al: Value of oropharyngeal Mallampati classification in predicting difficult laryngoscopy among obese patients. Eur J Anaesthesiol 1998;15:330-334.
54. Benumof JL: Obstructive sleep apnea in the adult obese patient: Implications for airway management. J Clin Anesth 2001;13:144-156.
55. Akashiba T, Kawahara S, Akahoshi T, et al: Relationship between quality of life and mood or depression in patients with severe obstructive sleep apnea syndrome. Chest 2002;122:861-865.
56. Flemons WW, Whitelaw WA, Brant R, et al: Likelihood ratios for a sleep apnea clinical prediction rule. Am J Respir Crit Care Med 1994;150(5 Pt 1):1279-1285.
57. Boushra NN: Anaesthetic management of patients with sleep apnoea syndrome. Can J Anaesth 1996;43:599-616.
58. Crapo RO, Kelly TM, Elliott CG, et al: Spirometry as a preoperative screening test in morbidly obese patients. Surgery 1986;99:763-768.
59. Hnatiuk OW, Dillard TA, Torrington KG: Adherence to established guidelines for preoperative pulmonary function testing. Chest 1995;107:1294-1297.
60. Roche N, Herer B, Roig C, et al: Prospective testing of two models based on clinical and oximetric variables for prediction of obstructive sleep apnea. Chest 2002;121:747-752.
61. Berry RB, Parish JM, Hartse KM: The use of auto-titrating continuous positive airway pressure for treatment of adult obstructive sleep apnea. An American Academy of Sleep Medicine review. Sleep 2002;25:148-13333373.
62. Waldhorn RE, Herrick TW, Nguyen MC, et al: Long-term compliance with nasal continuous positive airway pressure therapy of obstructive sleep apnea. Chest 1990;97:33-38.
63. Rennotte MT, Baele P, Aubert G, et al: Nasal continuous positive airway pressure in the perioperative management of patients with obstructive sleep apnea submitted to surgery. Chest 1995;107:367-374.
64. Tkacova R, Rankin F, Fitzgerald FS, et al: Effects of continuous positive airway pressure on obstructive sleep apnea and left ventricular afterload in patients with heart failure. Circulation 1998;98:2269-2275.
65. Wilcox I, Grunstein RR, Hedner JA, et al: Effect of nasal continuous positive airway pressure during sleep on 24-hour blood pressure in obstructive sleep apnea. Sleep 1993;16:539-544.
66. Drummond GB, Stedul K, Kingshott R, et al: Automatic CPAP compared with conventional treatment for episodic hypoxemia and sleep disturbance after major abdominal surgery. Anesthesiology 2002;96:817-826.
67. Eagle KA: ACC/AHA Guideline Update for Perioperative Cardiovascular Evaluation for Noncardiac Surgery: Executive summary. J Am Coll Cardiol 2002;39:542-553.
68. Lanfranchi P, Somers VK: Obstructive sleep apnea and vascular disease. Respir Res 2001;2:315-319.
69. Leung RS, Bradley TD: Sleep apnea and cardiovascular disease. Am J Respir Crit Care Med 2001;164:2147-2165.
70. Mooe T, Franklin KA, Wiklund U, et al: Sleep-disordered breathing and myocardial ischemia in patients with coronary artery disease. Chest 2000;117:1597-1602.
71. Chan J, Sanderson J, Chan W, et al: Prevalence of sleep-disordered breathing in diastolic heart failure. Chest 1997;111:1488-1493.
72. Cherniack NS: Apnea and periodic breathing during sleep. N Engl J Med 1999;341:985-987.
73. Harbison J, O'Reilly P, McNicholas WT: Cardiac rhythm disturbances in the obstructive sleep apnea syndrome: Effects of nasal continuous positive airway pressure therapy. Chest 2000;118:591-595.
74. Blaszyk H, Bjornsson J: Factor V Leiden and morbid obesity in fatal postoperative pulmonary embolism. Arch Surg 2000;135:1410-1413.
75. Blaszyk H, Wollan PC, Witkiewicz AK, et al: Death from pulmonary thromboembolism in severe obesity: Lack of association with established genetic and clinical risk factors. Virchows Arch 1999;434:529-532.
76. Kakkar VV, Howe CT, Nicolaides AN, et al: Deep vein thrombosis of the leg: Is there a "high risk" group? Am J Surg 1970;120:527-530.
77. Scholten DJ, Hoedema RM, Scholten SE: A comparison of two different prophylactic dose regimens of low molecular weight heparin in bariatric surgery. Obes Surg 2002;12:19-24.
78. Schwartz AE, Matteo RS, Ornstein E, et al: Pharmacokinetics of sufentanil in obese patients. Anesth Analg 1991;73:790-793.
79. Weinstein JA, Matteo RS, Ornstein E, et al: Pharmacodynamics of vecuronium and atracurium in the obese surgical patient. Anesth Analg 1988;67:1149-1153.
80. Vaughan RW, Bauer S, Wise L: Effect of position (semirecumbent versus supine) on postoperative oxygenation in markedly obese subjects. Anesth Analg 1976;55:37-41.
81. Fraser CG, Preuss FS, Bigford WD: Adrenal atrophy and irreversible shock associated with cortisone therapy. J Am Med Assoc 1952;149:1542-1543.
82. Esteban NV, Loughlin T, Yergey AL, et al: Daily cortisol production rate in man determined by stable isotope dilution/mass spectrometry. J Clin Endocrinol Metab 1991;72:39-45.
83. Coursin DB, Wood KE: Corticosteroid supplementation for adrenal insufficiency. JAMA 2002;287:236-240.
84. Marik PE, Zaloga GP: Adrenal insufficiency in the critically ill: A new look at an old problem. Chest 2002;122:1784-1796.

85. Salem M, Tainsh RE Jr, Bromberg J, et al: Perioperative glucocorticoid coverage: A reassessment 42 years after emergence of a problem. Ann Surg 1994;219:416-425.

86. Lamberts SW, Bruining HA, de Jong FH: Corticosteroid therapy in severe illness. N Engl J Med 1997;337:1285-1292.

87. Bromberg JS, Alfrey EJ, Barker CF, et al: Adrenal suppression and steroid supplementation in renal transplant recipients. Transplantation 1991;51:385-390.

88. Cooper MS, Stewart PM: Corticosteroid insufficiency in acutely ill patients. N Engl J Med 2003;348:727-734.

89. Beishuizen A, Thijs LG: Relative adrenal failure in intensive care: An identifiable problem requiring treatment? Best Pract Res Clin Endocrinol Metab 2001;15:513-531.

90. Annane D, Sebille V, Troche G, et al: A 3-level prognostic classification in septic shock based on cortisol levels and cortisol response to corticotropin. JAMA 2000;283:1038-1045.

91. Kay J, Findling JW, Raff H: Epidural triamcinolone suppresses the pituitary-adrenal axis in human subjects. Anesth Analg 1994;79:501-505.

92. Udelsman R, Goldstein DS, Loriaux DL, et al: Catecholamine-glucocorticoid interactions during surgical stress. J Surg Res 1987;43:539-545.

93. Connery LE, Coursin DB: Assessment and therapy of selected endocrine disorders. Anesthesiol Clin North America 2004;22:93-123.

94. Klemperer JD: Thyroid hormone and cardiac surgery. Thyroid 2002;12:517-521.

95. Wood KE, Becker BN, McCartney JG, et al: Care of the potential organ donor. N Engl J Med 2004;351:2730-2739.

96. Adrogue HJ, Madias NE: Hyponatremia. N Engl J Med 2000;342:1581-1589.

97. Cohen JD, Neaton JD, Prineas RJ, et al: Diuretics, serum potassium and ventricular arrhythmias in the Multiple Risk Factor Intervention Trial. Am J Cardiol 1987;60:548-554.

98. Dyckner T, Wester PO: Ventricular extrasystoles and intracellular electrolytes before and after potassium and magnesium infusions in patients on diuretic treatment. Am Heart J 1979;97:12-18.

99. Aldinger KA, Samaan NA: Hypokalemia with hypercalcemia: Prevalence and significance in treatment. Ann Intern Med 1977;87:571-573.

100. Surawicz B: Relationship between electrocardiogram and electrolytes. Am Heart J 1967;73:814-834.

101. Hirsch IA, Tomlinson DL, Slogoff S, et al: The overstated risk of preoperative hypokalemia. Anesth Analg 1988;67:131-136.

102. Vitez TS, Soper LE, Wong KC, et al: Chronic hypokalemia and intraoperative dysrhythmias. Anesthesiology 1985;63:130-133.

103. Lawson DH, Hutcheon AW, Jick H: Life threatening drug reactions amongst medical in-patients. Scott Med J 1979;24:127-130.

104. Wahr JA, Parks R, Boisvert D, et al: Preoperative serum potassium levels and perioperative outcomes in cardiac surgery patients. Multicenter Study of Perioperative Ischemia Research Group. JAMA 1999;281:2203-2210.

105. Holland OB, Nixon JV, Kuhnert L: Diuretic-induced ventricular ectopic activity. Am J Med 1981;70:762-768.

106. Duke M: Thiazide-induced hypokalemia: Association with acute myocardial infarction and ventricular fibrillation. JAMA 1978;239:43-45.

107. James MF: Clinical use of magnesium infusions in anesthesia. Anesth Analg 1992;74:129-136.

108. Tong GM, Rude RK: Magnesium deficiency in critical illness. J Intensive Care Med 2005;20:3-17.

109. Gries A, Bode C, Gross S, et al: The effect of intravenously administered magnesium on platelet function in patients after cardiac surgery. Anesth Analg 1999;88:1213-1219.

110. Carsten ME, Miller JD: A new look at uterine muscle contraction. Am J Obstet Gynecol 1987;157:1303-1315.

111. Kotlikoff MI, Wang YX: Calcium release and calcium-activated chloride channels in airway smooth muscle cells. Am J Respir Crit Care Med 1998;158(5 Pt 3):S109-114.

112. MacLennan DH, Kranias EG: Phospholamban: A crucial regulator of cardiac contractility. Nat Rev Mol Cell Biol 2003;4:566-577.

113. Mehta JL: Influence of calcium-channel blockers on platelet function and arachidonic acid metabolism. Am J Cardiol 1985;55:158B-164.

114. Morgan JP, Perreault CL, Morgan KG: The cellular basis of contraction and relaxation in cardiac and vascular smooth muscle. Am Heart J 1991;121(3 Pt 1):961-968.

115. Slomp J, van der Voort PH, Gerritsen RT, et al: Albumin-adjusted calcium is not suitable for diagnosis of hyper- and hypocalcemia in the critically ill. Crit Care Med 2003;31:1389-1393.

116. Wang S, McDonnell EH, Sedor FA, et al: pH effects on measurements of ionized calcium and ionized magnesium in blood. Arch Pathol Lab Med 2002;126:947-950.

117. Wong HR, Chundu KR: Metabolic alkalosis in children undergoing cardiac surgery. Crit Care Med 1993;21:884-887.

118. Brito D, Pedro M, Bordalo A, et al: Dilated cardiomyopathy due to endocrine dysfunction. Rev Port Cardiol 2003;22:377-387.

119. Riggs JE: Neurologic manifestations of electrolyte disturbances. Neurol Clin 2002;20:227-239, vii.

120. Schouten EG, Dekker JM, Meppelink P, et al: QT interval prolongation predicts cardiovascular mortality in an apparently healthy population. Circulation 1991;84:1516-1523.

121. Urban P, Scheidegger D, Buchmann B, et al: Cardiac arrest and blood ionized calcium levels. Ann Intern Med 1988;109:110-113.

122. Bashour T, Basha HS, Cheng TO: Hypocalcemic cardiomyopathy. Chest 1980;78:663-665.

123. Stulz PM, Scheidegger D, Drop LJ, et al: Ventricular pump performance during hypocalcemia: Clinical and experimental studies. J Thorac Cardiovasc Surg 1979;78:185-194.

124. Vered I, Vered Z, Perez JE, et al: Normal left ventricular performance documented by Doppler echocardiography in patients with long-standing hypocalcemia. Am J Med 1989;86:413-416.

125. Cote CJ, Drop LJ, Daniels AL, et al: Calcium chloride versus calcium gluconate: Comparison of ionization and cardiovascular effects in children and dogs. Anesthesiology 1987;66:465-470.

126. Denlinger JK, Nahrwold ML, Gibbs PS, et al: Hypocalcaemia during rapid blood transfusion in anaesthetized man. Br J Anaesth 1976;48:995-1000.

127. Duarte CG, Winnacker JL, Becker KL, et al: Thiazide-induced hypercalcemia. N Engl J Med 1971;284:828-830.

128. Price LH, Heninger GR: Lithium in the treatment of mood disorders. N Engl J Med 1994;331:591-598.

129. Bilezikian JP: Management of acute hypercalcemia. N Engl J Med 1992;326:1196-1203.

130. Rehm M, Orth V, Scheingraber S, et al: Acid-base changes caused by 5% albumin versus 6% hydroxyethyl starch solution in patients undergoing acute normovolemic hemodilution: A randomized prospective study. Anesthesiology 2000;93:1174-1183.

131. Prough DS, White RT: Acidosis associated with perioperative saline administration: dilution or delusion? Anesthesiology 2000;93:1167-1169.

132. Waters JH, Gottlieb A, Schoenwald P, et al: Normal saline versus lactated Ringer's solution for intraoperative fluid management in patients undergoing abdominal aortic aneurysm repair: An outcome study. Anesth Analg 2001;93:817-822.

133. Brill SA, Stewart TR, Brundage SI, et al: Base deficit does not predict mortality when secondary to hyperchloremic acidosis. Shock 2002;17:459-462.

Chapter

41 Pain, Delirium, and Anxiety

Winston C. V. Parris and Lesco Rogers

For all in happiness mankind can gain, it is not in
pleasure but in rest from pain.

JOHN DRYDEN

After all systemic illnesses are cured, after all metabolic
imbalances are corrected, after all diseased organs are
removed and broken bones repaired, chronic pain may emerge
and continue to persist. The variety of chronic pain syndromes is protean, and the etiologic bases for persisting pain
may be obvious in some cases but vague in others. Despite
the diverse etiology or complicated pathogenetic bases for
persistent (chronic) pain, patients with chronic pain tend to
share some common characteristics—depression, disability,
dependency, disuse atrophy, despair, disillusionment, doctor
shopping, and drug misuse or abuse.[1] Triage of the patient
with chronic pain begins with thorough pain assessment and
application of appropriate supporting disciplines, usually
within the structure of a pain clinic. Modalities that can be
used to control or eliminate chronic pain include pharmacologic management, physical therapy, psychological assessment with relevant interventions (biofeedback, relaxation
training, individual counseling, group therapy), occupational
therapy, vocational therapy, and a host of alternative therapies
including acupuncture, acupressure, massage therapy, and
intercessional prayer. In most cases, a plan of management
is designed and appropriate pain management strategies are
implemented. In this chapter, we discuss selected pain topics
and offer specific recommendations of care; we hope to
support our recommendations with clinical evidence and to
conclude each topic with a proposed algorithm for care based
on published evidence. A similar schema is used to discuss
delirium and anxiety.

As a result of the contributions of the late John J. Bonica,[2]
medical professionals have an increased awareness of the
major inadequacies of pain management, and almost simultaneously the general population has recognized that effective pain management is no longer optional but mandatory.
Bonica and others are largely responsible for the formation
of pain organizations that have highlighted pain management
at the organizational level of the medical community. In
fact, pain medicine currently has a seat in the House of
Delegates of the American Medical Association (AMA).
Furthermore, the dissemination of knowledge from these
organizations, along with the increased research activities
and interactions with various governmental institutions and
regulatory bodies, has contributed to securing a place for
pain medicine in the U.S. health system. In addition to
Bonica, Steve Brena, Harold Carron, Ron Melzack, Prithvi

Raj, Benjamin Crue, Sam Lipton, Terry Murphy, and many
others have made notable contributions to the field of pain
medicine.

Thus, the treatment of pain syndromes has developed
rapidly and together with patient demands has produced
many therapeutic modalities, drugs, and procedures, some of
which have not always been supported by evidence-based
clinical studies and investigations. The withdrawal of rofecoxib (Vioxx) and valdecoxib (Bextra) from the U.S. market
is representative of some of the problems that occur when
demands for effective remedies outpace the due diligence
that should be done before and after releasing new drugs. Of
the procedures that have been used to treat chronic pain
syndromes, some are anecdotally effective and others have
no evidence-based merit. Helping patients with chronic pain
and determining the scientific efficacy of the treatment are
equally important. Performing randomized, double-blind,
placebo-controlled studies and evaluating outcome studies
produce data that can help endorse or refute a claim of the
therapeutic efficacy of a pain-treatment modality.[3] Practice
guidelines issued by professional organizations help maintain
the high standards necessary in the discipline of pain
medicine.

A review of modalities used to treat all chronic pain
syndromes is beyond the scope of this chapter, so we will
limit our evaluation to four major chronic pain syndromes:
chronic back pain (lumbar degenerative disc disease, lumbar
facetogenic disease, lumbar spinal stenosis, sacroiliac joint
arthropathy, and myofascial pain syndrome), cancer pain
(pancreas, breast, and prostate), cervicogenic headache, and
postoperative (acute) pain. We will recommend treatment
strategies and suggest an algorithm for implementing therapy
for each syndrome.

■ CHRONIC BACK PAIN

I love the majesty of human suffering.

ALFRED DE VIGNY (1844)

Chronic low back pain exerts a heavy toll on emotional,
economic, occupational, and financial resources.[4] The costs
of treating chronic low back pain continue to rise, and the
suffering associated with continuing pain and time lost from
work, and the impact of that lost time on business, the
economy, the family, society, and the individual make the
true cost staggering.

Evaluating chronic low back pain involves a complete
physical examination, a history of past medical and surgical

events and drug use (including allergies), and a focused examination of the central nervous system and the musculoskeletal system. Some of the following may be indicated: lumbosacral radiographs, psychological screening, myelography, computed tomography (CT), CT-myelography, bone scintigraphy, magnetic resonance imaging (MRI), electromyography (EMG), nerve conduction studies, needle electrode examination, somatosensory evoked potential, diagnostic nerve blocks, and provocative lumbar discography.

Appropriate use and perceptive interpretation of these investigations contribute to precise diagnosis and effective treatment of chronic back pain syndromes. Interpretation requires appreciating that a patient may have multiple pain generators.[5] For example, a patient with chronic low back pain may have an MRI scan showing disc herniation at L4-L5 and L5-S1, but that patient may also have severe osteoarthritis of the left hip along with left sacroiliac joint arthropathy and a compression fracture of the L3 vertebral body. Thus, this patient has at least five potential pain generators, and reassessment of the history, physical examination, and other investigations may help to pinpoint the pain generator that is the most significant focus of pain and therefore the one most likely to provide pain relief after treatment.

It is useful to remember that 22% of asymptomatic patients less than 60 years old have MRI evidence of a herniated disc. With increasing age, the incidence of asymptomatic patients with disc herniation based on MRI findings increases. A thorough neuromuscular physical examination is necessary to correlate those findings (or the absence thereof) with the imaging and other relevant data obtained from the patient. Some patients have normal lumbar spine imaging and yet present with excruciating chronic low back pain. MRI and CT-myelography are both accurate in identifying aberrations of the intervertebral foramen, and both show, with consistent accuracy, central spinal stenosis, foraminal stenosis, disc bulges, osteophytes, lateral recess, and disc protrusions. MRI is superior to CT-myelography[6] in highlighting disc degeneration associated with spinal stenosis, but MRI technology has inherent limitations based on the physics associated with image generation. During MRI, an external magnet polarizes hydrogen protons contained in water molecules in the tissues of the spine and paraspinous structures, and a specific radiofrequency is pulsed into the body. Different images are generated depending on the number of mobile hydrogen ions (and thus water molecules) present in the tissues. These intrinsic characteristics may produce false-positive or exaggerated images that lead to erroneous diagnoses, so caution is warranted in the interpretation of the MRI findings, especially in certain disease states associated with inflammatory changes in paraspinous tissues.

Lumbar Degenerative Discogenic Disease

Patients with back pain may present with a relatively short history of pain for less than 6 months, and there may be a specific event that triggered the pain or an event that aggravated a prior prolonged history of chronic but tolerable back pain. Patients may be of any age, sex, race, or economic stratification. Most patients have seen a primary care provider and been treated with weak opioid analgesics, nonsteroidal anti-inflammatory drugs (NSAIDs), or muscle relaxants; some patients may be receiving physical therapy, massage therapy, or other physical modalities. Approximately 30% to 50% of these patients do not improve and the back pain may, in fact, get worse. The chronic axial low back pain may develop a radicular component, and the activities of daily living may become severely compromised. At this time, many patients have an MRI or a CT scan. Patients with positive MRI or CT findings and in whom the symptoms continue may be diagnosed with lumbar degenerative discogenic disease. The MRI may show loss of disc height, disc bulge, disc protrusion, disc herniation, or disc extrusion at multiple levels, and the clinician should correlate the clinical and neurologic findings with the MRI findings.

A reasonable recommendation would be for the patient to have a series of up to three lumbar transforaminal epidural steroid injections (TFESIs)[7] at the affected levels (ideally, three levels—e.g., L4, L5, S1) on the side (right or left) where the pain is greatest. When a patient has bilateral pain, the injections can be on alternating sides, and when the degenerative process is confined to one disc space (e.g., L4), a bilateral TFESI at L4 and L5 may be performed. If patients do not improve noticeably by the second TFESI, a third can be performed along with a percutaneous neuroplasty[8] for lysis of adhesions (i.e., adhesiolysis of epidural fibrosis using 10% hypertonic saline[9] and hyaluronidase[10] with a caudal epidural catheter). In these cases, the catheter is directed to the side of greatest pain and as close to the affected nerve roots as possible. Catheter positioning is confirmed using fluoroscopic guidance and epidurography (Fig. 41-1).

In our practice, betamethasone (Celestone) is the preferred steroid, and triamcinolone acetonide (Kenalog) is the second choice. Methylprednisolone (Depo-Medrol) was the popular and preferred agent when translaminar ESIs were common 6 to 10 years ago, but TFESI[11] appears to be superior for controlling radicular pain associated with degenerative disc disease and by virtue of its proximity to the neuraxis and, more specifically, the nerve roots. Serious complications are possible (though not common) even when the procedures are performed by experienced pain physicians. A serious complication that may result with methylprednisolone[12] is paraplegia, which occurs when particulate matter present in the methylprednisolone is inadvertently injected into the anterior spinal artery of Adamkiewicz, especially in anatomic aberrations that involve an abnormal takeoff of that vessel. This complication may be avoided or minimized by not using methylprednisolone and using either betamethasone or triamcinolone acetonide while carefully monitoring distribution of the contrast after injection.[13] If a vascular confirmation or washout of the contrast is observed, it is prudent to reestablish the needle position to avoid an intravascular injection with potentially disastrous complications.[14]

Neuroplasty appears to be very effective in producing satisfactory pain relief in patients who have not responded to initial TFESI. Preinjection studies of the epidurogram may identify the affected nerve roots, and when the catheter is

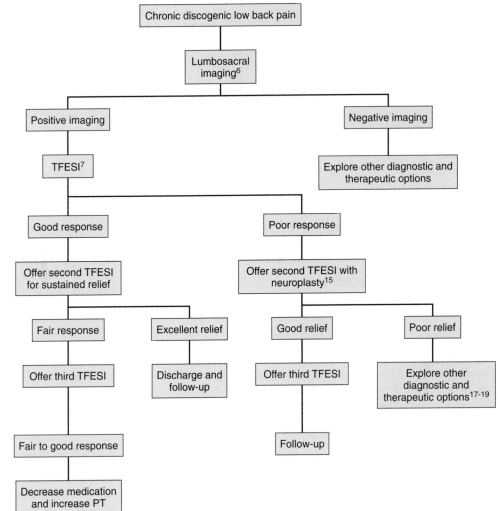

Figure 41-1 ▪ Algorithm for discogenic back pain. PT, physical therapy; TFESI, transforaminal epidural steroid injection.

placed closed to those nerve roots, satisfactory pain relief may occur. Our preference is to inject 8 mL of 10% hypertonic saline[15] through a caudal epidural catheter in the recovery area after verifying that no motor block exists after intraoperative caudal epidural injection of local anesthetics. If profound motor block exists 30 minutes after intraoperative injection, the catheter tip may be intrathecal. The catheter is then withdrawn and the percutaneous neuroplasty is aborted on the premise that 10% hypertonic saline may have neurolytic effects on the spinal cord if injected intrathecally. The actual epidural injection of hypertonic saline is usually painful, and the administration should be slow. Intravenous fentanyl (50 to 150 mEq) may be administered to minimize the discomfort associated with the injection. The patient should be kept in the lateral position with the painful side (and the side where the caudal epidural catheter is located in proximity to the nerve roots) dependent during the injection and for 15 to 20 minutes after the injection.

Neuroplasty may be also performed using a spinal endoscope (myeloscope)[16] for patients with intractable back pain associated with discogenic disease, and also for patients with failed back surgery syndrome. As in the case of percutaneous

epidural adhesiolysis (neuroplasty), the primary purpose of neuroplasty is to diminish or if possible eliminate the deleterious effects of epidural scar tissue, which may be a primary pain generator or may be physically preventing drugs from being deposited where they could be effective in reducing pain. Other potential mechanisms of action of epidural adhesiolysis with spinal endoscopy include the alteration of the pressure–volume relationships in the epidural space, and activation (stimulation) of dorsal column fibers. Although only a few controlled studies address the efficacy of adhesiolysis, the published clinical reports are exciting and encouraging. Our experience with this modality endorses the favorable reports; currently, in our institution, double-blind, randomized, placebo-controlled studies are addressing the issue of clinical efficacy of neuroplasty.

Some patients with chronic low back pain secondary to discogenic disease confirmed by MRI may not respond to epidural steroid injections or neuroplasty. In the absence of spinal stenosis (when lumbar facets may be the pain generators), discography may be useful in targeting the specific degenerated discs that may be responsible for the persisting chronic low back pain. Provocative discography may be useful in determining which patients might benefit from the following therapies: intradiscal electrothermal therapy (IDET),[17] nucleoplasty using bipolar radiofrequency coagulation,[18] minimally invasive surgery of the affected disc,[19] or orthopedic or neurosurgical discectomy.

It is often advisable to prevent or delay open surgical intervention because the postoperative results are not always very encouraging.[20] Many patients with postoperative pain (e.g., after discectomy or laminectomy) complain of more postprocedure pain than preprocedure pain. A common explanation for this phenomenon is the uncontrolled and unpredictable accumulation of epidural fibrosis and scar tissue in a very tight (i.e., restrictive) area. Properly selected patients with traumatized or inflamed annulus fibrosis and nucleolus pulposus respond to IDET[21] or nucleoplasty,[18] respectively. Recent studies suggest that these discogenic interventions are useful in relieving chronic low back pain in selected patients with discogenic pain.

Lumbar Facetogenic Disease

Chronic low back pain that originates in the facet or zygapophyseal joints may give rise to lumbar facet syndrome,[22] typically seen as mechanical low back pain that may be localized or may radiate to the buttocks and upper posterior thighs. The pain seldom radiates below the knees. There are significant variations in both clinical presentation and physical findings. Provocation of pain may be useful but usually does not produce reliable findings. Nevertheless, the elicitation of pain of rotation or twisting of the lumbar spine (the flexion test) appears to correlate with the presence of lumbar facetogenic disease. The lumbar facet joints are paired synovial joints with variable shapes and are innervated by the medial branches of the dorsal rami of L1, L2, L3, and L4 and by the dorsal ramus of L5. Unlike the medial branches of the dorsal rami of L1 through L4, which cross the base of the superior articular process at its junction with the transverse process, the dorsal ramus of L5 crosses the ala of the sacrum.[23] This variation is important when considering diagnostic and therapeutic lumbar facet blocks.

The lumbar facets may be blocked by fluoroscopically guided intra-articular injection[24] or by blocking the medial branches of the dorsal rami of L2 through S1. The efficacy of one procedure over another is unclear. The procedure chosen is usually based on the clinician's preference and expertise. However, an unsubstantiated clinical impression is that in the presence of a positive flexion test, intra-articular injection appears to be more effective than medial branch lumbar facet blocks, especially in the older population (older than 70 years). These blocks serve as diagnostic blocks,[25] and if pain relief is obtained, radiofrequency thermocoagulation lesioning[26] is performed for more definitive and sustained pain relief (Fig. 41-2). As with all neuraxial procedures, precautions for patients on anticoagulant and antiplatelet therapy must be observed. Most of these drugs are discontinued for 7 to 10 days before the procedure, and the relevant coagulation tests (prothrombin time; partial thromboplastin time; the International Normalized Ratio for drugs such as Coumadin, Plavix, and Lovenox; and bleeding time or platelet function assays for aspirin and related drugs) are performed

immediately before or the day before the procedure. Recent studies suggest that this approach for treating facetogenic back pain is highly efficacious in controlling pain.[27]

Lumbar Spinal Stenosis

In the middle to later decades of life (between 50 and 80 years of age), patients may present with lumbar spinal stenosis.[28] These patients usually have chronic low back pain, which is usually (but not always) associated with radiculopathy. The pathogenetic features of spinal stenosis involve an anatomic alteration of the intervertebral foramen, resulting in increased pressure on the lumbosacral nerve roots,[29] and this may be associated with thecal sac compression producing discrete neurologic changes. The contiguous structures surrounding the intervertebral foramen, including the ligamentum flavum, may be altered. In most MRI reports, the changes are referred to as ligamentum flavum hypertrophy—a misnomer because the true pathologic process is really buckling (and not hypertrophy) of the ligamentum flavum, which, together with the intervertebral disc, forms the posterior boundary of the intervertebral foramen. The resultant changes occurring in the intervertebral foramen cause alteration in the structural relationships of the lumbar facet joint, with painful consequences. This same process is accelerated when there is concomitant discogenic degeneration. Thus, the typical patient with lumbar spinal stenosis may have both discogenic and facetogenic pathology. Furthermore, the pain generators may be in one structure or in both. A full neuromuscular examination and a discerning review of the lumbosacral imaging data are useful in outlining an effective treatment plan.

Usually, a series of three transforaminal lumbar ESIs are planned at 2-week intervals with neuroplasty for lysis of epidural adhesions[30] and epidural fibrosis using 10% hypertonic saline, with hyaluronidase (Wydase) administered if the first or second epidural injections are not effective. If the pain generators are primarily discogenic, most patients obtain modest to significant pain relief. When pain relief is not evident, the possibility of facetogenic pain is very high. At that time and after clinical correlation, a diagnostic lumbar facet medial branch block is performed. If pain relief then becomes satisfactory from the patient's perspective, radiofrequency thermocoagulation lesioning of the medial branches of the posterior primary rami of L2 through S1 may be performed (Fig. 41-3).

The treatment of lumbar spinal stenosis may involve treating both discogenic and facetogenic pain.[31] Some patients may have other pain generators responsible for persistent low back pain in the presence of spinal stenosis. Fortunately, most of the pain in these patients is effectively controlled when the discogenic and facetogenic factors are treated. It is imperative to stress that ancillary support services including physical therapy, acupuncture, psychological services, occupational therapy, and a variety of pharmacologic agents including analgesics, NSAIDs, anticonvulsant drugs, and other analgesic adjuvants may be needed to effect pain control.

Sacroiliac Joint Arthropathy

The sacroiliac joint (SIJ) is a large joint that may produce low back pain when it is affected by degenerative or

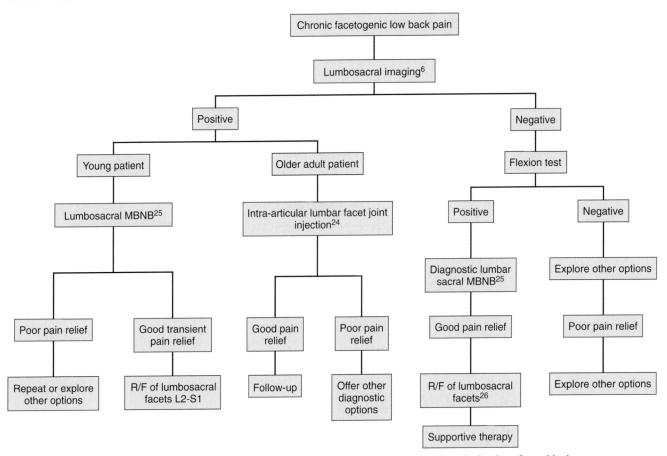

Figure 41-2 ■ Algorithm for facetogenic back pain. MBNB, medial branch lumbar facet block; R/F, radiofrequency thermocoagulation lesioning.

inflammatory disease processes. SIJ arthropathy[32] may mimic pain in the hip joint or low back pain of discogenic or facetogenic origin. Some patients even have radiculopathy associated with back pain. The clinical features of pain associated with SIJ arthropathy are not usually aggravated by hip flexion or by adduction or abduction of the hip joint, and there is usually well-localized tenderness over the SIJ itself. Radiography of the posterior lumbosacral area may show the degenerative characteristics of SIJ arthropathy, or the radiographs may appear normal.

Diagnostic SIJ blocks alone may be useful in controlling back pain associated with SIJ arthropathy. We have found that when the SIJ intra-articular injection was associated with transforaminal blocks of the anterior primary rami of S1 and S2, the resulting pain relief was more dramatic and longer-lasting than with SIJ blocks alone.[33] The rationale for this untested assumption was that branches from S1 and S2 directly innervate the SIJ joint on the ipsilateral side, and thus SIJ injection associated with the blocking of S1 and S2 provides better-quality and more sustained pain relief. For more sustained pain relief, radiofrequency thermocoagulation lesioning of the SIJ and S1 and S2[34] are implemented (Fig. 41-4). If both SIJs are involved and therefore painful, they

may be injected simultaneously without any significant complications.

Myofascial Pain Syndrome

Some patients have chronic low back pain that is characterized by generalized areas of pain that is nonspecific, nonradicular, and diffuse; intermittent in frequency; and, at times, migratory.[35] The etiologic basis of this pain, which can be referred to as myofascial pain syndrome, is chronic inflammation of the muscles, ligaments, tendons, and aponeuroses of the lumbar interspinous and paraspinous structures. Many patients with myofascial pain syndrome have other causes of chronic low back pain, including discogenic disease, facetogenic disease, spinal stenosis, and SIJ arthropathy. Furthermore, other systemic illnesses (e.g., collagen vascular disease, fibromyalgia, various myopathic syndromes, multiple myeloma, diabetic neuropathy, and other metabolic dysfunctional states) may mimic myofascial pain syndromes. The patients exhibit muscle spasm, muscle tension, muscle deficiency, and trigger points, all of which share an underlying inflammation of musculoskeletal paraspinous and supraspinous tissues of the lumbar spine.[36] Diagnosing myofascial pain syndrome involves a thorough history and physical

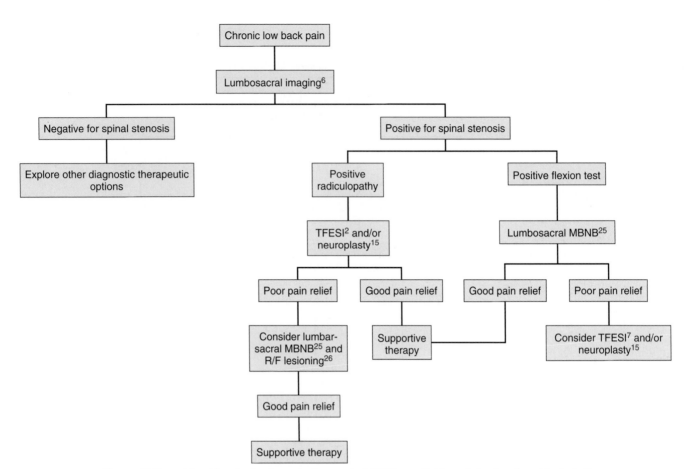

Figure 41-3 ■ Algorithm for lumbar spinal stenosis. MBNB, medial branch lumbar facet block; R/F, radiofrequency; TFESI, transforaminal epidural steroid injection.

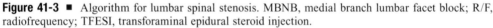
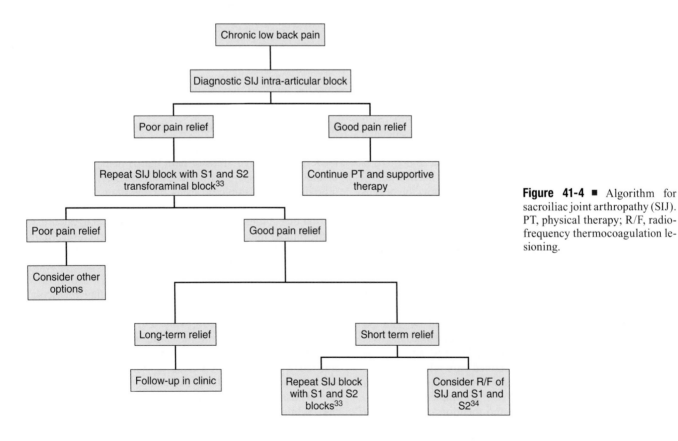

Figure 41-4 ■ Algorithm for sacroiliac joint arthropathy (SIJ). PT, physical therapy; R/F, radiofrequency thermocoagulation lesioning.

examination to exclude many of the systemic illnesses mentioned. Neurologic testing, laboratory investigation, lumbar radiographs, and lumbar spine imaging (MRI or CT scans, bone scans) are usually required to confirm or exclude a clinical impression before commencing treatment.

Treatment consists of trigger point injections (used widely when trigger points are identified), regenerative injection therapy (prolotherapy), acupuncture, acupressure, physical therapy, ice massage, heat, ethyl chloride spray, tetanizing currents, iontophoresis, stretching exercises, relaxation therapy, and the stretch-and-spray combination. When joints are involved in the pain syndrome, joint manipulation and mobilization, corrective and preventive measures, neuromuscular reeducation, and comprehensive exercise programs may be implemented.[37] The classic clinical features of trigger points include a palpable nodule, a positive "jump" sign, skin-fold hyperesthesia, and an increased hyperemia at the palpation site. When a muscle group (e.g., piriformis, longus colli, gluteal muscles) may be involved in the pain complex, selected peripheral nerve blocks (e.g., sciatic nerve block) may be effectively administered.

Generally, myofascial pain syndromes respond favorably to a number of therapeutic physical modalities. The most effective promote physical activity, relieve muscle tension, decrease muscle spasm, diminish tissue vasoconstriction, correct muscle deficiency, and decrease myofascial pain. The choice of modality depends on the patient and is reached with good clinical practice and sound judgment. A disadvantage of uni-disciplinary clinics is that a single modality may be used for all patients, and this is not appropriate in pain medicine.

Patients may present with back pain as a common denominator, but chronic low back pain has a variety of etiologies. Detailed history taking and meticulous neuromuscular examination with focused lumbar spine imaging usually produce a definitive diagnosis. When the diagnosis is not clear, an algorithm is useful for the logical evaluation and treatment of these patients.

■ CANCER PAIN

> We all must die. But that I can save him from days of torture, that is what I feel as my great and ever new privilege. Pain is a more terrible Lord of mankind than even death itself.
>
> ALBERT SCHWEITZER (1875-1965)

Cancer pain carries with it not only the pain and suffering[38] caused by the pathophysiologic and neurologic consequences of the tissue damage resulting from the cancer and cancer therapy but also the psychological and emotional trauma that is associated with the word *cancer*. Patients have fear of death and the possibility of prematurely ending relationships with family and friends; anxiety over surgery, chemotherapy, and radiotherapy to treat cancer (side effects of which may be worse than the cancer); concern over the spiritual and religious implications of death; and, if survival results, preoccupation over the morbidity of cancer and the complications of cancer therapy.

Cancer patients' pain can be caused by invasive pressure on surrounding nerves and plexuses, infiltration of mucosal and serosal membranes, secondary infection, lymphatic obstruction, vascular occlusions, thromboembolic phenomena, invasion of contiguous visceral organs, and involvement of periosteal structures. Cancer pain is usually classified as neuropathic[39] (lancinating, sharp, severe, and following a specific dermatomal distribution), as visceral (dull, vague, diffuse, and usually associated with nausea, vomiting, or bowel or urinary dysfunction), as somatic (musculoskeletal in origin, intermittent, fluctuating, aggravated by activity and relieved by rest), or as any combination of these.

Correctly identifying the location of the cancer is critical for determining and implementing appropriate pain therapy and producing satisfactory patient comfort. In this chapter, we explore the therapeutic options for cancer pain management in patients with pancreas carcinoma, breast carcinoma, and prostate carcinoma, as these affect patients of both sexes and all ethnic groups and ages.

Pain is the prevalent symptom in 40% to 60% of patients actively undergoing cancer therapy and may in fact be caused by the therapy,[40] whether it is surgery (neuroma-induced pain and phantom pain, somatic pain after autologous bone-marrow transplantation), chemotherapy (neuropathic pain), radiation (radiation plexopathy), or biological therapy. Familiarity with these cancer-related pain syndromes helps in making an accurate diagnosis and an optimal pain management plan. Herpes zoster and postherpetic neuralgia are other cancer-related syndromes that must be understood to optimize effective pain management in these patients. Furthermore, 80% to 90% of cancer patients with advanced carcinomatosis have significant pain.

The World Health Organization (WHO) and many other governmental agencies in the United States and abroad have recognized the importance of effective cancer pain management and have approved various guidelines, initiatives, and recommendations for managing cancer pain. The WHO three-step ladder recommendation remains a sound therapeutic structure for treating cancer pain patients. The three-step protocol is as follows[41]:

Step 1: Analgesic adjuvants (e.g., NSAIDs, cyclooxygenase [COX]-II inhibitors, anticonvulsants, tricyclic antidepressants, and other analgesic adjuvants)

Step 2: Weak opioids (e.g., oxycodone, codeine)

Step 3: Strong opioids (e.g., MS Contin, OxyContin, methadone, Kadian)

This protocol is effective in controlling pain in approximately 70% to 80% of cancer pain patients. However, the remaining 20% to 30% whose pain is not well controlled should not be left to suffer without hope, which does happen in facilities where cancer pain is not optimally managed. This situation is unnecessary, unkind, and rapidly becoming medicolegally unacceptable. However, most if not all oncologists have accepted the WHO recommendations or some variation of the three-step ladder and are implementing those recommendations fairly effectively. The current proposal of the pain community (not WHO) is that patients whose cancer pain is not controlled by the three-step ladder should be offered, when necessary and appropriate, interventional pain modalities—a fourth step of the WHO three-step ladder. When judiciously applied, these modalities may produce satisfactory pain relief and reduce the unnecessary suffering that patients with cancer pain have to bear. This is a noble, desirable, and attainable goal. Box 41-1 shows interventional pain modalities[42] that may be effective in controlling pain in cancer patients.

Interventional procedures for cancer pain patients, though intrinsically invasive, carry a relatively low risk of morbidity and mortality for several reasons: the adequate training and credentialing of most pain physicians, the preoperative monitoring associated with the procedures, the use of fluoroscopic guidance for precise needle placement, and proper patient selection and screening. When the end of the satisfactory quality of life is near, it is appropriate to introduce hospice interventions and palliative care.

A new direction in cancer pain management that may reduce the morbidity and perhaps the mortality associated with cancer pain management involves the study of the molecular mechanisms[43] of cancer pain. As a result, newer and possibly less invasive therapies may evolve. Recent progress in tumor detection, tumor markers, and tumor therapy will lead to newer therapies for control of the pain that follows tumor growth. Nociceptors and other specialized sensory neurons have a role in the transmission of sensory information from cancer-affected peripheral tissue to the brain and spinal cord. The impact of environmental factors (e.g., intracellular pH of solid tumors, cytokines, bradykinins, prostaglandins, endothelins, substance P, tumor growth factor, tumor necrosis factor, interleukin, platelet-derived growth factor, epidermal growth factor,[44] and others) is not clear. Many pathways and modes of action have been proposed for mechanisms that may initiate or aggravate cancer pain. Animal models of cancer pain are now available[45] and are already producing valuable data about the mechanisms that generate and maintain various kinds of cancer pain. Thus, a new generation of drugs and techniques may become available to effectively treat pain in cancer patients.

41-1	**Interventional Pain Modalities**

- Neuraxial and major plexus blocks
- Neurolytic blocks
- Systemic radioisotopes (brachytherapy)
- Palliative radiation therapy
- Radiofrequency thermocoagulation lesioning
- Neuroaugmentation techniques including opioid pump implantable devices
- Neurostimulation techniques including dorsal column and peripheral nerve stimulation
- Injection of agents that inhibit specific molecular and neurobiological targets on cancer cells
- Palliative surgery
- Intravenous, epidural, intrathecal, intraventricular, and dermoclytic infusion of both opioid and nonopioid agents

From Manchikanti L, Heavner J, Racz GB, et al: Pain Physician 2003;6:89-111.

Cancer of the Pancreas

Patients with cancer of the pancreas may present with nausea, vomiting, abdominal distention, flatulence, jaundice, and general malaise. Lesions of the body and tail of the pancreas may not be associated with pain until the disease is very advanced. Tumors involving the head of the pancreas are usually painful as a result of involvement of the many structures in close proximity to the pancreatic head. In most cases of pancreas cancer, life expectancy is diminished (6 months to 3 years) and the prognosis is poor.

When a tumor is identified early and in patients with a fair prognosis, pain management begins with the three-step WHO recommendation, and strong opioids are used earlier rather than later. Intravenous opioid infusion via patient-controlled analgesia (PCA)[46] may be used. The definitive treatment is diagnostic celiac plexus block using a two-needle technique. If adequate pain relief is obtained, a neurolytic celiac plexus block[47] with 6% phenol in 10% glycerin or with absolute alcohol is performed. If that procedure is unsuccessful in relieving pain, and if the prognosis is greater than 3 months, a permanent morphine pump (preceded by a 24-hour in-patient trial of intrathecal or epidural morphine) is implanted (Fig. 41-5). For patients with a poor prognosis, a continuous epidural morphine infusion using a micro-jet pump is used for pain control. Supplemental pain control may be attained using Duragesic patch, Actiq (fentanyl lollipop), and other analgesic adjuvants, depending on the clinical presentation and the symptoms.

Cancer of the Breast

The oncologic treatment of cancer of the breast has improved dramatically. Life expectancy and breast cancer survival continue to be lengthened for many reasons: early detection through routine mammography and via intraductal sampling technologies, awareness of the role of family history in the epidemiology of breast cancer, revised surgical techniques, aggressive radiotherapeutic protocols, increased understanding of angiogenesis, new chemotherapy agents, enhanced awareness of cancer-prevention techniques and beneficial lifestyle changes (in diet, exercise, smoking), promotion of regular self-examination, and improved mammography techniques.[48] Early and aggressive therapy is individualized to the patient and ultimately produces a decrease in the pain that used to be associated with breast cancer.

Pain becomes an issue in patients who develop bony metastases and infiltration to contiguous structures (e.g., lungs, mediastinum, pleura) and in those who develop hematogenous or lymphatic spread to the brain, liver, or other organs. Pain in patients with breast cancer may come not from the cancer per se but as a consequence of radiation, surgery, or chemotherapy. Breast cancer patients who have had radiation may develop brachial plexopathy, radiation neuritis, osteoradionecrosis, and pathologic fractures. Patients who receive chemotherapy may develop peripheral neuropathy and chemotherapy-induced immune suppression, which may result in herpes zoster[49] infection with associated postherpetic neuralgia.[50]

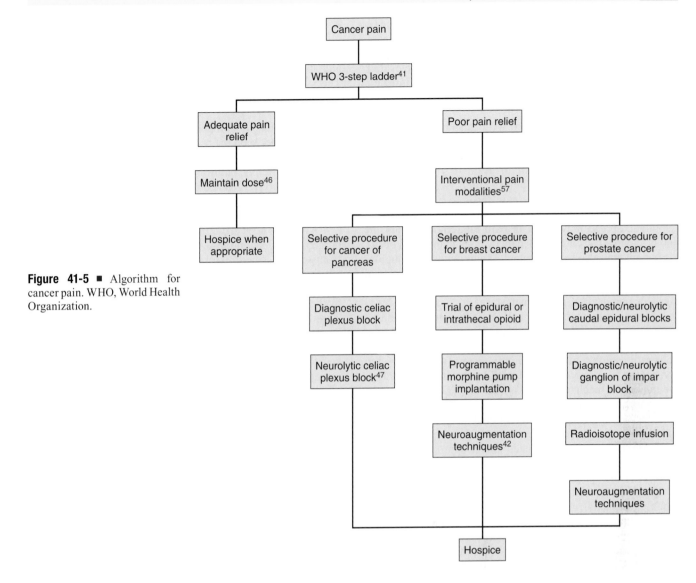

Figure 41-5 ■ Algorithm for cancer pain. WHO, World Health Organization.

The treatment of pain associated with breast cancer depends on the clinical presentation. As in most cancer patients, the first line of therapy is to initiate the WHO three-step ladder recommendation. Specific attention should be paid to diagnosis of the pain-related syndromes that are associated with breast cancer and its therapy. The use of strong opioids is warranted and application of opioid delivery systems is usually indicated—for example, intravenous, epidural, intrathecal, intraventricular, intranasal, subcutaneous, dermoclysis, and sublingual routes. Controlled-release opioids[51] (e.g., MS Contin, OxyContin, Kadian, Avinza), supplemented with breakthrough immediate-release opioids, are a good therapeutic option. A good scheme for opioid administration is as follows:

1. By mouth (whenever possible)
2. By the clock (not using the as-needed [PRN] approach)
3. By the WHO ladder

Neuroaugmentation techniques including morphine intrathecal pump implants should always be available for patients who have a prognosis of more than 3 months and for whom more conservative therapies have failed to adequately control pain (see Fig. 41-5).

Cancer of the Prostate

Although the prostate cancer rate appeared to increase toward the end of the 1900s, prognosis and survival have modestly improved in recent years. The reasons for this improvement include early diagnosis, routine prostatic specific antigen (PSA) screening, enhanced health awareness, improved techniques for treatment, decreased morbidity associated with surgery (e.g., use of nerve-sparing procedures for prostatectomy has decreased the incidence of postprostatectomy impotence), and, probably more importantly, changes in lifestyle (smoking, diet, exercise). Prostate cancer, like cancers of the breast, thyroid, lung, and kidney, commonly metastasize to bony structures, and patients often present with back pain. Lumbosacral metastases are frequent. When unexplained low back pain occurs in men older than 45 years, prostate cancer or multiple myeloma should be ruled out. When routine screening reveals that PSA levels are elevated, tumors of the prostate are diagnosed long before the prostatic capsule is infiltrated and usually before bony metastases have occurred.

Most of the pain associated with cancer of the prostate is caused by pelvic and perineal infiltration. These infiltrations may be associated with bowel and urinary obstruction or dysfunction and also with invasion of the contiguous osseous structures (sacrum, pubis, ilium, ischium, femoral head, and femoral neck). The pain tends to be more severe when periosteal involvement is extensive. Hematogenous and lymphatic spread may result in pain far removed from the pelvis and low back area. When metastases to the skull occur, the patient may also have sphenoidal sinus metastases, jugular foramen syndrome, clivus metastases, orbital and periorbital pain, fractures of the odontoid process, middle fossa metastases, or parasagittal region metastases.

Effective therapies for pain secondary to these metastatic deposits include the use of NSAIDs, strong opioids, and PCA with morphine or hydromorphone (Dilaudid). Intravenous radioisotope infusion and radiotherapy are also used to control the pain of bony metastases. As new developments in the molecular mechanisms of pain develop, newer drugs and newer techniques should evolve.

There is a role for interventional pain modalities[7] in the management of prostate cancer. As in other cancer pain syndromes, the WHO three-step ladder approach to pain is used first, and 70% to 80% of patients obtain satisfactory pain relief. For patients who do not respond, an alternative is diagnostic caudal epidural block followed by neurolytic block with phenol. As perineal involvement becomes widespread, ganglion impar block (both diagnostic and neurolytic) may be used. Intrathecal morphine trials with subsequent implantation of a programmable morphine pump with an intrathecal catheter may be used in patients with a life expectancy of greater than 3 months. In patients with a life expectancy of less than 3 months, an epidural catheter is inserted and the distal end of the catheter is tunneled approximately 5 to 6 inches away from the midline. A micro-jet pump can be used to infuse morphine or hydromorphone to facilitate delivery of the drug. In these circumstances, the implanted catheter can be kept in place without infection for several weeks. Prophylactic antibiotics can also be used to prevent infection and allow prolonged catheter use (see Fig. 41-5).

Several cancer-related pain syndromes[52] may develop in the course of cancer therapy, especially in patients who have received immunosuppressing chemotherapy. These include herpes zoster and postherpetic neuralgia, peripheral neuropathy secondary to chemotherapy, perineal dysesthesia, osteonecrosis, and a variety of postradiation syndromes including lumbar plexopathy, radiation neuritis, radiation myopathy, meralgia paresthetica, and radiation-induced peripheral nerve tumors. Most of these syndromes involve neuropathic pain, and appropriate therapy (especially steroids) is initiated.

■ CERVICOGENIC HEADACHE

Cervicogenic headache[53,54] involves a pattern of headaches, and its diagnosis and prospective therapies are evolving. The syndrome occurs as a result of nociceptive structures within the neck that precipitate neck pain and subsequent headache.

The headache component reflects the neuroanatomic relationship between the neck and the trigeminal nerve pathways, which involves the upper three cervical roots and the trigeminal afferent pathways.[55] The neurophysiologic pathways at this convergence of the cervical and trigeminal pathways explain the occipito-frontotemporal expression of symptoms in this group of patients.

Although neck structures are believed to be the primary progenitor of symptoms, these symptoms could originate from several structures in the neck, and imaging studies do not show the cause of the neck pain and headache.[56] The difficulty in diagnosing cervicogenic headache is compounded by the evolving description of the headache pattern. The early classification of this headache pattern, like that of the primary headache disorders, was based on clinical presentation, as no specific diagnostic parameters (e.g., underlying pathology, neurobiological markers) were available. Furthermore, on initial evaluation, there appears to be some clinical overlap of cervicogenic headache and the primary headache disorders.

The clinical presentation of cervicogenic headache is a unilateral (side-locked) pattern.[54,57] The pain tends to have a dull and aching pattern associated with headache with specific postural movements of the head. Additional but less common features include nausea, photophobia, and phonophobia, so the presentation may appear migrainous in nature.

The two major classification schemes come from the International Association for the Study of Pain (IASP) and the International Headache Society.[58] The major difference between the two classifications is that the IHS criteria require the presence of pathology. This requirement is not readily satisfied, even when the clinical picture is satisfied and there is a positive response to a nerve block.

If the primary basis of the pattern of pain is injury to the small fibers (A-delta and C), demonstration of injury is difficult, which results in a lower prevalence rate of cervicogenic headache. The different populations examined and the different methodologies and diagnostic criteria used result in a wide range of prevalence rates.

The differential diagnosis for cervicogenic headache includes migraine, hemicrania continua, and cluster and tension headache. Although there are overlapping features, distinguishing elements include the indomethacin response exhibited by cluster headache and hemicrania continua. The strict definitions of cervicogenic headache require that it be side locked. Migraine, on the contrary, tends to be unilateral with side shift, and tension headache tends to be bilateral.

Among the many criteria for the diagnosis of cervicogenic headache, the critical one is the presence of neck pain, which can be further divided into traumatic and nontraumatic etiologies. This may provide additional insight into the mechanisms of injury and thus direct medical management.

Epidemiology

The presence of neck pain in the general population is quite variable, with a lifetime prevalence of 13% to 50%.[59] Neck pain is not consistently linked to pathology in the cervical spine and may occur in the absence of significant neck pathology. In fact, significant spinal pathology may occur without any neck pain. The inability to confidently relate neck pain to underlying radiologic abnormalities causes difficulties in choosing among therapeutic treatment schemes. It helps to be able to determine whether there was a traumatic event.

Pathophysiology

Cervicogenic headache presents a significant clinical challenge. These patients may have a history of associated injury, with wide variation in the expression of underlying pathology, or none at all. The crux of the dilemma is a lack of a corroborating anatomic or neurophysiologic testing scheme.

There are two possible mechanisms that might account for the paradox of pain without clear injury. If tissue injury is presumed to be an important mechanism, the associated inflammatory milieu is presumed to be the trigger for the nociceptive response involving A-delta and C fibers. The primary etiology of the clinical presentation stems from the relationship between the C1 through C3 nerve roots, which mediate sensory input from the proximal cervical structures believed to contribute to this syndrome. These proximal cervical nerve roots converge on the descending trigeminal tracts to create the trigeminal cervical pathway, which readily facilitates the conduction of bidirectional nociceptive impulses between the neck and head. It is this convergence of the cervical and trigeminal afferent fibers that sets the stage for headache patterns that mimic the primary headache syndromes.

Furthermore, the relationship between the peripheral and central afferent pathways[60] sets the stage for central remodeling based on peripheral input, leading to persistent pain despite resolution of the initial tissue-injuring event. The injury leads to a series of physiologic events that culminate in a chronic pain state.

Several structures in the neck are sites of pain generation. Knowing the most likely site of tissue injury leads to a rational approach to treating the symptoms. Neurophysical testing of the injury reveals differences in thermal patterns in patients with cervicogenic injury and can help predict the prognosis for recovery. If the injury cannot be documented and the patient's course cannot be followed qualitatively or quantitatively, giving appropriate care is challenging. Sites that may represent sites of nociception include the atlanto-occipital joint, atlantoaxial joint, C2-3 facet joint, C2-C3 disc, C1 through C3 spinal nerve roots, and the musculature of the neck.

Psychological factors can confound the treatment path. One goal is to determine whether the patient has a mixed (or singular) pattern of persistent nociceptive input, or this is combined with a psychological element, or the pattern is predominantly psychological.

Unilateral Headaches

Identifying cervicogenic headache with the strictest criteria for unilateral headache is difficult, because symptoms in these patients are similar to symptoms in patients with primary headache. Up to 18% of patients with cervicogenic headache share a pattern of unilateral pain, nausea, neck and scalp tenderness, photophobia, and phonophobia with patients who have migraine without aura (Table 41-1).

The differential diagnosis for cervicogenic headache includes migraine, cluster headaches, hemicrania continua, and tension headache.[61,62] Each of these headache patterns possesses a clinical and epidemiologic pattern that may facilitate making the diagnosis (see Table 41-1).

Noninterventional Treatment Schemes

Physical therapy is the least aggressive therapy and is commonly used first.[63,64] Patients' responses to physical therapy are quite variable, and few randomized controlled trials have had adequate follow-up. The difficulty in blinding the patient to therapy contributes to the lack of studies with the statistical power to support outcomes.

Many treatment schemes for neck pain, alone or associated with headache, have become part of the standardized

41-1 **Unilateral Headache Patterns**				
	Cervicogenic Headache	**Migraine**	**Cluster Headache**	**Hemicrania Continua**
Sex	M:F 1.4	M:F 1.3	M:F 4.1	M < F
Headache location	Fixed (Side shift)	Side shift	Fixed	Fixed
Pain location	Occiput Frontoparietal	Frontal, orbital	Temporal, orbital	Occipitofrontal
Precipitating factor	Neck movement Neck triggers	Not neck	None	Not neck
Standard therapies	M, I	M	M	M
Evolving therapies	Bion ONS	Bion ONS	DBS	—

Bion, microstimulator; DBS, deep brain stimulator; I, interventional; M, medical. ONS, occipital nerve stimulator.

approach to management even though there are few randomized controlled studies that demonstrate their efficacy. Common modes of therapy include medical management with NSAIDs, muscle relaxants, opioids, physical therapy, manipulation, and soft collars. Despite the paucity of data, this stepwise and conservative approach is useful for the early management of these patients. When data from randomized controlled trials are available, clinical outcomes will improve because efforts will focus on the effective therapies.

Noninterventional management of cervicogenic headache typically progresses in a stepwise fashion, beginning with a pharmaceutical approach. NSAIDs are frequently used in conjunction with muscle relaxants, tricyclic antidepressants, and membrane-stabilizing agents. Few studies have shown positive outcomes with these drugs, although they have become a standard part of care.

Electrotherapy via a transcutaneous electrical nerve stimulation (TENS) unit[65] has demonstrated significant efficacy in a heterogeneous population of patients with headache and neck pain. Central to this therapy is the gate control theory of pain developed by Melzack and Wall.[66] Transcutaneous stimulation results in the inhibition of afferent A-delta and C nociceptive fibers. Significant efficacy has been demonstrated, although the subsequent development of tolerance leads to a decline in the therapeutic response within several months.

Interventional Therapies

Interventional therapies are directed at the structures in the neck believed to cause the pain.[67] The structures that could contribute to cervicogenic pain include the musculature of the cervical spine, ligaments, joints, cervical nerve roots, dorsal root ganglion, and peripheral nerves of the neck. An appropriate procedure is chosen on the basis of the history, examination, and presenting clinical picture. The treatment paradigm begins with the least invasive therapy and progresses to more invasive therapies, depending on the patient's response. Very few randomized controlled trials have been performed to determine the effectiveness or timing of these therapies.

Nerve or field blocks are the first-line interventional therapies. The goals are to localize the site of pain. Although the patient who gets optimal analgesia exhibits relief, the clinician cannot be sure whether this was the result of interrupting nociceptor conduction at the pain site or along the path of pain. Interpretation is further confounded by the possibility of false-positive and false-negative responses. The double-block paradigm (two blocks separated in time and consisting of a long- and a short-acting anesthetic) helps to define the response. The structure targeted is based on the ease of access, degree of patient risk, and the physical examination and history.

Occipital Nerve Blocks

The occipital nerves originate from the dorsal rami of C2 (greater occipital) and C3 (lesser occipital). Occipital neuralgia is often described in headache patients but is more commonly associated with trauma. Patients describe a paroxysmal pattern of paresthesias radiating from the occiput to the frontal regions.

The several techniques suggested for the performance of this block have varied responses because of the inconsistent nerve anatomy. Infiltration of 3 to 5 mL of local anesthetic in proximity to the nuchal ridge results in sensory blockade along the distribution of the occipital nerve. The typical response rate of 60% to 70% (in the personal experience of author LR) suggests that this may be an efficacious starting point in terms of interventional therapies. Unfortunately, the block often needs to be repeated.

Cryoanalgesia is a reversible neurolytic option that readily extends the benefit of a nerve block for up to 6 months. This procedure can be readily repeated with no significant adverse outcome. Radiofrequency (RF) is another option for treatment of this region. Experience has been rather limited with RF, but the primary concern is the risk of neuritis. Pulse RF,[67,68] an alternative that uses an electromagnetic field with a cool lesion at 42°C, appears to have some promise, but long-term studies will better assess its utility.

Zygapophyseal Joints

The zygapophyseal joints, which are formed by the superior articular surface of one vertebra and the inferior articular surface of the vertebra above, are implicated in the initiation and prolongation of cervicogenic headache.[69] Their primary functions are to limit extreme range of motion of the cervical spine and distribute excessive mechanical forces throughout the cervical spine.

Innervation of the zygapophyseal joints consists of the medial branch nerve of the joint at its level with an additional level of innervation from the joint below. The C2-3 level is an exception, as innervation there is supplied by the third occipital nerve, which has a deep and a superficial branch. The large superficial branch supplies the bulk of the innervation, and there is a smaller contribution from the C2 medial branch nerve.

Treatment of the cervicogenic headache via the facet joints involves primarily the C2-3 through the C7-T1 facets.[70] The atlanto-occipital and atlantoaxial joints have been implicated to a lesser degree in these headaches. The C2-3 joint and possibly the C3-4 joint are the most important in the management of cervicogenic headache. Each has been demonstrated to refer pain to a characteristic region of the head and neck; the C2-3 region produces the most stereotypical pattern associated with headache.

Both medial branch nerve block and intra-articular block have been associated with headache relief. However, double-blind, placebo-controlled, randomized studies have been conducted only with medial branch nerve block.[68,71] This demonstrated significant efficacy with cervical facet joints. Utilizing the double-block paradigm, patients with a positive response are ideal candidates for nerve thermocoagulation via radiofrequency ablation. This coagulative process can extend the therapeutic benefit of the local anesthetic block by several months.

Atlanto-occipital and Atlantoaxial Joints

Neural blockade of the atlanto-occipital and atlantoaxial joints requires considerable expertise because of their proximity to critical brain structures. Although procedures were defined for destruction of the sensory innervation of the facet joints, this has not been done for these joints.

Cervical Nerves

Cervical epidural steroid injections can be administered via a generalized translaminar approach. The steroid is typically diluted with saline and injected in a manner that spreads the mixture in a diffuse, nonspecific manner.[72] Alternatively, the transforaminal approach (or selective nerve root injection) involves directed injections to specific nerve roots. The response to epidural steroid injection is quite variable. Although it was once believed that patients whose pain had a radicular component would be more responsive to epidural injections, it is now evident that both somatic and radicular patterns respond.

The major limitation of this therapeutic modality is that injections should not be administered too frequently. The inherent risk associated with an excessive steroid load typically limits the injection schemes to two to three injections per 6-month period.

Cervical Disc

The cervical disc has been implicated in up to 40% of cervicogenic headache and neck pain syndromes.[73] MRI and CT may be somewhat helpful, but for many of these patients the optimal testing scheme is physiologic, using provocative discography. The discogenic etiology of the symptoms may be revealed in the setting of normal radiologic imaging.

Experimental schemes have involved treatment of the disc with radiofrequency lesioning. Although no randomized controlled trials have been performed with this therapy, some positive results have been seen. Management of cervical discogenic pain without surgery is a significant challenge. Figure

41-6 shows an interventional algorithm for cervicogenic headache.

Neuromodulation

Neuromodulation is evolving as an effective treatment for cervicogenic headache and migraine. Weiner and Reed[68] demonstrated that a wide range of cervical pathology is responsive to occipital nerve stimulation.[74] There are both peripheral and central elements to the therapy.[75]

Clinical and basic science efforts continue to reveal the neurophysiologic relationship between the trigeminal and cervical pathways and lead to therapeutic advances.

Peripheral nerve stimulation, which is an extension of treatments used for other chronic neuropathic pain states, can be directed toward patients who have failed conventional medical and nerve block therapies. It therapy requires a subcutaneous lead with electrodes and a combined power source–programming unit (off-label use of spinal cord stimulation devices). Anecdotal experience has demonstrated that up to 80% of patients with migraine or cervicogenic headaches that are refractory to conventional medical and interventional therapies have experienced a significant positive response.[76]

A limitation of these lead-based devices is that wires must traverse the neck, and they are connected to the pulse generator (power source). The leads are prone to migration because of the mobility of the neck, and cases of lead fracture have been noted. Nevertheless, the therapy has the potential to be quite efficacious, and three U.S. Food and Drug Administration trials are under way to explore the full utility of this treatment.

Peripheral nerve stimulation has evolved as a therapy with the introduction of the Bion microstimulator (Advanced Bionics Corp., Sylmar, Calif). This new device (27 mm in length and 3 mm in diameter) is a self-contained microstimulator with a rechargeable battery. The absence of leads reduces the risk of migration and fracture and enables patients to return to full activity with essentially no restrictions

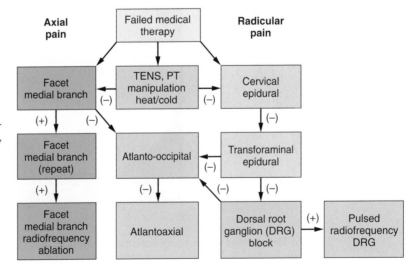

Figure 41-6 ■ An interventional algorithm for cervicogenic headache. PT, physical therapy; TENS, transcutaneous electronic nerve stimulation.

(personal experience of author LR with 13 patients). The monopolar device is placed percutaneously in proximity to the occipital nerve with specialized tools that involve an injection mechanism, which has been well accepted by patients in preliminary feasibility studies. Figure 41-7 demonstrates the Bion device being implanted into a patient.

The management of cervicogenic headache is evolving rapidly as we gain greater understanding of trigeminocervicogenic pathways. The management of this disease process will certainly include interventional therapies and microimplant technologies to treat headaches with cervicogenic etiology.[77]

■ POSTOPERATIVE PAIN

The management of postoperative pain is a critical perioperative element for the surgical patient.[78] Preoperatively, many patients are anxious about having significant and uncontrolled postoperative pain. The literature is quite full of pain management schemes,[79] and in this chapter we will only highlight the salient features of current management schemes.

Acute pain in the postoperative setting tends to be more easily defined than chronic pain. The region of the injury and its mechanism are identifiable, whether it originated with a surgical insult, was a preexisting injury, or is a combination of both. It begins with a maximal state of discomfort, which diminishes over time. On the other hand, chronic pain has a poorly defined etiology and progresses with incremental requirements for more aggressive treatment. In the postoperative setting, the treatment of acute pain is thus aggressive at the onset of and/or anticipation of pain, and the requirement for therapy diminishes as the initiating insult resolves.

The primary goals of postoperative acute pain management are to reduce physiologic and psychological discomfort associated with the insult, and to reduce the risk of having the acute conditions evolve into a chronic pain syndrome. Effective management of the acute pain state requires therapy tailored to the patient's specific requirements as dictated by site, surgical intervention, and the patient's ability to delineate an ideal choice.

In a dedicated pain service, the providers (physician and nursing staff) appreciate the fundamental principles of postoperative interventional treatment. Involvement of the patient is ideal to facilitate optimal management. When surgery is elective, staff members can educate patients about therapeutic options, learn what their expectations are, and find out about their past experiences, which may adversely impact their current expectations. Postoperative pain management begins with preoperative assessment. The anticipated procedure and the patient's comorbid medical conditions, psychological state, and age are factors that contribute to finding the best option for the individual patient.

The best options for pain management fall into four categories[80]:

- Intravenous PCA
- Epidural PCA
- Regional anesthesia
- Pharmacologic adjuvant therapies

The first three have shown significant efficacy in managing postoperative pain. The selection is based on patient-related factors, practitioner skill in performing regional and neuraxial procedures, and any associated mitigating factors. Published treatment algorithms can show the ideal management scheme for a given region undergoing surgery.[81]

In the healthy elective surgical patient, challenges to postoperative pain are readily defined, but several groups of patients have special requirements[82]:

- Children
- Older adults

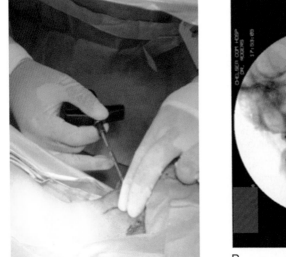
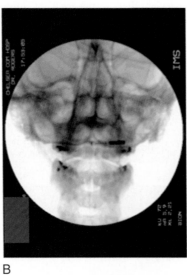
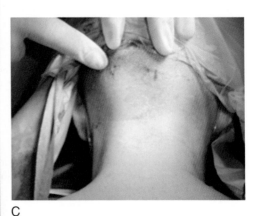

A

B

C

Figure 41-7 ■ Bion device being implanted in a patient. **A,** The introducer tool is placed into the subcutaneous tissue. **B,** The Bion in proximity to the nerve. **C,** The fully deployed Bion. *(Photos courtesy of Anne Traywick.)*

- Patients with cognitive impairment
- Patients with a preexisting chronic pain condition
- Patients with a previous history of substance abuse

For children, the surgical arena may precipitate significant anxiety. The distress associated with needles can be significant, particularly if a prior exposure was negative. Postoperative evaluation of the pediatric patient can be challenging. The disruption of the normal psychosocial environment for children can be so distressing that it can be difficult to determine whether that or the surgical insult is the primary cause of distress. The tendency to undermedicate pediatric patients arises partly from concern about opioid complications. When applicable, neuraxial anesthesia is initiated via the caudal route.

Older adults may have comorbid conditions in addition to sensitivity to the central effects of medications, and these two factors may contribute to less than satisfactory analgesia. For some patients, the extent of the associated comorbid medical conditions may limit the options for post-surgical care. The preoperative assessment will provide insights to plan the most efficacious and safe mode of management.

A history of substance abuses can pose a significant challenge in the recovery room.[83] Many of these patients have preexisting chronic pain and are being treated with opioids. There is a tendency to undermedicate patients in this group, but they may have low pain thresholds, and their opioid requirements may increase postoperatively. Their current medication regimen should be reviewed with a view toward opioid supplementation for the acute surgical insult. The opioid level can then be titrated until the patient is comfortable. When feasible, regional or neuraxial analgesia should be explored. Consultations with specialists in psychiatry, addiction medicine, and chronic pain may be required.

■ DELIRIUM

> Everywhere I see bliss from which I alone am irrevocably excluded.
>
> MARY SHELLEY (1797-1851)

Delirium is an acute confusional state that occurs in many systemic illnesses. It is characterized by an alteration in the level of consciousness and a diminished ability to maintain and focus attention on activities of normal daily living. The result is a cognitive or perceptual disturbance that is not associated with a predetermined clinical condition (e.g., stroke, brain tumor). Its duration is unpredictable, and it may have diurnal variations. It may be caused by a medical condition (e.g., hepatic encephalopathy, drug or alcohol intoxication) or it may be a side effect of narcotic, sedative, or psychoactive agents. Many of the disease entities associated with delirium are predictable. However, its occurrence is often unanticipated, and the clinician must be vigilant for these circumstances and be able to provide a diagnosis and an effective treatment.

Definition

The American Psychiatric Association's Diagnostic and Statistical Manual—Fourth edition (DSM-IV)[84] lists the following features that characterize delirium:

1. There is a change in the cognition or the development of a perceptual disturbance that is not better accounted for by a preexisting established or evolving dementia.
2. There is a disturbance of consciousness with diminished ability to focus, sustain, or shift attention.
3. There is evidence from history, physical examination, or laboratory findings that the disturbance is caused by a medical condition, substance intoxication, or medication side effects.
4. The disturbance develops over a short period of time and tends to fluctuate during the course of the day.
5. There are psychomotor behavioral disturbances, such as hypoactivity, hyperactivity, and increased sympathetic activity, and impairment in sleep duration or architecture.
6. There are variable emotional disturbances including, fear, depression, euphoria, and perplexity.

Although delirium is considered by most experts to be a variation of the confusional state,[85] not all confusional states can be called delirium. Elements of confusional states that are not necessarily associated with delirium include agitation, tremor, and hallucinations. However, there is not a generally accepted distinction between delirium and confusional states, and some terms (metabolic encephalopathy, toxic encephalopathy, acute brain syndrome, acute confusional state) have been used loosely to describe both. Patients described as having an acute confusional state may in fact have an acute state of altered consciousness, characterized by disordered attention, diminished clarity and coherence of thought, and diminished speed of performing and ability to perform basic tasks. Although this characterization may include some patients with delirium, patients with an acute confusional state have reduced alertness and psychomotor activity. On the other hand, patients with delirium may have, in addition to the essential characteristics of an acute confusional state, increased vigilance with psychomotor[86] and autonomic overactivity while displaying agitation, excitement, tremulousness, hallucinations, fantasies, and delusions.

Pathogenesis

The pathophysiology of either acute confusional state or of delirium is not well understood. There are several theories, but none offers a substantive explanation of the clinical condition. Because so many etiologic factors could produce delirium, it is very unlikely that a single mechanism is the cause. The molecular basis of delirium is not clearly understood, but investigations involving techniques based on brain imaging, neurotransmitter assays, and innovative electrophysiologic tests are ongoing and may provide some clues. The following factors may contribute to the pathogenesis of delirium.

Cortical Mechanisms. Electroencephalographic studies[87] in acutely ill patients have established that there is a disturbance of global cortical function, characterized by slowing of the dominant posterior alpha rhythm and the appearance of abnormal slow-wave activity. The findings were consistent with the observed clinical behavior and also the level of consciousness shown in the patients studied, regardless of the underlying etiology. These observations suggested that there is a final common neural pathway in the elicitation of delirium. However, when delirium was associated with alcohol or sedative drug withdrawal, the electroencephalographic findings were different: there was fast-wave activity that was associated with low voltage. Further investigations focusing on the brainstem auditory evoked potentials, neuroimaging studies, and, more recently, somatosensory evoked potentials have tended to suggest a subcortical basis for the clinical presentation of delirium. Potential subcortical sites include the pontine reticular formation, basal ganglia, and thalamus.[88] Some theories suggest that both cortical and subcortical structures may be involved in the general pathogenesis of delirium.

Neurotransmitter and Humoral Mechanisms. The role of acetylcholine in the pathogenesis of delirium is well established. Anticholinergic drugs may cause delirium in healthy volunteers, especially in older adults or cachectic patients whose systemic metabolism may be compromised.[89,90] Also, cholinesterase inhibitors (e.g., physostigmine) may reverse the effects induced by anticholinesterase drugs. Some clinical conditions (e.g., hypoglycemia, hypoxia, thiamine deficiency) are characterized by delirium, and the precipitating factor may very well be a decreased synthesis of acetylcholine in the central nervous system. Patients with Alzheimer's disease have been shown to have a decreased level of cholinergic neurons, and the risk of delirium may decrease when anticholinergic medications are administered. Thus, the anticholinergic mechanism may be a pathway for the production of delirium in patients with a variety of clinical conditions, because many drugs have a muscarinic binding effect on cholinergic receptors.

Signs of Attention. Judgment and insight depend on a high[8] level of integrated cortical function. When this system is dysfunctional, delirium and, in some cases, confusional states occur. The result is disruption of arousal and attention at the levels of the ascending reticular activation system and the pons.

Risk Factors. Factors that increase the risk of delirium and confusional states[91] include brain disease (e.g., stroke, dementia, and Parkinson's disease), advancing age, and sensory impairment. Each factor may coexist with others, compounding the clinical appearance of delirium.

Precipitating Factors. Factors that may precipitate the onset of delirium, or that may aggravate mild clinical symptoms of delirium, include polypharmacy, dehydration, malnutrition, systemic infection, immobility, and the prolonged use of bladder catheters. Polypharmacy is a factor because the side effects and potential drug interactions of some newer drugs may not be anticipated.

Related Clinical Syndromes

Several clinical syndromes are closely related to delirium, or delirium is an important part of their clinical manifestation. Patients with advanced cancer may develop delirium; it is usually underdiagnosed, and many patients may die in a state of delirium that has not been diagnosed or treated. The delirious state associated with alcohol and sedative withdrawal may produce significant pathophysiologic conditions that may even result in death. Hepatic encephalopathy is also associated with state of delirium; usually, this is a premorbid condition that forecasts hepatic failure.

Epidemiology

Delirium and acute confusional state have been studied primarily in the controlled environment of the hospital setting. Most cases of delirium occur outside the hospital: in nursing homes and assisted living facilities. Acute confusional state and delirium may occur perioperatively, particularly in the postanesthesia care unit.[92]

Delirium is also seen in the emergency department, where patients may arrive with a drug overdose or in the setting of psychotropic drug and recreational drug abuse. In the hospice environment, where patients are in advanced stages of cancer, chemotherapy, radiotherapy, or analgesic or psychoactive drugs may all contribute to delirium.

The economic impact of delirium can be considerable. Patients are usually admitted to the hospital, and the cost of investigations and the subsequent treatment add to the cost of health care.[93] Delirium is associated with a high incidence of mortality, and although it is potentially reversible, it may represent a decline in cerebral and general systemic function.

Clinical Features

The onset of delirium is characterized by a disturbance of consciousness and the appearance of altered cognition, which may fluctuate during the course of a day. It is associated with the loss of mental clarity and an inability to focus, and it may be subtle at first but then worsen. The symptoms are usually observed by family members and caregivers. Part of evaluating the patient is to question family members and caregivers about the patient's behavior and any subtle behavioral changes. Some patients initially present with drowsiness, which may progress to lethargy and a semicomatose state. Others present with hypervigilance, agitation, and enhanced autonomic and psychomotor function. This is usually seen in patients with alcohol and sedative withdrawal syndromes. A few patients present with cognitive and perceptual problems, including memory loss, dysphasia, dysarthria, and disorientation. Formal testing of the mental status, including an objective evaluation of the patient's general cognitive ability, may contribute to early diagnosis and treatment.

Symptoms may develop acutely and may persist for a period of a few hours to several days or even months. The severity of the presentation varies significantly, and it is not unusual for patients to appear relatively lucid at one point in the day and to be totally disoriented at another. Thus, when the diagnosis is suspected or anticipated, especially in older adult patients, evaluation should be performed at several times during the day.

Diagnosis

Evaluating for delirium depends first on recognizing the possibility that it may exist and then using appropriate tests to confirm or exclude the diagnosis. A detailed history should be obtained not only from the patient but also from the family. A history of organ failure, new and old medications, a recent febrile illness, alcohol or drug abuse, and recent depression may be helpful. Even if a comprehensive physical examination is not possible, a focused neurologic assessment concentrating on vital signs, state of hydration, skin condition, and potential sites of infection should be performed. The patient's general appearance could highlight a precipitating factor (e.g., jaundice for hepatic failure, needle tracks associated with drug abuse, cherry red lips associated with carbon monoxide poison, alcoholic facies and the odor of alcohol on the breath associated with chronic alcoholism, uremic facies associated with chronic kidney failure). Assessment of the level of consciousness and evaluation of the cranial nerves could help distinguish between delirium and other organic states such as a cerebrovascular accident.

The confusion assessment method (CAM)[94] is a simple tool that may be used to assess for the presence of delirium. The CAM is a standard screening device that can be used at the bedside in the clinical setting. It has a sensitivity of 94% to 100% and a specificity of 90% to 95%. The CAM-ICU[95] instrument has been modified to screen patients for delirium in the intensive care unit. Brain and spinal cord imaging and other biochemical serum and urinary investigations are conducted to identify other systemic syndromes that may have delirium as a component.

Delirium may be associated with the following:

- Infections, usually of the respiratory tract, urinary tract, skin, and soft tissue
- Drug and alcohol toxicity
- Fluid and electrolyte disturbances, including dehydration, hypernatremia, and hyponatremia
- Alcohol withdrawal
- Withdrawal from barbiturates, benzodiazepines, and selective serotonin reuptake inhibitors
- Metabolic disorders, including hypoglycemia, hypocalcemia, uremia, and liver failure
- Low profusion states, including heart failure and peripheral vascular shock
- Postoperative state

A list of the patient's medications is reviewed to exclude drug toxicity. Drug screens are performed to determine the blood levels of prescribed medications as well as the presence of medications that were not prescribed. The screen should include over-the-counter medications, as these may interact with prescribed medications to produce side effects such as delirium.

The differential diagnosis of patients with delirium is quite extensive. The common differential diagnoses would include focal neurologic syndromes such as temporal and parietal lesions, occipital lesions, and frontal lobe lesions. Nonconvulsive status epilepticus, dementia, Alzheimer's disease, and primary psychiatric illnesses including depression and dysphoria may mimic delirium. Some patients with bipolar disease may present with delirium. Some patients exhibit sundowning,[96] a syndrome in which they display lucidity in the mornings but behavioral deterioration in the evenings.

Laboratory testing includes analyses for serum electrolytes, creatinine, glucose, and calcium, along with a complete blood count, urinalysis, and the aforementioned drug screens. Blood gases are determined, particularly in hyperventilating patients and those who have metabolic acidosis.

Neuroimaging[97] is used to rule out any cerebral or spinal lesions. Lumbar punctures help to rule out bacterial meningitis and other neuraxial infections or degenerative states. Electroencephalography is useful in patients with altered consciousness to exclude seizures or to confirm the diagnosis of certain metabolic encephalopathies. Patients with a remote history of trauma, seizures, cerebrovascular accidents, or focal brain lesions may be at risk of developing convulsive or nonconvulsive seizures. These conditions must be differentiated from delirium.

Prophylaxis

Prevention is important in the management of delirium. For older adult and very ill patients who might be at risk of developing cerebrovascular accidents, dementia, or Parkinson's disease, and whose sensory function is deteriorating, care must be exercised to avoid precipitating or aggravating delirium.[98] Dehydration and infection must be avoided or treated vigorously. Immobility and disuse predispose to delirium. Malnutrition and prolonged bladder catheterization may lead to systemic infections, which may predispose to delirium. The use of multiple pharmaceutical agents including psychoactive drugs can produce side effects that may lead to delirium. Perioperatively, pain should be effectively treated because untreated pain (inadequate analgesia) can lead to delirium. Furthermore, inadequate sedation can produce a state of excitation that mimics delirium.

One consequence of strong opioids is an increased risk of encephalopathy and delirium, which results from the mu effect of opioids.[99] In the older adult patient, the balance between adequate analgesia and delirium is delicate, particularly in the presence of other sedative or psychoactive drugs. In the intensive care or in the nursing home setting, studies have shown that sensory deprivation may contribute to delirium in older patients. The situation is even more pronounced in patients who depend on reading glasses, hearing devices, and other devices that are not normally available to them in those settings. Thus, the presence of calendars, windows with views, clocks, and other objects requiring sensory interaction help prevent the development of delirium.

Treatment

The treatment of delirium is based on the following basic principles:

1. Avoid the factors known to cause or aggravate delirium.
2. Identify and treat underlying medical conditions (e.g., infections, fluid and electrolyte imbalances, drug toxicity, metabolic disorders, low perfusion states, alcohol and sedative withdrawal).
3. Provide supportive measures and restorative care to prevent further physical and cognitive decline.
4. Control dangerous and disruptive behaviors, so that definitive therapy can be implemented.

Approximately 30% of all cases of delirium are caused by drug toxicity. Determining the therapeutic levels of drugs such as digoxin, quinidine, and lithium is very important in assessing and treating the patient with delirium. Perioperatively, patients with anticholinergic effect or intoxication should be treated immediately with intravenous administration of physostigmine (1 to 2 mg intravenously) to reverse the anticholinergic effects of other drugs. This can be repeated as the duration of action is relatively short. However, side effects of physostigmine include bradycardia, bronchial spasm, and, in some cases, seizures.

Flumazenil is used to reverse drug-induced delirium and the mental dysfunction associated with hepatic encephalopathy.[100] It is particularly effective in reversing the delirium and disorientation created by several sedative drugs such as the benzodiazepines, especially in the postoperative period.

Supportive Care

The delirious patient may develop a variety of other conditions including altered mental state and altered consciousness. Thus, before functional decline occurs, an aggressive protocol to provide support and care, as well as to restore function, is an important general measure to combat the effects of delirium.[101] It is appropriate to consider delirium in the patient with cancer. Delirium is a common neuropsychiatric disorder that occurs in the advanced stages of cancer. Adequate pain control should be provided, but the administration of strong opioids and sedatives may lead to delirium. Thus, the effective therapeutic window is very narrow.

In patients with advanced cancer, factors that contribute to the development of delirium include brain tumor or metastases, opioid-induced neurotoxicity, chemotherapy and radiation therapy, psychotropic drugs (e.g., tricyclic antidepressants, benzodiazepines), metabolic factors (e.g., hypocalcaemia, hyponatremia, renal failure), paraneoplastic syndromes, and sepsis.

Some agents are used specifically to treat delirium. For example, haloperidol may be used, particularly in patients with hyperactive forms of delirium, including delusions and hallucinations. However, with adequate supportive care and effective pain management, such therapies are usually unwarranted if susceptible patients are managed early and judiciously.

■ ANXIETY

No grand inquisitor has in readiness such terrible tortures as has anxiety, and no spy knows how to attack more artfully the man he pursues, choosing the instant when he is weakest, nor knows how to lay traps where he will be caught and ensnared, as anxiety knows how.

SOREN KIERKEGAARD

Anxiety,[102] a common phenomenon experienced by all individuals, is a response to potentially or perceived harmful situations. The response takes on a pathologic role when the level of behavioral reaction is excessive in relationship to the threat, or if the response becomes protracted with associated impairment of normal levels of functioning. Acute and chronic medical conditions often have a significant comorbid contribution from anxiety disorders. The presence of anxiety disorders may occur more frequently than mood disorders such as depression in these settings.

The DSM-IV divides anxiety disorders[103,104] into subcategories. They may share similar features, but each has defining characteristics that set it apart. The common subcategories of this disease include the following:

- Anxiety resulting from general medical conditions
- Substance-induced anxiety
- Generalized anxiety
- Panic disorder
- Acute stress disorder
- Post-traumatic stress disorder
- Adjustment disorder with anxious features
- Social phobias
- Obsessive-compulsive disorders
- Specific phobias

This chapter will focus on the diagnosis and therapy of anxiety disorders as they relate to medical conditions and pain.[105] *Anxiety* is derived from the Latin word *angere,* meaning "to choke," a common symptom felt during panic attacks. Anxiety and fear are related and appear to share some clinical similarities in terms of their presentation. The primary difference is that fear typically has a well-defined external threat locus, whereas anxiety tends to be an internally generated phenomenon with poorly defined etiology of the inciting threat. Anxiety may represent a symptom of a serious underlying condition for which the etiology must be determined to optimally facilitate optimal clinical resolution of symptoms that can be quite debilitating.

The differential diagnosis for anxiety is extensive,[106] primarily because a wide range of medical and psychiatric conditions can precipitate this syndrome. Anxiety in these settings may be a primary disorder, a condition that is comorbid with acute or chronic disease, or a secondary condition. The challenge is to determine which it is without undertreating or too aggressively treating the patient. The patient often focuses on the anxiety-associated physical symptoms and thus presents with somatic complaints. This confounds the initial workup when underlying medical conditions are present. Patient–practitioner interaction in this setting involves significant dialogue and a full description of the symptoms in the context of the current circumstances. Box 41-2 shows symptoms common to anxiety disorders.

41-2	**Symptoms Common to Anxiety Disorders**

- Palpitations and rapid heart rate
- Trembling or shaking
- Chest pain
- Difficulty breathing
- Dizziness
- Fear of losing control, passing out
- Sweating
- Dry mouth
- Feeling of choking
- Nausea
- Feeling that objects are unreal or self-distant
- Fear of dying
- Hot flashes or cold chills

There is significant variability in anxiety prevalence rates between ethnicities and countries. The epidemiologic rates in the United States have been evaluated by two studies, the Epidemiological Catchment Area (ECA) and the National Comorbid Survey (NCS). The lifetime prevalence rate for anxiety disorders from these studies were panic disorder (2.3% to 2.7%), generalized anxiety disorder (4.1% to 6.6%), obsessive-compulsive disorder (2.3% to 2.6%), post-traumatic stress disorder (1% to 9.3%), and social phobias (2.6% to 13.3%). Anxiety disorders appear to correlate with chronic medical conditions, and anxiety rarely exists alone.

Evaluation of the patient with anxiety begins with a thorough history and physical examination. Laboratory investigations can be helpful early in the process, as are psychological screening tests, which may provide insights to associated comorbid conditions. Preliminary laboratory studies include a complete blood cell count, hematocrit, thyroid studies, and a urine drug screen. More extensive evaluations are required if a secondary etiology of the anxiety disorder is suspected. A cardiovascular, pulmonary, organic brain, and or substance abuse etiology should be ruled out.

Effective communication with the patient about the condition is warranted once primary medical conditions are ruled out or resolved. Reassurance about both symptoms and therapy is central to all communication, although reassurance may not be an effective tool for all patients. For those with pathologic levels of anxiety, reassurance is of little or no value. In such cases, a behavioral and or pharmaceutical approach facilitates short- and long-term resolution.

Mild anxiety readily responds to moderate levels of intervention, but severe anxiety carries a risk for potential morbidity and mortality resulting from hypertension and associated cardiac events. Depression may also contribute to morbidity and mortality via suicidal behavior. Thus, it is important to understand the triggers that may have precipitated the anxiety, and to explore the risk of suicidality. Anxiety disorders have a fairly low cure rate, and they tend to be chronic and subject to acute worsening with environmental and physical stressors. Anxiety disorders are commonly associated with chronic pain conditions and should be aggressively addressed as a component of care in this patient population.[107]

Cognitive behavioral therapy (CBT) can be an extremely effective long-term solution for many patients.[108] Its primary focus is to change the patient's interpretation of the anxiety-provoking circumstances from maladaptive to more positive adaptive thought processes.

The relationship between pain and anxiety is well established, but the mechanism has not been clearly delineated. The autonomic nervous system may be the primary link between pain and anxiety. A reduction in painful conditions often results in a reduction in associated anxiety, and vice versa. After any secondary etiology has been addressed, the focus of therapy should be on the anxiety disorder and any associated mood disorders.

Of the several classes of drugs that have been used to treat anxiety disorders, the most common for acute management has been the benzodiazepines.[109] However, although they are effective, they have been falling out of favor. They have a rather rapid therapeutic onset, but they are associated with significant potential impairment of the patient's level of cognitive functioning and psychomotor skills. They are also associated with an increased risk of addiction and are difficult to taper. Their removal from a therapeutic regimen is often associated with withdrawal symptoms similar to the original complaints, which bodes poorly for long-term use.

Nonspecific beta blockers have been advocated for anxiety associated with performance. Current clinical trials demonstrate minimal efficacy for resolution of the anxiety, but there is resolution of sympathetically mediated symptoms such as rapid heart rate and hypertension. Additional drug classes that have demonstrated effectiveness include the selective serotonin reuptake inhibitors (SSRIs) and older drugs such as the tricyclic antidepressants and monoamine oxidase inhibitors (MAOIs).

■ REFERENCES

1. Brena SF, Chapman SL: Chronic pain: An algorithm for management. Postgrad Med 1982;72:111.
2. Bonica JJ: Cancer pain. In JJ Bonica (ed): The Management of Pain. Philadelphia, Lea & Febiger, 1990, p 400.
3. Manchikanti L, Staats PS, Singh V, et al: Evidence-based practice guidelines for interventional techniques in the management of chronic spinal pain. Pain Physician 2003;6:3-80.
4. Waddell G: The Problem in the Back Pain Revolution. New York, Churchill Livingstone, 1998, pp 1-8.
5. Edgar MA, Ghadially JA: Innervation of the lumbar spine. Clin Orthop Rel Res 1976;115:35-41.
6. Bell GR, Rothman RH, Booth RE, et al: A study of computer-assisted tomography: II. Comparison of metrizamide myelography and computed tomography in the diagnosis of herniated lumbar disc and spinal stenosis. Spine 1984;9:552-556.
7. Manchikanti L, Singh V, Kloth D, et al: Interventional techniques in the management of chronic pain: Part 2.0. Pain Physician 2001;4:24-98.
8. Racz GB, Heavner JE, Raj PP: Percutaneous epidural neuroplasty: Prospective one-year follow-up. Pain Digest 1999;9:97-102
9. Racz GB, Holubec JT: Lysis of adhesions in the epidural space. In Racz GB (ed): Techniques of Neurolysis. Boston, Kluwer Academic, 1989, pp 57-72.
10. Anderson SR, Racz G, Heavner J: Evolution of epidural lysis of adhesions. Pain Physician 2000;3:262-270.

11. Manchikanti L, Pakanati RR, Pampati V: Comparison of three routes of epidural steroid injections in low back pain. Pain Dig 1999;9: 277-287.

12. Huntoon MA, Martin DP: Paralysis after transforaminal epidural injection and previous spinal surgery. Reg Anesth Pain Med 2004;29: 494-495.

13. Huntoon MA, Martin DP: Transforaminal injection of steroids. Reg Anesth Pain Med 2004;29:397-399.

14. Baker R, Dreyfuss P, Mercer S. Bogduk N: Cervical transforaminal injection of corticosteroids into a radicular artery: A possible mechanism for spinal cord injury. Pain 2003;103:211-215.

15. Wittenberg RH, Greskotter KR, Steffen R, et al: [Is epidural injection treatment with hypertonic saline solution in intervertebral disk replacement useful?] Z Orthop Ihre Grenzgeb 1990;128: 223-226.

16. Manchikanti L, Saini B, Singh V: Spinal endoscopy and lysis of epidural adhesions in the management of chronic low back pain. Pain Physician 2001;4:240-265.

17. Saal JA, Saal JS: Intradiscal electrothermal treatment for chronic discogenic low back pain. Spine 2000;25:2622-2627.

18. Sharps LS, Issac Z: Percutaneous disc decompression using nucleoplasty. Pain Physician 2002;5:121-126.

19. Schmidt UD: Microsurgery of lumbar disc prolapse: Superior results of microsurgery as compared to standard and percutaneous procedures. Nervenarzt 2000;71:265-274.

20. Weisel SW: The multiply operated lumbar spine. Instr Course Lect 1985;34:68-77.

21. Pauza KJ, Howell S, Dreyfuss P: A randomized, placebo-controlled trial of intradiscal electrothermal therapy for the treatment of discogenic low back pain. Spine J 2004;4:27-35.

22. Dreyfuss P, Kaplan M, Dreyer SJ: Zygapophyseal joint injection techniques in the spinal axis. In Lennard TA (ed): Pain Procedures in Clinical Practice, ed 2. Philadelphia, Hanley & Belfus, 2000, pp 276-308.

23. Suseki K, Takahashi Y, Takahashi K, et al: Innervation of the lumbar facet joints. Spine 1997;22:477-485.

24. Raymond J, Dumas JM: Intraarticular facet block: Diagnostic tests or therapeutic procedure? Radiology 1989;151:333-336.

25. Revel ME, Listrat VM, Chevalier XJ, et al: Facet joint block for low back pain: Identifying predictors of a good response. Arch Phys Med Rehabil 1992;73:824-828.

26. North RB, Han M, Zahurak M, et al: Radiofrequency lumbar facet denervation: Analysis of prognostic factors. Pain 1994;57:77-83.

27. Geurts JW, van Wijk RM, Strolker RJ, Groen GJ: Efficacy of radiofrequency procedures for the treatment of spinal pain: A systematic review of randomized clinical trials. Reg Anesth Pain Med 2001;26:394-400.

28. Arnold CC, Brodsky AE, Cauchoix J, et al: Lumbar spinal stenosis and nerve root entrapment syndromes. Clin Orthop 1776;115:4.

29. Vad V, Bhat A, Lutz G, et al: Transforaminal epidural steroid injections in lumbosacral radiculopathy: A prospective randomized study. Spine 2002;27:11-16.

30. Racz GB, Heavner JE, Raj PP: Epidural neuroplasty. Semin Anesth 1997;302:312.

31. Pawl RP: Arachnoiditis and epidural fibrosis: The relationship to chronic pain. Curr Rev Pain 1998;2:93-99.

32. Bernard TN Jr, Cassidy JD: The sacroiliac joint syndrome: Pathophysiology, diagnosis, and management. In Frymoyer JW, Ducker TB, Hadler NM, et al (eds): The Adult Spine: Principles and Practice. New York, Raven Press, 1991, pp 2107-2130.

33. Slipman CW, Isaac Z: The role of diagnostic selective nerve root blocks in the management of spinal pain. Pain Physician 2001;4: 214-226.

34. Ferrante FM, King LF, Roch EA, et al: Radiofrequency sacroiliac joint denervation for sacroiliac syndrome. Reg Anesth Pain Med 2001;26:137-142.

35. Sola AE, Bonica JJ: Myofascial pain syndromes. In Bonica JJ (ed): The Management of Pain. New York, Lea & Febiger, 1990, pp 352-367.

36. Bogduk N (ed): Low Back Pain: Clinical Anatomy of Lumbar Spine and Sacrum, ed 3. New York, Churchill Livingstone, 1997, pp 187-213.

37. Travell JG, Simons DG: Myofascial Pain and Dysfunction: The Trigger Point Manual, vol 2. Baltimore, Lippincott Williams & Wilkins, 1999.

38. Portenoy RK, Payne R, Jacobsen P: Breakthrough pain: Characteristics and impact in patients with cancer pain. Lancet 1999;353: 1695-1700.

39. Payne R: Mechanisms and management of bone pain. Cancer 1997;80:1608-1613.

40. Mercadante S: Malignant bone pain: Pathophysiology and treatment. Pain 1997;69:1-18.

41. Meuser T, Pietruck C, Radbruch L, et al: Symptoms during cancer pain treatment following WHO-guidelines: A longitudinal follow-up study of symptom prevalence, severity and etiology. Pain 2001;93: 247-257.

42. Manchikanti L, Heavner J, Racz GB, et al: Methods for evidence synthesis in interventional pain management. Pain Physician 2003;6: 89-111.

43. Julius D, Basbaum AI: Molecular mechanisms of nociception. Nature 2001;413:203-210.

44. Honore P, Schwei J, Rogers SD, et al: Cellular and neurochemical remodeling of the spinal cord in bone cancer pain. Prog Brain Res 2000;129:389-397.

45. Schwei MJ, Honore P, Rogers SD, et al: Neurochemical and cellular reorganization of the spinal cord in the murine model of bone cancer pain. J. Neurosci 1999;19:10886-10897.

46. Bruera E, Brenneis C, Micahud M, et al: Patient-controlled subcutaneous hydromorphone versus continuous subcutaneous infusion for the treatment of cancer pain. J Natl Cancer Inst 1988;80: 152.

47. Brown DL, Bulley CK, Quiel EL: Neurolytic celiac plexus block for pancreatic cancer pain. Anesth Analg 1987;66:869-873.

48. Monnin S, Schiller MR: Nutrition counseling for breast cancer patients. J Am Diet Assoc 1993;93:72.

49. Hope-Simpson RE: The nature of herpes zoster: A long-term study and a new hypothesis. Proc R Soc Med 1965;58:9.

50. Loeser JD: Herpes zoster and postherpetic neuralgia. Pain 1986;25: 149-164.

51. Levy MH: Oral controlled-release morphine: Guidelines for clinical use. In Benedetti C, Chapman CR, Moricca G (eds): Advances in Pain Research and Therapy, vol. 14. New York, Raven Press, 1900, p 285.

52. Parris WCV: Cancer pain syndromes and their management. In Parris WCV (ed): Cancer Pain Management: Principles and Practice. Boston, Butterworth Heinemann, 1997, pp 279-292.

53. Martelletti P, van Suijlekom H: Cervicogenic headache: Practical approaches to therapy. CNS Drugs 2004;18:793-805.

54. Antonaci F, Fredriksen TA, Sjaastad O: Cervicogenic headache: Clinical presentation, diagnostic criteria, and differential diagnosis. Curr Pain Headache Rep 2001;5:387-392.

55. Biondi DM: Cervicogenic headache: Diagnostic evaluation and treatment strategies. Curr Pain Headache Rep 2001;5:361-368.

56. Silverman SB: Cervicogenic headache: Interventional, anesthetic, and ablative treatment. Curr Pain Headache Rep 2002;6:308-314.

57. Dumas JP, Arsenault AB, Boudreau G, et al: Physical impairments in cervicogenic headache: Traumatic vs. nontraumatic onset. Cephalalgia 2001;21:884-893.

58. Taylor FR: Distinguishing primary headache disorders from cervicogenic headache: Clinical and therapeutic implications. Headache Currents 2005;2:37-41.

59. Guez M, Hildingsson C, Nilsson M, Toolanen G: The prevalence of neck pain: A population-based study from northern Sweden. Acta Orthop Scand 2002;73:455-459.

60. Bartsch T, Goadsby PJ: Increased responses in trigeminocervical nociceptive neurons to cervical input after stimulation of the dura mater. Brain 2003;126(Pt 8):1801-1813.

61. Sjaastad O, Fredriksen TA: Cervicogenic headache: Criteria, classification and epidemiology. Clin Exp Rheumatol 2000;18(2 Suppl 19): S3-6.

62. Bono G, Antonaci F, Dario A, et al: Unilateral headaches and their relationship with cervicogenic headache. Clin Exp Rheumatol 2000;18(2 Suppl 19):S11-15.

63. Bronfort G, Nilsson N, Haas M, et al: Non-invasive physical treatments for chronic/recurrent headache. Cochrane Database Syst Rev 2004;(3):CD001878.

64. Mills Roth J: Physical therapy in the treatment of chronic headache. Curr Pain Headache Rep 2003;7:482-489.

65. Bogduk N: The neck and headaches. Neurol Clin 2004;22:151-171.

66. Melzack R, Wall PD: Pain mechanisms: A new theory. Science 1965;150:971-979.

67. Ahadian FM: Pulsed radiofrequency neurotomy: Advances in pain medicine. Curr Pain Headache Rep 2004;8:34-40.

68. Mikeladze G, Espinal R, Finnegan R, et al: Pulsed radiofrequency application in treatment of chronic zygapophyseal joint pain. Spine J 2003;3:360-362.

69. Speldewinde GC, Bashford GM, Davidson IR: Diagnostic cervical zygapophyseal joint blocks for chronic cervical pain. Med J Aust 2001;174:174-176.

70. Inan N, Ceyhan A, Inan L, et al: C2/C3 nerve blocks and greater occipital nerve block in cervicogenic headache treatment. Funct Neurol 2001;16:239-243.

71. Blume HG: Cervicogenic headaches: Radiofrequency neurotomy and the cervical disc and fusion. Clin Exp Rheumatol 2000;18(2 Suppl 19):S53-58.

72. Peloso P, Gross A, Haines T, et al: Medicinal and injection therapies for mechanical neck disorders. Cochrane Database Syst Rev 2005;(2):CD000319.

73. Ohnmeiss DD, Guyer RD, Mason SL: The relation between cervical discographic pain responses and radiographic images. Clin J Pain 2000;16:1-5.

74. Weiner RL, Reed KL: Peripheral neurostimulation for control of intractable occipital neuralgia. Neuromodulation 1999;2:217.

75. Matharu MS, Bartsch T, Ward N, et al: Central neuromodulation in chronic migraine patients with suboccipital stimulators: A PET study. Brain 2004;127(Pt 1):220-230.

76. Popeney CA, Alo KM: Peripheral neurostimulation for the treatment of chronic, disabling transformed migraine. Headache 2003;43:369-375.

77. Arcos I, Davis R, Fey K, et al: Second-generation microstimulator. Artif Organs 2002;26:228-231.

78. Rosenquist R, Rosenberg J, U.S. Veterans Administration: Postoperative pain guidelines. Reg Anesth Pain Med 2003;28:279-288.

79. Dolin SJ, Cashman NJ, Bland MJ: Effectiveness of acute postoperative pain management: I. Evidence from published data. Br J Anesth 2002;89:409-423.

80. American Society of Anesthesiologists Task Force on Acute Pain Management: Practice Guidelines for Acute Pain Management in the Perioperative Setting. Anesthesiology 2004;100:1573-1581.

81. Department of Defense, Veterans Health Administration: Clinical Practice Guideline for the Management of Postoperative Pain, version 1.2. Washington, DC, DoD, VHA, 2002.

82. Australian and New Zealand College of Anaesthetists and Faculty of Pain Medicine: Guidelines on Acute Pain Management. PS41 (2000).

83. Mitra S, Sinatra RS: Perioperative management of acute pain in the opioid-dependent patient. Anesthesiology 2004;101:212-227.

84. American Psychiatric Association: Diagnostic and Statistical Manual, ed 4. Washington, DC, APA Press, 1994.

85. Adams RD, Victor M, Ropper AH: Delirium and other acute confusional states. In Principles of Neurology, ed 6. New York, McGraw-Hill, 1997, p 405.

86. Francis J: Delirium in older patients. J Am Geriatr Soc 1992;40:829.

87. Romano J, Engel GL: Delirium: I. Electroencephalographic data. Arch Neurol Psychiatr 1944;51:356.

88. Trzepacz PT: The neuropathogenesis of delirium: A need to focus our research. Psychosomatics 1994;35:374.

89. Tune L, Carr S, Hoag E, Cooper T: Anticholinergic effects of drugs commonly prescribed for the elderly: Potential means for assessing risk of delirium. Am J Psychiatry 1993;149:1393.

90. Mach JR, Dysken MW, Kuskowski M, et al: Serum anticholinergic activity in hospitalized older persons with delirium: A preliminary study. J Am Geriatr Soc 1995;43:491.

91. Lundstrom M, Edlund A, Bucht G, et al: Dementia after delirium in patients with femoral neck fractures. J Am Geriatr Soc 2003;51:1002.

92. Inouye SK, Rushing JT, Foreman MD, et al: Does delirium contribute to poor hospital outcomes? A three-site epidemiologic study. J Gen Intern Med 1998;13:234.

93. McCusker J, Cole M, Dendukuri N, et al: The course of delirium in older medical inpatients: A prospective study. J Gen Intern Med 2003;18:696.

94. Inouye SK, Van Dyck CH, Alessi CA, et al: Clarifying confusion: The confusion assessment method, a new method for detection of delirium. Ann Intern Med 1990;113:941.

95. Ely EW, Inouye SK, Bernard GR, et al: Delirium in mechanically ventilated patients: Validity and reliability of the confusion assessment method for the intensive care unit (CAM-ICU). JAMA 2001;286:2703.

96. Bliwise DL: What is sundowning? J Am Geriatr Soc 1994;42:1009.

97. Koponen H, Hurri L, Stenback U, et al: Computed tomography findings in delirium. J Nerv Ment Dis 1989;177:226.

98. Elie M, Cole MG, Primeau FJ, Bellavance F: Delirium risk factors in elderly hospitalized patients. J Gen Intern Med 1998;13:204.

99. Morrison RS, Magaziner J, Gilbert M, et al: Relationship between pain and opioid analgesics on the development of delirium following hip fracture. J Gerontol A Biol Sci Med Sci 2003;58:76.

100. Bostwick JM, Masterson BJ: Psychopharmacological treatment of delirium to restore mental capacity. Psychosomatics 1998;39:112.

101. Francis J, Kappor WN: Prognosis after hospital discharge of older medical patients with delirium. J Am Geriatr Soc 1992;40:601.

102. Cramer V, Torgersen S, Kringlen E: Quality of life and anxiety disorders: A population study. J Nerv Ment Dis 2005;192:106-202.

103. Zimmerman M, Chelminski I, Young D: On the threshold of disorder: A study of the impact of the DSM-IV clinical significance criterion on diagnosing depressive and anxiety disorders in clinical practice. J Clin Psychiatry 2004;65:1400-1405.

104. Ballenger JC: Treatment of anxiety disorders to remission. J Clin Psychiatry 2001;62(Suppl 12):5-9.

105. Surtees PG, Wainwright NW, Khaw KT, Day NE: Functional health status, chronic medical conditions and disorders of mood. Br J Psychiatry 2003;183:299-303.

106. Skodol AE: Anxiety in the medically ill: Nosology and principles of differential diagnosis. Semin Clin Neuropsychiatry 1999;4:64-71.

107. Eisendrath SJ: Psychiatric aspects of chronic pain. Neurology 1995;45(12 Suppl 9):S26-34; discussion S35-36.

108. Foa EB, Franklin ME, Moser J: Context in the clinic: How well do cognitive-behavioral therapies and medications work in combination? Biol Psychiatry 2002;52:987-997.

109. Bourin M, Lambert O: Pharmacotherapy of anxious disorders. Hum Psychopharmacol 2002;17:383-400.

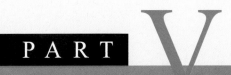

Conflicting Outcomes

42 Economic Analysis of Perioperative Optimization

Tom Archer, Steve Mannis, and Alex Macario

The goal of this chapter is to make the following points:

1. Taxpayers, employers, and employees are demanding that medicine deliver better value. Physicians need evidence-based medicine to establish which interventions are truly beneficial, and they need modern management techniques to minimize the costs of implementing those interventions.

2. Perioperative interventions are investments, each with its costs and, it is hoped, its benefits. The benefits of perioperative interventions are often non-monetary and difficult to quantify (e.g., pain relief).

3. Three ways of measuring the non-monetary benefits of health-care interventions are by improved clinical results (i.e., effects), by increased quality-adjusted life-years, or QALYs, and by benefit (i.e., the monetary equivalent of non-monetary benefit).

4. Interventions must be evaluated in comparison to alternatives. The fundamental concept is the incremental cost-to-effectiveness ratio, which is defined later.

5. Because of the multiplicity of players in health care (i.e., patients, providers, payers, and society as a whole), an economic study in health care must specify, and be consistent in, its point of view.

6. Costs of perioperative interventions are direct, indirect, and intangible. Direct costs are the easiest to define and quantify, but they are only estimates and can vary widely depending on the costing method used. The good news about costs is that they tend to decrease over time, because of competition, the learning curve, technological progress, work process redesign, and the bundling of interventions.

7. Much more attention is now being directed toward barriers to implementation of beneficial interventions. These barriers include (1) absence of clarity about what works and what it costs, (2) absent or perverse incentives for providers, and (3) cumbersome and inefficient work processes.

8. Over time, health outcomes will probably improve because of (1) increased scrutiny, publicity, and competition, (2) alignment of incentives (a nice way of saying "pay for performance" [see Chapter 43]), (3) increased use of evidence-based medicine (EBM) to know which interventions produce real benefits, (4) increased use of cost–effectiveness analysis, and (5) work process redesign.

With the aging of the post-war baby boomers and the explosion of technological options at medicine's disposal, health-care systems around the world are struggling to increase the quality and decrease the cost of care. As the movement for EBM gathers steam, health-care providers are scrambling to find out what really works and what does not. But it is not just physicians' intellectual honesty that is driving the search for better treatments and better outcomes. The ultimate payers of health-care costs—taxpayers, employers, and employees—are demanding that physicians provide better value for the money spent. Those who pay for health care have formed organizations such the Leapfrog Group, the Institute of Medicine, and the Centers for Medicare and Medicaid Services to set goals for health-care performance, and some payers have begun to "pay for performance." The unspoken implication is that there will soon be reduced or no pay for poor performance. The public is demanding the biggest bang for its health-care buck.

Physicians must first of all know which perioperative interventions actually benefit patients and then apply those interventions at the lowest possible cost. This is a moving target, as the economic attractiveness of perioperative interventions changes with time, as new interventions are introduced (e.g., ultrasound for central venous catheter placement) or old interventions evolve (e.g., adding anti-infective substances to central venous catheters). In this chapter, we aim to present the conceptual framework that is used for the economic analysis of perioperative interventions so the reader can critically appraise economic studies of perioperative optimization.

■ HEALTH-CARE INTERVENTIONS AS INVESTMENTS

Economics describes how people in societies satisfy their needs and wants in an environment of limited resources. During the 19th and 20th centuries, economists, political scientists, and politicians debated the merits of free-market capitalism, with individual freedom of choice versus central planning and state ownership of the means of production. For normal goods, the individualistic free market approach has won the day. In medicine, however, much of the central planning approach still seems to be in vogue, and perhaps with some justification, because the consumer (the patient) usually does not directly pay the full cost of the care and is often not able to fully judge the quality of the health-care product. Also, a global, or societal, perspective (which crosses institutional financial boundaries) appears to have merit to taking best care of the patient. In other words, medicine is still—and perhaps always will be—somewhat paternalistic. Physicians are called on to take care of people who are not fully able to take care of themselves. In economic language, physicians are asked to invest on behalf of their patients.

Costs and (We Hope) Benefits

Health-care interventions are investments, very similar to financial investments, in that there is a *cost* of the intervention, and then there is an *outcome*—and, one hopes, a *benefit*. Unfortunately, many medical practices have not been studied adequately to find out whether they are really beneficial, so some of our therapy is of uncertain value. The motivation of EBM is to find out whether our costly interventions really do, in fact, produce benefits. Once we know that an intervention actually provides a benefit to the patient, we have to decide whether the increased benefit is worth the increased cost.

No medical intervention can be considered cost effective in isolation but must be compared with an alternative treatment (usually, the standard therapy). This is hugely important. For example, if a new analgesic technique costs $100 and reduces postoperative pain scores by 50%, then its value needs to be compared with the best current treatment to determine if it is worthy of implementation.

In health care—as in any type of management—we manage at the margin, constantly analyzing *marginal, or incremental, benefits* and comparing them with the *marginal, or incremental, costs*. The fundamental analytical concept of managing at the margin is the *incremental cost–effectiveness ratio (ICER)*, defined as

$$(C_2 - C_1) \div (E_2 - E_1),$$

where C_2 and E_2 are the cost and effectiveness of the new intervention being evaluated, and C_1 and E_1 are the cost and effectiveness of the standard therapy.

Known perioperative interventions that appear to be underused and cost effective (i.e., relatively inexpensive in relationship to their known benefits) are the maintenance of normothermia and normoglycemia, deep vein thrombosis (DVT) prophylaxis, the use of beta-blockers, prevention of central venous catheter–related infection and ventilator-associated pneumonia, the provision of daily "sedation vacations" for intensive care unit (ICU) patients, surgical wound infection prophylaxis, and the elimination of unnecessary laboratory studies.

If it should occur that a new technique achieves a *better outcome at lower cost* (e.g., polio vaccination compared with polio treatment), the new cost-saving technique is said to *dominate* the old technique, and it should become the new standard treatment. For example, the use of beta-blockers dominates not using them in patients undergoing abdominal aortic aneurysm repair.[1] Once the value of beta-blockers has been demonstrated, the challenge is for providers to change patient care processes to ensure that patients in fact

consistently receive the medication. How to do this is not entirely clear, as is suggested by low compliance with this intervention.

The Agency Problem—Providers as Fiduciaries

Doctors are not the primary beneficiaries of the interventions they choose for their patients, and their compensation is usually not tied to patient outcomes (although this may be changing). Furthermore, doctors often benefit from the performance of interventions *regardless* of patient outcomes (e.g., because of direct monetary compensation or teaching benefit).

Within provider systems, parochial budgetary concerns may interfere with the simple goal of maximizing benefits to the patient. For example, a hospital pharmacy committee may not want to burden the hospital pharmacy budget by spending extra money on low-molecular-weight heparin (LMWH), despite evidence of better patient outcomes with LMWH than with unfractionated heparin.

Perverse incentives can be a problem as well. For example, a hospital that receives revenue from the treatment of heart failure exacerbation has reduced incentive to spend money on heart failure prevention.

In summary, health care suffers from the agency problem that is often seen in large corporations: Will the CEO and other members of top management (the providers and payers) act in the interest of the shareholders (the patients), or will they enrich themselves first, and only later think about what is best for the shareholders?

A Major Difference from Financial Investments

Health-care interventions differ from financial investments in one key respect. The primary benefits of health care for the patient—such as improved health, improved function, and pain relief—are non-monetary and, as such, are hard to quantify.

■ HEALTH-CARE ECONOMIC STUDIES OFFER CHALLENGES

The Point of View Must Be Clear and Consistent

Because there are multiple actors in health care, it is essential that we remain consistent in the *point of view* of our analysis. Are we looking at an issue from the point of view of the patient, the entity paying the bills, the provider (the physician, hospital, or clinic), or perhaps society as a whole?

Our Goal Is to Know What Works and How Much It Costs

If we were able to surmount the difficulties involved in quantifying the monetary and non-monetary costs and benefits of our perioperative interventions, and *if* we were able to clearly specify from whose point of view we were analyzing the issue, we might be able to construct a chart such as that in Figure 42-1. Such a comprehensive chart for the perioperative period, however, is still in the future—although cost–effectiveness studies of anesthetic and analgesic agents and techniques have been performed.[2-13]

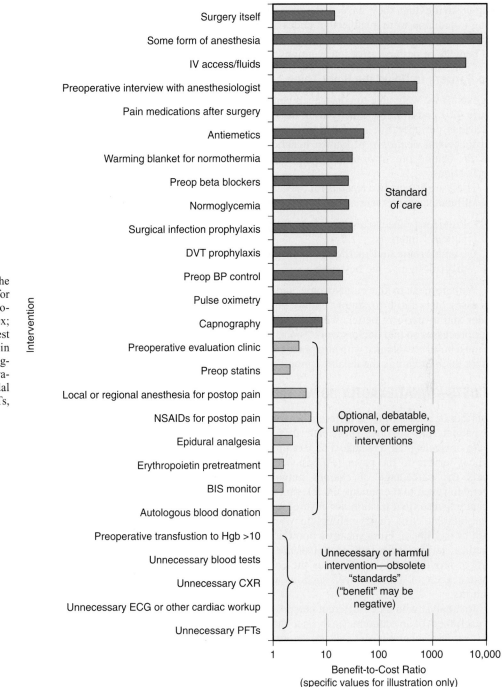

Figure 42-1 ■ A goal for the future: benefit-to-cost ratios for perioperative interventions (hypothetical). BIS, bispectral index; BP, blood pressure; CXR, chest radiography; DVT, deep vein thrombosis; ECG, electrocardiography; Hgb, hemoglobin; IV, intravenous; NSAIDs, nonsteroidal anti-inflammatory drugs; PFTs, pulmonary function tests.

Economic studies in health care often have serious methodological problems. Of roughly 1600 medical cost–utility studies in a Harvard database, only 118 met the following recommendations of the U.S. Public Health Service Panel on Cost Effectiveness in Health and Medicine.[14]

- Adopt a societal perspective.
- Use community- or patient-derived preference weights for utilities (as opposed to expert opinion).
- Use net costs (cost of intervention minus savings in future medical costs).
- Use appropriate incremental comparisons.
- Discount costs and QALYs at the same rate.

Cost-effectiveness analysis—like evidence-based medicine—is in its infancy in health care, in part because health care has been relatively immune from systematic scrutiny. Doctors have been able to defend their varying practices by simply saying that they have different practice styles, as though medicine were a subjective endeavor. Over the next decade, we can hope to see many more studies of the costs and benefits of perioperative interventions.

Two Barriers to Doing the Right Thing

But even if we were able to construct a chart such as that in Figure 42-1 and to know exactly what the costs and benefits of various perioperative interventions were, we would still find that *implementation* of known beneficial interventions lags far behind our *awareness of the effectiveness* of the interventions.

There are at least two reasons for the gap between awareness of beneficial interventions and their implementation?

- Providers' incentives are not fully aligned with patients' interests.
- Cumbersome and inefficient work processes make it difficult to give the best care.

With respect to the cumbersome and inefficient work processes, it is futile to simply exhort physicians to work harder and to perform better. We have to redesign medical work processes so that doctors work "smart" as well as hard. We must build compliance with best practices into the system, so that the best care is the default option.

■ COSTS—WHAT EXACTLY DO WE MEAN?

Costs can be analyzed from different points of view—that of the patient, the provider (physician, hospital, clinic), the payer, or society as a whole. For example, the cost of a medical service to the payer (e.g., an insurance company) equals the percentage of charges actually paid by the payer. However, to the patient, the relevant cost is the out-of-pocket expense (that portion not covered by insurance) plus other indirect costs (e.g., inability to work) incurred as a result of the illness. From society's point of view, the cost of a medical service is the total cost of all the different components of providing the service, plus the costs of any future consequences of that service, such as complications or disability.

An analyst who takes different perspectives complicates the usefulness of an economic analysis to different audiences. For example, pharmacists may be more focused on the hospital or provider perspective. The physician should give greatest weight to the patient's perspective, whereas the health economist is likely to focus on the analysis from society's perspective.

Aside from the difficulties presented by the different points of view, the term *costs* has many different meanings.

Direct Costs

Direct costs are the value of resources used to prevent, detect, and treat a health impairment. The adjective *direct* indicates that there is a clear matching of the expenditure with a patient. For example, an antibiotic administered to a patient is a direct medical cost because the antibiotic can easily be ascribed to the particular patient who received the medication.

In economic analyses, direct costs should be estimated on a net basis—that is, they are calculated as the cost of the intervention minus any savings in future medical costs. For example, if an antibiotic can be shown to prevent future wound infections, then the cost of the antibiotic for purposes of a cost–utility analysis should be reduced by probable future savings of medical costs. As another example, most published studies do not include the full scope of costs associated with intravenous (IV) patient-controlled analgesia. Cost drivers include nurse and pharmacy labor, pump and disposables, intangible costs (e.g., adverse events from programming errors), and potential events such as analgesic gaps from malfunctioning pumps or IV line failures.[15] As a third example, aprotinin may reduce future medical costs in coronary artery bypass graft (CABG) surgery.[16]

With respect to reducing net cost, Fischer[17] and Ferschl and colleagues[18] have shown that preoperative patient evaluation clinics can reduce future costs related to laboratory testing, specialty consults, and delayed or cancelled surgery.

A conceptual, financial, and political problem with this net-cost approach is that it may be difficult within an institution to spend money (or budget) in one area in order to save money in another area. Proponents of preoperative clinics (and of other efforts to redesign patient care) need to point out to administration that *investing* in a preoperative clinic may produce large financial returns elsewhere in the hospital, which may more than pay for the expense of running the clinic.

Costs versus Charges

Costs are not the same as charges. For example, a hospital's cost for giving a medication is usually interpreted to equal the acquisition cost of the medication, plus the true cost of delivering it to the patient. In contrast, charge refers to the amount of money the doctor or the facility bills the insurance company for the medication. Charges often bear little or no relation to acquisition cost, as anyone can attest who has heard about $10 aspirins and $40 plastic bedpans.

Cost-Estimation Techniques

To estimate costs, either a top-down or a bottom-up approach can be used. One top-down method of estimating costs uses cost-to-charge ratios, such as those that all U.S. hospitals supply to Medicare. These ratios are then used to convert hospital billing (charge) data to estimated costs. The biggest advantage of the cost-to-charge ratio method is that charge data are commonly available, and their use is well accepted.

The biggest disadvantage of the cost-to-charge ratio method is that charge data may not reflect the true cost to the facility of providing care, particularly when hospitals mark up charges for services in one area in order to invest in poorly reimbursed departments (e.g., medical records) or to pay for the development of new clinical programs. This cost-shifting is common—for example, areas of the hospital with low cost-to-charge ratios are used to subsidize areas that have high costs in relation to their charges.

Differing cost-to-charge ratios produce inaccurate cost estimates. For example, estimates of the savings from percutaneous transluminal coronary angioplasty (PTCA) procedures compared with CABG surgery range from $1935 to $10,087 depending on the type of cost assumptions used.[19]

Another top-down method of estimating costs uses Medicare diagnosis-related groups (DRGs) to classify episodes of care. Although simple and efficient, this method is limited because it does not account for variations of care within a DRG, or between hospitals of varying efficiency.

Bottom-up costing is an attempt to measure costs more precisely, because, in theory, resources are tracked as care occurs.[20] Bottom-up costing separates costs into fixed and variable components.[21] Fixed costs (e.g., rental of the building that houses the surgery suite) do not change in proportion to the volume of activity, whereas variable costs—such as the price of a disposable anesthesia circuit—are closely tied to the volume of production. The majority of the costs of providing hospital care are related to buildings, equipment, and salaried or full-time hourly labor, all of which are fixed over the short term.

A misleading overstatement of costs can occur when a portion of fixed costs is allocated to what appears to be a variable cost. It is because of this fixed-cost allocation that accountants and managers often make statements such as, "Operating room time costs $20 per minute," implying—incorrectly—that if we got a patient out of the operating room 10 minutes sooner, we could save $200. The truth is that the mortgage, the administrators, and the nurses all have to be paid, whether the patient is physically in the OR or not!

The same fallacy frequently occurs in discussions of medications such as propofol, which get patients out of the OR or the postanesthesia care unit (PACU) more rapidly than alternatives. Such drugs are frequently promoted by implying that they can decrease labor costs because of more rapid patient throughput. However, this would happen only if a marginally decreased PACU census could be translated into decreased staffing levels.

Indirect Costs

Indirect costs are the value of production lost to society as a result of a patient's absence from work, disability, or death. Because indirect costs are "opportunity" costs and do not directly influence expenditures for treating disease, they are not easily measurable.[22] According to the human-capital approach, indirect costs are estimated as the income lost while the patient is absent from work.

Intangible Costs

Intangible costs represent another category of costs that—like indirect costs—are difficult to measure. These are the costs of pain, suffering, grief, and other nonfinancial outcomes of disease and medical care. They are not usually included in economic evaluations but are captured indirectly through quality-of-life scales. For example, epidural analgesia provides better relief of labor pain than IV analgesia. The additional expected cost to society of epidural analgesia for labor pain ranges from $259 to $338 per patient (depending on whether nursing costs are assumed to increase as the number of epidurals increases), relative to the expected cost of IV analgesia for labor pain.[23] Patients, physicians, and society need to weigh the intangible value of improved pain relief from epidural analgesia versus the increased cost.

Skewness in Cost Data

A distinctive feature of cost data in health care is its asymmetrical distribution (skewed to the right) and large variance (Fig. 42-2). The three measures of central tendency or "average" value of a distribution are mode, median, and mean. High-cost patients (the right-skewed tail) increase the mean to a greater extent than the median. When information about the costs of alternative treatments is to be used to guide health-care policy decision making, it is the total budget needed to treat patients with the disease that is relevant. For example, health-care planners may need information about the total annual budget involved in providing a treatment at a particular hospital. An estimate of this total cost is obtained from data in a trial by multiplying the arithmetic mean (average) cost in a particular treatment group by the total number of patients to be treated. It is therefore the arithmetic mean that is the informative measure for cost data in pragmatic clinical trials.[24]

Future Costs Need to Be Discounted to Present Values

A cost today is not equivalent to a cost in the future. Even when inflation is taken into account, a cost or an outcome today is not equivalent in value to the same cost or outcome in the future. Since people prefer to have something today instead of having it in the future, a future value must be discounted to the present, typically at 3% to 7% per year.

Good News about Costs: Marginal Costs and the Learning Curve

Despite all the difficulties in defining and estimating costs, there is some good news. Marginal costs (the cost of the next unit of production) normally decline over time. Both individuals and institutions learn and get better at tasks over time. When a technique becomes routine, people develop ways of performing the technique easily. The following are examples:

- An outside clinical laboratory establishes a blood-drawing station right next to the office of a busy surgeon, thereby saving patients time and travel.
- Anesthesia technicians skillfully assist anesthesiologists in performing invasive line placement.
- Both arthroscopic meniscectomy and laparoscopic cholecystectomy were slow and cumbersome when surgeons and their OR teams were first learning the techniques. With experience, the duration of surgery decreased, and surgeons' productivity increased.
- Larger-volume hospitals and surgeons provide superior short-term outcomes from intracranial tumor surgery.[25,26]

Medical Costs are "Right-skewed"

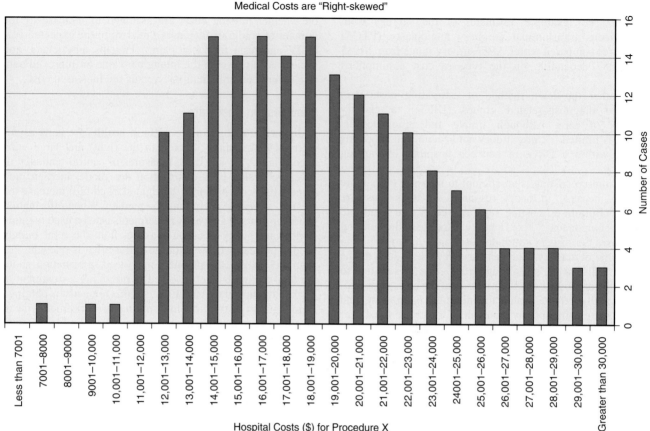

Hospital Costs ($) for Procedure X

Figure 42-2 ■ Hospital costs plotted by frequency do not follow a normal distribution. They usually exhibit skewness at the high-cost end of the distribution because there is an irreducible minimal cost even for uncomplicated cases, but there is no limit on the resources that can be consumed by complicated cases.

• System design, appropriate personnel, and an ongoing educational program are of key importance in the success of an acute pain service.[27]

Competition and the freedom to innovate produce the following "virtuous cycle" of process improvement in medicine:

Problem identification → Invention of a new treatment → Expensive and difficult implementation → Skill acquisition → Increased volume of treatment → Increased competition on the part of suppliers and caregivers → Drop in costs → A new standard of care is established at a lower marginal cost.

Because of this learning curve, truly beneficial interventions should be performed even if initial costs seem high, because we can count on costs coming down over time as a result of increased volume, experience, and competition. When curare was proposed as a new intervention to prevent fractures during electroconvulsive therapy, it might have been rejected as too expensive. Fortunately, the innovation was made despite the high initial costs.

■ BENEFITS—CLINICAL EFFECTIVENESS, UTILITY, AND "BENEFIT"

Three types of benefits are commonly studied in health-care economics:

• Desirable clinical results (i.e., effect)
• Increased utility (quality and duration of life)
• Benefit

Desirable clinical effects are desirable outcomes or results that can be measured. Examples include prolonged survival, reductions in complication rates, improved function, quicker discharge from the hospital, and decreased incidence of postoperative nausea and vomiting. Absolute risk reduction (ARR) is a way of expressing a reduction in the rate of a complication; for example, if an intervention decreased the rate of perioperative acute myocardial infarction from 5% to 2% in a selected group of patients, the resulting ARR would be 3%.

Increased Utility (Quality and Duration of Life)

Health is more than repairing injury, alleviating pain, and eliminating illness. As long ago as 1948, the World Health Organization expanded the boundaries of health to include complete physical, mental, and social well-being. We now consider the impact of a disease and its treatment on patients' daily lives.

For cost–utility analyses, quality of life has to be quantified—that is, converted into units that can be compared among different conditions. Utilities are numerical ratings, or preference weights, of the desirability of health states that reflect a person's preferences on a linear scale from 0.00 (death) to 1.00 (perfect health). It may be that some states (e.g., "recall with pain") are worse than death, but this is not easily taken into account with the utility metric. Preference values for health states are commonly obtained using valuation techniques such as the standard gamble, the time trade-off, or the visual analog scale.[28,29] Some examples of utility values for health conditions are shown in Table 42-1.

QALYs are now widely used in medical decision making and health economics as a useful outcome measure that reflects both quality of life and duration of survival. This single-score summary measure is obtained by multiplying the utility value for a given health condition by its duration. For example, the QALY score for an individual in perfect health (with a utility of 1.0) for 1 year (QALY = 1) is considered equivalent to 2 years in a health state with a utility of 0.5 (QALY = 1).

"Benefit"

The word *benefit* is used in a limited sense in the phrase *cost–benefit analysis* to mean an assigned monetary equivalent for a non-monetary benefit.

42-1 Examples of Utility Values of Health States

Health State	Utility Value
Best possible state of health	1
Postphlebotic syndrome, severe	0.93
>25 mo after lung transplantation	0.9
After kidney transplantation	0.9
Post–myocardial infarction, no congestive heart failure	0.88
Permanent colostomy without complications	0.85
Chronic hepatitis C	0.82
Angina: severe, chronic, stable	0.67
Hemodialysis	0.66
Rheumatoid arthritis, baseline	0.55
Chronic hypoxemia before oxygen therapy	0.53
Liver transplantation, first year	0.5
Stroke, moderate to severe residua	0.39
Multiple sclerosis, able to ambulate indoors with help	0.39
End-stage lung disease, 1-3 mo before death	0.3
Multiple sclerosis, confined to bed	0.26
Death	0

Data from the CEA Registry, Tufts-New England Medical Center, Institute for Clinical Research and Health Policy Studies.

■ TYPES OF ECONOMIC ANALYSIS

The three major types of economic analysis in health care are cost-identification (or cost-minimization) analysis, cost–effectiveness analysis (which includes cost–utility analysis), and cost–"benefit" analysis.

Cost-Identification (or Cost-Minimization) Analysis

Cost-identification analysis simply asks, What is the cost of a given intervention? By calculating the cost of delivering a drug, or by computing the total cost of the medical services used to treat a condition, the costs of alternative therapies can be compared. Cost-identification analysis is sometimes referred to as cost-minimization analysis, because it is often used to identify which of several therapies has the lowest cost. Cost-identification analysis assumes that the outcomes of the therapies are equivalent, so the goal is to find the least expensive way of achieving a standard outcome. For example, one study found the pharmacy cost of delivering postoperative analgesia to patients undergoing joint replacement surgery represents approximately 3.3% of the total costs of surgery.[30] No statement can be made from that study about how well the analgesia worked.

Cost-Effectiveness Analysis (Which Includes Cost-Utility Analysis)

Cost-effectiveness analyses are the most accepted economic evaluations in health care because they measure benefits in patient-oriented terms (clinical effects or quality of life). They permit comparison between different interventions by standardizing the denominators (clinical effects or utility).

Cost-effectiveness analysis, in contrast to cost-identification analysis, incorporates both cost and effect. It measures the incremental net cost of performing an intervention (expenditures for the intervention minus savings in future health-care costs) and compares it to the marginal, or incremental, benefit obtained. As described earlier (see Costs and Benefits), the incremental cost–effectiveness ratio is defined by the equation

$$ICER = (C_2 - C_1) \div (E_2 - E_1),$$

where C_2 and E_2 are the net cost and the effectiveness of the new intervention being evaluated and C_1 and E_1 are the net cost and the effectiveness of the standard therapy. In cost–utility analysis, outcomes are reported as $ per QALY. In other types of cost–effectiveness analysis, results are reported as $ per desirable clinical effect.

Medical interventions are considered to be cost effective when they produce health benefits at a cost comparable to that of other commonly accepted treatments. A general guide is that interventions that produce 1 QALY (equivalent to 1 year of perfect health) for under $50,000 are considered cost effective. Those that cost $50,000 to $100,000 per QALY are of questionable cost effectiveness, and those above $100,000 per QALY are not considered cost effective. A detailed database of cost–utility analyses is available over the internet.[31] Some examples of cost per QALY estimates from this database are shown in Table 42-2.

42-2	Examples of Cost per QALY Estimates for Interventions Compared with Alternatives				
Intervention	Alternative to Intervention	Cost* Per QALY	Year of Study	Ref. No.
Warfarin in nonvalvular atrial fibrillation, high risk for stroke	No warfarin	Cost-saving (better outcomes at lower cost)	1995	46
HIV antibody testing of blood donations	No testing	$440	1991	47
Ultrasonic screening for AAA and Rx, 60-yr-old men	No screening	$1,000	1990	48
Rx with nasal CPAP in patients with moderate to severe OSA	No Rx with nasal CPAP	$3,400	1994	49
CABG for left main CAD, good LV function, angina	Medical management	$7,500	1982	50
Antihypertensive Rx, 60-yr-old men with diastolic BP 110 mm Hg	No antihypertensive Rx	$52,000	1977	51
PA catheterization in acute COPD exacerbation, with mechanical ventilation	No PA catheter	$99,000	1994	52
Lung transplantation, patients with end-stage pulmonary disease	Standard care	$210,000	1995	53
Autologous blood donation, patients undergoing hysterectomy	Allogeneic blood donation	$1,700,000	1995	54
Annual carotid Doppler screening high-risk group	One-time screening	Dominated (worse outcomes at higher cost)	1996	55

*Cost is in 2002 dollars.

AAA, abdominal aortic aneurysm; BP, blood pressure; CABG, coronary artery bypass surgery; CAD, coronary artery disease; COPD, chronic obstructive pulmonary disease; CPAP, continuous positive airway pressure; HIV, human immunodeficiency virus; LV, left ventricular; OSA, obstructive sleep apnea; PA, pulmonary artery; Rx, treatment.

From Sa Rego MM, Inagaki Y, White PF: Anesth Analg 1999;88:723-728.

Cost–"Benefit" Analysis

Cost–"benefit" analysis, a third type of economic assessment of medical outcomes, forces an explicit decision about whether the benefit is worth the cost by quantifying benefit in dollar terms, estimated as the individual's maximal willingness to pay for the benefit. Because translating the value of health-care benefits (decreased pain and suffering, for example) into monetary terms is tricky, cost–benefit studies are done less often than cost–effectiveness studies. For example, if an analgesic provides pain relief but costs $20, a cost–benefit analysis would have the difficult methodological challenge of placing a dollar value on analgesia.

Decision Trees

Decision trees are used to evaluate costs and benefits when outcomes are uncertain but the probabilities of the outcomes can be estimated. Table 42-3 is a hypothetical decision tree analysis (DTA) of the net costs and benefits of beta blockers in patients undergoing abdominal aortic aneurysm repair. The decision tree shows the costs of the beta-blocker medication and of the three outcomes under consideration, uncomplicated recovery, acute myocardial infarction, and death, along with their probabilities, with and without perioperative beta-blocker treatment.

Despite their apparent mathematical precision, decision trees are only as good as the assumptions on which they are based. For a decision tree to be meaningful, we have to ask ourselves the following questions[32]:

1. Have we considered all relevant perioperative interventions to help the patient?
2. Have we considered all possible benefits and complications that each intervention might cause?
3. Have we accurately assessed what each possible perioperative outcome would cost the patient, both in monetary and in non-monetary terms?
4. Have we properly estimated the probabilities of the various outcomes with and without the contemplated intervention?

Sensitivity Analysis

Sensitivity analyses are necessary to evaluate the impact of changing key determining variables on the final result of the model.[33] When doing an economic modeling study, two distinct approaches are possible: frequentist and Bayesian. In the frequentist approach, unknown parameters are assumed to be fixed and nonrandom (but unknown) quantities that do not have associated probability distributions. The usual tactic for dealing with this uncertainty is to carry out a sensitivity analysis by varying the estimate within the ranges for the parameter reported in clinical trials or published literature and observing the effect of this variation on the result. This is cumbersome because it is difficult to present the results of varying three or more estimates simultaneously.

The alternative and now commonly used method is the Bayesian framework in which the parameters in a model are random variables, each with its own probability distribution.

42-3   Cost–Utility Analysis of Hypothetical Beta-Blocker

Procedure	Intervention/ Alternative	Possible Outcomes	Cost of Outcome (C)	Probability of Outcome (P)	Utility of Outcome (U)	Years Survival (S)	QALYs (P × U × S)	Cost (C × P)
AAA repair	Standard care + beta blocker	Uncomplicated recovery	20,300	.95	1	10	9.5	19,285
		AMI	31,300	.04	0.7	5	0.14	1,252
		Death	37,300	.01	0	0	0	373
		C_2 = Total cost of outcomes ($300 for beta blocker < other future medical costs)						**20,910**
		U_2 = Total QALYs					**9.64**	
	Standard care, no beta blocker	Uncomplicated recovery	20,000	.86	1	10	8.6	17,200
		AMI	31,000	.1	0.7	5	0.35	3,100
		Death	37,000	.04	0	0	0	1,480
		C_1 = Total cost of outcomes (future medical costs)						21,780
		U_1 = Total QALYs					8.95	

Conclusion: Incremental cost–utility ratio for beta blockers = $(C_2 - C_1) \div (U_2 - U_1) = -\$1,261$ per QALY. Using beta blockers *dominates* not using them. Cost/QALY is negative.

Assumptions: Total cost of administering beta blocker perioperatively = $300. Future cost savings from perioperative beta blocker use are assumed to be limited to current hospitalization.

AAA, abdominal aortic aneurysm; AMI, acute myocardial infarction.

Adapted from Fleisher LA, Corbett W, Berry C, Poldermans D: J Cardiothorac Vasc Anesth 2004;18:7-13.

For example, in a decision tree cost–utility analysis, the probability, cost, and utility of each outcome and the duration of survival are all assumed to be variables, each with a range of possible values in a probability distribution. A computer program is written to randomly select a value from the distribution of values of each parameter. In what is called Monte Carlo analysis, this process is repeated a large number of times and the mean and the variance of all the final results from all the runs are computed. This probabilistic sensitivity analysis normally assumes that the values of the parameters are independent of one another. The Bayesian framework is particularly helpful in considering uncertainties in all parameters simultaneously.[34] Importantly, this Bayesian model may produce results that are different from a simple analysis based on point estimates of probability and cost.

■ VERY HUMAN FACTORS: DIFFICULTIES IN IMPLEMENTING KNOWN BENEFICIAL INTERVENTIONS

We have attempted to outline an analytic framework for deciding what we should do in the perioperative period. This perspective highlights the need to quantify costs and benefits and then to choose the interventions that give the greatest bang for the buck, or benefit per dollar of net cost.

With relevant and reliable information about net monetary costs and rates of complications with and without our interventions, and with good estimates of what those complications cost the patient in non-monetary terms, we can, in theory, decide which of our interventions have benefits that justify their net costs. But what determines whether beneficial perioperative interventions are actually adopted or not? Are interventions with high benefit-to-cost ratios adopted

quickly? Or are forces at work other than sheer utilitarianism? We must look at human behavior to understand why adoption of beneficial perioperative interventions is not automatic and why the rate of adoption is probably not proportional to the benefit-to-cost ratio.

Incentives for Third-Party Payers

From the patient's point of view, it would be beneficial to first adopt those interventions with the highest benefit-to-cost ratios. But what are the incentives of the situation if the patient reaps the non-monetary benefit of the intervention, but a third-party payer is paying the monetary cost of the intervention?

A payer has an incentive to promote and pay for an intervention only if it will lower its own future costs. Hence, it is incumbent on doctors to demonstrate that perioperative interventions save future monetary costs as well as producing non-monetary benefits for the patient.

Incentives for Providers

Incentives are an under-recognized factor in health care because of the assumption that everyone is working for the patient's benefit. It is human nature to respond to incentives, and doctors are human. Incentives make us do things. They make us change, work harder, or work in new ways. They make us master new skills and undertake new responsibilities. They are particularly important when it is not clear who should be doing something, and also when health-care interventions are optional, exceptional, or new, and especially when they require special effort on the part of the practitioner.

We must also acknowledge when appropriate incentives are absent, as in the following examples:

- Who will take ownership of an effort to get more perioperative patients on beta blockers? The surgeon may say that it is the internist's problem, and the anesthesiologist may say that it is the surgeon's problem. If there were appropriate incentives for getting patients on beta blockers, someone might take ownership of the problem and solve it.
- Who will take ownership of DVT prophylaxis, surgical wound infection prophylaxis, or the elimination of unnecessary preoperative workups? Who has the incentive to expend time and energy to intervene across disciplinary lines, or to shake up a comfortable (and lucrative) routine?
- Substantial variation exists between hospitals in central venous catheter (CVC) insertion practices and in prevention of catheter-related bloodstream infections.[35] A meta-analysis of 11 studies demonstrated that chlorhexidine is better than povidone-iodine for site care, reducing catheter infection risk by 49%.[36] Chlorhexidine also appears to be cost effective.[37] Who has the incentive to make a systems change, such as routinely stocking chlorhexidine in ICUs and providing it in CVC trays, to ensure availability and use of chlorhexidine?

Can we be trusted to start doing things of value that we have not done before—especially if we do not get paid for them? Can we be trusted to stop doing things that have no value—especially when we have been getting paid for them?

A recent survey on the quality of health care delivered to adults in the United States revealed that the adults studied received only 54.9% of recommended care, and that the percentage of recommended care delivered varied substantially depending on the type of medical condition, ranging from 78.7% for senile cataracts to 10.5% for alcohol dependence.[38] Fee-for-service payment methods increase the performance of invasive procedures in a number of specialties, when compared with capitation and salary.[39]

Our purpose is not to disparage the profit motive in medicine, because money is a powerful motivator for most practitioners, and competition is a potent force for improvement. To be realistic about perioperative interventions and their implementation, however, we have to ask, Who makes money and who loses money with new interventions?

Ease of Performance—The Hassle Factor

Furthermore, which interventions are easy to introduce and which are a time-consuming hassle? Could ease of use be an important factor in the rate of adoption of new interventions and technologies?

Pulse oximetry and capnography were adopted rapidly in the OR because they made our jobs easier and could be installed once in an anesthetizing location and used readily for all patients. In contrast, giving DVT prophylaxis, for example, is a new effort for each patient—unless such therapy is built into the system of care.

We speculate that ease of use may help to explain differential rates of adoption of various interventions. For example, national evidence-based guidelines updated in 2002[40] recommend maximal barrier precautions (i.e., head cap, mask, sterile gloves and gown, and large sterile drape) and the Agency for Healthcare Research and Quality (AHRQ) listed these precautions as a high priority.[41] Nevertheless, compliance is low.[42] Explanations for low adherence to maximal barrier precautions include the following: (1) practitioners are not aware of the recommendations, (2) they judge that the studies were performed at sites with high infection rates, unlike their own, so the results do not apply to them, (3) they perceive the precautions to be cumbersome and time consuming, (4) they do not have the resources readily available to follow the recommendations, and (5) they do not believe the precautions are effective.[43]

To ensure the highest compliance of physicians with current best practices, we must either make sure that they have appropriate incentives for compliance or that compliance is very easy. It is the role of work-process redesign to make it easy to do the right thing! Figure 42-3 summarizes incentives and barriers to practicing the best medicine.

■ CONCLUSION: WHY OUTCOMES WILL IMPROVE

Medicine is a mixed economy, with some elements of central planning and some elements of individual freedom of choice. How do we allocate scarce resources under such circumstances? Do we build a new ICU or do we vaccinate children? And who are "we" to be deciding what society should do?

In medicine, suppliers may influence demand (e.g., a new doctor in town increases the number of surgical cases performed), patients are cost unconscious because of insurance, patients are shielded from the true cost of insurance because benefits are nontaxable, and uncertainty exists about the optimal services needed to treat patients.

Despite all these philosophical and financial cross-currents—or perhaps because of them—the reasons to be optimistic that outcomes will improve over the next decade are abundant, as shown in Figure 42-4. Some of the impetus for this improvement will come from improved technology and from physicians themselves, but much of it will come from forces outside traditional medicine: the competitive marketplace, consumer choice, and the watchdogs.

Technological Innovation

Technological innovation and the trend from invasive to noninvasive monitoring (e.g., pulse oximetry versus arterial blood gas, cardiac echocardiography versus catheterization, noninvasive cardiac output measurement versus thermodilution) will continue to increase the ease and decrease the expense of evaluating and monitoring the perioperative patient.

Physicians Get the Message of Evidence-Based Medicine

Impelled both by the demand for improved outcomes and by their intellectual honesty, doctors are embracing EBM. Whereas 20 years ago, we may have simply said that different doctors had different practice styles—as though medicine

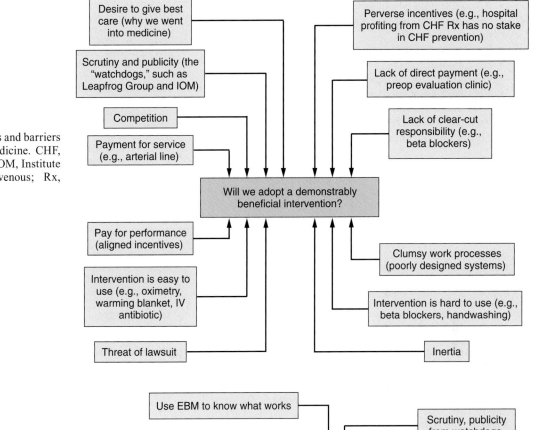

Figure 42-3 ■ Incentives and barriers to practicing the best medicine. CHF, congestive heart failure; IOM, Institute of Medicine; IV, intravenous; Rx, treatment.

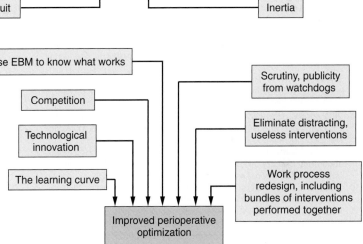

Figure 42-4 ■ How perioperative optimization gets easier, better, and cheaper. EBM, evidence-based medicine.

were a subjective discipline—today we are forced to face the fact that some of us simply practice better medicine than others.

Competition

Competition is needed to spur improvement and innovation. Competition also lowers prices in medicine, as in other areas.[44] With the end of the customary fee-for-service era, the future belongs to the lean, efficient, and effective practitioner.

The Watchdogs

Because physicians have not consistently taken ownership of significant medical problems in the realm of care delivery, a myriad of watchdog organizations, such as the Institute of Medicine, the Institute for Healthcare Improvement, and the Leapfrog Group have sprung up to provide incentives for us to do the right things in the right ways. Rather than digging in our heels and resisting change, physicians need to work with these organizations to make sure that they select worthy and achievable goals. The watchdogs will publicize our results to consumers, and physicians need to watch the watchdogs to make sure that they do a fair job of evaluating our performance.

Within general medicine the watchdogs have already set goals for management of acute myocardial infarction, heart failure, total knee replacement, and community-acquired pneumonia. With respect to the perioperative period, the watchdogs have identified the following high-priority areas[45]:

- Normothermia maintenance
- Glycemic control in the ICU and perioperative period
- Prophylaxis of deep vein thrombosis
- Beta blockers
- Central venous catheter–related infection
- Ventilator-associated pneumonia
- "Sedation vacation" for ICU patients
- Prophylaxis of surgical wound infections
- Elimination of unnecessary laboratory studies

■ REFERENCES

1. Fleisher LA, Corbett W, Berry C, Poldermans D: Cost-effectiveness of differing perioperative beta-blockade strategies in vascular surgery patients. J Cardiothorac Vasc Anesth 2004;18:7-13.
2. Lichtenberg ES, Hill LJ, Howe M, et al: A randomized comparison of propofol and methohexital as general anesthetics for vacuum abortion. Contraception 2003;68:211-217.
3. Eberhart LHJ, Eberspaecher M, Wulf H, Geldner G: Fast-track eligibility, costs and quality of recovery after intravenous anaesthesia with propofol-remifentanil versus balanced anaesthesia with isoflurane-alfentanil. Eur J Anaesthesiol 2004;21:107-114.
4. Bartha E, Carlsson P, Kalman S: Evaluation of costs and effects of epidural analgesia and patient controlled intravenous analgesia after major abdominal surgery. Br J Anaesth 2006;96:111-117.
5. Sungurtekin H, Sungurtekin U, Erdem E: Local anesthesia and midazolam versus spinal anesthesia in ambulatory pilonidal surgery. J Clin Anesth 2003;15:201-205.
6. Caron E, Bussieres JF, Lebel D, et al: Ondansetron for the prevention and treatment of nausea and vomiting following pediatric strabismus surgery. Can J Ophthalmol 2003;38:214-222.
7. Meiser A, Sirtl C, Bellgardt M, et al: Desflurane compared with propofol for postoperative sedation in the intensive care unit. Br J Anaesth 2003;90:273-280.
8. Nielsen KC, Steele SM: Outcome after regional anaesthesia in the ambulatory setting: Is it really worth it? Best Pract Res Clin Anaesthesiol 2002;16:145-157.
9. Pieri M, Meacci L, Santini L, et al: Control of acute pain after major abdominal surgery in 585 patients given tramadol and ketorolac by intravenous infusion. Drugs Exp Clin Res 2002;28:113-118.
10. Smith I: Cost considerations in the use of anaesthetic drugs. Pharmacoeconomics 2001;19(5 Pt 1):469-481.
11. Williams BA, Kentor ML, Williams JP, et al: Process analysis in outpatient knee surgery: Effects of regional and general anesthesia on anesthesia-controlled time. Anesthesiology 2000;93:529-538.
12. White PF: Pharmacoeconomic issues related to selection of neuromuscular blocking agents. Am J Health Syst Pharm 1999;56(11 Suppl 1):S18-21.
13. Sa Rego MM, Inagaki Y, White PF: The cost-effectiveness of methohexital versus propofol for sedation during monitored anesthesia care [see comment]. Anesth Analg 1999;88:723-728.
14. Tufts–New England Medical Center: Cost Effectiveness Analysis (CEA) Registry. Available at www.tufts-nemc.org/cearegistry.
15. Macario A: Systematic literature review of economics of IV patient controlled analgesia. Pharm Ther 2005;30:392-399.
16. Robinson D, Bliss E: A model of the direct and indirect effects of aprotinin administration on the overall costs of coronary revascularization surgery in a university teaching hospital cardiothoracic unit. Clin Ther 2002;24:1677-1689.
17. Fischer SP: Development and effectiveness of an anesthesia preoperative evaluation clinic in a teaching hospital [see comment]. Anesthesiology 1996;85:196-206.
18. Ferschl MB, Tung A, Sweitzer B, et al: Preoperative clinic visits reduce operating room cancellations and delays. Anesthesiology 2005;103:855-885.
19. Hlatky MA, Lipscomb J, Nelson C, et al: Resource use and cost of initial coronary revascularization: Coronary angioplasty versus coronary bypass surgery. Circulation 1990;82(Suppl 4):IV208-213.
20. Macario A, Vitez T, Dunn B, et al: Hospital costs and severity of illness in three types of elective surgery. Anesthesiology 1997;86:92-100.
21. Macario A, Vitez T, Dunn B, McDonald T: What does perioperative care really cost? Analysis of hospital costs and charges for inpatient surgical care. Anesthesiology 1995;83:1138-1144.
22. Liljas B: How to calculate indirect costs in economic evaluations. Pharmacoeconomics 1998;13(1, Pt 1):1-7.
23. Macario A, Scibetta W, Navarro J, Riley E: Analgesia for labor pain: An economic model. Anesthesiology 2000;92:841-850, .
24. Thompson SG, Barber JA. How should cost data in pragmatic randomized trials be analyzed? BMJ 2000;320:1197-1200.
25. Barker FG 2nd, Klibanski A, Swearingen B: Transsphenoidal surgery for pituitary tumors in the United States, 1996-2000: Mortality, morbidity, and the effects of hospital and surgeon volume. J Clin Endocrinol Metab 2003;88:4709-4719.
26. Long DM, Gordon T, Bowman H, et al: Outcome and cost of craniotomy performed to treat tumors in regional academic referral centers. Neurosurgery 2003;52:1056-1063.
27. Breivik H: How to implement an acute pain service. Best Pract Res Clin Anaesthesiol 2002;16:527-547.
28. Froberg DG, Kane RL: Methodology for measuring health-state preferences-II: Scaling methods. J Clin Epidemiol 1989;5:459-471.
29. Torrance GW: Social preferences for health states: An empirical evaluation of three measurement techniques. Socio-Econom Plann Sci 1976;10:129-136.
30. Macario A, McCoy M: The pharmacy cost of delivering postoperative analgesia to patients undergoing joint replacement surgery. J Pain 2003;4:22-28.
31. Harvard Center for Risk Analysis: The cost-effectiveness analysis registry. Boston, Harvard School of Public Health. Available at www.tufts-nemc.org/cearegistry.
32. Strauss SE, Richardson WS, Glasziou P, Haynes RB: Evidence-Based Medicine: How to Practice and Teach EBM, ed 3. New York, Churchill Livingstone, 2005.
33. Mullahy J, Manning W: Valuing health care: Costs, benefits, and effectiveness of pharmaceuticals and other medical technologies. In Sloan FA (ed): Statistical Issues in Cost-Effectiveness Analyses. New York, Cambridge University Press, 1995, pp 149-184.
34. Doubilet P, Begg C, Weinstein M, et al: Probabilistic sensitivity analysis using Monte-Carlo simulation. Med Dec Making 1985;5:157-177.
35. Braun BI, Kritchevsky SB, Wong ES, et al: Preventing central venous catheter-associated primary bloodstream infections: Characteristics of practices among hospitals participating in the Evaluation of Processes and Indicators in Infection Control (EPIC) study. Infect Control Hosp Epidemiol 2003;24:926-935.
36. Chaiyakunapruk N, Veenstra DL, Lipsky BA, Saint S: Chlorhexidine compared with povidone-iodine solution for vascular catheter-site care: A meta-analysis. Ann Intern Med 2002;136:792-801.
37. Chaiyakunapruk N, Veenstra DL, Lipsky BA, et al: Vascular catheter site care: The clinical and economic benefits of chlorhexidine gluconate compared with povidone iodine. Clin Infect Dis 2003;37:764-771.
38. McGlynn EA, Asch SM, Adams J, et al: The quality of health care delivered to adults in the United States. N Engl J Med 2003;348:2635-2645.
39. Saver BG, Ritzwoller DP, Maciosek M, et al: Does payment drive procedures? Payment for specialty services and procedure rate variations in 3 HMOs. Am J Manag Care 2004;10:229-237.
40. O'Grady NP, Alexander M, Dellinger EP, et al: Guidelines for the prevention of intravascular catheter-related infections. Centers for Disease Control and Prevention. MMWR Recomm Rep 2002;51(RR-10):1-29.
41. Shojania KG, Duncan BW, McDonald KM, Wachter RM: Making Health Care Safer: A Critical Analysis of Patient Safety Practices: Evidence Report/Technology Assessment No. 43. Rockville, Md, Agency for Healthcare Research and Quality, 2001, Publ 01-E058.
42. Rubinson L, Haponik EF, Wu AW, Diette GB: Internists' adherence to guidelines for prevention of intravascular catheter infections. JAMA 2003;290:2802.

43. Rubinson L, Wu AW, Haponik EE, Diette GB: Why is it that internists do not follow guidelines for preventing intravascular catheter infections? Infect Control Hosp Epidemiol 2005;26:525-523.

44. Gift TL, Arnould R, DeBrock L: Is healthy competition healthy? New evidence of the impact of hospital competition. Inquiry 2002;39: 45-55.

45. Maurer WG: Improving Quality and Safety in Perioperative Medicine, Cleveland Clinic Perioperative Medicine Summit, September 22, 2005.

46. Gage BF, Cardinalli AB, Albers GW: Cost-effectiveness of warfarin and aspirin for prophylaxis of stroke in patients with non-valvular atrial fibrillation. JAMA 1995;274:1839-1845.

47. Freedberg KA, Tosteson AN, Cohen CJ, Cotton DJ: Primary prophylaxis for *Pneumocystis carinii* pneumonia in HIV-infected people with CD4 counts below 200/mm^3: A cost-effectiveness analysis. J Acquir Immune Defic Syndr 1991;4:521-531.

48. Russell JG: Is screening for abdominal aortic aneurysm worthwhile? Clin Radiol 1990;41:182-184.

49. Tousignant P, Cosio MG, Levy RD, Groome PA: Quality adjusted life years added by treatment of obstructive sleep apnea. Sleep 1994; 17:52-60.

50. Weinstein MC, Stason WB: Cost-effectiveness of coronary artery bypass surgery. Circulation 1982;66:III56-66.

51. Stason WB, Weinstein MC: Public-health rounds at the Harvard School of Public Health: Allocation of resources to manage hypertension. N Engl J Med 1977;296:732-739.

52. Smith KJ, Pesce RR: Pulmonary artery catheterization in exacerbations of COPD requiring mechanical ventilation: A cost-effectiveness analysis. Respir Care 1994;39:961-967.

53. Ramsey SD, Patrick DL, Albert RK, et al: The cost-effectiveness of lung transplantation: A pilot study. University of Washington Medical Center Lung Transplant Study Group [comment]. Chest 1995;108: 1594-1601.

54. King JT Jr, Glick HA, Mason TJ, Flamm ES: Elective surgery for asymptomatic, unruptured, intracranial aneurysms: A cost-effectiveness analysis. J Neurosurg 1995;83:403-412.

55. Derdeyn CP, Powers WJ: Cost-effectiveness of screening for asymptomatic carotid atherosclerotic disease. Stroke 1996;27:1944-1950.

Chapter

43 Pay for Performance: An Incentive for Better Outcomes*

Ronald A. Gabel

The term *pay for performance* is generally used to mean financially rewarding health-care providers for superior performance in the care of patients.*

■ ORIGINS OF PAY FOR PERFORMANCE

Pay for performance originated with and is being driven by health-care purchasers and payers. The idea has been fueled by a relentless rise in the costs of health care. When those costs began to become a prohibitive part of the operating expenses of U.S. companies trying to compete in a global market, businesses that purchased health-care benefits for their employees began looking for ways to control costs. Many of the largest purchasers of health care are manufacturers of hard goods, who, when they purchased parts or raw materials, reasoned that they had to pay top dollar only when products met the highest specifications. In contrast, when purchasing health care, they were paying top dollar even though they had virtually no control over the quality of the product.

Payers for health care—insurance companies and health plans, looking after the interests of their primary customers, the purchasers of health care—have reasoned that money should be used as an incentive to optimize the value of their products. Whether from the purchasers' or the payers' perspective, pay for performance is driven by an effort to control health-care costs. Cynics hold that quality of care is at best a secondary consideration. On a positive note, pay for performance has energized a host of performance improvement initiatives that have languished in the absence of compelling incentives. Whether monetary rewards will actually improve the outcomes of patient care remains to be seen.

The federal government, as both a purchaser and a payer for health care, has become an enthusiastic supporter of pay for performance. The National Voluntary Hospital Reporting Initiative was started in 2003, and the Physician Voluntary Reporting Program (PVRP) was announced in October 2005. Both programs will be described here.

Pay for performance (P4P) has quickly become an integral part of health-care financing. This was documented by a 2005 survey showing that 52% of the health maintenance

organizations in 40 randomly selected U.S. markets used some form of pay for performance in their provider contracts.[1]

■ CONSUMER-DIRECTED HEALTH CARE

Pay for performance is related to consumer-directed health care, a movement based on the premise that a better-informed health-care consumer will benefit from increased knowledge about the performance of physicians and health-care organizations (hospitals, clinics, ambulatory surgery centers, and so on). Most pay-for-performance programs make the basic assumption that performance measures for which incentive bonuses are paid are "accountability measures," and those measures are fair game for public reporting. Rationale for public reporting includes the following:

- Public disclosure may motivate providers whose performance is lower than that of their peers to improve.
- Consumer choice of higher-quality health care may stretch limited health-care dollars by increasing the likelihood of favorable clinical outcomes.
- Consumer knowledge about the costs of care provided by different providers, coupled with out-of-pocket expenses (e.g., co-payments), might direct patients toward lower-cost providers.

■ VARIANTS OF PAY FOR PERFORMANCE

Many constructs of pay for performance exist:

- *Clinical processes:* Health-care providers who can document that they comply with acknowledged best practices are paid more than those who cannot so document.
- *Clinical outcomes:* Health-care providers whose clinical outcomes are superior are paid more than those who have less favorable outcomes.
- *Process improvement:* Health-care providers who can document that they engage in a program of self-improvement are financially rewarded for their efforts. This variant of pay for performance is sometimes called pay for participation.
- *Outcomes improvement:* In this variation of pay for participation, providers are paid incentive bonuses only if their quality improvement processes lead to improved patient-care outcomes.

*Because of the rapidity with which pay for performance is maturing, this chapter should be viewed as a snapshot taken in late 2006.

687

- *Processes reporting:* At least one major pay-for-performance program—the Centers for Medicare and Medicaid Services (CMS) National Voluntary Hospital Reporting Initiative—rewards providers for *reporting* whether they have complied with a set of clinical process measures, not for actually complying with the measures. (Hospitals are rewarded whether the performance is good or bad.) Results of the reporting are published on the CMS website as an adjunct to consumer-directed health care. This variant of P4P is sometimes called pay for reporting.
- *Information technology:* Many payers consider implementation of information technology to be worthy of financial reward. This approach is based on solid evidence that clinical outcomes are improved when electronic records are used to prompt for appropriate clinical processes and to flag intended actions having potential for harm (such as prescribing an inappropriate medication).
- *Patient experience:* As time goes on, payers are increasingly recognizing the importance of patient satisfaction as an indicator of quality.
- *"Efficiency":* In the lexicon of P4P, "efficiency" is a euphemism for cost (at a given level of quality). Using this metric, some payers are rewarding providers for using less expensive diagnostic and therapeutic measures, or for other forms of cost saving.
- *Appropriateness:* In the context of pay for performance, *appropriateness* refers to issues such as overuse and misuse of health-care resources. Appropriateness measures are primarily designed to control health-care costs, although some benefit may accrue to quality of patient care.

Most pay-for-performance initiatives in 2006 are focused on process-of-care measures—incentive bonuses rewarded for either reporting on or adhering to best clinical practices. In a perfect world, providers would be rewarded when their patients experience improved outcomes. However, measuring outcomes requires accounting for the considerable diversity in patient populations and severity of illness. "My patients are sicker than your patients" often provides a reasonable explanation for less favorable outcomes. Unfortunately, the science of risk adjustment is not yet sufficiently robust to be used for accurately (and fairly) comparing outcomes among different providers, either physicians or health-care organizations. Consequently, clinical processes are used as a (second-best) surrogate for outcomes.

■ MEDICARE PAYMENT ADVISORY COMMISSION

The Medicare Payment Advisory Commission (MedPAC) was established by the Balanced Budget Act of 1997 to advise the U.S. Congress on financial and quality issues related to the Medicare program. In 2003, MedPAC recommended that financial quality incentives should be built into Medicare payment policies for both individual physicians and health plans. MedPAC reasoned that higher-quality health care might ultimately lead to an overall reduction in health-care costs. The pay-for-performance system recommended by MedPAC would be revenue neutral. That is, the Medicare P4P

program should be funded through a redistribution of existing Medicare funds based on quality measurement. This would be accomplished by withholding a percentage of existing Medicare payments, thus creating a system in which some providers would be winners and some losers.[2]

In its March 2005 Report to Congress, MedPAC was specific in its recommendations, devoting a 43-page chapter to "Strategies to Improve Care: Pay for Performance and Information Technology." MedPAC explained, "We come to this year's recommendations by determining that quality measures can be used to distinguish among hospitals, home health agencies, and physicians. In each of these settings, there is some consensus on a core set of measures. Where necessary, adequate risk adjustment is available. Data needed to take these measurements can be collected without undue burden on providers or the program. Generally, there is room for improvement on the dimensions of quality we can measure. Expanded use of IT [information technology] would also increase the ability to measure and reward good performance. In sum, adequate measurement tools are available to begin paying for performance in these three settings."[3]

Many experts in quality measurement would question the optimism reflected in these statements, particularly the one regarding risk adjustment.

■ HOSPITAL QUALITY ALLIANCE

The Hospital Quality Alliance (HQA) is a collaborative representing hospitals, clinicians, consumer groups, purchasers, accrediting bodies, and government agencies. Major members include the American Hospital Association (AHA), Association of American Medical Colleges (AAMC), American Medical Association (AMA), Joint Commission on Accreditation of Healthcare Organizations (JCAHO), National Quality Forum (NQF), Agency for Healthcare Research and Quality (AHRQ), and CMS. Launched in late 2002, HQA's primary goal was to develop an infrastructure for the public reporting of quality measures by hospitals.

Box 43-1 shows HQA's original set of hospital performance measures.[4] These measures are supported and endorsed by CMS and the U.S. Congress. Medicare's operating payments to hospitals are increased annually by a factor determined in part by the projected annual change in the hospital "market basket." The 2003 Medicare Prescription Drug Improvement and Modernization Act (MMA) contains a provision that acute-care hospitals would have to submit data on the above 10 HQA measures to receive their full Medicare inpatient prospective payment system (PPS) market-basket update for fiscal years 2005-2007. Hospitals failing to submit data on these measures would have their market-basket updates reduced by 0.4%.[5] CMS referred to this reporting requirement as the National Voluntary Hospital Reporting Initiative.

Reinforcing that the Congress was in earnest when establishing a penalty for failure of hospitals to participate in this program, the Deficit Reduction Act of 2005 specified, "for fiscal year 2007 and each subsequent fiscal year . . . a hospital that does not submit, to the Secretary . . . data required to be submitted on measures selected . . . , the appli-

43-1	The Original Set of Hospital Quality Alliance Performance Measures

Heart Attack

- Did the patient receive aspirin within 24 hours before or after hospital arrival?
- Did the patient receive a beta blocker within 24 hours after hospital arrival?
- Was aspirin prescribed at hospital discharge?
- Was a beta blocker prescribed at hospital discharge?
- Was either an angiotensin-converting enzyme inhibitor (ACEI) or an angiotensin-receptor blocker (ARB) prescribed at hospital discharge?

Heart Failure

- Was left ventricular function (LVF) assessed before arrival or during hospitalization, or was assessment planned for after discharge?
- Was either an angiotensin-converting enzyme inhibitor (ACEI) or an angiotensin-receptor blocker (ARB) prescribed at hospital discharge for patients with left ventricular systolic dysfunction (LVSD)?

Pneumonia

- Did the patient receive a first dose of antibiotics within 4 hours after hospital arrival?
- Was the patient's arterial oxygenation assessed by arterial blood gas measurement or pulse oximetry within 24 hours prior to or after arrival at the hospital?
- Was the patient screened for pneumococcal vaccine status and administered the vaccine prior to hospital discharge if indicated?

From Department of Health and Human Services, Centers for Medicare and Medicaid Services: The Hospital Quality Alliance (HQA) Ten Measure "Starter Set." November 22, 2005. Available at www.cms.hhs.gov/HospitalQualityInits/downloads/HospitalStarterSet200512.pdf.

43-2	The Current Set of Hospital Quality Alliance (HQA) Measures

Heart Attack

- Aspirin at arrival
- Aspirin at discharge
- Beta blocker at arrival
- Beta blocker at discharge
- ACE inhibitor or angiotensin-receptor blocker (ARB) for left ventricular systolic dysfunction (LVSD)
- Thrombolytic agent received within 30 minutes of hospital arrival
- Percutaneous coronary intervention (PCI) received within 120 minutes of hospital arrival
- Adult smoking cessation advice/counseling

Heart Failure

- Left ventricular function (LVF) assessment
- ACE inhibitor or angiotensin-receptor blocker (ARB) for left ventricular systolic dysfunction (LVSD)
- Discharge instructions
- Adult smoking cessation advice/counseling

Pneumonia

- Initial antibiotic timing
- Pneumococcal vaccination status
- Oxygenation assessment
- Blood culture performed before first antibiotic received in hospital
- Appropriate initial antibiotic selection
- Adult smoking cessation advice/counseling

Surgical Infection Prevention

- Prophylactic antibiotic received within 1 hour prior to surgical incision
- Prophylactic antibiotics discontinued within 24 hours after surgery end time

From Department of Health & Human Services, Centers for Medicare & Medicaid Services. Overview of Specifications of Measures Displayed on Hospital Compare as of December 15, 2005. Available at www.cms.hhs.gov/HospitalQualityInits/downloads/HospitalOverviewOfSpecs200512.pdf.

cable percentage increase . . . for such fiscal year shall be reduced by 2.0 percentage points."[6] For reference, 2% of the annual PPS market-basket update could amount to as much as $750,000 for a hospital having an average daily occupancy of 200 patients.

In 2005, the HQA measurement set was ramped up to include the 20 measures shown in Box 43-2. From CMS's standpoint, the additional measures were voluntary, because only the initial 10 measures were linked to payment by the enabling legislation. However, other agencies, such as the Joint Commission, encouraged hospitals to collect and report on the expanded set of measures.

CMS has worked closely with the JCAHO in developing the measures associated with CMS's National Voluntary Hospital Reporting Initiative. In September 2004, CMS announced, "In an effort to help consumers make the best decisions about their health care, the Centers for Medicare & Medicaid Services (CMS) and the Joint Commission on the Accreditation of Healthcare Organizations (JCAHO) are adopting standardized performance measures for hospitals to report how well they provide health care services. . . . CMS and JCAHO today issued a technical manual for hospital quality measures that provides common definitions for each of the quality measures that are being collected and reported.

Hospitals will use these common definitions to report on their quality for both the National Voluntary Hospital Reporting Initiative and for JCAHO accreditation, beginning with January 2005 discharges."[7]

The 2005 Deficit Reduction Act ensured that the performance of all participating hospitals on each of the measures would be publicly reported: "The Secretary shall establish procedures for making data submitted under this clause available to the public. Such procedures shall ensure that a hospital has the opportunity to review the data that are to be made public with respect to the hospital prior to such data being made public. The Secretary shall report quality measures of process, structure, outcome, patients' perspectives on care, efficiency, and costs of care that relate to services furnished in inpatient settings in hospitals on the Internet website of the Centers for Medicare & Medicaid Services."[6]

Data reported through the National Voluntary Hospital Reporting Initiative are available to the public at www.hospitalcompare.hhs.gov.

■ PHYSICIAN VOLUNTARY REPORTING PROGRAM

The PVRP is a prelude to a Medicare pay-for-performance program for physicians. It was introduced through a CMS press release on October 28, 2005, which stated, "To help support better health outcomes for people with Medicare at a lower cost, CMS is working closely and collaboratively with medical professionals and Congress to consider changes to increase the effectiveness of how Medicare compensates physicians for providing services to Medicare beneficiaries, while avoiding increases in overall Medicare costs. As part of this effort, the Physician Voluntary Reporting Program will begin to phase in voluntary reporting of performance measures developed in collaboration with physicians and physician organizations, as well as other stakeholders."[8]

The initial plan was for physicians to submit information on their performance on a set of 36 measures. After sufficient data were aggregated, CMS would provide feedback to participating physicians on how their performance compares with other physicians. This pattern is similar to the manner in which CMS introduced the National Voluntary Hospital Reporting Initiative. In fact, the October 2005 press release on PVRP stated, "The Physician Voluntary Reporting Program is similar to previous CMS quality initiatives such as the hospital voluntary reporting program, which, after an initial collaborative process of evaluating and refining hospital data submission, resulted in the launch of www.HospitalCompare.hhs.gov in April, 2005."[8]

Many physicians and medical organizations viewed the PVRP with skepticism. Some felt that "incentive payments" represented only diversionary and token mitigation for continuing reductions in Medicare physician reimbursement. Others expressed serious concern about the administrative burden of reporting the measures and the resulting disincentive to caring for Medicare beneficiaries. Still others criticized the 36 performance measures chosen by CMS to be reported in the program.

Responsive to concerns expressed by physician organizations, CMS announced in December 2005, "Continued interaction with physicians after the announcement of PVRP has indicated significant interest in participation among physician practices. However, suggestions have also been made by several physician organizations to identify a starter set in order to lessen the potential reporting burden for physicians and better align the PVRP with other quality measurement activities affecting physicians. CMS has decided to adopt the suggestion of a smaller core starter set of PVRP measures. The core set consists of 16 measures which will significantly reduce the number of measures applicable to any individual physician practice specialty."[9]

CMS subsequently made several incremental changes in the specifications for the 16 performance measures in the PVRP "starter set." However, the measures themselves, which are listed in Box 43-3, remained stable between December 2005 and July 2006.[10]

The U.S. Congress will have to pass enabling legislation before pay for performance can be incorporated into the Medicare payment system for physicians. Two bills containing provisions for physician pay for performance were introduced during the 109th Congress:

- Medicare Value-Based Purchasing for Physicians' Services Act of 2005 (H.R. 3617) sponsored by Congresswoman Nancy L. Johnson (Connecticut)[11]
- Medicare Value Purchasing Act of 2005 (S. 1356) sponsored by Senator Chuck Grassley (Iowa)[12]

Neither of these bills had been voted into law by early December 2006.

■ COMMERCIAL PAY-FOR-PERFORMANCE PROGRAMS

Many commercial health-care insurers have enthusiastically embraced pay for performance for physicians. California is in the national vanguard, with Massachusetts running a strong second. To date, the most serious incentive payments for physicians have been directed toward large multiple-specialty group practices and primary care doctors.

A 2005 survey of health plans offering HMO (health maintenance organization) products in 40 randomly selected U.S. markets in which at least 100,000 persons were enrolled in HMOs showed that 52% of the HMOs studied (126 of 242) used some form of pay for performance in their provider contracts. Of the 126 health plans utilizing pay for perfor-

---

43-3	The 16-Measure "Starter Set" for the Physician Voluntary Reporting Program

1. Aspirin at arrival for acute myocardial infarction
2. Beta blocker at time of arrival for acute myocardial infarction
3. Hemoglobin A_{1c} control in patient with type I or type II diabetes mellitus
4. Low-density lipoprotein control in patient with type I or type II diabetes mellitus
5. High blood pressure control in patient with type I or type II diabetes mellitus
6. Angiotensin-converting enzyme inhibitor or angiotensin-receptor blocker therapy for left ventricular systolic dysfunction
7. Beta-blocker therapy for patient with prior myocardial infarction
8. Assessment of elderly patients for falls
9. Dialysis dose in end-stage renal disease patient
10. Hematocrit level in end-stage renal disease patient
11. Receipt of autogenous arteriovenous fistula in end-stage renal disease patient requiring hemodialysis
12. Antidepressant medication during acute phase for patient diagnosed with new episode of major depression
13. Antibiotic prophylaxis in surgical patient
14. Thromboembolism prophylaxis in surgical patient
15. Use of internal mammary artery in coronary artery bypass graft surgery
16. Preoperative beta blocker for patient with isolated coronary artery bypass graft

From Department of Health & Human Services, Centers for Medicare & Medicaid Services: Physician Voluntary Reporting Program (PVRP) 16 Measure Core Starter Set G-Code Specifications and Instruction. July 1, 2006. Available at www.cms.hhs.gov/PVRP/Downloads/PVRPCoreStarterSetSpecificationsAndInstruction200607.pdf.

mance, 90% had a physician P4P program and 38% a hospital program.[1]

California is a leader in P4P largely because about 50% of California's population belongs to an HMO. Integrated Health Association (IHA)—a pay-for-performance consortium of health plans, physician groups, health care systems, business groups, and consumer groups—plays a dominant role. IHA's pay-for-performance program, the largest in the nation, encompasses seven major health plans: Aetna, Blue Cross, Blue Shield, Cigna, Health Net, PacifiCare, and Western Health Advantage. IHA's P4P data are collected and aggregated by the National Committee on Quality Assurance (NCQA). In 2005, IHA paid more than $88 million to 235 medical groups involving about 35,000 physicians participating in California Pay for Performance.[13]

In 2006, the largest health-care insurer in Massachusetts, Blue Cross Blue Shield (BCBS), reported that it planned to increase the incentive-based portion of its payments to about 5200 primary-care physicians from 10% in 2005 to as much as 13%. That could amount to $10,000 per physician, and a total annual outlay of $52 million. Additionally, Massachusetts BCBS is developing ways to assess the performance of 9100 cardiologists, oncologists, and other specialists, planning eventually to use P4P scores to allocate 5% to 10% of its payments to specialists.[14]

■ PAY-FOR-PERFORMANCE PRINCIPLES AND GUIDELINES

The AMA has developed sets of principles and guidelines for pay for performance. The principles assert that P4P should do the following[15]:

- Ensure quality of care
- Foster the patient–physician relationship
- Offer voluntary physician participation
- Use accurate data and fair reporting
- Provide fair and equitable program incentives

The AMA "Guidelines for Pay-for-Performance Programs" augment the AMA's "Principles for Pay-for-Performance Programs," and they "provide AMA leaders, staff and members with operational boundaries that can be used in an assessment of specific PFP programs."[16]

Similarly, the JCAHO has developed "Principles for the Construct of Pay-for-Performance Programs," which declare (in part) the following[17]:

- The goal of pay-for-performance programs should be to align reimbursement with the practice of high quality, safe health care for all consumers.
- Programs should include a mix of financial and non-financial incentives (such as reduction of administrative and regulatory burdens and public acknowledgment of performance) that are designed to achieve program goals. Rewards should be great enough to drive desired behaviors and support consistently high quality care.
- When selecting the areas of clinical focus, programs should strongly consider consistency with national and regional efforts to leverage change and reduce conflicting or competing measurement.
- Programs should be designed to ensure that metrics upon which incentive payments are based are credible, valid and reliable.

■ DESIGN PRINCIPLES FOR PAY-FOR-PERFORMANCE MEASURES

The following set of six design principles for pay-for-performance measures were reported in the proceedings of a Disease Management Outcomes Summit held in November 2004[18]:

- *Volume:* The process or outcome being measured should be common or frequently experienced.
- *Gravity:* Changes in the performance being measured should have a substantial impact on health, functioning, or well being.
- *Evidence:* Empirical evidence should link changes in measures with clinically important changes in health, functioning, or well being.
- *Gap in care:* Measures should deal with discrepancies between current practice and what can be achieved.
- *Prospects:* The prospects for improvement in the performance being measured should be substantial.
- *Reliability-validity-feasibility:* Measures should produce consistent results over time and across observers ("reliability"); they should be consistently associated with desired outcomes ("validity"); and methods should exist for efficient and minimally burdensome acquisition of data ("feasibility").

■ PERFORMANCE MEASURES

Performance measures form the foundation of pay for performance, in that health-care providers are paid an incentive bonus based on meeting the specifications of a performance measure when providing patient care. The example in Box 43-4 is a process measure that could be used by physicians to document their compliance with a "best clinical practice."

Denominator exclusions are an important way for process measures to be applied fairly in pay for performance. Denominator exclusions are to process measures what risk adjustment is to outcome measures. That is, they compensate for factors that are not under direct control of the physician. Following are the types of denominator exclusions used for Category II Current Procedural Terminology (CPT) performance measurement codes[19]:

- *Medical reasons:* Not indicated (absence of organ/limb, already received/performed, other); contraindicated (patient allergic history, potential adverse drug interaction, other)
- *Patient reasons:* Patient declined; economic, social, or religious reasons; other patient reasons
- *System reasons:* Resources to perform the services not available; insurance coverage/payer-related limitations; other reasons attributable to health care delivery system

43-4	**Typical Physician Process Performance Measure***
Name of measure	Timely administration of prophylactic antibiotics
Clinical recommendation	Prophylactic antibiotics should be given within 1 hour prior to the surgical incision to ensure adequate concentration in the targeted tissues.
Rationale	Prophylactic antibiotics administered within 1 hour prior to the surgical incision have been demonstrated to reduce the incidence of surgical wound infections.
Level of evidence for rationale	Prospective cohort study involving 2800 patients in one medical center**
Gap in care	Available evidence suggests that although most surgical patients receive a prophylactic antibiotic, many do not receive the drug within one hour before incision as recommended.
Level of evidence for gap in care	Retrospective cohort study involving random sample of 34,000 patients**
Numerator	Surgical patients to whom administration of a prophylactic antibiotic was initiated within 1 hour prior to the surgical incision (or start of procedure when no incision is required)
Denominator	All surgical patients 18 years and older who have an order for an antibiotic to be given within 1 hour prior to the surgical incision (or start of procedure when no incision is required)
Denominator instruction	An order (written order, verbal order, or standing order/protocol) must be documented specifying that an antibiotic should be given within 1 hour prior to the surgical incision (or start of procedure when no incision is required).
Denominator exclusion	None
Population feedback	Percentage of patients who were given a prophylactic antibiotic within 1 hour prior to the surgical incision (or start of procedure when no incision is required) when so ordered

*This example is based loosely on a measure developed by the American Medical Association's Physician Consortium for Performance Improvement (available at www.physicianconsortium.org).

**Many methods exist for ranking strength of evidence. This example describes major studies rather than a standing in a ranking system.

43-5	**Performance Measurement Sets of the AMA Physician Consortium for Performance Improvement (December 2006)**

1. Adult diabetes
2. Asthma
3. Chronic obstructive pulmonary disease
4. Chronic stable coronary artery disease
5. Colorectal cancer screening
6. Community-acquired bacterial pneumonia
7. End-stage renal disease
8. Eye care
9. Heart failure
10. Hypertension
11. Influenza immunization
12. Major depressive disorder
13. Mammography screening
14. Melanoma
15. Osteoarthritis
16. Osteoporosis
17. Pediatric acute gastroenteritis
18. Prenatal testing
19. Perioperative care
20. Problem drinking
21. Stroke and stroke rehabilitation
22. Tobacco use

From American Medical Association: Consortium measures. Available at http://www.ama-assn.org/ama/pub/category/4837.html.

Consequently, the strength of evidence does not have to be as rigorous as for accountability measures, which are designed for public disclosure. Pay-for-performance measures are, by definition, accountability measures and therefore should meet a high standard for strength of evidence.

■ DEVELOPMENT AND ENDORSEMENT OF PERFORMANCE MEASURES

The Hospital Quality Alliance has developed the most influential hospital performance measures, as described earlier. Most physician performance measures have been developed by medical specialty societies, CMS, or NCQA, often working collaboratively. Technically, NCQA develops performance measures for health plans, but the measures are relevant to the physicians working in those plans.

The AMA in 2001 convened the Physician Consortium for Performance Improvement, a collaborative of medical societies dedicated to developing physician performance measures. By December 2006, the Consortium had grown to include 78 medical specialty societies and 19 state medical societies, and had developed 130 performance measures in the 22 measurement sets listed in Box 43-5. The Consortium has developed many of its measures in collaboration with CMS and NCQA for use in the Physician Voluntary Reporting Program.

NCQA was an early leader in the development of physician performance measures for use in its accreditation program for health plans. NCQA's HEDIS (Health Plan Employer Data and Information Set), first developed in 1991,

Performance measures may reflect differing thresholds for the strength of scientific evidence supporting them. Measures are sometimes dichotomized into two major categories: quality improvement and accountability. Quality improvement measures are usually designed for the private use of health-care providers and are not expected to be made public.

"is a set of standardized measures that specifies how organizations collect, audit and report performance information across the most pressing clinical areas, as well as important dimensions of customer satisfaction and patient experience."[20] Note that in this description, NCQA indicates that HEDIS is a measurement set for organizations, not for individual physicians.

The Ambulatory Care Quality Alliance (AQA) was founded in September 2004 by the American Academy of Family Physicians (AAFP), the American College of Physicians (ACP), America's Health Insurance Plans (AHIP), and the Agency for Healthcare Research and Quality. The goal of the founding organizations was to improve physician-level performance measurement, data aggregation, and reporting mechanisms. After starting with a relatively narrow focus, AQA broadened its mission to address all areas of physician practice—not just ambulatory care—and grew rapidly. By September 2006, representatives of 114 providers, consumers, payers, and purchasers of health care were participating in AQA activities.[21] In 2005, AQA compiled a "starter set" of 26 ambulatory care measures composed of physician performance measures that were developed by other organizations.[22] AQA does not develop performance measures itself. The AQA starter set formed a foundation for the CMS Physician Voluntary Reporting Project.[8-10]

Endorsement by the National Quality Forum (NQF) is considered by many to be an essential stamp of approval for performance measures. The NQF was founded on recommendation of the 1998 President's Advisory Commission on Consumer Protection and Quality in the Healthcare Industry.[23] The NQF is organized into four large Councils: (1) Consumer, (2) Health Professional, Provider, and Health Plan, (3) Purchaser, and (4) Research and Quality Improvement. On balance, the voice of health-care providers in the NQF is widely perceived to be subordinate to that of consumers and purchasers of health care. Emblematic of that balance is the NQF's official position on public reporting: "Underlying all of the NQF's activities is a philosophy that health care quality data are a public good and should be in the public domain, and when joining the NQF, member organizations acknowledge a statement of principle, indicating their willingness to use indicators of health care quality and to publicly disclose the results."[24] This philosophy tends to preclude NQF from endorsing physician-developed performance measures designed primarily for physician self-improvement, which may not have attributes permitting fair comparison among physicians.

METHODS FOR REPORTING PERFORMANCE

Providers rendering clinical care meeting the criteria of specific performance measures can report their eligibility for an incentive bonus either retrospectively or concurrently with the rendering of clinical services. The method used depends largely on the type of provider doing the reporting. Physicians are more likely to gather and report performance measures as an integral part of their care of patients, often using a coding system integrated into their billing systems. Healthcare organizations, on the other hand, are more likely to report performance measures based on retrospective review of medical records.

Concurrent reporting has a substantial advantage over retrospective reporting in terms of its ability to modify behavior. When quality management is integrated into clinical practice management, the quality process can drive appropriate practice. Paper-based flow sheets and electronic medical records designed to collect quality data can concurrently prompt the physician to meet quality standards. Retrospective data gathering does not have this benefit.

Two national coding systems exist for reporting compliance with the specifications of performance measures. The Healthcare Common Procedure Coding System (HCPCS) is maintained by CMS. G-codes, which appear in HCPCS in the form "Gxxxx" (where xxxx is a number), have traditionally been used as temporary billing codes until more permanent codes could be developed. However, CMS has designated certain G-codes to be used for pay for performance.[10]

CPT codes form the foundation for physician billing in the United States. In 2001, the AMA, which maintains the CPT coding system, added Category II codes to the CPT system. In contrast to Category I codes, which are used to report clinical services for which payment is sought, Category II codes are used to report performance. By December 2006, the CPT coding system contained more than 250 numerator and denominator codes for performance measures.[19] Category II CPT codes are more widely applicable than HCPCS G-codes, because they encompass a wider range of performance measures and are not limited to those applicable to the Medicare population. The specifications for the PVRP performance measures list both CPT-II and G-codes, where applicable.[10]

PERIOPERATIVE PERFORMANCE MEASURES

Perioperative performance measures exist for both hospitals and physicians. The expanded set of Hospital Quality Alliance measures in Box 43-2 contains two perioperative measures under the heading of Surgical Infection Prevention:

- Prophylactic antibiotic received within 1 hour prior to surgical incision
- Prophylactic antibiotics discontinued within 24 hours after surgery end time

These measures are similar to the first four measures in the following set of physician perioperative performance measures promulgated by the AMA Physician Consortium[25]:

- Timing of prophylactic antibiotics—ordering physician
- Timing of prophylactic antibiotics—administering physician
- Discontinuation of prophylactic antibiotics (noncardiac procedures)
- Discontinuation of prophylactic antibiotics (cardiac procedures)
- Selection of prophylactic antibiotic
- Venous thromboembolism (VTE) prophylaxis

As is evident from the first two *physician* measures, some physician measures include an attribute that hospital measures do not have—designation of the person responsible for ensuring compliance with the measure. The surgeon is expected to write the order or be responsible for ensuring that an order is written for the timely administration of prophylactic antibiotics. The anesthesiologist is expected to administer the antibiotics or ensure that they are administered in timely fashion. In contrast, hospital measures display no such specificity, because the hospital will be rewarded or penalized based on compliance with the measures (or reporting on them) no matter who ensures that the best practices embodied in the measures are followed.

Another difference between the hospital and physician perioperative measures is the method of reporting. As noted earlier (see Methods for Reporting Performance), physicians gather data concurrently with providing the clinical service, and they report on the measures when submitting financial claims for their services. In contrast, hospitals gather data on the HQA measures through retrospective chart review and report them to the JCAHO and CMS through an independent process unrelated to hospital billing. When the first sets of perioperative physician measures were developed, concern was expressed about minor inconsistencies between the physician measures and the HQA hospital measures (which had been developed first). In retrospect, this was not a problem, because the measures are complementary and not contradictory. Overlapping hospital and physician measures do not have to be identical to ensure compliance with best clinical practices.

EFFICIENCY PERFORMANCE MEASURES

In support of the hypothesis that pay for performance is as strongly related to cost as to quality, "efficiency measures" are increasingly being added to the pay-for-performance mix. *Efficiency of care* refers to achieving a specified level of quality of care at the lowest possible cost. Included in the definition are considerations of waste, misuse, and overuse.

The Executive Director of the MedPAC recommended the following action during Congressional testimony in March 2005: "The Secretary should use Medicare claims data to measure fee-for-service physicians' resource use and share results with physicians confidentially to educate them about how they compare with aggregated peer performance. The Congress should direct the Secretary to perform this function. Educating physicians about their resource use should encourage those who practice significantly differently than their peers to reconsider their practice patterns."[26]

CMS has not yet initiated such a program, largely because of the enormity of the task and its associated costs. In contrast, many commercial insurers have liberally incorporated "efficiency measures" into their pay-for-performance programs.

Care must be taken to look at *efficiency* and *cost of care* in the context of quality. Clearly, resource use that does not lead to patient benefit should be critically scrutinized. However, increased quality of patient care is often dependent on increased resource utilization. Consequently, high rates of utilization are not appropriate surrogates for waste, misuse, or overuse. The development of efficiency performance measures that are meaningful and contribute to quality is not a trivial task. In fact, without the ability to measure clinical outcomes reliably, "efficiency measures" could lead to serious unintended consequences.

FINANCIAL INCENTIVES

Participation in P4P involves both benefits and costs to health-care providers. The cost and effort required to gather and transmit necessary data to the payers can be substantial. Payers are trying to determine how high the financial rewards need to be to modify provider behavior. Current conventional wisdom suggests that incentive payments of about 10% of revenues might be necessary to entice physicians to participate.[14]

Indifference to the rewards of P4P is exhibited in the following statement titled "Primary Care—Will It Survive?" that appeared in a 2006 article: "Pay-for-performance programs appear to be insufficient to make a substantial difference; physicians could increase their income more-with less additional work-by adding one or two patient visits each day than by meeting all the quality standards in current performance-based payment programs."[27] This statement challenges the designers of payment systems who seek to alter the balance between performance-based and volume-based reimbursement.

Financial incentives can be positive or negative. That is, better performers can be rewarded, or providers at the low end of the continuum can be penalized, for their performance. An example of the latter is the CMS National Voluntary Hospital Reporting Initiative, in which annual payment updates are reduced for hospitals that do not meet certain reporting requirements.

THE BRITISH EXPERIENCE

The British National Health Service (NHS) was an early adopter of pay for performance, having initiated its first program in 1991. After the success of increasingly more ambitious efforts, the NHS in 2004 introduced a large-scale pay-for-performance program for family practitioners that is being supported over the first 3 years by £1.8 billion ($3.2 billion) in new funding. The program is capable of increasing the income of family practitioners by up to 25%, depending on their performance on 146 quality indicators covering clinical care for 10 chronic diseases, organization of care, and patient experience.[28]

An analysis of the first year of the program showed that the gross income of the average practitioner was increased by £23,000 ($40,200) for achieving a median of 95.5% of the total number of points available. The incremental income was offset to an unknown extent by the costs of meeting the targets and reporting the data. Roughly half of the incentive points were allocated to clinical quality indicators, and the remainder to organizational quality and patient experience. The median achievement on the clinical indicators was 83.4%

overall, with scores for individual diseases ranging from 80.1% for diabetes to 96.0% for hypothyroidism.[28]

The NHS program permits practitioners to exclude certain patients for indicators associated with inappropriate treatment, such as cholesterol management in terminally ill patients. "Exception reports" represented a median of 6% of all reports during the first year of the program. However, the range was from 0% to 86%, with 91 practices (1.1%) excluding more than 15% of their patients. This suggests "gaming," because exception reporting provides an opportunity to obtain incentive income by inappropriately excluding patients for whom quality targets have not been reached.[28]

■ UNCERTAINTIES AND POTENTIAL PITFALLS

Pay for performance is at an early stage of development in the United States. Consequently, little scientific evidence is available to answer important questions:

- Does P4P lead to improved health status of patients whose health-care providers are rewarded for meeting certain quality targets?
- Does P4P produce unintended consequences, such as increased costs of care or even patient harm resulting from financially rewarding behavior that is based on a set of predetermined rules?
- What are the absolute and relative costs of gathering, reporting, and processing P4P data? What proportion of the incentive payments represents overhead costs for gathering and reporting data?

A scientific article published in 2005 found that P4P rewarded practitioners who had high performance at baseline but did little to improve quality of care.[29] An accompanying editorial appealed for increased research on pay for performance and outlined a set of research priorities.[30]

Financial incentives have considerable power to modify human behavior. However, a potential downside exists when health care is the object of the behavioral modification. Many aspects of the care of patients may be too complex to be subject to a set of rules that simply state, in essence, "Do this and be financially rewarded. Do that, and be penalized." For the system to work safely in the best interests of all patients, performance measures must be structured so their application is very unlikely to produce patient harm.

Another potential pitfall is related to the rapidity with which the scientific foundations of health care change. Compounding that potential problem is the relative slowness with which bureaucracies modify rules they have established. P4P programs must be under continuous reassessment to ensure that the actions rewarded are, in fact, the most clinically appropriate and up-to-date.

■ THE FUTURE

The growth of pay-for-performance initiatives in both number and variations has not yet reached its pinnacle. Current trends forecast increasing pressures for (1) the public accountability of health-care providers, (2) continued growth in consumer-directed health care, and (3) increasing financial rewards for providers who meet certain performance targets related to both quality and "efficiency." Currently available performance measures tend to be narrowly defined and applicable to only a limited patient population and a small number of health-care issues. Future measures are likely to become more broadly based so as to be more representative of overall quality and cost of care. Some observers even predict that the current provider payment system based on units of service may eventually be replaced by a system based largely on performance.

■ REFERENCES

1. Rosenthal MB, Landon BE, Normand ST, et al: Pay for performance in commercial HMOs. N Engl J Med 2006;355:1895-1902.
2. Milgate K, Cheng SB: Pay-for-performance: The MedPAC perspective. Health Affairs 2006;25:413-419.
3. MedPAC Report to the Congress: Medicare Payment Policy. March 2005. Available at www.medpac.gov/publications/congressional_reports/Mar05_EntireReport.pdf (accessed December 4, 2006).
4. Department of Health and Human Services, Centers for Medicare and Medicaid Services: The Hospital Quality Alliance (HQA) Ten Measure "Starter Set." November 22, 2005. Available at www.cms.hhs.gov/HospitalQualityInits/downloads/HospitalStarterSet200512.pdf (accessed December 4, 2006).
5. CMS Legislative Summary of H.R. 1 Medicare Prescription Drug, Improvement, and Modernization Act of 2003, Public Law 108-173. Sec. 501: Revision of Acute Care Hospital Payment Updates, p 69. April 2004. Available at www.cms.hhs.gov/relevantlaws/downloads/legislativesummaryforMMAof2003.pdf (accessed December 4, 2006).
6. Deficit Reduction Act of 2005, Conference Report 109-362 [to accompany S. 1932]. December 19, 2005, pp 26-27. Available at frwebgate.access.gpo.gov/cgi-bin/getdoc.cgi?dbname=109_cong_reports&docid=f:hr362.pdf (accessed December 4, 2006).
7. Department of Health and Human Services, Centers for Medicare and Medicaid Services: Press release: CMS and JCAHO make it easier for consumers to assess hospital quality. Medicare teams with hospital accrediting organization on national measures for hospital performance. September 15, 2004. Available at www.cms.hhs.gov/apps/media/press/release.asp?Counter=1201 (accessed December 4, 2006).
8. Department of Health and Human Services, Centers for Medicare and Medicaid Services: Press release: Medicare takes key step toward voluntary quality reporting for physicians. October 28, 2005. Available at www.cms.hhs.gov/apps/media/press/release.asp?Counter=1699 (accessed December 4, 2006).
9. Department of Health and Human Services, Centers for Medicare and Medicaid Services: PVRP Core Starter Set Background and General Information, as of December 27, 2005. Available at www.cms.hhs.gov/PhysicianFocusedQualInits/Downloads/PFQIPVRP_Starter_Set_Information.pdf (accessed December 4, 2006).
10. Department of Health and Human Services, Centers for Medicare and Medicaid Services: Physician Voluntary Reporting Program (PVRP) 16 Measure Core Starter Set G-Code Specifications and Instruction. July 1, 2006. Available at www.cms.hhs.gov/PVRP/Downloads/PVRPCoreStarterSetSpecificationsAndInstruction200607.pdf (accessed December 4, 2006).
11. Medicare Value-Based Purchasing for Physicians' Services Act of 2005 (H.R. 3617). July 29, 2005. Available at http://frwebgate.access.gpo.gov/cgi-bin/getdoc.cgi?dbname=109_cong_bills&docid=f:h3617ih.txt.pdf (accessed December 4, 2006).
12. Medicare Value Purchasing Act of 2005 (S.1356). June 30, 2005. Available at http://frwebgate.access.gpo.gov/cgi-bin/getdoc.cgi?dbname=109_cong_bills&docid=f:s1356is.txt.pdf (accessed December 4, 2006).
13. Lauer G: California pay-for-performance programs draws national attention. California Healthline, February 8, 2006. Available at www.californiahealthline.org/index.cfm?action=dspItem&itemID=118603 (accessed December 4, 2006).

14. Rowland C: A better tool to fight rising health costs? Blue Cross to double its spending on incentives tied to performance by doctors and hospitals, raising fears patient care could suffer. Boston Globe, May 10, 2006. Available at www.boston.com/business/globe/articles/2006/05/10/a_better_tool_to_fight_rising_health_costs?mode=PF (accessed December 4, 2006).

15. American Medical Association: Principles for Pay-for-Performance Programs. June 25, 2005. Available at www.ama-assn.org/ama1/pub/upload/mm/368/principles4pay62705.pdf (accessed December 4, 2006).

16. American Medical Association: Guidelines for Pay-for-Performance Programs. June 25, 2005. Available at www.ama-assn.org/ama1/pub/upload/mm/368/guidelines4pay62705.pdf (accessed December 4, 2006).

17. Joint Commission on Accreditation of Healthcare Organizations: Principles for the Construct of Pay-for-Performance Programs. Available at www.jointcommission.org/PublicPolicy/pay.htm (accessed December 4, 2006).

18. American Healthways and Johns Hopkins University: Outcomes-based compensation: Pay-for-performance design principles. November 2004. Available at www.rewardingquality.com/resources/PFPDocumentFinal022805.pdf (accessed December 4, 2006).

19. American Medical Association: Category II CPT Codes: Appendix H—Alphabetic Index of Performance Measures by Clinical Condition or Topic. Available at www.ama-assn.org/ama1/pub/upload/mm/362/appendixh4406.pdf (accessed December 4, 2006).

20. National Committee on Quality Assurance: HEDIS: Health Plan Employer Data and Information Set. Available at www.ncqa.org/publications/hedispub.htm (accessed December 4, 2006).

21. Ambulatory Care Quality Alliance: Mission statement. Available at www.ambulatoryqualityalliance.org/default.htm (accessed December 4, 2006).

22. Ambulatory Care Quality Alliance: Press release: Ambulatory performance measures "major step" in improving quality of health care. Broad-based coalition reaches consensus on "starter set" for physicians. May 3, 2005. Available at www.ambulatoryqualityalliance.org/files/Aqapressrelease.Doc (accessed December 4, 2006).

23. President's Advisory Commission on Consumer Protection and Quality in the Healthcare Industry: Quality First: Better Health Care for All Americans. Chapter 5: Creating Public-Private Partnerships. March 12, 1986. Available at www.hcqualitycommission.gov/final/ (accessed December 4, 2006).

24. Kizer KW: Establishing health care performance standards in an era of consumerism. JAMA 2001;286:1213-1217.

25. American Medical Association: Consortium measures. Available at www.ama-assn.org/ama/pub/category/4837.html (accessed December 4, 2006).

26. Medicare Payment Advisory Commission: MedPAC recommendations on imaging services. Statement of Mark E. Miller, Ph.D., Executive Director, Medicare Payment Advisory Commission, before the Subcommittee on Health, Committee on Ways and Means, U.S. House of Representatives. March 17, 2005. Available at www.medpac.gov/publications/congressional_testimony/031705_TestimonyImaging-Hou.pdf (accessed December 4, 2006).

27. Brodenheimer T: Primary care: Will it survive? N Engl J Med 2006;355:861-864.

28. Doran T, Fullwood C, Gravelle H, et al: Pay-for-performance programs in family practices in the United Kingdom. N Engl J Med 2006;355:375-384.

29. Rosenthal MB, Frank RG, Li Z, Epstein AM: Early experience with pay-for-performance: From concept to practice. JAMA 2005;294:1788-1793.

30. Dudley RA: Pay-for-performance research: How to learn what clinicians and policy makers need to know. JAMA 2005;294:1821-1823.

Index

Note: Page numbers followed by b, f, and t indicate boxed text, figures, and tables, respectively.